SECOND EDITION

ANATOMY AND PHYSIOLOGY

FOR HEALTH PROFESSIONALS

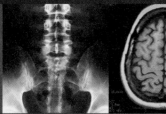
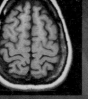
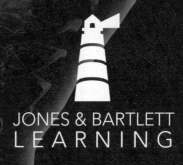

JAHANGIR MOINI, MD, MPH

Professor of Science and Health
Eastern Florida State College
Palm Bay, Florida

JONES & BARTLETT
LEARNING

World Headquarters
Jones & Bartlett Learning
5 Wall Street
Burlington, MA 01803
978-443-5000
info@jblearning.com
www.jblearning.com

Jones & Bartlett Learning books and products are available through most bookstores and online booksellers. To contact Jones & Bartlett Learning directly, call 800-832-0034, fax 978-443-8000, or visit our website, www.jblearning.com.

05787-4

Production Credits

Chief Executive Officer: Ty Field
President: James Homer
Chief Product Officer: Eduardo Moura
VP, Executive Publisher: Vernon Anthony
Executive Editor: Rhonda Dearborn
Associate Editor: Sean Fabery
Production Assistant: Talia Adry
Marketing Manager: Grace Richards
Rights and Photo Research Coordinator: Amy Rathburn
Art Development Editor: Joanna Lundeen
Art Development Assistant: Shannon Sheehan

VP, Manufacturing and Inventory Control: Therese Connell
Composition: Cenveo® Publisher Services
Cover Design: Kristin E. Parker
Cover Images: From left to right: © IxMaster/Shutterstock,
© Allison Herreid/Shutterstock, © Michelangelus/Shutterstock,
© Pan Xunbin/Shutterstock, © Guzel Studio/Shutterstock,
© Vshivkova/Shutterstock, © Mopic/Shutterstock,
© Praisaeng/Shutterstock, © Mopic/Shutterstock
Printing and Binding: RR Donnelley Companies
Cover Printing: RR Donnelley Companies

Library of Congress Cataloging-in-Publication Data
Moini, Jahangir, 1942- , author.
[Anatomy and physiology for health professionals]
Anatomy & physiology for health professionals / Jahangir Moini. — Second edition.
    p. ; cm.
Preceded by Anatomy and physiology for health professionals / Jahangir Moini. c2012.
Includes index.
ISBN 978-1-284-03694-7
I. Title.
[DNLM: 1. Anatomy. 2. Allied Health Personnel. 3. Physiological Phenomena. QS 4]
QP34.5
612—dc23
                                                    2014028797

6048

Printed in the United States of America
20 19 18 17 16   10 9 8 7 6 5 4 3

This book is dedicated to my wonderful and amazing wife, Hengameh, and two beautiful daughters, Mahkameh and Morvarid.

It is also dedicated to my granddaughters, Laila Jade and Annabelle Jasmine Mabry.

BRIEF CONTENTS

TABLE OF CONTENTS

Contents   **vii**

PREFACE

In 24 years of teaching anatomy and physiology, I have utilized numerous books related to the subject. Some were very high-level while others were very low-level, and I couldn't find a "middle ground" book that really taught the subject to allied health students—surprising, given that this is a time when the field is growing exponentially. Therefore, I undertook the writing of this book for all allied health professionals. Anatomy and physiology are two of the major core subjects for almost all allied health professionals; they must understand the structures and normal functions of the body in the simplest possible terms. This book strives to make that possible.

Organization of This Text

This text is based on levels of organization within the body and becomes more multifaceted as the student incorporates the understanding of basic, then intermediate, and finally more complex subjects.

In total, the text consists of six units. Unit I, "Levels of Organization," begins by providing a general introduction to human anatomy and physiology, along with the organization levels through which the body is understood. The unit then delves into the atomic, molecular, and chemical interactions on which life is based before moving on to discussions of the cells and tissues that comprise the body.

As the title implies, Unit II, "Support and Movement," focuses on the body systems that support the body and allow for a range of motion. The unit first considers the integumentary system, composed of the skin and its accessory structures: These are the body's first line of defense against the environment. The text then approaches the bones and joints that comprise the skeletal system before discussing the muscular system.

Unit III, "Control and Coordination," tackles the critical components of the body that control all body functions. The text considers the all-important nervous system across four chapters on neural tissue, the central nervous system, the peripheral nervous system, and the senses. The unit then ends with a chapter on the endocrine system, which works along with the nervous system to regulate the functions of the human body to maintain homeostasis.

Unit IV, "Transport," focuses on the cardiovascular and lymphatic systems, which keep the body running. The first three chapters discuss the major components of the cardiovascular system: the heart, blood, and blood vessels. The last chapter in this unit focuses on the lymphatic system. Like the cardiovascular system, it transports fluids through a network of vessels; without the lymphatic system, fluid would accumulate in tissue spaces.

Unit V, "Environmental Exchange," considers the systems and processes that balance what the body intakes with what it expels. The unit first examines the respiratory system, which intakes oxygen and removes carbon dioxide from the body, before shifting focus to the urinary system, which eliminates wastes and maintains homeostatic regulation of the volume and solute concentration of blood plasma. The text then surveys fluid, electrolyte, and acid-base balance before moving on to the digestive system, which in simplest terms supplies nutrients for body cells.

Finally, in Unit VI, "Continuity of Life," the focus shifts to the male and female reproductive systems, which, while not essential to the survival of an individual, are needed to ensure the continued existence of the human species. The final chapter then discusses pregnancy before delving into a brief discussion of genetics.

In addition to the recurring features that guide the student through each chapter (of which an overview is given in the "How to Use This Book" section), the body systems chapters contained in this text address the effects of aging on each specific system, information that is especially critical at a time when the number of older adults is on the rise.

New to This Edition

This second edition has been updated to take into account both advancements in medical knowledge in the last several years as well as feedback from valued users of the *First Edition*.

For the *Second Edition*, the text was expanded from 20 to 24 chapters. Changes include the following:

- Chapter 8, "Articulations," is new to this edition and provides an overview of the classifications of joints, types of joint movements, intervertebral joints and ligaments, and joint injuries.
- The content in the "Nervous System" chapter has been expanded and divided into three chapters: Chapter 10, "Neural Tissue"; Chapter 11, "The Central Nervous System"; and Chapter 12, "The Peripheral Nervous System."
- The content in the "Cardiovascular System" chapter has also been expanded and divided into two chapters: Chapter 16, "The Heart," and Chapter 17, "The Vascular System."
- *Focus on Pathology* boxes have been added throughout the chapters, incorporating explanation of abnormal conditions relating to the body systems.
- *Essay Questions* have been added to the end of each chapter, while the *Critical Thinking Questions* have been expanded.

New tables and figures have been added as appropriate, particularly ones that focus on diagnostic imaging.

Instructor Resources

Qualified instructors can receive a full suite of extensive Instructor Resources, including:

- Slides in PowerPoint format, featuring more than 2,000 slides
- Test Bank, containing more than 800 questions
- Instructor's Manual, including teaching strategies, lecture outlines, discussion topics, and answers to end-of-chapter questions

- Image Bank, supplying key figures from the text
- Sample Syllabus, showing how a course can be structured around this text
- Transition Guide, providing guidance in switching from the previous edition

To gain access to these valuable teaching materials, contact your Health Professions Account Specialist at go.jblearning.com/findarep.

Jahangir Moini, MD, MPH

HOW TO USE THIS BOOK

Anatomy and Physiology for Health Professionals, Second Edition incorporates a number of engaging pedagogical features to aid in the student's understanding and retention of the material. A colorful and engaging layout enables easy reading and supports the retention of important concepts. More than 450 full-color photographs and medically accurate illustrations provide valuable insight into human anatomy and physiology.

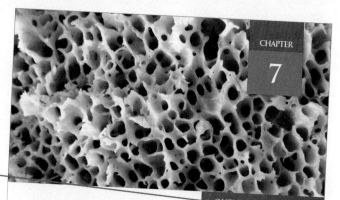

Chapter Objectives and Outline

Each chapter begins with a framework for learning the most important topics by presenting *Objectives* that list the chapter's desired outcomes and an *Outline* indicating the material to be discussed.

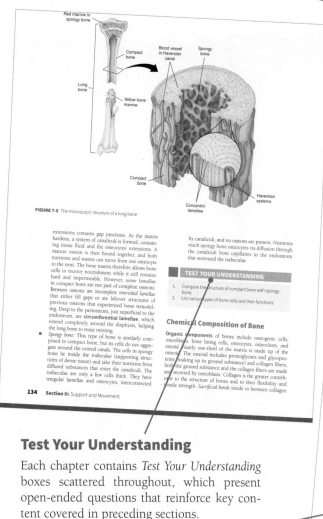

FIGURE 7-5 The microscopic structure of a long bone

extensions contains gap junctions. As the matrix hardens, a system of canaliculi is formed, containing tissue fluid and the osteocytes' extensions. A mature osteon is then bound together, and both nutrients and wastes can move from one osteocyte to the next. The bone matrix therefore allows bone cells to receive nourishment while it still remains hard and impermeable. However, some lamellae in compact bone are not part of complete osteons. Between osteons are incomplete *interstitial lamellae* that either fill gaps or are leftover structures of previous osteons that experienced bone remodeling. Deep to the periosteum, just superficial to the endosteum, are **circumferential lamellae**, which extend completely around the diaphysis, helping the long bone to resist twisting.

- *Spongy bone:* This type of bone is similarly composed to compact bone, but its cells do not aggregate around the central canals. The cells in spongy bone lie inside the *trabeculae* (supporting structures of dense tissue) and take their nutrients from diffused substances that enter the canaliculi. The trabeculae are only a few cells thick. They have irregular lamellae and osteocytes, interconnected

by canaliculi, and no osteons are present. Nutrients reach spongy bone osteocytes via diffusion through the canaliculi from capillaries in the endosteum that surround the trabeculae.

TEST YOUR UNDERSTANDING

1. Compare the structure of compact bone with spongy bone.
2. List various types of bone cells and their functions.

Chemical Composition of Bone

Organic components of bones include osteogenic cells, osteoblasts, bone lining cells, osteocytes, osteoclasts, and *osteoid*. Nearly one-third of the matrix is made up of the *osteoid*. The osteoid includes proteoglycans and glycoproteins (making up its ground substance) and collagen fibers, both the ground substance and the collagen fibers are made and secreted by osteoblasts. Collagen is the greater contributor to the structure of bones and to their flexibility and tensile strength. *Sacrificial bonds* inside or between collagen

134 Section II: Support and Movement

Test Your Understanding

Each chapter contains *Test Your Understanding* boxes scattered throughout, which present open-ended questions that reinforce key content covered in preceding sections.

Focus on Pathology

Focus on Pathology boxes connect the book's coverage of anatomy and physiology to important topics in pathology, or the study of disease.

Bone Tissues and the Skeletal System

OBJECTIVES

After studying this chapter, readers should be able to:

1. Discuss the major functions of bones.
2. Discuss bone classifications and give examples of each.
3. Distinguish between the axial and appendicular skeletons.
4. Identify the major features of the bones that compose the thoracic cage and the upper limbs.
5. Distinguish the major parts of a long bone.
6. List the substances normally stored in bone tissue.
7. Name each of the bones of the cranium.
8. Explain how the structures of cervical, thoracic, and lumbar vertebrae differ.
9. Name each of the bones of the lower limbs.
10. List the bones of the ankle and identify the largest of these.

128

CHAPTER 7

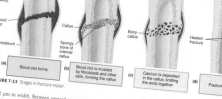

FIGURE 7-13 Stages in fracture repair.

(a) Blood clot forms
(b) Blood clot is invaded by fibroblasts and other cells, forming the callus
(c) Calcium is deposited in the callus, knitting the ends together
(d) Fracture is repaired

to 12 μm in width. Between osteoid seams and older bone, an abrupt transition point exists, known as the *calcification front*. The osteoid seams mature for about 1 week before calcification occurs. Mechanical signals are involved in this calcification. In the endosteal cavity, nearby concentrations of calcium and phosphate ions are needed for calcification to occur. When this calcium–phosphate product is sufficient, tiny crystals of hydroxyapatites are formed. They catalyze continued crystallization of calcium salts. Additional factors include matrix proteins (which bind and concentrate calcium) and *alkaline phosphatase*, an enzyme that is lost in matrix vesicles by osteoblasts, and which is critical for mineralization. Eventually, calcium salts are deposited at one time throughout the matured matrix in an ordered manner.

Bone Resorption

Bone resorption occurs because of osteoclast activities, including the creation of grooves or depressions as bone matrix is broken down. Osteoclast borders use their irregular shape to stick to the bone and seal off areas of bone destruction. They secrete lysosomal enzymes, digesting protons and the organic matrix. In the resorption bays, the high acidity converts calcium salts into soluble forms. Dead osteocytes and demineralized matrix may be phagocytized by the osteoclasts. Endocytosis occurs to the digested growth factors, matrix end products, and dissolved minerals. These are moved, via transcytosis, across the osteoclasts to be released at the opposite end, entering the interstitial fluid and blood. Osteoclasts undergo apoptosis after a certain bone area has been resorbed. Both parathyroid hormone (PTH) and protein from the immune system's T cells play a role.

Control of Bone Remodeling

Bone remodeling is controlled by genetic factors, a negative feedback hormonal loop, and in response to gravitational and mechanical forces. The negative feedback hormonal loop maintains calcium ion homeostasis in the blood. Ionic calcium is essential for nerve impulse transmission, blood coagulation, muscle contraction, cell division, and secretion

by glands as well as nerve cells. More than 99% of the body's 1,200 to 1,400 g of calcium is present in the bones. The remainder is primarily in the cells, and a small amount is in the blood. Hormonal controls keep blood calcium ions in a range between 9 and 11 mg/dL (100 mL) of blood. Vitamin D metabolites control calcium absorption from the intestine. Children under age 10 need 400 to 800 mg of calcium in their daily diet, whereas people between ages 11 and 24 require 1,200 to 1,500 mg.

PTH, released by the *parathyroid glands*, is the primary hormonal controller of bone remodeling, although *calcitonin* is also involved to a lesser degree. The parathyroid glands are embedded in the thyroid gland in the neck. PTH is released when blood levels of ionic calcium decline, stimulating osteoclasts to resorb bone and releasing calcium into the blood. Osteoclasts break down old as well as new bone matrix. Rising blood calcium causes PTH release to stop, reversing its effects and lowering blood calcium. Blood calcium homeostasis is therefore maintained. However, if blood calcium levels are low for a long time, the bones lose minerals and develop large, irregular holes.

FOCUS ON PATHOLOGY

Calcium ion levels must be strictly controlled by the body and usually only change within 10% of their normal amounts. If they decrease by 35%, convulsions may occur. If they increase by 30%, muscle cells and neurons become unresponsive. If they reduce to 50%, death usually occurs. Hypercalcemia is the condition of sustained high blood levels of calcium. This can lead to dangerous calcium salt deposition in the blood vessels and soft organs such as the kidneys, which results in kidney stones. This deposition can harm their function in many different ways.

Chapter 7: Bone Tissues and the Skeletal System **141**

Summary

A number of features appear at the end of each chapter. The *Summary* recaps the most important points in the chapter and connects it to the student's overall journey.

Key Terms

Key Terms list the most important new terms covered in the chapter; correlating definitions can be found in the end-of-text glossary.

Learning Goals

Learning Goals encapsulate how each *Objective* has been addressed over the course of the chapter.

Critical Thinking Questions

A range of questions are also included at the end of each chapter; the student can use these for self-study or submit their answers to the instructor. A case is presented at the end of each chapter, with *Critical Thinking Questions* that cause the student to reflect on the situation described.

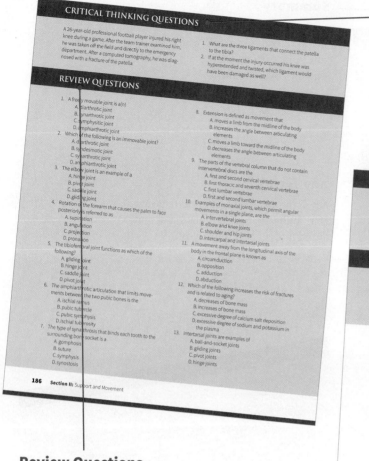

REVIEW QUESTIONS (CONTINUED)

14. Which of the following are examples of saddle joints?
    A. elbow joints
    B. shoulder joints
    C. wrist joints
    D. carpometacarpal joints
15. Moving the ankle so the top of the foot comes closer to the tibial bone is called
    A. hyperextension
    B. plantar flexion
    C. dorsiflexion
    D. abduction

ESSAY QUESTIONS

1. Describe articulation.
2. Define the terms nonaxial, biaxial, and multiaxial.
3. Classify the various types of joints.
4. Discuss types of joint movements.
5. List the six characteristics of synovial joints.
6. Classify the various types of synovial joints.
7. Compare the elbow joints with the hip joints.
8. Define circumduction and pronation.
9. Describe the intervertebral ligaments.
10. Explain the effects of aging upon the joints.

Review Questions

Review Questions provide students with a chance to answer multiple choice questions.

Essay Questions

Finally, *Essay Questions* ask students to delve deeply into the content.

ACKNOWLEDGMENTS

I would like to acknowledge the following individuals for their time and efforts in aiding with this book:

Morvarid Moini, Designer, Dental Student
Nova Southeastern University

Greg Vadimsky, Author's Assistant
Melbourne, Florida

I would like to thank the entire staff of Jones & Bartlett Learning, especially Rhonda Dearborn, Sean Fabery, Talia Adry, Amy Rathburn, Joanna Lundeen, Shannon Sheehan, and Grace Richards.

I would also like to thank the reviewers who gave their time and guidance in helping me complete this book.

ABOUT THE AUTHOR

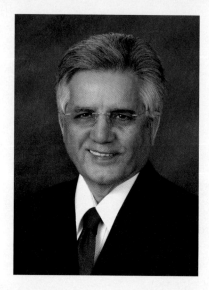

Dr. Jahangir Moini is currently a professor at Eastern Florida State College, where he teaches anatomy and physiology as well as other science courses. He was previously assistant professor at Tehran University School of Medicine for nine years, where he taught medical and allied health students. The author is a former professor and director (for 15 years) of allied health programs at Everest University.

As a physician and instructor for the past 42 years, he advocates that all health professionals must understand the structures and functions of the human body. Other sciences such as pathology, pharmacology, and chemistry are correlated with the knowledge of anatomy and physiology.

Dr. Moini is actively involved in teaching and helping students prepare for service in various health professions. He has been an internationally published author of various allied health books since 1999.

REVIEWERS

Raheleh Ahangari, MD,
Assistant Professor
College of Medicine
University of Central Florida
Orlando, Florida

Gina Buldra, BS, RRT, RCP
Respiratory Therapy Program Director
Division of Health
Eastern New Mexico University-Roswell
Roswell, New Mexico

Stephen C. Enwefa, PHD, CCC-SLP, ND
Professor
College of Sciences
Southern University and A & M College
Baton Rouge, Louisiana

Stasha Kathryn Fulton, MS, RT(R)(VI)
Assistant Professor
Radiologic Technology & Medical Imaging Programs
Clarkson College
Omaha, Nebraska

Terri King, BS, MA, NREMT-P
Adjunct Professor
Emergency Medical Services Professions Department
Austin Community College
Cedar Park, Texas

Anita Lane, MEd, OTR
Instructor
Occupational Therapy Assistant Program
Navarro College
Corsicana, Texas

Alice Nakatsuka, MS
Senior Health Sciences Instructor
ITT Technical Institute
Indianapolis, Indiana

Marilyn E. Thompson Odom, Ph.D.
Professor
College of Pharmacy
Belmont University
Nashville, Tennessee

Eva Oltman, MEd
Professor and Chair
Allied Health Division
Jefferson Community and Technical College
Louisville, Kentucky

Linda Parks, MA-HIM, RHIT, CCS, CTR
Assistant Professor
Health Information Management Programs
Dakota State University
Madison, South Dakota

Robin A. Reedy, BA, I/C, NR-AEMT
Adjunct Faculty
Emergency Medical Services Program
Eastern New Mexico University-Roswell
Roswell, New Mexico

Mohtashem Samsam, MD, PhD
Associate Professor
College of Medicine
University of Central Florida
Orlando, Florida

Richard C. Shok, BSN, RN, EMS-I
Owner and Director
Code One Training Solutions, LLC
East Hartford, Connecticut

Almos Bela Trif, MD, PhD, JD, MS
Associate Professor
College of Medical Sciences
Nova Southeastern University
Fort Lauderdale, Florida

Ashley Underhill, MS, ExSc, EMT
Program Director
Boyd H. Anderson High School
Lauderdale Lakes, Florida

Brenda Williams
Instructor
Baton Rouge Community College—Jackson
Jackson, Louisiana

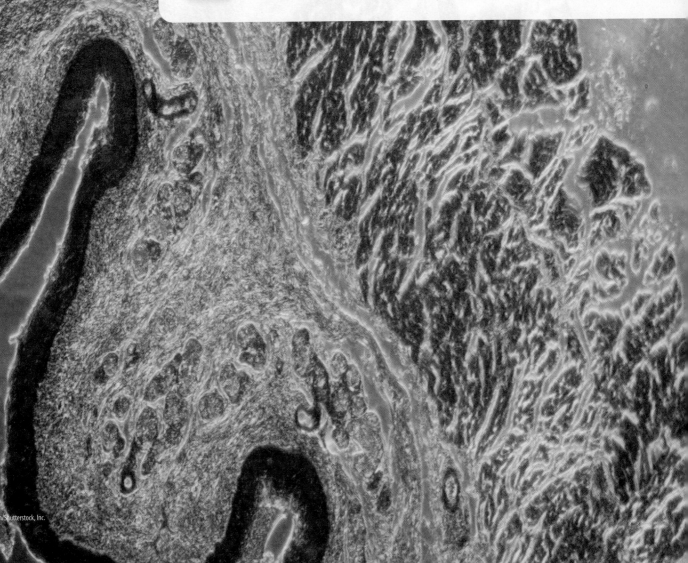

UNIT 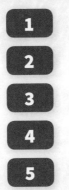 I

LEVELS OF ORGANIZATION

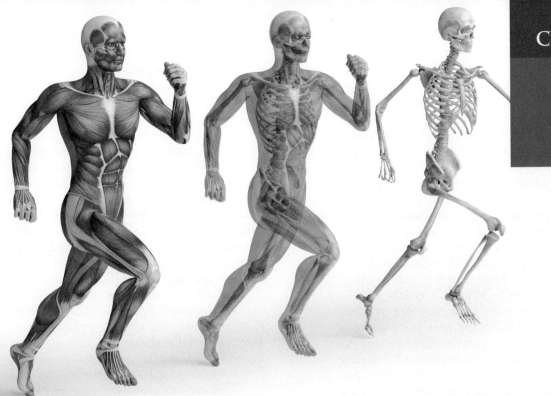

Introduction to Human Anatomy and Physiology

OBJECTIVES

After studying this chapter, readers should be able to

1. Define anatomy and physiology.
2. Name the components that make up the organization levels of the body.
3. Describe the major essentials of life.
4. Define *homeostasis* and describe its importance to survival.
5. Describe the major body cavities.
6. List the systems of the body and give the organs in each system.
7. Describe directions and planes of the body.
8. Discuss the membranes near the heart, lungs, and abdominal cavity.
9. List the nine abdominal regions.
10. Compare positive and negative feedback mechanisms.

Overview

The study of anatomy and physiology is vital for all health professionals and involves many different areas of science to understand how the human body works as well as how it is structured. The study of anatomy and physiology provides answers to many questions about the functions of the body in both health and disease. As a result of this understanding, it is possible to see what happens to the body when it is injured, stressed, or contracts a disease or infection. It is important that all allied health students become familiar with the terminology used in anatomy and physiology. In this chapter, the focus is on a complete introduction to anatomy and physiology.

The structures and functions of the human body are closely related. **Anatomy** is the study of the structure of body parts and how they are organized. This term is derived from the Greek words meaning *to cut apart*. **Physiology** is the study of how body parts work. Every body part functions to assist the human body in different ways. It is not easy to separate the topics of anatomy and physiology because the structures of body parts are so closely associated with their functions. Each part has its own unique substructures that allow it to perform its needed functions. **Pathophysiology** is the study of changes associated with or resulting from disease or injury. It is also concerned with biologic and physical manifestations of disease as they relate to underlying abnormalities and physiologic disturbances. Pathophysiology explains the processes within the body that result in disease signs and symptoms but does not focus directly on the treatment of disease.

The human body has been studied for hundreds of years. Even though its inner workings are well understood, new discoveries are still being made even today. In 2003 the human genome (instructions that allow the body to operate) was deciphered for the first time. There are more than 20,000 genes in the human body, so this substantial discovery took many years to complete. Researchers frequently discover new information about physiology, particularly at the molecular level, but basic human anatomy changes very slowly as time progresses.

Classifications of Anatomy

The many subdivisions of anatomy include gross (macroscopic) anatomy, microscopic anatomy, and developmental anatomy. These can be further broken down as follows:

- **Gross (macroscopic) anatomy:** The study of large body structures that can been seen without a microscope. These include the brain, heart, kidneys, lungs, and skin. Studies performed to understand gross anatomy used dissected animals and their organs.
  - **Regional anatomy:** All structures in a certain body region are examined at the same time. For example, if an arm were being examined, structures would include skin, muscles, bones, nerves, blood vessels, and others.
    - **Systemic anatomy:** Each body system is examined. For example, the heart would be examined when studying the cardiovascular system, but so would all the blood vessels of the whole body.
    - **Surface anatomy:** This is the examination of internal structures related to overlying skin surfaces. Surface anatomy is used, for example, to locate the correct blood vessels used for phlebotomy.
- **Microscopic anatomy:** The study of small body structures that require a microscope to be seen. This requires making thin slices of tissues, which are then stained and affixed (mounted) to glass slides for microscopic examination.
  - **Cytology:** A subdivision of microscopic anatomy that focuses on body cells.
  - **Histology:** A subdivision of microscopic anatomy that focuses on body tissues.
- **Developmental anatomy:** The study of structural changes in anatomy throughout the life span.
  - **Embryology:** A subdivision of developmental anatomy that focuses on developmental changes occurring before birth.

For medical diagnosis, scientific research, and other highly specialized needs, *pathological* or *radiographic* anatomy may be used. Pathological anatomy focuses on disease and the structural changes that result, whereas radiographic anatomy focuses on internal structures via the use of x-rays or specialized scanning equipment such as magnetic resonance imaging (MRI) or computed tomography (CT). *Molecular anatomy* focuses on the structure of chemical substances (biological molecules). Although formally considered a branch of *biology*, molecular anatomy is still considered part of the overall study of anatomy as it focuses on subcellular particles of the body.

Anatomical studies require a combination of many different skills. These include anatomic terminology, observation, *auscultation* (using a stethoscope to listen to organ sounds), manipulation, and *palpation* (feeling body organs for normal or abnormal conditions by using the hands).

Classifications of Physiology

Physiology is concerned with how the body functions, often focusing on cellular or molecular activities. There are also many subdivisions of physiology, which are primarily focused on certain organ systems. Examples of physiology classifications are as follows:

- *Respiratory physiology:* focuses on the functions of the respiratory system
- *Cardiovascular physiology:* focuses on the heart and blood vessels
- *Neurophysiology:* focuses on the nervous system
- *Renal physiology:* focuses on the functions of the kidneys, including urine production

The physiology of the human body is based on chemical reactions that affect the actions of cells or the molecular level.

Physiology is also linked to the study of physics, which takes into account body functions such as blood pressure, electrical currents, and muscular movement.

Organization Levels of the Body

Every body structure is made up of smaller structures, which are, likewise, made up of even smaller components. Chemicals compose every material found in the human body. They contain microscopic **atoms** combined into structures known as **molecules**. Many molecules may be combined into macromolecules. These macromolecules, in turn, form **organelles**, which help to complete the intended functions of a **cell**, the basic unit of both structure and function in the human body.

Cells are microscopic structures that may be quite different in size, shape, and function. Cells are grouped together to form **tissues**, which in turn are grouped together to form **organs**. Groups of similarly functioning organs form **organ systems**, which then combine to form a living **organism** (**FIGURE 1-1**). Body parts are organized into different levels of complexity, including the atomic level, molecular level, and cellular level. Atoms are the most simple in structure, with complexity increasing in molecules, organelles, tissues, and organs.

TEST YOUR UNDERSTANDING

1. What is an organism?
2. Explain the organization levels of the body.

Essentials for Life

Humans and other animals share many similar traits. All body cells are interdependent as we are multicellular organisms. Vital body functions occur over various organ systems, which contribute to overall body health.

Boundaries

The body's boundaries are maintained to keep the internal environment distinct from the external environment. All body cells are surrounded by selectively permeable membranes. The skin encloses and protects the body as a whole from factors such as dryness, bacteria, heat, sunlight, and chemicals.

Movement

Movement of the body is achieved via the muscular and skeletal systems. Inside the body, the cardiovascular, digestive, and urinary systems also use movement to transport blood, food materials, and urine. Even cells move, such as when muscle cells move by shortening, which is known as *contractility*.

Responsiveness

The ability to sense and respond to environmental stimuli (changes) is known as *responsiveness*, which is also referred to as *excitability*. An example is the way we quickly withdraw our hands from a hot saucepan on the stove. Nerve cells are highly excitable. They communicate with rapid electrical impulses, and therefore the nervous system is the most responsive of all body systems. However, all body systems have some degree of excitability.

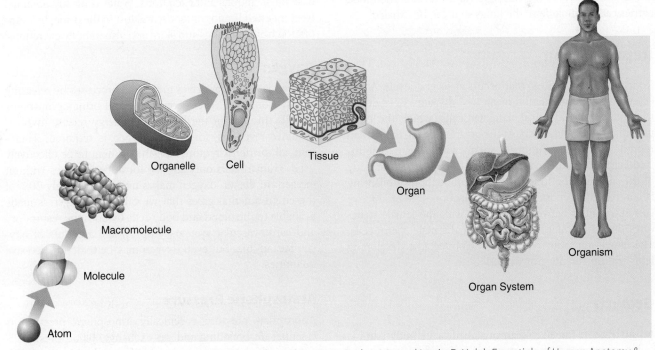

Organelle   Cell   Tissue   Organ

Macromolecule

Molecule

Organism

Organ System

Atom

FIGURE 1-1 Organization levels of the body. (Adapted from Shier, D. N., Butler, J. L., and Lewis, R. Hole's Essentials of Human Anatomy & Physiology, Tenth edition. McGraw Hill Higher Education, 2009.)

Digestion

Humans require specific nutrients to remain healthy and to grow and develop normally. Energy is gained from the breakdown, digestion, absorption, and assimilation of food. Digestion breaks down food materials to simple, more easily absorbed molecules. Absorbed nutrients move throughout the body's circulation. Nutrient-rich blood is distributed, via the cardiovascular system, to the entire body. Respiration brings in oxygen that works with nutrients to grow and repair body parts. The unusable parts of these processes are then excreted as waste.

Metabolism

The body's **metabolism** controls all these processes. It includes all chemical reactions inside body cells, the breaking down of substances into simpler forms (*catabolism*), creating more complex cellular components from simpler substances (*anabolism*), and the use of nutrients and oxygen to produce energy-rich ATP molecules (via *cellular respiration*). In metabolism, nutrients and oxygen from the digestive and respiratory systems are circulated to all body cells. Hormones from endocrine system glands have strong regulatory control over metabolism.

Excretion

The process of removing wastes from the body is known as *excretion*. Non-useful substances that are produced during digestion and metabolism must be removed. The digestive system removes food components that cannot be digested in the feces. The urinary system removes urea and other metabolic wastes containing nitrogen via the urine. The blood carries carbon dioxide to the lungs so it can be exhaled.

Reproduction

Reproduction is a process that occurs at several levels. At the cellular level, reproduction means cell division. Cells divide to produce two identical daughter cells, which the body uses for growth and repair. At the organism level, the human reproduction system unites a sperm with an egg. A fertilized egg is formed, developing into a baby inside the body of the mother. The function of the production of offspring is controlled by endocrine system hormones. Reproductive structures differ between the sexes, with the female structures providing a fertilization site for the male sperm cells. The female reproductive structures protect the developing fetus and nurture its growth until birth.

Growth

An increase in the size of an organism or its body parts is called *growth*. Most often, growth is achieved by an increase in the amount of cells. Even when they do not divide, however, cells can increase in size. True growth occurs when constructive activities occur more quickly than destructive activities.

Survival

Human beings need several substances for survival: food (nutrients), water, oxygen, pressure, and heat in specific quantities and with specific qualities.

Nutrients

Food provides nutrients for energy, growth, and regulation of the chemical reactions in the body. Some of these chemicals are used as energy sources or supply the raw materials needed for building new living matter. Others help to regulate vital chemical reactions. Plant-based foods contain high levels of carbohydrates, vitamins, and minerals. Carbohydrates are the primary energy fuel for body cells. Certain vitamins and minerals are needed for chemical reactions inside cells and for oxygen transport in the blood. Calcium is a mineral that assists in making bones harder and is needed for blood clotting. Animal-based foods contain high levels of proteins and fats. Proteins are the most essential component required for building cell structures. Fats also assist in this and are a great source of energy-providing fuel for the body.

Water

Water is required for metabolic processes and makes up most of the body's actual structure, transporting substances and regulating temperature. It makes up 60% to 80% of body weight and is the most abundant chemical in the body. Water allows chemical reactions to occur and is also the fluid base for secretions and excretions. Water is mostly obtained from ingested liquids or foods, and lost in the urine, by evaporation from the lungs and skin, and also in body excretions.

Oxygen

Oxygen is a gas that drives metabolic processes by releasing energy from food that is consumed and bringing nutrients to cells throughout the body. This energy release involves *oxidative* reactions, for which oxygen is required. Therefore, all nutrients require oxygen for them to be effectively used. Human cells only survive for a few minutes without oxygen. In the air, oxygen makes up approximately 20% of the environmental gases that we breathe. Oxygen is made available to the blood and body cells by both the respiratory and cardiovascular systems. Appropriate amounts of oxygen sustain life, but even oxygen may be toxic in excessive quantities.

Atmospheric Pressure

Appropriate pressure, specifically atmospheric pressure, is essential for breathing and gas exchange. Blood pressure is a form of hydrostatic pressure that forces the blood through the veins and arteries. Atmospheric pressure may be defined as the force that air exerts upon the body's surface. Gas exchange, in higher altitudes, may be insufficient to support cellular metabolism because at these altitudes atmospheric pressure is lower and the air is thinner. At sea level, the average atmospheric pressure is 760 mm Hg.

Body Temperature

Heat is produced as energy from metabolic reactions, influencing their speed, with the muscular system generating the most body heat. Body heat is measured as temperature. Normal body temperature must be maintained if chemical reactions are to continually sustain life. If the temperature is too high, chemical reactions occur very quickly, and proteins in the body change shape and cease functioning. If body temperature drops below 98.6°F (37°C), metabolic reactions slow down and eventually stop. Death may occur because of either variation in temperature.

TEST YOUR UNDERSTANDING

1. What factors are necessary to sustain life in humans?
2. What elements are needed by the body for survival?

Homeostasis

The internal environment of the human body must stay relatively stable for the person to survive. **Homeostasis** is a term that describes a stable internal body environment. It requires a constant balance, or normal concentrations of nutrients, oxygen, and water to be normal and balanced and for heat and pressure to be regulated at tolerable levels. **Homeostatic mechanisms** regulate the body by negative or positive feedback.

Homeostatic Control

For homeostasis to occur, the body primarily uses the nervous and endocrine systems. These systems allow forms of communication to occur that control homeostasis. The nervous system uses neural electrical impulses for these activities, whereas the endocrine system uses blood borne hormones. The event or factor that is being controlled (regulated) is referred to as the *variable*. All mechanisms used for homeostatic control involve at least three components:

- *Receptors:* These are "sensors" that monitor the internal body environment and respond to stimuli. Receptors send information to the *control center* along the *afferent pathway.* You can remember this more easily because the afferent pathway carries information that is "approaching" the control center.
- *Control center:* This is a point in the body that determines the *set point* (the range or level at which a variable must be maintained). It analyzes the input from the receptors to determine appropriate

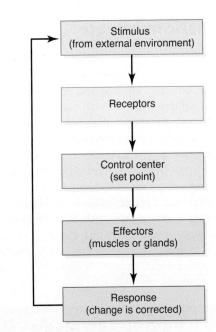

FIGURE 1-2 Homeostatic mechanism

responses or actions. It then sends information to *effectors* via the *efferent pathway.* You can remember this more easily because the efferent pathway carries information that is "exiting" the control center (**FIGURE 1-2**). The set point for the average body temperature, for example, is 98.6°F (37°C). Another set point is the one for normal adult blood pressure, which is ideally below 120 (systolic) and under 80 (diastolic).

- *Effectors:* These are components of homeostatic control that allow the control center to respond to stimuli. The control center's response involves negative (reducing) or positive (enhancing) feedback. Basically, negative feedback shuts off the control process, whereas positive feedback makes it occur at a faster rate.

Positive and Negative Feedback

The body uses positive and negative feedback systems to regulate various activities. A positive feedback mechanism is one that makes conditions move away from the normal state to stimulate further changes. They are usually short-lived and extremely specific actions. A positive feedback mechanism is defined as one that results in or responds in an enhanced way to the original stimulus, accelerating the result or response. Examples of positive feedback are the onset of contractions before childbirth, the process of blood clotting, lactation, the secretion of estrogen during the follicular phase of menstruation, and the generation of nerve signals. A negative feedback mechanism is one that prevents the correction of deviations from doing too much (which could possibly harm the body). Most of the feedback mechanisms of the human body use negative feedback. Examples of negative feedback are blood pressure regulation, erythropoiesis (the production of red blood cells), body temperature regulation, and control of blood glucose levels.

Homeostatic Imbalance

Most diseases occur because of *homeostatic imbalance* (meaning the disturbance of homeostasis). Aging causes body systems to become less efficient and more uncontrollable, resulting in instability in the internal body environment and increasing the risk for illness. Also, when helpful negative feedback mechanisms become overwhelmed, certain destructive positive feedback mechanisms can dominate (such as seen in some forms of heart failure). Additional examples of homeostatic imbalance include abdominal injury due to physical trauma (and lack of protective bones in this body region), sepsis (resulting in severe pain, such as in **peritonitis**), and metabolic acidosis or alkalosis (which can affect all body systems and lead to death). Trauma may involve hemorrhage and perforation of abdominal organs. Any cause of homeostatic imbalance can result in death if untreated.

FOCUS ON PATHOLOGY

The abdominopelvic organs are frequently damaged because of physical trauma, such as in a car accident. The organs of the upper chest or pelvis are protected by bones, but only the abdominal muscles form the walls of the abdominal cavity.

TEST YOUR UNDERSTANDING

1. Why is homeostasis essential to survival?
2. Describe two homeostatic mechanisms.

Organization of the Body

The human body is composed of distinct body parts, cavities, membranes, and organ systems that include various body systems, discussed in greater detail in the following sections.

Body Cavities and Membranes

The body is divided into two main cavities, the dorsal cavity and the ventral cavity. These two main cavities are divided into smaller subcavities. The dorsal cavity protects the organs of the nervous system. Its two subdivisions include the *cranial cavity* of the skull, which encases the brain, and the *vertebral (spinal) cavity*, located inside the vertebral column, which encases the spinal cord. The vertebral cavity is also referred to as the *vertebral canal*. The cranial and spinal cavities are continuous with each other.

The ventral cavity contains most of the body's organs. More anterior and larger than the dorsal cavity, it houses the viscera (visceral organs). The ventral cavity is divided into the *thoracic* cavity and the *abdominopelvic* cavity. The thoracic cavity is larger and is surrounded by the chest muscles and ribs. It is subdivided into lateral *pleural cavities*, which each surround one lung, and the medial *mediastinum*.

The thoracic cavity is separated from the inferior abdominopelvic cavity by the diaphragm. This muscle is dome-shaped and very important for respiration. There are two parts in the abdominopelvic cavity, but these are not separated by a membrane or muscle. The superior portion is called the *abdominal cavity*. It contains the stomach, spleen, liver, pancreas, gallbladder, most of the intestines, kidneys, and other organs. The inferior *pelvic cavity* lies within the pelvic bones. It contains the urinary bladder, various reproductive organs, and the rectum. The abdominal and pelvic cavities are not aligned, with the pelvis "tipping" away in a perpendicular fashion.

Both the dorsal and ventral cavities, like all other body cavities, are lined by a **serous membrane** (or *serosa*) composed of two layers: a *parietal membrane* and a *visceral membrane*. The parietal membrane folds in upon itself to form the visceral membrane, which covers the organs inside the cavity. The parietal membrane is not exposed and is fused to the cavity walls. Between these membranes is a lubricating *serous fluid* that reduces friction when organs move. Serous fluid is secreted by both the parietal and visceral membranes. There is a thin, slit-like cavity between these membranes that contains the serous fluid, allowing the organs to slide across the cavity walls and each other without friction. This ability to "slide" is very important for organs such as the stomach (as it digests) and the heart (as it pumps).

Other body cavities are smaller than these cavities. The head contains the oral cavity (housing the teeth and tongue), nasal cavity (inside the nose, divided into right and left portions), sinuses, orbital cavities (housing the eyes and related structures), and middle ear cavities (housing the middle ear bones). These cavities are located in the head and are opened to the exterior of the body. Other examples include the *synovial cavities* that surround various joints in the body.

The **viscera** are the internal organs within the thoracic and abdominopelvic cavities. The **mediastinum** separates the thoracic cavity into right and left halves and contains the heart, trachea, esophagus, and thymus gland. The lungs lie outside the mediastinum yet are still contained within the thoracic cavity. The major cavities of the body are shown in **FIGURE 1-3, A** and **B**. The inner thoracic and abdominopelvic cavities are lined with connective membranes. For example, the heart is surrounded by a double-walled sac known as the pericardium, which has a superficial, loose-fitting section known as the fibrous pericardium. This protects the heart, connects it to surrounding structures, and keeps it from overfilling with blood. Below the fibrous pericardium is the serous pericardium, which is a thin, double-layered membrane that forms a closed sac containing the heart. It has a parietal layer, which lines the internal surface of the fibrous pericardium, and a visceral layer (epicardium) that continues to cover the external heart surface. All these structures are housed in the pericardial cavity. The lungs are lined with the **parietal** pleura and covered by the **visceral** pleura. There is no

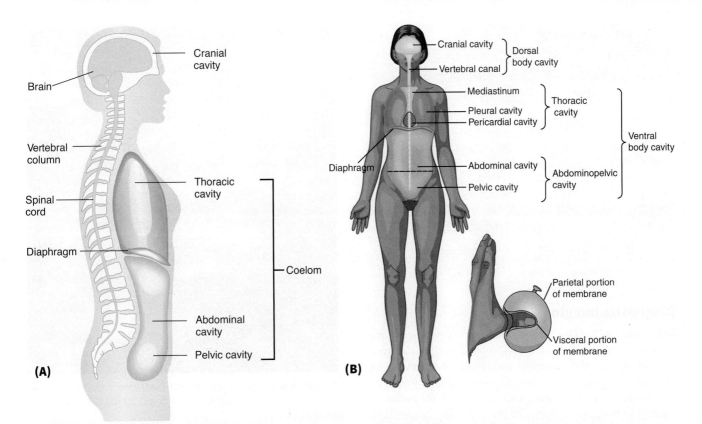

FIGURE 1-3 (A) Lateral view of the body cavities. (B) Anterior view of the body cavities. (© Jones & Bartlett Learning)

actual space between these pleural membranes, but the region between them is still referred to as the pleural cavity.

The abdominopelvic cavity is lined with **peritoneal membranes**, including the *parietal peritoneum* lining the walls and the *visceral peritoneum* covering each organ. Between these membranes, the potential space is called the peritoneal cavity (**FIGURE 1-4**). Organs in the abdominopelvic cavity are located either inside the peritoneum (**intraperitoneal**) or behind the peritoneum (**retroperitoneal**). Intraperitoneal and retroperitoneal organs are listed in **TABLE 1-1**.

FOCUS ON PATHOLOGY

Pleurisy is the inflammation of the tissue that covers the lungs and chest wall. The primary symptoms are chest pain associated with breathing. It may be caused by infections such as tuberculosis, toxins such as ammonia, rheumatoid arthritis, lupus, lung or breast cancer, and mesothelioma. *Peritonitis* is the sudden inflammation of the peritoneal membranes that causes abrupt abdominal pain. Its most serious causes include perforation of the esophagus, stomach, duodenum, gallbladder, bile duct, bowel, and appendix.

TEST YOUR UNDERSTANDING

1. List the cavities of the head.
2. Which body cavity will be opened if an incision is made just inferior to the diaphragm?

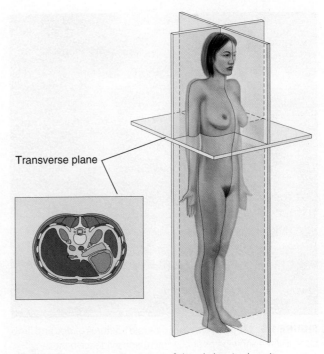

FIGURE 1-4 Transverse section of the abdominal cavity showing the peritoneal cavity.

TABLE 1-1

Intraperitoneal and Retroperitoneal Organs

Intraperitoneal Organs	Retroperitoneal Organs
Stomach	Kidneys
Liver	Adrenal glands
Gallbladder	Pancreas
Spleen	Urinary bladder
Uterus	Ureters
Ovaries	Duodenum
Jejunum	Ascending colon
Ileum	Descending colon
Transverse colon	Rectum
Sigmoid colon	Inferior vena cava
	Abdominal aorta

Diagnostic Imaging

Diagnostic or "medical" imaging was developed over time in order to view the internal organs and body structures, in both normal and abnormal conditions. It began in the first decade of the 1900s when physicist Wilhelm Roentgen discovered x-rays. Until the 1950s, x-rays were the exclusive method of imaging available. In the beginning, x-rays took much longer to produce and exposed the patient to significantly higher amounts of radiation. An example of an x-ray is shown in **FIGURE 1-5**.

Additional medical imaging developments are as follows:

■ The development of fluorescent screens that were used with special glasses allowed real-time viewing of x-ray images but also exposed physicians to radiation.

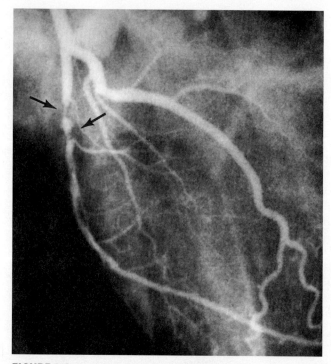

FIGURE 1-6 A coronary angiogram illustrating segmental narrowing (arrows). (Courtesy of Leonard V. Crowley, MD, Century College.)

■ Contrast agents barium and iodine help to improve viewing of the esophagus, stomach, coronary arteries, and other structures. Examples of procedures that use contrast agents include intravenous pyelogram and angiogram (**FIGURE 1-6**).

■ In 1955, x-ray image intensifiers allowed moving x-rays to be viewed by using television cameras and monitors.

■ Radionuclide scanning, or *nuclear medicine*, was developed in the 1950s. This type of scan uses special gamma cameras and low-level radioactive chemicals introduced into the body, allowing the evaluation of functional activity of organs. Results of nuclear medicine are recorded as a *nuclear isotope scan* (**FIGURE 1-7**).

■ Ultrasound scanning appeared in the 1960s, using high-frequency sound waves to penetrate the body, bounce off the internal structures, and then be reconstructed into live pictures by a computer (**FIGURE 1-8**). Ultrasound is most useful for soft tissues and body fluids and is commonly used to view the gallbladder, urinary bladder, and uterus.

■ Digital imaging came along in the 1970s with the development of CT. All preexisting technologies were upgraded to digital forms. Digital x-ray detectors are replacing previous analog technologies, allowing better imaging and less health risks. CT acquires an image in less than a second and instantly reconstructs it. It offers detailed cross-sectional

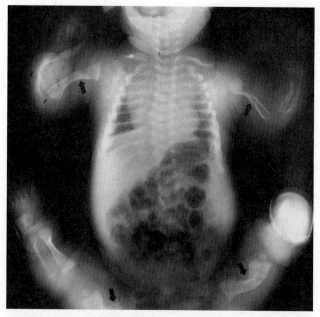

FIGURE 1-5 X-ray film showing multiple fractures of ribs and limb bones, some showing poor alignment and evidence of healing. Arrows indicate the location of four fractures. (Courtesy of Leonard V. Crowley, MD, Century College.)

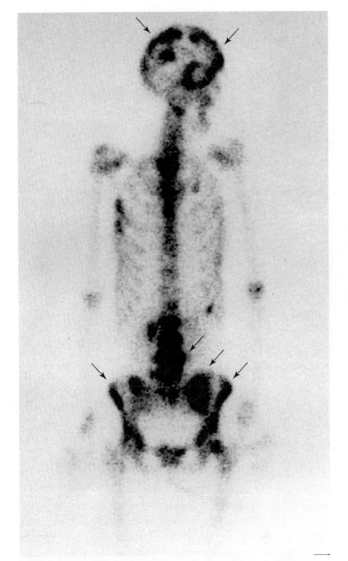

FIGURE 1-7 Radioisotope bone scan of head, chest, and pelvis. Dark areas (arrows) indicate the concentration of radioisotope around tumor deposits in bone. (Courtesy of Leonard V. Crowley, MD, Century College.)

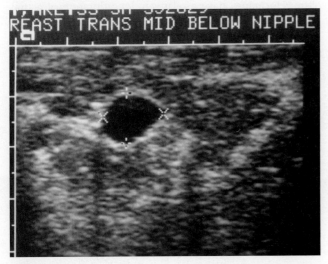

FIGURE 1-8 An ultrasound examination of breast, revealing a breast cyst (a dark area near the center of the photograph). (Courtesy of Leonard V. Crowley, MD, Century College.)

images of body structures. **FIGURE 1-9** shows a CT machine, and **FIGURE 1-10** shows a CT scan of the abdomen.

- *MRI*, first offered in 1984, allows detailed imaging without exposure to radiation (**FIGURE 1-11**). Images are produced by displacing protons in atomic nuclei with radiofrequency signals. However, it cannot be used on any patient who has any metal implants because of its extremely powerful magnetization. Also, the person must remain completely still for a long period of time in a small, confined space. MRI is often used for bone, joint, brain, and nerve imaging.

Organ Systems

In each organ system of the human body, organs work together to maintain homeostasis. These organ systems include the integumentary, skeletal, muscular, nervous, endocrine, cardiovascular, lymphatic, digestive, respiratory, urinary, and reproductive systems (**FIGURE 1-12**).

Integumentary System

The integumentary system includes the skin, hair, nails, sebaceous (oil) glands, and sweat glands. It functions to protect the underlying tissues of the body, assist in the regulation of body temperature, contain various sensory receptors, and manufacture certain substances (such as vitamin D).

Skeletal System

The skeletal system supports and protects the soft tissues of the body and helps the body move. It consists of bones, which are bound together by ligaments and cartilages. The skeletal system shields soft tissues and attaches to muscles. The bones also help in blood formation and provide storage of mineral salts.

Muscular System

The muscular system works with the skeletal system in helping the body to move. Body parts are moved by muscle contraction. Posture and body heat are maintained by the muscular system. The muscular system also includes the tendons.

Nervous System

The nervous and endocrine systems control and coordinate various organ functions, helping to maintain homeostasis. The nervous system consists of the brain, spinal cord, nerves, and sensory organs. *Nerve impulses* are electrochemical signals used by nerve cells to communicate with each other and with the glands and muscles of the body. Certain nerve cells (called *sensory receptors*) detect internal

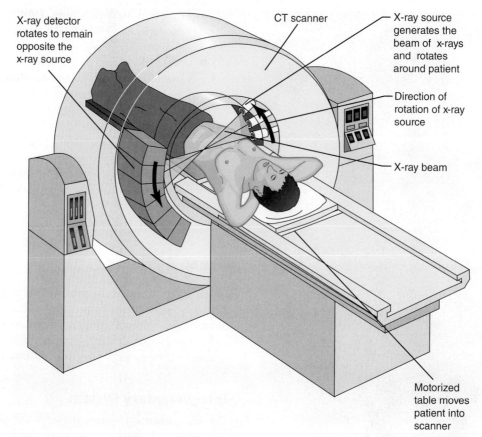

X-ray detector rotates to remain opposite the x-ray source

CT scanner

X-ray source generates the beam of x-rays and rotates around patient

Direction of rotation of x-ray source

X-ray beam

Motorized table moves patient into scanner

FIGURE 1-9 CT scan. The patient lies on a table that is gradually advanced into the scanner. An x-ray tube mounted in the scanner rotates around the patient, and radiation detectors also rotate so that detectors remain opposite the x-ray source. Data from the radiation detectors generate computer-reconstructed images of the patient's body at multiple levels.

and external changes that affect the body. Other nerve cells interpret and respond to these stimuli. Additional nerve cells carry impulses from the brain or spinal cord to the glands and muscles. These nerves are able to stimulate the muscles to contract and cause the glands to secrete their products.

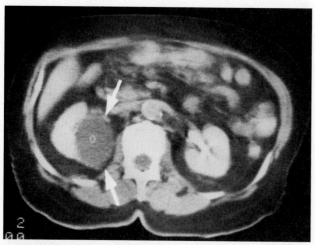

FIGURE 1-10 CT views of the abdomen at the level of the kidneys, illustrating a fluid-filled cyst in the kidney (arrow). The cyst appears less dense than surrounding renal tissue. The opposite kidney (right side of photograph) appears to be normal. (Courtesy of Leonard V. Crowley, MD, Century College.)

The characteristics of the nervous system include short-term effects, rapid responses, and very specific responses, as well as a variety of other responses.

Endocrine System

The endocrine system consists of hormone-secreting glands. Hormones affect specific target cells, altering their metabolism. Hormones have a relatively long duration of action compared with nerve impulses, lasting for days or longer. The endocrine system also produces a slower response regarding body changes than the nervous system. The organs of the endocrine system include the hypothalamus (in the brain), pituitary gland, pineal gland, thyroid gland, parathyroid glands, adrenal glands, pancreas, and thymus. Other organs with endocrine function include the ovaries and testes, which also are part of the reproductive system. The endocrine system can produce effects involving several organs or tissues at the same time.

Cardiovascular System

The cardiovascular system includes the heart, blood, arteries, veins, and capillaries. The heart muscle pumps blood through the arteries, transporting gases, hormones, nutrients, and wastes. Blood returns to the heart via the veins. Oxygen is carried from the lungs to the body, and nutrients are carried from the digestive system. The blood also

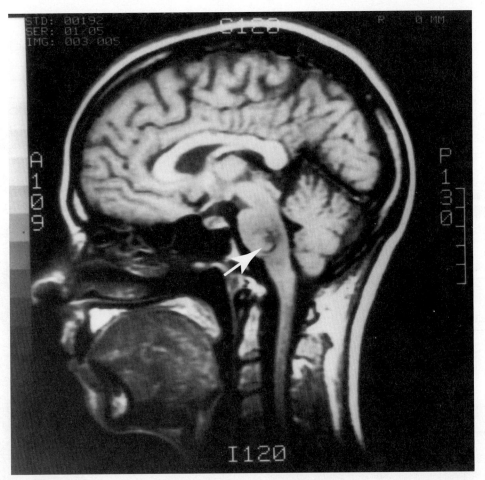

FIGURE 1-11 MRI view of brain, which is clearly visible because skull bones are not visualized by MRI. The white line surrounding the brain represents scalp tissue. The arrow indicates a malformation composed of blood vessels within the brainstem. (Courtesy of Leonard V. Crowley, MD, Century College.)

transports biochemicals required for metabolism. Wastes are carried in the blood from body cells to the excretory organs.

Lymphatic System

The lymphatic system is composed of the lymphatic vessels, lymph nodes, thymus, spleen, and lymph fluid. It works with the cardiovascular system, transporting tissue fluid back into the bloodstream. It also carries specific fats from digestive organs into the bloodstream. Lymphatic cells (lymphocytes) defend the body against infection. The lymphatic vessels have two ducts in the chest, known as the thoracic duct and the right lymphatic duct.

Digestive System

The digestive system takes in food from outside the body, breaking down and absorbing nutrients. It then excretes wastes from its various processes. The digestive system also produces certain hormones and works in conjunction with the endocrine system. The structures of the digestive system include the mouth, teeth, salivary glands, tongue, esophagus, stomach, liver, gallbladder, pancreas, small intestine, large intestine, rectum, and anus. The pharynx is part of both the digestive and respiratory systems.

Respiratory System

The respiratory system takes in and expels air, exchanging oxygen and carbon dioxide via the lungs and bloodstream. The structures of the respiratory system include the nose, nasal cavity, larynx, trachea, bronchi, and lungs. Again, the pharynx is part of both the respiratory and digestive systems.

Urinary System

The urinary system functions to remove liquid wastes from the body. It consists of the kidneys, ureters, urinary bladder, and urethra; it is through the urethra that urine is expelled. The female urethra is located just above the vagina, while the male urethra runs through the penis. The kidneys filter wastes from the blood and maintain electrolyte concentrations. The urinary bladder stores urine, and the urethra carries it outside of the body.

Reproductive System

The reproductive system in females consists of the ovaries, uterine tubes, uterus, vagina, clitoris, and vulva. The female sex cells are called *oocytes* or *eggs*. They are fertilized

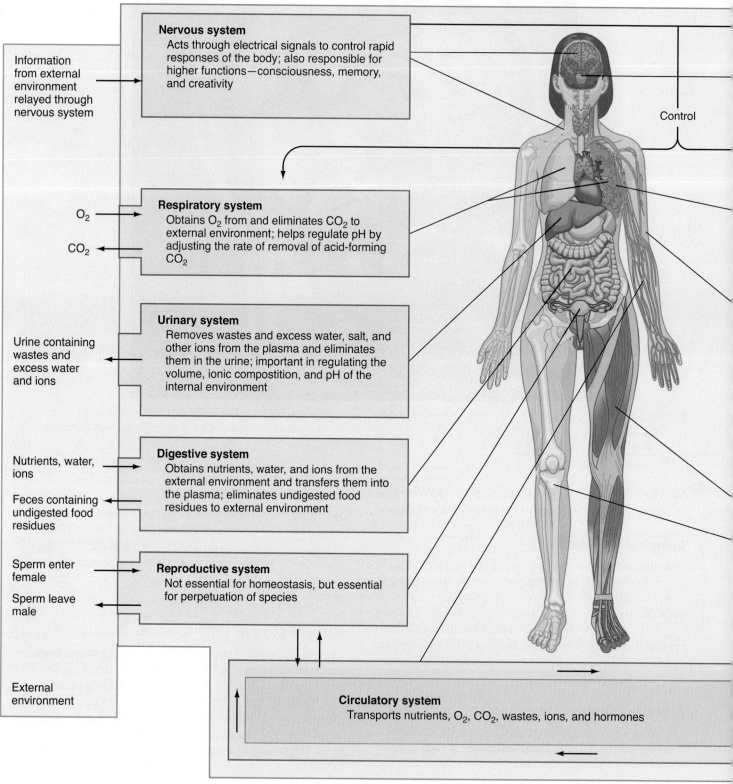

BODY SYSTEMS
Made up of cells organized by specialization to maintain

Nervous system
Acts through electrical signals to control rapid responses of the body; also responsible for higher functions—consciousness, memory, and creativity

Information from external environment relayed through nervous system

Control

O_2

Respiratory system
Obtains O_2 from and eliminates CO_2 to external environment; helps regulate pH by adjusting the rate of removal of acid-forming CO_2

CO_2

Urine containing wastes and excess water and ions

Urinary system
Removes wastes and excess water, salt, and other ions from the plasma and eliminates them in the urine; important in regulating the volume, ionic compostition, and pH of the internal environment

Nutrients, water, ions

Digestive system
Obtains nutrients, water, and ions from the external environment and transfers them into the plasma; eliminates undigested food residues to external environment

Feces containing undigested food residues

Sperm enter female

Reproductive system
Not essential for homeostasis, but essential for perpetuation of species

Sperm leave male

External environment

Circulatory system
Transports nutrients, O_2, CO_2, wastes, ions, and hormones

FIGURE 1-12 Systems of the body

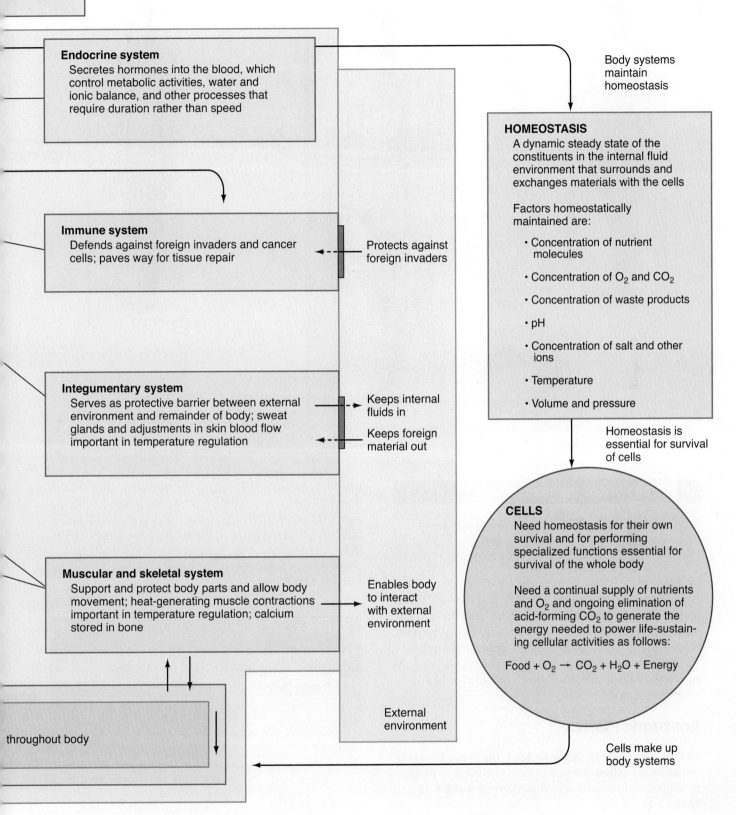

Endocrine system
Secretes hormones into the blood, which control metabolic activities, water and ionic balance, and other processes that require duration rather than speed

Immune system
Defends against foreign invaders and cancer cells; paves way for tissue repair

Protects against foreign invaders

Integumentary system
Serves as protective barrier between external environment and remainder of body; sweat glands and adjustments in skin blood flow important in temperature regulation

Keeps internal fluids in

Keeps foreign material out

Muscular and skeletal system
Support and protect body parts and allow body movement; heat-generating muscle contractions important in temperature regulation; calcium stored in bone

Enables body to interact with external environment

External environment

throughout body

Body systems maintain homeostasis

HOMEOSTASIS
A dynamic steady state of the constituents in the internal fluid environment that surrounds and exchanges materials with the cells

Factors homeostatically maintained are:

• Concentration of nutrient molecules

• Concentration of O_2 and CO_2

• Concentration of waste products

• pH

• Concentration of salt and other ions

• Temperature

• Volume and pressure

Homeostasis is essential for survival of cells

CELLS
Need homeostasis for their own survival and for performing specialized functions essential for survival of the whole body

Need a continual supply of nutrients and O_2 and ongoing elimination of acid-forming CO_2 to generate the energy needed to power life-sustaining cellular activities as follows:

$$Food + O_2 \rightarrow CO_2 + H_2O + Energy$$

Cells make up body systems

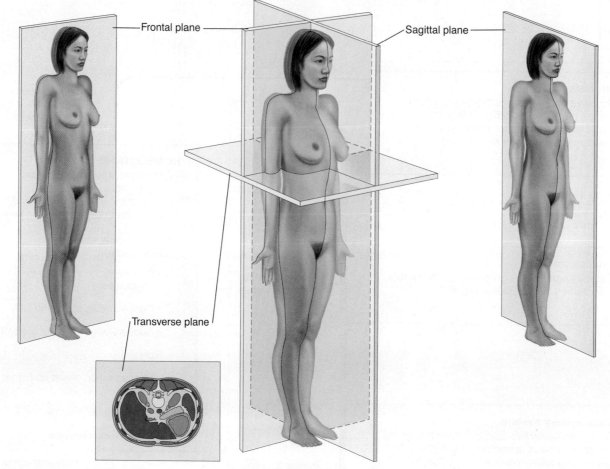

FIGURE 1-13 Anatomic planes

by male sex cells (*sperm* or *spermatozoa*). When a female is impregnated, the embryo normally develops within the uterus. The male reproductive system includes the scrotum, testes, epididymides, ductus deferentia, seminal vesicles, prostate gland, bulbourethral glands, penis, and urethra.

Reproduction is the process of producing offspring. As embryonic cells divide, they grow and produce new cells, which continue the process.

Anatomic Planes

The body can be visually divided into specific areas, called *planes*. These planes "divide" the body at particular angles and in particular directions (**FIGURE 1-13** and **TABLE 1-2**).

Directional Terms

Directional terms used in the study of anatomy include words that describe relative positions of body parts as well as

imaginary anatomical divisions. The term *anatomical position* describes the body standing erect, facing forward, with the arms held to the sides of the body, palms of the hands facing forward. When the terms *right* and *left* are used, they refer to those specific sides of the body when it is in the anatomical position. Important directional terms used in anatomy are listed in **TABLE 1-3**.

TABLE 1-2	
Anatomic Planes	
Anatomic Plane	**Meaning**
Coronal (frontal)	A plane dividing the body into anterior and posterior portions.
Sagittal	A plane dividing the body lengthwise into right and left portions. A median (midsagittal) plane passes along the midline, dividing the body into equal parts. A parasagittal plane divides the body similarly but is lateral to the midline.
Transverse (horizontal)	A plane that divides the body into superior and inferior portions.

TABLE 1-3

Directional Terms

Directional Term	Meaning	Example
Inferior	A body part is below another body part or is located toward the feet	The neck is inferior to the head.
Superior	A body part is above another body part or is located toward the head	The thoracic cavity is superior to the abdominopelvic cavity.
Anterior (ventral)	Toward the front	The eyes are anterior to the brain.
Posterior (dorsal)	Toward the back	The pharynx is posterior to the mouth.
Lateral	Toward the side as related to the midline of the body	The ears are lateral to the eyes.
Bilateral	Refers to paired structures, with one on each side of the body	The lungs are bilateral.
Contralateral	Refers to structures on the opposite side	If the right leg is injured, the patient may have to put most of his or her weight on the contralateral leg instead of using both equally.
Ipsilateral	Refers to structures on the same side	The right kidney and right lung are ipsilateral.
Medial	Refers to an imaginary midline that divides the body into left and right halves	The nose is medial (closer to the body's midline) to the eyes.
Distal	A body part is *farther* from the point of attachment to the trunk than another part	The fingers are distal to the wrist.
Proximal	A body part is *closer* to the point of attachment to the trunk than another part	The elbow is proximal to the wrist.
Deep	A body part is more *internal* than another part	The dermis is the deep layer of the skin.
Superficial	A body part is more *external* than another part	The epidermis is the superficial layer of the skin.

Abdominal Regions

Anatomists have divided the abdomen and pelvis into nine imaginary regions, which are helpful in identifying the location of particular abdominal organs. They are also useful for describing the location of abdominal pain. **FIGURE 1-14** shows the nine abdominal regions, identified from the left to the right and moving from top to bottom one row at a time. The abdomen may also be divided into four quadrants, as shown in **FIGURE 1-15**. **TABLE 1-4** explains each abdominal region in greater detail.

Body Regions

The remainder of the body is classified into various regions that clinically describe them. For example, *carpal tunnel syndrome* refers to the carpal area—the wrist—where acute pain can occur from the development of this syndrome. The most common body regions are listed in **TABLE 1-5**.

TEST YOUR UNDERSTANDING

1. Name the nine abdominopelvic regions.
2. Describe the anatomic planes of the body.

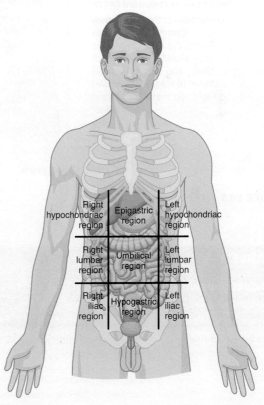

FIGURE 1-14 Abdominal regions. (Adapted from Shier, D. N., Butler, J. L., and Lewis, R. Hole's Essentials of Human Anatomy & Physiology, Tenth edition. McGraw Hill Higher Education, 2009.)

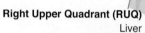

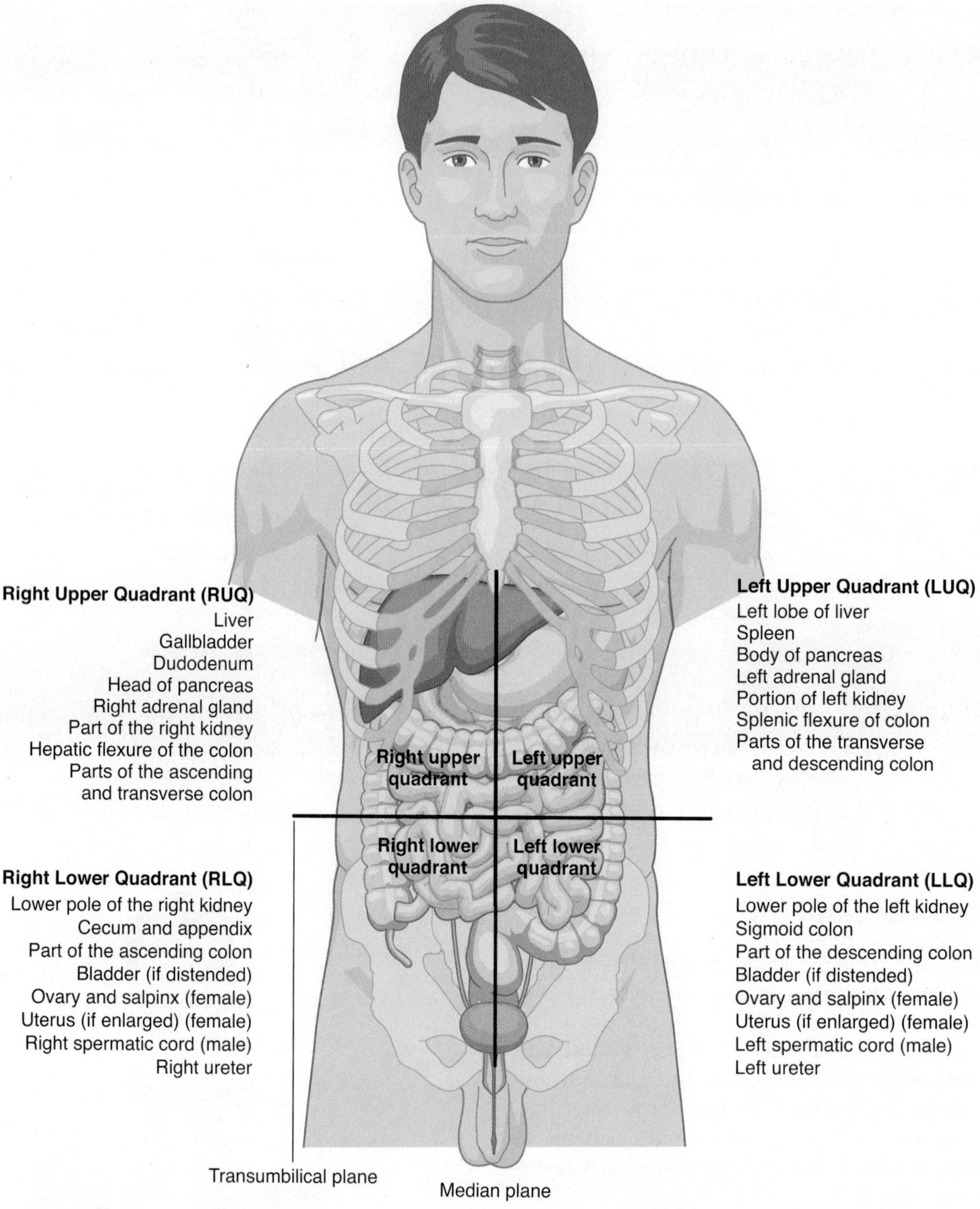

Right Upper Quadrant (RUQ)
Liver
Gallbladder
Dudodenum
Head of pancreas
Right adrenal gland
Part of the right kidney
Hepatic flexure of the colon
Parts of the ascending
and transverse colon

Left Upper Quadrant (LUQ)
Left lobe of liver
Spleen
Body of pancreas
Left adrenal gland
Portion of left kidney
Splenic flexure of colon
Parts of the transverse
and descending colon

Right upper quadrant | Left upper quadrant

Right lower quadrant | Left lower quadrant

Right Lower Quadrant (RLQ)
Lower pole of the right kidney
Cecum and appendix
Part of the ascending colon
Bladder (if distended)
Ovary and salpinx (female)
Uterus (if enlarged) (female)
Right spermatic cord (male)
Right ureter

Left Lower Quadrant (LLQ)
Lower pole of the left kidney
Sigmoid colon
Part of the descending colon
Bladder (if distended)
Ovary and salpinx (female)
Uterus (if enlarged) (female)
Left spermatic cord (male)
Left ureter

Transumbilical plane

Median plane

FIGURE 1-15 Four quadrants

TABLE 1-4	
Abdominopelvic Regions	
Region	**Meaning**
Left hypochondriac	The upper left abdominal region, under the angle of the ribs and diaphragm; this region contains a small portion of the stomach, a portion of the large intestine, and the spleen.
Epigastric	The upper middle abdominal region, between the left and right hypochondriac regions and under the cartilage of the lower ribs; this region contains parts of the liver and most of the stomach.
Right hypochondriac	The upper right abdominal region, under the angle of the ribs and diaphragm; this region contains the right lobe of the liver and the gallbladder.

TABLE 1-4

Abdominopelvic Regions (continued)

Left lumbar	The middle left abdominal region, beneath the left hypochondriac region; this region contains part of the small intestine and part of the colon.
Umbilical	The middle center portion of the abdomen, where the navel is located; it lies between the left and right lumbar regions and contains part of the transverse colon, small intestine, and pancreas.
Right lumbar	The middle right abdominal region, beneath the right hypochondriac region; this region contains parts of the small and large intestines.
Left iliac (inguinal)	The lower left abdominal region, beneath the left lumbar region; this region contains parts of the colon, small intestine, and left ovary (in women).
Hypogastric	The lower middle abdominal region, between the left and right iliac regions; this region contains the urinary bladder, parts of the small intestine, and uterus (in women).
Right iliac (inguinal)	The lower right abdominal region, beneath the right lumbar region; this region contains parts of the small intestine, cecum, appendix, and right ovary (in women).

TABLE 1-5

Body Regions and Terms

Region	Meaning	Region	Meaning
Abdominal	Between the thorax and pelvis	Femoral	Thigh
Acromial	Point of the shoulder	Frontal	Forehead
Antebrachial	Forearm	Genital	Reproductive organs
Antecubital	Space in front of the elbow	Gluteal	Buttocks
Axillary	Armpit	Inguinal	Groin (depressions of abdominal wall near thighs)
Brachial	Arm	Lumbar	Loin (lower back, between ribs and pelvis)
Buccal	Cheek	Mammary	Breast
Carpal	Wrist	Mental	Chin
Celiac	Abdomen	Nasal	Nose
Cephalic	Head	Occipital	Lower posterior region of the head
Cervical	Neck	Oral	Mouth
Costal	Ribs	Orbital	Eye cavity
Coxal	Hip	Otic	Ear
Crural	Leg	Palmar	Palm of the hand
Cubital	Elbow	Patellar	Front of the knee (kneecap)
Digital	Finger or toe	Pectoral	Chest
Dorsal	Back	Pedal	Foot

TABLE 1-5

Body Regions and Terms (continued)

Region	Meaning	Region	Meaning
Pelvic	Pelvis	Sternal	Anterior middle of the thorax
Perineal	Perineum; between the anus and external reproductive organs	Sural	Calf of the leg
Plantar	Sole of the foot	Tarsal	Instep of the foot
Pollex	Thumb	Umbilical	Navel
Popliteal	Area behind the knee	Vertebral	Spinal column
Sacral	Posterior region between the hipbones		

SUMMARY

Anatomy is the science of body structures and the relationships among these structures. Physiology is the science of body functions. The human body consists of six levels of structural organization: the chemical, cellular, tissue, organ, system, and organism levels. Certain processes that distinguish life processes from nonliving things include metabolism, responsiveness, movement, growth, differentiation, and reproduction. Essentials for life include body boundaries, movement, responsiveness, digestion, metabolism, excretion, reproduction, and growth. Survival requires nutrients, water, oxygen, atmospheric pressure, and the maintenance of adequate body temperature. Homeostasis of the body is controlled by receptors, effectors, and a set point that is achieved by the control center of the body (which primarily uses the nervous and endocrine systems).

The abdomen and pelvis are divided into nine abdominopelvic regions as follows: left hypochondriac, epigastric, right hypochondriac, left lumbar, umbilical, right lumbar, left iliac (inguinal), hypogastric, and right iliac (inguinal). Body cavities are mainly divided into two sections: the dorsal and ventral cavities. The dorsal cavity is subdivided into the cranial cavity (which contains the brain) and the vertebral cavity or canal (which contains the spinal cord). The meninges are protective tissues that line the dorsal body cavity.

The ventral body cavity is subdivided by the diaphragm into a superior thoracic cavity and an inferior abdominopelvic cavity. The viscera are organs within the ventral cavity. A serous membrane lines the wall of the cavity and adheres to the viscera. The thoracic cavity is subdivided into three smaller cavities, the pericardial cavity, the mediastinum, and the pleural cavity. The body's organ systems work together to maintain homeostasis. These systems include the integumentary, skeletal, muscular, nervous, endocrine, cardiovascular, lymphatic, digestive, respiratory, urinary, and reproductive systems. The body's anatomic planes include the coronal (frontal), sagittal, and transverse (horizontal) planes.

KEY TERMS

Anatomists
Anatomy
Atoms
Cell
Cytology
Developmental anatomy
Embryology

Gross (macroscopic) anatomy
Histology
Homeostasis
Homeostatic mechanisms
Intraperitoneal
Mediastinum

Metabolism
Microscopic anatomy
Molecules
Organ systems
Organelles
Organism
Organs

Parietal
Pathophysiology
Peritoneal membranes
Peritonitis
Pleurisy

Physiology
Regional anatomy
Retroperitoneal
Serous membrane
Surface anatomy

Systemic anatomy
Tissues
Viscera
Visceral

LEARNING GOALS

The following learning goals correspond to the objectives at the beginning of this chapter:

1. Anatomy is defined as the study of body parts, forms, and structures. Physiology is defined as the study of body functions.
2. The organization levels of the body include the atoms, molecules, macromolecules, organelles, cells, tissues, organs, organ systems, and the living organism.
3. Essentials for life include specific nutrients such as food, water, and oxygen as well as pressure and heat.
4. Homeostasis is defined as a stable internal body environment. It requires concentrations of nutrients, oxygen, and water as well as heat and pressure. Homeostatic mechanisms regulate the body.
5. The major body cavities are the cranial cavity (housing the brain), thoracic cavity (inside the chest), and abdominopelvic cavity (inside the abdomen and pelvic areas).
6. The systems of the body and their organs are as follows:
   Integumentary: skin, hair, nails, sebaceous (oil) glands, sweat glands
   Skeletal: bones, ligaments, cartilages
   Muscular: muscles, tendons
   Nervous: brain, spinal cord, nerves, sensory organs
   Endocrine: hypothalamus, pituitary, thyroid, parathyroid glands, pancreas, pineal gland, adrenal glands, thymus
   Cardiovascular: heart, blood, arteries, veins, capillaries
   Lymphatic: lymphatic vessels, lymph nodes, thymus, spleen, lymph fluid
   Digestive: mouth, teeth, salivary glands, tongue, pharynx, esophagus, stomach, liver, gallbladder, pancreas, small intestine, large intestine, rectum, anus
   Respiratory: nose, nasal cavity, pharynx, larynx, trachea, bronchi, lungs
   Urinary: kidneys, ureters, urinary bladder, urethra, penis

   Reproductive: ovaries, uterine tubes, uterus, vagina, clitoris, and vulva in the female and scrotum, testes, epididymides, ductus deferentia, seminal vesicles, prostate gland, bulbourethral glands, penis, and urethra in the male
7. Inferior, below another body part; superior, above another body part; anterior (ventral), toward the front; posterior (dorsal), toward the back; lateral, toward the side; bilateral, refers to paired structures; contralateral, refers to structures on opposite sides; ipsilateral, refers to structures on the same side; medial, refers to an imaginary body midline; distal, farther from the point of attachment to the trunk; proximal, closer to the point of attachment to the trunk; deep, more internal; superficial, more external. Body planes include coronal (frontal), dividing the body into anterior and posterior portions; sagittal, dividing the body lengthwise into right and left portions; and transverse (horizontal), dividing the body into superior and inferior portions.
8. The heart is surrounded by pericardial membranes, including the visceral pericardium over the heart's surface. The lungs are lined with a membrane called the parietal pleura and covered by a membrane called the visceral pleura. The abdominopelvic cavity is lined with peritoneal membranes. The parietal peritoneum lines its walls, and the visceral peritoneum covers each organ.
9. The nine abdominal regions are the left hypochondriac, epigastric, right hypochondriac, left lumbar, umbilical, right lumbar, left iliac (inguinal), hypogastric, and right iliac (inguinal) regions.
10. A positive feedback mechanism is one that makes conditions move away from the normal state, stimulating further changes. They are usually short-lived and extremely specific actions. A negative feedback mechanism is one that prevents the correction of deviations from doing too much, which could potentially harm the body. Most feedback mechanisms of the human body use negative feedback.

CRITICAL THINKING QUESTIONS

An 8-year-old boy had severe abdominal pain, a low fever, nausea, and vomiting. He was brought to the emergency department. His parents explained that his pain had started about 14 hours before. After physical examination on the boy's abdomen, the physician located the site of pain and then suspected the boy had appendicitis.

1. Explain the nine abdominal regions.
2. Explain which abdominal region contains the appendix.

REVIEW QUESTIONS

1. The maintenance of a relatively constant internal environment in the human body is termed
   - A. positive feedback
   - B. negative feedback
   - C. homeostasis
   - D. effector control

2. The lungs are to the respiratory system as the spleen is to the
   - A. lymphatic system
   - B. cardiovascular system
   - C. digestive system
   - D. urinary system

3. The pituitary and thyroid glands are components of the
   - A. respiratory system
   - B. endocrine system
   - C. lymphatic system
   - D. cardiovascular system

4. Support, protection of soft tissue, mineral storage, and blood formation are functions of which system?
   - A. nervous
   - B. muscular
   - C. skeletal
   - D. integumentary

5. The chemical or molecular level of organization begins with _____ and forms _____?
   - A. cells; tissues
   - B. molecules; atoms
   - C. organs; systems
   - D. atoms; molecules

6. Which sectional plane divides the body so the face remains intact?
   - A. midsagittal plane
   - B. coronal plane
   - C. sagittal plane
   - D. parasagittal plane

7. Which of the following cavities are spaces for joints?
   - A. orbital
   - B. synovial
   - C. oral
   - D. nasal

8. Which of the following terms indicates the front (anterior) of the body?
   - A. ventral
   - B. dorsal
   - C. posterior
   - D. proximal

9. The navel is located between which of the following?
   - A. left and right lungs
   - B. left and right lumbar regions
   - C. left and right iliac regions
   - D. left and right hypochondriac regions

10. Which of the following is an example of positive feedback?
    - A. blood pressure regulation
    - B. control of blood glucose
    - C. contractions before childbirth
    - D. body temperature regulation

11. A cut passing through the midline of the body that divides it into equal left and right halves is referred to as which of the following planes?
    - A. coronal
    - B. midsagittal
    - C. transverse
    - D. frontal

12. Skin, hair, and nails are associated with the
    - A. digestive system
    - B. endocrine system
    - C. lymphatic system
    - D. integumentary system

13. Which of the following is/are lateral to the nose?
    A. forehead
    B. chin
    C. eyes
    D. chest
14. The chest is _____ to the mouth.
    A. inferior
    B. posterior
    C. superior
    D. anterior

15. The thoracic cavity contains the
    A. cranium
    B. pelvic cavity
    C. abdominal cavity
    D. pericardial cavity

ESSAY QUESTIONS

1. How does anatomy relate to physiology?
2. Define homeostasis.
3. Briefly describe five external factors that help to sustain life.
4. List various systems of the body, and name three organs from each system.
5. Compare the operation of positive and negative feedback mechanisms in maintaining homeostasis.
6. Why is the anatomical position important?
7. Define the terms "plane" and "section."
8. Describe the lateral view of the body cavities.
9. List as many directional terms as you can, and define them.
10. Name two organs that are located in each of the named body regions.

Chemical Basics of Life

OBJECTIVES

After studying this chapter, readers should be able to

1. Describe the relationships between atoms and molecules.
2. Explain chemical bonds.
3. Describe how an atomic number is determined.
4. List the major groups of inorganic chemicals common in cells.
5. Explain acids, bases, and buffers.
6. Define the characteristics of lipids and proteins.
7. Define pH.
8. Describe the functions of various types of organic chemicals in cells.
9. List four examples of steroid molecules.
10. Explain nucleic acids.

OUTLINE

Overview

Chemistry is the science that deals with the structure of matter, and the study of the human body begins with chemistry. It is essential for other sciences, including physiology, pathology, pharmacology, and microbiology. Life is based on atomic, molecular, and chemical interactions. Each cell of the body contains organelles made up of macromolecules. The cells then compose tissues and organs. The chemical basics of life require the interactions of all these components.

Basic Chemistry

Studying basic chemistry and its relation to anatomy and physiology is extremely important as the entire human body is made up of chemicals. Basic chemistry takes into account matter, the states of matter, and **energy** in all its various types. This chapter focuses on both basic chemistry and biochemistry.

Matter is a term that describes all things occupying space and having *mass*. Most types of matter can be sensed in various forms. Mass is not exactly the same as *weight*. An object's mass is equal to its actual amount of matter. Mass remains constant regardless of where the object is located. Weight is different because it varies with gravity. For example, because of differences in gravitational pull, your body weighs slightly more at extremely low sea levels and slightly less at extremely high sea levels. However, your body's mass is exactly the same at both levels. Chemistry studies the nature of matter and how chemical building blocks interact and how they are constructed.

The various *states* of matter are *gaseous, liquid,* and *solid.* The human body contains examples of all three states. Gases have no shape or definite volume. An example is the air that we breathe. *Liquids* have definite volume but are "shaped" by the structure containing them. An example is blood plasma, which assumes the shape of the blood vessels. *Solids* have a definite shape and volume. Examples include teeth and bones.

Atoms, Molecules, and Chemical Bonds

The composition of matter and changes in its composition are the focuses of the study of chemistry. If you understand chemistry, your understanding of anatomy and physiology will be improved. Chemical changes within cells influence body functions and the status of the body's structures. Chemicals of the body include water, proteins, carbohydrates, lipids, nucleic acids, and salts, as well as foods, drinks, and medications.

Elements are fundamental substances that compose matter. Copper, iron, gold, silver, aluminum, carbon, hydrogen, and oxygen are all examples of elements. Most living organisms need about 20 elements to survive. **TABLE 2-1** lists the major and trace elements required by the human body. The *periodic table of elements* is a tabular arrangement of the chemical elements. It is organized on the basis of atomic numbers, electron configurations, and recurring chemical properties. The elements are presented in order of increasing atomic number, which is the number of protons in the nucleus (**FIGURE 2-1**).

Atoms are tiny particles that compose elements, and are the smallest complete units of an element that retain its properties, and vary in size, weight, and interaction with other atoms. The characteristics of living and nonliving objects result from the atoms they contain and how those atoms combine and interact. Thus, by forming chemical bonds, atoms can combine with other atoms that are not similar to them.

Atomic Structure

Atoms are composed of subatomic particles. Each atom consists of protons, neutrons, and electrons. Protons and neutrons are similar in size and mass; however, **protons** bear a positive electrical charge, whereas **neutrons** are electrically

TABLE 2-1	
Elements of the Human Body	
	Percentage in the Body
Major elements (totaling 99.9%)	
Oxygen (O)	65%
Carbon (C)	18.5%
Hydrogen (H)	9.5%
Nitrogen (N)	3.2%
Calcium (Ca)	1.5%
Phosphorus (P)	1%
Potassium (K)	0.4%
Sulfur (S)	0.3%
Chlorine (Cl)	0.2%
Sodium (Na)	0.2%
Magnesium (Mg)	0.1%
Trace elements (totaling 0.1%)	
Chromium (Cr)	—
Cobalt (Co)	—
Copper (Cu)	—
Fluorine (F)	—
Iodine (I)	—
Iron (Fe)	—
Manganese (Mn)	—
Zinc (Zn)	—

neutral (uncharged). **Electrons** bear a negative electrical charge. An atom's mass is determined mostly by the number of protons and neutrons in its **nucleus**. The nucleus contains approximately the entire mass (99.9%) of the atom. The mass of a larger object, such as the human body, is the sum of the masses of all its atoms. **FIGURE 2-2** shows the components of an atom and its nucleus.

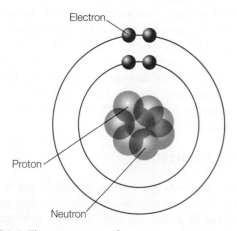

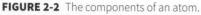

FIGURE 2-2 The components of an atom.

Electrons orbit an atom's nucleus at high speed, forming a spherical electron cloud. Atoms normally contain equal numbers of protons and electrons. The number of protons in an atom is known as its **atomic number**. Thus, hydrogen (H), the simplest atom, has one proton, giving it the atomic number 1, whereas magnesium, with 12 protons, has the atomic number 12.

The **atomic weight** of an element's atom equals the number of protons and neutrons in its nucleus. For example, oxygen has eight protons and eight neutrons, so its atomic weight is 16. An **isotope** is defined as when an element's atoms have nuclei containing the same number of protons but different numbers of neutrons. Isotopes may or may not be radioactive. Radioactivity is the emission of energetic particles known as *radiation*, which occurs because of instability of the atomic nuclei.

The nuclei of certain isotopes (**radioisotopes**) spontaneously emit subatomic particles or radiation in measurable amounts. The process of emitting radiation is called *radioactive decay*. Strongly radioactive isotopes are dangerous because their emissions can destroy molecules, cells, and living tissue. For diagnostic procedures, weaker radioactive isotopes are used to diagnose structural and functional characteristics of internal organs. Radiation is basically identified as one of three common forms: alpha (α), beta (β), or gamma (γ). Gamma radiation is the most penetrating type and is similar to x-ray radiation.

Health professionals and researchers use radioactive isotopes for clinical applications because they are easily detected and measured. All isotopes of a certain element have the same atomic number. For example, two types of iodine, 125-iodine and 131-iodine, can substitute for 126-iodine in chemical reactions. Iodine may be used in diagnostic procedures involving the thyroid gland to detect thyroid cancer.

| **TEST YOUR UNDERSTANDING** |

1. Differentiate between atomic weight and atomic number.
2. Describe the locations of electrons, protons, and neutrons.

Molecules and Compounds

The term **molecule** is defined as any chemical structure that consists of atoms held together by covalent bonds (involving the sharing of electrons between atoms). When two atoms of the same element bond, they produce molecules of that element, such as hydrogen, oxygen, or nitrogen molecules. Most atoms are chemically combined with other atoms. For example, when two oxygen atoms combine, a molecule of O_2 (oxygen gas) is formed.

When two different kinds of atoms combine, they form molecules of a *compound* (discussed in more detail under Covalent Bonds, below). **Compounds** are chemically pure, with identical molecules. A molecule is the smallest particle of a compound that still has the specific characteristics of that compound. Examples of compounds include water (a compound of hydrogen and oxygen), dry ice (frozen carbon dioxide), table sugar, baking soda, alcohol (as used in beverages), natural gas, and most medicinal drugs. A molecule of a compound has specific types and amounts of atoms (see Hydrogen Bonds, below).

Mixtures

Mixtures are substances containing two or more components that are physically *intermixed*. They do not chemically combine and may not occur in fixed (specific) proportions. An example is the various powders combined together in a capsule with an active drug. The individual characteristics of the components of a mixture are not lost. They may be separated from each other if this is required. The three basic types of mixtures are colloids, solutions, and suspensions. In nature, most matter exists in the form of mixtures. Colloids, solutions, and suspensions are each found in both living and nonliving systems. Living material is the most complex mixture of all, containing colloids, solutions, and suspensions—all of which interact with each other.

Colloids

Colloids are also known as *emulsions*. Their composition differs in various areas of their mixtures, meaning they are referred to as *heterogeneous mixtures*. Colloids have solute particles that are larger than the particles in true solutions and do not settle. The appearance of a colloid is often milky or translucent. Light is scattered when shown through a colloid, meaning the path of the light beam is visible.

Colloids often have the ability to undergo *sol-gel transformations*. This means they can change (reversibly) from a sol (fluid) state to a gel (more solid) state. An example of a nonliving colloid that undergoes a sol-gel transformation (when refrigerated) is a gelatin product such as Jell-O. Also, the reverse process occurs when these products are heated, such as by sunlight, with their state returning to a liquid. In living cells the semifluid material known as cytosol undergoes sol-gel transformations. **Cytosol** has many dispersed proteins, and these transformations are the basis for cell division, cell shape changes, and other important activities.

Solutions

Solutions may be gases, liquids, or solids and are homogeneous mixtures of these components. This means the mixture has exactly the same composition throughout, in terms of the atoms or molecules it contains. One sample of any part of the mixture will reveal an identical composition to any other sample of the mixture. Examples include ocean water (which is a mixture of water and salts) and environmental air (which is a mixture of gases). In a mixture, the **solvent** is the substance that is present in the largest amount. A solvent is also known as a *dissolving medium* and is usually a liquid. The substances present in a mixture in smaller amounts are called **solutes**.

In the human body, water is the primary solvent. Most body solutions are called *true solutions*, which are usually transparent. They contain gases, liquids, or solids dissolved in water. True solutions are exemplified by mineral water, glucose/water, and saline solution (which is a mixture of sodium chloride and water). In true solutions the solutes are minute, usually consisting of individual atoms and molecules. These microscopic solutes do not scatter light (allow a beam of light to pass through) or settle.

True solutions are described by their *concentration*, which is often described in parts per 100 (percent), of the solute in the total solution. Water is usually assumed to be the solvent. True solutions may also be described in *milligrams per deciliter* (mg/dL). Another way to describe true solutions is **molarity** (M), which is defined as *moles per liter*. This is a complicated, but more chemically useful, method. A **mole** is equal to an element or compound's atomic weight or **molecular weight**, in grams. For example, glucose is written as a combination of 6 carbon atoms, 12 hydrogen atoms, and 6 oxygen atoms ($C_6H_{12}O_6$). To find its molecular weight, you must multiply the number of atoms of each component by its atomic weight. Then, you must add the total atomic weights of the three components to find the total atomic weight of glucose. In this example, carbon's 6 atoms

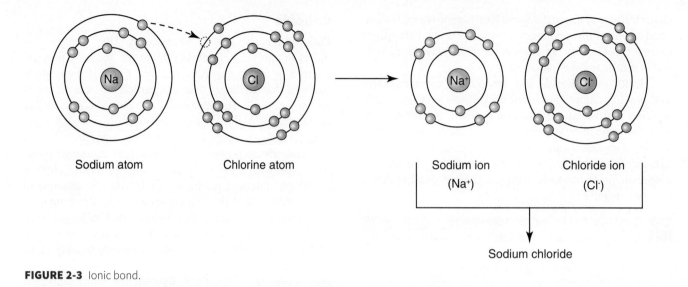

FIGURE 2-3 Ionic bond.

multiplied by its atomic weight of 12.011 equals a total atomic weight of 72.066. Using the same formula, the total atomic weights of hydrogen (12.096) and oxygen (95.994) are added together to find that the total atomic weight of glucose is 180.156. Overall, it is most important to understand that 1 mole of any substance always contains exactly the same number of solute particles. This is referred to as *Avogadro's number* and is calculated, in molecules of the substance, as 6.02×10^{23}. In body fluids, because solute concentrations are very low, their values are usually described in terms of *millimoles* (Mmol, or 1/1,000 mole).

Suspensions

Suspensions, known as *heterogeneous mixtures*, have large, often visible solutes that usually settle. In the blood, living blood cells are *suspended* in the fluid portion of the blood (the blood plasma). When a blood sample is left still for a period of time, the suspended cells settle unless they are mixed or shaken. In the body, they do not settle because of blood circulation.

> ### TEST YOUR UNDERSTANDING
>
> 1. Define the terms *molecule, compound,* and *mixture.*
> 1. List examples of *true solutions* in the body.
> 1. Define the terms *mole, molarity,* and *molecular weight.*

Chemical Bonds

Atoms can bond with other atoms by using chemical bonds that result from interactions between their electrons. During this process the atoms may either gain, lose, or share electrons. Chemically inactive atoms are known as *inert* atoms. An example of a chemical that is made up of inert atoms is helium. Atoms that either gain or lose electrons are called **ions**. These atoms are electrically charged. An example of an electrically charged atom, or ion, is sodium. The three important types of chemical bonds are ionic, covalent, and hydrogen.

Ionic Bonds

Ionic bonds form between ions. They are chemical bonds between atoms that form because of the transfer of electrons. The atom gaining one or more electrons is referred to as the *electron acceptor.* Ions that acquire a net positive charge are called **cations**, and those that acquire a net negative charge are called **anions**. Oppositely charged ions attract each other to form an *ionic bond.* This is a chemical bond that forms arrays (indiscreet molecules) such as crystals. An example is when sodium forms an ionic bond with chloride to create sodium chloride (or table salt). An ionic bond is shown in **FIGURE 2-3**. Sodium has an atomic number of 11 and only has one electron inside its valence shell (its outermost energy level that contains electrons). If this electron is lost, the second shell (with eight electrons) becomes the valence shell. The loss of the single electron in the third (outer) shell causes sodium to become stable, meaning it is then a cation. Oppositely, chlorine (with an atomic number of 17) only needs one electron to fill its valence shell. When it gains one electron, it becomes stable and is then an anion.

The interaction of sodium and chlorine involves sodium donating one electron to chlorine. Oppositely charged ions then attract each other to form sodium chloride. Examples of ionic bonds include atoms that have one or two valence shell electrons and atoms that have seven valence shell electrons. Those with one or two valence shell electrons include calcium, potassium, and sodium (all are metallic elements), and those with seven valence shell electrons include chlorine, fluorine, and iodine.

In this category, most ionic compounds are referred to as *salts.* They do not exist as individual molecules in their dry state but instead form **crystals**. These are large collections of cations and anions held together by ionic bonds. Sodium chloride gives us an example of a compound that is very different from the atoms that make it up individually. Separately, sodium is a metal that is silver-white in color. Chlorine is a green-colored gas. Mixed together to become sodium chloride, the result is a white crystalline solid (table salt).

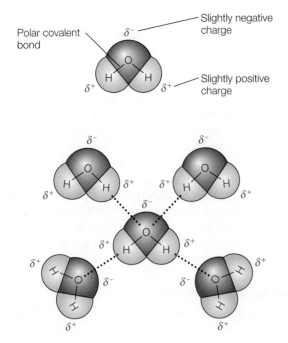

Polar covalent bond

δ⁻ Slightly negative charge

δ⁺ δ⁺ Slightly positive charge

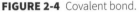

FIGURE 2-4 Covalent bond.

Covalent Bonds

For atoms to achieve stability, electrons do not have to be completely transferred. They may be shared, meaning each atom can fill its outer electron shell for part of the time. When electrons are shared, this produces molecules in which the shared electrons are located in a single orbital that is common to both atoms. This makes up a **covalent bond**. Hydrogen has only one electron. It can fill its only shell, labeled as *Shell 1*, when a pair of electrons from another atom is shared. If a hydrogen atom shares with another hydrogen atom, a molecule of hydrogen gas is formed. Therefore, the shared electron pair orbits around the molecule *as a whole* to make each atom achieve stability. An example of a covalent bond is when two hydrogen atoms bond to form a hydrogen molecule (**FIGURE 2-4**).

Each atom has different needs in terms of bonding to achieve stability. Shared electrons orbit and become part of the whole molecule, which ensures the stability of each atom. Hydrogen has only its one electron but needs two. Carbon has four electrons in its outer shell but needs eight for stability. For a methane molecule (CH_4), carbon shares four pairs of electrons with four hydrogen atoms, meaning one pair with each hydrogen atom. A single covalent bond is formed when two atoms share one pair of electrons. A double covalent bond occurs when two electron pairs are shared. Likewise, a triple covalent bond occurs when three electron pairs are shared. When written, the amount of covalent bonds present are signified by using single, double, or triple horizontal lines, as follows (using oxygen as the example): O—O, O═O, or O≡O.

In covalent bonds, molecules may be either polar or nonpolar. *Nonpolar molecules* are electrically balanced. They do not have separate positive and negative poles of charge. However, this does not always occur. Covalent bonds always have a specific three-dimensional shape to their molecules.

The bonds are formed at definite angles. The shape helps to determine with which other atoms or molecules the original molecule can interact. However, it may also cause unequal electron pair sharing. This creates a **polar** molecule. This is most common in nonsymmetric molecules that contain atoms with different electron-attracting abilities.

Oxygen, nitrogen, and chlorine are examples of electro-hungry atoms that attract electrons strongly. This is a capability of atoms known as **electronegativity**. These small atoms have six or seven valence shell electrons. However, most atoms that have only one or two valence shell electrons are **electropositive**. Their ability to attract electrons is so low that, most often, they lose their own valence shell electrons to other atoms. Potassium and sodium each have one valence shell electron and are examples of electropositive atoms.

Whether a covalently bonded molecule will be polar or nonpolar is determined by the molecular shape and related electron-attracting ability of each atom. For example, in the carbon dioxide (CO_2) molecule, four electron pairs of carbon are shared with two oxygen atoms, meaning two pairs are shared with each oxygen. Because oxygen is extremely electronegative, it attracts the shared electrons more strongly than carbon is able to. Even so, because the carbon dioxide molecule is symmetric and linear, the ability of one oxygen atom to pull electrons is offset by the other oxygen atom. Therefore, the shared electrons continue to orbit the entire molecule, and carbon dioxide is a nonpolar compound.

A different example exists in the water (H_2O) molecule, which is V-shaped, or bent. On the same end of this molecule are located two electropositive hydrogen atoms. The extremely electronegative oxygen atom is at the opposite end. Therefore, oxygen can pull the shared electrons away from the two hydrogen atoms. The electron pairs are not shared equally. Instead, they are closer to the oxygen for most of the time. Because of the negative charges of electrons, the oxygen end is slightly more negative and the hydrogen end slightly more positive. Water is a polar molecule with two poles of charge, which is also called a **dipole**.

Polar molecules are essential for chemical reactions in body cells. They orient themselves toward charged particles (ions, certain proteins, etc.) or other dipoles. Various molecules have different degrees of polarity. There is a gradual change from ionic to nonpolar covalent bonding. Complete electron transfer is referred to as an *ionic bond*. Equal electron sharing is known as a *nonpolar covalent bond*. These are extremes compared with each other. There are various degrees of unequal electron sharing in between these two extremes.

Hydrogen Bonds

When the positive hydrogen end of a polar molecule is attracted to the negative nitrogen or oxygen end of another polar molecule, the attraction is called a **hydrogen bond** (**FIGURE 2-5**). Hydrogen atoms already covalently linked to one electronegative atom (such as oxygen or nitrogen) are attracted by an atom requiring electrons, forming a "bridge." These bonds are weak at body temperature. In environmental

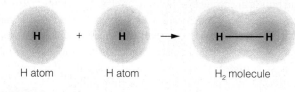

H atom   H atom H_2 molecule

FIGURE 2-5 Hydrogen bond.

extremes they may change form, from water to ice and back again. Hydrogen bonds are important in protein and nucleic acid structure, forming between polar regions of different parts of a single, large molecule. Hydrogen bonding commonly occurs between *dipoles*, an example of which is the water molecule. It occurs because the (slightly) negative oxygen atoms of a certain molecule attract the (slightly) positive hydrogen atoms of another molecule. Therefore, because of hydrogen bonding, water molecules usually cling together. They form *films*, and this formation process is referred to as *surface tension*. As a result, water beads into spheres when it is on a hard surface such as a countertop. This is also the reason that certain small insects are able to walk on the surface of a body of water.

Hydrogen bonds are too weak to bind atoms together and form molecules. However, they are important *intramolecular bonds*, holding different parts of one large molecule in a specific three-dimensional shape. Proteins and DNA are examples of large biologic molecules that have many hydrogen bonds helping to maintain and stabilize their structures. The water molecule is one excellent example of a hydrogen bond. It consists of two hydrogen atoms and one oxygen atom. Another example occurs when two hydrogen atoms bind with two oxygen atoms, forming hydrogen peroxide.

Because the properties of compounds are usually different from the properties of their contained atoms, it is difficult to tell which atoms are contained without a chemical analysis (e.g., water, which is made up of hydrogen and oxygen). The numbers and types of atoms in a molecule are represented by a *molecular formula*. The molecular formula for water is H_2O, signifying the two atoms of hydrogen and the one atom of oxygen. *Structural formulas* are used to signify how atoms are joined and arranged inside molecules. Single bonds are represented by single lines, and double bonds are represented by double lines. When structural formulas are represented in three-dimensional models, different colors are used to show different types of atoms.

Chemical Reactions

A **chemical reaction** occurs when a chemical bond is formed, broken, or rearranged. Chemical reactions are written using symbols, which are known as *chemical*

equations. Any number that is written in a smaller letter that appears below the level of the main text (a *subscript*) indicates the atoms are joined by chemical bonds. A number written as a *prefix* shows the number of unjoined atoms or molecules. For example, for H_2O the number "2" indicates that two hydrogen atoms are bonded together with one oxygen atom to form the water molecule. If an equation used the term "2H," it would mean there were two unjoined hydrogen atoms. A chemical equation contains the kinds and number of reacting substances (*reactants*), the chemical composition of the results (*products*), and, if the equation is *balanced*, the relative proportion of each reactant and each product. Four types of chemical reactions are important to the study of physiology: synthesis reactions, decomposition reactions, exchange reactions, and reversible reactions.

Synthesis Reactions

Chemical reactions change the bonds between atoms, molecules, and ions to generate new chemical combinations. **Synthesis** is a reaction that occurs when two or more reactants (atoms) bond to form a more complex product or structure. The formation of water from hydrogen and oxygen molecules is a synthesis reaction. Synthesis always involves the formation of new chemical bonds, whether the reactants are atoms or molecules. Synthesis requires energy, and it is important for growth and the repair of tissues. Synthesis is symbolized as follows: $A + B \rightarrow AB$.

Decomposition Reactions

Decomposition is a reaction that occurs when bonds within a reactant molecule break, forming simpler atoms, molecules, or ions. For example, a typical meal contains molecules of sugars, proteins, and fats that are too large and too complex to be absorbed and used by the body. Decomposition reactions in the digestive tract break these molecules down into smaller fragments before absorption begins. Decomposition is symbolized as follows: $AB \rightarrow A + B>$

Exchange Reactions

In an *exchange reaction*, parts of the reacting molecules are shuffled around to produce new products. An example of an exchange reaction is the reaction of an acid with a base, which forms water and a salt. Exchange reactions are symbolized as follows: $AB + CD \rightarrow AD + CB$.

Reversible Reactions

A *reversible reaction* is one wherein the products of the reaction can change back into the reactants they originally were. These reactions can proceed in opposite directions, depending on the relative proportions of reactants and products, as well as how much energy is available.

So, if $A + B \rightarrow AB$, then $AB \rightarrow A + B$. Many important biological reactions are freely reversible. Such reactions can be represented as the equation $A + B \rightarrow AB$.

1. Describe four kinds of chemical reactions.
2. What are the structural formulas for synthesis reactions and exchange reactions?

FOCUS ON PATHOLOGY

The kidneys play a very important role in maintaining homeostasis, balancing ions and fluids. In serious kidney disorders, this balance can be disturbed, resulting in physiological disturbances in the body. Complications of these imbalances include hyperkalemia, hypernatremia, and overhydration.

Acids, Bases, and the pH Scale

Electrolytes are substances that release ions in water. When they dissolve in water, the negative and positive ends of water molecules cause ions to separate and interact with water molecules instead of each other. The resulting solution contains electrically charged particles (ions) that conduct electricity. **Acids** are electrolytes that release hydrogen ions in water. An example of an acid is hydrochloric acid, made up of hydrogen and chloride ions. **Bases** are electrolytes that release ions that bond with hydrogen ions. An example of a base is sodium hydroxide, made up of sodium, oxygen, and hydrogen ions. In body fluids the concentrations of hydrogen and hydroxide ions greatly affect chemical reactions. These reactions control certain physiological functions such as blood pressure and breathing rates.

Hydrogen ion concentrations can be measured by a value called **pH**. The hydrogen ion concentration in body fluids is vital. It is expressed in a type of mathematical shorthand based on concentrations calculated in moles per liter (with a mole representing an amount of solute in a solution). The pH of a solution is defined as the level of acidity or basicity. The pH scale ranges from 0 to 14, with 7 being the midpoint (meaning it has equal numbers of hydrogen and hydroxide ions). Pure water has a pH of 7, and this midpoint is considered to be neutral (neither acidic nor basic). Therefore, a solution containing an equal number of hydrogen ions and hydroxide ions is neutral. Measurements of less than 7 pH are considered acidic, meaning there are more hydrogen ions than hydroxide ions. Measurements of more than 7 pH are considered basic, also known as alkaline, meaning there are more hydroxide ions than hydrogen ions.

The pH of blood usually ranges from 7.35 to 7.45. Abnormal fluctuations in pH can damage cells and tissues, change the shapes of proteins, and alter cellular functions. *Acidosis* is an abnormal physiological state caused by blood pH that is lower than 7.35. If pH falls below 7, coma may occur. The two different types of acidosis are *metabolic* and *respiratory*. Metabolic acidosis is a condition in which the kidneys are not able to remove ketone bodies, which are metabolites of fats. In patients with type 1 diabetes, the body may be producing too many ketone bodies. Respiratory acidosis occurs in patients suffering from chronic lung diseases such as emphysema or chronic bronchitis. Higher carbon dioxide concentrations in the blood results in blood pH decreasing.

Alkalosis results from blood pH that is higher than 7.45. If pH rises above 7.8, it generally causes uncontrollable and sustained skeletal muscle contractions. Alkalosis also may be metabolic or respiratory. Metabolic alkalosis involves elevations of tissue pH, either as a result of decreased hydrogen ion concentration or a direct result of increased bicarbonate concentrations. Respiratory alkalosis is caused by increased respiration, which elevates the blood pH. It may be caused by pneumonia, stroke, meningitis, fever, and pregnancy.

Chemicals that resist pH changes are called *buffers*. They combine with hydrogen ions when these ions are excessive and contribute hydrogen ions when these ions are reduced. **FIGURE 2-6** shows the pH values of acids and bases. An example of a buffer that is important in body fluids is *sodium bicarbonate*.

1. Define electrolytes, acids, and bases.
2. What does pH measure?

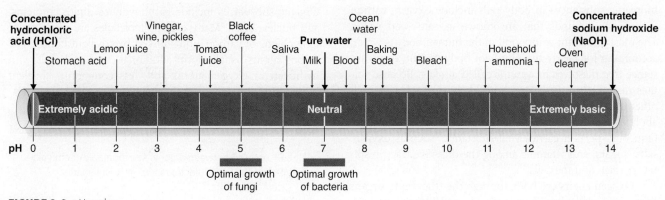

FIGURE 2-6 pH scale.

TABLE 2-2

Inorganic Substances in Cells

Formula or Symbol	Molecule or Ion	Function
H_2O	Water molecule	Major component of body fluids, biochemical reactions, chemical transport, and temperature regulation
O_2	Oxygen molecule	Used for energy release from glucose molecules
CO_2	Carbon dioxide	Metabolic waste product; forms carbonic acid via reaction with water
HCO_3^-	Bicarbonate ions	Assists in acid–base balance
Ca^{+2}	Calcium ions	Used in bone development, muscle contraction, and blood clotting
CO_3^{-2}	Carbonate ions	Important for formation of bone tissue
Cl^-	Chloride ions	Assists in maintaining water balance
Mg^{+2}	Magnesium ions	Important for formation of bone tissue and certain metabolic processes
PO_4^{-3}	Phosphate ions	Used in ATP, nucleic acid, and other vital substance synthesis; important for formation of bone tissue and to maintain cell membrane polarization
K^+	Potassium ions	Needed for cell membrane polarization
Na^+	Sodium ions	Needed for cell membrane polarization and to maintain water balance
SO_4^{-2}	Sulfate ions	Assists in cell membrane polarization

Biochemistry

The term "biochemistry" is also known as *biological chemistry*, which is the study of chemical processes within and relating to living organisms. Chemicals can basically be divided into two main groups: organic and inorganic. **Organic** chemicals are those that always contain the elements carbon and hydrogen and generally oxygen as well. **Inorganic** chemicals are any chemicals that do not. Inorganic substances release ions in water and are also called electrolytes. Although many organic substances also dissolve in water, they dissolve to great effect in alcohol or ether. Organic substances that dissolve in water usually do not release ions and are known as *nonelectrolytes*.

Inorganic Substances

Inorganic substances in body cells include oxygen, carbon dioxide, compounds that are known as salts, and water. The most abundant compound in the human body is water, accounting for nearly two-thirds of body weight. Any substance that dissolves in water is called a *solute*. Because solutes dissolved in water are more likely to react with each other as they break down into smaller particles, most metabolic reactions occur in water. In the blood, the watery (aqueous) portion carries vital substances such as oxygen, salts, sugars, and vitamins among the digestive tract, respiratory tract, and the cells.

Oxygen enters the body through the respiratory organs and is transported in the blood. The red blood cells bind and carry the largest amount of oxygen. Organelles inside the cells use oxygen for energy release from nutrients such as glucose (sugar) to drive cellular metabolic activities. Carbon dioxide is an inorganic compound produced as a waste product when some metabolic processes release energy. It is exhaled via the lungs.

Salts are compounds of oppositely charged ions that are abundant in tissues in fluids. Many ions required by the body are supplied in salts, including sodium, chloride, calcium, magnesium, phosphate, carbonate, bicarbonate, potassium, and sulfate. Salt ions are important for transporting substances to and from the cells and for muscle contractions and nerve impulse conduction. Common inorganic molecules are summarized in **TABLE 2-2.**

Organic Substances

Organic substances include carbohydrates, lipids, proteins, and nucleic acids. Many organic molecules are made up of long chains of carbon atoms linked by covalent bonds. The carbon atoms usually form additional covalent bonds with hydrogen or oxygen atoms and, less commonly, covalent bonds with nitrogen, phosphorus, sulfur, or other elements.

TEST YOUR UNDERSTANDING

1. Distinguish between organic and inorganic chemicals.
2. Define the term "biochemistry" and list its other descriptive title.

Carbohydrates

Carbohydrates provide much of the energy required by the body's cells and help to build cell structures. Carbohydrate molecules consist of carbon, hydrogen, and oxygen molecules. The carbon atoms they contain join in chains that vary with the type of carbohydrate. The hydrogen and oxygen atoms usually occur in a 2:1 ratio, which is the same as in water. In most cases the overall carbon to hydrogen to oxygen ratio is 1:2:1. Carbohydrates with shorter chains are called *sugars*. Carbohydrates also include *starches*. Collectively, carbohydrates represent 1% to 2% of cell mass in the body. The term *carbohydrate* actually means "hydrated carbon." Usually, the larger the carbohydrate molecule, the less soluble it is in water. Simple sugars have 6 carbon atoms, 12 hydrogen atoms, and 6 oxygen atoms ($C_6H_{12}O_6$). They are also known as **monosaccharides**. Simple sugars include glucose, fructose, galactose, ribose, and deoxyribose. Ribose and deoxyribose differ from the others in that they each contain five atoms of carbon. Monosaccharides are single-chain or single-ring structures. They may contain between three and seven carbon atoms. Monosaccharides are generally named based on the number of carbon atoms they contain. In the human body the most important ones are the pentose (five-carbon) and hexose (six-carbon) sugars (**FIGURE 2-7**).

Complex carbohydrates include sucrose (table sugar) and lactose (milk sugar). Some of these carbohydrates are double sugars or **disaccharides** and are formed when two monosaccharides are joined by *dehydration synthesis*. A water molecule is lost as the bond is made. Another important disaccharide is *maltose* (malt sugar). Disaccharides cannot pass through cell membranes because of their size so instead are digested to simple sugar units for absorption from the digestive tract. They decompose via *hydrolysis*, which is basically the reverse process of dehydration synthesis. A water molecule is added, which breaks the bond and releases the simple sugar units.

Other types of complex carbohydrates contain many simple joined sugar units, such as plant starch, and are known as **polysaccharides**. They are polymers of simple sugars, linked together via dehydration synthesis, and function as storage products because they are large and fairly insoluble. They are less sweet than the simple and double sugars. Humans and other animals synthesize a polysaccharide called glycogen.

Glycogen is the storage carbohydrate of animal tissues. It is mostly stored in skeletal muscle and the liver and is highly branched (like starch) and made up of large molecules. When the blood sugar level drops quickly, the liver cells break down glycogen, releasing its glucose units into the blood. Because of many branch ends that can release glucose at the same time, body cells can have almost immediate stores of glucose to use as fuel.

Only glycogen and starch are of major importance in the human body. They are glucose polymers with different forms of *branching*. *Starch* is the storage carbohydrate that is formed by plants, with high and variable amounts of glucose units. Starches include potatoes and grain products. In order for absorption, the starch must be digested. Humans cannot digest *cellulose*, which is another polysaccharide found in plants, but it functions as *bulk*, a form of fiber, which aids in peristalsis of feces.

Carbohydrates are primarily used by the body for ever-ready, easy to use cellular fuel. Glucose is the primary form of fuel used by most cells, which in general can only use a few types of other simple sugars. Remember that glucose is broken down and oxidized inside cells, during which time electrons are transferred. This releases the bond energy that is stored in the glucose, and adenosine triphosphate (ATP) can be synthesized. When ATP is sufficiently present, carbohydrates from the diet can be converted to glycogen (or fat) and stored in the body. For structural needs, only tiny amounts of carbohydrates are used. There are some sugars in human genes, whereas others are attached to external cell surfaces and used to guide interactions between cells.

Lipids

Lipids are insoluble in water but may dissolve in other lipids, oils, ether, chloroform, or alcohol. Lipids include a variety of compounds, such as triglycerides, phospholipids, and steroids, with vital cell functions. Fats are the most common type of lipids. Like carbohydrates, fat molecules also contain carbon, hydrogen, and oxygen but have far fewer oxygen

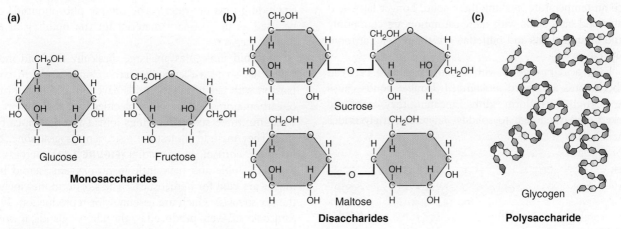

FIGURE 2-7 (A) Monosaccharide, (B) disaccharide, and (C) polysaccharide.

atoms than do carbohydrates. Some complex lipids also contain phosphorus.

Fatty acids and glycerol are the building blocks of fat molecules. A single fat molecule consists of one glycerol molecule bonded to three fatty acid molecules. These fat molecules are known as *triglycerides* (neutral fats), a subcategory of lipids that includes fats (when solid) and oils (when liquid). These molecules are formed by the condensation of one molecule of glycerol, which is a three-carbon sugar alcohol (a modified simple sugar). Glycerol contains three fatty acid molecules. Triglycerides contain different saturated and unsaturated fatty acid combinations. Those with mostly saturated fatty acids are called *saturated fats*. Those with mostly unsaturated fatty acids are called *unsaturated fats*. In general, the ratio of fatty acids to glycerol in a triglyceride is 3:1. Via dehydration synthesis, fat synthesis involves the attachment of three fatty acid chains to just one glycerol molecule. An E-shaped molecule is developed. The fatty acid chains vary, but the glycerol is always the same in all triglycerides.

Fatty acids are linear chains of carbon and hydrogen atoms, known as *hydrocarbon chains*, with an organic acid group located at one end. They consist of a long hydrocarbon *tail* and a smaller area consisting of a carboxyl group, known as the *head* (**FIGURE 2-8**). Triglycerides may be made up of hundreds of atoms. Fats and oils, after being consumed, must be broken down to their simpler building blocks before they can be absorbed. Nonpolar molecules are made from their hydrocarbon chains. Oils (fats) and water cannot mix because polar and nonpolar molecular molecules cannot interact. Triglycerides provide the body's best type of stored energy. Upon oxidizing, they release large amounts of energy. Deeper body tissues are protected from heat loss and mechanical trauma by triglycerides, which are mostly found beneath the skin. Women have a thicker subcutaneous fatty layer than men, which helps to insulate them from colder temperatures.

Saturated fat is defined as containing carbon atoms that are bound to as many hydrogen atoms as possible, becoming saturated with them. The degree of saturation determines how solid the molecule is at various temperatures. Saturated fats have fatty acid changes with single covalent bonds between carbon atoms (**FIGURE 2-9**). These straight fatty acid chains have saturated fat molecules packed closely together at room temperature, making them solid. Longer fatty acid chains and fatty acids with more saturation are commonly found in animal fats and butterfat, which are solid at room temperature.

Fatty acid molecules with one double bond between carbon atoms are called *unsaturated*. Double bonds cause fatty acid chains to form "kinks," meaning they cannot be packed closely enough to solidify. Therefore, triglycerides

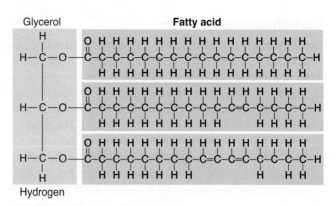

FIGURE 2-9 Saturated fats.

with either short fatty acid chains or unsaturated fatty acids are oils. They are liquid at room temperature, which is a typical factor of plant lipids. Examples include oils from corn, olives, peanuts, safflowers, and soybeans. Unsaturated fats (especially olive oil) are healthier. Fatty acid molecules with many double-bonded carbon atoms are called *polyunsaturated*. **FIGURE 2-10** compares the differences between saturated and unsaturated fats.

Many types of margarines and baked products contain **trans fats**, which are oils solidified by adding hydrogen atoms at the sites of carbon double bonds. Trans fats are now known to increase risks for heart disease even more significantly than solid animal fats. Oppositely, the **omega-3 fatty acids** from cold-water fish are known to decrease the risk of heart disease and certain inflammatory diseases.

Similar to a fat molecule, a **phospholipid** consists of a glycerol portion with fatty acid chains. Phospholipids are structurally related to glycolipids and are actually modified triglycerides. Human cells can synthesize both types of lipids, primarily from fatty acids. A phospholipid includes a phosphate group that is soluble in water and a fatty acid portion that is not. Phospholipids are an important part of cell structures. The distinctive chemical properties of phospholipids come from the phosphorus-containing group. The tails of these molecules (the hydrocarbon portion) are nonpolar. They react only with nonpolar molecules. The heads of these molecules (the phosphorus-containing part) are polar, attracting other polar or charged particles (including ions or water). The unique phospholipids can be used as the primary material for the building of cell membranes.

Steroid molecules are large, basically flat lipid molecules that share a distinctive carbon framework, in comparison with fats or oils. Steroids have four connected rings of carbon atoms. All steroid molecules have the same basic structure: three six-carbon rings joined to one five-carbon ring. They include cholesterol, estrogen, progesterone, testosterone, cortisol, and estradiol (**FIGURE 2-11**). Steroids are also fat soluble and have little to no oxygen. Steroid hormones are vital for homeostasis. The sex hormones include the *sex steroids*, which are essential for reproduction. If no *corticosteroids* were produced by the adrenal glands, it would be fatal.

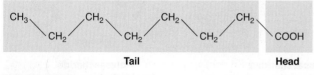

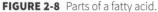

FIGURE 2-8 Parts of a fatty acid.

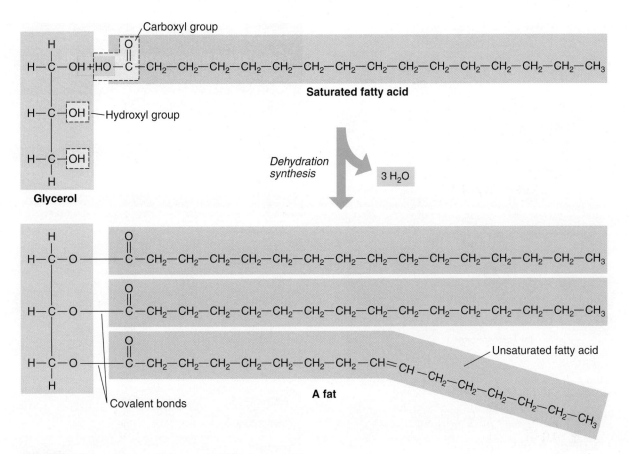

FIGURE 2-10 Saturated versus unsaturated fats.

Cholesterol is the most important steroid and is ingested in animal foods such as cheese, eggs, and meat. The liver also produces certain amounts of cholesterol. Although essential for human life, excessive cholesterol participates in atherosclerosis and related disease. In the cell membranes, cholesterol is the raw material that helps to synthesize vitamin D, bile salts, and steroid hormones.

Eicosanoids are lipids that are mostly derived from **arachidonic acid**, a 20-carbon fatty acid existing in all cell membranes, the most important of which are the *prostaglandins* and related acids. Eicosanoids are important for blood clotting, inflammation, labor contractions, regulation of blood pressure, and many other body processes. Prostaglandin synthesis and inflammatory effects are blocked by medications such as the cyclooxygenase inhibitors and nonsteroidal anti-inflammatory drugs.

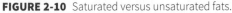

TEST YOUR UNDERSTANDING

1. Explain the most common type of lipids and list the components their molecules contain.
2. Distinguish between saturated and unsaturated fats.
3. Define the terms *phospholipid* and *steroid*.

Proteins

Proteins are the most abundant organic components of the human body and in many ways the most important. They make up between 10% and 30% of cell mass and are the basic structural materials of the body. Proteins are vital for many body functions, including structures and their functions, energy, defense (antibodies), and hormonal requirements. On cell surfaces some proteins combine with carbohydrates to become glycoproteins. They allow cells to respond to certain molecules that bind to them. Proteins include biologic **catalysts** (enzymes), contractile proteins of muscles, and the hemoglobin of the blood.

There are more than 200,000 types of proteins in the human body, the full set known as the *proteome*. Antibodies are proteins that detect and destroy foreign substances. All proteins contain carbon, hydrogen, oxygen, and nitrogen atoms, with small quantities of sulfur also present. Proteins always contain nitrogen atoms. Twenty common amino acids, both essential and nonessential, make up the proteins that exist in humans and most other living organisms (**TABLE 2-3**). Amino acids are the building blocks of proteins, with two primary groups: *amines* and *organic acids*. Amino acids act as either bases (proton acceptors) or acids (proton donors). All amino acids are exactly the same except for one group of atoms, known as the amino acid's *R group*. Differences in the R group determine the chemical uniqueness of each amino acid (**FIGURE 2-12**).

Protein molecules consisting of amino acids held together by peptide bonds are called *peptides*. They are joined together via dehydration synthesis. The amine end of one amino acid is linked to the acid end of the next amino acid. This forms the characteristic atomic arrangement of a *peptide bond*. Each type of peptide is named for the amount of amino acids that are

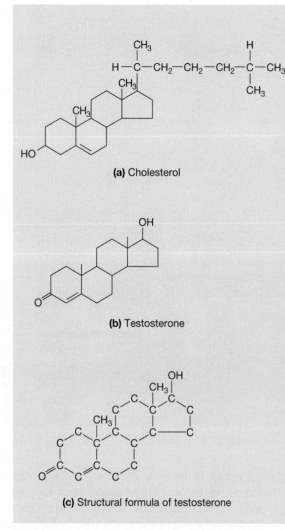

(a) Cholesterol

(b) Testosterone

(c) Structural formula of testosterone

FIGURE 2-11 Various types of steroid molecules.

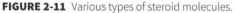

TABLE 2-3

Essential and Nonessential Amino Acids

Amino Acid	Abbreviation
Alanine	Ala
Arginine	Arg
Asparagine	Asn
Aspartic acid	Asp
Cysteine	Cys
Glutamic acid	Glu
Glutamine	Gln
Glycine	Gly
Histidine	His
Isoleucine	Ile
Leucine	Leu
Lysine	Lys
Methionine	Met
Phenylalanine	Phe
Proline	Pro
Serine	Ser
Threonine	Thr
Tryptophan	Trp
Tyrosine	Tyr
Valine	Val

united: *dipeptide* (2), *tripeptide* (3), *polypeptide* (10 or more), and so on. Although most proteins are *macromolecules*, polypeptides that contain more than 50 amino acids are called proteins. *Macromolecules* are large and complex molecules with as few as 100 to over 10,000 amino acids.

Every type of amino acid has its own distinct properties. The way they bind determines how the proteins they produce are structured and how they function. A change in one amino acid that is linked to others produces an entirely unique function. Such a change can also make the protein become nonfunctional.

There are thousands of different proteins in the body, with different functions. All of them are made up of different combinations of the common amino acids. Various types of proteins include structural proteins such as collagen, which gives strength to ligaments and connective tissues, and keratin, which functions to prevent water loss through the skin. More active proteins include antibodies and enzymes. Cell membrane proteins may serve as receptors and carriers for specific molecules. Most hormones are proteins. Examples include insulin, oxytocin, and glucagon (**FIGURE 2-13**).

Types of Proteins Proteins are generally classified as either fibrous or globular. **Fibrous proteins** are longer and resemble "strands" and are highly stable and insoluble in water. They provide mechanical support and tensile strength for body tissues. **Collagen**, the most abundant protein in the body, is a fibrous protein, as are elastin, keratin, and some contractile proteins found in muscles. Because of their supporting functions, they are also called *structural proteins*.

Globular proteins are more compact than fibrous proteins and spherical in shape. They are chemically active and water-soluble. Globular proteins are important in almost all biologic processes and are therefore also referred to as *functional proteins*. Examples of globular proteins are antibodies,

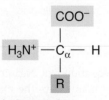

FIGURE 2-12 General amino acid.

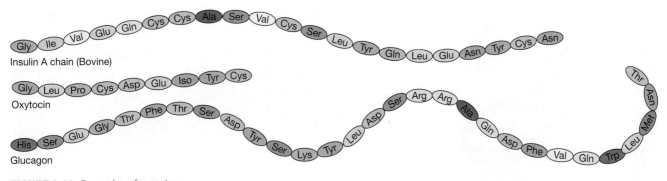

FIGURE 2-13 Examples of proteins.

protein-based hormones, and enzymes. Antibodies function in immunity, whereas protein-based hormones control growth and development. Enzymes are catalysts for nearly every chemical reaction taking place in the body.

TEST YOUR UNDERSTANDING

1. List some of the functions of proteins in the human body.
2. Explain how a peptide bond forms.
3. Differentiate between fibrous and globular proteins.

Nucleic Acids (DNA and RNA)

Nucleic acids are large organic molecules (macromolecules) that carry genetic information or form structures within cells. They are composed of carbon, hydrogen, oxygen, nitrogen, and phosphorus. Nucleic acids are actually the largest molecules in the body. Nucleic acids store and process information at the molecular level, inside the cells. The two classes of nucleic acids are **deoxyribonucleic acid (DNA)** and **ribonucleic acid (RNA)**. Nucleic acids are found in all living things, cells, and viruses. Individual strands of DNA and RNA have a similar structure (**FIGURE 2-14**).

Nucleotides are the structural units of nucleic acids. These complex units consist of a nitrogen-containing base, a pentose sugar, and a phosphate group. The nucleotide structure is based on five major types of nitrogen-containing bases:

- *Adenine (A):* a large, two-ring base (purine)
- *Guanine (G):* also a purine
- *Cytosine (C):* a smaller, single-ring base (pyrimidine)
- *Thymine (T):* also a pyrimidine
- *Uracil (U):* also a pyrimidine

The DNA in our cells determines our inherited characteristics, including hair color, eye color, and blood type. DNA affects all aspects of body structure and function. DNA molecules encode the information needed to build proteins. By directing structural protein synthesis, DNA controls the shape and physical characteristics of the human body.

Several forms of RNA cooperate to manufacture specific proteins by using the information provided by DNA. Important structural differences distinguish RNA from DNA. An RNA molecule consists of a single chain of nucleotides. Human cells have three types of RNA:

1. Messenger RNA, or mRNA
2. Transfer RNA, or tRNA
3. Ribosomal RNA, or rRNA

A DNA molecule consists of a pair of nucleotide chains (**FIGURE 2-15A**). The two DNA strands twist around each other in a **double helix** that resembles a spiral staircase. **TABLE 2-4** compares the characteristics of DNA and RNA.

TEST YOUR UNDERSTANDING

1. List three types of RNA.
2. Distinguish between DNA and RNA.

Enzymes

Enzymes are globular proteins that promote chemical reactions by lowering the **activation energy** requirements. Activation energy is the energy that must be overcome for a chemical reaction to occur. Therefore, they make chemical reactions possible and catalyze the reactions that sustain life. This means that enzymes belong to a class of substances called *catalysts* (compounds that accelerate chemical reactions without themselves being permanently changed or consumed). Enzyme molecules are manufactured by cells to promote a specific reactions. Enzymes are among the most important of all the

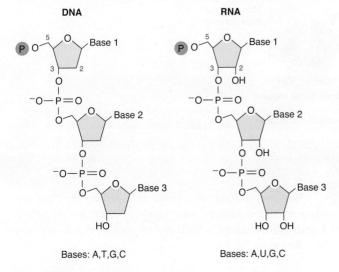

FIGURE 2-14 Strand structures of DNA and RNA.

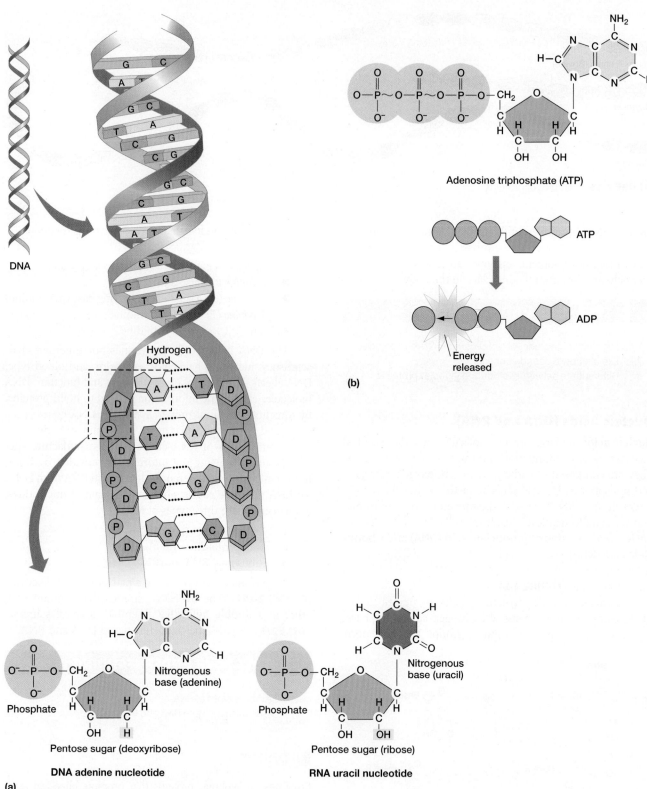

FIGURE 2-15 (A) Nucleic acids, DNA, a DNA nucleotide, and an RNA nucleotide. (B) ATP.

body's proteins. Nearly everything that occurs in the human body relies on a specific enzyme. In the body, enzymes assist in the digestion of food, drug metabolism, protein formation, and many other types of reactions. Enzymes make metabolic reactions possible inside cells by controlling temperature conditions that otherwise would be too mild for them to occur.

Enzymes are complex molecules. When they are not used in the reactions they catalyze, they are recycled. Enzymatic reactions, which are reversible, can be written as follows:

$$A + B \rightleftarrows AB$$

TABLE 2-4

Characteristics of DNA and RNA

Characteristic	DNA	RNA
Structure	Double stranded and coiled into a *double helix*	Single stranded, either straight or folded
Major functions	Genetic material, direction of protein synthesis; it self-replicates before cell division	Synthesizes proteins based on genetic instructions
Major site in the cells	Nucleus	Cytoplasm (the cell area outside the nucleus)
Sugar	Deoxyribose	Ribose
Bases	Adenosine, cytosine, guanine, thymine	Adenine, cytosine, guanine, uracil

Enzymes cannot cause a chemical reaction between molecules that would not react without them. They increase the speed of enzymatic reactions greatly, between 100,000 to more than 1 billion times the rate of a reaction that is uncatalyzed. Otherwise, biochemical reactions would occur extremely slowly, almost to no effect. Enzymes are vital in making these reactions occur at an adequate pace.

Enzyme Characteristics

Enzymes differ in their makeup. Some are only made of protein, whereas others have a two-part structure, consisting of a protein portion (the *apoenzyme*) and a **cofactor**. Collectively, these two parts are referred to as the **holoenzyme**. Enzyme cofactors may be either a metal element ion (such as iron or copper) or an organic molecule that assists the reaction. Most organic cofactors are derived from B (or other) vitamins, in which case they are referred to as **coenzymes**.

Enzymes have chemical-specific actions. Some control one chemical reaction, whereas others regulate a small group of similar reactions by binding to molecules that are only slightly different. Enzymes act on substances referred to as **substrates**. Certain enzymes, when present, determine which reactions are sped up and which reactions will occur. If there is no enzyme, there is no reaction. Enzymes are often named after their substrates, using the suffix *-ase*. For example, a lipid is catalyzed by an enzyme called a *lipase*. Another enzyme, called a *catalase*, breaks down hydrogen peroxide into water and oxygen. Hydrogen peroxide is a toxic substance that results from certain metabolic reactions.

Every cell holds hundreds of various enzymes, each of which recognizes its specific substrates. Enzyme molecules have three-dimensional shapes (conformations) that allow them to identify their substrates. The coiled and twisted polypeptide chain of each enzyme fits the shape of its substrate. The **active site** of an enzyme molecule combines with portions of its substrate molecules temporarily. This forms an enzyme–substrate complex (**FIGURE 2-16**).

When enzyme–substrate complexes are formed, some chemical bonds within the substrates are distorted or strained. Requiring less energy as a result, the enzyme is released as it

was originally configured. Enzyme-catalyzed reactions can be summarized as follows:

$$\text{Substrate molecules} + \text{Enzyme molecule} \Rightarrow \text{Enzyme-substrate complex} \Rightarrow \text{Produce (changed substrates)} + \text{Enzyme molecule}$$

These reactions are often reversible. Sometimes, the same enzyme catalyzes the reaction in both directions. The reactions occur at differing rates, based on the number of molecules of

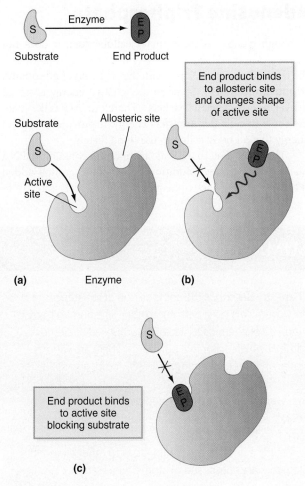

FIGURE 2-16 Enzyme-catalyzed reaction.

the enzyme and its substrate. Some enzymes process a few substrate molecules every second, whereas others can process thousands in the same length of time.

TEST YOUR UNDERSTANDING

1. Define enzymes and explain their functions.
2. Define the terms *cofactor, holoenzyme,* and *coenzymes.*

FOCUS ON PATHOLOGY

Metabolic disorders are genetic disorders that result in biochemical defects, such as enzyme deficiencies. They cause the body to be unable to catabolize or efficiently use the nutrients required for growth, repair, and energy. Newborns are routinely screened for metabolic disorders, because they can harm early physical and mental development. The most common metabolic disorders include **phenylketonuria, maple syrup urine disease, galactosemia**, and **homocystinuria**.

Adenosine Triphosphate

Although glucose is the primary cellular fuel, it does not directly power cellular work. When glucose is catabolized, the released energy is paired with the synthesis of **adenosine triphosphate** (ATP). Some of the released energy is stored by ATP bonds in small "packets." Therefore, ATP is the main molecule in cells that transfers energy. It provides a type of energy that all body cells can use immediately.

The structure of ATP is an adenine-containing RNA nucleotide, with two additional phosphate groups added (**FIGURE 2-15B**). The triphosphate "tail" of ATP is ready to chemically release enormous amounts of energy. ATP is a highly unstable molecule that stores energy. This is because its three phosphate groups are negatively charged and closely packed. They repel each other, and when the terminal high-energy phosphate bonds are hydrolyzed, the molecule becomes more stable.

The ATP bond energy is taken by the cells during coupled reactions. The cells use enzymes to transfer terminal phosphate groups from ATP to various compounds. The newly *phosphorylated* molecules temporarily have higher energy and can perform various types of cellular work. During this work, the molecules lose the phosphate group. The amount of energy needed for most biochemical reactions is closely related to the amount of energy released and transferred during the hydrolysis of ATP. Therefore, the cells are not damaged by an excessive energy release, and very little energy is wasted.

When the terminal phosphate bond of ATP is cleaved, a molecule is given off that has two phosphate groups: *adenosine diphosphate (ADP)* and an inorganic phosphate group. There is a transfer of energy. ADP accumulates as ATP is hydrolyzed for cellular energy needs. When the terminal phosphate bond of ADP is cleaved, a similar amount of energy is liberated. This produces *adenosine monophosphate.*

As glucose and other fuel-providing molecules are oxidized, their bond energy is released, and ATP supplies in the cells are replenished. The same amount of energy is needed to be acquired as is released when the terminal phosphates of ATP are cleaved. This energy must be used to reverse the reaction, reattaching phosphates and reforming energy-transferring phosphate bonds. Molecules cannot be made or degraded without ATP. Also, without ATP cells cannot transport substances across boundaries, muscles cannot shorten to pull on other body structures, and the process of life will cease.

Certain compounds may be lethal because they interfere with the mitochondrial production of ATP. An example is cyanide, which when inhaled or absorbed has extreme effects on the brain and heart. When the cells do not have sufficient ATP, they die because they lack the energy needed for anabolic chemical reactions, active transport, and other cell processes.

SUMMARY

Chemistry describes the composition of substances and how chemicals react with each other. The human body is made up of chemicals. Matter is composed of elements, some of which occur in a pure form. There are various states of matter, including gaseous, liquid, and solid states. Energy is different from matter, taking up space, having no mass, and only being measured by how it affects matter. Energy is the capacity to put matter into motion or to perform "work."

Many elements are combined with other elements. Elements are composed of atoms, which are the smallest complete units that still have the properties of the elements they form. Atoms of different elements have characteristic sizes, weights, and ways of interacting. An atom consists of one or more electrons surrounding a nucleus, which contains one or more protons and usually one or more neutrons. Electrons are negative, protons are positive, and neutrons are uncharged. When atoms combine they gain, lose, or share electrons. Atoms of the same element may bond to form a molecule of that element. Compounds that release ions when they dissolve in water are known as electrolytes. A molecule is any chemical structure that consists of atoms held together by covalent bonds. Compounds are chemically pure, with identical molecules.

Mixtures are substances containing two or more components that are physically intermixed and include colloids, solutions, and suspensions. Chemical bonds are energy exchanges between electrons of reacting atoms and include ionic, covalent, and hydrogen bonds. Ionic bonds form between ions. Covalent bonds are formed when electrons are shared, producing molecules in which the shared electrons are located in a single orbital common to both atoms. When the positive hydrogen end of a polar molecule is attracted to the negative nitrogen or oxygen end of another polar molecule, the attraction is called a hydrogen bond. A chemical reaction occurs when a chemical bond is formed, broken, or rearranged. The four types of chemical reactions are synthesis, decomposition, exchange, and reversible reactions. Catalysts can increase the rate of chemical reactions without becoming chemically changed themselves or without becoming a part of the product.

Acids are electrolytes that release hydrogen ions in water. Bases are electrolytes that release ions that bond with hydrogen ions. Hydrogen ion concentrations can be measured by a value called pH. Biochemistry (biologic chemistry) is the study of chemical processes within and relating to living organisms. Organic chemicals are those that always contain the elements carbon and hydrogen and generally oxygen as well. Inorganic chemicals do not contain these elements. Inorganic substances include water, oxygen, carbon dioxide, and salts. Organic substances include carbohydrates, lipids, and proteins. Carbohydrates provide much of the energy required by the body's cells and help to build cell structures. They include various types of sugars, including monosaccharides, disaccharides, and polysaccharides. Lipids are insoluble in water and may dissolve in other lipids, oils, ether, chloroform, or alcohol. Fats are the most common type of lipids. Unsaturated fats are safer than saturated or trans fats. Proteins are the most abundant organic components of the human body and are the basic structural materials of the body. Nucleic acids are large organic molecules that carry genetic information or form structures within cells. They include DNA and RNA.

In the body, enzymes promote chemical reactions by acting as catalysts to accelerate these reactions without themselves being permanently changed or consumed. Some enzymes are only made of protein, whereas others have a protein portion (apoenzyme) and a cofactor. Most organic cofactors are derived from B complex (or other) vitamins and are known as coenzymes. ATP pairs with catabolized glucose to power the body. ATP is the main molecule in cells that transfer energy and provides a type of energy that all body cells can use immediately.

KEY TERMS

Acids
Activation energy
Active site
Adenosine triphosphate
Anions
Arachidonic acid
Atomic number
Atomic weight
Atoms
Bases
Carbohydrates
Catalysts
Cations
Chemical reaction
Chemistry
Coenzymes
Cofactor
Collagen

Colloids
Compounds
Covalent bond
Crystals
Cytosol
Decomposition
Deoxyribonucleic acid (DNA)
Dipole
Disaccharides
Double helix
Eicosanoids
Electrolytes
Electronegativity
Electrons
Electropositive
Elements
Energy
Enzymes

Fibrous proteins
Galactosemia
Globular proteins
Holoenzyme
Homocystinuria
Hydrogen bond
Inorganic
Ions
Isotope
Lipids
Maple syrup urine disease
Matter
Mixtures
Molarity
Mole
Molecular weight
Molecule
Monosaccharides

Neutrons
Nucleic acids
Nucleus
Omega-3 fatty acids
Organic
pH
Phenylketonuria
Phospholipid

Polar
Polysaccharides
Proteins
Protons
Radioisotopes
Ribonucleic acid (RNA)
Solutes
Solutions

Solvent
Steroid
Substrates
Suspensions
Synthesis
Trans fats

LEARNING GOALS

The following learning goals correspond to the objectives at the beginning of this chapter:

1. Atoms are tiny particles that compose elements. A molecule is formed when two or more atoms bond. When two atoms of the same element bond, they produce molecules of that element, such as hydrogen, oxygen, or nitrogen molecules.

2. Atoms can bond with other atoms by using chemical bonds that result from interactions between their electrons. The atoms may gain, lose, or share electrons. Atoms that either gain or lose electrons are called ions.

3. Each atom consists of a central nucleus and one or more electrons continually moving around it. Inside the nucleus are one or more protons and neutrons. The number of protons in an atom is known as its atomic number.

4. The major groups of inorganic chemicals common in cells are oxygen, carbon dioxide, salts, and water. Other inorganic substances in cells include the ions of bicarbonate, calcium, carbonate, chloride, magnesium, phosphate, potassium, sodium, and sulfate.

5. Acids are electrolytes that release hydrogen ions in water (such as hydrochloric acid). Bases are electrolytes that release ions that bond with hydrogen ions (such as sodium hydroxide). Buffers are chemicals that resist pH changes. They combine with hydrogen ions when these ions are excessive and contribute hydrogen ions when these ions are reduced.

6. Lipids are not soluble in water; they may dissolve in other lipids, oils, ether, chloroform, or alcohol. Proteins are vital for many body functions. They can combine with carbohydrates or lipids, and always contain carbon, hydrogen, oxygen, and nitrogen atoms.

7. The term *pH* is defined as the measurement of hydrogen ion concentration. The pH scale ranges from 0 to 14, with 7 being the midpoint (an equal number of hydrogen and hydroxide ions) or "neutral"—neither acidic nor basic.

8. Organic substances in cells include carbohydrates, lipids, proteins, and nucleic acids. Carbohydrates provide much of the energy required by the body's cells and help to build cell structures. Lipids are vital for many cell functions such as the building of the cell membrane, and include fats, phospholipids, and steroids. Proteins are vital for body structures, functions, energy, enzymatic functions, defense (antibodies), and hormonal requirements. Nucleic acids carry genetic information or form structures within cells, and include DNA and RNA.

9. Steroid molecules include cholesterol, estrogen, progesterone, testosterone, cortisol, and estradiol.

10. Nucleic acids are macromolecules that carry genetic information or form structures within cells. They are composed of carbon, hydrogen, oxygen, nitrogen, and phosphorus. Nucleic acids are found in all living things, cells, and viruses.

CRITICAL THINKING QUESTIONS

A 65-year-old man who has had diabetes for two decades was brought to the emergency department. He appeared confused and said he was feeling weak. His blood tests revealed elevation of ketone bodies.

1. Explain whether the physician should suspect alkalosis or acidosis, and why.
2. Explain the various types of alkalosis and acidosis.

REVIEW QUESTIONS

1. Which of the following represents an atomic number?
   A. protons in an atom
   B. protons and neutrons
   C. electrons in an ion
   D. neutrons in an atom
2. Which of the following is an important buffer in body fluids?
   A. hydrochloric acid
   B. sodium bicarbonate
   C. sodium chloride
   D. water
3. A solution containing an equal number of hydrogen ions and hydroxide ions is
   A. basic
   B. alkaline
   C. acidic
   D. neutral
4. Which of the following statements about water is false?
   A. It has a relatively low heat capacity.
   B. It contains hydrogen bonds.
   C. It dissolves many compounds.
   D. It is responsible for about two-thirds of the mass of the human body.
5. Which of the following is the most important high-energy compound in cells?
   A. glucose
   B. protein
   C. fructose
   D. adenosine triphosphate
6. The molecules that store and process information at the molecular level are the
   A. steroids
   B. carbohydrates
   C. nucleic acids
   D. lipids

7. An unstable isotope that emits subatomic particles spontaneously is referred to as
   A. a proton
   B. an atom
   C. a radioisotope
   D. a neutron
8. Which of the following is the smallest particle of an element that has the properties of that element?
   A. an electron
   B. an atom
   C. a neutron
   D. a proton
9. The building blocks of fat molecules are
   A. fatty acids
   B. triglycerides
   C. glycerols
   D. fatty acids and glycerol
10. Nucleic acids are composed of units called
    A. fatty acids
    B. nucleotides
    C. amino acids
    D. adenosines
11. Which of the following is a true statement about lipids?
    A. They provide roughly twice the energy of carbohydrates.
    B. They provide roughly twice the energy of proteins.
    C. They help to cushion delicate organs from damage.
    D. All of the above.
12. A fatty acid that contains many double covalent bonds in its carbon chain is said to be
    A. polyunsaturated
    B. monounsaturated
    C. hydrogenated
    D. saturated

13. Which of the following is the most important metabolic fuel molecule in the body?
    A. starch
    B. protein
    C. glucose
    D. sucrose
14. Ions with a negative charge are called
    A. cations
    B. anions
    C. polyatomic ions
    D. radicals
15. The atomic weight of an element includes which of the following?
    A. protons and neutrons in the nucleus
    B. protons and electrons in an atom
    C. electrons in the outer shells
    D. neutrons in the nucleus

ESSAY QUESTIONS

1. Provide the atomic symbols for sodium, potassium, hydrogen, oxygen, nitrogen, calcium, iron, and carbon.
2. Define radioisotopes.
3. Describe ionic and covalent bonds with two examples for each.
4. What are hydrogen bonds, and how are they important in the body?
5. What are the four types of chemical reactions?
6. Define electrolytes, acids, and bases.
7. Define chemical equilibrium.
8. What is the mechanism of enzyme action?
9. List six examples of steroids.
10. Define the characteristics of the nucleic acids.

Cells

OBJECTIVES

After studying this chapter, readers should be able to

1. Explain the parts of a cell's structure.
2. Describe the structure and function of the cell membrane.
3. Describe the structure and function of cytoplasm and cytosol.
4. Describe the parts of the cell nucleus and their functions.
5. Describe the "powerhouses" of the cell.
6. Describe the processes that transport substances across the plasma membrane.
7. Compare and define cilia and flagella.
8. Compare passive and active cell mechanisms.
9. Describe the parts of the cell cycle.
10. Explain cell division and cancer.

Overview

Cells are the building blocks of all plants and animals. All cells come from the division of preexisting cells. They are the smallest units of the body that perform all vital physiological functions. Approximately 75 trillion cells exist in an adult human being. Each cell maintains homeostasis at the cellular level. Cells have different sizes, shapes, and forms, depending on their functions. Today, the study of cellular structure and function, or **cytology**, is part of the broader discipline of *cell biology*, which includes aspects of biology, chemistry, and physics.

Structure of the Cell

The human body contains two general classes of cells: sex cells and somatic cells. **Sex cells** (also called *germ cells* or *reproductive cells*) are either the sperm of males or the oocytes of females. **Somatic cells** (derived from the term *soma*, meaning "body") include all other cells in the human body. This chapter focuses on somatic cells.

The three major parts to a cell are the cell membrane, the nucleus, and the cytoplasm. The cell membrane encloses the cell, its nucleus, various organelles, and its cytoplasm. The nucleus contains the cell's genetic material and controls its activities. The cytoplasm fills out the cell and its shape. Organelles are microscopic, specialized cell structures that perform specific functions required by the cell (**FIGURE 3-1**).

The organelles fulfill functions and processes that are vital to the life of cells, tissues, and organisms.

Cell Membrane

The **cell membrane** (also called the *plasma membrane*) controls movement of substances both into and out of the cell. The cell membrane allows selective communication between the intracellular and extracellular compartments while aiding in cellular movement. It gives form to the cell and is also where much of the cell's biological activities are conducted. Molecules in the cell membrane form pathways that allow the signals from outside the cell to be detected and transmitted inside. When cells form tissues, the cell membrane assists by adhering the cell to other cells.

Each cell's membrane is extremely thin and delicate, able to stretch to differing degrees. There are usually tiny folds on the surface, which help to increase its surface area. Only certain substances can enter or leave each cell (a condition known as *selective permeability*). Cell membranes can be differentially permeable or **semipermeable**. A semipermeable membrane allows certain elements to pass through but not others.

Lipids and proteins are the primary substances that make up cell membranes, usually in a double layer of phospholipid molecules (**FIGURE 3-2**). The phosphate portion forms the outer surface, with the fatty acid portion forming the inner surface. Substances such as oxygen and carbon dioxide, which are soluble in lipids, can easily pass through

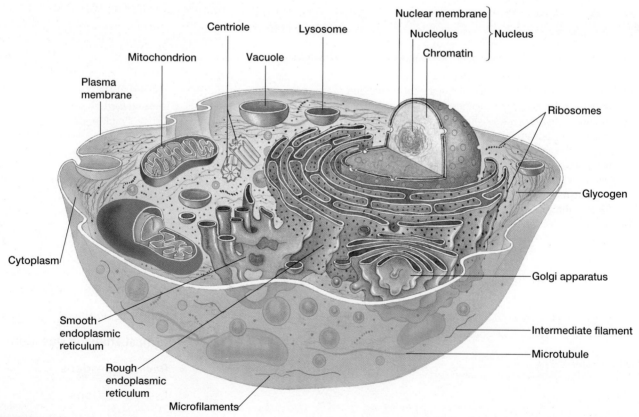

FIGURE 3-1 The cell.

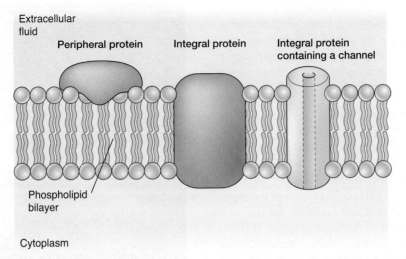

FIGURE 3-2 Membrane associated proteins.

this double layer (also called a *bilayer*). Other substances, such as amino acids, proteins, nucleic acids, certain ions, and sugars, cannot pass through this layer. Cholesterol in the inner cell membrane helps to keep the membrane stable. The phospholipids organize themselves in a bilayer to hide their hydrophobic tail regions and expose the hydrophilic regions to water. This process does not require energy and forms a layer that is the wall between the inside and outside of the cell.

The proteins in a cell membrane are classified according to where they are positioned. They also may have different shapes, such as fibrous, globular, or rod-like. Proteins can move in the cell membrane because they are enclosed in an oily background. Cell membrane proteins may form receptors for hormones or growth factors, transport substances across the cell membrane, and form selective channels that determine which types of ions can enter or leave the cell. On the cell membrane's outer surface, proteins may extend outward, marking the cell as a component of a particular tissue or organ. Many proteins are attached to carbohydrates to form glycoproteins.

Membrane Lipids

The basic fabric of the cell membrane is formed by the lipid bilayer. It is most made up of phospholipids but also contains glycolipids, cholesterol, and lipid rafts.

Phospholipids   Phospholipids are lipids that have both charged and uncharged sections. They are shaped similar to lollipops, with a polar "head" portion that is charged and *hydrophilic* (water-attracting). The uncharged, nonpolar "tail" portion is *hydrophobic* (water-repelling). Because the polar

heads are attracted to water, they are positioned on the inner and outer surfaces of the cell membrane. The nonpolar tails are aligned in the center of the cell membrane. All plasma membranes and biological membranes are composed of two parallel sheets of phospholipid molecules lying tail to tail. The polar heads are exposed to water on either side of both the membranes and organelles. Because phospholipids are self-orienting, they encourage biological membranes to form closed, mostly round structures that reseal when torn.

The plasma membrane is similar to olive oil in consistency. It is constantly changing, with lipid molecules moving from side to side, parallel to the membrane surface. Polar–nonpolar interactions keep molecules from moving from one half of the bilayer to the other. There are varieties of different lipids (and their amounts) in various membranes. These differences help to determine structure and function. Most membrane phospholipids are unsaturated. This makes their tail portions kink, to increase space between them, increasing membrane fluidity.

Glycolipids   Glycolipids are lipids that have sugar groups attached and are found only in the outer plasma membrane surface. They make up approximately 5% of total membrane lipids. Like the phosphate-containing groups of phospholipids, their sugar groups cause that end of the glycolipid molecule to become polar. Their fatty acid tails are nonpolar.

Cholesterol   Similarly, cholesterol also has a polar region and a nonpolar region. The polar region is its hydroxyl group, whereas the nonpolar region is its fused ring system. Cholesterol has plate-like hydrocarbon rings that are wedged between phospholipid tails. These rings serve to both stabilize the membrane and decrease mobility of phospholipids and membrane fluidity. Approximately 20% of the cell membrane lipid is cholesterol.

Membrane Proteins

Cell membrane proteins are numerous, allowing the cell to communicate with its environment. Approximately half of the mass of the plasma membrane is made up of proteins, which are responsible for most specialized membrane functions. The proteins differ in that some of them float freely and others are bound to intracellular structures making up the cell's *cytoskeleton*. The two distinct types of membrane proteins are termed *integral* and *peripheral*.

Integral Proteins **Integral proteins** are inserted into the lipid bilayer, with some protruding from one face of the membrane. However, most of them are *transmembrane proteins* that protrude on both sides. All integral proteins have hydrophobic and hydrophilic regions. Therefore, they can interact with the nonpolar lipid tails embedded in the membrane and with the water inside and outside of the cell.

Certain transmembrane proteins are engaged in transport. They are clustered, forming pores (*channels*). Small ions or water-soluble molecules move through them and bypass the lipid portion of the membrane. Other transmembrane proteins are *carriers*. They move a substance through the membrane by binding to it. Still others are enzymes or receptors for hormones (or other chemical messengers). These receptor proteins relay messages to the cell interior, which is known as *signal transduction*.

Peripheral Proteins **Peripheral proteins** differ in that they are not embedded in the lipid bilayer but rather are loosely attached to integral proteins, being easily removed without disrupting the cell membrane. The cytoplasmic side of the membrane is partially supported by a network of filaments, a formation of peripheral proteins. Others are enzymes, motor proteins, or have cell-linking functions. Motor proteins are involved in changing cell shape during muscle cell contraction and cell division.

Lipid Rafts

Lipid rafts are dynamic structures of saturated phospholipids packed tightly together. Approximately 20% of the outer cell membrane surface contains lipid rafts. They are associated with unique lipids (*sphingolipids*) and large amounts of cholesterol. Lipid rafts resemble quilts. They are more stable yet less fluid than the remainder of the cell membrane, including or excluding certain proteins. They are therefore believed to concentrate certain receptor molecules or protein molecules required for membrane invagination (infolding), cell signaling, or other activities.

TEST YOUR UNDERSTANDING

1. Contrast and compare glycolipids, cholesterol, and lipid rafts.
2. What are the differences between integral and peripheral proteins?

Cytoplasm

Cytoplasm is the substance that contains all the cellular contents between the cell membrane and the nucleus. It serves as a matrix substance in which chemical reactions occur.

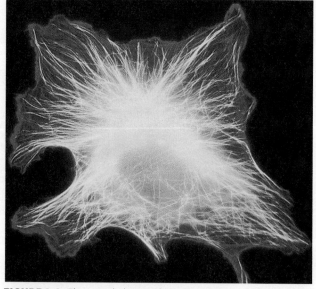

FIGURE 3-3 The cytoskeleton. Photomicrograph of the cytoskeleton of a human fibroblast (connective tissue cell). The microtubules are yellow, and the microfilaments are red. (© M. Schliwa/Visuals Unlimited)

Cytoplasm makes up most of each cell's volume and is a gel-like material suspending the cell's organelles. It usually appears clear with scattered "specks," although more powerful magnification reveals that it contains membranous networks, protein frameworks, and a **cytoskeleton** (**FIGURE 3-3**).

Cytoplasm consists of **cytosol** and organelles (excluding the nucleus), which are subcellular structures that perform specific functions. Cytosol is the fluid portion of cytoplasm, containing mostly water as well as glucose, amino acids, fatty acids, ions, lipids, proteins, adenosine triphosphate (ATP), and waste products. Cytosol is the site of many chemical reactions that are required for cells to exist. It is the part of the cytoplasm that cannot be removed by centrifugation.

The most important differences between cytosol and extracellular fluid are as follows:

- Cytosol contains higher amounts of suspended proteins than does extracellular fluid. Many of these proteins are enzymes that regulate metabolic operations; others are involved with the various organelles.
- Cytosol also contains higher amounts of potassium ions than does extracellular fluid; however, the concentration of sodium ions is much lower in cytosol than in extracellular fluid.
- Cytosol usually contains small amounts of lipids, carbohydrates, and amino acids.

The cytoplasm receives, processes, and uses nutrients. It contains various types of organelles (nonmembranous or membranous). Organelles perform most of the tasks that keep the cell alive and functioning normally. Each organelle accomplishes specific tasks related to cell structure, growth, maintenance, and metabolism. An organelle's membrane often allows it to unite with the interactive, intracellular *endomembrane system*. The following organelles have specific actions that help the cell to carry out its activities:

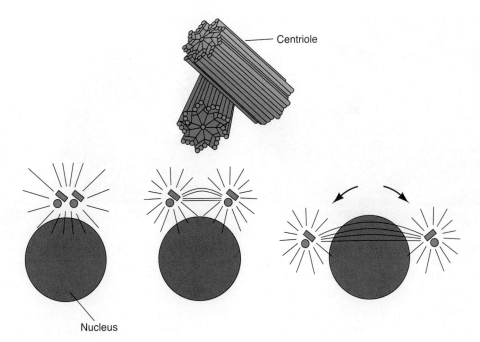

Centriole

Nucleus

FIGURE 3-4 Centrioles

■ *Centrioles:* Cell division requires a pair of centrioles, which are cylindrical structures composed of short microtubules (**FIGURE 3-4**). During cell division, the centrioles form the spindle-shaped structure needed for movement of DNA strands. Cardiac muscle cells, skeletal muscle cells, mature red blood cells, and typical neurons have no centrioles; therefore, these cells are incapable of dividing. The **centrosome** is the cytoplasm surrounding the centrioles. Microtubules of the cytoskeleton usually begin at the centrosome and radiate through the cytoplasm. The centrosome is also known as the *cell center*. It consists of nine microtubule *triplets* that are arranged like a pinwheel. Each microtubule is connected to the next one by nontubulin proteins. The microtubules are arranged to form a hollow tube. The centrioles also form the bases of cilia and flagella.

■ *Cilia and flagella:* These structures extend from certain cell surfaces. Cilia are short, hair-like structures that move in a coordinated sweeping motion to propel fluids over the surface of tissues (**FIGURE 3-5**). They are found in large numbers on cells lining the respiratory and reproductive tracts. Cilia are formed when centrioles multiply, lining up beneath the plasma membrane at the cell's exposed (free) surface. The microtubules emerge from each centriole to form the ciliary projections. They accomplish this by causing pressure on the plasma membrane. During this time, the centrioles are referred to as *basal bodies*. As a cilium moves, it experiences propulsive *power strokes* and *recovery strokes*, which bend and return it to its initial position. It can repeat these two strokes between 10 and 20 times per second. When

one cilium bends, it is soon followed by the bending of the next cilium, and so forth. This creates a cell surface "current." Flagella are longer than cilia and often exist as only a single flagellum. The only example of a flagellum is the "tail" of a sperm cell (**FIGURE 3-6**). The key difference between cilia and flagella is that cilia propel other substances, whereas flagella propel the cells to which they are attached. There are also *nonmotile cilia* (*primary cilia*), which are actually present just as one single cilium on the surface of most cells in the body. Primary cilia act as antennae, which examine the external environment for recognizable molecules. They coordinate various intracellular pathways regulating embryonic development and maintain healthy tissues in later life.

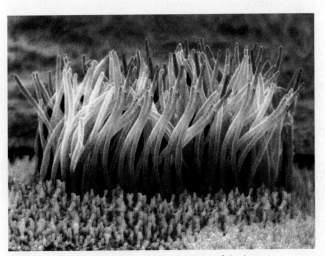

FIGURE 3-5 Cilia on cells lining the trachea of the human respiratory tract. (© Dr. David Phillips/Visuals Unlimited)

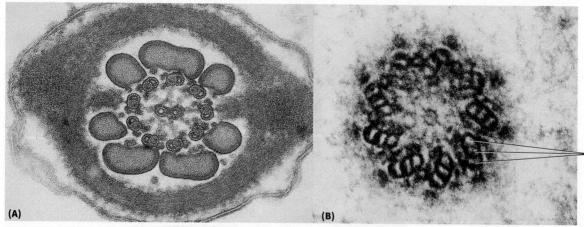

FIGURE 3-6 (A) A sperm flagellum, showing the 9 + 2 arrangement and additional fibers thought to provide support and strength to the vigorously beating tail. (B) A basal body is found at the base of each cilium and flagellum. It consists of nine sets of triplets that give rise to the microtubule doublets of the flagellum and cilium. (© Dr. David Phillips/Visuals Unlimited)

■ *Microvilli:* These are tiny, finger-like extensions of the plasma membrane. They project from exposed cell surfaces, increasing the plasma membrane surface area to a large degree. Microvilli are usually found on absorptive cell surfaces, such as in the kidney tubules and intestines. A core of actin filaments, in bundles, extend into the *terminal web* of the cytoskeleton. In the microvilli, actin appears to have a mechanically stiffening function.

■ *Endoplasmic reticulum (ER):* The ER is a network of intracellular membranes connected to the nuclear envelope, which surrounds a cell's nucleus. It has interconnected tubules and parallel membranes that enclose fluid-filled **cisterns** (cavities). The ER coils and twists through the cytosol and is continuous with the outer nuclear membrane. Nearly 50% of the cell's membranes are made up of the ER. The two types of ER are the *smooth endoplasmic reticulum* (SER) and the *rough endoplasmic reticulum* (RER). The SER does not have ribosomes on its outer surface, whereas fixed ribosomes appear on the RER's outer surface, giving it a "studded" appearance (**FIGURE 3-7**). Proteins on these ribosomes are threaded into the ER cisterns. The SER can synthesize phospholipids and cholesterol, which are needed for the cell membrane's growth and maintenance. It is continuous with the RER, consisting of a network of looped tubules. Its enzymes catalyze many different reactions. These reactions are used for many functions, including metabolizing lipids, synthesizing steroid-based hormones, detoxification of drugs and chemicals, breaking down stored glycogen to form free glucose, and for fat absorption, synthesis, and transport. Cardiac and skeletal muscle cells have an elaborate SER (the *sarcoplasmic reticulum*) that helps to store and release calcium during muscle contraction. Overall, most body cells contain very little SER. The RER can synthesize proteins, and newly made proteins are enclosed in vesicles when they move to the Golgi apparatus for additional processing. In most secretory cells, liver cells, and antibody-producing plasma cells,

the RER is very well developed. The RER is the cell's *membrane factory*, manufacturing integral proteins and phospholipids that form parts of cellular membranes. On the external face of the ER membrane, enzymes required for lipid synthesis have active sites. Both free and fixed ribosomes synthesize proteins via instructions from messenger RNA.

■ *Golgi apparatus:* This apparatus, also called the *Golgi complex*, consists of a stack of several flattened sacs. These "pancake-like" structures are hollow, with cavities called *cisternae* inside them. The flattening of these sacs is caused by a protein complex that pulls them, when they contain newly synthesized proteins, off of the Golgi. Vesicles from the RER fuse with the convex

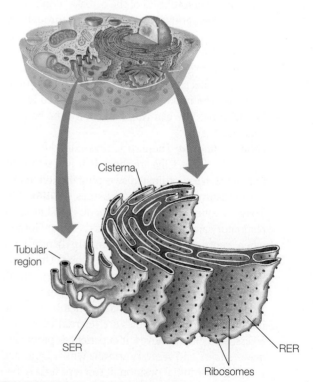

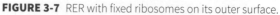

FIGURE 3-7 RER with fixed ribosomes on its outer surface.

receiving side of the Golgi, which is known as the *cis face*. Glycoproteins are modified inside, with sugar groups being added or deleted and, sometimes, with phosphate groups being added. Three or more types of vesicles bud from the concave *trans face* of the Golgi apparatus. Those that contain proteins to be exported pinch off as *secretory vesicles* (*granules*). They migrate to the plasma membrane, discharging their contents from the cell via exocytosis. The enzyme-producing pancreatic cells are examples of specialized secretory cells that have a prominent Golgi apparatus. Other vesicles that contain lipids and transmembrane proteins are pinched off by the Golgi apparatus and sent to the plasma membrane or other membranous organelles. Digestive enzymes are packaged by the Golgi apparatus into membranous lysosomes that remain in the cell (**FIGURE 3-8**). The Golgi apparatus has three main functions: (1) modifying and packaging secretions (such as hormones or enzymes) that are released via exocytosis, (2) packaging special enzymes inside vesicles for use in the cytosol, and (3) renewing or modifying the cell membrane.

- **Lysosomes:** These tiny spherical sacs begin as endosomes with inactive enzymes. Lysosomes dispose of cell wastes, using enzymes to break down nutrients or foreign particles (such as bacteria). They also destroy older parts of the cell. This breakdown process requires the use of powerful enzymes. It often generates toxic chemicals capable of damaging or killing the cell. Lysosomes are specialized vesicles that provide an isolated environment for potentially dangerous chemical reactions. They are produced close to the Golgi apparatus and contain digestive enzymes. In phagocytes, lysosomes are large and plentiful, able to digest nearly every type of biological molecule. They are most effective in acidic conditions and are known as *acid hydrolases*. The lysosomal membrane contains hydrogen proton pumps. These ATPases collect hydrogen ions from surrounding cytosol that maintain the acidic pH of the organelle. The lysosomal membrane also traps dangerous acid hydrolases as it allows final digestive product to leave for use by the cell or excretion. Because of lysosomes, sites are provided where digestion can occur safely inside a cell. The many functions of lysosomes also include digestion of bacteria, viruses, toxins, and other particles taken in by endocytosis; performing glycogen breakdown and release and other metabolic functions; breaking down bone to release calcium into the blood; degrading organelles that are nonfunctional or "worn out"; and breaking down nonuseful tissues, an example of which is the uterine lining during menstruation. Although mostly stable, the lysosomal membrane becomes fragile when the cell is deprived of oxygen, has too much vitamin A, or is injured. Rupture of lysosomes causes the cell to digest itself (*autolysis*), which assists in desirable destruction of cells.

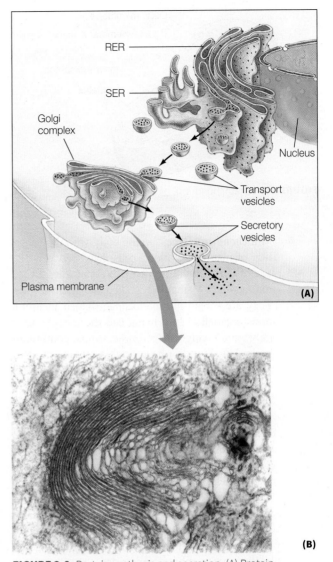

FIGURE 3-8 Protein synthesis and secretion. (A) Protein packed in lysosomes and secretory granules (for later export) is synthesized on the RER and then transferred in tiny transport vesicles to the Golgi complex. Protein is sometimes chemically modified in the cisternae of both the RER and the Golgi complex. The Golgi complex separates protein by destination and repackages it into secretory granules, which remain in the cytoplasm until secreted by exocytosis. (B) Transmission electron micrograph of the Golgi complex. (Courtesy of Prof. Constantin Craciun from Electron Microscopy Center, Babes-Bolyai University, Cluj-Napoca, Romania.)

- **Microfilaments:** The smallest of the cytoskeletal elements, microfilaments are composed of the proteins actin and myosin. Similar, larger cytoskeletal elements include the intermediate filaments and microtubules. They are typically found in muscle cells. Microfilaments provide cell movement and contraction via interaction with actin and myosin. This process can also change the shape of the entire cell. Microfilaments, as well as intermediate filaments, and microtubules are also discussed in their relation to the cytoskeleton later in this chapter.

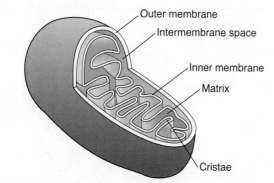

FIGURE 3-9 A mitochondrion.

■ **Mitochondria:** All cells in the body, with the exception of mature red blood cells, have between 100 and a few thousand complex organelles called mitochondria (singularly called a *mitochondrion*). They are thread-like or lozenge-shaped membranous organelles. In a living cell the mitochondria move and change shape on an almost continuous basis. Mitochondria have double membranes that play the central role in the production of energy (via ATP). Mitochondria are the "powerhouses" of cells (**FIGURE 3-9**). Mitochondria are usually clustered where most cellular activity is occurring. The liver, kidneys, and muscles have a large number of mitochondria in their cells because they use ATP at a high rate. A mitochondrion is surrounded by two membranes that are similar in structure to the plasma membrane. The outer mitochondrial membrane is smooth. The inner mitochondrial membrane has a series of folds called *cristae* that protrude into the central fluid-filled cavity (the *matrix*), which is enclosed by the inner membrane and cristae.

  ● The number of mitochondria in a particular cell varies, based on the cell's energy demands. They can migrate through the cytoplasm of a cell and are able to reproduce themselves. Mitochondria contain their own DNA but in a more primitive form than that found within the cell nucleus. They also contain their own RNA and ribosomes.

  ● Glucose and other food fuel products are broken down by enzymes to water and carbon dioxide. Some of these dissolve in the mitochondrial matrix, whereas others form part of the crista membrane. During oxidization of metabolites, some released energy is captured and then used to form ATP by attaching phosphate groups to adenosine diphosphate molecules (a process known as *aerobic cellular respiration*).

  ● Approximately 37 mitochondrial genes control synthesis of 1% of the proteins needed for mitochondrial function. The remaining proteins needed for cellular respiration are encoded by the DNA of the cell nucleus. As the cell requires more ATP, the mitochondria either halve themselves (*fission*) or synthesize more cristae. This increases their number, and they grow to their former size. Mitochondria are similar to the purple bacteria phylum. Mitochondrial DNA is also bacteria-like.

■ **Peroxisomes:** These spherical sacs have enzymes (primarily, oxidases and catalases) that speed up many biochemical reactions. They are abundant in the liver and kidney cells, and their diverse actions include synthesis of bile acids, detoxification of hydrogen peroxide or alcohol, and breaking down lipids and biochemicals. Oxidases use molecular oxygen to detoxify alcohol, formaldehyde, and other harmful substances. Most important, oxidases neutralize *free radicals*, which are highly reactive chemicals. Free radicals have unpaired electrons that can ruin the structure of biological molecules. Oxidases convert free radicals to hydrogen peroxide, which catalyzes quickly into water. Although hydrogen peroxide, as well as free radicals, are normal cellular metabolic byproducts, they can greatly harm cells if they accumulate in excessive numbers. Peroxisomes also aid in energy metabolism via the breakdown and synthesis of fatty acids. They appear similar to small lysosomes that usually form by budding off of the ER via special processes.

■ **Ribosomes:** These occur on the outer membrane of the ER where protein synthesis occurs; they may also be scattered through the cytoplasm. Ribosomes are composed of protein and RNA. Their functions involve the formation of proteins, and they are therefore called the "protein factories" of the cell. Ribosomes are small, dark-staining granules. They are made up of *ribosomal RNAs* and proteins. They have globular subunits (two per ribosome) that fit together to form structures that resemble acorns. Protein synthesis is shared by two different types of ribosomes. *Free ribosomes* float freely in cytoplasm, making soluble proteins that function, whereas other proteins are transported to the mitochondria and certain organelles. *Membrane-bound ribosomes* form the *RER* and synthesize proteins that will be incorporated into cell membranes or lysosomes. These proteins may also be exported out of the cell. Subtypes of ribosomes can change functions. They can attach to ER membranes as well as detach from them, based on the type of protein they are making.

■ *Thick filaments:* Relatively massive bundles of subunits composed of the protein **myosin**. Thick filaments appear in muscle cells only, where they interact with actin filaments to produce powerful contractions.

■ **Vesicles:** Also known as *vacuoles*, these sacs are formed when a part of a cell membrane folds inward, establishing a bubble-like structure within the cytoplasm. Vesicles contain various liquid or solid materials that formerly existed outside of the cell membrane.

TABLE 3-1 summarizes the structures and functions of organelles.

FOCUS ON PATHOLOGY

When lysosomal enzymes are nonfunctional, certain diseases may result. Several genetic disorders, such as *Pompe disease*, *mucopolysaccharidoses*, and *familial hyperlipoproteinemia*, that are linked to nonfunctional lysosomal enzymes. Pompe disease is the accumulation of large amounts of glycogen in the heart, liver, and skeletal muscles. Mucopolysaccharidoses (such as Hurler syndrome) involve the inability to break down mucopolysaccharides, causing them to accumulate, which leads to mental retardation and skeletal deformities. Familial hyperlipoproteinemia occurs because lipid droplets cannot be broken down, leading to abdominal pain, hepatomegaly, splenomegaly, and yellow skin nodules.

TABLE 3-1

Structures and Functions of Organelles

Organelles	Structure	Function
Centrioles	Paired cylindrical bodies that are each made up of nine triplets of microtubules.	During mitosis (cell division), they organize a microtubule network to form the spindle and asters. They form the bases of cilia and flagella.
RER	A membranous system that encloses a cavity (cistern). It coils through the cytoplasm, and is externally studded with ribosomes.	Within the cisterns, sugar groups are attached to proteins. The proteins are bound in vesicles so they can be transported to the Golgi apparatus and other sites. Their external faces synthesize phospholipids.
SER	A membranous system of sacs and tubules that lack ribosomes.	The site of steroid (cholesterol) and lipid synthesis, lipid metabolism, and drug detoxification.
Golgi apparatus	Located close to the nucleus, it is a stack of flattened membranes and associated vesicles.	It packages, changes, and separates proteins for secretion from the cell, to be included in lysosomes, and to be incorporated into the plasma membrane.
Lysosomes	Membranous sacs that contain acid hydrolases.	The sites of intracellular digestion.
Microfilaments	Fine filaments composed of actin, a protein.	Aid in muscle contraction and other intracellular movement and help to form the cell's cytoskeleton.
Intermediate filaments	Protein fibers of various composition.	They are stable cytoskeletal elements that resist mechanical forces acting upon the cell.
Microtubules	Cylindrically shaped structures made of tubulin proteins.	They support the cell, giving it shape, and are involved in intracellular and cellular movements. Microtubules form centrioles and, if present, cilia and flagella. They form the mitotic spindles during cell division, binding to the chromosomes and separating the two strands.
Mitochondria	Double-membrane structures that are rod-like in appearance; they are folded into projections (cristae).	The site of ATP synthesis. The mitochondria are the powerhouses of cells.
Peroxisomes	Membranous sacs of the enzymes catalase and oxidase.	Their enzymes detoxify many substances. Catalase is the most important enzyme, which breaks down hydrogen peroxide.
Ribosomes	Dense particles made up of two subunits that are each composed of ribosomal RNA and protein. They may be free, or attached to the RER.	The sites of protein synthesis.

Endomembrane System

The *endomembrane system* consists of organelles that collectively produce and degrade biologic molecules (also storing and exporting them) and that degrade substances that may be harmful. This system is made up of the ER, Golgi apparatus, secretory vesicles, lysosome, and the nuclear membrane. Its components include all membranous organelles or elements that are structurally continuous or that arise due to fusing or forming transport vehicles. Continuities exist between the nuclear envelope, the RER, and the SER. Although not an actual *endomembrane*, the plasma membrane is also part of the endomembrane system. Throughout this system, many indirect interactions occur. Certain vesicles that begin in the ER are eventually fused with the Golgi apparatus or plasma membrane. Vesicles from the Golgi apparatus can become part of the lysosomes, plasma membrane, or secretory vesicles.

Cytoskeleton

The *cytoskeleton* is a network of many rods and hundreds of proteins. The rods run through the cytosol, whereas the proteins link them to other structures of the cell. The cytoskeleton therefore functions as the cell's skeleton, muscles, and ligaments. Various cell movements are also generated by the cytoskeleton. The three types of rods in the cytoskeleton, all of which lack covering membranes, are **microfilaments,** *intermediate filaments,* and *microtubules.*

Microfilaments are the thinnest type of cytoskeletal rods, are semiflexible, and are made of *actin,* a protein. Because no two cells are identical, each has its own unique microfilaments. However, almost all cells have a cross-linked microfilament network (the *terminal web*) that is attached to the cytoplasmic side of the plasma membrane. The cell surface is strengthened by this web, which also acts against compression and transmits force during shape changes and cellular movements.

Microfilaments are usually involved in cell movement and shape changes. Actin filaments interact with *unconventional myosin,* another protein, to generate contractile cellular forces. It is by this mechanism that cells are "pinched" into two cells during cell division. Microfilaments are used for the motion of amoeba and when membranes change during exocytosis and endocytosis. In most cells except for muscle cells, actin filaments break down regularly and reform from smaller subunits as needed.

Intermediate filaments resemble ropes and are made of strong, insoluble protein fibers. Twisted *tetramer fibrils* form intermediate filaments, which are thicker (in diameter) than microfilaments but thinner than microtubules. Intermediate filaments have high tensile strength and of all cytoskeletal elements are the most permanent and stable. They attach to desmosomes to resist pulling forces that may be exerted on the cell. Their protein composition differs in various cell types. Therefore, they are named differently based on the cells they exist in. For example, in nerve cells, the intermediate filaments are referred to as *neurofilaments.*

Microtubules are hollow organelles, made up of spherical *tubulins,* which are protein subunits. They usually radiate from a small area of cytoplasm near the nucleus (the *centrosome* or *cell center*). Microtubules are always active, growing from the centrosome, then disassembling, and then reassembling in either different sites or the same site. They are stiff but bendable and determine the cell's overall shape as well as how cellular organelles are distributed. From the microtubules, structures appear to "hang." These include lysosomes, mitochondria, and secretory vesicles. Tiny *motor proteins* constantly move and reposition organelles along the microtubules. These motor proteins include *dyneins, kinesins,* and others. They function by changing shape, energized by ATP. Some move substances along the microtubules evenly, whereas others grip and release the microtubule, repeating these actions again and again.

Nucleus

The **nucleus** is usually the largest, most visible organelle inside a cell. The nucleus serves as the control center for cellular operations. It contains DNA, or genetic material, that controls cell activities. A single nucleus stores all required information that directs the synthesis of the 100,000 proteins in the human body. A cell without a nucleus cannot repair itself, disintegrating within 3 to 4 months. The nucleus contains the genetic instructions needed to synthesize the proteins that determine cell structures and functions. These instructions are stored in the chromosomes. These structures consist of DNA and various proteins that control and access genetic information. Most cells contain a single nucleus, with the exception of skeletal muscle cells (with numerous nuclei) and mature red blood cells (with no nuclei).

The nucleus of a cell is usually round and is enclosed in a double nuclear envelope, with inner and outer lipid membranes. This envelope also has a protein lining, allowing certain molecules to exit the nucleus. Communication between the nucleus and cytosol occurs through nuclear pore complexes, which are large protein complexes that have a central channel. Ions and small molecules move freely through the central channel while it is open. However, large molecules (proteins, RNA, etc.) require energy for their transport process. Inside the nucleus is a fluid called *nucleoplasm* that suspends the following structures:

- *Nucleolus:* A "mini-nucleus" made up mostly of RNA and protein molecules, with no surrounding membrane. Ribosomes form in the nucleolus and migrate out to the cell's cytoplasm.
- *Chromatin:* Loosely coiled DNA and protein fibers that condense, forming **chromosomes (FIGURE 3-10)**. The DNA controls protein synthesis, and when the cell starts to divide, the chromatin fibers coil tightly to form the chromosomes.

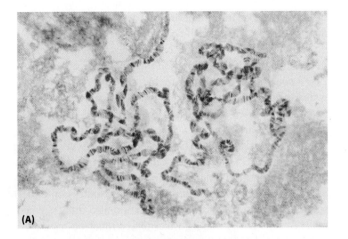

(A)

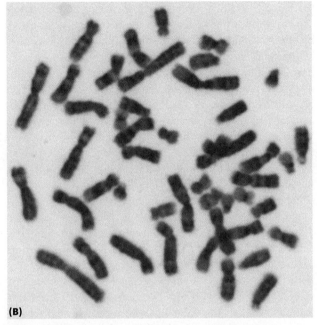

(B)

FIGURE 3-10 Chromosomes. (A) The threadlike chromosomes, made of chromatin fibers consisting of protein and DNA, must condense before the nucleus can divide. (B) Condensed chromosomes. Can you think of any advantages to this strategy?

Movements Through Cell Membranes

The cell membrane controls which substances can enter and leave the cell. It does this by using passive and active mechanisms. Passive mechanisms do not require cellular energy, whereas active mechanisms do.

Passive Cell Mechanisms

Passive cell mechanisms include diffusion, osmosis, and filtration. Diffusion (also known as *simple diffusion*) is the process by which substances spontaneously move from regions of higher concentration to regions of lower concentration (the *concentration gradient*). Molecules and ions in various substances move very quickly, colliding with many other types of particles. These collisions occur at the rate of a million times per second. The speed of diffusion is influenced by kinetic energy, molecular size, and temperature. Once particles have diffused to be evenly distributed throughout a substance such as water, they have achieved a state of **equilibrium**. Examples of diffusion include ion movement across cell membranes, and neurotransmitter movement between nerve cells.

Cells allow substances to diffuse into or out of them only if the cell membrane is permeable to the substance and if the concentration of a substance is higher on one side of the membrane than the other (**FIGURE 3-11**). A molecule or ion will diffuse through the cell membrane if it is lipid soluble, assisted by a carrier molecule, or small enough to pass through membrane channels. *Simple diffusion* is further defined as unassisted diffusion of very small or lipid-soluble particles. Nonpolar and lipid-soluble substances are diffused through the lipid bilayer. These substances include carbon dioxide, fat-soluble vitamins, and oxygen. Oxygen continuously diffuses from the blood into the cells because its concentration is always higher in the blood than in tissue cells. Oppositely, because carbon dioxide is in higher concentration within the cells, it diffuses from tissue cells into the blood.

Some substances cannot pass through the lipid bilayer of a cell membrane, requiring proteins in the membrane to assist them. This process is known as **facilitated diffusion**, which is also known as *assisted diffusion*. It is similar to simple diffusion

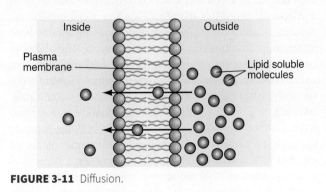

FIGURE 3-11 Diffusion.

because it only moves molecules from areas of higher concentration toward areas of lower concentration. Substances that require facilitated diffusion include certain amino acids, ions, and molecules such as glucose and other sugars. Facilitated diffusion is a passive transport process. Transported substances either bind to protein carriers in the membrane (and then move across it) or move through water-filled protein channels.

Therefore, the two types of facilitated diffusion are called *carrier mediated* and *channel mediated*. *Carriers* are proteins that are described as *transmembrane integral*. They are specific for the transport of certain polar molecules or types of molecules such as sugars and amino acids (which cannot pass through membrane channels because of their size). Therefore, the carrier alters its shape to envelop and later release the transported substance. The carrier shields the substance as it is moved, from the nonpolar membrane regions. Basically, these carrier changes move the binding site from one location on the membrane to the other.

Just as in simple diffusion, substances transported by carrier-mediated facilitated diffusion move down their concentration gradients. For example, glucose is usually in higher concentrations in the blood than in the cells. Therefore, its transport is usually *unidirectional*—into the cells. Carrier-mediated transport is limited by how many protein carriers are present. When all glucose carriers are engaged (*saturated*), glucose transport occurs at its fastest rate.

Channels are transmembrane proteins that move ions, water, and other substances through aqueous channels from one side of a membrane to the other. Because of pore size and amino acid charges in the lining of the channel, they act selectively. *Gated channels* are opened or closed by chemical or electrical signals. *Leakage channels* are always open. They allow water or ions to move through based on concentration gradients. Similar to carriers, channels can also be inhibited by some molecules, be specific, and show saturation. The concentration gradient is also followed in channels. As substances cross the membrane by simple diffusion, the diffusion rate is not controlled because the lipid solubility of the membrane is not immediately changeable. However, the facilitated diffusion rate is controllable, because membrane permeability may be altered by regulating the number or activity of individual channels (or carriers).

Osmosis is a special type of diffusion that occurs when water molecules diffuse from an area of higher water concentration to an area of lower water concentration. This requires a selectively permeable membrane such as a cell membrane. Solutions containing higher concentrations of solutes have lower concentrations of water, and vice versa. The ability of osmosis to create enough pressure to raise a volume of water is called **osmotic pressure**. Water always diffuses toward solutions of greater osmotic pressure. Via osmosis, water equilibrates throughout the body so the concentration of water and solutes in both intracellular and extracellular fluids is nearly the same. Surprisingly, although highly polar, water passes via osmosis through the lipid bilayer. This may occur because of random movements of membrane lipids, which open small gaps in the membrane that allow water to move through.

Osmosis is very important in the determination of water distribution in the cells, blood, and other fluid-containing body compartments. It basically continues until osmotic and hydrostatic pressures acting upon the membrane are equal.

Aquaporins are transmembrane proteins that construct water-specific channels that allow water to move freely and reversibly and water molecules to be diffused in a single-file manner. Although believed to exist in all cell types, they are most prevalent in red blood cells and cells involved in water balance (kidney tubule cells and others). Whenever water concentration differs on opposite sides of a membrane, osmosis occurs. If the solute concentration differs on either side of a membrane, water concentration also differs. *When solute concentration increases, water concentration decreases.*

The number (not the type) of solute particles determines the extent to which solutes decrease water concentration. This is because one water molecule is (basically) displaced by one molecule or one ion of solute. **Osmolarity** is defined as the total concentration of all solute particles in a solution. Net diffusion of both solute and water occurs, moving down their concentration gradients, when the same volumes of aqueous solutions of different osmolarity are separated by a membrane that is permeable to *all molecules* in the system. When the water and solute concentration on both sides of the membrane is the same, *equilibrium* is reached. Osmolarity is based only on a solution's total solute concentration. It is expressed as *osmoles per liter* (osmol/L). One osmol is equal to 1 mole of nonionizing molecules.

If a membrane is impermeable to solute particles, water diffuses quickly from the left to the right compartment. This continues until the concentration is the same on both sides of the membrane. In this example, equilibrium results only from the movement of water because the solutes are prevented from moving. The movement of water causes dramatic changes in the volumes of both compartments. This is similar to *osmosis* across plasma membranes of living cells. In a living plant cell, different from the previous example, the rigid cell wall outside the plasma membrane will eventually reach a point where water that is diffusing in will cause its **hydrostatic pressure** to equal its *osmotic pressure*. There will then be no further net water entry. In general, the higher the amount of *nonpenetrating* (nondiffusible) solutes in a cell, the higher the osmotic pressure. Also, this means that a greater hydrostatic pressure must occur to resist additional net water entry. The hydrostatic pressure pushes water out, whereas the osmotic pressure pulls water in.

In living animal cells, these major hydrostatic versus osmotic changes do not occur, because cell walls are not as rigid. When an osmotic imbalance causes an animal cell to swell or shrink, one of two things occurs. Either the solute concentration will be the same on both sides of the plasma membrane, or the membrane will stretch until it breaks. *Tonicity* refers to a solution's ability to change the shape or tone of cells by altering their internal water volume. This is not the same as osmolarity, because tonicity is based on how a solution affects cell volume. This is based on two factors: the solute concentration and the solute permeability of the plasma membrane.

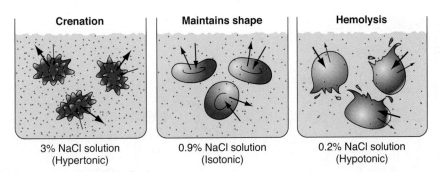

Crenation	Maintains shape	Hemolysis
3% NaCl solution (Hypertonic)	0.9% NaCl solution (Isotonic)	0.2% NaCl solution (Hypotonic)

FIGURE 3-12 Various osmotic pressures in body fluids.

Any solution with the same osmotic pressure as body fluids is called **isotonic**. The concentrations of nonpenetrating solutes are the same as those found in the cells (5% glucose or 0.9% saline). When a cell is exposed to an isotonic solution, it retains its normal shape, with no net gain or loss of water. The body's extracellular fluids and most intravenous solutions are isotonic.

Any solution with a higher osmotic pressure than body fluids is called *hypertonic*. This type of solution has a higher concentration of nonpenetrating solutes than in the cells. Cells that receive hypertonic solutions lose water and crenate (shrink). A strong saline solution is an example of a hypertonic solution. Likewise, any solution with a lower osmotic pressure than body fluids is called *hypotonic* (**FIGURE 3-12**). A hypotonic solution is more dilute, with a lower concentration of nonpenetrating solutes, than cells. A cell receiving a hypotonic solution swells quickly. The most extreme example of a hypotonic solution is distilled water, which contains zero solutes. It causes cells to eventually lyse (burst).

Filtration forces molecules through membranes and is commonly used to separate solids from water. Inside the body, tissue fluid is formed by forcing out water and small dissolved substances through capillary walls. The force of this action comes from the blood pressure, although impermeable proteins usually hold water inside blood vessels via osmosis. This action prevents excess tissue fluid formation (edema). Filtration in the kidneys is the process that cleans the blood.

Hypertonic solutions are commonly given intravenously to patients who are swollen (edematous) because water is retained in their tissues. These solutions cause the excess water to be drawn out of the extracellular space. It is then moved into the blood to be eliminated by the kidneys. Hypotonic solutions rehydrate tissues that have become dehydrated. When dehydration is mild, the patient is usually given hypotonic fluids such as apple juice or a "sports drink," and rehydration usually results.

Active Cell Mechanisms

Particles sometimes move from a region of lower concentration to a region of higher concentration. When this occurs, energy is required. This energy comes from the cellular metabolism, specifically from the molecule known as ATP, which is created in the mitochondria of cells. Active cell mechanisms include active transport, endocytosis, and exocytosis.

Active transport is the movement of particles through membranes from regions of lower concentration to regions of higher concentration. Similar to carrier-mediated facilitated diffusion, it also requires carrier proteins, which combine with transported substances both specifically and reversibly. This process is similar to facilitated diffusion because of its use of specific carrier molecules in the cell membranes (**FIGURE 3-13**). These carrier molecules are proteins that have binding sites that combine with the particles they are carrying. However, active transport differs from facilitated diffusion in that ATP is required. Active transport moves sugar, amino acid, sodium, potassium, calcium, and hydrogen particles across cell membranes. Active transporters (*solute pumps*) move solutes, mostly ions, *against* the concentration gradient, requiring energy.

There are two types of active transport. In *primary active transport*, required energy comes directly from the hydrolysis of ATP. In *secondary active transport*, the process indirectly uses energy that is stored in ionic gradients. These are created by primary active transport pumps. Secondary active transport is a *coupled system* that moves more than one substance at a time. There are two subforms. In a *symport system*, the two substances are transported in the same direction. In an *antiport system*, they cross the membrane in opposite directions.

In *primary active transport*, hydrolyzed ATP causes phosphorylation of the transport protein, changing its shape so it pumps the bound solute across the membrane. Calcium and hydrogen pumps are primary active transport systems. However, perhaps the best studied of these systems is the *sodium-potassium pump*, which uses the enzyme *sodium-potassium ATPase* (Na⁺-K⁺ ATPase). Remember that the concentration of potassium inside cells is much higher than outside of them (by about 10 times), and the reverse is true of sodium. These balances are used for essential muscle and nerve cell function and to maintain normal fluid volume

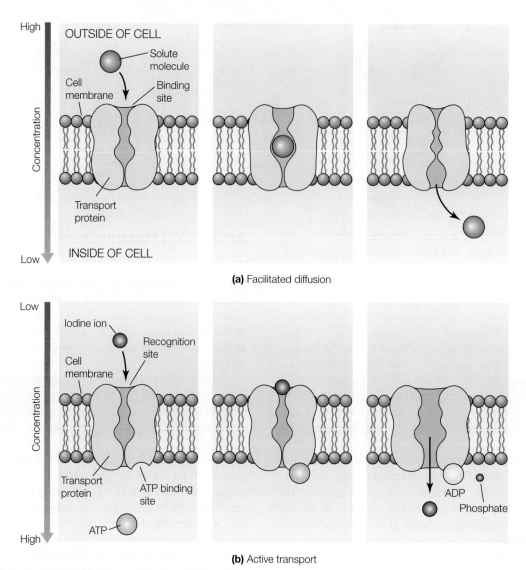

(a) Facilitated diffusion

(b) Active transport

FIGURE 3-13 A comparison of facilitated diffusion to active transport.

in all body cells. Sodium and potassium leak continuously yet slowly through leakage channels in the plasma membrane. They cross more quickly in stimulated muscle and nerve cells. Therefore, the sodium-potassium pump acts as a nearly continuous antiporter. It drives sodium out of cells, against a large concentration gradient, as it pumps potassium back into them.

Ions driven by a concentration gradient may be slowed in their movement by the negative or positive charges of certain plasma membranes. Ions realistically diffuse according to *electrochemical gradients*. Therefore, these gradients used by the sodium-potassium pump are the basis for most secondary active transport of ions as well as nutrients, of vital importance to cardiac, neuronal, and skeletal muscle function.

One ATP-powered pump can indirectly drive the *secondary active transport* of a few other solutes. The pump stores energy in the ion gradient by moving sodium against its concentration gradient, across the plasma membrane. A substance pumped across a membrane can accomplish work as it leaks back, down along its concentration gradient.

Therefore, other substances are cotransported as sodium moves back into the cell via carrier proteins (a symport system). An example is the secondary active transport of certain sugars, amino acids, and ions into the cells that line the small intestine. Because the concentration gradient of the ion is used for energy, the ion has to be pumped out of the cell in order to maintain its diffusion gradient.

Antiport systems can also be driven by ion gradients. An example of such an antiport system is one that helps regulate intracellular pH by using the sodium gradient for the expulsion of hydrogen ions. Each membrane pump or cotransporter transports only specific substances, no matter how energy is acquired to do so. When substances cannot pass by diffusion, the cell uses active transport systems to be selective. If there is no pump, nothing can be transported.

Vesicular transport involves the transportation of fluids with large particles and macromolecules across cellular membranes inside *vesicles* (membranous sacs). It is similar to active transport in that it also moves substances into the cell and out of the cell. Vesicular transport is also used for *transcytosis*, in which substances are moved into, across, and out of cells.

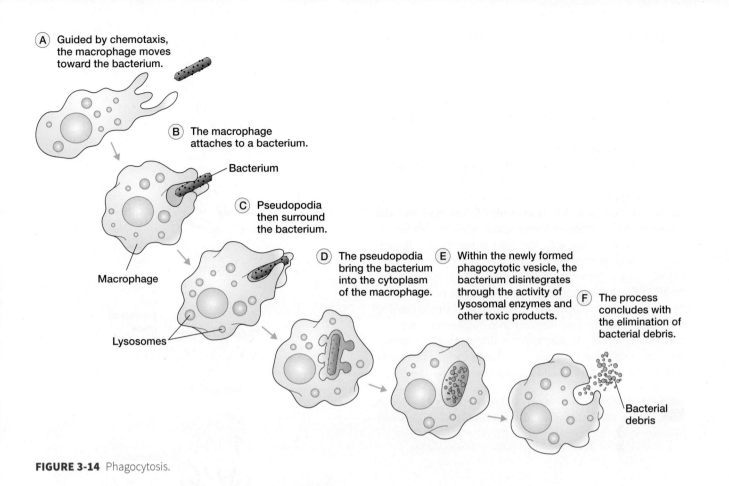

FIGURE 3-14 Phagocytosis.

Vesicular trafficking is a process of movement of substances from an area (or membranous organelle) to another. ATP is required for vesicular transport processes, but another compound (guanosine triphosphate) may also be used. For transcytosis and endocytosis, protein-coated vesicles allow for movement of bulk solids, fluids, and most macromolecules.

Endocytosis and **exocytosis** both use energy from the cell to move substances into or out of the cell without crossing the cell membrane. The opposite process to endocytosis is exocytosis, in which a substance stored in a vesicle is secreted from the cell. In endocytosis, a secretion from the cell membrane moves particles too large to enter the cell by other processes within a vesicle of the cell. The three forms of endocytosis are pinocytosis, phagocytosis, and receptor-mediated endocytosis.

Pinocytosis ("cell drinking") involves cells taking in small liquid droplets from the surrounding cell environment with a small indentation of the cell membrane. It is also known as *fluid-phase endocytosis*. Infolding plasma membrane surrounds extracellular fluid that contains dissolved molecules. This small droplet enters the cell, fusing with an endosome. It is a routine activity of most cells, which differs from phagocytosis. Therefore, they can sample the extracellular fluid, which is an important function of cells that absorb nutrients, such as those in the intestines. The parts of the plasma membrane that are removed during the internalization of the membranous sacs are recycled back via exocytosis. Therefore, the plasma membrane's surface area can remain very constant.

Phagocytosis ("cell eating") involves cells taking in solids instead of liquids (**FIGURE 3-14**). Receptor-mediated endocytosis involves the movement of specific kinds of particles into the cell, with protein molecules extending through part of the cell membrane to the outer surface. This process is triggered when a particle binds to receptors on the cell's surface. *Pseudopods* (cytoplasmic extensions) form and flow around the particle. A *phagosome* (endocytotic vesicle) is formed, which usually fuses with a lysosome as the contents are digested. Exocytosis is then used to eject any indigestible contents from the cell. The primary cells used for phagocytosis are the macrophages and certain white blood cells, commonly referred to as *phagocytes*. These cells ingest and dispose of bacteria, other foreign substances, and dead tissue cells. Their disposal is important because dead cell remnants can trigger inflammation or stimulate an unwanted immune response. Phagocytes usually move via *amoeboid motion*, with their cytoplasm flowing into temporary extensions that allow them to propel forward.

Receptor-mediated endocytosis is the primary mechanism for specific endocytosis and transcytosis of most macromolecules. Cells use it to focus just on material present in tiny amounts in the extracellular fluid. Plasma membrane proteins that bind specific substances are used. The receptors and their attached molecules are internalized in a pit coated with a bristled protein (**clathrin**). Then, pinocytosis or phagocytosis occurs. Receptor-mediated endocytosis is used to take up enzymes, insulin and other hormones, iron, and low-density lipoproteins such as cholesterol. However, this process can be used to enter cells by cholera toxins, diphtheria, and the influenza virus. For other types of vesicular transport, coating proteins such as *caveolae* may be used. These are flask-shaped or tubular pockets of the plasma membrane. They capture certain molecules in coated vesicles and used forms of transcytosis.

In exocytosis, stimulation occurs via binding of a hormone to a membrane receptor or because of a change in membrane voltage. Exocytosis is involved in hormone secretion, mucous secretion, neurotransmitter release, and, sometimes, waste ejection. A *secretory vesicle* forms, enclosing the substance to be removed from the cell. Usually, this vesicle migrates to and fuses with the plasma membrane. It then ruptures, and its contents are spilled outside of the cell. Exocytosis uses a process wherein transmembrane proteins (v-SNAREs) on the vesicles recognize specific plasma membrane proteins (t-SNAREs). They bind with them, causing the membranes to fuse together in a "corkscrew" pattern. Lipid monolayers are rearranged without mixing together with the transmembrane proteins. Material added by exocytosis is then removed by endocytosis.

TEST YOUR UNDERSTANDING

1. Distinguish between phagocytosis and pinocytosis.
2. Explain the three active cell mechanisms.

Cell Life Cycle

The cell's life cycle is regulated via stimulation from hormones or growth factors. Disruption of the cycle can affect the health of the body. Most human cells divide from 40 to 60 times before they die. The life cycle of a cell includes the following steps:

- *Interphase:* The cell obtains nutrients to grow and duplicate. This is actually the period from cell formation to cell division. This step may be better understood as being a metabolic or growth phase.
- *Cell division (mitosis):* The nucleus divides.
- *Cytoplasmic division (cytokinesis):* The cytoplasm divides.
- *Differentiation:* The cell becomes specialized.

Interphase

A cell must grow and duplicate most of its contents before it can actively divide (**FIGURE 3-15**). *Interphase* describes this period of the cell getting prepared to divide. During interphase the cell manufactures new living material, duplicating membranes, lysosomes, mitochondria, and ribosomes. It also replicates its own genetic material. Interphase is divided into an initial growth phase (G_1 phase), a synthesis phase (S phase), and a final growth phase (G_2 phase). Chromatin is produced only during the S phase.

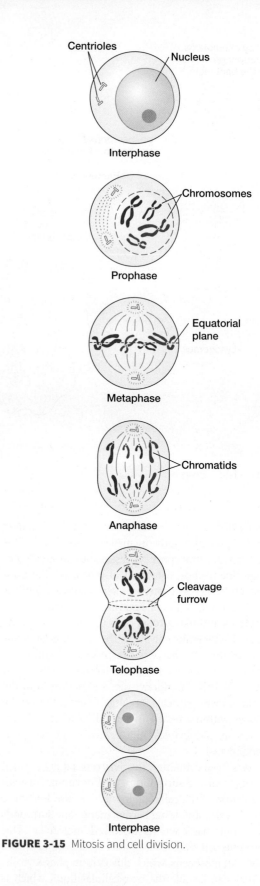

FIGURE 3-15 Mitosis and cell division.

In the G_1 phase, the cell is metabolically active, with rapid protein synthesis and growth. This phase may vary widely in its length. Cells that divide rapidly may do so in minutes to hours, but cells that divide slowly may last for days to years. Any cell that permanently stops dividing is described as being in the G_0 phase. Nearly no cell division activities occur during the G_1 phase. As this phase ends, the centrioles begin replication, preparing for cell division.

In the S phase, DNA is replicated so identical copies of genetic material are received by the two future cells. Chromatin is assembled by the making of new *histones* (basic alkaline proteins). There can be no correct mitotic phase without the S phase also being correctly accomplished. The process of DNA replication involves enzymes attaching to origins or replication. The DNA strands separate, with *replication bubbles* forming. A Y-shaped *replication fork* on the end of each bubble is where helical parental DNA strands are unwound. These strands help to make complementary DNA strands. However, new nucleotides can only be added to preexisting strands and cannot be manufactured newly. Therefore, a short *RNA primer* is formed by a *primase enzyme*. The enzyme *DNA polymerase* aligns complementary nucleotides along the strand and links them together using covalent bonds, only in one direction. The *leading strand* is synthesized continuously once it has been primed, according to the movement of the replication fork. Another *lagging strand* is made in segments in the opposite direction. It requires that a primer replicates each segment. Short segments of DNA are spliced together by *ligase enzymes*. The primers are then replaced by DNA polymerases with DNA nucleotides.

In the very brief G_2 phase, cell division-influencing enzymes and other proteins are synthesized and moved to their required sites. Centriole replication finishes, and the cell is now ready to divide. The cell has continued to grow through this phase as well as the S phase and also has been functioning normally.

Ultimately, two DNA molecules are formed from the original template strands (DNA helix), which are identical to their parents. Each new molecule has one old and one new nucleotide strand, a process known as *semiconservative replication*. Histones then work with the DNA to make two new chromatin strands that are joined by a centromere. Via a protein complex called *cohesin*, they remain together until the anaphase stage of mitotic cell division. Distribution then occurs to the daughter cells, with identical genetic information. If any DNA damage has occurred during the entire process, the cell cycle often stops until the DNA is repaired. However, the cell cycle may also cause a cellular change to occur or even develop into cancer.

Cell Division and Cytoplasmic Division

The two types of cell division are *meiosis* and *mitosis/cytokinesis*. Meiosis is part of gametogenesis (the formation of egg or sperm cells depending on gender). Meiosis reduces by half the number of chromosomes, from 46 to 23, in eggs and sperm so when they unite the fertilized egg will have the proper total of 46 chromosomes.

In the rest of the body, cell numbers are increased by **mitosis**, the division of the nucleus of a cell, and cytokinesis, the division of the cytoplasm of a cell. All cells except egg and sperm cells can be divided by mitosis. When the nucleus divides, it must be precise so an accurate copy of

the DNA information can be made by the new cell. There are several stages of mitosis:

- *Prophase:* The two new centriole pairs move to opposite ends of the cell. The chromatin becomes shorter and thicker. Spindle fibers develop, whereas the nucleolus and nuclear membrane disappear.
- *Metaphase:* The chromosomes line up near the middle portion (the *equator* of the cell), between the centrioles, and spindle fibers attach to them.
- *Anaphase:* The centromere sections of each chromosome are pulled apart to become individual homologous chromosomes and move toward opposite ends (poles) of the cell.
- *Telophase:* The spindle fibers disappear, and the chromosomes lengthen and unwind, with a nuclear envelope forming around them and nucleoli appearing in each newly formed nucleus (the beginning of cytokinesis).

Cytoplasmic division (cytokinesis) begins during anaphase, when the cell membrane constricts down the middle portion of the cell. This continuous process is completed through telophase to divide the cytoplasm. The two newly formed nuclei are then separated, and nearly half of the organelles are distributed into each new cell.

TEST YOUR UNDERSTANDING

1. Explain the steps in the cell life cycle.
2. Why must division of DNA during mitosis be precise?

Differentiation

Differentiation, the process of specialization of a cell, makes each cell unique. New cells must be generated for growth and tissue repair to occur. **Stem cells** are those that can divide repeatedly without specializing. They can divide either into two identical daughter cells or so that one daughter cell becomes partially specialized (progenitor cells). In the human body, all differentiated cell types are created because of the variance of stem and progenitor cells.

Stem cells in certain organs may have the ability to heal the body in the future, even though they were differentiated when the organism was still an embryo or fetus. As the body continually develops, cells use different parts of complete genetic instructions so they can become specialized. Genes may be activated in various types of cells.

Cell Division and Cancer

Cell division and growth normally occur at approximately the same rate as cell death. However, when cell division and growth are higher than the cell death rate, tissues enlarge. A neoplasm or *tumor* is a mass of tissue produced by abnormal cell growth and division. A tumor is called *benign* when it remains within the epithelium or a capsule made of connective tissue. This type of tumor seldom becomes life threatening and can usually be surgically removed if it affects tissue function.

Malignant tumors spread into surrounding tissues in a process called *invasion*. The primary tumor may result in malignant cells traveling to other organs or tissue to establish secondary tumors. This process, called *metastasis*, is not easily controlled. *Cancer* develops, as shown in **FIGURE 3-16**, and exhibits mutations disrupting normal cell growth. Usually, all tumor cells are daughter cells of just one malignant cell. Malignancy often occurs when a normal gene mutates. These modified genes are called *oncogenes*. Genes that promote cell division are called *proto-oncogenes*, and oncogenes are created by these genes. Oncogenes often code for the proteins controlling cell division.

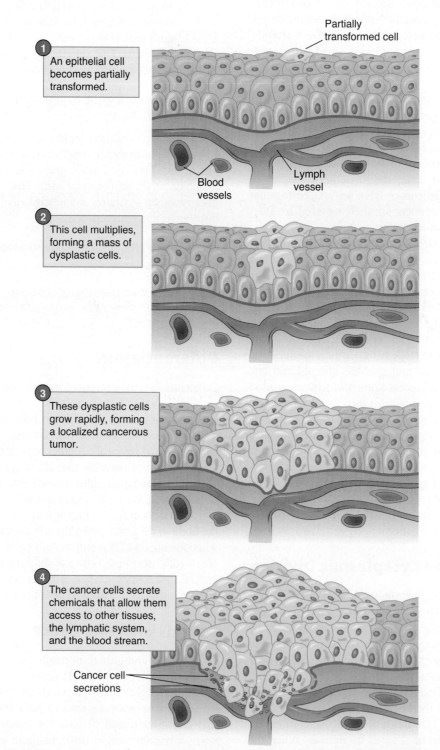

1. An epithelial cell becomes partially transformed.

Partially transformed cell

Blood vessels

Lymph vessel

2. This cell multiplies, forming a mass of dysplastic cells.

3. These dysplastic cells grow rapidly, forming a localized cancerous tumor.

4. The cancer cells secrete chemicals that allow them access to other tissues, the lymphatic system, and the blood stream.

Cancer cell secretions

FIGURE 3-16 How cancer develops.

Most cancers are caused by mutations of the genes inside *somatic cells*. This is linked to mutations occurring during cell division. A small number of errors occur while DNA is being replicated before cell division. A *mutation* is defined as a DNA sequence with replication errors inside it. Mutations may also be caused by chemicals, toxins, radiation, and viruses. Cancer most commonly develops in tissues that experience frequent cell divisions, such as epithelial cells. Multiple mutations, occurring over many cell generations, result in cancer. This is why older people more commonly develop cancer than younger people.

Cancer cells change shape as they grow and gradually resemble normal cells less and less. Tumor cells escape the primary tumor to invade surrounding tissue—this is the manner in which metastasis begins. If tumor cells penetrate blood vessels, they circulate throughout the body. If they enter the lymphatic system, they accumulate in lymph nodes. The presence of tumor cells stimulates the growth of new blood vessels where the cells situate themselves. This supplies them with more nutrients and accelerates their growth and further metastasis.

As metastasis increases, organ function changes. Cancer cells grow and multiply by taking nutrients and space from normal cells, causing weight loss in most cancer patients as the normal cells deteriorate. When cancer cells compress vital organs or have replaced healthy cells in vital organs, death may occur. Cancer often begins where stem cells divide, because a greater chance of error occurs the more frequently that chromosomes are copied for cell division.

To prevent the development of cancer in cells, the body uses two major mechanisms. The first involves DNA repair enzymes, which detect and correct errors that occurred during replication. If these enzymes are made less effective because of their controlling genes becoming mutated, this first mechanism of fighting against cancer cannot be effective. The second mechanism is *apoptosis*, which is a self-destructive process that destroys cells containing abnormal DNA. Therefore, mutated cells are made to self-destruct before cancer can develop. Apoptosis also occurs in normal cells that have a limited life span. However, mutations of genes that influence apoptosis may result in persistently mutated cells, which can continue to divide and proliferate.

Tumor suppressor genes are normal genes that slow or even stop cell division. They can be affected by mutations that cause them to have reduced actions. In human cancer cells, many types of oncogenes and altered tumor suppressor genes have been identified. Cancer therapy focuses on the confinement of malignant cells and then their destruction. Cancerous tissue is killed by lasers, x-rays, and drugs (chemotherapy) and removed by surgery. However, many cancers cannot be completely destroyed. Some of the adverse effects of cancer therapies include the destruction of normal cells in rapidly growing tissues such as bone marrow. This can lead to anemia, because of reduced numbers of red blood cells.

SUMMARY

The cell is the basic unit that performs all the vital physiologic functions in the body. The three parts of the cell are the semipermeable cell membrane, the cytoplasm, and the nucleus. The cell membrane is mostly made up of lipids and proteins, usually in a double layer of phospholipid molecules. The cytoplasm is a gel-like material suspending the cell's organelles. The organelles in the cytoplasm each have specific actions that help to carry out the cell's activities. They are vital to the life of the cell, tissue, and organism.

The cell nucleus is the control center for cellular operations. Inside the nucleus, a fluid called nucleoplasm suspends the nucleolus and chromatin. The nucleus also contains chromosomes. The DNA controls protein synthesis in the nucleus.

The cell membrane uses passive and active mechanisms to allow various substances to enter or leave the cell. Passive cell mechanisms include diffusion, osmosis, and filtration. Active cell mechanisms require energy and specific carrier molecules and include active transport, endocytosis, and exocytosis. A neoplasm is a mass of tissue produced by abnormal cell growth and division. The two types of tumors are benign or malignant. Tumors that are malignant spread into surrounding tissues in a process known as metastasis.

KEY TERMS

Active transport	Chromosomes	Cytoplasm
Cell membrane	Cilia	Cytoskeleton
Centrioles	Cisterns	Cytosol
Centrosome	Clathrin	Endocytosis
Chromatin	Cytology	Endoplasmic reticulum (ER)

Equilibrium
Exocytosis
Facilitated diffusion
Flagella
Golgi apparatus
Glycolipids
Hydrostatic pressure
Integral proteins
Isotonic
Lipid rafts

Lysosomes
Microfilaments
Mitochondria
Mitosis
Myosin
Nucleolus
Nucleus
Osmolarity
Osmotic pressure
Peripheral proteins

Peroxisomes
Phospholipids
Ribosomes
Semipermeable
Sex cells
Somatic cells
Stem cells
Vesicles

LEARNING GOALS

The following learning goals correspond to the objectives at the beginning of this chapter:

1. There are three major parts to a cell: the cell membrane, the nucleus, and the cytoplasm. The cell membrane encloses the cell, its nucleus, and its cytoplasm. The nucleus contains the cell's genetic material and controls its activities. The cytoplasm fills out the cell and its shape.

2. The cell (plasma) membrane controls movement of substances both into and out of the cell. It is also where much of the cell's biologic activities are conducted. Molecules in the cell membrane form pathways that allow the detection of signals from outside the cell to be transmitted inside. Each cell's membrane is thin, delicate, and able to stretch. There are usually tiny folds on the surface, which help to increase its surface area. Cell membranes can be differentially permeable or semipermeable.

3. Cytoplasm is a substance that contains all the cellular contents between the plasma membrane and the nucleus. It makes up most of each cell's volume and is a gel-like material suspending the cell's organelles. Cytoplasm consists of cytosol and a cytoskeleton. Cytosol is the fluid portion of cytoplasm.

4. The cell nucleus serves as the control center for cellular operations. Inside the nucleus is a fluid called nucleoplasm that suspends the following structures:
   - *Nucleolus:* A mini-nucleus made up of mostly RNA and protein, with no surrounding membrane
   - *Chromatin:* Loosely coiled DNA and protein fibers that condense, forming chromosomes

5. The mitochondria are the "powerhouses" of each cell. They are organelles with double membranes that play a central role in the production of ATP. There may be hundreds or thousands of mitochondria in each cell. Cells that use more ATP have more mitochondria (such as liver, kidney, and muscle cells).

6. Passive cell mechanisms include diffusion, osmosis, and filtration. Active cell mechanisms include active transport, endocytosis, and exocytosis.
   - Diffusion is the process by which substances spontaneously move from regions of higher concentration to regions of lower concentration.
   - Osmosis is a special type of diffusion that occurs when water molecules diffuse from an area of higher water concentration to an area of lower water concentration.
   - Filtration forces molecules through membranes.
   - Active transport is the movement of particles through membranes from regions of lower concentration to regions of higher concentration.
   - Endocytosis involves a secretion from the cell membrane moving particles too large to enter the cell by other processes within a vesicle of the cell.
   - Exocytosis is the opposite process of endocytosis, in which a substance stored in a vesicle is secreted from the cell.

7. Cilia and flagella extend from certain cell surfaces. Cilia are hair-like, moving in a coordinated sweeping motion to move fluids over the surface of tissues. Flagella are longer than cilia and often exist as only a single flagellum, such as the tail of a sperm cell.

8. Passive cell mechanisms do not require energy, whereas active cell mechanisms do.

9. The life cycle of a cell includes the following:
   - *Interphase:* The cell obtains nutrients to grow and duplicate.
   - *Mitosis:* The nucleus divides.
   - *Cytoplasmic division (cytokinesis):* The cytoplasm divides.
   - *Differentiation:* The cell becomes specialized.
10. Cell division and growth normally occur at approximately the same rate as cell death. However, when cell division and growth are higher than the cell death rate, tissues enlarge. A neoplasm or tumor is a mass of tissue produced by abnormal cell growth and division. Cancer develops in a process called metastasis, wherein malignant cells travel to other organs or tissue to establish secondary tumors. Cancer exhibits mutations disrupting normal cell growth.

CRITICAL THINKING QUESTIONS

A 63-year-old woman was diagnosed with carcinoma of the thyroid. Unfortunately, it had metastasized to her vertebral bones.

1. Explain the cell division in relation to cancer.
2. Describe the term *metastasis* and the most common cause of cancer.

REVIEW QUESTIONS

1. Which of the following is the control center for cellular operations?
   - A. cell membrane
   - B. lysosomes
   - C. nucleus
   - D. mitochondria
2. Which of the following organelles is involved in the digestion of foreign material?
   - A. ribosomes
   - B. lysosomes
   - C. mitochondria
   - D. Golgi apparatus
3. Where is most of the ATP required to power cellular operations produced?
   - A. mitochondria
   - B. nucleoli
   - C. Golgi apparatus
   - D. centrioles
4. Where does synthesis of lipids take place?
   - A. lysosomes
   - B. nucleoli
   - C. rough endoplasmic reticulum
   - D. smooth endoplasmic reticulum
5. A solution that contains a higher solute concentration than the cytoplasm of a cell is referred to as
   - A. hypertonic
   - B. isotonic
   - C. hypotonic
   - D. semitonic
6. Which of the following is true about cell membranes?
   - A. They are impermeable.
   - B. They are freely permeable.
   - C. They are differentially permeable or semipermeable.
   - D. They are actively permeable.
7. The movement of oxygen from an area of high concentration to an area of low concentration is an example of
   - A. filtration
   - B. diffusion
   - C. osmosis
   - D. active transport
8. The fluid-filled cavity within mitochondria is called the
   - A. matrix
   - B. cristae
   - C. vesicle
   - D. anticodon

9. The basic structural and functional unit of the human body is the
   A. tissue
   B. cell
   C. organ
   D. chromosome

10. Which organelles are responsible for protein synthesis?
    A. mitochondria
    B. ribosomes
    C. lysosomes
    D. Golgi apparatus

11. The cell membrane is also called the
    A. cutaneous membrane
    B. serous membrane
    C. mucous membrane
    D. plasma membrane

12. The primary substances that make up cell membranes are
    A. proteins
    B. carbohydrates
    C. lipids
    D. both A and C

13. The clear liquid portion of the cytoplasm is known as the
    A. centrosome
    B. cytosol
    C. microfilament
    D. vesicle

14. Which of the following is made up mostly of RNA and protein and has no surrounding membrane?
    A. nucleolus
    B. vesicles
    C. mitochondria
    D. lysosomes

15. Which of the following is not a passive cell mechanism?
    A. diffusion
    B. osmosis
    C. endocytosis
    D. filtration

ESSAY QUESTIONS

1. What are the lipid and protein membranes of a cell?
2. Compare hydrophilic and hydrophobic lipids.
3. How many membrane proteins are found in the cell membrane? Describe them.
4. What are lipid rafts? Give two examples.
5. Compare cilia with flagella.
6. Contrast the roles of the ER-bound ribosomes with those that are free in the cytosol.
7. Compare and contrast active and passive cell membranes.
8. Name the cell life cycle and its four phases.
9. Explain the structure and functions of the Golgi apparatus and the microtubules.
10. Define the structures of DNA and RNA, and identify their locations.

Cellular Metabolism

OBJECTIVES

After studying this chapter, readers should be able to

1. Define metabolism, catabolism, and anabolism.
2. Describe what takes place in an oxidation-reduction reaction.
3. Explain cellular respiration.
4. Compare and contrast glycogenesis, gluconeogenesis, and lipolysis.
5. Discuss hydrolysis of a water molecule.
6. Describe glycolysis in the cellular respiration.
7. Describe oxidation of glycerol and fatty acids.
8. Explain the oxidation of amino acids.
9. Discuss metabolic pathways.
10. Define oxidation and energy.

Overview

The chemical reactions involved in cellular metabolism release energy because of the breakdown of nutrients. Molecules are built to store energy. As cells divide, they use energy to copy their genetic material. They build proteins from amino acids. *Enzymes* are proteins required for cellular metabolism and to control metabolic reactions. Nutrients in body cells are used for biochemical reactions that collectively are described as *metabolism*, during which time substances are built up and broken down continuously.

Metabolic Reactions

Metabolism consists of the chemical changes that take place inside living cells. As a result of metabolism, organisms grow, maintain body functions, release or store energy, produce and eliminate waste, digest nutrients, or destroy toxins. These reactions alter the chemical nature of a chemical substance, maintaining homeostasis.

Two major types of metabolic reactions control how cells use energy. The buildup of larger molecules from smaller molecules is called **anabolism**. An example of anabolism is when amino acids bond together and form proteins. The breakdown of larger molecules into smaller ones is called **catabolism**. An example of catabolism is when foods are hydrolyzed in the digestive tract. Both anabolism and catabolism require the use of energy.

Anabolism

Anabolism is the process of building complex molecules in the body from simpler materials. When a person is healthy and has adequate nutrition, simple nutrients (such as amino acids, fats, and glucose) are used by the body to build the basic chemicals that support cellular functioning and sustain life.

Anabolism supplies biochemicals needed for cells to grow and repair themselves. An example of anabolism is when simple sugar molecules called *monosaccharides* are linked to form a chain, making up molecules of glycogen (a carbohydrate). This anabolic process is called **dehydration synthesis**. As the links in this chain are formed, an OH (hydroxyl group) is removed from one molecule, whereas an H (hydrogen atom) from another is removed. Together the OH and H produce a water molecule (H_2O). The monosaccharides are then joined by a shared oxygen atom, making the chain grow (**FIGURE 4-1**).

Dehydration synthesis, which links glycerol and fatty acid molecules in adipose (fat) cells, forms fat molecules (triglycerides). This occurs when three hydrogen atoms are removed from a glycerol molecule. An OH group is removed from each of three fatty acid molecules (**FIGURE 4-2**). This creates three water molecules and one fat molecule. Oxygen atoms are then shared between the glycerol and fatty acid portions.

Cells also use dehydration synthesis to join amino acid molecules, eventually forming protein molecules. As two amino acids unite, one OH molecule is removed from one of them, whereas one H molecule is removed from the NH_2 group of another. This forms a water molecule. The amino acid molecules are then joined by a bond created between a nitrogen atom and a carbon atom, called a *peptide bond*, shown in **FIGURE 4-3**.

A *dipeptide* is formed from two amino acids bound together, and a *polypeptide* is formed from many amino acids bound into a chain. Polypeptides usually have specialized functions. When a polypeptide has more than 100 molecules, it is considered to be a protein. Certain protein molecules have more than one polypeptide.

The three primary stages involved in processing nutrients for energy release are as follows:

- *Stage 1:* Digestion in the gastrointestinal tract. Absorbed nutrients are transported to the tissue cells by the blood.

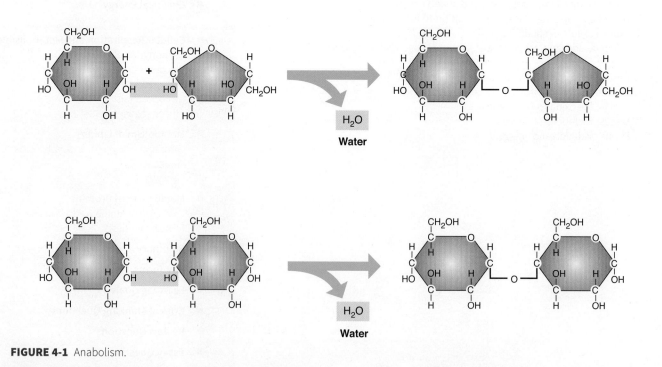

FIGURE 4-1 Anabolism.

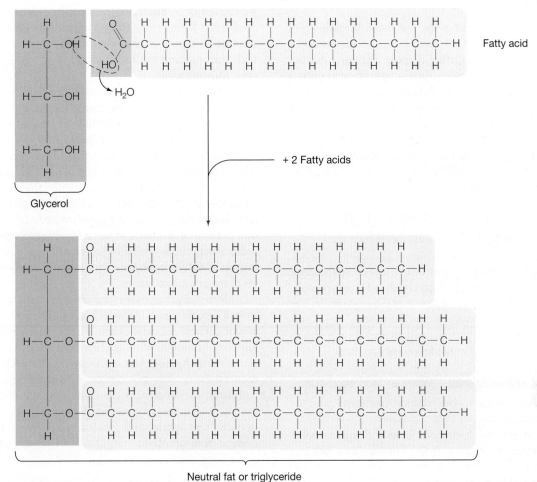

FIGURE 4-2 Dehydration synthesis.

- *Stage 2:* In the tissue cells, nutrients are built into glycogen, lipids, and proteins or are broken down to *pyruvic acid* and *acetyl coenzyme A (CoA)* in the cell cytoplasm.
- *Stage 3:* In the mitochondria, there is much catabolic activity, requiring oxygen. This finalizes food breakdown, produces water and carbon dioxide, and collects large amounts of adenosine triphosphate (ATP). Carbohydrates such as glucose combine with oxygen to produce large amounts of ATP.

The glycolysis occurring in stage 2 and all events in stage 3 make up *cellular respiration,* which is discussed in detail later in this chapter.

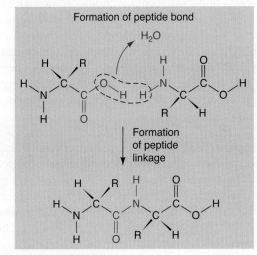

FIGURE 4-3 Peptide bond.

FOCUS ON PATHOLOGY

Mitochondrial disease is a term that actually describes a variety of neuromuscular diseases caused by damage to the mitochondria of cells. Symptoms involve weak or spontaneous muscle contractions, arrhythmias, dementia, seizures, and heart failure. Most forms of mitochondrial disease are progressive and can cause death. Although there is no specific treatment, physical therapy and vitamin supplementation may help improve energy levels and prevent fatigue.

Catabolism

Catabolism can be defined as the metabolic breakdown of stored carbohydrates, fats, or proteins to provide energy. It occurs continuously to differing degrees. Excessive catabolism leads to wasting of tissues. An example of catabolism is the process of **hydrolysis**, which is actually the opposite of dehydration synthesis. This involves the decomposition of carbohydrates, lipids, and proteins.

Hydrolysis splits a water molecule; for example, hydrolysis of sucrose (a disaccharide) gives off glucose and fructose (two monosaccharides) as the water molecule splits. The equation is as follows:

$$C_{12}H_{22}O_{11} + H_2O \rightarrow C_6H_{12}O_6 + C_6H_{12}O_6$$
$$\text{(Sucrose)} \quad \text{(Water)} \quad \text{(Glucose)} \quad \text{(Fructose)}$$

As shown in the equation, inside the sucrose molecule the bond between the simple sugars breaks. The water molecule supplies a hydrogen atom to one of the sugar molecules while supplying a hydroxyl group to the other.

Both dehydration synthesis and hydrolysis are reversible and are summarized in the following equation:

Hydrolysis $\rightarrow$ Disaccharide + Water $\leftrightarrow$ Monosaccharide

+ Monosaccharide $\leftarrow$ Dehydration synthesis

During digestion, hydrolysis breaks down carbohydrates into monosaccharides. It also breaks down fats into glycerol and fatty acids, nucleic acids into nucleotides, and proteins into amino acids.

TEST YOUR UNDERSTANDING

1. What are the functions of catabolism and anabolism?
2. Explain the differences between dehydration synthesis and hydrolysis.

Control of Metabolic Reactions

Nerve, muscle, and blood cells are specialized to carry out distinctive chemical reactions; however, every type of cell performs basic chemical reactions. These include the buildup and breakdown of carbohydrates, lipids, nucleic acids, and proteins. Enzymes coordinate hundreds of rapid chemical changes to control metabolic reactions.

Oxidation-Reduction Reactions

Inside the cells, many reactions are described as *oxidation reactions*. *Oxidation* is the gain of oxygen or the loss of hydrogen. The oxidized substance always loses, or nearly loses, electrons as they move either toward or to a substance with a strong attraction for them. Nearly all oxidation of

food fuels requires removal or pairs of hydrogen atoms as well as pairs of electrons from substrate molecules. This eventually leaves only carbon dioxide behind. The final electron acceptor is molecular oxygen, which combines with the removed hydrogen atoms at the end of the process, forming water.

When a substance loses electrons, meaning it is oxidized, another substance gains electrons, meaning it is reduced. Therefore, oxidation and reduction are *coupled reactions* that are referred to as *oxidation-reduction (redox) reactions*. It is important to understand that oxidized substances lose energy, whereas reduced substances gain energy. Oxidation of food fuels transfers their energy to many other molecules, then to adenosine diphosphate (ADP), which forms the energy-rich ATP. Redox reactions are catalyzed by enzymes, just like all other chemical reactions in the body. Enzymes that catalyze redox reactions, in which hydrogen atoms are removed, are known as **dehydrogenases**. Enzymes that catalyze the transfer of oxygen are **oxidases**.

Most dehydrogenases and oxidases require assistance from a certain coenzyme, which is usually derived from a B vitamin. These enzymes cannot accept the hydrogen, meaning they cannot bond to it. However, their *coenzymes* can act as either hydrogen or electron acceptors. They become reduced every time a substrate is oxidized. For oxidative pathways, two important coenzymes are derived from two specific B vitamins: *nicotinamide adenine dinucleotide* (NAD^+), derived from niacin, and *flavin adenine dinucleotide* (*FAD*), derived from riboflavin.

Chemical Energy

The ability to do work and to change or move matter is called **energy**. Most metabolic processes use chemical energy, which is the type of energy stored in the bonds of chemical substances. Other forms of energy include heat, light, electrical energy, mechanical energy, and sound.

Chemical Energy Release

When the bonds between the atoms of molecules are broken, chemical energy is released. When a substance is burned, for example, bonds break and energy escapes as both light and heat. During the process of **oxidation**, cells "burn" molecules of glucose to release chemical energy that fuels the process of anabolism; however, oxidation is different from the burning of substances that exist outside cells.

Inside the cells, enzymes reduce the amount of activation energy needed for oxidation as part of cellular respiration. Energy is released in the bonds of nutrient molecules. The cells then transfer about 40% of the released energy to special energy-carrying molecules. The remaining energy escapes as heat, helping the body to remain at normal temperature. When the body gains more heat than it is able to lose, *hyperthermia* develops.

Hyperthermia is elevated body temperature, which can develop when the body cannot lose heat as rapidly as the amount of heat it gains. This may result from a variety of factors, which include excessive exercise, fever, hot and humid environments, and anesthesia. Exercising in a hot, humid environment may cause a decrease in the evaporation of sweat, which can lead to overheating. This can lead to states such as heat exhaustion and heat stroke.

Cellular Respiration and Metabolism of Carbohydrates

Cellular respiration is a process that releases energy from organic compounds. This process requires three types of reactions: glycolysis, the citric acid cycle, and the electron transport chain. In cellular respiration, glucose and oxygen are needed. The products of these reactions include carbon dioxide, water, and energy. Therefore, in cellular respiration the presence of oxygen is vital to produce a significant amount of energy. During cellular respiration, food fuels (primarily glucose) are broken down in the cells. Glucose enters tissue cells via facilitated diffusion, which is largely enhanced by insulin. It is then immediately phosphorylated to *glucose-6-phosphate* by transfer of a phosphate group to its sixth carbon as part of a coupled reaction with ATP. Glucose is basically trapped inside the cells because they have a lack of enzymes required to reverse this reaction. Intracellular glucose levels are kept low, which maintains a concentration gradient for glucose entry. The only cells that can reverse this **phosphorylation** reaction are intestinal mucosa cells, kidney tubule cells, and liver cells. For carbohydrates, catabolism and anabolism both begin with glucose-6-phosphate.

In cellular respiration, some of the released energy is captured for the formation of ATP, which links catabolic reactions to the work of the cells. Enzymes shift the high-energy phosphate groups of ATP to other molecules, which are then termed *phosphorylated*. This process causes molecules to increase activity, have movement, or perform work. Important steps in metabolic pathways are catalyzed when phosphorylation activates regulatory enzymes.

Two mechanisms by which the cells capture part of the energy that is released during cellular respiration to manufacture ATP molecules are *substrate-level phosphorylation* and *oxidative phosphorylation*. When high-energy phosphate groups are directly transferred from phosphorylated substrates to ADP, substrate-level phosphorylation occurs. Phosphorylated substrates are identified as metabolic intermediates, of which glyceraldehyde 3-phosphate is an example. This process basically occurs because of high-energy bonds attaching phosphate groups to the substrates. They are highly unstable, even more so than the bonds of ATP. During glycolysis (see below), ATP is synthesized twice by this process and once during each phase of the *Krebs cycle*. The enzymes that catalyze these processes are found in the cytosol and in the watery matrix of the mitochondria.

The second mechanism is known as oxidative phosphorylation, which also releases most of the energy captured in ATP bonding during cellular respiration. It occurs because of electron transport proteins that form portions of the inner mitochondrial membranes. It is a *chemiosmotic process*, which couples chemical reactions with substance movements across membranes. Some energy released when food fuels are oxidized helps to pump protons across inner mitochondrial membranes into the intermembrane space. A steep concentration gradient for protons is therefore created across the membrane. When hydrogen ions flow back across it, through the membrane channel protein *ATP synthase*, a portion of this gradient energy is captured and aids in the attachment of phosphate groups to ADP.

The process of oxidative phosphorylation may be disrupted by poisons such as cyanide. This occurs when cyanide gas binds to cytochrome *c*-oxidase (also known as enzyme complex IV). This blocks the electron transport from cytochrome *c*-oxidase, inhibiting it from releasing oxygen. The proton gradient is destroyed when the inner mitochondrial membrane becomes permeable to hydrogen ions. Without controlled movement of hydrogen ions through ADP synthase, ATP is not formed. Although the electron transport chain still operates at a high rate and oxygen consumption rises, no ATP can be made.

Glycolysis

Glycolysis is a process that involves a series of enzymatically catalyzed reactions in which glucose is broken down to yield lactic acid or pyruvic acid. The breakdown releases energy as **ATP** (**FIGURE 4-4**). The six-carbon sugar glucose is broken down in the cytosol; it becomes two three-carbon pyruvic acid molecules, gaining two ATP and releasing high-energy electrons. Remember: *glucose is the most important fuel molecule in the oxidative pathways, which produce ATP.*

Glycolysis, also referred to as *the glycolytic pathway*, begins the process of cellular respiration. It occurs in the cytosol (the liquid portion of the cytoplasm) and has 10 chemical steps.

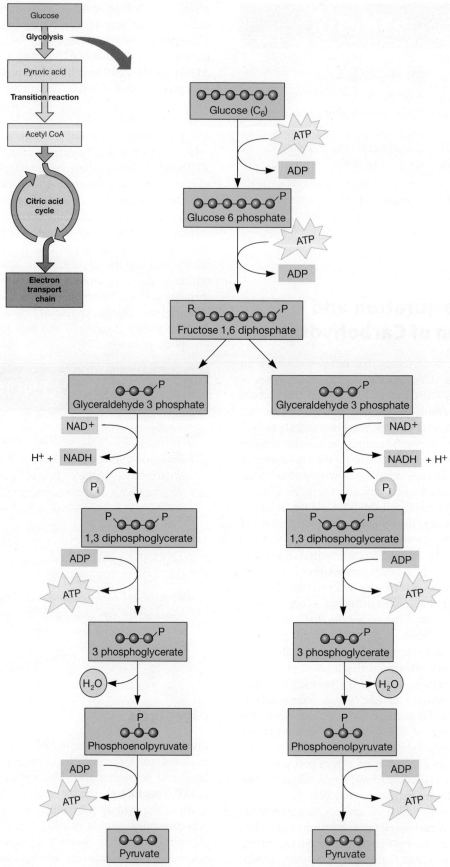

FIGURE 4-4 Glycolysis.

Except for the first step (when glucose that enters the cell is phosphorylated to glucose-6-phosphate), all steps are reversible. Glycolysis does not require oxygen and is occasionally referred to as the **anaerobic** phase, because it occurs whether or not oxygen is present. If oxygen is present in the right amounts, pyruvic acid, which is generated by glycolysis, can enter the more energy-efficient pathways of **aerobic respiration**. These pathways are located in the mitochondria.

The three major phases of glycolysis are *sugar activation,* *sugar cleavage,* and *sugar oxidation with ATP formation:*

- *Phase 1 (sugar activation):* Glucose is phosphorylated, converted to fructose-6-phosphate, and phosphorylated a second time. This process requires two ATP molecules, which are recovered later, and releases fructose-1,6-bisphosphate. The two reactions provide *activation energy,* which is required for the later pathway stages. Therefore, phase 1 may be described as the *energy investment phase.*
- *Phase 2 (sugar cleavage):* Fructose-1,6-bisphosphate is cleaved into two three-carbon fragments, which are reversible isomers of dihydroxyacetone phosphate or glyceraldehyde 3-phosphate.
- *Phase 3 (sugar oxidation with ATP formation):* This phase is separated into six steps, during which two major events occur. The first event is the oxidization of the two three-carbon fragments (via hydrogen removal), which are picked up by NAD+. Some of the energy from glucose is transferred to NAD+. The second event is the attachment of inorganic phosphate groups (P_i) to each oxidized fragment, via high-energy bonds. When the terminal phosphates are eventually cleaved off, four ATP molecules can be formed from the captured energy (*substrate-level phosphorylation*).

When glycolysis is complete, there will be two molecules of pyruvic acid and two molecules of reduced NAD+, which is described as NADH + H+. Each glucose molecule has a net gain of two ATP molecules. Four ATP molecules are produced, but two of these are consumed in phase 1, as previously explained. What will happen to the pyruvic acid is based on the availability of oxygen. Because of limited NAD+, glycolysis continues only if the reduced coenzymes (NADH + H+) are relieved of extra hydrogen.

When oxygen is not sufficiently present, NADH + H+ releases its hydrogen atoms back onto pyruvic acid, which reduces it. *Lactic acid* is then yielded, some of which diffuses out of cells for transport to the liver (for processing). When oxygen becomes available, lactic acid is oxidized back to pyruvic acid. It enters the *aerobic pathways* and is completely oxidized to carbon dioxide and water. The aerobic pathways are defined as the Krebs cycle and electron transport chain within the mitochondria.

Aerobic reactions yield as many as 36 ATP molecules per glucose molecule. Completely decomposed glucose molecules can produce up to 38 molecules of ATP. Most result from the aerobic phase, with only two resulting from glycolysis. Approximately half of the released energy is used for ATP synthesis, whereas the rest becomes heat. The oxidation of glucose also produces carbon dioxide (which is exhaled) and water (which is absorbed into the internal body environment). The volume of water produced by metabolism is lower than the requirements of the body, so the drinking of water is necessary for survival.

FOCUS ON PATHOLOGY

Glycolysis is very important process for health. Several diseases are linked to aerobic glycolysis, including genetic diseases, Alzheimer's disease, cancer, and immune-related diseases that usually cause anemia. High amounts of aerobic glycolysis in the brain are linked to deposition of plaques in later life, which results in Alzheimer's disease. Beta-amyloid pieces stick together to form plaques in the brain. They damage brain cells by blocking cell-to-cell signaling at synapses and may activate immune system cells, triggering inflammation and phagocytosis of disabled brain cells.

Citric Acid Cycle (Krebs Cycle)

The *citric acid cycle* is also called the *tricarboxylic acid cycle* or the *TCA cycle.* It is a sequence of enzymatic reactions involving the metabolism of carbon chains of glucose, fatty acids, and amino acids to yield carbon dioxide, water, and high-energy phosphate bonds (ATP). The three-carbon pyruvic acids enter the mitochondria, each losing a carbon. They then combine with a coenzyme to form a two-carbon acetyl CoA and release more high-energy electrons; then, each acetyl CoA combines with a four-carbon *oxaloacetic acid* to form a six-carbon *citric acid.* During the eight steps of this cycle, citric acid atoms are rearranged to produce various intermediate molecules, most of which are *keto acids.* Eventually, the acetic acid will be totally disposed of, and the pickup molecule (*oxaloacetic acid*) will be regenerated. The citric acid (Krebs) cycle produces two carbon dioxide molecules and four molecules of reduced coenzymes.

A series of reactions removes two carbons, synthesizes one ATP, and releases more high-energy electrons (**FIGURE 4-5**). When food is ingested, large macromolecules are broken down to simple molecules. Proteins are broken down into amino acids, carbohydrates are broken down into simple sugars (glucose), and fats are broken down into both glycerol and fatty acids. In fact, all food carbohydrates are eventually transformed into glucose. The breakdown of simple molecules to acetyl CoA is accompanied by the production of limited amounts of ATP (via glycolysis) and high-energy electrons.

Glucose, through glycolysis, is converted into pyruvic acid. Glycerol and amino acids are also broken down into

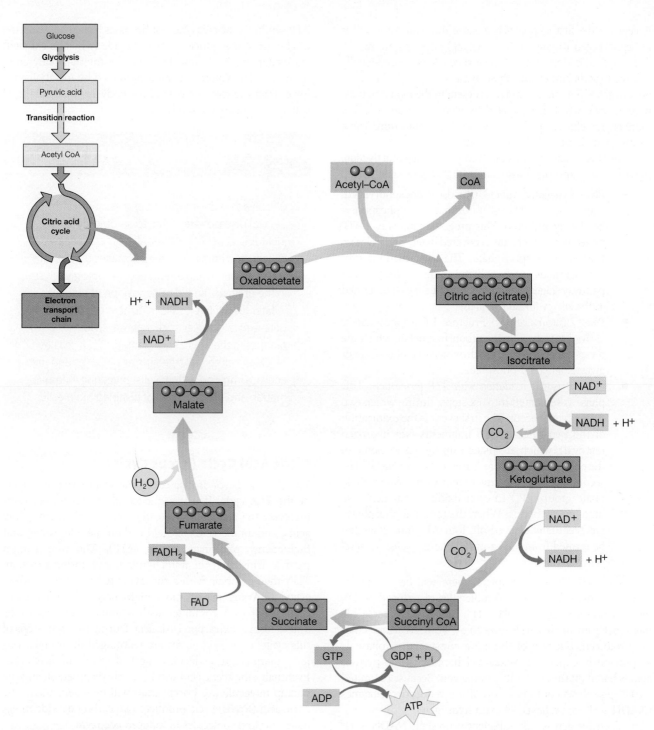

FIGURE 4-5 Citric acid cycle.

pyruvic acid. Actually, all of these processes result, in differing ways, in acetyl CoA. Complete oxidation of acetyl CoA to H_2O and CO_2 produces high-energy electrons, which yield greater amounts of ATP via the electron transport chain. In the TCA cycle, the process of oxidation provides more molecules of ATP. The following summarizes the citric acid (Krebs) cycle:

- *Decarboxylation:* A pyruvic acid carbon is removed and released as carbon dioxide gas. This diffuses into the blood, for expulsion by the lungs. This is

the first time carbon dioxide is released during cellular respiration.

- *Oxidation:* Acetic acid, the remaining 2C fragment, is oxidized via removal of hydrogen atoms. These atoms are picked up by NAD^+.

- *Acetyl CoA formation:* The final reactive product, *acetyl CoA*, is produced when acetic acid combines with coenzyme A. This coenzyme contains sulfur that is derived from vitamin B5.

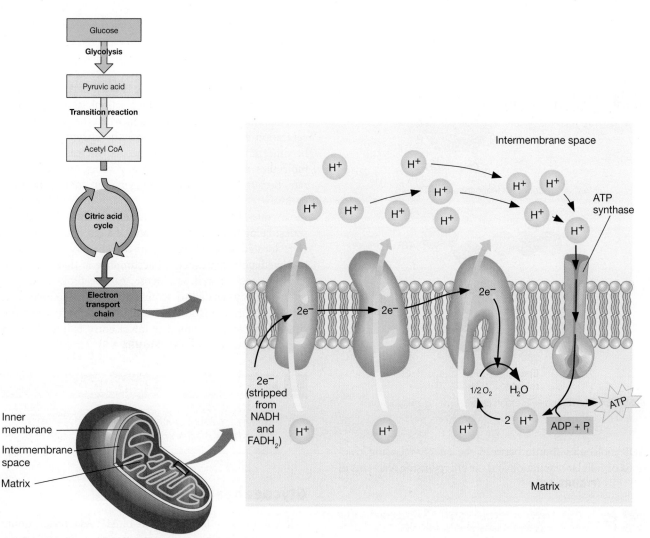

FIGURE 4-6 Electron transport.

Electron Transport Chain

In the *electron transport chain*, the high-energy electrons still contain most of the chemical energy of the original glucose molecule. Special carrier molecules bring them to enzymes that store most of the remaining energy in more ATP molecules; heat and water are also produced. Oxygen is the final electron acceptor in this step; hence, the overall process being termed *aerobic respiration* (**FIGURE 4-6**).

For cellular respiration, glucose and oxygen are required. This process produces carbon dioxide, water, and energy. Nearly half of the energy is recaptured as high-energy electrons stored in the cells through the synthesis of ATP. This process is an example of *oxidative phosphorylation*. Most of the involved components of the electron transport chain are proteins bound to *cofactors* (metal atoms). They form multiprotein complexes embedded in the inner mitochondrial membrane. Some of these proteins are *flavins* (from riboflavin), whereas others contain iron and sulfur. However, most of these proteins are *cytochromes* (iron-containing pigments). Four *respiratory enzyme complexes* are formed by nearby clustered carriers. These complexes are reduced and oxidized as they pick up electrons and move them on to the next complex in the chain.

The electron transport chain converts energy via release of electronic energy to pump protons (from the matrix) to the intermembrane space. An *electrochemical proton (H⁺) gradient* is created across the inner mitochondrial membrane. This gradient has potential energy and can perform work. The only parts of the membrane freely permeable to H⁺ are *ATP synthases*, which are large complexes consisting of enzymes and proteins. An electrical current is created, and ATP synthase uses it to catalyze attachment of a phosphate group to ADP, forming ATP.

Each ATP molecule has a chain of three chemical groups, called *phosphates*. Some of the energy is recaptured in the bond of the end phosphate. When energy is later needed, the terminal phosphate bond breaks to release the stored energy. Cells use ATP for many functions, including active transport and the synthesis of needed compounds.

When an ATP molecule has lost its terminal phosphate, it becomes an ADP molecule. ADP can be converted back into ATP by adding energy and a third phosphate. ATP and

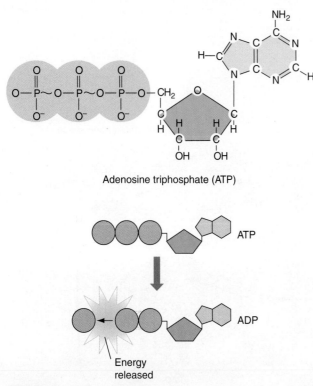

Adenosine triphosphate (ATP)

FIGURE 4-7 ATP and ADP molecules.

ADP molecules shuttle between the energy-releasing reactions of cellular respiration and the energy-using reactions of the cells (**FIGURE 4-7**).

TEST YOUR UNDERSTANDING

1. Explain oxidation-reduction reactions and dehydrogenases.
2. What are the end products of cellular respiration with the presence of oxygen?

Metabolic Pathways

There are a number of steps in each of the processes of cellular respiration, anabolic reactions, and catabolic reactions. A specific sequence of enzymatic actions control these reactions; therefore, the enzymes are organized in the exact same sequence as the reactions they control. Each sequence of enzyme-controlled reactions is called a *metabolic pathway* (**FIGURE 4-8**).

An enzyme-controlled reaction usually increases its rate if the number of substrate molecules or enzyme molecules increases; however, the rate is often determined by an enzyme that regulates one of the reaction's steps. Regulatory enzyme molecules are limited, and when the substrate concentration exceeds a certain level, the enzyme supply can become saturated. When this occurs, increasing substrate molecules will no longer have any effect on the reaction rate. Because of this, just one enzyme can control the entire pathway.

A *rate-limiting enzyme* is usually the first enzyme in a series. Being first is critical because if a rate-limiting enzyme were located somewhere else in the chemical pathway, an intermediate chemical could accumulate at that point. Fats and proteins, as well as glucose, can be broken down to release energy needed to synthesize ATP. In all three cases, aerobic respiration is still the result of these breakdown processes. The most common point of entry is into the citric acid cycle as *acetyl CoA* (see **FIGURE 4-9**).

TEST YOUR UNDERSTANDING

1. What is a metabolic pathway?
2. Why is being the first enzyme in a series critical?

Glycogenesis

Cells cannot store large amounts of ATP. As a result, unlimited amounts of glucose do not cause an unlimited amount of ATP to be synthesized. If there is excessive glucose available that cannot be oxidized immediately, glucose catabolism is soon inhibited by the increasing concentrations of ATP in the cells. Therefore, glucose is stored as either fat or glycogen. Fats make up 80% to 85% of stored energy because the body is able to store much more fat than glycogen. **Glycogenesis** is a process in which glucose molecules are joined (in long chains) to form glycogen. This occurs when ATP levels begin to stop glycolysis from occurring. Glucose enters the cells, to become phosphorylated to glucose-6-phosphate. It is then converted to its isomer, which is known as glucose-1-phosphate. As the enzyme *glycogen synthase* catalyzes glucose attachment to the glycogen chain,

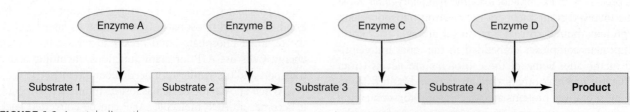

FIGURE 4-8 A metabolic pathway.

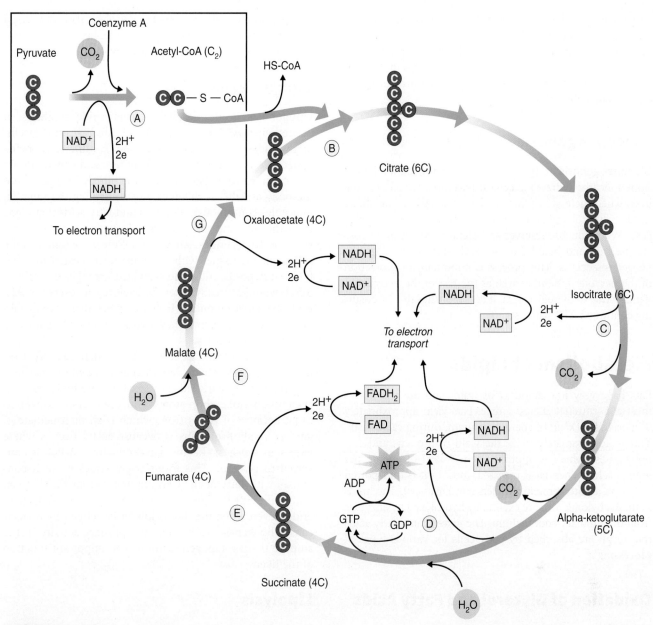

FIGURE 4-9 Acetyl CoA.

the terminal phosphate group is cleaved off. When glycogen is being synthesized and stored, the skeletal muscle and liver cells are at their most active states.

Glycogenolysis

Glycogen splitting or *lysis* occurs when blood glucose levels drop, in a process known as **glycogenolysis**. Glycogen is phosphorylated and cleaved to release glucose-1-phosphate. This is then converted to glucose-6-phosphate, which is able to enter the glycolytic pathway. Glucose-6-phosphate can then be oxidized for energy. The enzyme responsible for all this activity is *glycogen phosphorylase*. The glucose-6-phosphate is then trapped in muscle cells (and most other cells) because it cannot cross cell membranes. *Glucose-6-phosphatase* is an enzyme in liver cells and in certain intestinal and kidney cells, which removes the terminal phosphate to produce free glucose. Because glucose can easily diffuse into the blood, the liver uses its stores of glycogen to supply blood sugar for other body organs when there is a drop in glucose levels. Glycogen from the liver is very important for skeletal muscles that have been depleted of glycogen reserves.

A person who consumes many complex carbohydrates has more glycogen stored in the muscles. For sustaining intense muscle activity, this is a more effective method than consuming high-protein meals. This is not true for highly sugary foods such as candy. *Complex carbohydrates* are required to meet increased needs of growing muscles, along with extra protein. Complex carbohydrates function in this manner because they are protein-sparing. The loading of complex carbohydrates before an intense workout causes the muscles to store more glycogen than usual. A carbohydrate-rich diet, which consists of 75% of energy intake, must be eaten for 3 to 4 days before an intense physical event, while activity is decreased during this time. The muscles store approximately twice as much glycogen as normal, meaning the individual will have more endurance and better performance during his or her planned physical activity.

Gluconeogenesis

Gluconeogenesis is the process of forming new glucose from noncarbohydrate molecules. This process occurs in the liver, when there is insufficient glucose to supply metabolic needs. Glycerol and amino acids are then converted to glucose. When glucose reserves and dietary sources of glucose are used up and blood glucose levels start to drop, gluconeogenesis occurs. This process is important for protection of the nervous system, as well as the rest of the body, from damage due to hypoglycemia. It accomplishes this by ensuring continued ATP synthesis.

Metabolism of Lipids

Fats have very low amounts of water and are the body's most concentrated energy source. Fats yield approximately 9 kilocalories (kcal) of energy, per gram, during catabolism. This is approximately twice the yield of proteins and carbohydrates (which is approximately 4 kcal of energy per gram, each). When fat is digested, most of it is transported in lymph as fatty-protein droplets (*chylomicrons*). The lipids in these chylomicrons are eventually hydrolyzed by enzymes from the capillary endothelium. The glycerol and fatty acids that result are absorbed by body cells for various types of processing.

Oxidation of Glycerol and Fatty Acids

Although there are many lipids, triglycerides are the only type regularly oxidized for energy. This requires separate catabolism of glycerol and fatty acid chains. Glycerol is easily converted, by most body cells, to glyceraldehyde-3-phosphate. This acts as an intermediate substance during glycolysis. It soon enters the Krebs cycle. The ATP energy that is gained from the complete oxidation of glyceraldehyde is about half of the energy gained from glucose (15 ATP/glycerol). Glyceraldehyde is therefore equal to half of one glucose molecule.

The initial phase of fatty acid oxidation is called *beta oxidation*, which occurs in the mitochondria. Fatty acid chains are broken into two-carbon fragments of *acetic acid*. Also, the FAD and NAD+ coenzymes are reduced. The acetic acid molecules are fused to CoA. This forms acetyl CoA. During beta oxidation, carbon in the third (beta) position is oxidized. The fatty acid is cleaved between alpha and beta carbons. The acetyl CoA is picked up by oxaloacetic acid. This enters the aerobic pathways for oxidization to carbon dioxide and water. This is different from the oxidation of

glycerol, which instead enters the glycolytic pathway. Acetyl CoA cannot be used for gluconeogenesis because the metabolic pathway is irreversible past pyruvic acid.

Lipogenesis

Lipogenesis is also known as triglyceride synthesis. It occurs when ATP and glucose levels are high in the cells. Triglycerides in adipose tissue are continuously being cycled. New fats are stored for later use, and stored fats are broken down to be released into the blood. Fat pockets on the body are always different, not containing the same fat molecules continuously. Glycerol and fatty acids that come from the diet and are not needed quickly for energy are stored as triglycerides. About half of these are found in the subcutaneous tissue, with the remainder located in other body fat deposits. Although acetyl CoA and glyceraldehyde 3-PO$_4$ would normally enter the Krebs cycle, excessive ATP leads them to accumulate. However, when these two metabolites become excessive, they are moved into the pathways of triglyceride synthesis.

Fatty acid chains are formed by condensed acetyl CoA molecules. These chains lengthen at a rate of two carbons at a time, and nearly all fatty acids in the body have an even number of carbon atoms. Glucose is easily converted to fat because of acetyl CoA, which is an intermediate of glucose catabolism. This is because acetyl CoA is where fatty acid synthesis begins. Glyceraldehyde 3-PO$_4$ is converted to glycerol. This forms triglycerides when it condenses with fatty acids. Carbohydrates from the diet can always provide the basic materials needed to make triglycerides, even when the diet is low in fat. High blood sugar causes lipogenesis to become the primary activity in the adipose tissues. Lipogenesis is also an important function of the liver.

Lipolysis

Lipolysis is basically the opposite of lipogenesis. It is defined as the breakdown of stored fats into fatty acids and glycerol. These substances are then released to the blood, giving continuous supplies of fat fuels to the organs that is needed for aerobic respiration. Fatty acids are the preferred energy fuel for cardiac muscle, the liver, and the skeletal muscles when they are at rest. When carbohydrate intake is insufficient, lipolysis increases to fuel the body with fats. The availability of oxaloacetic acid to become a pickup molecule influences the ability of acetyl CoA to enter the Krebs cycle. Oxaloacetic acid is converted to glucose, to provide energy for the brain, when carbohydrates are lacking. Without this acid, acetyl CoA accumulates because fat oxidation is incomplete.

The liver converts acetyl CoA molecules to **ketones** (ketone bodies) during the process known as **ketogenesis**. Ketones are defined as organic compounds containing the carbonyl group *CdbondO*, whose carbon atom is joined to two other carbon atoms, with the carbonyl group occurring within the carbon chain. The produced ketones are then released into the blood. Examples of ketones include acetone, acetoacetic acid, and β-hydroxybutyric acid. These are not the same as the *keto acids* that cycle through the Krebs cycle or the *ketone bodies* that are produced during fat metabolism.

FOCUS ON PATHOLOGY

Accumulation of ketone bodies in the blood causes *ketosis*. Large amounts of ketone bodies are then excreted in the urine. This is a common result of diabetes mellitus, a diet that is severely low in carbohydrates, or starvation. Ketosis leads to *metabolic acidosis* because most ketone bodies are organic acids. The blood pH drops to dangerous levels. As acetone is vaporized from the lungs, the patient's breath smells like fruit. The breathing then becomes more rapid because the respiratory system attempts to reduce blood carbonic acid, via expelling carbon dioxide, to raise blood pH. If severe and untreated, the patient can enter a coma or die as the acidic pH depresses his or her nervous system.

Metabolism of Proteins

Proteins must also be broken down and replaced before they deteriorate. During their catabolism, contained amino acids are recycled for use in building new proteins. They may also be modified into different nitrogen-containing compounds. Active transport processes allow the cells to absorb newly ingested amino acids from the blood. The cells can then use the amino acids to replace tissue proteins. This occurs at a rate of approximately 100 grams in 24 hours. Excess protein *cannot be stored by the body*. When excess protein is present, amino acids are either oxidized for energy or converted to fat so they may be used for energy in the future.

Oxidation of Amino Acids

Amino acids must be *deaminated* before they can be oxidized for energy. To do this, their amine group (NH_2) must be removed. The molecule that results is then converted to pyruvic acid or to a keto acid intermediate during the Krebs cycle. These intermediates include acetyl CoA, α-ketoglutaric acid, fumaric acid, oxaloacetic acid, or succinyl CoA. With amino acids that contain sulfur (cysteine, methionine, etc.), sulfur is released before deamination occurs. *Glutamic acid* is the key molecule used in the oxidation of amino acids. The oxidation of amino acids occurs in the following steps:

- *Transamination:* The reversible exchange of amino groups between different amino acids. A variety of amino acids are able to transfer their amine group to the Krebs cycle keto acid known as α-*ketoglutaric acid*. Then, this acid is transformed to glutamic acid. The original amino acid therefore becomes a keto acid, having an oxygen atom in the place where the amine group used to be.
- *Oxidative deamination:* The oxidative breakdown of amino acids. Specialized enzyme systems carry out the process, such as *d-amino oxidase*. The amine group of glutamic acid is removed, in the liver, as **ammonia** (NH_3). Regeneration of α-ketoglutaric acid occurs. The freed ammonia molecules combine with carbon dioxide to yield **urea** and water. The urea enters the blood to be excreted from the body in urine. It is vital that glutamic acid can move the amine groups into the urea cycle, because ammonia is toxic. Therefore, this cycle removes ammonia that was produced by oxidative deamination and ammonia in the blood that was produced by intestinal bacteria.
- *Modification of keto acids:* As amino acids are degraded, molecules are produced that may be oxidized during the Krebs cycle or converted into glucose. Transamination produces keto acids that may be altered to form metabolites, which can enter the Krebs cycle. Pyruvic acid, acetyl CoA, α-ketoglutaric acid, and oxaloacetic acid are the most important of these metabolites. Deaminated amino acids converted to pyruvic acid can be reconverted to glucose, because glycolytic reactions are reversible. These converted amino acids can then act as part of gluconeogenesis.

Protein Synthesis

The most important anabolic nutrients are amino acids, which form all protein structures as well as most of the body's functional molecules. Protein synthesis occurs on ribosomes, where enzymes control formation of peptide bonds. These bonds link amino acids together, forming protein polymers. The amount and type of protein that is synthesized are regulated by growth hormone, sex hormones, thyroxine, and other hormones. The anabolism of protein is directly related to the individual's hormonal balance, which is different throughout the stages of life.

The human body easily forms the nonessential amino acids by removing keto acids from the Krebs cycle and transferring amine groups to them. Therefore, during an average lifetime the body synthesizes approximately 500 to 1,000 pounds of proteins (225–450 kg). This means that an individual is not required to consume, via the diet, the amount of protein required by the body. The liver is where most of these transformations occur. Nearly all nonessential amino acids are provided there, producing the small amount of protein synthesized by the body in a 24-hour period.

However, protein synthesis requires a complete set of amino acids to occur. The diet must provide all the essential amino acids. If it does not, the remainder is oxidized for energy. This occurs even if they are needed for anabolism. Therefore, the protein in the body is "consumed" to supply the essential amino acids required and it experiences a negative nitrogen balance.

TEST YOUR UNDERSTANDING

1. Explain when glycogenolysis occurs and include its definition.
2. List and define the three steps that occur during the oxidation of amino acids.

FOCUS ON PATHOLOGY

Carnitine is an amino acid that is required to transport the fatty acid called *CoA*, which enters the mitochondria to be oxidized to provide energy. *Carnitine deficiency* results from inadequate intake or inability to metabolize carnitine. This results in heterogeneous disorders that include myopathy, hypoglycemia, or cardiomyopathy. In infants, hypoglycemic, hypoketotic encephalopathy is usually present. Treatment includes dietary L-carnitine.

SUMMARY

The body's many chemical reactions constitute its metabolism. A chemical reaction stores and uses energy to maintain homeostasis and to perform all the body's essential functions. The two major types of metabolic reactions that control the use of energy by the cells are anabolism and catabolism. Anabolism is the building of larger and new molecules. Catabolism is the breakdown of larger molecules into smaller ones. Every type of cell in the body performs basic chemical reactions.

During oxidation, glucose burns in the cells to release energy that fuels the process of anabolism. Inside the cells, enzymes reduce the amount of activation energy needed for oxidation as part of cellular respiration. Oxidation-reduction reactions occur when one substance gains oxygen or loses hydrogen (the process of oxidation), causing another substance to gain electrons (the process of reduction). These are coupled reactions that are also referred to as redox reactions. When the bonds between the atoms of molecules are broken, chemical energy is released.

The process of cellular respiration requires three types of reactions: glycolysis, the citric acid cycle, and the electron transport chain. Glycolysis involves the breakdown of glucose to yield lactic acid or pyruvic acid, releasing energy as ATP. The citric acid cycle, or Krebs cycle, involves metabolism of carbon chains of glucose, fatty acids, and amino acids. It yields carbon dioxide, water, and high-energy phosphate bonds (ATP). In the electron transport chain, the high-energy electrons still contain most of the chemical energy of the original glucose molecule. Because oxygen is the final electron acceptor, this overall process is called aerobic respiration. Aerobic respiration generates energy in the mitochondria. Anaerobic respiration occurs outside of the mitochondria, releasing less energy than aerobic respiration.

Specific sequences of enzymatic actions control cellular respiration, anabolic reactions, and catabolic reactions. Each sequence is called a metabolic pathway. Glycogenesis joins glucose molecules in long chains to form glycogen. The splitting (lysis) of glycogen occurs when blood glucose levels drop, which is known as glycogenolysis. Gluconeogenesis is the process of forming new glucose from noncarbohydrate molecules. Fats are the body's most concentrated energy source, yet triglycerides are the only type of fats regularly oxidized for energy. Lipogenesis is also known as triglyceride synthesis, which occurs when ATP and glucose levels are high in the cells. Lipolysis is basically the opposite of lipogenesis and is defined as the breakdown of stored fats into fatty acids and glycerol. Because the body cannot store excess protein, it is broken down and replaced before it deteriorates. Amino acids must be deaminated before they can be oxidized for energy, with glutamic acid being the key molecule used for this purpose. The most important anabolic nutrients are amino acids, which form all protein structures and most of the body's functional molecules. Protein synthesis occurs on ribosomes, regulated by hormones such as growth hormone, sex hormones, thyroxine, and others.

KEY TERMS

Aerobic respiration
Ammonia
Anabolism
Anaerobic
ATP (adenosine triphosphate)
Catabolism
Dehydration synthesis
Dehydrogenases

Energy
Gluconeogenesis
Glycogenesis
Glycogenolysis
Glycolysis
Hydrolysis
Ketogenesis
Ketones

Lipogenesis
Lipolysis
Metabolism
Oxidases
Oxidation
Phosphorylation
Urea

LEARNING GOALS

The following learning goals correspond to the objectives at the beginning of this chapter:

1. *Metabolism:* A process consisting of chemical changes that take place inside living cells
   Catabolism: Breakdown of larger molecules into smaller ones
   Anabolism: Synthesis of larger molecules from smaller ones

2. In an oxidation-reduction reaction, the first thing that occurs is the gain of oxygen or the loss of hydrogen (oxidation). Electrons are usually lost from the oxidized substance. Carbon dioxide remains, and molecular oxygen is the final electron acceptor. It combines with the removed hydrogen at the end of the process to form water. After oxidation, another substance gains electrons, meaning it is reduced. Oxidation and reduction are, therefore, coupled reactions. They are also known as redox reactions. Oxidized substances lose energy, whereas reduced substances gain energy.

3. Cellular respiration is a process that releases energy from organic compounds. It requires glycolysis, the citric acid cycle, and the electron transport chain. Glucose and oxygen are required for cellular respiration.

4. Glycolysis is a process that involves a series of enzymatically catalyzed reactions in which glucose is broken down to yield lactic acid or pyruvic acid. The breakdown releases energy as ATP. Gluconeogenesis is the process of forming new glucose from noncarbohydrate molecules. This process occurs in the liver, when there is insufficient glucose to supply metabolic needs. Lipolysis is basically the opposite of lipogenesis and is defined as the breakdown of stored fats into fatty acids and glycerol. These substances are then released to the blood, giving continuous supplies of fat fuels to the organs, needed for aerobic respiration.

5. Hydrolysis splits a water molecule as in the following example. Hydrolysis of sucrose (a disaccharide) gives off glucose and fructose (two monosaccharides) as the water molecule splits. Inside the sucrose molecule, the bond between the simple sugars breaks. The water molecule supplies a hydrogen atom to one of the sugar molecules and a hydroxyl group to the other.

6. Glycolysis releases energy as ATP, which begins the process of cellular respiration, occurring in the cytosol. It does not require oxygen and is occasionally referred to as the anaerobic phase.

7. Although there are many lipids, triglycerides are the only type regularly oxidized for energy. This requires separate catabolism of glycerol and fatty acid chains. Glycerol is easily converted to glyceraldehyde-3-phosphate, which acts as an intermediate substance during glycolysis and soon enters the Krebs cycle. The initial phase of fatty acid oxidation is called beta oxidation, which occurs in the mitochondria. Fatty acid chains are broken into two-carbon fragments of acetic acid. The FAD and NAD^+ coenzymes are reduced. The acetic acid molecules are fused to CoA to form acetyl CoA. Carbon in the third (beta) position is oxidized. The fatty acid is cleaved between alpha and beta carbons. The acetyl CoA is picked up by oxaloacetic acid, entering the aerobic pathways, for oxidization to carbon dioxide and water.

8. Amino acids must be deaminated before they can be oxidized for energy. To do this, their amine group must be removed. The resulting molecule is converted to pyruvic acid or to a keto acid intermediate during the Krebs cycle. These intermediates include

acetyl CoA, α-ketoglutaric acid, fumaric acid, oxalo-acetic acid, or succinyl CoA. With amino acids that contain sulfur (such as cystine or methionine), sulfur is released before deamination occurs. Glutamic acid is the key molecule used in the oxidation of amino acids, which occurs in the steps known as transamination, oxidative deamination, and modification of keto acids.

9. A specific sequence of enzymatic actions control the steps involved in cellular respiration, anabolic reactions, and catabolic reactions. Enzymes are organized in the exact same sequence as the reactions they control. Each sequence of enzyme-controlled reactions is called a metabolic pathway. Just one enzyme can control the entire pathway.

10. *Oxidation:* The process by which oxygen combines with another chemical, is involved in the removal of hydrogen, or loses electrons

   Energy: An ability to move something and thus do work

CRITICAL THINKING QUESTIONS

An 87-year-old woman has had many signs and symptoms of Alzheimer's disease. She was unable to live by herself. Therefore, her relative took her to live at a nursing facility.

1. Explain how glycolysis may be linked to Alzheimer's disease.
2. What damage to brain cells occur as a result of glycolysis?

REVIEW QUESTIONS

1. Which of the following is the definition of metabolism?
   A. the number of calories it takes to run
   B. the sum of biochemical reactions involved in building up or breaking down molecules
   C. the length of time to digest and absorb proteins
   D. a measure of glucose to make calories

2. Which of the following is used for an anabolic process?
   A. dehydration synthesis
   B. hydrolysis
   C. oxidation
   D. activation energy

3. The process of breaking down triglycerides into glycerol and fatty acids is referred to as
   A. lipolysis
   B. lipogenesis
   C. glycolysis
   D. glycogenolysis

4. All chemical reactions that take place in an organism are collectively called
   A. catabolism
   B. metabolism
   C. hypermetabolism
   D. anabolism

5. The primary function of cellular respiration is to
   A. efficiently monitor the energy needs of the tissues
   B. determine the amount of energy needed by various organs
   C. break down food molecules and generate ATP
   D. supply enough vitamins for the body

6. Two bound amino acids form a(n)
   A. monopeptide
   B. dipeptide
   C. polypeptide
   D. enzyme

7. A sequence of enzyme-controlled reactions is called a
   A. rate-limiting enzyme
   B. oxidation
   C. glycolysis
   D. metabolic pathway

8. Which of the following is the outcome of ketosis?
   A. metabolic alkalosis
   B. glucogenesis
   C. metabolic acidosis
   D. glycolysis

9. Hydrolysis occurs during digestion breakdown of which of the following nutrients?
    A. carbohydrates, fats, and vitamins
    B. proteins, nucleic acids, and vitamins
    C. proteins, carbohydrates, and fats
    D. carbohydrates, nucleic acids, and vitamins

10. The breakdown of larger molecules into smaller ones, which releases energy, is called
    A. catabolism
    B. metabolism
    C. anabolism
    D. homeostasis

11. Aerobic reactions yield up to how many molecules of ATP per glucose molecule?
    A. 2
    B. 16
    C. 36
    D. 38

12. In addition to releasing energy, the complete oxidation of glucose produces
    A. carbon dioxide and water
    B. acetyl CoA and fat
    C. nucleic acid and water
    D. coenzyme and cofactor

13. Oxidation-reduction reactions may involve the loss of
    A. hydrogen
    B. electrons
    C. oxygen
    D. electrons and hydrogen

14. Which of the following is the outcome of oxidative deamination in the liver?
    A. ketone bodies
    B. ammonia
    C. acetyl CoA
    D. coenzyme A

15. Glucose can be obtained from which of the following processes?
    A. lipogenesis
    B. protein anabolism
    C. triglyceride anabolism
    D. glycogenolysis

ESSAY QUESTIONS

1. Explain cellular respiration.
2. Describe glycolysis and glycogenesis.
3. What substance is converted from pyruvic acid to enter the Krebs cycle?
4. Compare and contrast anabolism with catabolism.
5. What is the electron transport chain?
6. Define gluconeogenesis and glycogenolysis.
7. Describe lipogenesis and lipolysis.
8. Explain ketogenesis and ketones.
9. Describe oxidative deamination.
10. What is the meaning of transamination?

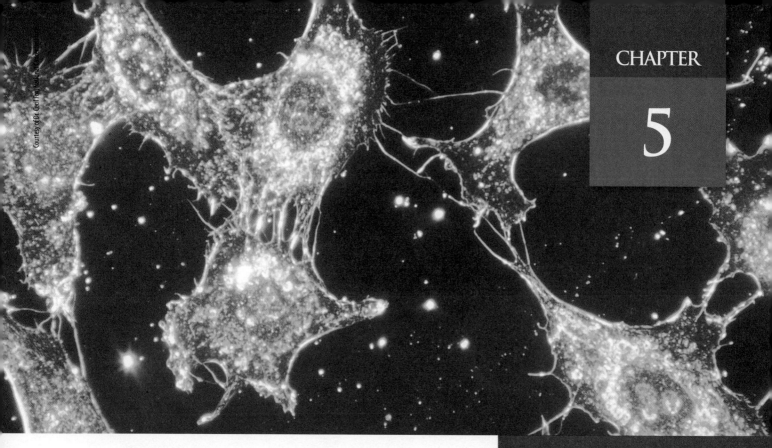

CHAPTER

5

Tissues

OBJECTIVES

After studying this chapter, readers should be able to

1. Describe the four major types of tissues.
2. Discuss the types and functions of epithelial tissue.
3. Identify endocrine and exocrine glands.
4. Explain the characteristics of mast cells, macrophages, and adipocytes.
5. Describe three types of connective tissue fibers.
6. Explain fluid connective tissues.
7. Describe the various types of cartilage.
8. Describe how bone tissue establishes the framework of the body.
9. Describe the three types of muscle tissue and their characteristics.
10. Discuss the basic structure and role of neural tissue.

Overview

There are trillions of cells in the human body, each with specialized functions. Cells are the body's basic units of structure and function, and their specialization enables the body to function in highly efficient ways. For this ability, several different types of cells must coordinate their efforts. The combination of different cell types, with similar structures and functions, creates **tissues.** The four basic tissue types are epithelial, connective, nervous, and muscle tissues. In general, epithelial tissues have covering functions, connective tissues have supporting functions, nervous tissues have controlling functions, and muscle tissues produce movement. However, most organs contain all four tissue types. The study of tissues is called **histology**.

Types of Tissues

The human body is primarily made up of four major types of tissue: epithelial, connective, muscle, and nervous tissues. **Epithelial tissues** cover body surfaces, cover and line internal organs, and make up the glands. **Connective tissues** are widely distributed throughout the body, filling internal spaces, and function to bind, support, and protect body structures. **Muscle tissues** are specialized for contraction and include the skeletal muscles of the body, the heart, and the muscular walls of hollow organs. Skeletal muscles are attached to bones and are used for movement of the body. **Nervous tissues** carry information from one part of the body to another via electrical impulses. They are found in the brain, spinal cord, and nerves (**TABLE 5-1**).

TEST YOUR UNDERSTANDING

1. Define histology.
2. Identify the four major types of tissue in the body.

Epithelial Tissues

Epithelial tissues include epithelia and glands. **Epithelium** covers the surface of the skin and organs, forms the inner lining of the body's cavities, and also lines hollow organs. Epithelial tissues throughout the body are anchored to connective tissue by a **basement membrane**. An epithelium is an **avascular** layer of cells that forms a barrier, providing protection and regulating permeability. Glands are secretory structures derived from epithelia.

Epithelial cells divide quickly, aiding in wound healing and replacement of cells when damage occurs. Tightly packed epithelial cells protect body structures such as the outer skin and the lining of body cavities such as the mouth. Epithelial tissues are involved in secretion, absorption, and excretion. They also provide sensation. They are classified according to the shape of their cells and the number of cell layers that exist (**FIGURE 5-1**). Different types of epithelial tissues are summarized in **TABLE 5-2**.

Epithelia perform many functions:

- *Physical protection:* Epithelia protect exposed and internal surfaces from abrasion, dehydration, and destruction from biologic or chemical agents. Smooth, tightly interlocked epithelial cells of the circulatory system reduce friction between the blood and the walls of the blood vessels.
- *Absorption:* Epithelia also control absorption, which is related to permeability (see below). Examples of epithelia that absorb or secrete substance are those that line the kidney tubules and intestine. In the intestine, certain epithelia absorb nutrients from the digestion of food.
- *Filtration:* Some epithelia have tiny, motile cilia that propel substance along free surfaces, as part of filtration. These include epithelia lining the trachea and other air passages. Also, a thin supporting sheet adjacent to the basal surface of an epithelium is called the *basal lamina*, which acts as a selective filter. It determines which molecules that diffuse from underlying connective tissue can enter the epithelium.
- *Excretion:* In the kidneys, epithelia excrete waste products and also reabsorb needed materials from the urine. In the skin, the epithelia of sweat glands excrete sweat.
- *Sensation:* Most epithelia are very sensitive to stimulation because they have a large sensory nerve supply. Sensory stimuli penetrate specialized epithelia. Such tissue is found in the eyes, ears, skin, nose, and on the tongue.
- *Specialized secretions:* Epithelial cells that produce secretions are called *gland cells*, and individual cells of this type are scattered among other types of cells in an epithelium. Most or all of the epithelial cells in a glandular epithelium produce secretions, which are either discharged onto the surface of the epithelium or released into the surrounding interstitial fluid and blood. These secretions include enzymes, hormones, and lubricating fluids.
- *Permeability:* Any substance entering or leaving the body must cross an epithelium, so the epithelia control permeability. Some epithelia are relatively impermeable, whereas others are crossed easily by compounds of various sizes. In response to stimuli, the epithelial barrier may be modified and regulated. Hormones can affect ion and nutrient transport through epithelial cells. Physical stress can also alter the structure and properties of epithelia. An example is the formation of calluses on the hands after repeated manual labor.
- *Regeneration:* Epithelia have a strong ability to regenerate because they are often exposed to friction, acids, bacteria, smoke, and other environmental substances or factors. They begin to reproduce quickly when their apical–basal polarity and lateral contacts are destroyed. Epithelia can replace lost cells (due to cell division) for as long as they receive enough nutrition.

TABLE 5-1

Tissue Classifications

Main Tissue	Classifications	Variations	Examples
Epithelium	Covers external body surfaces or lines internal body surfaces	*Simple* • Columnar	Gallbladder (nonciliated) Intestinal mucosa
		• Cuboidal • Squamous	Uterine tube (ciliated) Collecting tubule (kidney)
		Pseudostratified • Columnar	Glomerular capsule (kidney blood vessels)
		Stratified • Columnar • Cuboidal • Squamous	Male urethra (non-ciliated) Trachea (ciliated)
	Multicellular glands	*Transitional* *Endocrine* *Exocrine* • Compound • Simple	Male urethra Sweat glands and mammary glands Cornea Mouth, esophagus Vagina and Skin Urinary bladder and ureters Adrenal, thyroid Salivary Gastric, sweat
Connective	*General* • Dense • Loose *Special*	*Irregular* *Regular* *Adipose* *Areolar* *Mesenchyme* *Mucoid* *Reticular* *Blood* *Bone* • Cancellous • Compact *Cartilage* • Elastic • Fibrous • Hyaline *Hematopoietic* • Lymphoid • Myeloid *Lymph*	Dermis, organ capsules Cornea, tendons Subcutaneous tissue Most organs and tissues Embryonic and fetal tissues Umbilical cord (Wharton's jelly) Bone marrow, lymph nodes Epiphyses of long bones Shafts of long bones Epiglottis, external ear Intervertebral disc Costal cartilage, trachea Lymph nodes, spleen Bone marrow
Muscle	Cardiac (involuntary) Smooth (involuntary) Striated (voluntary)		Heart muscle Blood vessels, intestinal tract Skeletal muscle
Nervous		*Central nervous system* • Gray matter • White matter *Peripheral nervous system* • Gray matter • White matter *Special receptors*	Brain, spinal cord Nuclei Tracts Ganglia Non-myelinated nerves Myelinated nerves Cutaneous, ear, eye, nose

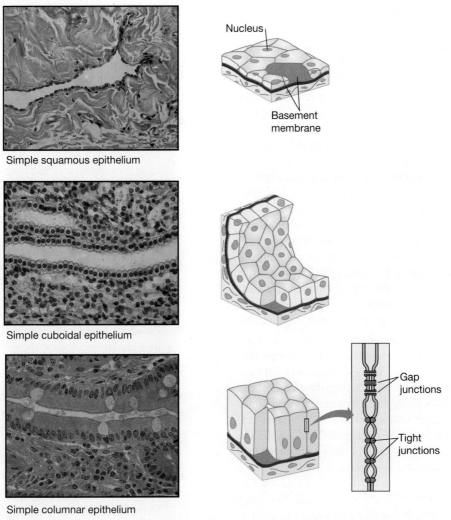

Simple squamous epithelium

Simple cuboidal epithelium

Simple columnar epithelium

Nucleus

Basement membrane

Gap junctions

Tight junctions

FIGURE 5-1 Shapes of epithelial cells. (Photos: © Donna Beer Stolz, PhD, Center for Biologic Imaging, University of Pittsburgh Medical School.)

TABLE 5-2

Types of Epithelial Tissues

Type	Location	Function
Simple squamous epithelium	Air sacs of lungs, capillary walls, linings of lymph, and blood vessels	Diffusion, filtration, osmosis, covering of surfaces
Simple cuboidal epithelium	Ovary surfaces, kidney tubule linings, linings of ducts of certain glands	Absorption, secretion
Simple columnar epithelium	Intestine, stomach, and uterus linings	Absorption, protection, secretion
Pseudostratified columnar epithelium	Respiratory passage linings	Movement of mucus, protection, secretion
Stratified squamous epithelium	Outer layer of skin, linings of anal canal, oral cavity, throat, and vagina	Protection
Stratified cuboidal epithelium	Linings of larger mammary gland ducts, pancreas, salivary glands, sweat glands	Protection
Stratified columnar epithelium	Part of male urethra and parts of the pharynx	Protection, secretion
Transitional epithelium	Inner urinary bladder lining, linings of ureters, and part of urethra	Distensibility, protection
Glandular epithelium	Endocrine, salivary, and sweat glands	Secretion

Classification of Epithelia

There are two names for each type of epithelium: one describes how many cell layers are present, and the other describes the shape of the cells that make up the epithelium. Simple epithelia have one cell layer and are usually found in areas where absorption, filtration, and secretion occur. In these areas, only a thin epithelial barrier is needed. Stratified epithelia are made of two or more cell layers stacked on each other. They are usually found in areas of high abrasion that require protection. Examples of these areas include the lining of the mouth and the skin surfaces. All stratified epithelial cells have six irregular sides, resembling the appearance of a honeycomb. As a result of their shapes, these cells can be loosely packed together. The shape of each epithelial cell's nucleus resembles the overall cell shape. Simple epithelia are easier to classify because of shapes that are nearly identical (Figure 5-1). The cell shape of stratified epithelia, however, is different based on each layer. Therefore, stratified epithelial are named based on how cells are shaped in their *apical* layer.

The following are the various forms of epithelial tissues:

- *Simple squamous epithelium:* Consists of a single layer of thin and laterally flattened cells with flattened, disc-like nuclei. It lines areas where filtration or rapid diffusion occur, including the alveoli of the lungs and in the kidneys. It forms capillary walls, lines blood and lymph vessels, and covers membranes that line body cavities. Squamous cells have a scale-like appearance. The cytoplasm of simple squamous epithelium is sparse and often permeable. In the kidneys it makes up part of the filtration membrane, and in the lungs it forms the walls of the alveoli. Two types of simple squamous epithelia are named according to their locations. *Endothelium* provides a slick lining in lymphatic vessels and in the hollow organs of the cardiovascular system, where it reduces friction. These organs include the blood vessels and heart. The capillaries are completely made up of endothelium. Its thin structure allows for efficient nutrient and waste exchanges between surrounding tissue cells and the bloodstream. The *mesothelium* is the epithelium inside serous membranes, which line the ventral body cavity and cover its organs.

- *Simple cuboidal epithelium:* Consists of a single layer of cube-shaped cells with round nuclei. When stained, these nuclei become dark, and the cell layer resembles a string of pearls. It covers the ovaries, lines many kidney tubules and glandular ducts, and functions in secretion and absorption. Cuboidal cells appear to be approximately the same size in height and width.

- *Simple columnar epithelium:* Consists of cells that are longer than wide, composed of a single cellular layer with elongated nuclei, located near the basement membrane, and may have cilia on their surfaces. It is found in the female reproductive tubes, uterus, and most digestive tract organs, being involved in secretion and absorption. Simple columnar cells, specialized for absorption, usually have tiny, cylinder-shaped processes (microvilli) that extend from their surfaces and increase the surface area of the cell membrane. Often, special flask-shaped glandular cells (**goblet cells**) are scattered among the columnar cells, secreting mucus on the tissue surface (Figure 5-1).

- *Pseudostratified columnar epithelium:* Appear as if they are layered (hence the word "pseudostratified") because the nuclei are located at different levels (**FIGURE 5-2**). The cells vary in shape and usually reach the basement membrane. Pseudostratified columnar epithelium usually has cilia and lines respiratory system passages, as well as being involved in secretion and absorption. Goblet cells are found throughout this tissue.

- *Stratified squamous epithelium:* A thick layer with cells that flatten as they are pushed outward. It forms the epidermis, with cells hardening as they age (keratinization). It also lines the mouth, esophagus, vagina, and anus, where the cells do not harden but remain soft and moist. Stratified epithelia regenerate from below, with basal cells dividing and pushing apically, replacing older surface cells. They are much more durable than simple epithelia. Stratified squamous epithelium is the most widespread of all stratified epithelia. Interestingly, the cells of its deeper layers are columnar or cuboidal. Although the epidermis is keratinized, other areas

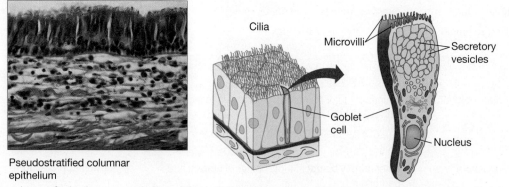

Cilia

Microvilli

Secretory vesicles

Goblet cell

Nucleus

Pseudostratified columnar epithelium

FIGURE 5-2 Pseudostratified columnar epithelium. (Photo: © Donna Beer Stolz, PhD, Center for Biologic Imaging, University of Pittsburgh Medical School.)

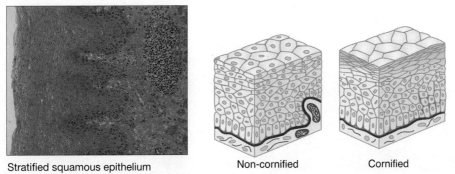

Simple squamous epithelium

Stratified squamous epithelium

Non-cornified   Cornified

FIGURE 5-3 Stratified squamous epithelium. (Photo: © Donna Beer Stolz, PhD, Center for Biologic Imaging, University of Pittsburgh Medical School.)

of stratified squamous epithelium in the body are nonkeratinized. This is also described as "cornified" or "noncornified" (**FIGURE 5-3**).

■ *Stratified cuboidal epithelium:* Consists of usually two but may have up to three layers of cubed cells. It lines the mammary gland ducts, sweat glands, salivary glands, pancreas, and the developing ovaries and seminiferous tubules. This type of epithelium is rare in the body compared with other types.

■ *Stratified columnar epithelium:* Consists of several layers of either columnar or cubed shapes. It is found in the male urethra, ductus deferens, and areas of the pharynx but in few other areas of the body. It occurs at junctions or transition areas between two other types of epithelia. In this type, only the apical layer of cells is columnar.

■ *Transitional epithelium:* Changes in appearance in response to tension. It lines the urinary bladder, ureters, and superior urethra and prevents urinary tract contents from diffusing back into the internal body environment. The cells of its basal layer are columnar or cuboidal. Apical cells have different appearances, based on how much distention occurs in the specific organ in which they are found. For example, distention of the bladder with urine causes it to thin from approximately six cell layers to only three, with the dome-like apical cells flattening to appear like squamous cells (**FIGURE 5-4**).

This transitional ability allows for greater volumes of urine to be stored in the bladder, or in tube-like organs, for more urine to flow through.

■ *Glandular epithelium:* Consists of specialized cells that produce and secrete substances into ducts or body fluids. It is usually found in **exocrine glands** (which open onto surfaces or into the digestive tract) or in **endocrine glands** (which secrete into tissue fluid or blood). The basic term *gland* is defined as one or more cells making and secreting a certain product (*secretion*). Most secretions are water-based (aqueous) fluids, often containing proteins. However, some contain lipids or steroids.

● The three types of exocrine glands are merocrine, apocrine, and holocrine (**FIGURE 5-5**). **Merocrine glands** release fluid by exocytosis, **apocrine glands** lose parts of their cell bodies during secretion, and **holocrine glands** release entire cells that disintegrate to release secretions. *Exocrine glands* always secrete onto body surfaces or into body cavities. When the gland is unicellular, exocytosis is the process used for secretion. When the gland is multicellular, an epithelium-walled duct is used to transport secretions to the epithelial surface. The products of exocrine glands include

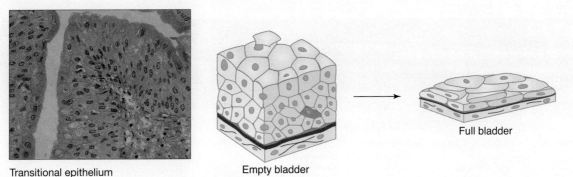

Transitional epithelium

Empty bladder   Full bladder

FIGURE 5-4 Transitional epithelium. (Photo: © Donna Beer Stolz, PhD, Center for Biologic Imaging, University of Pittsburgh Medical School.)

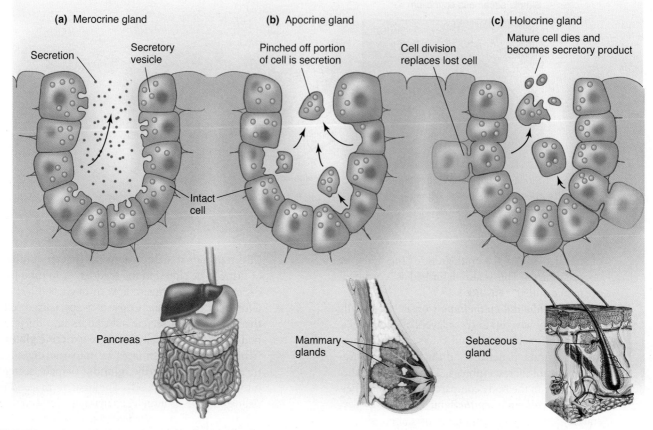

(a) Merocrine gland

Secretion

Secretory vesicle

Intact cell

Pancreas

(b) Apocrine gland

Pinched off portion of cell is secretion

Mammary glands

(c) Holocrine gland

Cell division replaces lost cell

Mature cell dies and becomes secretory product

Sebaceous gland

FIGURE 5-5 Merocrine, apocrine, and holocrine glands. (Adapted from Shier, D. N., Butler, J. L., and Lewis, R. Hole's Essentials of Human Anatomy & Physiology, Tenth edition. McGraw-Hill Higher Education, 2009.)

mucus, oil, sweat, saliva, bile (in the liver), digestive enzymes (in the pancreas), and many others. Unicellular exocrine glands are only exemplified by goblet and mucus cells. They are found in the linings of the respiratory and intestinal tracts, near columnar cells that have different functions. They produce *mucin*, which is a complex glycoprotein. It dissolves in water when secreted, forming mucus, which protects and lubricates surfaces with its slimy texture. Although most multicellular epithelial glands are formed by inward growth (invagination) of an epithelial sheet into underlying connective tissue, unicellular glands are simply scattered inside epithelial sheets. Most glands have ducts (initially), which are connections to epithelial sheets. These connections are tube-like in appearance. **TABLE 5-3** lists the types of exocrine secretions. Secretion is an active process that occurs as glandular cells obtain needed blood substances and then chemically transform them. These substances are then discharged. The term *secretion* refers to the products of glands as well as the processes of these products

TABLE 5-3

Types of Exocrine Gland Secretions

Type	Example	Secretions
Apocrine	Ceruminous glands in the external ear canal, mammary glands	Cellular product and portions of the free ends of glandular cells pinched off during secretion
Holocrine	Sebaceous glands in the skin	Disintegrated whole cells filled with secretory products
Merocrine	Pancreatic glands, salivary glands, sweat glands in the skin	A fluid product released through cell membranes via exocytosis

being manufactured and released. Multicellular exocrine glands are more complex, with a duct derived from epithelium and an *acinus* (secretory unit) made up of secretory cells. Supportive connective tissue usually surrounds the secretory unit, supplying it with nerve fibers and blood vessels. This forms a *fibrous capsule*, extending into the gland to divide it into *lobes*. The merocrine type produces their secretions without any structural alteration, such as in the pancreas, salivary glands, and most sweat glands. In the holocrine glands, the secretory cells collect their secretions until they rupture. The only true examples of holocrine glands are the oil (sebaceous) glands of the skin. Apocrine glands also accumulate their products, but just beneath their free surfaces, with apex pinching off to release secretory granules and tiny amounts of cytoplasm.

Endocrine glands eventually lose their ducts and are therefore termed *ductless glands*. They produce **hormones**, secreted by exocytosis, directly into the extracellular space. The hormones then enter the lymphatic fluid or blood, traveling to specific target organs to prompt them to act in a certain way. For example, intestinal hormones such as *secretin* may cause the pancreas to release digestive enzymes. Endocrine glands are usually compact and multicellular but also consist of individual hormone-producing cells, such as in the brain or mucosa of the digestive tract. This is described as the *diffuse endocrine system*. Endocrine secretions range from glycoproteins to steroids and from amino acids to peptides. Not all endocrine glands derive from epithelia.

TEST YOUR UNDERSTANDING

1. List five important characteristics of epithelial tissue.
2. Describe the type of epithelial organization that exists in the mouth, esophagus, anus, and vagina.

FOCUS ON PATHOLOGY

The most common disorders affecting the epithelia of the body are various types of cancers, ulcers, burns, infections, inflammation, and necrosis. In the skin, examples include basal cell carcinoma, squamous cell carcinoma, and malignant melanoma. In the stomach, common examples include peptic ulcer, which are usually gastric or duodenal. Diabetes mellitus may also result in necrosis of the epithelia of the extremities because of poor circulation.

FOCUS ON PATHOLOGY

Stomach carcinoma is not common in the United States but is prevalent in other countries such as Korea, Mongolia, and Japan. It is more common in men after the age of 40. The primary cause is infection with *Helicobacter pylori*, followed by smoking, and certain foods such as those that are smoked, high in salt content, or pickled. Red or processed meats are also linked to stomach carcinoma. Genetics plays a role in the development of stomach cancer.

FOCUS ON PATHOLOGY

Merocrine glands include salivary glands, pancreatic glands, and the eccrine and apocrine sweat glands. Salivary gland disorders include mumps, Sjögren's syndrome, and graft-versus-host disease. Diabetes mellitus is an example of a serious disorder affecting the glands of the pancreas. The most common sweat gland disorder is hyperhidrosis (excessive sweating).

Connective Tissues

The cells that make up connective tissues are farther apart than those of epithelial tissues. These tissues bind body structures, provide support and protection, create frameworks, fill body spaces, store fat for reserve fuel, insulate the body, produce blood cells, transport fluids and dissolved materials, repair damaged tissues, and protect the body from infection. Connective tissues usually contain a large amount of matrix. This matrix is composed of fibers and ground substance.

Components of Connective Tissues

Connective tissues vary greatly in appearance and function but have three basic components:

- Specialized cells.
- Extracellular protein fibers.
- A fluid known as a **ground substance**, which is the unstructured material filling spaces between cells and containing fibers. It is made up of cell adhesion proteins, interstitial fluid, and proteoglycans. Cell adhesion proteins include **fibronectin**, **laminin**, and others. They attach connective tissue cells to elements of the matrix. Proteoglycans have a protein core that is attached to glycosaminoglycans. These are strand-like polysaccharides that include *chondroitin sulfate* and *hyaluronic acid*, emerging from the core like spikes.

Together, the extracellular protein fibers and ground substance constitute the **matrix**, which surrounds the cells. Although cells make up most epithelial tissue, the matrix usually accounts for most connective tissue. Connective tissues vary in amount per organ but overall are the most widely distributed and abundant of primary body tissues.

Connective Tissue Cells

Most connective tissue cells divide, have good blood supply, and require large amounts of nourishment. Connective tissues include those of bone, cartilage, and fat. Connective tissues contain different types of cells, including those that are fixed or wandering. Connective tissue cells exist in both immature (undifferentiated) and mature forms. Immature cells are described using the suffix -blast, which means "forming." These actively mitotic cells secrete the ground substance and the fibers that make up their portion of the matrix. The most common type of fixed cell is the star-shaped **fibroblast**, which produces fibers via protein secretion into the extracellular matrix. Other cells include *chondroblasts* (which produce cartilage) and *osteoblasts* (which produce bone). Blood cells are produced by *hematopoietic stem cells*, which are not located in the blood and do not make the matrix of the blood, which is known as the *plasma*. **TABLE 5-4** summarizes the major cells and tissue fibers of connective tissue.

Connective Tissue Fibers

Connective tissue fibers provide support. Fibroblasts produce three connective tissue fibers:

- *Collagenous fibers:* Important for body parts that hold structures together (**ligaments** and **tendons**), collagenous fibers are also called *dense connective tissue* or *white fibers*. They are the strongest and most abundant type of connective tissue fibers.

Constructed mostly of the fibrous protein *collagen*, these fibers are very tough and resist being pulled apart, providing *tensile strength* to the matrix. If steel fibers existed at the same size, the collagenous fibers would be stronger. The fibers are formed as the extracellular space receives secreted collagen molecules, which assemble into fibrils that have a cross-linked organization. These are then bundled into thicker collagen fibers.

- *Elastic fibers:* Common in body parts that are often stretched, such as the vocal cords, large blood vessel walls (such as those leaving the heart), lungs, and skin. They are composed of a protein called *elastin* and are also called *yellow fibers*. Elastic fibers are long and thin. In the extracellular matrix, they form branching networks. Elastin allows these fibers to stretch and then recoil, which then causes the connective tissue to return to its normal length and shape.

- *Reticular fibers:* Form delicate supporting networks in the spleen and other tissues. They are short and fine in structure, made up of collagen, but in a different form than the collagenous fibers. However, the reticular fibers are continuous with the collagenous fibers. They form delicately branched networks that extensively surround small blood vessels, providing soft organ tissue support. They are highly abundant where connective tissue meets other types of tissue, such as the epithelial tissue basement membranes and in the areas that surround capillaries. Here, the reticular fibers form net-like structures that provide more "give and take" than larger collagenous fibers are able to provide.

The other types of cells found in connective tissue include mast cells, macrophages, adipocytes (fat cells), neutrophils, eosinophils, lymphocytes, and melanocytes. **Mast cells** are distributed throughout connective tissues, usually near blood vessels, and release both heparin (to prevent blood clotting) and histamine (for the inflammatory and allergic response). Mast cells are oval-shaped and cause the inflammatory response against foreign microorganisms when they are detected. The cytoplasm of mast cells contains secretory granules of heparin, histamine, proteases, and various other enzymes. **Macrophages** are responsible for phagocytosis, are large and irregularly shaped, and are able to ingest many different foreign materials, including entire bacteria, dust particles, and dead tissue cells. Macrophages are the primary cellular components of the immune system. They are found throughout bone marrow, loose connective tissue, and lymphatic tissue. Adipocytes store body fat. Melanocytes are specialized cells in the deeper epithelium of the skin that are responsible for the production of melanin.

TABLE 5-4	
Connective Tissue Cells and Tissue Fibers	
Tissue Cell Type	**Action**
Fibroblasts	Produce fibers
Macrophages	Engulf and devour many microorganisms as well as dust particles and dead tissue cells
Mast cells	Secrete histamine, heparin, and proteases; initiate inflammatory and allergic responses
Tissue Fiber Type	**Action**
Collagenous	Bind structures together with high tensile strength
Elastic	Allow stretching of connective tissues
Reticular	Give delicate support

TEST YOUR UNDERSTANDING

1. List the components of connective tissues.
2. Explain the three connective tissue fibers produced by fibroblasts.

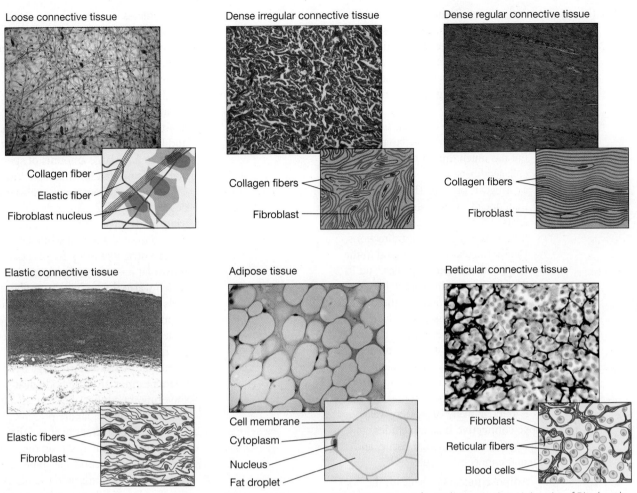

FIGURE 5-6 Types of typical connective tissues. (Photos: © Donna Beer Stolz, PhD, Center for Biologic Imaging, University of Pittsburgh Medical School.)

Classifications of Connective Tissue

Connective tissues are classified based on their physical properties. The three general categories of connective tissue are connective tissue proper, supporting connective tissues, and fluid connective tissues.

- *Connective tissue proper* includes those connective tissues with many types of cells and extracellular fibers in a syrup-like ground substance. This includes fat and the fibrous tissue of ligaments. All mature connective tissues, except for bone, cartilage, and blood, are connective tissue proper. Connective tissue proper is divided into dense connective tissue and loose connective tissue (**FIGURE 5-6**).
  - **Dense connective tissue** contains many collagenous fibers and appears white. Its fine network of elastic fibers contains few cells and is very strong. The forms of dense connective tissue include dense regular, dense irregular, and elastic. In the tendons and ligaments, dense connective tissue binds muscles to bones and bones to other bones. It also exists in the eyeballs and deep skin layers. Dense connective tissue has a poor blood supply

and is repaired very slowly as a result. Because it has prominent fibers, dense connective tissue is also known as *fibrous connective tissue*.

- *Dense regular connective tissue* has tightly packed collagen fiber bundles that run in the same direction, pulling in one parallel direction. These bundles appear as flexible white structures that have great resistance to any tension. Between the collagen fibers are lines of fibroblasts. These cells manufacture the fibers continually as well as small amounts of ground substance. Collagen fibers are wavy in appearance and allow a small amount of tissue stretching. They have few cells (except for fibroblasts) and poor vascularization. However, they have high tensile strength and form the *tendons* (cords attaching muscles to bones), *aponeuroses* (flat tendons that attach muscles to each other or to bones), and *ligaments* (which bind bones together at the joints). There is more elastin in ligaments, meaning they stretch to a greater degree than tendons. Dense regular connective tissue forms *fascia*, the fibrous membrane around muscles, muscle groups, nerves, and blood vessels.

- *Dense irregular connective tissue* resembles dense regular connective tissue but has much thicker bundles of collagen fibers, which are arranged in an irregular pattern. They run in more than one plane, forming sheets in areas of the body where tension occurs from a variety of different directions. Dense irregular tissue is found in the *dermis*, fibrous joint capsules, and in the fibrous coverings of the bones, cartilages, kidneys, muscles, and nerves.

- *Elastic connective tissue* actually describes the dense regular connective tissue of certain ligaments, which are able to stretch extensively. These include the ligaments connecting adjacent vertebrae. Also, this type of connective tissue is found in many large artery walls.

- **Loose connective tissue** includes adipose (fat) tissue, areolar tissue, and reticular connective tissue.

  - **Adipose tissue** lies beneath the skin, between muscles, around the kidneys, behind the eyes, in certain membranes of the abdomen, on the heart's surface, and around some of the body's joints. It functions as a cushion for these body parts and, in total, comprises approximately 18% of an average adult's body weight. Up to 50% of body weight can be that of the adipose tissue before the person is termed *morbidly obese*. Adipose tissue is also important for storing energy in fat molecules (triglycerides). *Adipocytes* (fat cells) make up approximately 90% of its mass. Adipose tissue has a simple matrix, with its cells packed together tightly, resembling a wire fence. Most of each adipocyte's volume is filled with nearly pure triglyceride, which displaces its nucleus to one side. In the entire human body, the mature adipocyte is one of the largest cells. They become "plump" as they take up fat and more wrinkled when they release it. Adipose tissue has high metabolic activity because of its rich vascularization. It usually

accumulates in subcutaneous tissue but may develop anywhere in the body that has adequate areolar tissue. Under the skin, abundant fat supplies general nutrients to the body. Small fat deposits supply nutrients to highly active organs, such as the heart, lymph nodes, certain muscles, and bone marrow. Often, these local deposits have large amounts of special lipids needed for their activities. This type of adipose tissue is also described as *white adipose tissue* or *white fat*. It differs from *brown adipose tissue (brown fat)* in that white fat stores nutrients mostly for other cells. Brown fat has many mitochondria, which warm the body by using lipid fuels to heat the bloodstream, instead of producing adenosine triphosphate molecules. Brown fat is richly vascular. It is found mostly on the backs of infants, as at this early stage of life infants cannot produce body heat by shivering. In adults, only very small amounts of brown fat are present. This is located primarily above the collarbones, on the neck, on the abdomen, and around the spine.

- **Areolar tissue** binds skin to underlying organs and fills in spaces between muscles. It is found beneath most layers of the epithelium and is similar to adipose tissue in both structure and function but lacks the nutrient-storing capability of adipose tissue. It also supports other tissues, holds body fluids, defends against infection, and stores nutrients as fat. Fibroblasts, mast cells, and macrophages are the primary cells in areolar tissue that act as barriers to pathogens. Fat cells are either single or in clusters, and mast cells are present as large, darkly stained cytoplasmic granules. Other cell types are also present, but in lower concentrations. Areolar tissue has loose fibers, and the remainder of its matrix appears "empty," containing only its ground substance. This looseness allows the tissue to act as a water and salt reservoir for nearby body tissues. It can hold about the same amount of fluid as is present in the entire bloodstream. Basically, all body cells get nutrients from this tissue fluid and release their wastes into it. Hyaluronic acid is present in high concentrations, which makes its ground substance thick (viscous), slowly cellular movement through it. Certain white blood cells therefore secrete *hyaluronidase*, an enzyme that liquefies the ground substance somewhat so they can pass through it more easily. Certain bacteria can also do this. Inflammation in a body region causes the areolar tissue to absorb excess fluids, so the area becomes swollen (the condition known as *edema*). There is more areolar connective tissue throughout the body than any other type. It holds body parts together while letting them move freely over each other; encases glands, nerves, and small blood vessels; and forms the subcutaneous tissue. Most epithelia rest on areolar tissue, and it is also present in all mucous membranes.

- **Reticular connective tissue** helps to create a framework inside internal organs such as the spleen and liver and in the lymph nodes and bone marrow. It appears similar to areolar tissue but only has reticular fibers in its matrix, forming a delicate network containing scattered reticular cells (fibroblasts). Even though reticular fibers are found throughout the body, reticular tissue is only found in certain areas. Reticular tissue forms an internal framework (*stroma*) supporting free lymphocytes and other blood cells.

- *Supporting connective tissue* differs from connective tissue proper because it has a less diverse cell population and a matrix that contains many more densely packaged fibers. Supporting connective tissue protects soft tissues and some or all of the body's weight. The two types of supporting connective tissue are cartilage and bone.

- **Cartilage** is a tough but flexible connective tissue with a gelatinous matrix that contains an abundance of fibers. It supports, frames, and attaches to many underlying tissues and bones. Mature cartilage cells, known as **chondrocytes**, lie totally inside the extracellular matrix, within cavities called *lacunae*. Cartilage is enclosed in a covering called the *perichondrium*, which provides nutrients via diffusion. It has no direct blood supply, so cartilage heals very slowly. Cartilage protects the body from excessive tension and compression and is harder than dense connective tissue but softer than bone. It also lacks nerve fibers. The ground substance of cartilage has great amounts of chondroitin sulfate and hyaluronic acid bound firmly within its collagen (and elastic) fibers. There is a large amount of tissue fluid in its matrix. Surprisingly, cartilage is made up of about 80% water, which allows it to recover after being compressed and nourishes its cells.

- The three major types of cartilage are as follows:

  - *Hyaline cartilage:* This type is found on the ends of bones in many joints, the soft portion (tip) of the nose, and in the respiratory passages' supporting rings. It is important for bone growth. Hyaline cartilage is the most common type of cartilage in the body (**FIGURE 5-7**). Hyaline cartilage is commonly referred to as *gristle*. Its matrix appears "glassy," with a bluish white color. However, under a microscope a large number of collagen fibers are seen. Only 1% to 10% of its volume is made up of chondrocytes. Hyaline cartilage is partially pliable and provides firm support. On the ends of long bones, it is known as *articular cartilage*, because it absorbs

Hyaline cartilage

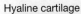
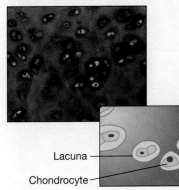

Lacuna
Chondrocyte

Fibrocartilage

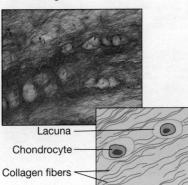

Lacuna
Chondrocyte
Collagen fibers

Elastic cartilage

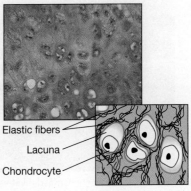

Elastic fibers
Lacuna
Chondrocyte

FIGURE 5-7 Types of cartilage. (Photos: © Donna Beer Stolz, PhD, Center for Biologic Imaging, University of Pittsburgh Medical School.)

compression at the joints. It also connects the ribs to the sternum. Most of the skeletons of human embryos consist of hyaline cartilage before the formation of the bones. During childhood, skeletal hyaline cartilage persists as the *epiphyseal plates*, which are continually growing regions near the ends of the long bones.

- **Elastic cartilage:** This flexible cartilage provides framework for the *pinna* of the ear and the *epiglottis* of the larynx. Although nearly identical to hyaline cartilage, elastic cartilage has much more elastin. It is mostly located where a large amount of stretching capacity is needed, but it also supplies significant strength to various body structures.

- **Fibrocartilage:** This tough form of cartilage absorbs shock in the intervertebral discs of the spinal column, spongy cartilages (menisci) of the knees, and in the pelvic girdle. It is a structural "halfway point" between hyaline cartilage and dense regular connective tissues. Fibrocartilage contains rows of chondrocytes that alternate with rows of thick collagen fibers. It is able to be compressed and also to resist tension. Fibrocartilage is located wherever there is a need for extreme support or to withstand heavy pressure.

- **Bone** (osseous tissue) is the most rigid type of connective tissue, with a high mineral content that makes it harder than other types. Bone tissue establishes the framework of the body. Bone consists of a matrix of connective tissue, blood vessels, and minerals (particularly calcium and phosphorus). The bone matrix is more rigid and harder than other types of connective tissue matrices, because of two elements: increased amounts of collagen fibers and the presence of bone salts, which are inorganic calcium salts. The bones also store fat and synthesize blood cells. Bones attach to muscles and protect and support vital body structures.

  - *Bone marrow* is the soft tissue that fills the inside of bones and is the site of production of red blood cells, platelets, and most white blood cells.
  - Bone cells, or **osteocytes**, contain a small amount of ground substance but actually consist of a dense and mineralized matrix. These cells are located in the lacunae of the bone matrix. The osteocytes and layers of the extracellular matrix form a cylinder-shaped **osteon** (also called a *Haversian system*) (**FIGURE 5-8**). They have concentric rings of bony matrix (*lamellae*) that surround central canals. These canals contain blood vessels and nerves. Many osteons that are cemented together form the substance of bone. Bone is well supplied by blood vessels, unlike cartilage. The organic portion of the matrix is formed by *osteoblasts*, followed by deposition of bone salts on and between the fibers.

- *Fluid connective tissues* have distinctive populations of cells suspended in a water matrix. This contains

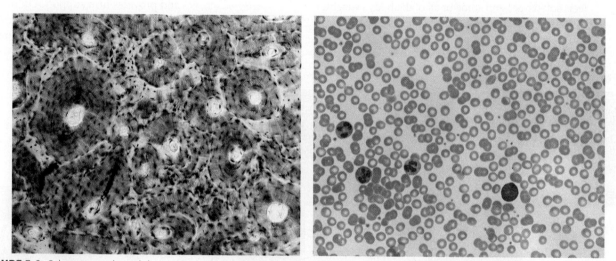

FIGURE 5-8 Other mesenchymal derivatives include bone (left) and blood (right). (© Donna Beer Stolz, PhD, Center for Biologic Imaging, University of Pittsburgh Medical School)

dissolved proteins and may be of two types: blood or lymph. **Blood** and **lymph** are fluid connective tissues that contain distinctive collections of cells in a fluid matrix. They transport many materials between interior body cells and other cells that exchange substances with the external environment, maintaining a stable internal environment. Blood contains formed elements (red blood cells, white blood cells, and platelets) that are suspended in a liquid extracellular matrix known as *blood plasma*. Together, the formed elements and blood plasma make up the blood. Most blood cells are formed in the red bone marrow. Red blood cells (erythrocytes) are the most prevalent type of blood cells. Blood is classified as a connective tissue because it develops from mesenchyme. During blood clotting, the fibers of blood (soluble protein molecules) form visible fiber-like structures. Lymph forms as interstitial fluid entering the lymphatic vessels, which return the lymph to the cardiovascular system. Unlike other connective tissues, blood and lymph do not connect structures or provide any mechanical support.

FOCUS ON PATHOLOGY

When cartilage is injured, it heals very slowly. This is because it is avascular and also because aging cartilage cells stop dividing. In later life, some cartilage calcifies or even ossifies. This causes the chondrocytes to die from lack of nutrition.

TEST YOUR UNDERSTANDING

1. What are the functions of connective tissue?
2. What are the primary blast cell types of connective tissue?
3. What are the three types of cartilage?
4. Name the three types of fibers that make up connective tissues.
5. Which types of connective tissue have a fluid matrix?

FOCUS ON PATHOLOGY

More than 200 disorders involve connective tissue. The most common include cellulitis, Ehlers-Danlos syndrome, osteogenesis imperfecta, scleroderma, and Marfan's syndrome. Injuries can also cause connective tissue disorders, such as scars. Disorders may be of genetic origin, from infections, or of unknown cause.

FOCUS ON PATHOLOGY

An inherited connective tissue disorder, known as *Marfan's syndrome*, affects many different parts of the body. The glycoprotein *fibrillin* is defective in this disorder. The most visible signs of Marfan's syndrome are skeletal, with the affected person having a very tall height and abnormally long fingers and limbs. However, the most severe effects of this syndrome are related to the connective tissues of the cardiovascular system, which can lead to bursting of a major artery and death from excessive blood loss.

Muscle Tissues

Muscle tissues can contract by shortening their elongated muscle fibers. This action moves body parts. *Myofilaments* in muscle cells are responsible for the muscles' ability to move or contract. The three types of muscle tissue are skeletal muscle tissue, smooth muscle tissue, and cardiac muscle tissue.

- *Skeletal muscle tissue:* Known as voluntary muscle tissue because it is found in muscles controlled by conscious effort, it attaches to bones and is composed of long thread-like cells that have light and dark markings called *striations* (**FIGURE 5-9**). These multinucleated muscle cells contract when stimulated by nerve cells. Skeletal muscle tissue moves the head, trunk, and limbs, allowing all voluntary movements in these body areas. Skeletal muscle cells are also called *muscle fibers*. They are long and cylindrical, containing many peripherally located nuclei.

- *Smooth muscle tissue:* Composed of elongated, spindle-shaped cells in muscles not under voluntary control. Smooth muscle fibers are shorter than striated fibers, having only one nucleus per spindle-shaped fiber. They are also called *nonstriated involuntary*

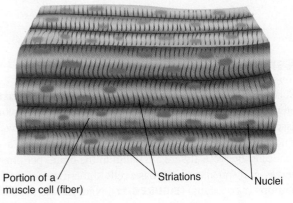

Portion of a muscle cell (fiber) — Striations — Nuclei

FIGURE 5-9 Skeletal muscle tissue with striations.

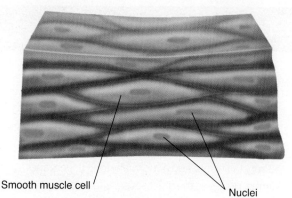

FIGURE 5-10 Smooth muscle tissue.

muscles or *unstriated muscles* (**FIGURE 5-10**). Smooth muscle cells can divide; therefore, they regenerate after being injured. Smooth muscle tissue composes hollow internal organ walls (such as the intestines, stomach, urinary bladder, blood vessels, and uterus). Smooth muscle cannot, in most cases, be controlled by conscious effort. This type of tissue moves food through the digestive tract, empties the urinary bladder, and constricts blood vessels. It accomplishes these tasks by either contracting or relaxing.

- *Cardiac muscle tissue:* Also called *myocardium*, this is a thick contractile middle layer of the heart wall. The contractile tissue of the myocardium is composed of fibers with the characteristic cross-striations of muscular tissue. These striations branch frequently and are interconnected, forming a network. Myocardial muscle contains less connective tissue than skeletal muscle and is usually uninucleate (having one nucleus, located centrally). Cardiac muscle is involuntary and makes up most of the heart. Cardiac muscle relies on pacemaker cells for regular contraction. Cardiac muscle cells are branched and fit together tightly at junctions known as *intercalated discs.*

TEST YOUR UNDERSTANDING

1. What type of muscle cells are striated?
2. Explain which muscles are voluntary and involuntary.

Nervous Tissues

Nervous tissues are specialized for the conduction of electrical impulses from one region of the body to another. Nervous tissues contain two basic types of cells: **neurons** and several kinds of supporting cells, collectively called neuroglia or glial cells. Nervous tissues are found in the brain, peripheral nerves, and spinal cord; the basic cells of these tissues are the neurons (nerve cells) (**FIGURE 5-11**). Neurons are the basic

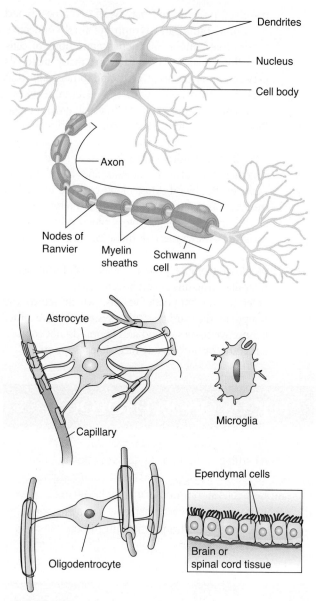

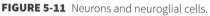

FIGURE 5-11 Neurons and neuroglial cells.

structures of neural tissue that respond to environmental changes by transmitting impulses along *axons* (cellular processes) to other neurons, muscles, or glands. They respond to stimuli via processes called *dendrites*. Neurons coordinate, integrate, and regulate a wide variety of functions in the body. **Neuroglial cells** are crucial to neuronal functioning. These cells divide and support nervous tissue components. Neuroglial cells also phagocytize other cells, supply nutrients to neurons, and help in communications between cells. The four types of neuroglia are astrocytes, oligodendroglia, microglia, and ependymal cells.

TEST YOUR UNDERSTANDING

1. What are the functions of the neurons?
2. What are the major functions of the neuroglia?

Tissue Membranes

Membranes form a barrier or an interface. There are many different types of anatomical membranes. **Epithelial membranes** are thin structures made up of epithelium and underlying connective tissue. They cover body surfaces and line body cavities. There are four types of membranes:

- *Serous membranes:* Line body cavities that lack openings to the outside of the body. Serous membranes consist of simple squamous epithelium (a mesothelium) and loose connective (areolar) tissue and secrete serous fluid, which lubricates membrane surfaces. *Serosae* are moist membranes. The mesothelium cells mix hyaluronic acid with a fluid from the capillaries of related connective tissue to produce thin, clear *serous fluid* or *transudate*. This lubricates opposing surfaces of the visceral and parietal layers so they can slide across each other with ease. The serosae are named for their locations. Examples include the *pericardium* (which encloses the heart), *peritoneum* (which encloses the abdominopelvic viscera), and the *pleurae* (which line the thoracic wall and cover the lungs).

- *Mucous membranes:* Also known as *mucosae*, these membranes line body cavities that open to the outside of the body, including the nose and mouth, as well as digestive, respiratory, urinary, and reproductive tubes. Mucous membranes consist of epithelium above loose connective tissue (the *lamina propria*), with goblet cells that secrete mucus. In some mucosae, the lamina propria lies over a third, deeper layer of smooth muscle cells. Mucous membranes are always wet or moist membranes. The cell composition of mucous membranes actually varies, but most contain either simple columnar epithelia or stratified squamous epithelia. Mucous membranes may be adapted for absorption and secretion. Many, but not all, secrete mucus. The urinary tract is an example of mucosae that do not secrete mucus.

- *Cutaneous membrane:* The skin, which covers the body surface, consists of a keratinized stratified squamous epithelium, known as the *epidermis*. This is firmly attached to a thick connective tissue layer known as the *dermis*. The epidermis differs from other epithelial membranes in that it is dry and exposed to the air.

- *Synovial membrane:* Forms an incomplete lining within the cavities of the synovial joints and is entirely made up of loose connective tissues. Synovial membranes may be the inner of the two layers of the articular capsule of a synovial joint, with a free smooth surface lining the joint cavity. They may also be either the superior or inferior membranes lining the articular capsule of the temporomandibular joint. Synovial fluid is the clear, viscid, lubricating fluid secreted by synovial membranes. It is similar in consistency to that of an *egg white*. Synovial membranes often have an outer *subintima* layer (that may be fibrous, fatty, or loosely areolar) and an inner *intima* layer that consists of a sheet of cells that is thinner than a sheet of paper. When the subintima is loose, the intima sits on a pliable membrane.

TEST YOUR UNDERSTANDING

1. List the four types of tissue membranes in the body.
2. Which cavities in the body are covered by serous membranes?
3. Define synovial membranes.

Tissue Repair

The steps of tissue repair are based on division and migration of cells. These activities are controlled by growth factors, also known as *wound hormones*, which are released by injured cells. Destroyed tissue is replaced, with the same type of tissue, in a process called *regeneration*. When *fibrosis* occurs, fibrous connective tissue is produced in greater quantities, forming *scar tissue*. Regeneration or fibrosis occurs as a result of two factors: the type of tissue that was damaged and the severity of the injury. When the skin is injured, both regeneration and fibrosis occur for tissue repair.

Inflammation begins the process of tissue repair. The capillaries dilate and become highly permeable. White blood cells and plasma fluid (containing strong clotting proteins, antibodies, and other helpful substances) reach the injured area to construct a clot. This holds the wound edges together to isolate the injured area. Bacteria, toxins, and other harmful agents are prevented from spreading to the surrounding tissues. The exposed part of the clot dries and hardens, forming a *scab*. Lymphatic vessels or macrophages eventually remove debris, parts of destroyed cells, and excess fluid that may be left behind.

A phase called *organization* begins wherein the blood clot is replaced by *granulation tissue*. This delicate pink tissue contains capillaries in the formation of a new capillary bed. It is granular in appearance due to the presence of the capillaries and bleeds easily if disturbed. Fibroblasts proliferate to produce growth factors and new collagen fibers. Certain fibroblasts contract to pull the wound margins together or to pull existing blood vessels into the wound. Macrophages digest the original blood clot. Collagen fibers continue to be deposited. Granulation tissue is very resistant to infection (because it produces substances that inhibit bacteria) and eventually becomes scar tissue. When sufficient matrix has accumulated, the fibroblasts either return to resting or die.

The surface epithelium regenerates and grows under the scab, which soon detaches. Underneath, the fibrous tissue matures and contracts. The epithelium eventually looks like the surrounding skin and is fully regenerated, with an underlying area of scar tissue. Based on the wound's severity, the scar tissue may be invisible, appear as a thin white line, or may appear more substantially. This entire process describes how a skin cut, scrape, or puncture heals. Simple infections heal only by regeneration (such as a sore throat or a pimple). Severe and destructive infections cause clot formation or scarring.

FOCUS ON PATHOLOGY

Some organs may be severely harmed by scar tissue formation. Examples include the heart and urinary bladder. Internal volume of such organs may be reduced, or the related fluids may not be able to move through the organ normally. Scar tissue in the heart interferes with its contracting ability, leading to progressive heart failure. In a visceral organ that has been operated on, an *adhesion* may form, in which scar tissue connects adjacent organs together. If an adhesion develops in the intestine, peristalsis may be compromised, with dangerous outcomes.

Effects of Aging on Various Tissues

As body tissues age, they are repaired more slowly and much less effectively. Hormone secretion slows down, and, in general, physical activity becomes less regular. Connective tissues become more fragile, epithelial tissues thin, bones become brittle, and skin bruising occurs more easily. Continual damage to the body can lead to cardiovascular disease, deterioration of mental function, and other major health problems. The effects of aging may be genetic, as in the condition known as *osteoporosis*, which is also related to reductions in sex hormones, lack of exercise, and low dietary calcium. However, healthy bones can be maintained by correcting these deficiencies, and other types of tissue degeneration can be temporarily slowed or even reversed with supplements, hormone (and other) therapies, and regular exercise.

TEST YOUR UNDERSTANDING

1. List the steps of tissue repair.
2. Explain the reason behind the name of "granulation tissue."

SUMMARY

Tissues are made up of groups of specialized cells. The four tissue types are epithelial, connective, muscle, and neural tissue. Histology is the study of tissues. Epithelial tissue includes epithelia and glands. An epithelium is an avascular layer of cells that forms a barrier that provides protection.

Glands are secretory structures derived from epithelia. Epithelial tissue provides physical protection, absorbs, filters, excretes, provides sensation, produces specialized secretions, is permeable, and regenerates. Epithelia are classified on the basis of the number of cell layers and the shape of the cells. A simple epithelium has a single layer of cells, whereas a stratified epithelium has several layers.

Exocrine glands discharge secretions onto the body surface or into ducts. Endocrine glands secrete hormones into the blood circulation. A glandular epithelial cell may release its secretions by merocrine, apocrine, or holocrine modes. Connective tissue is internal tissue with many important functions. It transports fluids and dissolved materials, establishes a structural framework, protects organs, stores fat for reserve fuel, insulates the body, and defends the body from microorganisms. All connective tissue contains specialized cells and a matrix, composed of extracellular protein fibers and a ground substance. Connective tissue contains fibers and various types of cells.

Muscle tissue is specialized for contraction. The three types of muscle tissue are skeletal, cardiac, and smooth muscle. The cells of skeletal muscle tissue are multinuclear.

Skeletal muscle is also known as striated voluntary muscle. Cardiac muscle tissue is found only in the heart. It is striated involuntary muscle, relying on pacemaker cells for regular contraction. Smooth muscle tissue, which is involuntary muscle tissue, is not striated.

Neural tissue conducts electrical impulses, conveying information from one area of the body to another. Cells in neural tissue are either neurons or neuroglia. Neurons transmit information as electrical impulses. The basic functions of neuroglia include supporting neural tissue and helping to supply nutrients to neurons. Epithelial membranes cover body surfaces and line body cavities. The four types of membranes are serous, mucous, cutaneous, and synovial membranes. Tissue repair is based on the processes of regeneration and fibrosis. As body tissues age, they are repaired more slowly. Connective tissues become more fragile, bones become brittle, and skin bruising occurs more easily.

KEY TERMS

Adipose tissue
Apocrine glands
Areolar tissue
Avascular
Basement membrane
Blood
Bone
Cardiac muscle tissue
Cartilage
Chondrocytes
Connective tissues
Cutaneous membrane
Dense connective tissue
Elastic cartilage
Epithelial membranes
Epithelial tissues
Epithelium
Endocrine glands
Exocrine glands
Fibroblast

Fibrocartilage
Fibronectin
Glandular epithelium
Goblet cells
Ground substance
Histology
Holocrine glands
Hormones
Hyaline cartilage
Laminin
Ligaments
Loose connective tissue
Lymph
Macrophages
Mast cells
Matrix
Merocrine glands
Mucous membranes
Muscle tissues
Nervous tissues

Neuroglial cells
Neurons
Osteocytes
Osteon
Pseudostratified columnar epithelium
Reticular connective tissue
Serous membranes
Simple columnar epithelium
Simple cuboidal epithelium
Simple squamous epithelium
Skeletal muscle tissue
Smooth muscle tissue
Stratified columnar epithelium
Stratified cuboidal epithelium
Stratified squamous epithelium
Synovial membrane
Tendons
Tissues
Transitional epithelium

LEARNING GOALS

The following learning goals correspond to the objectives at the beginning of this chapter:

1. The four major types of tissues are as follows:
   - *Epithelial:* Cover organs, form inner linings, line hollow organs
   - *Connective:* Bind, support, protect, frame, and fill body structures
   - *Muscle:* Contractile tissue with filaments of actin and myosin
   - *Nervous:* Neurons and neuroglia

2. The types and functions of epithelial tissue are as follows:
   - *Simple squamous epithelium:* Lines alveoli, forms capillary walls, lines blood and lymph vessels, covers body cavity membranes
   - *Simple cuboidal epithelium:* Covers ovaries, lines kidney tubules and glandular ducts, functions in secretion and absorption
   - *Simple columnar epithelium:* Found in female reproductive tubes, uterus, and most digestive tract organs; involved in secretion and absorption
   - *Pseudostratified columnar epithelium:* Lines respiratory passages and is involved in secretion
   - *Stratified squamous epithelium:* Forms the epidermis and lines the mouth, esophagus, vagina, and anus
   - *Stratified cuboidal epithelium:* Lines mammary gland ducts, sweat glands, salivary glands, pancreas, and the developing ovaries and seminiferous tubules
   - *Stratified columnar epithelium:* Found in the male urethra, ductus deferens, and areas of the pharynx
   - *Transitional epithelium:* Lines the urinary bladder, ureters, and superior urethra; prevents urinary tract contents from diffusing back into the internal body environment
   - *Glandular epithelium:* Usually found in exocrine glands or endocrine glands

3. Endocrine glands secrete into tissue fluid or blood. Exocrine glands open onto surfaces or into the digestive tract.

4. *Mast cells:* Distributed throughout connective tissues, usually near blood vessels; release heparin and histamine
   Microphages: Responsible for phagocytosis
   Adipocytes: Store body fat

5. Three types of connective tissue fibers are the following:
   - *Dense connective tissue:* Many collagenous fibers; appears white
   - *Loose connective tissue:* Includes adipose tissue, areolar tissue, and reticular connective tissue
   - *Reticular connective tissue:* Helps to create a framework inside internal organs such as the spleen and liver

6. Blood and lymph are fluid connective tissues that contain distinctive collections of cells in a fluid matrix. They transport many materials between interior body cells and other cells that exchange substances with the external environment, maintaining a stable internal environment.

7. Types of cartilage are as follows:
   - *Hyaline cartilage:* On the ends of bones in many joints, the soft portion of the nose, and in the respiratory passages' supporting rings
   - *Elastic cartilage:* Provides the framework for the ears and larynx
   - *Fibrocartilage:* Absorbs shock in the spinal column, knees, and pelvic girdle

8. Bone, the most rigid type of connective tissue, establishes the framework of the body. Bone consists of a matrix of connective tissue, blood vessels, and minerals (particularly calcium and phosphorus).

9. The three types of muscle tissue are as follows:
   - *Skeletal muscle tissue:* Known as voluntary muscle tissue because it is found in muscles controlled by conscious effort
   - *Smooth muscle tissue:* Composed of elongated, spindle-shaped cells in muscles not under voluntary control
   - *Cardiac muscle tissue:* Also called *myocardium*, a thick contractile middle layer of the heart wall

10. Neurons are the basic structures of neural tissue. They respond to environmental changes by transmitting impulses along axons (cellular processes) to other neurons, to muscles, or to glands. Neurons coordinate, integrate, and regulate a wide variety of functions in the body.

CRITICAL THINKING QUESTIONS

A 17-year-old girl delivered her baby but lost a lot of blood during the process. She was anemic, and the physician prescribed some supplements to treat the anemia.

1. What are the major components of blood?
2. Explain the main four types of tissues in the body, and the one that blood is considered to be.

REVIEW QUESTIONS

1. Which of the following tissues binds structures and provides protection?
    A. epithelial
    B. muscle
    C. nervous
    D. connective
2. A matrix is a characteristic of which of the following types of tissues?
    A. neural
    B. epithelial
    C. connective
    D. muscle
3. The most common type of cartilage is
    A. hyaline
    B. fibrocartilage
    C. elastic
    D. collagenous
4. Stratified squamous epithelium covers or lines which of the following parts of the body?
    A. vagina
    B. mouth
    C. skin
    D. all of the above
5. Epithelium is connected to underlying connective tissue by
    A. intracellular glue
    B. a basement membrane
    C. a fibrous netting
    D. reticular fibers
6. Simple cuboidal epithelium is found
    A. lining the trachea
    B. lining the esophagus
    C. lining glandular ducts
    D. lining the blood vessels
7. Which of the following tissues is specialized for the conduction of electrical impulses?
    A. epithelial tissue
    B. areolar tissue
    C. nervous tissue
    D. muscle tissue
8. Which of the following muscle tissues is multinucleated?
    A. smooth muscle
    B. skeletal muscle
    C. involuntary muscle
    D. cardiac muscle
9. Which of the following is not a type of epithelial tissue?
    A. glandular
    B. cartilage
    C. pseudostratified columnar
    D. transitional
10. Which of the following statements is true about cardiac muscle?
    A. It can contract independently of neuronal stimulation.
    B. It has multiple nuclei.
    C. It forms muscle fibers.
    D. It contains visible striations.
11. Another term for skeletal muscle tissue is
    A. involuntary tissue
    B. smooth voluntary tissue
    C. striated voluntary tissue
    D. smooth tissue
12. The urinary bladder contains which of the following types of tissue?
    A. stratified squamous
    B. transitional epithelium
    C. simple cuboidal
    D. pseudostratified columnar epithelium

13. Heparin and histamine are released from
    A. macrophages
    B. fibroblasts
    C. lymphocytes
    D. mast cells
14. Which of the following is not one of the four types of membranes in the human body?
    A. serous
    B. cartilage
    C. mucous
    D. cutaneous

15. Which of the following are apocrine glands?
    A. salivary glands
    B. sweat glands
    C. mammary glands
    D. pancreatic glands

ESSAY QUESTIONS

1. What are the classifications of epithelial tissues?
2. Describe connective tissues and compare them with nervous tissues.
3. List various types of connective tissue cells.
4. Classify and explain the characteristics of muscle tissues.
5. Explain the anatomy of the neuron.
6. Discuss the types of exocrine gland secretions, and give one example for each.
7. Describe the major types of cartilage.
8. Define the terms "mast cells," "goblet cells," and "macrophages," and explain their functions.
9. What are the functions of simple cuboidal epithelium and stratified squamous epithelium?
10. Discuss the four types of membranes in the body.

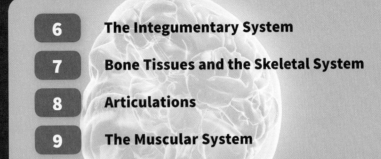

Integumentary System

OBJECTIVES

After studying this chapter, readers should be able to

1. Explain the structure of the dermis and epidermis.
2. Describe the normal and pathological colors skin can have.
3. List the functions of the skin.
4. Describe the structure of nails.
5. Discuss the various kinds of glands in the skin and the secretions of each.
6. Explain how the sweat glands play a major role in regulating body temperature.
7. Describe the three most common forms of skin cancer.
8. Describe the location and function of sebaceous and ceruminous glands.
9. Explain the anatomic parts of a hair.
10. Describe the effects of aging on the integumentary system.

Overview

The **integumentary system**, which consists of the skin (cutaneous membrane) and accessory structures, accounts for approximately 16% of the total body weight of an adult. Its surface area covers from 1.5 to 2 m². The skin, which is the largest organ of the body in surface area and weight, is continually bombarded by all sorts of environmental components, including attack by microorganisms, radiation from sunlight, and exposure to chemicals. The accessory integumentary system structures include hairs, nails, sweat glands, and oil glands. The integumentary system is the first line of defense against the environment. The skin, as well as the deeper *hypodermis*, has many functions, such as protection, excretion, temperature maintenance, melanin production, keratin production, vitamin D₃ (cholecalciferol) synthesis, lipid storage, and sensory detection.

Skin

The skin is also known as the *integument*, which means "covering." This is where the name *integumentary system* is derived. The skin varies in thickness between 1.5 and 4 mm,

depending on which part of the body it covers. The two main layers of skin are the epidermis and dermis. The **epidermis**, the outer layer, is made up of keratinized stratified squamous epithelium (**FIGURE 6-1**). The epidermis is also called the *superficial epithelium*. It has four primary cell types and four or five layers, depending on body location (four layers in most body areas and five layers on the palms, fingertips, and soles of the feet). Unlike the dermis, the epidermis is not vascularized. Nutrients must diffuse through dermal blood vessels and tissue fluid to reach the epidermis. The **dermis**, the inner layer, is much thicker than the epidermis and consists of papillary and reticular regions. The papillary region contains fine elastic fibers and dermal papillae. The reticular region is composed of connective tissue containing collagen, elastic fibers, fat tissue, hair follicles, nerves, sebaceous (oil) glands, and the ducts of sweat glands. The epidermis is connected to the dermis by a basement membrane.

Loose connective tissue below the dermis binds the skin to the organs underneath. This tissue, which is predominantly adipose (fatty), forms the **subcutaneous layer**, also known as the *hypodermis* or *superficial fascia*. It is deep below the dermis and not actually part of the skin. This adipose tissue insulates the body, conserving inner heat and helping to keep excessive heat from outside the body from entering.

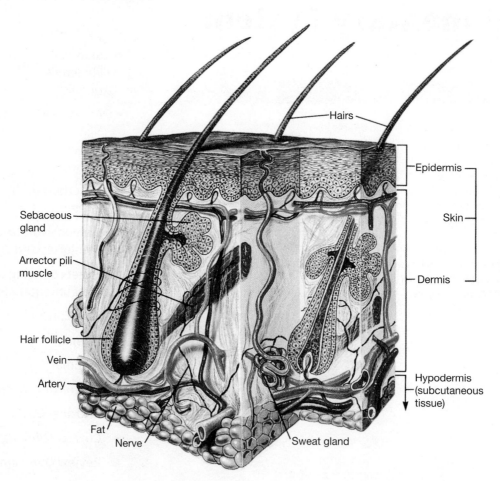

FIGURE 6-1 Anatomy of the skin.

The major blood vessels that supply the skin and adipose tissue are contained within the subcutaneous layer. The hypodermis is loose enough that the skin slides with ease over its underlying structures. It also acts as a shock absorber and becomes much thicker when weight is gained. This tissue first accumulates in the anterior abdomen in males and in the thighs and breasts in females. The hypodermis lends its name to the term "hypodermic," which is where subcutaneous injections are made via *hypodermic needles*.

FOCUS ON PATHOLOGY

Liposuction is a procedure that removes excessive amounts of adipose tissue. Because of the obesity epidemic, it has become a relatively common procedure. Liposuction is also called *lipoplasty*. Subcutaneous adipose tissue is removed through a tube inserted deep to the skin. The complications of liposuction include bleeding, infection, fluid loss, sensory loss, and risks related to anesthesia.

Epidermis

The epidermis is the outermost layer of the skin and is composed of stratified squamous epithelium. The epidermis does not contain blood vessels, although its deepest layer, the stratum basale, receives blood via the dermal blood vessels. Epidermal cells require diffusion of oxygen and nutrients from the capillaries within the dermis. Cells that have a higher metabolic demand are located closer to the basement membrane. Cells in this layer of the epidermis divide and grow, moving toward the skin surface and away from the dermis below. As they move upward, they receive fewer nutrients and eventually die. Older cells are called **keratinocytes**, which harden with age in the process known as *keratinization*. Keratin protein fills the cytoplasm of these skin cells, which collectively form a layer called the *stratum corneum*. Dead skin cells in this layer are eventually shed from the body.

Epidermis Layers

There are basically five layers of the epidermis: stratum germinativum (stratum basale), stratum spinosum, stratum granulosum, stratum lucidum, and stratum corneum. Most of the body surface is covered by *thin skin*, consisting of four layers of keratinocytes that total only 0.08 mm in thickness. Areas of *thick skin* (the palms and soles) contain a fifth layer, the stratum lucidum, and the stratum corneum in these areas is much thicker. Therefore, on the palms and soles, the epidermal layers total about 0.5 mm in thickness. The five individual layers are explained as follows:

- The **stratum germinativum** (the "germinative or basal layer") is the innermost epidermal layer and is also known as the **stratum basale** (basal layer).

It is interlocked with the underlying dermis via *hemidesmosomes*, which are tiny pin-like structures. This layer forms the epidermal ridges, extending into the dermis, which are adjacent to dermal projections (dermal papillae). The attachment of the stratum basale to the dermis is along a wavy borderline. Epidermal ridges are important because the strength of the attachment of the layer is proportional to the surface area of the **basal lamina**. Ridge shapes are genetically determined, and the pattern of epidermal ridges does not change during the entire life span of an individual (**FIGURE 6-2**). The ridge patterns on the tip of each finger are instrumental in the forming of fingerprints. Each person's fingerprints are unique, including those of identical twins. As a result, fingerprints are commonly used in criminal cases to identify individuals. Large basal (germinative) cells dominate the stratum germinativum. Stem cells are usually in single rows, with divisions that replace superficial keratinocytes that are lost or shed on the epithelial surface. When a stem cell divides into daughter cells, they are pushed from the stratum germinativum upward into the next layer, the stratum spinosum. There are many mitotic cell nuclei in this layer, reflecting rapid cell division. Approximately 10% to 25% of these cells are melanocytes that reach into the stratum spinosum. The ridges on the palms and soles also increase the surface area of the skin and help us to grip objects due to the increased friction. In areas where the skin surface does not have hair, there are specialized epithelial cells known as *Merkel* or *tactile* cells. They are sensitive to touch, releasing chemicals that stimulate sensory nerve endings when they are compressed. The brownish color of the skin comes from *melanocytes*, distributed in the stratum germinativum. They have cell processes that extend into the more superficial layers.

- The **stratum spinosum** (the "spinous or prickle cell layer") is made up of 8 to 10 layers of keratinocytes that are bound together by **desmosomes**. It contains cells that look like tiny pin cushions because of exposure to chemicals that caused the keratinocyte cytoplasm to shrink slightly. However, the desmosomes and elements of the cytoskeleton remained intact. Some entering cells from the stratum basale continue dividing, which increases the thickness of the epithelium. This layer also contains Langerhans cells, also known as *dendritic cells*, which stimulate immune defenses against microorganisms and superficial skin cancers.

- The **stratum granulosum** (the "granular layer") is the third layer and consists of only three to six layers of keratinocytes. Cells in this layer have mostly stopped dividing and begin to make the proteins keratin and keratohyalin. Keratin is tough and fibrous, making up hairs and nails. Developing keratin fibers become flatter and thinner, as their

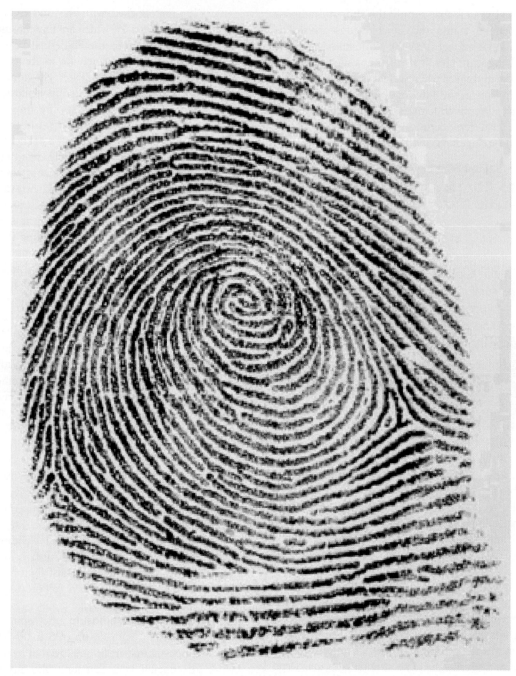

FIGURE 6-2 A fingerprint. (© AbleStock)

membranes thicken and lose permeability. Keratohyalin forms cytoplasmic granules that dehydrate cells and aggregate and cross-link keratin fibers. The cells die as the nuclei and other organelles disintegrate. Continued dehydration causes this layer to become extremely interlocked. Nutrients are brought via capillaries in the dermis. However, above this layer, the cells are too distant from the dermal capillaries and glycolipids coating them keep nutrients from being supplied, hence their normal death.

- The **stratum lucidum** (the "clear layer") is the fourth region, which is only found on the palms of the hands and soles of the feet, with a glassy

or clear appearance. Therefore, the overall skin of the palms and soles is thicker than on other parts of the body. In this layer, the cells are flattened and densely packed, have few organelles, and are filled with keratin. The stratum lucidum is microscopically viewed only in thick skin, appearing as a thin translucent band above the stratum granulosum. It consists only of two or three rows of flat and dead keratinocytes that have indistinct boundaries.

- The **stratum corneum** (the "horny layer") makes up the surface of the skin and contains 15 to 30 layers of keratinized cells that are protective and filled with keratin. The process of keratinization is also known as *cornification*. It occurs on all exposed body surfaces except the anterior eye surfaces. The dead cells of the stratum corneum are tightly interconnected by desmosomes. Because of this interconnection, keratinized cells of this layer are shed in large sheets rather than individually. Cells move from the stratum germinativum to the stratum corneum in 7 to 30 days, remaining in the stratum corneum for about 2 weeks before being washed away or naturally shed. The dryness of the stratum corneum reduces the amount of potential microbial growth, and this layer is coated with lipid secretions from the sebaceous glands. This layer is water resistant but not waterproof. Water from the interstitial fluids eventually penetrates to the surface. About 500 mL of water is lost from this layer via evaporation every day in a process known as *insensible perspiration*. This differs from *sensible perspiration*, which is produced by active sweat glands. The rate of insensible perspiration may be increased when the epidermis is damaged and sometimes can be dangerous, such as when severe burns excessively damage the epidermis. Oppositely, being immersed in fresh (hypotonic) water for a long time causes the epidermal cells to swell up to four times their normal volume. This is most noticeable on the palms and soles. Immersion in ocean (hypertonic) water causes water to leave the epidermal cells, eventually resulting in dehydration. **FIGURE 6-3** shows how healthy skin balances the production of epidermal cells with the loss of dead cells. The stratum corneum makes up nearly three-fourths of the total epidermal thickness. Keratin protects it against abrasion, and glycolipids cause its water resistance. Approximately 50,000 dead cells are shed from this layer every minute. In an average lifetime, you will lose 40 pounds of these dead skin cells.

FOCUS ON PATHOLOGY

Psoriasis is a chronic inflammatory autoimmune condition of the skin characterized by thickened areas of silver-colored scales. The epidermal cells proliferate, and the condition is most common on the knees, elbows, scalp, lower back, face, palms, and soles. Psoriasis is most prevalent in Caucasians between the ages of 15 and 25, with one in three patients having a family member with the condition. Physicians can diagnose psoriasis simply by visualizing the lesions. Psoriasis may seem similar to eczema, but its scales have well-defined edges.

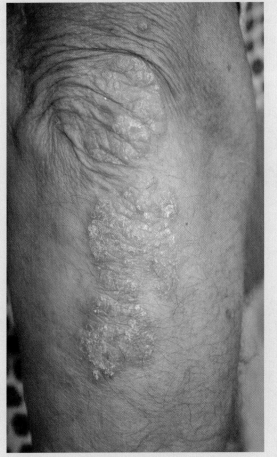

Psoriasis. (Courtesy of Yale Residents' Slide Collection, Dermatology Department, Yale University School of Medicine.)

Epidermal Cells

The epidermis protects the underlying tissues against the effects of harmful chemicals, excess water loss, mechanical injury, and pathogenic microorganisms. Layers of pigment in the epidermis help protect both epidermal and dermal tissues. **Melanin** is a brown, yellow-brown, or black pigment produced by spider-shaped **melanocytes** located in the stratum germinativum, either between or deeply rooted in the epithelial cells (**FIGURE 6-4**). It is made of tyrosine amino acids and has two forms that range in color (from red-yellow to brown-black). Synthesis of melanin is based on an enzyme called **tyrosinase**. Melanin accumulates in granules that are bound to membranes, called *melanosomes*. Lysosomes eventually break down **melanosomes**, meaning that melanin pigment is found only in the deeper layers of the epidermis. Motor proteins move down actin filaments to reach the ends of each melanocyte's processes. They then move to nearby keratinocytes, accumulating on the superficial side of the keratinocyte nucleus. Normal exposure of the skin to sunlight causes the keratinocytes to secrete chemicals that stimulate the melanocytes. Melanin absorbs *ultraviolet (UV) radiation* from sunlight, protecting the epidermis and dermis from its harmful effects. It builds up from sun exposure, absorbing rays, dissipating this energy as heat, and protecting DNA of viable skin cells from UV radiation. However, sunlight contains extremely significant amounts of UV radiation. Although small amounts of UV radiation are beneficial because they stimulate the epidermal production

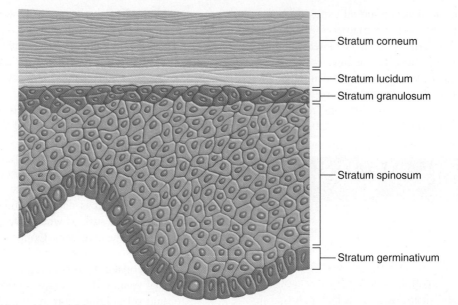

— Stratum corneum

— Stratum lucidum
— Stratum granulosum

— Stratum spinosum

— Stratum germinativum

FIGURE 6-3 The epidermal layers of the skin.

of a compound required for calcium ion homeostasis (the production of vitamin D), larger amounts damage DNA. This causes mutations, promoting the development of cancer. UV radiation can also produce burns. When severe, they can damage the epidermis and the dermis.

Keratinocytes produce *keratin*, which is the fibrous protein that aids the epidermis in protecting the body. Most epidermal cells are keratinocytes, which arise in the stratum

basale. Upon reaching the skin surface, they are already dead. At this time, they have a scale-like appearance and are basically plasma membranes filled with keratin. Every day, millions of dead keratinocytes rub off. Therefore, the epidermis is totally replaced every 25 to 45 days.

Star-shaped **dendritic cells**, or *Langerhans cells,* from the bone marrow eventually move to the epidermis. They consume foreign substances and play a key role in activating

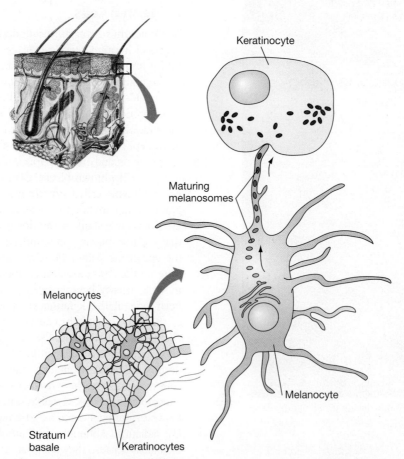

Keratinocyte

Maturing
melanosomes

Melanocytes

Stratum
basale

Keratinocytes

Melanocyte

FIGURE 6-4 Melanocytes produce melanin, the pigment of skin, package it in melanosomes, and transfer it to keratinocytes.

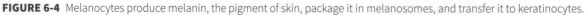

the immune system. **Tactile cells**, or *Merkel cells,* are located at the epidermal–dermal junction. They have spiked shapes and combine with disc-like sensory nerve endings to form *tactile discs,* which are receptors for the sense of touch.

Differences in skin color are based on the amount of melanin produced and how it is distributed throughout the skin. Skin color is based on a person's genetics, which regulates the amount of melanin produced by the melanocytes. Other factors that affect skin color include sunlight, UV light, and x-rays. Dermal vessel blood also affects the color of the skin. Well-oxygenated blood makes light-skinned people appear pinker, whereas poorly oxygenated blood makes them appear bluer, as in the condition known as *cyanosis.* Diet also affects skin color, as do biochemical imbalances. For example, the buildup of the substance known as *bilirubin* makes the skin appear yellowish, as in the condition called *jaundice.*

Also contributing to skin color are the pigments *carotene* and *hemoglobin.* Carotene is a yellow to orange pigment that primarily accumulates in the stratum corneum and the hypodermic fatty tissue. It is also found in plant products such as carrots and other orange-colored vegetables. The color of carotene is most easily seen in the palms and soles, especially in lighter skinned individuals, where the stratum corneum is present in thicker cellular levels. It intensifies in the body when large amounts of foods rich in carotene are consumed. Carotene can be converted to vitamin A (essential for normal vision), which aids in the health of the epidermis. Carotene, along with variations in melanin, contributes to the skin color of people from certain Asian countries. *Hemoglobin* is the red pigment inside

red blood cells. As it circulates throughout the dermal capillaries, it gives off a pink color that is easily seen in people with fairer skin.

Dermis

The *dermis* lies between the epidermis and the subcutaneous layer and has two major components: a superficial papillary layer and a deeper reticular layer. The dermis also contains all cells of connective tissue proper. Epidermal accessory organs extend into the dermis, and both the papillary and reticular layers of the dermis contain many blood vessels, lymph vessels, and nerve fibers. The dermis is the second major skin structure and is a strong and flexible connective tissue. Dermal cells contain fibroblasts, macrophages, and smaller amounts of mast cells and white blood cells. The major portions of hair follicles, oil glands, and sweat glands are found in the dermis, even though they derive from epidermal tissue.

The **papillary layer** consists of areolar tissue and contains capillaries, lymphatics, and sensory neurons. The papillary layer is named for the dermal papillae that project between the epidermal ridges. It is thin and superficial areolar connective tissue with interwoven collagen and elastic fibers. The papillary layer is loose, allowing phagocytes and various defensive cells to move freely, searching for bacteria that have gotten through the skin. Dermal papillae often contain loops of capillaries or may contain pain receptors and touch receptors. In the thicker skin of the palms or soles, these papillae are above larger *dermal ridges,* which then cause the epidermis to form its *epidermal ridges.* These ridges leave pressure marks that are commonly referred to as *fingerprints,* unique to every individual human being.

The deeper *reticular layer* is made up of connective tissue containing collagen and elastic fibers. The boundary between the papillary and reticular layers is not distinct. The reticular layer makes up approximately 80% of the overall thickness of the dermis. It is nourished by the *cutaneous plexus.* Collagen fibers mostly run parallel to the skin surface, with less dense regions known as *separations* forming **cleavage lines** in the skin. Also known as *tension lines,* these lines are used for surgeries to make parallel incisions, meaning better healing afterward. A third type of skin marking, **flexure lines**, occur close to joints, where the dermis is more tightly secured to deeper structures. Examples include the creases on the palms of the hands. In the papillary layer, small arteries form a branched network known as the *papillary plexus,* which provides arterial blood to the capillaries along the epidermis–dermis boundary.

The collagenous and elastic fibers of the dermis make it both tough and elastic. The skin's water content helps it to be flexible and resilient, which is known as *skin turgor.* A sign of dehydration is the loss of skin turgor. Processes from nerve cells are located throughout the dermis. Motor processes carry impulses to the dermal glands and muscles, whereas sensory processes carry impulses back to the brain and spinal cord. Cutaneous sensations include touch, hot, cold, and pain.

TEST YOUR UNDERSTANDING

1. List and discuss the five layers of the epidermis.
2. Explain melanin, melanocytes, and melanosomes.
3. Which layer of the epidermis is vascular?

FOCUS ON PATHOLOGY

The skin is eventually damaged by excessive sun exposure, regardless of the protective abilities of melanin. Elastic fibers clump together, and the skin becomes "leathery." The immune system is depressed, which can lead to skin cancer by altering skin cell DNA. Dark-skinned people get skin cancer less often than light-skinned people, and when they develop it, cancerous lesions usually occur on areas of lighter skin, such as the palms or soles. UV radiation also destroys stores of folic acid in the body, which can lead to developmental defects in pregnant women.

FOCUS ON PATHOLOGY

Excessive stretching of the skin can tear the dermis, leaving silver-white scars known as *striae* or "stretch marks." These are often due to events such as pregnancy. Also, acute trauma that is short term may cause a *blister*, a fluid-filled pocket between the epidermal and dermal layers.

FOCUS ON PATHOLOGY

Petechiae are small hemorrhages in the skin caused by decreased amounts of platelets, resulting in bleeding from capillaries. Sometimes, petechiae occur after application of a tourniquet. Petechiae may be caused by platelet abnormalities such as thrombocytopenia or platelet dysfunction, vasculitis, and infections such as meningococcemia or Rocky Mountain spotted fever.

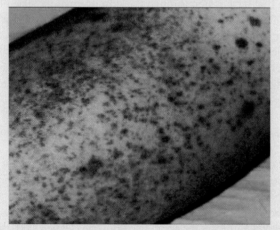

Petechiae.

TEST YOUR UNDERSTANDING

1. Describe the layer of the dermis that determines a person's fingerprints.
2. What forms cleavage lines in the skin?

Accessory Structures

The accessory structures of the integumentary system include nails, hair and hair follicles, and sebaceous and sweat glands. These glands are multicellular and have exocrine functions. Most accessory structures are located in the dermis and protrude through the epidermis to reach the surface of the skin.

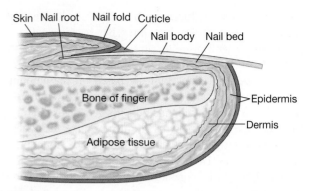

FIGURE 6-5 Fingernail anatomy.

Nails

Nails protect the ends of the fingers and toes, consisting of a nail plate above a skin surface called the *nail bed*. A *nail* is a modification of the epidermis that contains hard keratin. The part of the *nail plate* (*nail body*) that grows most actively is covered by a whitish, half-moon–shaped *lunula* or *lunule*, where epithelial cells divide and become keratinized. The nail cells push forward over the *nail bed*, causing the nail body to continually grow outward. The nail bed is surrounded on each side by depressions known as the *lateral nail grooves*. The thickened proximal part of the nail bed is called the *nail matrix*, which is the part that causes nail growth. The nail of the middle finger grows fastest, whereas the nail of the thumb grows slowest (**FIGURE 6-5**).

The free edge of each nail is the part that is trimmed when it extends to a sufficient length, with the thicker region underneath where dirt accumulates called the **hyponychium** or the "quick." The hyponychium secures the nail plate's free edge at the fingertip. Skin folds called **nail folds** overlap the proximal and lateral borders of each nail. The proximal nail fold attaches to the nail body as the **cuticle** (eponychium).

Nails begin growing at the nail root, which lies very close to the bone of the fingertip. A part of the stratum corneum forms the cuticle, with underlying blood vessels that give the nail a pinkish color. The nail body consists of dead, compressed cells packed with keratin. Changes in the nails can help to diagnose many different body conditions. Nails normally appear pink in color because of underlying capillaries, with the white crescent-shaped *lunula* above the nail matrix. Discoloration of a nail may indicate respiratory, thyroid, or immune disorders. A yellow tinge may indicate a respiratory or thyroid gland condition. Pitting or distortion of the shapes of the nails may indicate psoriasis, and a concave shape may indicate a blood disorder. Thickened yellow nails may indicate a fungal infection. If the nail is outwardly concaved (*spoon nail*), an iron deficiency may exist. Horizontal *Beau's lines* across the nails may signify malnutrition.

TEST YOUR UNDERSTANDING

1. Describe the substance that makes nails "hard."
2. Define the nail folds, cuticle, and lunula.

Paronychia is a condition wherein abscesses occur around the nails. When acute, the edges of the nails may swell because of a collection of pus. When chronic, paronychia is usually caused by jobs in which the hands remain wet on a regular basis. Chronic paronychia is also caused by diabetes or immunocompromised states. The condition may be an irritant dermatitis, with secondary fungal colonization.

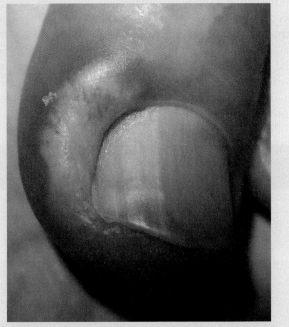

Paronychia. (Courtesy of Yale Residents' Slide Collection, Dermatology Department, Yale University School of Medicine.)

Hairs

Hairs (*pili*) project above the skin surface over most of the body, except for the sides and soles of the feet, the palms of the hands, the sides of the fingers and toes, the lips, and parts of the external genitalia. They begin to form during embryologic development and are also known as *epidermal derivatives* because they arise from the epidermis. There are about 2.5 million hairs on the human body, of which over 75% is on the general body surface and not the head. Hairs are structures produced in organs called **hair follicles** (**FIGURE 6-6**). They consist of a large amount of dead keratinized cells, dominated by hard keratin. Hair follicles extend from the skin surface into the dermis, containing hair *roots* that are nourished with dermal blood. Each hair follicle is attached to an *arrector pili* muscle, which helps the hair *shaft* (in which keratinization is complete) to stand on end when it contracts. This occurs during emotional upset and cold temperatures. Hairs are pushed upward as epidermal hair cells divide and grow, becoming keratinized and then dying.

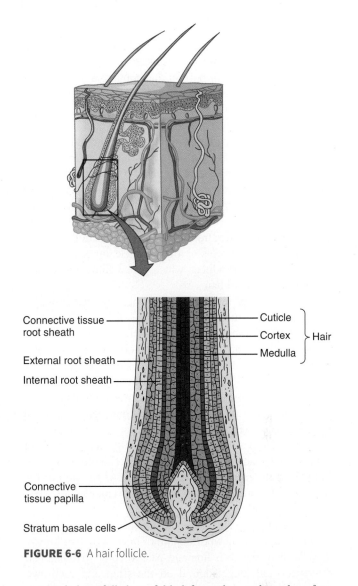

FIGURE 6-6 A hair follicle.

Each hair follicle is folded from the epidermal surface into the dermis. They may extend into the hypodermis of the scalp. Each follicle originates at about 4 mm below the skin surface, expanding to form a **hair bulb**. A *root hair plexus* or *hair follicle receptor* consists of a cluster of sensory nerve endings, wrapping around each hair bulb. When the hair is bent, these endings are stimulated, meaning that hairs act as touch receptors, with extreme sensitivity. Nipple-like dermal tissue makes up a *hair papilla*, which protrudes into each hair bulb. It contains a knot of capillaries that give nutrients to the growing hair. A *fibrous peripheral connective tissue sheath* makes up the wall of a hair follicle. This derives from the dermis. The other components of the hair follicle wall are the thickened basal *glassy membrane* and the inner *epithelial root sheath*. This sheath becomes thinner as it approaches the hair bulb, with only one layer of epithelial cells covering the papilla.

The **hair matrix** is the actively dividing part of the hair bulb that produces the hair. It originates in the *hair bulge*, just a small portion of 1 mm above the hair bulb. Chemical signals that reach the hair bulge cause certain cells to move to the papilla, divide, and produce new hair cells. The older part of each hair is then pushed upward, with the fused cells getting more keratin and dying.

Each hair has three concentric layers known as the *medulla, cortex,* and *cuticle.* The central core of a hair is the medulla. It is made up of air spaces and large cells. The medulla is the only hair portion that contains soft keratin. It does not exist in fine hairs. Surrounding the medulla is the bulky *cortex,* made up of a few layers of flat cells. A single layer of cells forms the outermost *cuticle* of a hair. In the cuticle, cells are overlapped like shingles, which helps keep each hair shaft from matting with others. Most hard keratin is in the cuticle, which provides strength to the hair shaft and keeps the inner layers compacted tightly together. The cuticle experiences the most abrasion and usually wears away at the tip. This causes what is commonly known as *split ends,* in which fibrils of keratin from the cortex and medulla become split. The rough surfaces of a hair cuticle are smoothed by hair conditioning products, which give a shiny appearance to a person's head of hair.

Hair color is reflected by genetics and variations in the pigment produced by melanocytes at the hair papilla. Darker hair has more eumelanin (which is brownish-black), whereas lighter hair has more pheomelanin (which is reddish-yellow). The different forms of melanin give hair a wide variety of shades, ranging from dark brown to yellow brown, to red. Albinos have white hair because their hair shafts completely lack melanin. Hormonal and environmental factors also influence the hair's condition. As pigment production decreases with age, hair color lightens. White hair results from a lack of pigment along with the presence of air bubbles in the medulla of the hair shaft. As the proportion of white hairs increases, the overall hair color is described as gray.

Hairs are basically classified as either *vellus* or *terminal.* Adult women and newborn children have body hair known as *vellus hair,* which is fine and pale in color. *Terminal hair* is coarser and longer, found on the scalp and eyebrows, and often darker than vellus hair. Terminal hairs appear in the axillary and pubic regions of males and females during puberty. On males at puberty, they also appear on the face, chest, and usually, the arms and legs. These hairs are stimulated to grow by androgens (primarily testosterone). Large amounts of male hormones cause thick terminal hair growth. Nutrition and hormones influence hair density and growth. Chronic physical inflammation or irritation may cause increased local hair growth. Hair growth that is not cosmetically attractive may be slowed or stopped by electrolysis or laser treatments.

Hair grows at an average rate of 2.5 mm per week, but this varies with sex, age, and body regions. Growth cycles occur in each hair follicle, including an active phase that ranges from weeks to years and a regressive phase, when hair matrix cells die. The hair follicle base and hair bulb then shrink, causing the hair papilla to be moved upward to touch the part of the follicle that does not regress. Then, a 1- to 3-month resting phase occurs. After this, the cycling area of the follicle is regenerated. Activated bulge cells migrate to the papilla. The matrix is then able to form a new hair. Many proteins control a hair's life span, and scalp hair follicles are active for up to 10 years before being inactivated for several months. Approximately 90 scalp hairs are lost per day. The eyebrows never reach the length of the scalp hair because each eyebrow follicle is active for only 3 to 4 months.

Each hair follicle of the body has a limited number of growth cycles, with growing being fastest between the teenage years and the forties. Hair thinning occurs after this time because shedding happens more quickly than hair replacement. Both sexes, beginning in middle age, experience a certain degree of hair thinning and/or *alopecia* (baldness), but it is more commonly seen in men. By age 35, approximately 40% of men have visible hair loss, and by age 60 the percentage is about 85%. Scalp hair loss usually begins at the anterior hairline, progressing posteriorly. The hair becomes thinner as vellus hairs being to replace the coarser terminal hairs. However, *true baldness* (most commonly, *male pattern baldness*) is not the same situation. It is sex-influenced and genetically determined, linked to a gene that activates during adulthood and changes how the hair follicles respond to dihydrotestosterone, (DHT), which is a metabolite of testosterone.

FOCUS ON PATHOLOGY

Albinism is a genetic disorder in which there is a lack of melanin. Most cases are autosomal recessive. Albinism affects the hair, skin, and eyes. The hair is usually white or very pale yellow, the skin extremely pale, and the eyes may range in color from blue to reddish, violet, hazel, or brown. As a result of albinism, eye conditions may include nystagmus, strabismus, or decreased vision. Patients must avoid skin damage from the sun by wearing sunscreen, hats, and protective clothing. For eye movement disorders, surgery may be helpful.

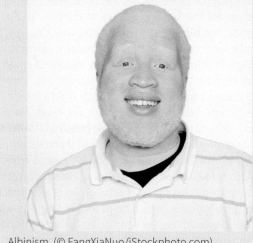

Albinism. (© FangXiaNuo/iStockphoto.com)

In women, excessive hair growth (*hirsuitism*) may result from an adrenal gland or ovarian tumor secreting abnormally large amounts of androgens. This condition is defined as excessive growth of thick or dark hair in women in locations that are typical of male hair growth patterns, including the face, chest, shoulders, lower abdomen, back, and inner thighs. Oppositely, hair thinning may be linked to surgery, very high fever, severe emotional trauma, excessive vitamin A, and medications (anabolic steroids, certain antidepressants or blood thinners, and most chemotherapy drugs). Other reversible causes of hair thinning include lactation and protein-deficient diets.

TEST YOUR UNDERSTANDING

1. Describe the mechanism that causes hairs to "stand on end."
2. Explain the tissue that comprises the hair papilla.
3. Describe the hair follicles, the root hair plexus, and the hair matrix.

Glands in the Skin

The skin contains two types of exocrine glands: sebaceous glands and sweat glands. The sebaceous (oil) glands are simple and branched alveolar glands covering the body, except on the palms and soles. The sweat (sudoriferous) glands are found all over the body except for the lips, nipples and certain parts of the external genitalia.

Sebaceous Glands

Sebaceous glands (oil glands) are made up of specialized epidermal cells and are primarily located near hair follicles. These glands are largest on the face, neck, and upper chest. They are actually holocrine glands, secreting **sebum**, which is an oily mixture of fatty material and debris from cells. The central alveoli cells accumulate lipids until they burst, and the combined lipids and cell fragments make up sebum. The sebum is secreted through small hair follicle ducts, helping to keep both hair and skin pliable and waterproof. The sebum is a mixture of cholesterol, triacylglycerides, proteins, and electrolytes. Sebum inhibits bacterial growth, protecting the keratin of the hair shafts. Sebum is forced out of hair follicles, to the skin surface, via arrector pili contractions. This lubricates the hair and skin, keeping the hair supple and slowing the loss of water from the skin during times of low environmental humidity. Sebum has a strong bactericidal action. Its secretion is stimulated by androgens primarily. Hence, sebaceous glands are less active until a human reaches puberty and androgen production rises.

Sebaceous follicles are large sebaceous glands that surround hair follicles. Their ducts discharge sebum directly onto the epidermis (**FIGURE 6-7**). They are found on the face, chest, nipples, back, and external genitalia. During the final phases of fetal development, their secretions, as well as epidermal cells that have been shed, coat the skin surface to form a protective layer. When the sebaceous glands become overactive, usually occurring on the scalp, an inflammation may develop around them. This is known as *seborrheic dermatitis*.

Sweat Glands

Sweat glands consist of a small tube originating as a coil in the deep dermis or superficial subcutaneous layers. The coiled portion is lined with sweat-secreting epithelial cells. Sweat is carried out of the skin by tubes called pores that

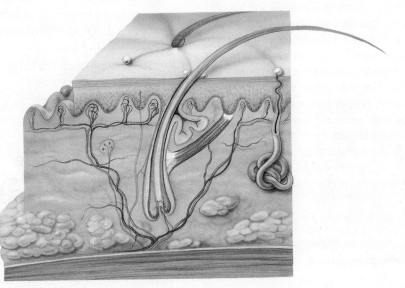

FIGURE 6-7 The structure of sebaceous glands and follicles.

open at the skin surface. Sweat is made up of 99% water as well as salts, which are primarily sodium chloride, ascorbic acid, or vitamin C; antibodies; and waste products, including urea, ammonia, and uric acid. Sweat also contains *dermicidin*, which is a peptide that kills microbes. Overall, sweat is a hypotonic filtrate of blood, passing through secretory cells via exocytosis. Its composition is based on diet, heredity, and, partially, certain drugs that are ingested. Sweat has a normal acidic pH of between 4 and 6. Sweating is regulated by the autonomic nervous system to prevent overheating. It begins on the forehead, spreading inferiorly to the rest of the body. When sweating is brought about by nervousness or fright (cold sweating), it starts on the palms, axillae, and soles before spreading throughout the body.

The skin contains two types of **sweat glands (sudoriferous glands)**: merocrine sweat glands and apocrine sweat glands. Merocrine (eccrine) glands are the predominant type of sweat glands, responding to body temperature, and are present at birth. They excrete water and electrolytes and also provide protection from hazards in the environment. Adult skin contains 2 to 5 million merocrine sweat glands. They are found on the forehead, neck, and back, although the palms and soles have the highest numbers. They are simple tubular glands with a coiled appearance. In the dermis is found the secretory portion, whereas the duct opens in a funnel-shaped *pore* at the surface of the skin. These pores are not the same as the "complexion pores," which are the outlets of hair follicles.

Apocrine glands are sweat glands that become active at puberty and number about 2,000. They are found mostly in the armpits and groin, with the sweat excreted at these places developing a scent as they come into contact with skin bacteria (**FIGURE 6-8**). This is the basis of body odor. Modified sweat glands include the **ceruminous glands** of the external ear (which produce earwax) and the mammary glands (which produce milk). *Cerumen* or earwax is believed to block entry of foreign materials or insects into the ear.

It should be noted that apocrine glands are still actually merocrine glands that produce their product in the same way as eccrine sweat glands. However, they are larger in size, are located in the dermis or hypodermis, and empty into hair follicles. Their secretions are similar to eccrine glands but also include proteins and fatty substances. The color of these secretions may be white or yellow. The function of apocrine glands is controlled by androgens, activated by sympathetic nerve fibers during stress and pain. In women they enlarge and recede along with the menstrual cycle. The secretory cells of apocrine glands are surrounded by *myoepithelial cells* that squeeze them to discharge accumulated sweat into the hair follicles.

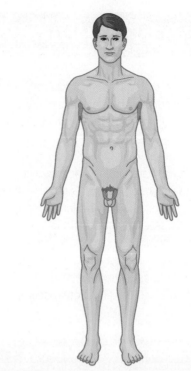

FIGURE 6-8 The locations of the apocrine sweat glands are shown in red. They include the axilla, areola, pubis, and circumanal region (not shown).

FOCUS ON PATHOLOGY

A sebaceous gland duct that is blocked by accumulated sebum is referred to as a *whitehead*, and when this material oxidizes and dries, it darkens, forming a *blackhead*. Active inflammation of the sebaceous glands accompanied by skin pustules or cysts is known as *acne*. These lesions are commonly referred to as *pimples*. Acne is usually caused by a staphylococci infection and can become severe enough to cause permanent scarring. *Seborrhea* is caused by overactive sebaceous glands. In infants, this is referred to as *cradle cap*.

Functions of the Integumentary System

The skin is constantly exposed to abrasion, microorganisms, chemicals, and extremes of temperature and has three primary barriers that protect the body: chemical, physical, and biological barriers. Chemical barriers include melanin and secretions from the skin. The low pH of skin secretions is described as the **acid mantle**, which slows the multiplication of microorganisms. Many bacteria are killed directly by

TEST YOUR UNDERSTANDING

1. Describe how hairs grow out of the skin.
2. Distinguish between eccrine and apocrine glands.

contact with bactericidal substances from the sebum and the **dermicidin** from the sweat. **Defensins** are natural substances secreted by skin cells that create holes in bacteria, helping to kill them. Protective peptides or *cathelicidins* are released by injured skin and are effective against many bacteria, but mostly against group A streptococci.

Physical barriers are created by skin continuity and hardened, keratinized cells. In the stratum corneum there are many layers of flat, dead cells surrounded by glycolipids along with the acid mantle and skin secretions to stop bacterial invasion. Water and water-soluble substances are largely kept from diffusing between cells by the glycolipids. Even so, a continual loss of small amounts of water occurs through the epidermis. In limited amounts, the following substances are able to penetrate the skin: lipid-soluble substances, oleoresins, organic solvents, heavy metal salts, certain drugs, and drug agents known as *penetration enhancers*. Lipid-soluble substances include carbon dioxide, oxygen, the fat-soluble vitamins (A, D, E, and K), and steroids such as estrogens.

Examples of *oleoresins* (plant resins) include poison oak and poison ivy. Organic solvents, which dissolve cell lipids, include acetone, dry-cleaning fluids, and paint thinner. Examples of heavy metal salts include lead and mercury. Drugs that can penetrate the skin include nicotine, nitroglycerine, and medications used to stop seasickness. Also, for at least 24 hours after being ingested, drinks containing alcohol enhance skin permeability to a large degree.

The body also has biologic barriers that act for its protection: the dendritic cells in the epidermis, the macrophages in the dermis, and the body's DNA. Dendritic cells are active immune system components that patrol the epidermis for *antigens* (foreign substances). The dendritic cells play the same role in the epidermis as the lymphocytes in the blood. The second line of biological barriers consists of the dermal macrophages, which function in much the same way as the dendritic cells. They dispose of bacteria and viruses that get past the epidermis. DNA is a fairly potent biologic sunscreen, and its electrons absorb UV radiation. This is transferred to the nuclei of DNA atoms, causing them to heat and vibrate quickly. The heat dissipates to nearby water molecules in an instant. Therefore, DNA converts possibly harmful UV radiation into heat, which has no negative effects in this example.

As mentioned previously, the skin is important in regulating body temperature. The deeper body parts are normally set at 98.6°F (which is equivalent to 37 degrees Celsius [°C]). Body heat is produced by cellular metabolism, with most body heat being produced by the skeletal and cardiac muscle cells as well as certain glandular cells (such as liver cells). As temperature rises, the body is stimulated to release body heat by relaxing dermal blood vessel walls. The eccrine sweat glands release sweat to the skin surface, which evaporates to cool the skin. The reverse process occurs when the body temperature drops. This holds heat in, and if the temperature continues to drop, the body signals certain muscles to contract. Shivering is the result, which helps to generate more body heat.

The sweat glands secrete about 17 ounces (500 mL) of sweat per day when the body is at rest and when the environmental temperature is below 88 to 90°F (31–32°C).

This normal, unnoticed sweating is described as *insensible perspiration*. The sweat glands greatly increase their activity when body temperature rises and the nervous system causes the dermal blood vessels to dilate. If the weather is hot, sweat becomes noticeable (*sensible perspiration*), accounting for up to 3 gallons (12 liters) of body water loss in a single day. As the sweat evaporates, the body is cooled and overheating is prevented. On cold days, dermal blood vessels constrict to cause the blood to temporarily bypass the skin. The skin temperature assumes the temperature of the external environment. Passive heat loss slows down, and the body conserves heat.

Sensory receptors are located in the dermis and are actually parts of the nervous system. They initiate nerve impulses that can reach our conscious awareness and are classified as *exteroceptors* because they respond to stimuli from outside the body. Nerve fibers in the skin control blood flow, adjust gland secretion rates, and monitor sensory receptors in the dermis and deeper layers of the epidermis. The epidermis also contains the extension of sensory neurons that provide sensations of pain and temperature. The dermis contains similar receptors and other, more specialized receptors (for example, sensations of touch and pressure). In the dermal papillae, *Meissner's (tactile) corpuscles* and *tactile discs* sense light surface touching. In the deeper dermis or hypodermis, *Pacinian* or *lamellar corpuscles* sense harder contacts that involve deep pressure. Even hair follicle receptors play a part in the sense of touch. Painful stimuli are sensed by free nerve endings located throughout the skin.

The skin also has many metabolic functions. It reacts to sunlight by converting modified cholesterol molecules to vitamin D precursors. These are carried by the blood to other areas of the body for conversion to vitamin D, which aids in calcium metabolism. Without vitamin D, calcium could not be absorbed from the gastrointestinal tract. Therefore, sunlight is essential so the bones can absorb calcium via the presence of vitamin D. The epidermis carries out chemical conversions that assist the liver. Keratinocyte enzymes play important roles related to cancer and inflammation. These enzymes can either convert harmless chemicals to carcinogens or disarm chemicals that are carcinogenic. They activate certain steroids, such as when they transform cortisone into hydrocortisone, which has strong anti-inflammatory properties. Other important proteins manufactured by skin cells include *collagenase*, which fights against wrinkling by stimulating the natural use and reuse of collagen.

The skin also acts as a blood reservoir and plays a role in excretion. Nearly 5% of the body's entire blood volume can be contained by the extensive vascular supply of the dermis. The nervous system constricts dermal blood vessels to supply more blood to other body organs that need this supply. More blood is moved into the general circulation by this constriction, and working muscles or other organs use it. Nitrogen-containing wastes are also eliminated through the sweat, although most of this elimination goes through the urine. These nitrogen-containing wastes include ammonia, urea, and uric acid. When sweating is profuse, water and sodium chloride (salt) are lost in large quantities.

TEST YOUR UNDERSTANDING

1.   What are the three types of skin protection?
2.   Explain metabolic skin functions.
3.   Describe the chemical agents that protect the skin.
4.   Why is sunlight essential for bone health?

Response of the Integument to Injuries and Wounds

The integument responds to injuries and wounds with inflammation, which causes redness, increased warmth, and painful swelling. The blood vessels of the wounded area dilate and allow fluids to leak into the damaged tissues. This provides more nutrients and oxygen to the tissues, aiding in healing. Shallow breaks in the skin cause epithelial cells to divide more rapidly, with the new cells filling the break.

A cut that extends into the dermis or subcutaneous layers breaks blood vessels. The escaping blood then forms a clot in the wound, eventually forming a *scab* as it dries. The scab protects the underlying tissues. Cells called *fibroblasts* move to the injury to form new collagenous fibers that bind the edges of the wound together. Large skin breaks may require suturing or other methods of closing them more completely, which actually helps to speed up the action of the fibroblasts in healing.

Wound healing proceeds as blood vessels extend into the area below the scab, with phagocytic cells removing dead cells and debris. As tissue is replaced, the scab eventually falls off. Extensive wounds may cause the newly formed tissue to appear on the skin surface as a *scar*. Large open wounds may develop small round masses called *granulations*, which consist of new blood vessel branches and clusters of fibroblasts. Once the fibroblasts eventually move away, the resultant scar is mostly composed of collagenous fibers.

If a wound is large or occurs in an area where the skin is thin, epithelial cells cannot cover the surface until dermal repairs are already under way. Circulation to the area is enhanced so that blood clotting, fibroblasts, and an extensive capillary network can combine to combat the injury. (Together, these components are known as *granulation tissue*.) Repairs do not restore the dermis to its original condition, and collagen fibers dominate with relatively few new blood vessels. *Scar tissue* is relatively inflexible and noncellular. Thickened, raised scar tissue is referred to as a *keloid*, featuring a shiny and smooth surface. Keloids are harmless but unsightly.

Effects of Aging on the Integumentary System

Damaged skin affects almost every body system. It leads to bone softening, impaired or accelerated metabolism, failure of the cardiovascular system, changes in immune function, and many other outcomes. Intact skin can greatly improve quality of life in later years. It protects the muscles, improving body temperature regulation and blood flow.

Nervous system organs such as touch receptors are protected by intact skin. It also protects endocrine organs, prevents fluid loss, regulates normal secretions, protects lymphatic organs to prevent edema, protects respiratory organs for adequate oxygen supply, protects digestive organs for nutrient absorption, protects urinary organs for proper excretion, and protects reproductive organ health.

The skin initially develops from either the embryonic ectoderm (epidermis) or the mesoderm (dermis and hypodermis). The skin is mostly formed by the end of the fourth month of gestation. The fetus is covered with delicate colorless hairs (the *lanugo coat*) during months 5 and 6 of gestation, but this coat disappears by the seventh month, replaced by vellus hairs. At birth, the newborn's skin is covered with *vernix caseosa*, a white substance that appears "cheese-like." It is produced by the sebaceous glands to protect the skin while the infant is still inside the mother's amnion. Small white spots appear on the forehead and nose (these are called *milia*), which are accumulations in the sebaceous glands. They usually disappear by the third week after birth. The skin thickens during infancy and childhood, with more subcutaneous fat being deposited. During adolescence, skin and hair both become oilier due to activation of the sebaceous glands. Acne may develop during this time, which usually subsides by early adulthood. The skin reaches its best appearance in a person's twenties and thirties. Later, when it shows the effects of abrasion, chemicals, sun, and wind, common conditions include scaling or *dermatitis* (skin inflammation). *Atopic dermatitis* or *eczema* is a genetic condition that is also exacerbated by environmental factors.

In older age, epidermal cells are replaced less quickly. The skin becomes thinner and is more susceptible to bruises and other injuries. It is less lubricated and often becomes dry and itchy. Clumping of elastic fibers occurs. There are less collagen fibers, and they also become stiffer. Older people are unable to tolerate colder temperatures as well because their subcutaneous fat layer diminishes. Fat distribution becomes more similar between men and women because they have lower levels of sex hormones than earlier in life. Wrinkling occurs due to decreased skin elasticity and less subcutaneous tissue. Incidence of skin cancer is higher because of decreased amounts of melanocytes and dendritic cells. Because they have less melanin than other people, fair-skinned and redheaded people usually show age-related changes more quickly. Hair thinning results by age 50, because active hair follicles are two-thirds less prevalent. The hair loses its luster, and the genes activate that trigger male pattern baldness and hair graying.

To slow skin aging, you should shield your skin from the aging UVA rays and the burning UVB rays of the sun. When protection from the sun is lifelong, aged skin will remain unwrinkled and unmarked, although it still thins and loses a certain amount of elasticity. Protective clothing and sunscreens or sunblocks of 15 (or higher) sun protection factors (SPFs) are encouraged. Although a nice tan may be appealing early in life, sunlight eventually causes the skin to sag, wrinkle, and become marked with pigmented "liver spots." UVA rays activate *matrix metalloproteinase* enzymes, degrading dermal components such as collagen. However, the skin aging process may be delayed by cleanliness, good nutrition, plenty of fluid consumption, and the drug *tretinoin* (Retin-A®). This agent is related to vitamin A and inhibits the matrix metalloproteinases. It is found in many skin creams designed to slow photo-aging.

In most people, signs of aging generally appear by their late forties. Signs of aging in the integumentary system include thinning, graying hair; dry hair and skin; thinning skin; sagging skin; bleeding within the skin; easier bruising; slower healing from injuries; and recurring infections. Body heat regulation varies because of atrophy of blood vessels, sweat glands, and subcutaneous fat. The skin may also show signs of yellowing, mottling, age spots, and wrinkling. The most serious condition affecting the skin during the aging process is skin cancer (discussed below). With age, germinative cell activity declines, Langerhans cells decrease, vitamin D_3 production decreases, melanocytes decline, glandular activity declines, dermal blood supply reduces, and many hormones reduce in level.

FOCUS ON PATHOLOGY

Eczema, or *atopic dermatitis,* is most common in patients with allergies or asthma and usually begins in infancy on the face, scalp, or knees. The condition spreads to other locations on the body with aging and causes severe itching, papules, and plaques. Eczema is an immune-mediated inflammation of the skin that is linked to both genetic and environmental factors. Diagnosis is by history and examination. Treatment involves moisturizers, topical corticosteroids, and avoidance of allergic and irritant triggers.

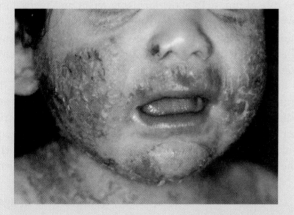

Eczema. (Courtesy of Dr. Richard Antaya, Dermatology Department, Yale University School of Medicine.)

TEST YOUR UNDERSTANDING

1. What is the vernix caseosa that covers the skin of a newborn baby?
2. Why are elderly people less able to tolerate cold temperatures?
3. Why do skin wrinkles develop because of the aging process?

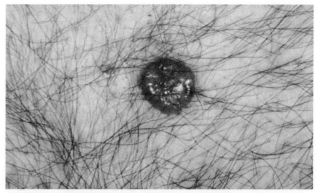

FIGURE 6-9 Basal cell carcinoma. (Courtesy of National Cancer Institute.)

Skin Cancer

Skin cancers originating from epithelial cells are called *cutaneous carcinomas* (squamous cell carcinomas or basal cell carcinomas), whereas those arising from melanocytes are *cutaneous melanomas* (melanocarcinomas or malignant melanomas). The UV rays of the sun can cause skin cancer, usually on the head and neck because they are the areas most exposed. Fair-skinned people and elderly people are the most likely candidates for skin cancer. The use of sunscreen or sunblock, minimum SPF-15, may protect against sunburn (including UVA and UVB rays) but not completely against skin cancer. Genetic factors and hormones may influence a person's chance for developing skin cancer. Although very common, skin cancer is one of the easiest forms of cancer to diagnose and treat. When detected and treated early, survival rates are high. The three types of skin cancer, named for the specific epidermal cells in which they originate, are as follows:

- *Basal cell carcinoma:* The most common yet least dangerous type, it begins in the stratum basale, invading the dermis. A small, shiny lesion appears as a "bump" on the skin, which enlarges to form a central depression with a beaded, pearl-like edge (**FIGURE 6-9**).
- *Squamous cell carcinoma:* It begins in the keratinocytes of the stratum spinosum; the lesion appears raised, reddened, and scaly, forming a concave ulcer with edges that are raised (**FIGURE 6-10**). Early detection

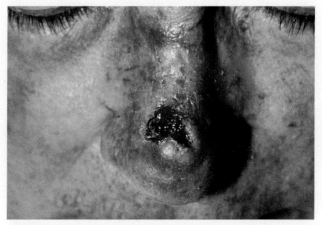

FIGURE 6-10 Squamous cell carcinoma. (Courtesy of National Cancer Institute.)

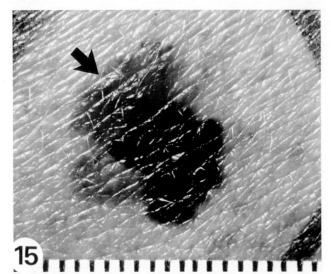

FIGURE 6-11 Malignant melanoma. (Courtesy of National Cancer Institute.)

TABLE 6-1

Rule of Nines

Surface Area of the Body	Percentage of Each Body Region
Anterior head and neck	4½
Posterior head and neck	4½
Anterior upper limbs	9
Posterior upper limbs	9
Anterior trunk	18
Posterior trunk	18
Anterior lower limbs	18
Posterior lower limbs	18
Perineum	1

and surgical removal raises the survival rate, but this cancer often metastasizes to the lymph nodes to become potentially fatal.

- *Malignant melanoma:* This much more serious form of skin cancer is increasing in incidence. It often starts in the melanocytes of a preexisting mole, metastasizing quickly. It is often fatal if not treated immediately. The lesion appears as a large, flat, dark-colored patch that spreads and has a "scalloped" border (**FIGURE 6-11**). According to the American Cancer Society, the *ABCD Rule* should be used for recognizing melanoma:

    Asymmetry: The two sides of a mole or pigmented spot do not match
    Border irregularity: The lesion's borders have indentations
    Color: There are several colors in the pigmented spot, such as black, brown, tan, and, occasionally, blue or red
    Diameter: The lesion is larger than a pencil eraser (approximately 6 mm in diameter)
    NOTE: Some cancer authorities also add an "E" to the ABCD Rule, which signifies "elevation" above the surface of the skin.

TEST YOUR UNDERSTANDING

1. What type of skin cancer is the most malignant?
2. What is the rule used for recognizing melanoma?

Burns

A **burn** is tissue damage caused by intense heat, chemicals, electricity, or radiation that kills cells and denatures cell proteins. The leading causes of accidental death are burns. They may occur because of fires, UV radiation, hot water, spills, radiation, strong acids or bases, or electrical shock. Burns may

cause death as a result of fluid loss, infection, and the toxic effects of burned tissue (known as *eschar*). A severely burned patient often dies from dehydration and electrolyte imbalance, which lead to renal failure and circulatory shock. Immediate intravenous infusion of lost fluids is required to save the lives of these patients.

In a burned adult, fluid loss volume is estimated by using the **rule of nines**, which assesses the percentage of the overall body that has been burned. The body is divided into 11 areas that basically each account for 9% of the overall body area, with an additional area accounting for the genital area (1%). **TABLE 6-1** summarizes an estimation of body burns by using the rule of nines. To allow for tissue repair and replace lost proteins, the burn patient requires thousands of daily food calories that are in excess of normal caloric requirements. This is provided by supplementary nutrition via intravenous and gastric tubing. Once stabilized, the next concern is infection. Widespread bacterial infection (sepsis) is the primary cause of death in burn victims. Although burned skin remains sterile for 24 hours, the destroyed skin barrier can then be easily penetrated by many different pathogens, which multiply quickly in this nutrient-rich environment. The immune system, by this point, has also become deficient.

Burns are classified into three types:

- *First-degree burns:* Involve only the epidermis; signified by redness, pain, and slight edema. These burns heal quickly and usually do not leave scars. Most sunburns are first-degree burns (**FIGURE 6-12**).
- *Second-degree (partial-thickness) burns:* Involve the epidermis and dermis but leave some of the dermis intact; they may appear red, tan, or white with blisters. Second-degree burns are very painful, are slow healing, and may leave scars. Serious sunburns and many scaldings are second-degree burns (**FIGURE 6-13**).
- *Third-degree (full-thickness) burns:* The epidermis and dermis are completely destroyed, and deeper

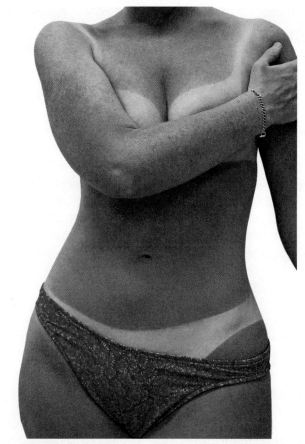

FIGURE 6-12 First-degree burn. (© Amy Walters/ShutterStock, Inc.)

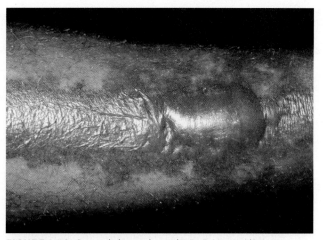

FIGURE 6-13 Second-degree burn. (© Dr P. Marazzi/Science Source)

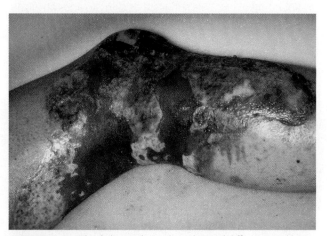

FIGURE 6-14 Third-degree burn. (© John Radcliffe Hospital/ Science Source)

tissue may even be damaged; the skin can repair itself only from the edges of the wound. These burns often require skin grafts, and if left to heal on their own may result in abnormal connective tissue fibrosis and severe disfigurement (**FIGURE 6-14**).

Burns are considered critical if over 25% of the body has second-degree burns, if over 10% of the body has third-degree burns, or if there are third-degree burns on the face, hands, or feet. A facial burn may include burning of the respiratory passageways, causing swelling and suffocation. Burned joints of the body can result in debilitating scar tissue, preventing mobility.

TEST YOUR UNDERSTANDING

1. Is sunburn *usually* an example of a first-degree, second-degree, or third-degree burn?
2. List the main causes of burns.

SUMMARY

The skin is also known as the *integument*, which means "covering." The integumentary system consists of the skin and its accessory structures (hair, nails, glands, muscles, and nerves). The skin is the largest organ of the body in surface area and weight. The major parts of the skin are the epidermis (which is not vascularized) and the dermis (which is highly vascularized). The subcutaneous layer (hypodermis) is deep below the dermis and not part of the skin.

Keratinocytes and melanocytes are the main cells in the epidermis. The keratinocytes produce keratin, which is the fibrous protein that aids the epidermis in protecting the body. The melanocytes produce melanin, which is the dark pigment that absorbs UV radiation from sunlight. The epidermal layers, from deep to superficial, are the stratum basale (also known as stratum germinativum), stratum spinosum, stratum granulosum, stratum lucidum, and stratum corneum. The stratum lucidum is located only on the soles and palms.

The dermis consists of papillary and reticular regions and lies between the epidermis and subcutaneous layer. The papillary region contains fine elastic fibers and dermal papillae. The reticular region is composed of connective tissue containing collagen, elastic fibers, fat tissue, hair follicles, nerves, sebaceous (oil) glands, and the ducts of sweat glands. The color of skin is due to melanin, carotene, and hemoglobin.

Skin functions include body temperature regulation, protection, sensation, excretion, absorption, and the synthesis of vitamin D. The skin participates in thermoregulation by liberating sweat at its surface. The skin provides physical, chemical, and biological barriers that help protect the body. Cutaneous sensations include touch, hot, cold, and pain.

Nails protect the ends of the fingers and toes and are modifications of the epidermis that contain hard keratin. Hairs (pili) project above the skin surfaces and are also dominated by hard keratin. Hairs are basically classified as either vellus or terminal, with terminal hairs being coarser, darker, and longer. Hair follicles have limited growth cycles and usually begin to slow their activity when a person is in his or her forties. The skin contains two types of exocrine glands: sebaceous (oil) and sudoriferous (sweat) glands.

The three primary skin barriers are the chemical, physical, and biological barriers. Chemical barriers include melanin and skin secretions. Skin continuity and hardened, keratinized cells create physical barriers. Biological barriers include the dendritic cells (epidermal), macrophages

(dermal), and the body's DNA. The skin is also important for regulating body temperature, providing touch reception, maintaining many metabolic functions, storing blood, and excreting a variety of substances.

The skin responds to injuries and wounds with inflammation, which causes redness, increased warmth, and painful swelling. Wound healing involves the processes of clotting, scabbing, collagenous fiber formation, revascularization, phagocytosis, scarring, and granulation tissue formation. Signs of skin aging usually appear when a person is in his or her late forties and include thinned gray hair, dry hair and skin, thin and sagging skin, bleeding inside skin, easier bruising, slower healing, and recurring infections. Protecting the skin from excessive UV radiation should continue throughout life to limit the amount of skin damage, wrinkling, sagging, and unsightly marking that might occur.

The three types of skin cancers are basal cell carcinoma, squamous cell carcinoma, and malignant melanoma. Malignant melanoma is the least common but most dangerous form because of its tendency to metastasize quickly. Burns are caused by intense heat, chemicals, electricity, or radiation that kills cells and denatures cell proteins. They are the leading causes of accidental death, which actually occurs after the burn due to dehydration, electrolyte imbalance, renal failure, and circulatory shock. First-degree burns most frequently occur from sunburns, whereas second-degree burns are often from scalding or severe sunburns. Third-degree burns often require skin grafts and usually cause severe disfigurement.

KEY TERMS

Acid mantle
Basal lamina
Burn
Ceruminous glands
Cleavage lines
Cuticle
Defensins
Dendritic cells
Dermicidin
Dermis
Desmosomes
Epidermis
Flexure lines

Hair bulb
Hair follicles
Hair matrix
Hyponychium
Integumentary system
Keratinocytes
Melanin
Melanocytes
Melanosomes
Nail folds
Papillary layer
Rule of nines
Sebaceous follicles

Sebaceous glands
Sebum
Sensory receptors
Stratum basale
Stratum corneum
Stratum germinativum
Stratum granulosum
Stratum lucidum
Stratum spinosum
Subcutaneous layer
Sweat glands (sudoriferous glands)
Tactile cells
Tyrosinase

The following learning goals correspond to the objectives at the beginning of this chapter:

1. The epidermis is the outer skin layer, made up of stratified squamous epithelium. The dermis is the inner layer and is much thicker than the epidermis. The dermis consists of papillary and reticular regions and is connected to the epidermis by a basement membrane.

2. Differences in skin color are based on the amount of melanin produced and how it is distributed throughout the skin. Well-oxygenated blood makes light-skinned people appear pinker, whereas poorly oxygenated blood makes them appear bluer. The build-up of bilirubin makes the skin appear yellowish.

3. The skin protects the body and helps to maintain homeostasis. It also aids in the regulation of body temperature, slows water loss from deep tissues, synthesizes biochemicals, excretes certain wastes, and contains sensory receptors. It also helps to produce vitamin D and to stimulate the development of white blood cells known as T lymphocytes.

4. Nails consist of a nail plate above a skin surface called the nail bed. The part of the nail plate that grows most actively is covered by a whitish, half-moon–shaped lunula, where epithelial cells divide and become keratinized. The nail cells push forward over the nail bed, causing the nail to continually grow outward.

5. Skin glands include sebaceous glands and sweat (sudoriferous) glands. Sebaceous glands are primarily located near hair follicles and secrete sebum, an oily mixture of fatty material and cell debris. Sebum helps to keep both hair and skin pliable and waterproof. Sweat (sudoriferous) glands originate in the deep dermis or superficial subcutaneous layers, and secrete sweat. The two types of sweat glands are merocrine (eccrine) and apocrine glands. Sweat is carried out of the skin through the pores and is made up of water, salt, and waste products such as urea and uric acid. Modified sweat glands include the ceruminous glands of the ear (which produce earwax) and the mammary glands (which produce milk).

6. The sweat glands help to regulate body temperature by releasing sweat to the skin surface, which evaporates to cool the skin.

7. The three most common forms of skin cancer are as follows:
   - *Basal cell carcinoma:* The least dangerous type, it appears as a small, shiny lesion and "bump" on the skin, which enlarges to form a central depression with a beaded, pearl-like edge.
   - *Squamous cell carcinoma:* The lesion appears raised, reddened, and scaly, forming a concave ulcer with edges that are raised. Early detection and surgical removal raises the survival rate, but this cancer often metastasizes to the lymph nodes to become potentially fatal.
   - *Malignant melanoma:* The least common yet most dangerous type, it metastasizes quickly and is often fatal if not treated immediately. The lesion appears as a large, flat, dark-colored patch that spreads and has a "scalloped" border.

8. Sebaceous glands are located near hair follicles and secrete sebum to lubricate the skin and hair. Ceruminous glands are located in the ears and secrete earwax.

9. A hair is made up of a root and a shaft. Hairs develop from epidermal cells at the base of tube-like hair follicles that extend from the skin surface into the dermis. The hair roots are nourished with dermal blood. Each hair follicle is attached to an arrector pili muscle, which helps the hair shaft to stand on end. Hairs are pushed upward, becoming keratinized and then dying. Hair shafts are actually composed of dead epidermal cells. Hair is found in most areas of the body.

10. Signs of aging in the integumentary system include the following:
    - The hair becomes thin, gray, and dry.
    - The skin becomes thinner, saggy, and less resistant to bleeding within the skin and bruising. It also heals more slowly from injuries and may experience recurring infections. The skin may also become yellowed, mottled, wrinkled, and marked with age spots.
    - Body heat regulation changes due to atrophy of blood vessels, sweat glands, and subcutaneous fat.

CRITICAL THINKING QUESTIONS

A 10-year-old boy who lived in Florida his entire life was diagnosed with melanoma. The boy previously had a mole that was ignored.

1. Why is melanoma the deadliest type of skin cancer?

2. List the methods that may be used to reduce likelihood of developing melanoma.

3. How is melanoma differentiated from the other types of skin cancer discussed in this chapter?

REVIEW QUESTIONS

1. Which of the following layers of the epidermis is found only on the skin of the soles of the feet and palms of the hands?
   A. stratum germinativum
   B. stratum granulosum
   C. stratum spinosum
   D. stratum lucidum

2. The most abundant cells in the epidermis are
   A. melanocytes
   B. keratinocytes
   C. adipocytes
   D. leukocytes

3. Which of the following glands discharge an oily secretion into the hair follicles?
   A. merocrine sweat glands
   B. sebaceous glands
   C. apocrine sweat glands
   D. ceruminous glands

4. The nail body covers the
   A. nail bed
   B. nail root
   C. free edge
   D. lunula

5. The highest concentration of merocrine sweat glands can be found
   A. on the palms of the hands
   B. on the chest
   C. on the upper back
   D. in the axillae

6. Which of the following vitamins is formed in the skin when it is exposed to sunlight?
   A. vitamin A
   B. vitamin B
   C. vitamin C
   D. vitamin D

7. Which of the following is a true statement about merocrine sweat glands?
   A. They primarily function in lubricating hairs.
   B. They secrete a watery fluid directly onto the surface of the skin.
   C. They increase in number and activity with aging.
   D. They produce a toxin that destroys bacteria.

8. An albino individual lacks the ability to produce
   A. carotene
   B. melanin
   C. keratin
   D. vitamin D

9. The cutaneous membrane includes which of the following components?
   A. epidermis and hypodermis
   B. integument and dermis
   C. epidermis and dermis
   D. epidermis and superficial fascia

10. Which layer of the epidermis undergoes cell division?
    A. stratum germinativum
    B. stratum granulosum
    C. stratum spinosum
    D. stratum corneum

11. Nails begin growing at the nail
    A. cuticle
    B. root
    C. body
    D. bed

12. A mammary gland is one type of
    A. ceruminous gland
    B. merocrine sweat gland
    C. apocrine sweat gland
    D. eccrine sweat gland

13. Which of the following layers of the skin provides initial protection against bacteria?
    A. subcutaneous layer
    B. dermis
    C. stratum corneum
    D. epidermis
14. The region of the dermis that is in direct contact with the epidermis is the
    A. papillary region
    B. stratum corneum
    C. hypodermis
    D. reticular region

15. Which of the following statements about the function of the skin is false?
    A. It helps regulate body temperature.
    B. It participates in the synthesis of vitamin D.
    C. It is waterproof.
    D. It detects stimuli related to temperature and pain.

ESSAY QUESTIONS

1. Distinguish between sensible and insensible perspiration.
2. Which layer of the epidermis is the thickest, and what is its role?
3. Describe the process of hair formation.
4. Explain melanin, carotene, and hemoglobin.
5. Which epidermal cells are referred to as prickle cells?

6. What is the cause of skin wrinkling?
7. Distinguish first-, second-, and third-degree burns.
8. What condition may cause horizontal Beau's lines across the nails?
9. Distinguish between vellus and terminal hair.
10. What is the role of the sebaceous glands in the skin?

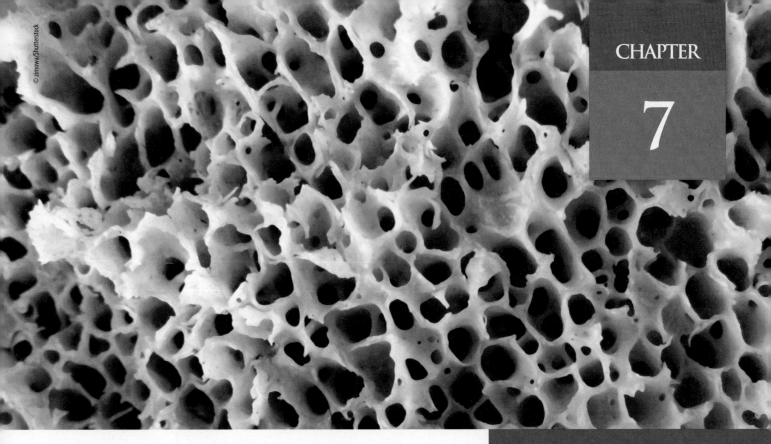

© zinowa/Shutterstock

Bone Tissues and the Skeletal System

OBJECTIVES

After studying this chapter, readers should be able to:

1. Discuss the major functions of bones.
2. Discuss bone classifications and give examples of each.
3. Distinguish between the axial and appendicular skeletons.
4. Identify the major features of the bones that compose the thoracic cage and the upper limbs.
5. Distinguish the major parts of a long bone.
6. List the substances normally stored in bone tissue.
7. Name each of the bones of the cranium.
8. Explain how the structures of cervical, thoracic, and lumbar vertebrae differ.
9. Name each of the bones of the lower limbs.
10. List the bones of the ankle and identify the largest of these.

OUTLINE

Overview

The skeletal system is made up of bone tissue, cartilage, blood, dense connective tissue, and nervous tissue. Bones function in many different ways and are made up of living tissue. Bones attach to muscles, protect softer tissues, contain cells that produce blood, store salts, and form blood vessels and nerve passageways. Bones support the weight of the body and also work with muscles to maintain body position and control precise movements. Muscle fibers could not make the body sit, walk, run, or stand if there was no skeleton to pull against.

Classifications of Bones

The bones of the skeleton are divided into the axial and appendicular groups. The **axial skeleton** makes up the body's long axis and includes the bones that comprise the skull, vertebral column, and rib cage, which function to protect and support various body parts. The **appendicular skeleton** is formed by the bones of the upper and lower limbs and the girdles (shoulder and hip bones), which attach the limbs to the axial skeleton (**FIGURE 7-1**). The sizes of bones vary greatly in the human body, from the tiny inner ear bones to the femur or thighbone, which may be approximately 2 feet in length. Each unique bone shape serves a certain function. Every adult skeleton contains 206 major bones, which are classified based on their individual shapes, as follows:

- *Flat bones*: These resemble plates, with broad surfaces, and include the ribs, sternum or breastbone, scapulae or shoulder blades, and most skull bones. They provide protection for underlying soft tissues and may be thin and slightly curved.
- *Irregular bones*: Irregular bones have different and complex shapes and are often connected to other bones. They include many facial bones and those that make up the vertebrae in the spine and the pelvis.
- *Short bones*: Small and often cube-shaped, short bones include the carpal (wrist) bones and tarsal (ankle) bones.
- *Long bones*: These have long bone shafts with expanded ends and are much longer than they are wide and are named for their elongated shape instead of their actual size. For example, the three bones of each finger are long bones, even though they are relatively small. All bones of the limbs are long bones, except for the patella (kneecap) and the bones of the wrists and ankles. Long bones are located in the arms, legs, palms, soles, fingers, and toes. The femur bone is an example of a long bone (**FIGURE 7-2**).
- *Sutural bones*: Also known as *Wormian bones*, these are the small, flat, and irregular bones between the flat bones of the skull. They range in size from as large as a quarter to as small as a grain of sand.

- *Sesamoid bones*: These are small, flat bones resembling sesame seeds that are most often located near joints of the hands, knees, and feet. The *patellae* are sesamoid bones. This type of bone may form in up to 26 locations in the body. Each individual has different numbers of sesamoid bones. Some help to control the directions in which tendons pull, and some have unknown functions.

FOCUS ON PATHOLOGY

The carpal tunnel is a narrow passageway formed from ligament and bones at the base of the hand, containing the median nerve and various tendons. Thickening or swelling due to tendon irritation from overuse narrows the tunnel, compressing the median nerve. Symptoms usually begin gradually but lead to tingling, numbness, and then sharp pain that becomes greatest at night. Grasping objects becomes difficult. These symptoms identify *carpal tunnel syndrome*. People who continually work with computer keyboards often develop the condition.

TEST YOUR UNDERSTANDING

1. Compare the structures and functions of the axial skeleton with the appendicular skeleton.
2. List the classifications of bones.
3. Give examples of long, short, flat, irregular, and sesamoid bones.

Structures of Bones

Bones are considered organs because they contain various types of tissue. They are dominated by osseous (bony) tissue but also contain nervous tissue, cartilage, fibrous connective tissue, and both muscle and epithelial tissues. Nervous tissue is found in bone nerves, whereas cartilage is found in articular cartilages. Fibrous connective tissue lines bone cavities, and both muscle and epithelial tissues are found in the blood vessels of bones.

Gross Anatomy

The external layer of bones is called **compact bone**, which contains **spongy bone** that is made up of small flat or needle-like pieces called **trabeculae** (**FIGURE 7-3**). It appears smooth and solid to the naked eye. Open spaces between trabeculae are filled with red and yellow bone **marrow**. Spongy bone is made up of open struts and plates, covered by a thin

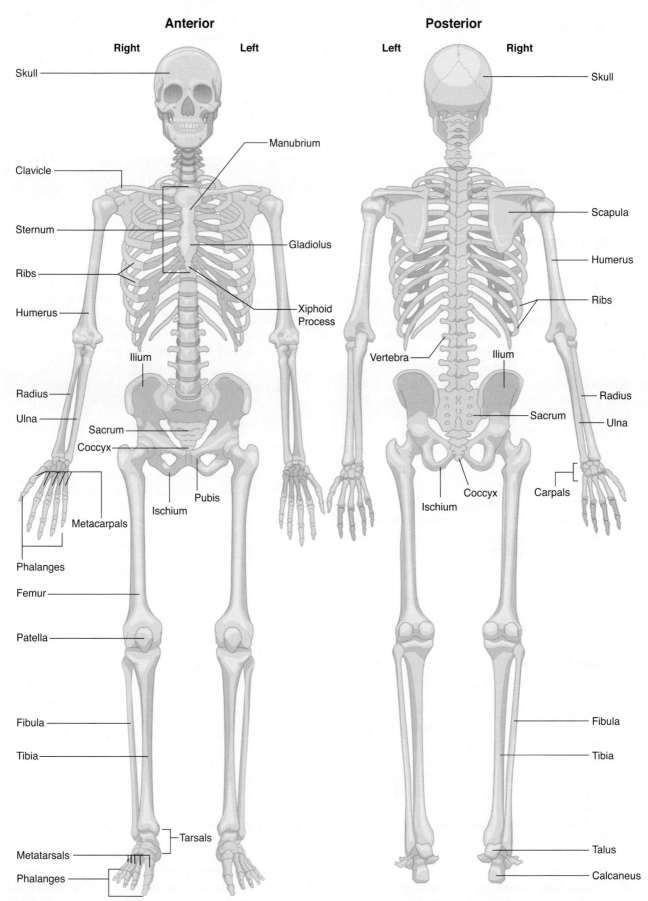

FIGURE 7-1 Anterior and posterior views of the human skeleton showing the normal position of each bone (© Jones & Bartlett Learning)

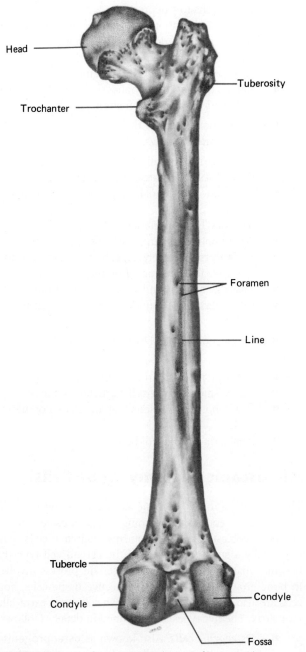

FIGURE 7-2 Femur showing general types of bone markings.

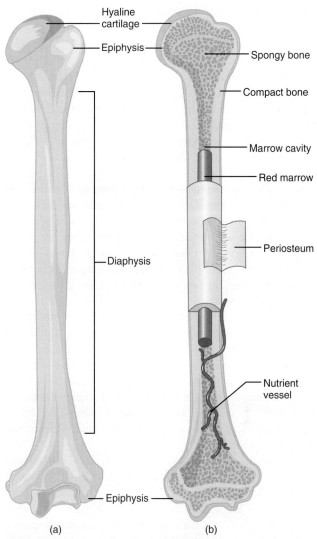

FIGURE 7-3 Anatomy of long bones. (A) Drawing of the humerus. Notice the long shaft and dilated ends. (B) Longitudinal section of the humerus showing compact bone, spongy bone, and marrow.

cortex of compact bone. This covering is also referred to as *cortical bone*.

Bones described as short, irregular, or flat are all made up of thin plates of spongy bone covered by compact bone. The plates are covered by connective tissue membranes (the *periosteum* outside and the *endosteum* inside). These bones have no shaft or epiphyses because they are not cylindrical. Inside, they have bone marrow between their trabeculae, although there is not a well-formed marrow cavity. Hyaline cartilage covers the surfaces of these bones where they form movable joints with nearby bones. The spongy bone in flat bones is called the **diploe**.

Nearly all long bones have the structure of a *shaft, bone ends,* and *membranes.* The shaft is known as the **diaphysis**.

It is a tubular structure forming the long bone axis, made of a thick collar of compact bone surrounding a central *medullary cavity.* This cavity is called the *yellow marrow cavity* in adults because it contains fat (yellow marrow).

The bone ends are called **epiphyses**, which are usually broader than the diaphysis. Inside, they have spongy bone, whereas their outer shell is made of compact bone. The joint surface of each epiphysis is covered by a thin layer of hyaline cartilage. This layer cushions opposing bone ends as they move and absorbs stress. Between the diaphysis and each epiphysis of long bones is an *epiphyseal line*, which is a leftover remnant of the **epiphyseal plate**. There is also a disc of hyaline cartilage that develops during childhood, lengthening the bone. At the point where the diaphysis and epiphysis meet is a flared portion that is sometimes referred to as the *metaphysis*.

The external surface of a bone, except for the joint surfaces, is covered by a shiny, white, and double-layered

periosteum, a membrane that is richly supplied with blood vessels and nerve fibers. Dense irregular connective tissue makes up the outer *fibrous layer*. Inside, an *osteogenic layer* touches the bone surface and is made up mostly of primitive stem cells known as *osteogenic cells*. These cells form all bone cells except for those that function in bone destruction. The blood vessels and nerve fibers of the periosteum pass through the bone shaft, entering the marrow cavity through openings known as *nutrient foramina*. Groups of collagen fibers called *perforating fibers* or *Sharpey's fibers* extend from the fibrous layer into the bone matrix and bind the periosteum to the underlying bone. The periosteum also serves to anchor tendons and ligaments in areas that are extremely dense. *Metaphyseal vessels* supply blood to the diaphyseal surface of the epiphyseal cartilages where they are being replaced by bone. *Periosteal vessels* provide blood to the superficial osteons of the bone shafts. During endochondral bone formation, they branch to enter the epiphyses and provide blood to the secondary ossification centers.

The **endosteum** is a delicate connective tissue membrane covering internal bone surfaces. In most trabecular cavities of spongy bone (in long bones) and in the diploe of flat bones is found hematopoietic **red marrow**. As a result, both of these cavities are referred to as *red marrow cavities*. The endosteum covers the trabeculae of spongy bone and lines canals that pass through compact bone. The endosteum also contains osteogenic cells, which may differentiate into various bone cells.

In the newborn, red bone marrow is found in the medullary cavity of the diaphysis as well as all areas of spongy bone. In adults, most long bones have a medullary cavity that contains fat, which extends a good length into the epiphysis. Very little red marrow is found in an adult's spongy bone cavities. As a result, red blood cell production in adult long bones usually occurs only in the heads of the femur and humerus. There is a greater amount of hematopoietic activity in the red marrow of the diploe of flat bones (such as the sternum) and certain irregular bones (such as the hipbones). **Yellow marrow** in the medullary cavity can convert back to red marrow if there is significant anemia, requiring more red blood cells.

Bone Markings

External surfaces of bones usually have depressions, projections, and openings. These *bone markings* are where ligaments, muscles, and tendons attach, or they may occur at joint surfaces. They also may serve as conduits for nerves and blood vessels. Projections bulge outward from bone surfaces, and include heads, spines, trochanters, and others. Each of these has its own unique features. Most bone projections show stresses caused by attached muscles or are modified surfaces where the bones meet and form articulations.

Depressions and openings in bones allow for passage of nerves and blood vessels and include the following:

- *Fissures:* narrow, slit-like openings
- *Foramina:* oval or round openings through bones

- *Grooves:* shallow depressions
- *Notches:* indentations at the edges of structures
- *Fossae:* shallow depressions in bones that often serve as articular surfaces
- *Meatuses:* passageways that resemble canals
- *Sinuses:* cavities inside bones that are filled with air and lined with mucous membranes

Bone projections that are the sites where muscles and ligaments attach are as follows:

- *Crests:* narrow, usually prominent ridges of bone
- *Epicondyles:* raised areas on or above condyles
- *Lines:* narrow ridges of bone that are not as prominent as crests
- *Processes:* bony prominences
- *Spines:* pointed, sharp, or slender projections
- *Trochanters:* extremely large, blunt, irregular shaped processes that only occur on the femurs
- *Tubercles:* small rounded projections or processes
- *Tuberosities:* large rounded projections that may be rough

Bone projections that help to form joints include the following:

- *Condyles:* rounded articular projections
- *Facets:* smooth, almost flat articular surfaces
- *Heads:* bony expansions that are carried on narrow necks
- *Rami:* arm-like bars of bone

Microscopic Anatomy (Bone Cells)

The five major types of bone cells are osteogenic cells, osteoblasts, osteocytes, bone lining cells, and osteoclasts. All except osteoblasts originate from mesenchymal cells. Each is basically a specialized form of the certain cell type that becomes mature or functions in a certain process involved in bone growth. Like various connective tissue cells, bone cells are also surrounded by their own self-made extracellular matrix. The five types are explained in detail as follows:

- *Osteogenic cells*: Also known as **osteoprogenitor cells**, these mitotically active stem cells are found in the periosteum and endosteum. They are squamous or flattened cells when bones are growing. Stimulation of these cells causes them to often differentiate into osteoblasts or bone lining cells. Others may remain osteogenic cells (**FIGURE 7-4**).
- *Osteoblasts*: These cells produce bone matrix and are related to osteoprogenitor cells, **osteocytes**, fibroblasts, and chondroblasts. They are mitotic and become active with connective tissue layers, depositing bony matrix around them. Spongy bone tissue forms in all directions within the layers of connective tissues. They secrete an unmineralized bone matrix, which includes collagen (which makes up the majority of bone protein) and calcium-binding proteins that form the original unmineralized bone (**osteoid**). They also aid in matrix

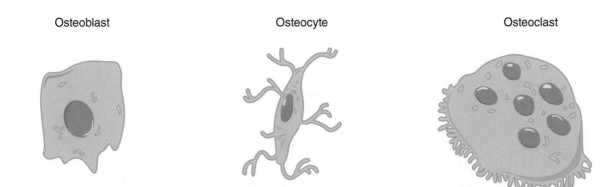

Osteoblast **Osteocyte** **Osteoclast**

FIGURE 7-4 Osteogenic cells

calcification. Osteoblasts are cube shaped when they are depositing matrix but appear similar to flattened osteogenic cells when inactive. They may also differentiate into bone lining cells. Osteoblasts become osteocytes when they are totally surrounded by the matrix they are secreting.

- *Osteocytes:* These are mature osteoblasts that have become embedded in the bone matrix. They occupy small cavities (**lacunae**) in the bone and have protoplasmic projections connected with the same structure of other osteocytes. The osteocytes conform to the shapes of the lacunae. These connections form a system of tiny canals within the bone matrix and act to maintain it as needed. When osteocytes die, the matrix surrounding them is resorbed. They also react to strain or stress and respond to stimuli such as bone deformation, bone loading, and weightlessness. The osteocytes alert the osteoblasts and osteoclasts to build up or degrade the bone matrix as needed. This preserves calcium homeostasis.
- *Bone lining cells:* These are flat cells on bone surfaces where bone remodeling does not occur and are believed to also help maintain the bone matrix. On external bone surfaces, they are also called *periosteal cells.* When they line internal surfaces, they are called *endosteal cells.*
- *Osteoclasts:* These are large, multinucleated bone cells found at sites of bone resorption, which is also called *osteolysis.* They form from the hematopoietic stem cells that also differentiate into macrophages. During fractures and bone healing and certain disease processes, osteoclasts use enzymes to excavate passages (*resorption bays*) through surrounding tissue, breaking down the calcified extracellular matrix. At this point, they have an *irregular border* that contacts bone directly. This border has deep plasma membrane infoldings that greatly increase the surface area for bone degradation via enzyme activity. The infoldings also close off the surface area from the matrix surrounding it. Osteoclasts are also known as *osteophages.* They secrete an acid that dissolves the matrix. Osteoclasts resorb bone matrix throughout life, replacing it with osteoblasts. These opposing

processes (resorption and deposition) are regulated by hormones that control blood calcium.

- *Compact bone:* Bone cells called osteocytes occupy small chambers (lacunae) that create concentric circles around central canals in bones (**FIGURE 7-5**). Cellular processes passing through canaliculi (microscopic canals) allow osteocytes to communicate with other cells. Bone tissue is mostly made up of collagen and inorganic salts such as calcium phosphate. Calcium phosphate interacts with calcium hydroxide to form crystals of *hydroxyapatite.* These crystals incorporate various calcium salts as well as ions, such as fluoride, magnesium, and sodium. Compact bones have a central canal that helps to make up cylinder-shaped osteons (**Haversian systems**). The **osteons** are parallel to the bone's long axis, aid in weight bearing, and are the structural units of compact bone. Each osteon consists of a group of hollow tubes of bone matrix that appear like the rings in a tree trunk. Each **lamella** (matrix tube) lends its name to the other description of compact bone, which is **lamellar bone**. The collagen fibers of each lamella run in one direction, whereas those in nearby lamellae run in different directions. This alteration of collagen fiber placement strengthens compact bone and resists twisting motions. Between collagen fibrils, bone salt crystals also are aligned with directional alterations. Each central canal contains nerve fibers, blood vessels, and surrounding connective tissue. The central canals are connected by perforating **Volkmann's canals**, which contain larger nerves and blood vessels. The Volkmann's canals lie at right angles to the long axis of the bone. They are not surrounded by concentric lamellae but are lined with endosteum. At the junctions of the lamellae are spider-shaped osteocytes occupying the *lacunae.* Thin, hair-like *canaliculi* connect lacunae to each other and to the central canal. During bone formation, the osteoblasts that secrete bone matrix surround blood vessels and stay in contact with each other, as well as nearby osteocytes, via projections that extend outward. Each of these

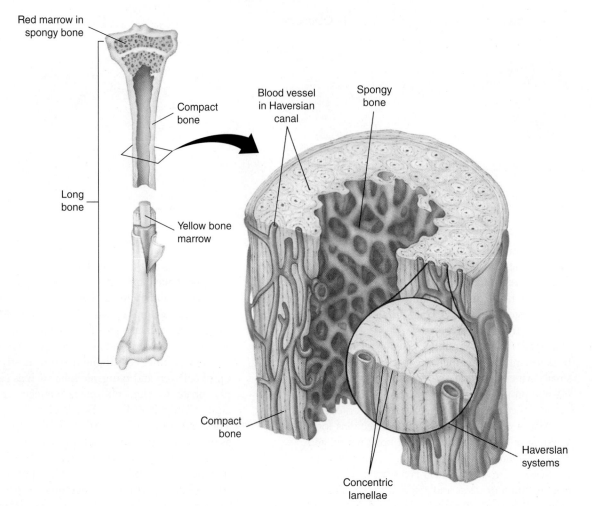

FIGURE 7-5 The microscopic structure of a long bone

extensions contains gap junctions. As the matrix hardens, a system of canaliculi is formed, containing tissue fluid and the osteocytes' extensions. A mature osteon is then bound together, and both nutrients and wastes can move from one osteocyte to the next. The bone matrix therefore allows bone cells to receive nourishment while it still remains hard and impermeable. However, some lamellae in compact bone are not part of complete osteons. Between osteons are incomplete *interstitial lamellae* that either fill gaps or are leftover structures of previous osteons that experienced bone remodeling. Deep to the periosteum, just superficial to the endosteum, are **circumferential lamellae**, which extend completely around the diaphysis, helping the long bone to resist twisting.

■ *Spongy bone:* This type of bone is similarly composed to compact bone, but its cells do not aggregate around the central canals. The cells in spongy bone lie inside the *trabeculae* (supporting structures of dense tissue) and take their nutrients from diffused substances that enter the canaliculi. The trabeculae are only a few cells thick. They have irregular lamellae and osteocytes, interconnected

by canaliculi, and no osteons are present. Nutrients reach spongy bone osteocytes via diffusion through the canaliculi from capillaries in the endosteum that surround the trabeculae.

| TEST YOUR UNDERSTANDING |

1. Compare the structure of compact bone with spongy bone.
2. List various types of bone cells and their functions.

Chemical Composition of Bone

Organic components of bones include osteogenic cells, osteoblasts, bone lining cells, osteocytes, osteoclasts, and *osteoid*. Nearly one-third of the matrix is made up of the osteoid. The osteoid includes proteoglycans and glycoproteins (making up its ground substance) and collagen fibers, both the ground substance and the collagen fibers are made and secreted by osteoblasts. Collagen is the greater contributor to the structure of bones and to their flexibility and tensile strength. *Sacrificial bonds* inside or between collagen molecules appear to aid in bone resilience. Because they can stretch and break easily when impacted, energy is exhausted. This helps to avoid an actual bone fracture. Most sacrificial bonds reform when trauma is discontinued, over time.

The **inorganic components** of bone are made up of *hydroxyapatites* or *mineral salts*, which make up 65% of bone mass. Mostly made of calcium phosphates, these components are needle-shaped crystals packed tightly in and around the collagen fibers of the extracellular matrix. They are responsible for bone hardness and the ability of bone to resist compression. Combined with organic components of bone, inorganic components provide strength while keeping bones from becoming brittle. Healthy bones may be more easily compressed when they are able to resist tension. They are as strong as steel in resisting tension. Mineral salts in bones make them able to retain their mass even after death, for many years. The long bones of a cadaver still display horizontal growth arrest lines, giving a visible proof of certain illnesses.

Growth and Development of Bones

Bones begin to form in utero during the first 8 weeks after fertilization. Intramembranous bones originate between layers of connective tissues that are sheet-like in appearance. Examples of intramembranous bones are the flat, broad bones of the skull. These bones, also called *dermal bones*, begin development when unspecialized connective tissues form at the sites where future bones will be developed. Bone-forming cells (osteoblasts) develop, depositing bony matrix around them. When extracellular matrix has surrounded the osteoblasts, they are termed *osteocytes*. The surrounding membranous tissues begin to form the periosteum of a bone. Inside the periosteum, the osteoblasts form a compact bone layer over the new spongy bone.

Endochondral bones begin as cartilaginous masses that are eventually replaced by bone tissue. These bones develop from hyaline cartilage that is shaped similarly to the bones they will become (**FIGURE 7-6**). They grow rapidly at first and then begin to change in appearance. When spongy bone begins to replace the original cartilage, a primary ossification center is created, with bone tissue developing outward toward the ends of the structure. Eventually, secondary ossification centers appear in the epiphyses, forming more spongy bone.

During the first 8 weeks of development, the skeleton is cartilaginous. The bones increase greatly in size as the fetus develops and throughout childhood (**FIGURE 7-7**). Bone growth continues through adolescence. The process of replacing other tissues with bone is called **ossification**, which involves the deposition of calcium salts. In embryos, ossification (as well as osteogenesis) leads to formation of the skeleton. Later in development, *bone growth* occurs until early adulthood. Throughout life, the bones can become thicker. *Osteogenesis* is defined as the formation of bone.

The skeleton of a human embryo, before week 8 of gestation, is made of fibrous membranes and hyaline cartilage.

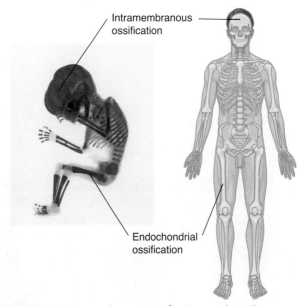

FIGURE 7-6 Intramembranous ossification results in the development of flat bones. Endochondral ossification results in the production of long bones. (Photo: © Ralph Hutchings/Visuals Unlimited)

At week 8 bone tissue begins to develop, replacing most existing cartilage or fibrous structures over time. For example, the long bones are first formed of hyaline cartilage and later replaced by bony tissue that becomes compact bone. This process begins with the diaphysis and ends with the epiphyses of each long bone. This process of bone formation is called *endochondral ossification*. Cartilage is also referred to as *endochondral bone*.

Nearly all bones below the base of the skull (except the clavicles) are formed by endochondral ossification. At month 2 of gestation, hyaline cartilages previously formed are used as models for actual bones. Endochondral ossification is more complicated than intramembranous ossification because hyaline cartilage is broken down while ossification is occurring. For long bones the center of a hyaline cartilage shaft (the *primary ossification center*) is where ossification begins. Blood vessels form in the perichondrium that covers the hyaline cartilage bone model and convert it to a vascularized periosteum. As nutrients become more plentiful, underlying mesenchymal cells specialize to become osteoblasts. This becomes the basis for ossification.

Bone collars form around the diaphysis of the hyaline cartilage models, as osteoblasts secrete osteoid against the hyaline cartilage diaphysis. They enclose it in a collar-like structure known as the *periosteal bone collar*. In the center of the diaphysis, the cartilage calcifies, developing cavities. Chondrocytes in the shaft enlarge (hypertrophy), which leads to surrounding cartilage matrix to calcify. Because this matrix cannot be penetrated by diffusing nutrients, chondrocytes die. The matrix deteriorates, opening up cavities. The bone collar stabilizes the hyaline cartilage model. In other locations the cartilage is still healthy, growing quickly, which lengthens the cartilage model.

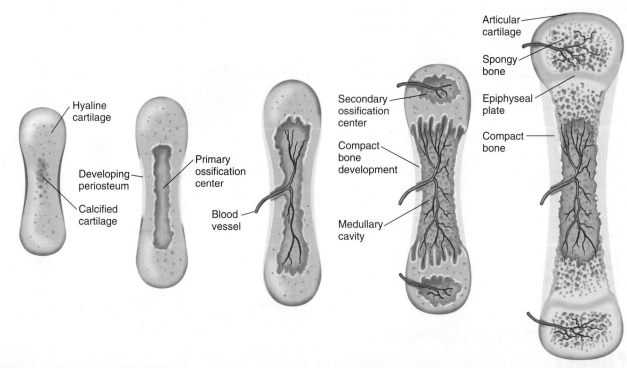

FIGURE 7-7 The major stages in the development of an endochondral bone. (Adapted from Shier, D. N., Butler, J. L., and Lewis, R. Hole's Essentials of Human Anatomy & Physiology, Tenth edition. McGraw-Hill Higher Education, 2009.)

By the third month, the cavities are invaded by elements collectively known as the *periosteal bud*. This contains a nutrient artery and vein, red marrow elements, nerve fibers, osteoclasts, and osteogenic cells. The calcified cartilage matrix is partially eroded by the osteoclasts. The osteogenic cells become osteoblasts, secreting osteoid around calcified fragment of hyaline cartilage. This forms a bone-covered cartilage trabeculae. Therefore, an early version of spongy bone develops in the long bone.

Osteoclasts break down the new spongy bone as the primary ossification center enlarges. A medullary cavity is opened in the center of the diaphysis. From week 9 until birth, the quickly growing epiphyses are made only of cartilage. The hyaline cartilage models continue lengthening via division of viable cartilage cells at the epiphyses. Down the length of the shaft, cartilage calcifies, erodes, and is replaced by spiked bone structures on epiphyseal surfaces that face the medullary cavity.

At birth, most long bones have a bony diaphysis that surrounds spongy bone remnants, a medullary cavity that is widening, and two epiphyses made of cartilage. *Secondary ossification centers* develop in one or both epiphyses just before or just after birth. Usually, secondary centers form in both epiphyses of larger long bones. In smaller long bones, usually only one secondary ossification center forms. The central cartilage of the epiphysis calcifies and deteriorates. Cavities open, allowing a periosteal bud to enter. Bone trabeculae appear similar to how they appeared in the primary ossification center. Short bones develop differently in that only the primary ossification center is formed, and most irregular bones have several distinct ossification centers from which they develop.

Secondary ossification is very similar to primary ossification, except for interior spongy bone being retained and the lack of a medullary cavity being formed in the epiphyses. Hyaline cartilage remains only on the epiphyseal surfaces (as articular cartilages) and at the junction of diaphyses and epiphyses (forming epiphyseal plates) when secondary ossification is complete.

Flat bones are not formed in the same way as long bones. Flat bones develop from fibrous connective tissue membranes (formed by mesenchymal cells) that are replaced by spongy bone and then compact bone in a process is called *intramembranous ossification*. The produced bones are also referred to as *membrane bones*. In the embryonic skeleton, membranes and cartilages allow for mitosis. Examples of flat bones formed via intramembranous ossification include the frontal, parietal, occipital, and temporal bones of the skull and the clavicles. Ossification begins at about week 8 of gestation.

When the bones are growing, the diaphyses meet the epiphyses at a structure called the *epiphyseal plate*. It is made of four cartilage layers: reserve cartilage, proliferating (hyperplastic) cartilage, hypertrophic cartilage, and the calcified matrix. Growth of long bones depends on good nutrition and several hormones, including human growth hormone. Interstitial growth of the epiphyseal plate cartilage, and then replacement by bone, is responsible for all long bone growth after birth. All bones grow in thickness by appositional growth. The other hormones involved in long bone growth include thyroid hormone, estrogen, and testosterone. Once the epiphyseal plate experiences closure, the long bones can no longer grow (**FIGURE 7-8**). Length of bone is balanced by increased bone width. Osteoblast and osteoclast activity is balanced in the body so bones grow with uniformity. Most bone growth stops during adolescence, although the bones of the nose and lower jaw (as well as other facial bones) may continue to grow in only tiny increments throughout life.

Bone development, growth, and repair are influenced by nutrition, hormones, and exercise. Vitamin D is required for the absorption of calcium in the small intestine. Without it, calcium is not absorbed well, softening bones and potentially causing deformity. Growth hormone from the anterior pituitary gland stimulates cell division in the epiphyseal plates. During infancy and childhood, *growth hormone* from the anterior pituitary gland determines epiphyseal plate growth activity. This hormone is modulated by thyroid hormones so the skeleton develops the proper proportions during growth. *Calcitriol*, synthesized from another steroid called *cholecalciferol* (vitamin D_3), is made by the kidneys. It is essential for normal phosphate and calcium ion absorption in the digestive tract. Cholecalciferol is produced in the skin or absorbed from the diet. Vitamin C must also be present in the diet, because it is needed for important enzyme reactions in collagen synthesis

and to stimulate osteoblast differentiation. Vitamin A stimulates osteoblast activity, and vitamins K and B_{12} are essential for synthesis of normal bone proteins.

At puberty, male and female sex hormones (testosterone and estrogen, respectively) stimulate ossification of these plates. Thyroid hormone modulates the activity of growth hormone. Exercise stresses the bones, stimulating them to become thickened and strong. Abnormal skeletal growth occurs because of excesses or deficits of these hormones. If growth hormone is excessively secreted, gigantism occurs. Similarly, hormone deficits result in various forms of dwarfism.

TEST YOUR UNDERSTANDING

1. Explain how bones begin to form.
2. Describe the location of the primary and secondary ossification centers in long bones.

Functions of Bones

Bone is a connective tissue that performs several basic functions: hemopoiesis, movement, support and protection, and storage of minerals and lipids.

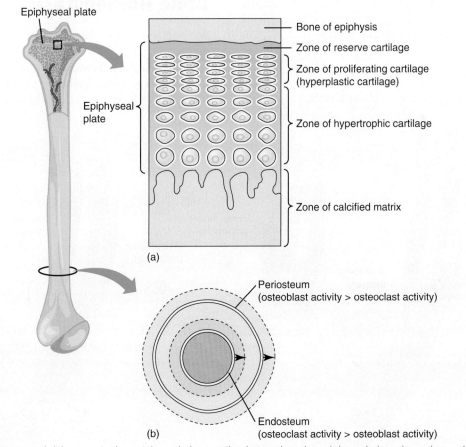

FIGURE 7-8 Lengthwise growth (A) occurs in the epiphyseal plate until puberty when the epiphyseal plate closes, becoming the epiphyseal line. Growth in diameter (B) involves altered rates of osteoclast and osteoblast activity at the periosteum and endosteum.

- *Hemopoiesis:* The process of blood cell production begins in the yolk sac of the developing embryo, which is also referred to as *hematopoiesis*. Later, this process occurs in the *red bone marrow*, which contains stem cells that form all blood cell types. Its color is derived from hemoglobin, which is the oxygen-carrying pigment of the red blood cells. The locations of red bone marrow differ between children and adults. In children, red bone marrow is in the spongy bone inside most of the bones of the body. As children mature into adults, much of the red bone marrow degenerates into a fatty tissue called *yellow bone marrow*. As a result, adults have red bone marrow only in certain portions of the axial skeleton, such as the flat bones of the skull, the vertebrae, the sternum, the ribs, and the hip-bones. Adults also have red bone marrow in the proximal epiphyses of the femur and **humerus**.
- *Movement:* The bones assist in body movement by providing attachments for skeletal muscles that pull on the bones, causing the bones to act as levers (**FIGURE 7-9**). For example, when the arm is bent and then straightened at the elbow, the bones and muscles are functioning together in a lever-like way. When the arm bends, the hand is moved against resistance provided by the weight of the arm, and the muscles on the anterior side of the arm (including the biceps brachii) supply force. When the arm is then straightened, the triceps brachii muscle on the posterior side of the arm supplies the force. The types of movements that are possible depend on the type of joints involved.
- *Support and protection:* The bones support and protect vital organs of the body such as the brain, spinal cord, lungs, and heart. They also protect other soft tissues of the body. The bones of the lower limbs support the trunk of the body during standing, whereas the rib cage supports the thoracic wall.
- *Storage of minerals and growth factor:* The bones store more than 90% of the minerals calcium and phosphorus, which are essential for many body processes. When these minerals are needed, some connective bone tissue is broken down so they can be released into the bloodstream. Phosphorus is important for the creation of organic phosphate, which provides adenosine triphosphate. Important growth factors are stored in the mineralized bone matrix.
- *Fat storage:* In fat, triglyceride is an energy source stored in bone cavities.
- *Hormone production:* The hormone *osteocalcin* is produced by bones. It helps to regulate bone formation and also protects against glucose intolerance, diabetes mellitus, and obesity.

TEST YOUR UNDERSTANDING

1. What is the function of red bone marrow?
2. What chemical substances are stored in the bones?

Bone Homeostasis

Bone homeostasis is the process of self-repair of the bones, which are active and dynamic types of tissue that undergo continual changes. Between 5% and 7% of bone mass is recycled every week. Each day, up to 500 mg of calcium may enter or leave the skeleton of an adult. Compact bone

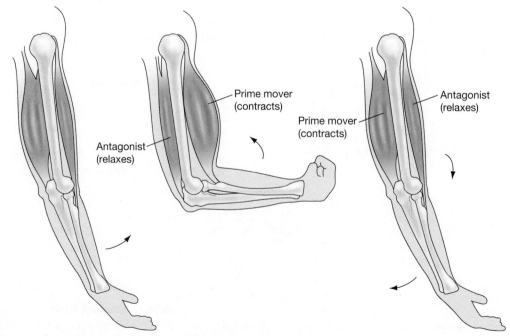

FIGURE 7-9 Bones and muscles form lever systems when they interact to move body parts.

is replaced every 10 years or so, whereas spongy bone is replaced every 3 to 4 years. These activities help to avoid bones becoming brittle, which occurs when calcium salts slowly crystallize over time. Brittle bones are much more likely to become fractured. Bone fracture is the most common disorder of bone homeostasis.

Bone Remodeling

The surfaces of a bone's periosteum and endosteum experience both bone deposit and resorption in adults. Bone deposit and resorption make up the process of *bone remodeling*. Groups of nearby osteoblasts and osteoclasts form *remodeling units*. These units control bone remodeling, assisted by osteocytes, which sense bone stressors. Total bone mass is constant in healthy, younger adults. This means that rates of bone deposit and resorption are in balance. Remodeling occurs in different amounts in various bones. Although the shaft of the femur (thighbone) is remodeled slowly, its distal area is completely replaced within 6 months.

Bone Fracture

Bone fractures are classified as positioning, completeness of the fracture, and penetration of the skin by the bones. Positioning of fractures includes classifications such as *nondisplaced fractures* and *displaced fractures*. A nondisplaced fracture means the bone ends remain in their normal position. A displaced fracture means the bones are out of their normal alignment. Regarding the completeness of the fracture, a *complete fracture* describes one in which the bone is broken completely through (**FIGURE 7-10**), whereas an *incomplete fracture* means the bone is not broken completely through. If a bone penetrates the skin, it is called an *open* or *compound fracture* (**FIGURE 7-11**). If not, it is called a *closed* or *simple fracture*. Fractures can also be described in terms of their location, their external appearance, and the manner in which the bone is broken:

- *Comminuted fracture*: The bone has fragmented into three or more pieces. This type is more common in elderly people, whose bones may be brittle.
- *Compression fracture*: The bone has been crushed. This type is common in porous bones, such as when the condition known as *osteoporosis* exists or when a person falls from a great height, causing extreme bone trauma.
- *Depressed fracture*: The broken bone portion is pressed inward, as often occurs in skull fractures.
- *Epiphyseal fracture*: The epiphysis has separated from the diaphysis along the epiphyseal plate. This type of fracture often occurs where cartilage cells are dying and the matrix is becoming calcified.
- *Greenstick fracture*: The bone breaks incompletely, with breakage occurring only on one side of the shaft, whereas the other side bends. This type of fracture is common in children, because their bones have more organic matrix, lending more flexibility than the bones of adults.

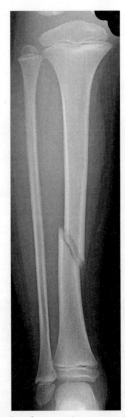

FIGURE 7-10 Complete fracture. (Courtesy of Dr. Kirkland W. Davis, MD, Department of Radiology, University of Wisconsin School of Medicine and Public Health)

- *Spiral fracture*: Because of excessive twisting forces, a ragged bone break occurs. This type of fracture commonly occurs due to sports activities.

Treatment of bone fractures requires *reduction*, which is the realignment of the broken bone ends. A *closed* or *external reduction* requires the physician to physically manipulate the bone ends into position. An *open* or *internal reduction* requires the bone ends to be pulled together surgically, using pins or wires. After reduction, the broken bones are immobilized by a cast or traction. In a young adult, a simple fracture

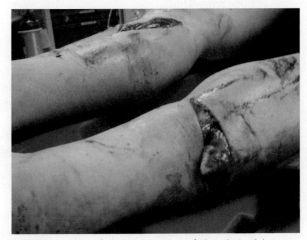

FIGURE 7-11 Open fracture. (Courtesy of Rhonda Beck.)

of a small or medium-sized bone will heal within 8 weeks. However, the break of a larger, weight-bearing bone requires a much longer time to heal. In an elderly person, because of their reduced circulation, bone fractures always take longer to heal compared with younger adults. Various classifications of fractures are shown in **FIGURE 7-12**.

FOCUS ON PATHOLOGY

A skull fracture is a break in one or more of the eight bones forming the cranium that usually occurs because of blunt force trauma. Excessive force may fracture the skull at or near the site of impact and damage the brain. It may also rupture blood vessels and result in severe hemorrhage.

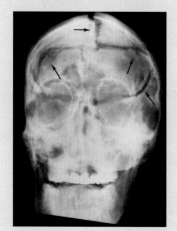

Large skull fracture. (Courtesy of Leonard V. Crowley, MD, Century College.)

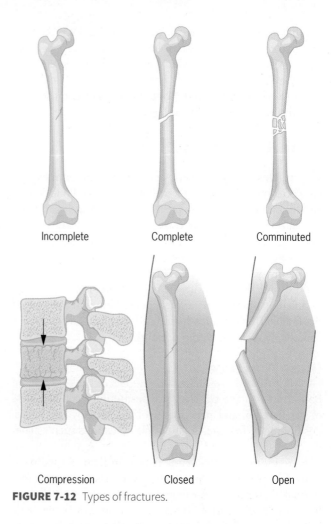

Incomplete   Complete   Comminuted

Compression   Closed   Open

FIGURE 7-12 Types of fractures.

Bone Repair

For simple bone fractures, bone repair involves four primary stages (**FIGURE 7-13**): hematoma formation, formation of a fibrocartilaginous callus, formation of a bony callus, and the process of bone remodeling:

- *Hematoma formation:* The fracture of a bone causes bone and periosteum blood vessels to hemorrhage. A *hematoma* (clotted blood mass) forms at the fracture site. This is also referred to as a *fracture hematoma*. Because of a lack of nutrients bone cells die, and the area of the fracture becomes inflamed, painful, and swollen.
- *Fibrocartilaginous callus formation:* A soft fibrocartilaginous callus (soft granulation tissue) forms in a few days, with capillaries growing into the hematoma. This is also known as an *internal callus*. Phagocytes engulf debris as fibroblasts, cartilage, and osteogenic cells begin bone reconstruction. Collagen fibers are produced by the fibroblasts, spanning the break and connecting the bone ends. Certain precursor cells differentiate into chondroblasts, secreting cartilage

matrix. Inside the tissue repair mass, osteoblasts start to form spongy bone. Cartilage cells at the furthest point from the capillaries secrete a cartilaginous matrix, which bulges, and eventually calcify. This entire repair tissue mass is called the *fibrocartilaginous callus* and splints broken bones.

- *Bony callus formation:* New bone trabeculae appear in the fibrocartilaginous callus within 1 week. They slowly convert it to a hard, *bony callus* of spongy bone. This is also known as an *external callus*. This process continues until a union has become firm and requires about 2 months. Basically, this process duplicates the events of endochondral ossification.
- *Bone remodeling:* The bony callus is remodeled during bony callus formation. This continues for several months. Excess material inside the medullary cavity and on the diaphysis is removed. Compact bone is laid down, rebuilding bone shaft walls. Eventually, the final repaired bone structure appears nearly identical to the original unbroken region because it responds to the same forms of mechanical stress.

Bone Deposition

Areas of new bone matrix deposits are signified by *osteoid seams*, unmineralized sections of thin bone matrix, only 10

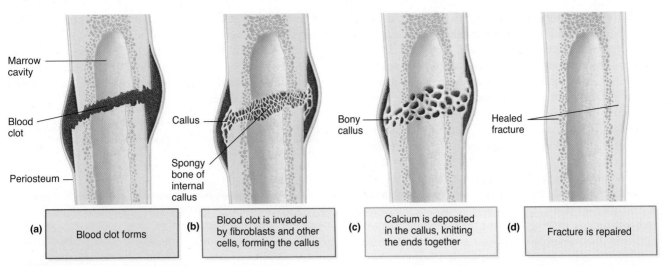

Marrow
cavity

Blood
clot

Periosteum

Callus

Spongy
bone of
internal
callus

Bony
callus

Healed
fracture

(a) Blood clot forms

(b) Blood clot is invaded by fibroblasts and other cells, forming the callus

(c) Calcium is deposited in the callus, knitting the ends together

(d) Fracture is repaired

FIGURE 7-13 Stages in fracture repair.

to 12 μm in width. Between osteoid seams and older bone, an abrupt transition point exists, known as the *calcification front*. The osteoid seams mature for about 1 week before calcification occurs. Mechanical signals are involved in this calcification. In the endosteal cavity, nearby concentrations of calcium and phosphate ions are needed for calcification to occur. When this calcium–phosphate product is sufficient, tiny crystals of hydroxyapatites are formed. They catalyze continued crystallization of calcium salts. Additional factors include matrix proteins (which bind and concentrate calcium) and *alkaline phosphatase*, an enzyme that is lost in *matrix vesicles* by osteoblasts, and which is critical for mineralization. Eventually, calcium salts are deposited at one time throughout the matured matrix in an ordered manner.

Bone Resorption

Bone resorption occurs because of osteoclast activities, including the creation of grooves or depressions as bone matrix is broken down. Osteoclast borders use their irregular shape to stick to the bone and seal off areas of bone destruction. They secrete lysosomal enzymes, digesting protons and the organic matrix. In the resorption bays, the high acidity converts calcium salts into soluble forms. Dead osteocytes and demineralized matrix may be phagocytized by the osteoclasts. Endocytosis occurs to the digested growth factors, matrix end products, and dissolved minerals. These are moved, via transcytosis, across the osteoclasts to be released at the opposite end, entering the interstitial fluid and blood. Osteoclasts undergo apoptosis after a certain bone area has been resorbed. Both parathyroid hormone (PTH) and protein from the immune system's T cells play a role.

Control of Bone Remodeling

Bone remodeling is controlled by genetic factors, a negative feedback hormonal loop, and in response to gravitational and mechanical forces. The negative feedback hormonal loop maintains calcium ion homeostasis in the blood. Ionic calcium is essential for nerve impulse transmission, blood coagulation, muscle contraction, cell division, and secretion

by glands as well as nerve cells. More than 99% of the body's 1,200 to 1,400 g of calcium is present in the bones. The remainder is primarily in the cells, and a small amount is in the blood. Hormonal controls keep blood calcium ions in a range between 9 and 11 mg/dL (100 mL) of blood. Vitamin D metabolites control calcium absorption from the intestine. Children under age 10 need 400 to 800 mg of calcium in their daily diet, whereas people between ages 11 and 24 require 1,200 to 1,500 mg.

PTH, released by the *parathyroid glands*, is the primary hormonal controller of bone remodeling, although *calcitonin* is also involved to a lesser degree. The parathyroid glands are embedded in the thyroid gland in the neck. PTH is released when blood levels of ionic calcium decline, stimulating osteoclasts to resorb bone and releasing calcium into the blood. Osteoclasts break down old as well as new bone matrix. Rising blood calcium causes PTH release to stop, reversing its effects and lowering blood calcium. Blood calcium homeostasis is therefore maintained. However, if blood calcium levels are low for a long time, the bones lose minerals and develop large, irregular holes.

FOCUS ON PATHOLOGY

Calcium ion levels must be strictly controlled by the body and usually only change within 10% of their normal amounts. If they decrease by 35%, convulsions may occur. If they increase by 30%, muscle cells and neurons become unresponsive. If they reduce to 50%, death usually occurs. Hypercalcemia is the condition of sustained high blood levels of calcium. This can lead to dangerous calcium salt deposition in the blood vessels and soft organs such as the kidneys, which results in kidney stones. This deposition can harm their function in many different ways.

Both bone density and bone turnover react to a variety of hormones. The adipose tissue releases the hormone *leptin*, which helps to regulate bone density, weight, and energy balance. Leptin appears to inhibit the actions of osteoblasts, via mediation by the hypothalamus, activating sympathetic nerves that serve bones. The balance between bone destruction and formation are regulated by interactive processes of the brain, skeleton, and intestine. *Serotonin* mediates these processes and is primarily manufactured in the intestine. It cannot enter the brain because of the blood–brain barrier. Serotonin is secreted during eating, circulating to the bones to interfere with osteoblast activity. Because bone turnover is reduced after eating, calcium may be held in bones while new calcium is moving into the bloodstream. Serotonin uptake inhibitors make excessive serotonin available to bone cells, resulting in lower bone density and higher potential for fracture.

Bone remodeling is also controlled by gravity and mechanical stressors. According to *Wolff's law*, bones grow or remodel in response to demands placed on them. The anatomy of a bone is related to its common stressors. A bone is stressed when muscles pull on it or weight bears down on it. These stressors are usually not centered and cause bending of the bone. On one side the bone is compressed by bending, whereas on the other side it experiences tension (stretching). Long bones are therefore thickest at the midpoint of the diaphysis because this is where bending stresses are strongest. Toward the center of the bone, compression and tension are lowest because of their opposition of each other's effects. Without causing any serious complications, a bone can be hollowed out for lightness, which means using spongy bone rather than compact bone. *Wolff's law* has several other points, as follows:

- Curved bones are thickest at the point where they are most likely to break
- Whether you are right or left handed (*handedness*) determines the bones of the most-used upper limb to be thicker than those of the less-used upper limb. Large increases in bone strength occur from vigorous exercise of the most-used upper limb.
- Where heavy and active muscles attach, large and bony projections develop.
- Spongy bone trabeculae form a supportive framework along compression lines.
- When bones are not stressed, such as in a fetus or an immobilized patient, the bones lack normal features.

Deformation of a bone causes an electrical current, with compressed and stretched regions having opposite charges. Therefore, it is believed by some experts that electrical signals are in control of bone remodeling. Within the canaliculi, the flowing of fluids appears to provide stimuli that control bone remodeling.

Both hormonal and mechanical factors affect the skeleton continuously. Hormonal controls, in response to changing levels of blood calcium, determine when (and if) remodeling occurs. The location where remodeling occurs is determined by mechanical stressors. When bone is required to be broken down to increase blood calcium, PTH is released, targeting osteoclasts. Mechanical forces determine which of the osteoclasts will be most sensitive to PTH. Therefore, bone in areas of lowest stress is broken down because it is temporarily not essential to the body.

TEST YOUR UNDERSTANDING

1. Describe the borders created by osteoclast activity and their significance.
2. For maintaining blood calcium levels needed for bone homeostasis, is PTH or mechanical stressors more important as a stimulus?
3. Differentiate between bone growth and bone remodeling.

Bone Homeostatic Imbalance

When imbalances occur between bone deposition and bone resorption, a variety of diseases can affect the skeleton, such as rickets (in children), osteomalacia (in adults), and osteoporosis (primarily in elderly women).

Rickets

Rickets is a disease in children that is nearly identical to *osteomalacia* in adults. However, rickets is more severe because the bones of children are actively growing. It usually causes bowing of the legs and deformities of the pelvis (**FIGURE 7-14**), rib cage, and skull. Because the epiphyseal plates are unable to calcify, they widen continually. Ends of long bones become abnormally long and visibly enlarged. Rickets, as well as osteomalacia, is caused by insufficient dietary calcium or by vitamin D deficiency. Both disorders can be cured by exposure to sunlight (which stimulates formation of vitamin D by the body) and drinking milk that is fortified with vitamin D. Rickets has become very uncommon in the United States because of improved diets and public education. However, if a mother develops osteomalacia due to sun deprivation, nursing her infant will pass her vitamin D deficiency through the breast milk, with the result of the infant developing rickets.

Osteomalacia

Osteomalacia actually describes a variety of disorders involving poor bone mineralization. Although osteoid is produced, there is inadequate deposition of calcium salts. The bones become soft and weak. The affected individual may feel pain when weight is put on affected bones (usually the lower spine, pelvis, hips, legs, and ribs). Soft bones are much more likely to fracture than strong, healthy bones. Osteomalacia is not the same as osteoporosis. When there are no actual symptoms in a person with osteomalacia, the condition may still be apparent on x-rays or other diagnostic procedures. Osteomalacia may also result in an abnormal gait, decreased muscle tone, weakness, and immobility.

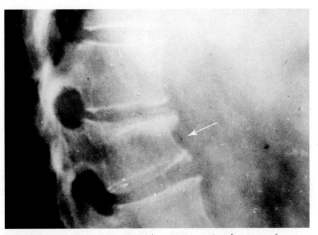

FIGURE 7-15 Osteoporosis with a compression fracture of vertebral body. Vertebral bodies are less dense than normal, and the front of one vertebral body has collapsed (arrow). Compare the compression fracture in this vertebral body with the vertebra above in which the anterior and posterior surfaces are the same height. (Courtesy of Leonard V. Crowley, MD, Century College.)

A postmenopausal woman is most likely to develop osteoporosis when these factors exist:

- She does not exercise sufficiently.
- She has a petite body form.
- She has abnormal vitamin D receptors.
- Her diet is low in calcium and protein.
- She has hormone-related conditions such as hyperthyroidism, diabetes mellitus, or low blood levels of thyroid-stimulating hormone.
- She smokes, which further reduces estrogen levels.

Also, a person at any age can develop osteoporosis because of immobility. Men with prostate cancer have a higher risk for osteoporosis because treatments for this cancer include androgen-suppressing drugs.

Skeletal Organization

The skeleton is divided into two major portions: the axial skeleton (**FIGURE 7-16**) and the appendicular skeleton. Including those of the middle ear, there are 206 bones in the human body.

Axial Skeleton

The axial skeleton supports and protects the head, neck, and trunk. It includes the skull, **hyoid bone** (a single bone in the neck that supports the tongue and its muscles), vertebral column, and thoracic cage.

Skull

The human **skull** is made up of 22 firmly interlocked bones. These are divided into the **cranium** (brain case) and the facial bones. The cranium is made up of 8 bones, and the face is made up of 14. The lines where the bones of the skull lock

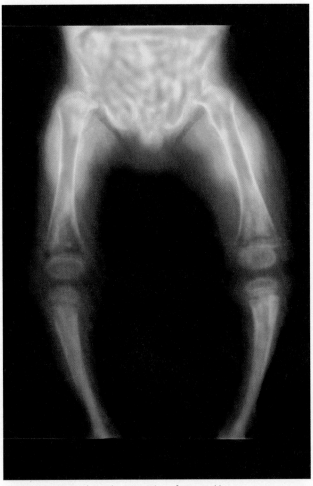

FIGURE 7-14 Rickets. (© DR LR/age fotostock)

Osteoporosis

Osteoporosis actually defines a group of diseases involving bone resorption that is quicker than bone deposition. The bones become extremely fragile, able to be fractured by walking down stairs or excessively hard sneezing. In osteoporosis, bone mass declines while the composition of the matrix remains the same. The bones become porous and light, with the spongy bone of the spine being most vulnerable. As a result, compression fractures of the vertebrae often occur (**FIGURE 7-15**). Also, the neck of the femur is very likely to fracture. This is referred to as a *broken hip*.

Osteoporosis is most common in postmenopausal women, although men develop it also. Between the ages of 60 and 70, nearly 30% of American women have osteoporosis. By age 80 as many as 70% will develop the disease. The most susceptible group for osteoporosis is Caucasian women, with 30% experiencing a bone fracture as a result. Normal bone density is maintained by the sex hormones (estrogens in females and androgens in males). Bone density is balanced by promoting deposit of new bone and by restraining the activities of osteoclasts.

In postmenopausal women, estrogen secretion normally slows. Its deficiency greatly contributes to osteoporosis.

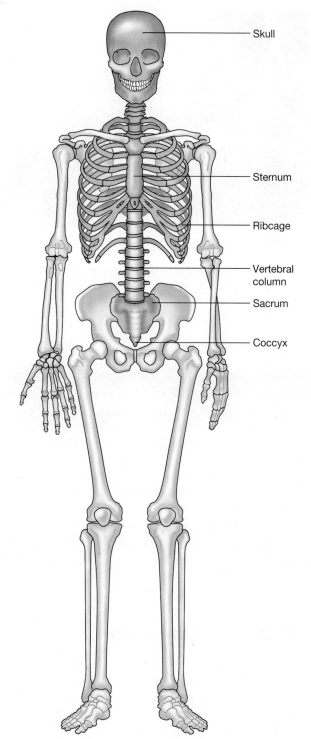

FIGURE 7-16 Major bones of the axial skeleton.

Skull

Sternum

Ribcage

Vertebral column

Sacrum

Coccyx

The bones of the cranium are as follows:

- **Frontal bone**: Forms the anterior skull above the eyes, with each eye orbit (the eye socket) having a *supraorbital foramen* or *notch*. Blood vessels and nerves pass through this structure to the forehead tissues. The frontal bone contains two *frontal sinuses* above the central part of the eyes. The *frontal squama* is also known as the *forehead*, forming the anterior, superior portion of the cranium. It provides a surface area where the facial muscles attach. The *lacrimal fossa* is a shallow depression marking the location of the *lacrimal (tear) gland*.

- **Parietal bones**: Located on each side of the skull behind the frontal bone, these two bones form the sides and roof of the cranium and are fused in the middle along the sagittal suture. They meet the frontal bone along the coronal suture.

- **Occipital bone**: Joining the parietal bones along the lambdoid suture, the occipital bone forms the back of the skull and base of the cranium. A large opening at the lower portion of this bone (the *foramen magnum*) allows nerve fibers to pass through from the brain into the spinal cord. The *jugular foramen* is between the occipital and temporal bones and allows the internal jugular vein to pass through. Rounded *occipital condyles* on each side of the foramen magnum articulate with the first vertebra of the spine. The *hypoglossal canals* begin at each occipital condyle's lateral base, ending on the inner surface of the occipital bone near the foramen magnum. The hypoglossal nerves pass through them. The *external occipital protuberance* is a small bump on the inferior surface, at the midline, of the occipital bone. The *external occipital crest* begins here, marking the attachment of a ligament that helps stabilize the neck vertebrae.

- **Temporal bones**: These two bones join the parietal bone on each side of the skull, along the squamous suture, and form parts of the sides and base of the cranium. An opening called the *external acoustic meatus* leads through each temporal bone to the inner ear. The *mandibular fossae* are depressions that articulate with the mandible. Two projections below each external acoustic meatus (the *mastoid process* and the styloid process) provide points of attachment. The mastoid process attaches to certain neck muscles, and the styloid process attaches to muscles of the tongue and pharynx. The *zygomatic process* projects from the temporal bone to join the zygomatic bone, helping to form the cheek at the *zygomatic arch*. The *squamous part (squama)* of the temporal bone is convex and irregular, bordering the squamous suture. The *petrous part* of the temporal bone encloses the structures of the inner ear. The *auditory ossicles* are located inside the tympanic cavity (middle ear). They transfer sound vibrations

together are called *sutures*. The only movable bone in the skull is the **mandible** (lower jaw), which is attached to the cranium by ligaments. The cranium houses and protects the brain. Air-filled spaces inside the cranial bones called *paranasal sinuses* help the voice to resonate and also reduce the weight of the skull. The cranial bones enclose the chamber that supports the brain, which is known as the *cranial cavity*. **FIGURE 7-17A and 17B** shows various views of the human skull and its bones.

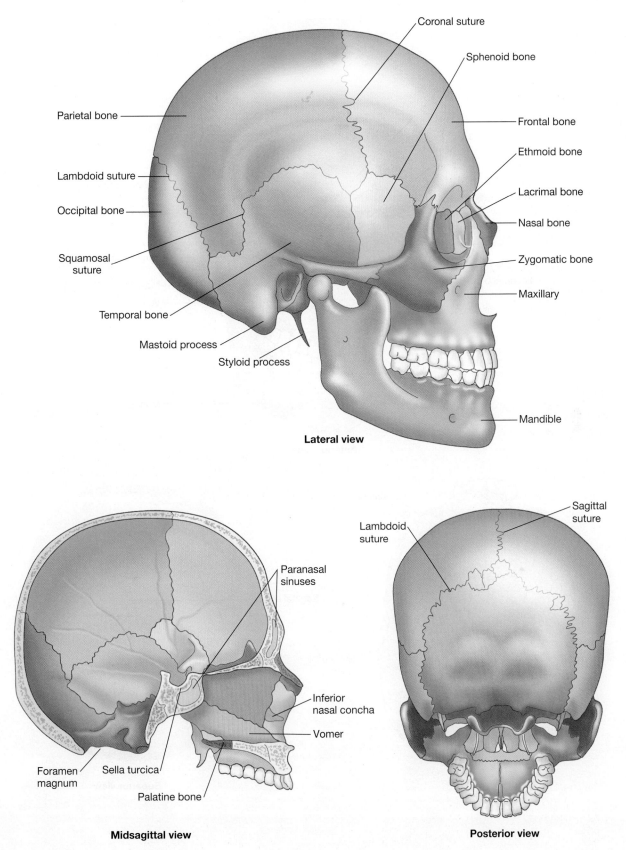

Lateral view

Coronal suture

Sphenoid bone

Parietal bone

Frontal bone

Lambdoid suture

Ethmoid bone

Occipital bone

Lacrimal bone

Nasal bone

Squamosal suture

Zygomatic bone

Maxillary

Temporal bone

Mastoid process

Styloid process

Mandible

Paranasal sinuses

Inferior nasal concha

Vomer

Foramen magnum

Sella turcica

Palatine bone

Midsagittal view

Lambdoid suture

Sagittal suture

Posterior view

FIGURE 7-17A Lateral, midsagittal, and posterior views of the skull.

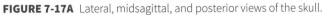

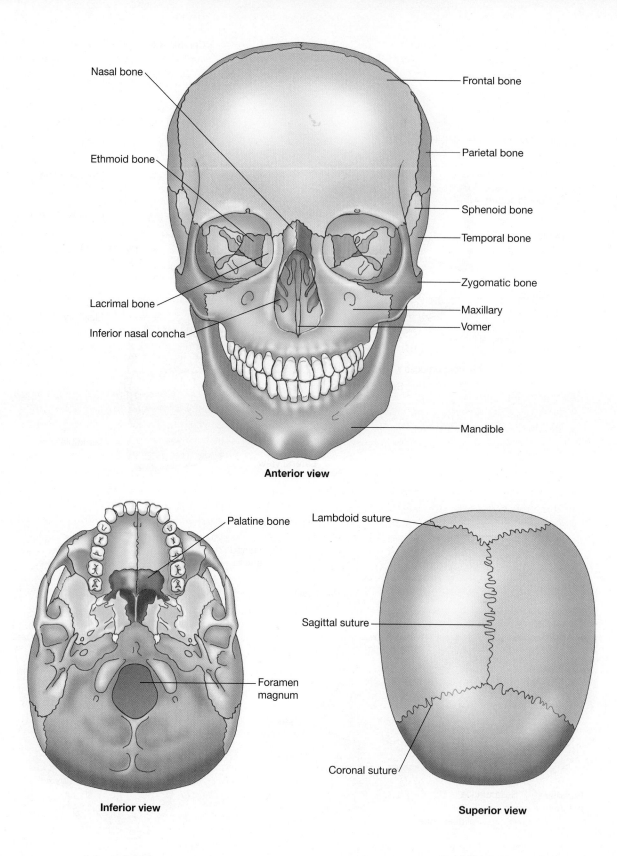

Nasal bone

Ethmoid bone

Lacrimal bone

Inferior nasal concha

Frontal bone

Parietal bone

Sphenoid bone

Temporal bone

Zygomatic bone

Maxillary

Vomer

Mandible

Anterior view

Palatine bone

Foramen
magnum

Inferior view

Lambdoid suture

Sagittal suture

Coronal suture

Superior view

FIGURE 7-17B Anterior, inferior, and superior views of the skull. (*Continued*)

from the eardrum to the inner ear. The *carotid canal* provides a passageway for the internal carotid artery of the brain. The *foramen lacerum* is thin, extending between the sphenoid and temporal bones, containing hyaline cartilage and small arteries supplying the inner surface of the cranium. The *stylomastoid foramen* is posterior to the base of the styloid process, allowing the facial nerve to pass through. The *internal acoustic meatus* is a canal that carries blood vessels and nerves to the inner ear as well as the facial nerve to the stylomastoid foramen.

- *Sphenoid bone*: This complex, bat-shaped bone forms part of the base of the cranium, sides of the skull, and floors and sides of the eye orbits (**FIGURE 7-18**). The eye orbits are actually formed by seven bones in total, known as the *orbital complexes*. Each orbital complex consists of portions of the sphenoid, frontal, maxilla, lacrimal, ethmoid, palatine, and zygomatic bones. The superior portion of the sphenoid bone has an indentation that forms the *sella turcica (Turk's saddle)*, which contains the pituitary gland in its "seat," known as the *hypophyseal fossa*. It is considered the cranium's *keystone* because it articulates with all other cranial bones. The sphenoid bone is described as having a *central body* and three pairs of processes known as the *greater wings, lesser wings,* and *pterygoid processes*. The body of the sphenoid bone houses two *sphenoidal sinuses*. The greater wings project laterally from the body of the sphenoid bone. They form parts of the middle cranial fossa, the posterior orbit walls, and the external skull wall. At this final point, they are flag-shaped areas medial to the zygomatic arch. The sphenoid bone's lesser wings resemble horns and form part of the anterior cranial fossa's floor as well as part of the orbits' medial walls. The pterygoid processes are narrow depressions, projecting inferiorly from where the body and greater wings join. They anchor the chewing-related *pterygoid muscles*. The sphenoid bone has many openings. The *optic canals*, anterior to the sella turcica, allow the optic nerves to reach the eyes. A crescent-shaped row of four openings lies on each side of the sphenoid body. The most anterior opening is the *superior orbital fissure*, which appears as a long slit between the greater and lesser wings. This fissure allows cranial nerves III, IV, and VI to enter the orbit. It can be most easily seen in an anterior skull view. Two other openings, the *foramen rotundum* and *foramen ovale*, create passageways for cranial nerve V to reach the face. The foramen rotundum is usually oval (not round) in shape, regardless of its name. The large foramen ovale lies posterior to the foramen rotundum and is also seen in an inferior view of the skull. The small *foramen spinosum* lies posterolateral to the foramen ovale and allows the *middle meningeal artery* to pass through, serving certain cranial bones.

- *Ethmoid bone*: Located in front of the sphenoid bone, the ethmoid bone forms a mass on each side of the nasal cavity that is joined by thin *cribriform plates* that partially form the roof of the nasal cavity. Between the cribriform plates, a triangular process (the **crista galli**) attaches to membranes that enclose the brain. Parts of the ethmoid bone form pieces of the cranial floor, walls of the eye orbits, and walls of the nasal cavity. A **perpendicular plate** forms most of the nasal septum. The *superior nasal conchae* and *middle nasal conchae* project inward toward the perpendicular plate, with the lateral ethmoid bone containing many ethmoidal sinuses (**FIGURE 7-19**). The *lateral masses* contain the *ethmoidal labyrinth*, which has interconnected *ethmoidal air cells* opening into the nasal cavity on either side. The *olfactory foramina* inside the cribriform plate allows passage of the olfactory nerves.

The **facial skeleton** consists of the following 14 bones (see Figures 17A and 17B):

- *Maxillae*: These two bones form the upper jaw, anterior roof of the mouth (hard palate), floors of the eye orbits, and the nasal cavity sides and floor. The maxillae contain the upper teeth sockets as well as the *maxillary sinuses*, which are the largest sinuses in the skull. The *orbital rim* protects the eye and other structures in the eye orbit. As the human body grows, *palatine processes* of the maxillae grow together and fuse to form the anterior *hard palate*. Along with the *alveolar process*, the alveolar arch (dental arch) is formed, where the teeth are bound via dense connective tissue. The *nasolacrimal canal* is formed by a maxilla and lacrimal bone, protecting the *lacrimal sac* and *nasolacrimal duct*, through which tears flow from the orbit to the nasal cavity. The *infraorbital foramen* allows passage of a major sensory nerve reaching the brain through the foramen rotundum of the

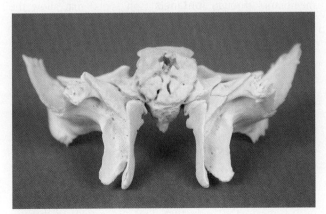

FIGURE 7-18 The sphenoid bone.

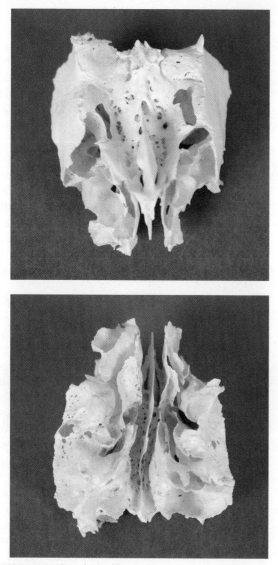

FIGURE 7-19 The ethmoid bone. (© Jones & Bartlett Learning. Specimen courtesy of the Biology Department, Northeastern University.)

bones that enclose the nasal cavities as well as the paranasal sinuses. These bones include the *frontal, sphenoid, ethmoid, maxilla, lacrimal, ethmoid, palatine,* and *inferior nasal conchae.*

■ **Vomer bone:** This thin, flat bone is found along the midline of the nasal cavity, joining the ethmoid bone to form the nasal septum.

■ **Inferior nasal conchae:** These two bones are scroll-shaped, attached to the lateral nasal cavity walls, and support the mucous membranes of the cavity.

■ **Lacrimal bones:** These two thin structures are located in the medial wall of each eye orbit between the maxillae and ethmoid bone. A groove along the anterior lateral surface, known as the *lacrimal sulcus,* marks the location of the lacrimal sac.

■ **Palatine bones:** Located behind the maxillae, the two L-shaped palatine bones form the posterior hard palate and nasal cavity floor as well as the nasal cavity lateral walls. The *horizontal plate* actually forms the posterior hard palate, whereas the *perpendicular plate* extends from the horizontal place to the *orbital process,* forming part of the floor of the orbit.

■ *Mandible:* This horseshoe-shaped bone projects upward at each end with the mandibular *condyle* and *coronoid process.* These processes are separated by the *mandibular notch.* The mandible articulates with the temporal bone and provides attachments for the muscles needed for chewing. The curved *alveolar arch* contains the hollow sockets for the lower teeth. The mandible is the only movable bone of the facial skeleton. The *body* of the mandible is its horizontal portion, whereas the *ramus* is the ascending portion beginning at the mandibular angle on each side. The *mental foramina* open to allow nerves to pass through that carry sensory information form the lips and chin to the brain. The *mandibular foramen* is where the mandibular canal begins, which allows blood vessels and nerves to pass that service the lower teeth.

In infants, the cranial bones are connected by fibrous membranes through **fontanels** (soft spots) that allow the cranium to slightly change shape. When the infant is born, the cranium compresses somewhat in order to pass through the birth canal. The fontanels eventually close as the cranium ossifies and the bones grow together. The skull of an infant fractures less easily than that of an adult. The two fontanels are termed anterior and *posterior.* The anterior fontanel closes at 18 months of age, and the posterior fontanel closes at 2 months of age.

The **hyoid bone** is unique in that it is not actually part of the skull and lies just below the mandible in the anterior neck. It actually resembles the mandible in shape but is much smaller (**FIGURE 7-20**). The hyoid bone is the only bone in the body that does not articulate directly

sphenoid bone. Between the maxillae and sphenoid, the *inferior orbital fissure* allows passage of blood vessels and cranial nerves.

■ **Zygomatic bones:** These two bones form the cheek prominences below the eyes as well as the lateral walls and floors of the eye orbits. A *temporal process* extends from the zygomatic bones to form a zygomatic arch. The *zygomaticofacial foramen* on each zygomatic bone's anterior surface allows passage of a sensory nerve that innervates the cheek.

■ **Nasal bones:** These two long, thin bones lie side by side, fusing at the midline to form the bridge of the nose. Flexible cartilages support the distal nose and extend along with soft tissues to the superior border of the *external nares,* which are the entrances to the nasal cavity. The *nasal complex* consists of the

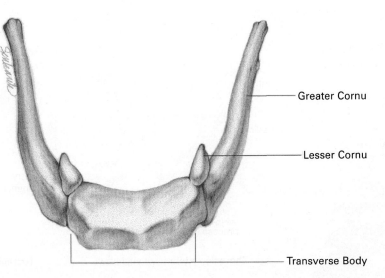

Greater Cornu

Lesser Cornu

Transverse Body

FIGURE 7-20 The hyoid bone, superior view.

with any other bone but is instead anchored by thin *sty-lohyoid ligaments* to the styloid processes of the tempo-ral bones. Its somewhat "horseshoe" shape consists of a *body* and two pairs of *cornua* (horns). The *greater horns* (cornua) help to support the larynx and attach to the tongue muscles. The *lesser cornua* are attached to the sty-lohyoid ligaments. The hyoid bone is a movable base for the tongue, serving to provide attachment points for neck muscles that control laryngeal movements during speech and swallowing.

FOCUS ON PATHOLOGY

One of the complications of otitis media is *mas-toiditis*, which is inflammation of the mastoid pro-cess of the temporal bones. The mastoid process contains sinuses, also known as *mastoid air cells*. There is a lack of blood circulation in this location, making antibiotic treatments much more difficult. If long-term treatment with antibiotics is not suc-cessful, surgery is require to remove part of the bone and drain the mastoid.

Spine

The vertical axis of the human skeleton is formed by the **vertebral column** (backbone), which extends from the skull to the pelvis. It is made up of 26 bony **vertebrae** sep-arated by intervertebral discs made of cushioning cartilage, connected by ligaments (**FIGURE 7-21**). Each vertebra has a drum-shaped body, making up the thick anterior portion of the bone.

The head and trunk are supported by the vertebral col-umn, which also protects the spinal cord. The spinal cord

passes through a *vertebral canal* created by openings in the vertebrae. At the bottom of the backbone, some vertebrae are fused to form the **sacrum** (a part of the pelvis) and the **coccyx** (tailbone), which is attached to the end of the sacrum.

The *vertebral body* (centrum) is the area of a vertebra that transfers weight along the vertebral column's axis. Two short stalks (pedicles) project from each drum-shaped ver-tebra, with two plates called laminae that fuse to become a *spinous process*. These structures collectively form a bony *vertebral arch* around the *vertebral foramen*, where the spinal cord passes through. A *transverse process* projects posteriorly, attached to ligaments and muscles. Superior and inferior *articular processes* project upward and downward with carti-lage coverings, joined to the vertebra above and below. Each articular process has a smooth concave surface known as an *articular facet*. Notches align with adjacent vertebrae forming openings (*intervertebral foramina*) through which the spinal nerves pass.

The vertebrae that make up the spine are listed below, beginning with those located at the top of the spine, with the others listed sequentially (moving down the spine):

- *Cervical vertebrae*: These seven structures com-prise the neck, with distinctive transverse processes and round *transverse foramina*, which allow the arteries leading to the brain to pass through. The forked processes of the second through fifth cervi-cal vertebrae provide attachments for muscles. The **atlas** (first vertebra) supports the head with two kidney-shaped facets articulating with the occipi-tal condyles. It is different from the other vertebrae because it lacks a body and spinous process and has a large, round vertebral foramen that is bounded by anterior and posterior arches. The **axis** (second vertebra) has a process (the *dens*) that projects upward into the ring of the atlas. When the head turns side to side, the atlas pivots around the dens. A notched spinous process, such as those on the C_2

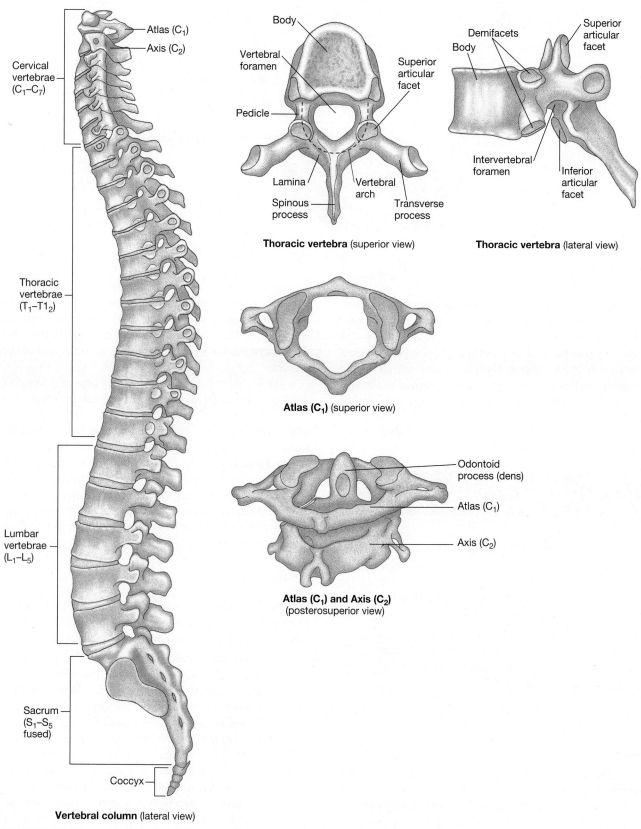

Thoracic vertebra (superior view)

Body

Vertebral foramen

Pedicle

Superior articular facet

Lamina

Spinous process

Vertebral arch

Transverse process

Thoracic vertebra (lateral view)

Demifacets

Body

Superior articular facet

Intervertebral foramen

Inferior articular facet

Atlas (C_1) (superior view)

Odontoid process (dens)

Atlas (C_1)

Axis (C_2)

Atlas (C_1) and Axis (C_2)
(posterosuperior view)

Atlas (C_1)

Axis (C_2)

Cervical vertebrae (C_1–C_7)

Thoracic vertebrae (T_1–$T1_2$)

Lumbar vertebrae (L_1–L_5)

Sacrum (S_1–S_5 fused)

Coccyx

Vertebral column (lateral view)

FIGURE 7-21 The vertebral column and features of skeletal vertebrae.

to C_6 vertebrae, is referred to as *bifid*. The transverse processes are fused laterally to the *costal processes*, originating near the ventrolateral portion of the vertebral body. A partial or complete dislocation of the cervical vertebrae may result from sudden acceleration or deceleration, such as in a car crash, causing an injury to the muscles, ligaments, and spinal cord that is referred to as *whiplash*. The last cervical vertebra (C_7) resembles the first thoracic vertebra (T_1). This rule is generally true where each different section of the vertebrae joins the next. C_7, the *vertebra prominens*, has a long, thin spinous process ending in a broad tubercle that can be felt through the skin at the base of the neck. The *ligamentum nuchae* is a thick elastic ligament that begins at C_7 and extends to insert along the skull's occipital crest.

■ ***Thoracic vertebrae***: These 12 structures are larger than the cervical vertebrae and have long processes that slope downward to articulate with the ribs. The thoracic vertebrae increase in size down the spine to bear increasing loads of body weight. Each thoracic vertebra articulates with ribs along the body's dorsolateral surfaces. The *costal facets* on the vertebral bodies articulate with the heads of the various ribs. The transverse processes of vertebrae T_1 to T_{10} are relatively thick. They contain *transverse costal facts* for rib articulation.

■ ***Lumbar vertebrae***: These five structures in the lower back are even larger than the thoracic vertebrae, supporting more body weight. The lumbar vertebrae do not have costal facts, but their slender transverse processes project dorsolaterally. They have a triangular vertebral foramen, with short spinous processes projecting dorsally. The superior articular processes face medially, whereas the inferior articular processes face laterally.

■ *Sacrum:* This triangular structure containing five fused vertebrae forms the vertebral column's base (**FIGURE 7-22**). A ridge of tubercles project outward with rows of openings (the posterior sacral foramina) through which nerves and blood vessels pass. The *sacral canal* continues through the sacrum to an opening called the *sacral hiatus*, where four pairs of anterior sacral foramina allow nerves and blood vessels to pass.

■ *Coccyx:* Also known as the *tailbone*, the coccyx is the lowest part of the vertebral column and is composed of four fused vertebrae. It is attached to the sacral hiatus by ligaments. The prominent laminae of the first coccygeal vertebrae are called the *coccygeal cornua*.

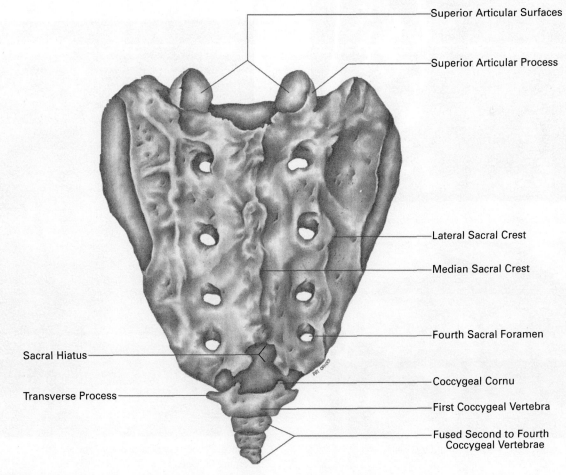

FIGURE 7-22 Sacrum and coccyx, posterior aspect.

Disc herniation in the lumbar area of the spine is very common. With aging, the intervertebral discs dry out and are prone to *herniation*, which is outward bulging. This results in severe lower back pain and nerve pressure that results in *radiculopathy* (pain in the tissues served by the affected spinal nerve).

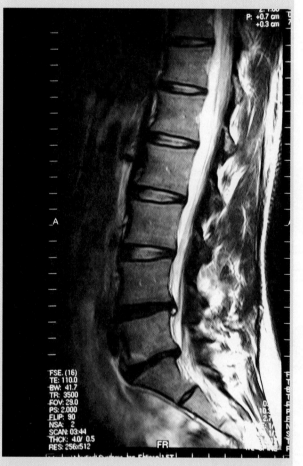

Herniated intervertebral discs. (© kourafas5/iStockphoto.com)

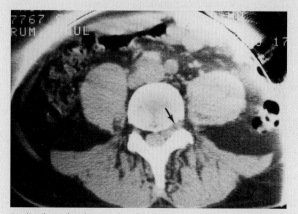

Radiculopathy. (Courtesy of Leonard V. Crowley, MD, Century College.)

Spinal Curvature

The vertebral column consists of four spinal curves: the cervical, thoracic, lumbar, and sacral curves. The thoracic and sacral curves are called *primary curves*. They are also called *accommodation curves* because they accommodate the thoracic and abdominopelvic viscera. The cervical and lumbar curves are called *secondary curves* (**FIGURE 7-23**). They are also called *compensation curves* because they help shift body weight to allow an upright posture.

Abnormal spinal curvatures include kyphosis, lordosis, and scoliosis. *Kyphosis* is an exaggeration of the dorsal curvature in the thoracic region. It is very common in elderly people due to osteoporosis, discussed above. *Lordosis* is an inward lumbar region curvature that is linked to osteomalacia or spinal tuberculosis. *Scoliosis* is an abnormal lateral curvature, usually in the thoracic region, that mostly affects females.

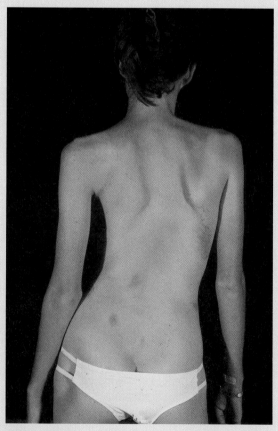

Scoliosis. (Courtesy of Leonard V. Crowley, MD, Century College.)

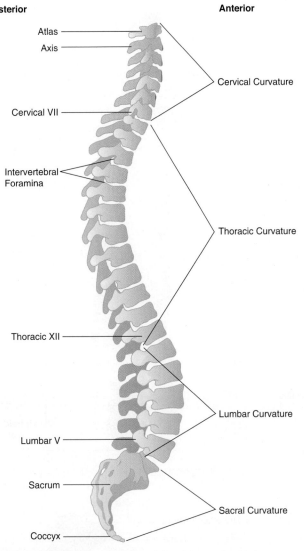

Posterior / **Anterior**

- Atlas
- Axis
- Cervical Curvature
- Cervical VII
- Intervertebral Foramina
- Thoracic Curvature
- Thoracic XII
- Lumbar Curvature
- Lumbar V
- Sacrum
- Sacral Curvature
- Coccyx

FIGURE 7-23 Normal curvatures of the human spinal column.

Thorax

The thorax is composed of the **thoracic cage**, which includes 12 pairs of **ribs** connected posteriorly to the thoracic vertebrae (**FIGURE 7-24**), the **sternum**, and the costal cartilages, which attach the ribs to the sternum anteriorly. The thoracic cage supports the pectoral girdle and upper limbs and protects the visceral organs inside the thoracic and upper abdominal cavities.

- *Sternum:* Also known as the *breastbone*, the sternum is located in the middle anterior thoracic cage. It is composed of an upper *manubrium*, a middle *body* or *gladiolus*, and a lower *xiphoid process* (**FIGURE 7-25**). The manubrium attaches to the clavicles. The *jugular notch* is a shallow indentation between the clavicular articulations, on the manubrium's superior surface.
- *Ribs:* One pair of ribs is attached to each of the 12 thoracic vertebrae, totaling 24 in all. The first seven pairs are *true ribs* (vertebrosternal ribs),

attached to the sternum via *costal cartilages*. The last five pairs are *false ribs* (meaning their cartilages do not reach the sternum directly). The cartilages of the upper three false rib pairs join the cartilages of the seventh true ribs. The final two false rib pairs are called floating ribs (vertebral ribs) because they do not attach to the sternum via cartilage at all. Ribs are curved with enlarged ends (*heads*), allowing them to attach to the sternum via facets (surfaces where bones meet). The transverse process of the vertebrae articulates with a *tubercle* (projection) close to the rib's head. The angle of a rib is where the tubular shaft (*body*) begins to curve toward the sternum. **FIGURE 7-26** illustrates the structure of the sixth rib in its anterior view.

TEST YOUR UNDERSTANDING

1. Distinguish between true, false, and floating ribs.
2. List the numbers of cervical, thoracic, and lumbar vertebrae.

Appendicular Skeleton

The appendicular skeleton contains the upper and lower limb bones and the bones anchoring the limbs to the axial skeleton. The appendicular skeleton includes the pectoral girdle, upper limbs, pelvic girdle, and lower limbs.

Pectoral Girdle

Also known as the *shoulder girdle*, the **pectoral girdle** is made up of a **clavicle** (collarbone) and a **scapula** (shoulder blade) on each side of the body. These structures aid in the movements of the arms. The pectoral girdle is actually an incomplete ring that opens in the back between the scapulae. It connects the upper limb bones to the axial skeleton. The sternum separates the bones of the pectoral girdle in the front. The pectoral girdle supports the upper limbs and is where the muscles that move the upper limbs attach.

- *Clavicles:* The collarbones are shaped like rods with an elongated S-shape (**FIGURE 7-27**). They are located at the base of the neck, running horizontally between the manubrium and the scapulae. These bones brace the scapulae to hold the shoulders in place and provide muscle attachment points for the upper limbs, chest, and back. Each clavicle curves laterally and posteriorly from its pyramidal *sternal end* to form a smooth posterior curve. The flat *acromial end* is wider than the sternal end.
- *Scapulae:* The shoulder blades are somewhat triangular bones on either side of the upper back (**FIGURE 7-28**). Each scapula is divided by a spine that leads to an *acromion process* (forming the tip of the shoulder) and a *coracoid process* (that curves to the clavicle). The acromion process provides muscle attachments for

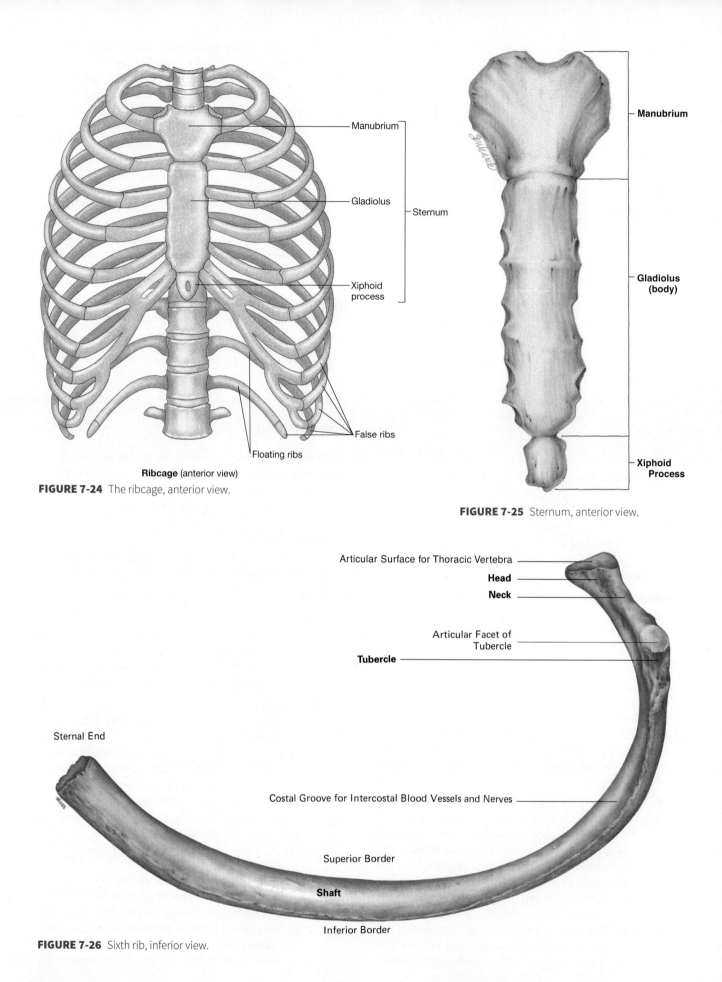

FIGURE 7-24 The ribcage, anterior view.

Manubrium

Gladiolus

Sternum

Xiphoid process

False ribs

Floating ribs

Ribcage (anterior view)

Manubrium

Gladiolus (body)

Xiphoid Process

FIGURE 7-25 Sternum, anterior view.

Articular Surface for Thoracic Vertebra

Head

Neck

Articular Facet of Tubercle

Tubercle

Sternal End

Costal Groove for Intercostal Blood Vessels and Nerves

Superior Border

Shaft

Inferior Border

FIGURE 7-26 Sixth rib, inferior view.

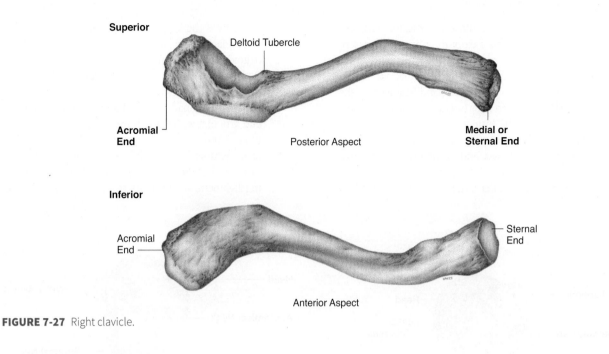

Superior

Deltoid Tubercle

**Acromial
End**

Posterior Aspect

**Medial or
Sternal End**

Inferior

Acromial
End

Sternal
End

Anterior Aspect

FIGURE 7-27 Right clavicle.

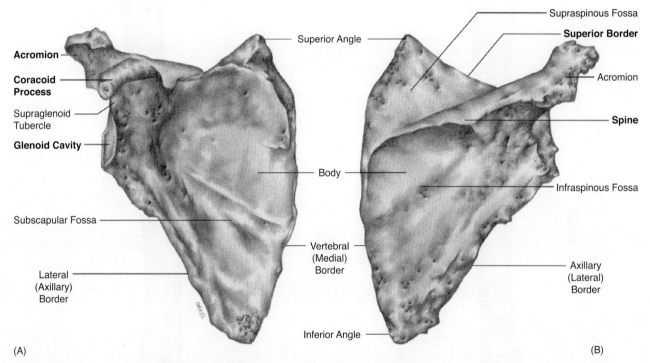

Acromion

**Coracoid
Process**

Supraglenoid
Tubercle

Glenoid Cavity

Subscapular Fossa

Lateral
(Axillary)
Border

(A)

Superior Angle

Body

Vertebral
(Medial)
Border

Inferior Angle

Supraspinous Fossa

Superior Border

Acromion

Spine

Infraspinous Fossa

Axillary
(Lateral)
Border

(B)

FIGURE 7-28 The scapulae, showing (A) anterior view of right scapula and (B) posterior view of right scapula.

the upper limbs and chest and is continuous with the scapular spine, a ridge crossing the posterior scapular surface and ending at the medial border. The coracoid process provides similar attachments. The *glenoid cavity* is a depression that articulates with the head of the humerus bone in the arm. A depression on each scapula's anterior surface is known as the *subscapular fossa*. The area superior to the scapular spine is the *supraspinous fossa*, whereas the area inferior to it is the *infraspinous fossa*.

Upper Limbs

The bones of the **upper limbs** include those of the arms, forearms, and hands. They provide muscle attachments and function to move limb parts. The bones of the upper limbs are as follows:

- *Humerus:* The upper arm bone extends from the scapula to the elbow. It has a smooth upper head that fits into the glenoid cavity, with two tubercles providing muscle attachment points (**FIGURE 7-29**). The lower portion of the humerus has two smooth condyles that articulate with the **ulna** and **radius**. The narrow depression in this area of the humerus that separates it from the greater and lesser tubercles is the *anatomical neck*. Structures called medial and lateral *epicondyles* attach to the muscles and ligaments of the elbow. The olecranon fossa is a depression on the posterior surface of the humerus that receives an ulnar olecranon process when the upper limb straightens at the elbow. At the lower end of the humerus are two smooth *condyles* (round projections) that articulate with the radius and ulna at the elbow joint. The *deltoid*

tuberosity is the large and rough elevation on the lateral surface of the shaft of the humerus, to which the deltoid muscle attaches.

■ *Radius:* Located on the thumb side of the forearm, this bone extends from the elbow to the wrist, crossing over the ulna when the hand is turned. Its upper end articulates with the humerus and a notch in the ulna. A process called the *radial tuberosity* serves as an attachment for the biceps brachii muscle. The distal end of the radius has a *styloid process* providing ligament attachments to the wrist. Fracture of

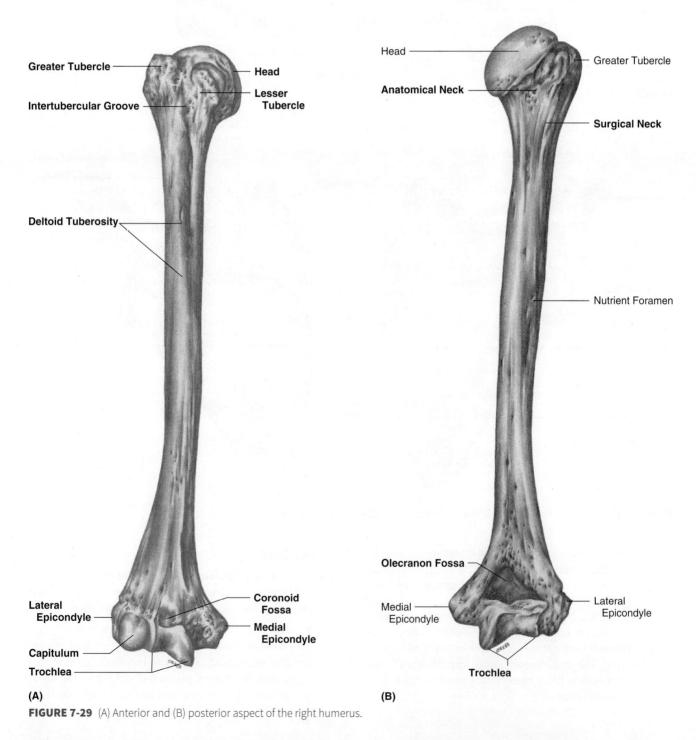

FIGURE 7-29 (A) Anterior and (B) posterior aspect of the right humerus.

the lower end of the radius is called *Colles fracture*. It is a common injury, consisting of fracture of the distal radial metaphyseal region. Colles fracture is often seen in people who play high impact sports or in elderly people who fall onto their hands.

- *Ulna:* Longer than the radius, the ulna overlaps the end of the humerus and has a trochlear notch at its proximal end that articulates with the humerus (**FIGURE 7-30**). The distal end of the ulna has a *head* that articulates with the notch of the radius. The *olecranon and coronoid processes*, located on each side of this notch, provide attachments for muscles.

A disc of fibrocartilage joins the triquetrum bone of the wrist.

- *Hand:* This part of the upper limb consists of the wrist, palm, and fingers. The wrist contains eight bones called **carpals**, in two rows of four bones each. They are the scaphoid, lunate, triquetrum, pisiform, trapezium, trapezoid, capitate, and hamate bones. This mass (the carpus) articulates with radius, ulna, and metacarpal bones. Five bones called **metacarpals** form the palm (metacarpus) of the hand. The rounded ends of these bones form the knuckles and are numbered from one to five, beginning with the thumb. The metacarpals

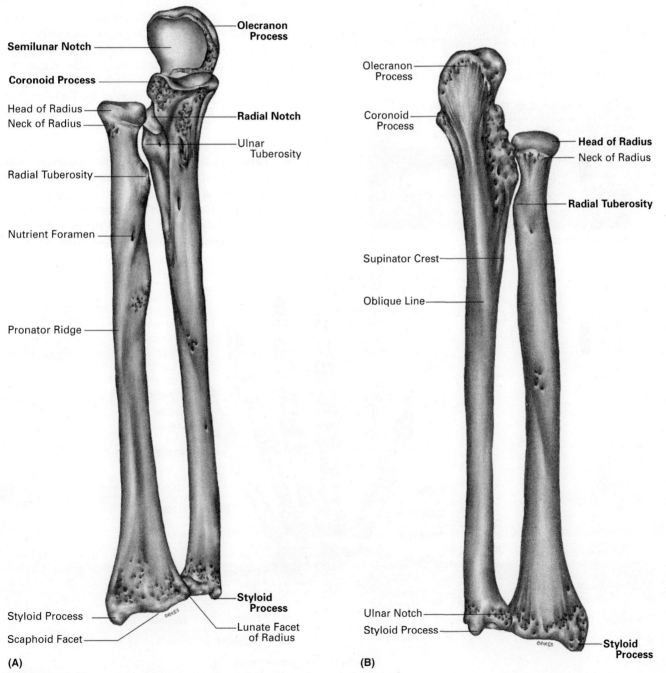

FIGURE 7-30 (A) Anterior and (B) posterior views of the right radius and ulna.

articulate with the carpals and **phalanges** (finger bones). Each finger except the thumb (pollex) has three phalanges (a proximal, middle, and distal phalanx). The thumb has only two phalanges because it lacks a middle phalanx (**FIGURE 7-31**).

FOCUS ON PATHOLOGY

Marfan syndrome is a condition caused by a gene mutation that results in the patient having a tall, thin stature with abnormally long limbs and fingers, as well as other nonskeletal manifestations. The skeletal abnormalities occur due to excessive cartilage formation at the epiphyseal cartilages. Connective tissue throughout the body is affected, which may result in life-threatening cardiovascular problems.

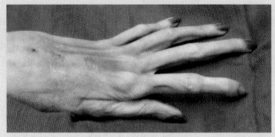

Marfan syndrome.

Pelvic Girdle

Two hipbones, which articulate with each other and the sacrum, make up the **pelvic girdle** (**FIGURE 7-32**). The hipbones are also called the *coxal* or *pelvic* bones. The pelvic girdle attaches the lower limbs to the axial skeleton. Together, the sacrum, coccyx, and pelvic girdle form the **pelvis**.

The pelvis of females is usually wider in all diameters than that of males. The pelvic girdle supports, protects, and/or articulates with the trunk, lower limbs, urinary bladder, large intestine, and reproductive organs. The hipbones each have three parts (the ilium, ischium, and pubis) fused together into an *acetabulum*, which houses the rounded head of the femur (thigh bone).

- *Ilium*: The largest portion of the hipbone, it forms the prominence of the hip. The margin of the prominence is called the *iliac crest*. The ilium joins the sacrum at the sacroiliac joint. A projection from the ilium provides attachments for ligaments and muscles. Ligaments from the *iliac tuberosity* stabilize the sacroiliac joint.
- *Ischium*: The lowest portion of the hipbone, it is L-shaped. It supports the weight of the body when sitting. Its angle, the ischial tuberosity, points downward and posteriorly.
- *Pubis*: The anterior portion of the hipbone, it forms an angle known as the *pubic arch*. The two pubic bones join at the *symphysis pubis*, the upper margin of which (the pelvic brim) separates the lower pelvis from the upper portion. A large opening, known as the *obturator foramen*, lies between the pubis and ischium.

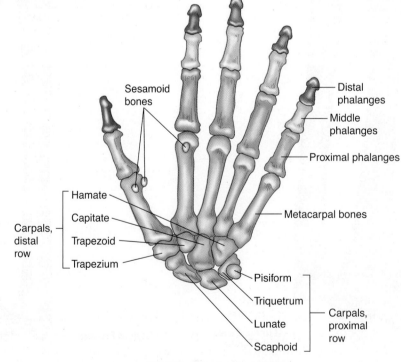

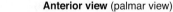

Anterior view (palmar view)

FIGURE 7-31 Anterior view of the bones of the left hand.

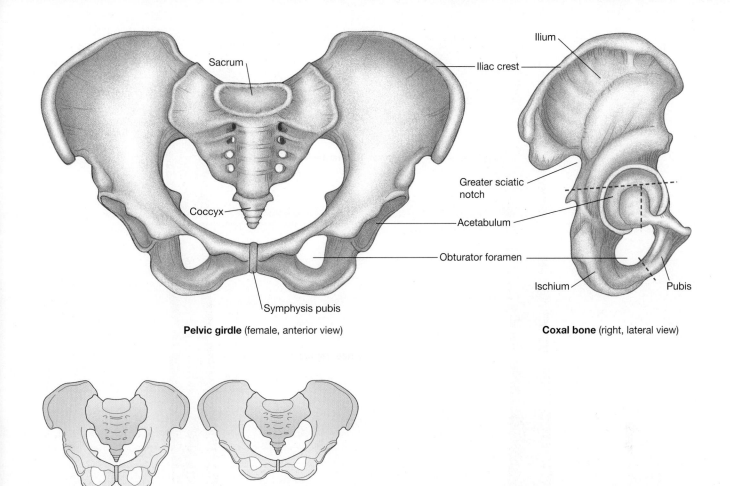

Sacrum

Coccyx

Symphysis pubis

Pelvic girdle (female, anterior view)

Ilium

Iliac crest

Greater sciatic notch

Acetabulum

Obturator foramen

Ischium

Pubis

Coxal bone (right, lateral view)

Male

Female

FIGURE 7-32 The pelvic girdle.

Lower Limbs

The **lower limbs** consist of the bones of the thigh, leg, and foot.

- *Femur*: The thighbone is the longest bone in the body, extending from the hip to the knee (**FIGURE 7-33**). Various processes from the femur provide attachments for muscles of the lower limbs and buttocks. A pit on the head of the femur capitis marks the point of attachment of the ligamentum capitis. Just below the head is a neck (constriction) and the large processes known as the lateral *greater trochanter* and the medial *lesser trochanter*, where muscles are also attached. The kneecap (**patella**) is a triangular-shaped bone that articulates with the femur and is located in a tendon passing over the knee. The patella has a convex, rough anterior surface and a broad base. The apex of the patella is connected to the tibia by the patellar ligament. The rough surface of the patella is where the anterior and superior surfaces of the quadriceps tendon and the patellar ligament attach. The femur articulates with the tibia via the lateral and medial condyle processes.

- *Tibia*: The shinbone is the larger of the two leg bones, located on the medial side. Its distal end expands to form a prominence on the inner ankle where ligaments attach (**FIGURE 7-34**). A depression on its lateral side articulates with the fibula. The tibial tuberosity is the process where the patellar ligament attaches. The distal end of the tibia has an inner prominence (the *medial malleolus*) where ligaments attach.

- *Fibula*: A slender bone located on the lateral side of the tibia, it does not enter into the knee joint and does not bear any body weight. The head of the fibula articulates with the tibia. The fibula has slightly enlarged ends, a proximal head and a distal *lateral malleolus*.

- *Foot*: This part of the lower limb consists of the ankle, instep, and toes. The ankle (*tarsus*) is made up of seven bones called **tarsals** that are arranged so the **talus** bone moves freely where it joins the leg bones. The tarsal bones connect the tibia and fibula to the foot. The other tarsal bones are firmly bound in a mass supporting the talus. The largest tarsal bone is the **calcaneus** (heel bone), which

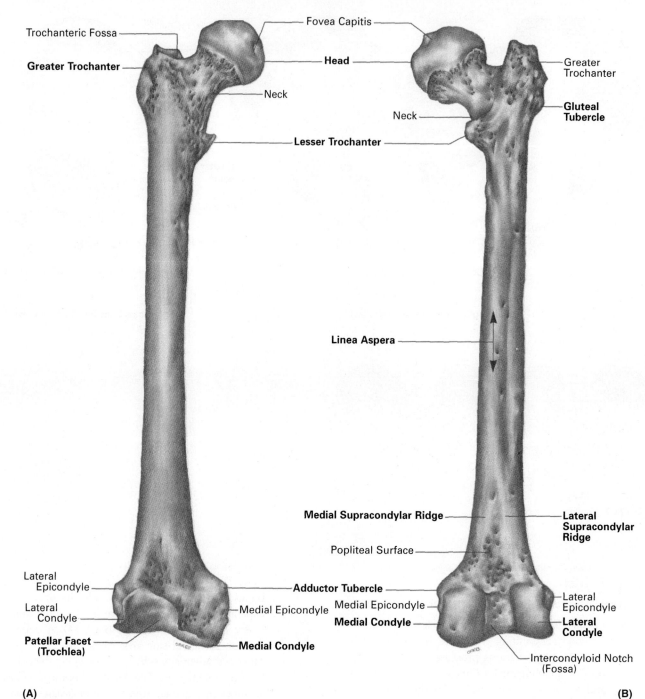

FIGURE 7-33 (A) Anterior and (B) posterior aspect of the right femur.

helps support body weight and provides muscle attachment for foot movement. The instep (metatarsus) is made up of five bones called **metatarsals** numbered one through five, beginning with the medial side. The phalanges of the toes, similar to those of the fingers, are aligned with the metatarsals. Each toe has three phalanges except the great toe, which has only two (**FIGURE 7-35**).

The *longitudinal arch* of the foot allows for weight transfer to occur and is maintained by the ligaments and tendons that bind the calcaneus to the distal portions of the metatarsal bones. The degree of curvature from the medial to lateral foot borders is called the *transverse arch*.

The bones of the adult skeleton are listed in **TABLE 7-1**. Terms describing skeletal structures are listed in **TABLE 7-2**.

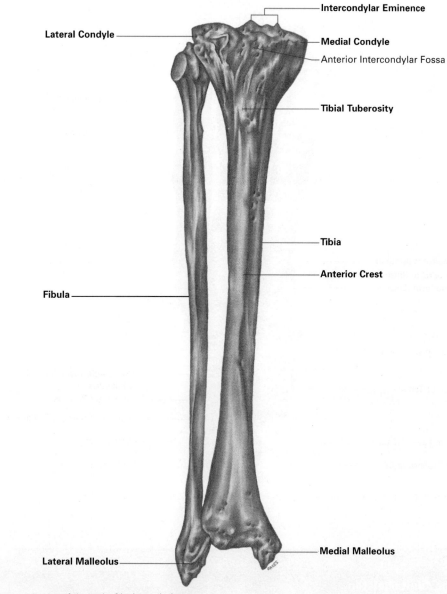

Intercondylar Eminence

Lateral Condyle

Medial Condyle

Anterior Intercondylar Fossa

Tibial Tuberosity

Tibia

Anterior Crest

Fibula

Medial Malleolus

Lateral Malleolus

FIGURE 7-34 Anterior aspect of the right fibula and tibia.

FOCUS ON PATHOLOGY

A common sports-related injury that occurs at the distal end of the fibula, tibia, or both is known as *Pott's fracture*. Because it occurs in similar ways to ankle sprains, it may be hard to distinguish between the two, at least soon after the injury. Pain is usually immediate and severe. The injured person cannot put any weight on the leg. Pott's fracture is followed by considerable swelling and bruising.

TEST YOUR UNDERSTANDING

1. List the bones of the upper limbs.
2. List the bones of the lower limbs.

Effects of Aging on the Skeletal System

Bone mass decreases and bones become weaker as we age. Inadequate ossification is referred to as *osteopenia*, and every adult becomes slightly osteopenic with increased aging. Fractures can occur when the bones are stressed

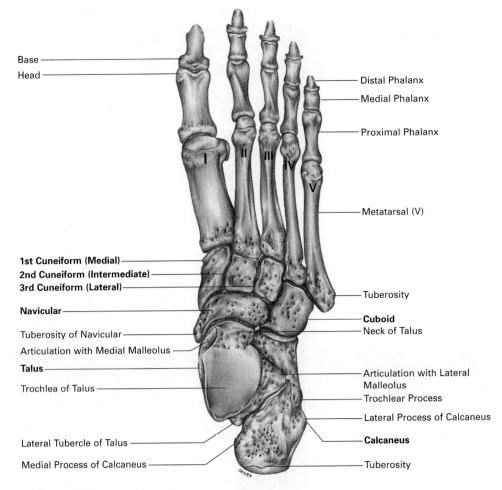

Base —
Head —

— Distal Phalanx
— Medial Phalanx

— Proximal Phalanx

I II III IV V

— Metatarsal (V)

1st Cuneiform (Medial) —
2nd Cuneiform (Intermediate) —
3rd Cuneiform (Lateral) —

Navicular —

Tuberosity of Navicular —
Articulation with Medial Malleolus —

Talus —

Trochlea of Talus —

— Tuberosity

— **Cuboid**
— Neck of Talus

— Articulation with Lateral
  Malleolus
— Trochlear Process

— Lateral Process of Calcaneus

— **Calcaneus**

Lateral Tubercle of Talus —

Medial Process of Calcaneus —

— Tuberosity

FIGURE 7-35 Bones of the right foot (superior view).

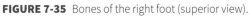

TABLE 7-1		
The 206 Bones of the Adult Skeleton		
Section of Skeleton	**Bone Sections**	**Individual Bones**
Axial skeleton	*Skull* (22) 8 cranial bones 14 facial bones	 Frontal (1), temporal (2), parietal (2), sphenoid (1), occipital (1), and ethmoid (1) Maxilla (2), lacrimal (2), zygomatic (2), nasal (2), palatine (2), vomer (1), inferior nasal concha (2), and mandible (1)
	Middle ear bones (6)	Malleus (2), incus (2), and stapes (2)
	Hyoid (1)	Hyoid bone (1)
	Vertebral column (26)	Cervical vertebra (7), thoracic vertebra (12), lumbar vertebra (5), sacrum (1), and coccyx (1)
	Thoracic cage (25)	Rib (24) and sternum (1)
Appendicular skeleton	*Pectoral girdle* (4)	Scapula (2) and clavicle (2)
	Upper limbs (60)	Humerus (2), radius (2), ulna (2), carpal (16), metacarpal (10), and phalanx (28)
	Pelvic girdle (2)	Hip bone (2)
	Lower limbs (60)	Femur (2), tibia (2), fibula (2), patella (2), tarsal (14), metatarsal (10), and phalanx (28)

TABLE 7-2

Skeletal Structure Terms

Skeletal Term	Description	Example
Canal	Passage through the substance of a bone	Semicircular canal in the inner ear
Condyle	Rounded process at the end of a bone that anchors muscle ligaments and articulates with another bone	Femur bone
Crest	Narrow, ridge-like projection	Crest of the ilium
Epicondyle	Projection above a condyle	Epicondyle of the humerus
Facet	Small, almost flat surface	Rib facet of thoracic vertebra
Fissure	Elongated cleft	Between the occipital and sphenoid bones
Fontanel	Soft spot in skull where membranes cover spaces between bones	Between frontal and parietal bones
Foramen	Opening through bone, usually for blood vessels, ligaments, or nerves	Foramen magnum of occipital bone
Fossa	Relatively deep depression or pit	Olecranon fossa of the humerus
Fovea	Relatively tiny depression or pit	Fovea capitis of the femur
Head	Enlargement on the end of a bone	Head of the humerus
Line	Low ridge	Attachment point for tendons and ligaments
Meatus	Tube-like passage within a bone	External acoustic meatus of the ear
Neck	Narrow connection between epiphysis and diaphysis	In a long bone such as the femur
Process	Prominent projection on a bone	Mastoid process of temporal bone
Ramus	Bone extension that creates an angle with remainder of the structure	Superior pubic ramus
Sinus (antrum)	Cavity within a bone	Frontal bone sinus
Spine	Thorny projection	Spine of the scapula
Sulcus	Narrow groove	Frontal/occipital/parietal sulcus
Suture	Interlocking line where bones unite	Lambdoid suture between occipital and parietal bones
Trochanter	Relatively large process	Trochanter of the femur
Trochlea	Smooth, grooved, pulley-shaped articular process	Trochlea of the humerus
Tubercle	Relatively small, knoblike process	Tubercle of the humerus
Tuberosity	A knob-like process that is larger than a tubercle	Tuberosity of the radius

in ways that would not cause fracture in younger people. The hips are common sites of fracture in the elderly, which may result in hip dislocation, pelvic fracture, and hip replacement procedures. Other commonly fractured bones include the neck of the femur and the vertebrae of the spine. The intervertebral discs of the spine become thinner and less hydrated because of aging. They lose elasticity, increasing the risk of disc herniation. By age 55, the average person is several centimeters shorter than earlier in life. Conditions that can cause even more shortening include kyphosis (known as *dowager's hump*; **FIGURE 7-36**) and osteoporosis. The vertebral column slowly resumes the initial arc-like shape that it had as a newborn. Osteoporosis is also linked to cancers of the breast, bone marrow, and other tissues. These cancers release *osteoclast-activating factor*, which increases the number and activity of osteoclasts, producing severe osteoporosis.

Aging also causes the thorax to become stiffer, mostly because of ossification of costal cartilages. Breathing, therefore, becomes shallower, and gas exchange is less efficient. The bones of the skeleton lose mass with age, and most of this loss occurs in noncranial bones. However, the jawbones are altered somewhat, becoming more similar to how they appeared in childhood. Loss of teeth causes an acceleration of bone loss from the jaws, because there is resorption of the alveolar region bone.

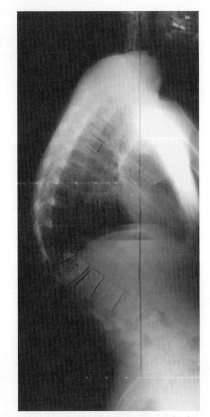

FIGURE 7-36 The vertebral column has a marked convex deformity on lateral x-ray. (Courtesy of Dr. Kenneth Noonan, Department of Pediatric Orthopedics, University of Wisconsin School of Medicine and Public Health.)

SUMMARY

The skeleton protects and supports other systems of the body. Bones are classified according to their shapes, such as flat, irregular, long, short, and sesamoid (round). Long bones consist of an epiphysis at each end and are covered with articular cartilage that connects with other bones. The shaft of bone is called the diaphysis. The three types of bone cells are osteoblasts, osteocytes, and osteoclasts (osteophages). The skeleton is divided into two major portions, the axial skeleton and the appendicular skeleton. The major parts of the axial skeleton include the skull (22 bones), vertebral column (24 movable vertebrae, the sacrum, and the coccyx), and thoracic cage (12 pairs of ribs, the sternum, and the thoracic vertebrae). All bones of the skull, except for the temporomandibular joints, are joined by immovable sutures. The cranium contains 8 bones, and the face contains 14 bones. The primary curvatures of the vertebral column are the thoracic and sacral

curvatures, whereas the secondary curvatures are the cervical and lumbar. The major parts of the appendicular skeleton include the pectoral girdle (one clavicle and one scapula on each side), upper limbs (30 bones each), pelvic girdle (2 hip bones and the sacrum), and lower limbs (37 bones each). Growth of the cranium after birth is based on brain growth, whereas growth of the face is based on enlargement of the nose and sinus cavities as well as tooth development. The vertebral column is C-shaped at birth, with only thoracic and sacral curvatures being present, and reverts back toward this shape in the elderly. Long bones continue to grow until late adolescence. In females, the pelvis changes during puberty to prepare for childbirth. Once an adult reaches full height, the skeleton remains mostly the same until late middle age. Aging leads to reductions in height because of changes in the intervertebral discs and osteoporosis.

Appendicular skeleton
Atlas
Axial skeleton
Axis
Bone lining cells
Calcaneus
Carpals
Cervical vertebrae
Circumferential lamellae
Clavicle
Coccyx
Compact bone
Cranium
Crista galli
Diaphysis
Diploe
Endosteum
Epiphyseal plate
Epiphyses
Ethmoid bone
Facial skeleton
Femur
Fibula
Flat bones
Fontanels
Frontal bone
Haversian systems
Hemopoiesis
Humerus
Hyoid bone
Ilium
Inferior nasal conchae

Inorganic components
Irregular bones
Ischium
Lacrimal bones
Lacunae
Lamella
Lamellar bone
Long bones
Lower limbs
Lumbar vertebrae
Mandible
Marrow
Maxillae
Metacarpals
Metatarsals
Nasal bones
Occipital bone
Organic components
Ossification
Osteoblasts
Osteoclasts
Osteocytes
Osteogenic cells
Osteoid
Osteoprogenitor cells
Osteons
Palatine bones
Parietal bones
Patella
Pectoral girdle
Pelvic girdle
Pelvis

Periosteum
Perpendicular plate
Phalanges
Pubis
Radius
Red marrow
Ribs
Sacrum
Scapula
Sesamoid bones
Short bones
Skull
Sphenoid bone
Spongy bone
Sternum
Sutural bones
Talus
Tarsals
Temporal bones
Thoracic cage
Thoracic vertebrae
Tibia
Trabeculae
Ulna
Upper limbs
Vertebrae
Vertebral column
Volkmann's canals
Vomer bone
Yellow marrow
Zygomatic bones

LEARNING GOALS

The following learning goals correspond to the objectives at the beginning of this chapter:

1. The major functions of bones include supporting and protecting the body, body movement, hemopoiesis, storage of minerals, and storage of energy reserves. Bones are the body's framework and are attachment sites for muscles, some organs, and certain soft tissues.

2. Bones are classified as follows:
   - *Flat:* ribs, scapulae, certain skull bones
   - *Irregular:* many facial bones, vertebrae of spine and pelvis
   - *Sesamoid (round):* inside tendons near joints in knees, hands, and feet
   - *Short:* wrists and ankles
   - *Long:* arms, forearms, thighs, legs, palms, soles, fingers, toes

3. The axial skeleton includes the skull, hyoid bone, vertebral column, and thoracic cage. The appendicular skeleton includes the pectoral girdle, upper limbs, pelvic girdle, and lower limbs.

4. The bones that compose the thoracic cage and the upper limbs include 12 pairs of ribs, the sternum, and costal cartilages (which attach the ribs to the sternum anteriorly). The thoracic cage supports the pectoral girdle and upper limbs while protecting the visceral organs. The upper limbs include the arms, forearms, and hands, including the humerus, radius, ulna, carpals, metacarpals, and phalanges.

5. The major parts of a long bone are the epiphysis, diaphysis, marrow cavity, endosteum, and periosteum.

6. Bone tissue stores more than 90% of the body's calcium and phosphorus. The shafts of long bones store yellow bone marrow (in adults), which contains lipids used for the body's energy needs. Red bone marrow is a connective tissue also stored inside the bones.

7. The bones of the cranium are the frontal bone, parietal bones, occipital bone, temporal bones, sphenoid bone, and ethmoid bone.

8. The structures of cervical, thoracic, and lumbar vertebrae differ as follows:
   - *Cervical vertebrae:* Distinctive transverse processes and transverse foramina, they have forked processes on the second through fifth cervical vertebrae.
   - *Thoracic vertebrae:* Larger than cervical vertebrae, they have long processes that slope downward to articulate with the ribs.
   - *Lumbar vertebrae:* Even larger than the thoracic vertebrae, they support more body weight.

9. The bones of the lower limbs are the femurs, patellae, tibiae, fibulae, tarsals, talus bones, calcaneus bones, metatarsals, and phalanges.

10. The bones of the ankle (tarsus) include the seven tarsal bones. They are arranged so the talus bone moves freely where it joins the leg bones. The tarsal bones connect the tibia and fibula to the foot. The other tarsal bones are firmly bound in a mass supporting the talus. The largest tarsal bone is the calcaneus (heel bone), which helps support body weight and provides muscle attachment for foot movement.

CRITICAL THINKING QUESTIONS

During a game, an 18-year-old football player was injured. He was suffering from severe pain in his lower forearm. He was taken to the emergency department, and x-rays showed a fracture of the radius.

1. Clinically, what medical term is used for this fracture?
2. Explain the articulations of the upper and lower parts of the radius.

1. Which of the following is a component of the axial skeleton?
    A. femur
    B. humerus
    C. hyoid
    D. scapula

2. Which of the following is a bone of the forearm?
    A. radius
    B. femur
    C. fibula
    D. humerus

3. The olecranon process is located on the
    A. femur
    B. tibia
    C. ulna
    D. radius

4. Which of the following bones is triangular in shape?
    A. sternum
    B. scapula
    C. clavicle
    D. hyoid

5. The first cervical vertebra is the
    A. sternum
    B. scapula
    C. axis
    D. atlas

6. The bones that form the wrist are the
    A. metacarpals
    B. metatarsals
    C. tarsals
    D. carpals

7. Which of the following is the longest bone in the body?
    A. tibia
    B. femur
    C. fibula
    D. humerus

8. Which of the following portions of the sternum articulates with the clavicles?
    A. manubrium
    B. xiphoid process
    C. body
    D. tuberculum

9. The ankle consists of how many bones?
    A. 3
    B. 5
    C. 7
    D. 8

10. Which of the following bones contains the external auditory meatus?
    A. parietal
    B. temporal
    C. occipital
    D. sphenoid

11. The spinal column of the thorax contains how many vertebrae?
    A. 5
    B. 7
    C. 12
    D. 26

12. Which of the following is the largest bone in the foot?
    A. cuneiform
    B. calcaneus
    C. navicular
    D. talus

13. The pituitary gland is housed in the
    A. foramen lacerum
    B. maxillae
    C. sinuses of the ethmoid bone
    D. sella turcica of the sphenoid bone

14. Which of the following cells of bone tissue are bone-forming cells that secrete the bone matrix?
    A. osteoclasts
    B. osteoblasts
    C. osteocytes
    D. bone lining cells

15. Which of the following is the structural unit of compact bone?
    A. lamella
    B. central canal
    C. osteon
    D. osteoclast

ESSAY QUESTIONS

1. Describe bone composition and its functions.
2. Which component of bone (organic or inorganic) makes it hard?
3. Compare osteoblasts with osteoclasts and describe their effects on the bones.
4. Why are fractures most common in elderly individuals?
5. Name the cranial and facial bones, and compare their functions.
6. Name the normal vertebral curvatures.
7. Explain true and false ribs.
8. List at least two of the largest foramens in the body and their locations.
9. List two processes of the temporal bone.
10. Name at least two bones in the body that are triangular and their locations.

Articulations

OBJECTIVES

After studying this chapter, readers should be able to

1. Define joints (articulations).
2. Classify joints by structure and function.
3. Describe the structures of synovial joints.
4. Name six types of synovial joints.
5. Name and describe common body movements.
6. Name the most common joint injuries.
7. Compare and contrast the common types of arthritis.
8. List the ligaments that accompany the knee joints.
9. Compare gliding and angular movements.
10. Describe the causes and complications of Lyme disease.

Overview

Joints, also referred to as *articulations*, act as junctions between bones and vary widely in structure and function. They are classified both as to how they move and according to the types of tissue that binds bones together at the joint. The two primary functions of joints are to hold the skeleton together (which offers a certain amount of protection) and to make the skeleton mobile. However, they are the weakest components of the skeleton. They resist tearing, crushing, and other forces that are able to force them out of alignment.

Classifications of Joints

Joints are functionally classified as immovable (**synarthrotic**), slightly movable (**amphiarthrotic**), or freely movable (**diarthrotic**). Less movable joints usually have more stability. They can also be structurally grouped according to the type of tissue binding them at their junctions, such as fibrous, cartilaginous, and synovial joints. In general, fibrous joints are immovable, whereas synovial joints are freely movable. Cartilaginous joints may be either rigid or slightly movable. **TABLE 8-1** shows functional classifications of joints.

TEST YOUR UNDERSTANDING

1. List the three types of joints as classified by their degrees of movement.
2. Compare amphiarthrotic with synarthrotic joints.

Fibrous Joints

Lying between bones that closely contact each other, **fibrous joints** are joined by thin, dense connective tissue (**FIGURE 8-1A**). They have no actual joint cavity. An example of a fibrous joint is a suture between flat bones of the skull. No real movement takes place in most fibrous joints, making them synarthrotic in classification. Those with limited movement (amphiarthrotic) include the joint between the distal tibia and fibula. The amount of movement they have depends on the length of the connective tissue fibers that unite the bones. There are three types of fibrous joints:

- *Sutures*: Seams that occur only between the bones of the skull, sutures have waved and articulated bone edges that interlock. Each junction is totally filled by a tiny amount of extremely short connective tissue fibers. These fibers are continuous with

TABLE 8-1

Functional Classifications of Joints

Category and Type	Comments	Example
Synarthrosis (no movement)		
Fibrous: suture	Fibrous connections and interlocking projections	Between skull bones
Fibrous: gomphoses	Fibrous connections and insertion in alveolar process	Between teeth and jaws; binding the teeth to their bony sockets
Cartilaginous: synchondrosis	Cartilage plate interposed	Epiphyseal cartilages, vertebrosternal ribs, and the sternum
Bony fusion: synostosis	Conversion of other joint forms to a solid bone mass	Parts of skull, epiphyseal lines
Amphiarthrosis (slight movement)		
Fibrous: syndesmosis	Connections of ligaments	Between the distal tibia and fibula
Cartilaginous: symphysis	Connections via a fibrocartilage pad	Between the two pubic bones of pelvis
Diarthrosis (free movement)		
Synovial	Complex joint in a joint capsule with synovial fluid	Numerous; subdivided according to range of movement
Synovial joint Monaxial	Allows movement in one plane	Elbows and ankles
Biaxial	Allows movement in two planes	Ribs and waist
Triaxial	Allows movement in all three planes	Shoulders and hips

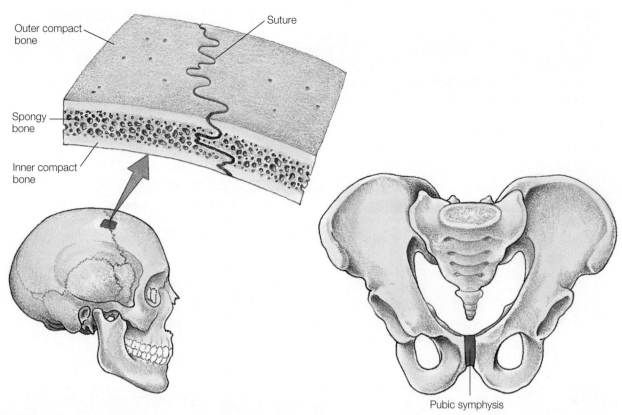

Outer compact bone

Suture

Spongy bone

Inner compact bone

Pubic symphysis

FIGURE 8-1 Fibrous joints.

the periosteum, creating rigid structures joining the bones together. However, they also allow the skull to expand during childhood, when the brain is growing. Closed sutures, during brain growth, are better described as **synostoses**. The immobility of the sutures helps to protect the brain.

- *Syndesmoses*: Ligaments connect the bones in these joints, and the connecting fibers are longer than those found in sutures. The varied lengths of these fibers control the amount of movement that can occur. Syndesmoses with shorter fibers have little or no allowed "give" (movement): an example is the ligament connecting the distal ends of the fibula and tibia. When they are longer, more movement is possible: an example is the interosseous membrane (similar to a ligament) that connects the ulna and radius.
- *Gomphoses*: These are fibrous joints with a peg-in-socket structure. In the human body, gomphoses are only exemplified by the articulation of the teeth in their alveolar sockets. The singular term *gomphosis* refers to how the teeth are embedded in their socket (as if they were hammered in). In gomphoses, the fibrous connects are the short *periodontal ligaments*.

Articulations of the axial skeleton are described in **TABLE 8-2**.

Cartilaginous Joints

Connected by hyaline cartilage, or fibrocartilage, **cartilaginous joints** include those that separate the vertebrae. Each intervertebral disc is an example of a cartilaginous joint and has slight flexibility. Cartilaginous joints also lack a joint cavity. The two types of cartilaginous joints are as follows:

- *Synchondroses*: These are plates or bars of hyaline cartilage uniting the bones. Nearly all synchondroses are synarthrotic. In children, the best example of synchondroses are the epiphyseal plates in the long bones. These plates are temporary joints, eventually becoming synostoses. The immovable joint between the manubrium of the sternum and the first rib's costal cartilage is another example.
- *Symphyses*: These are joints where fibrocartilage unites bones (**FIGURE 8-1B**). Fibrocartilage acts as a shock absorber because of its ability to be compressed and then recover its original shape. A limited amount of movement at the joint is allowed. Hyaline cartilage is also present in symphyses, as articular cartilage on bony surfaces. Symphyses are amphiarthrotic joints allowing flexibility but maintaining strength. Examples include the pubic symphysis of the pelvis and the symphyses of the intervertebral joints.

TABLE 8-2

Axial Skeleton Articulations

Area	Articulation	Type/Movements
Cranial–facial bones of skull	Various	Synarthroses (suture or synostosis)/none
Maxilla–teeth and mandible–teeth	Alveolar	Synarthrosis (gomphoses)/none
Temporal bone–mandible	Temporomandibular	Combined gliding joint and hinge diarthrosis/elevation, depression, lateral gliding
Occipital bone–atlas	Atlanto-occipital	Condylar diarthrosis/flexion, extension
Atlas-axis	Atlanto-axial	Pivot diarthrosis/rotation
Other vertebrae structures	Intervertebral, between vertebral bodies Intervertebral, between articular processes	Amphiarthrosis (symphysis)/slight movement Gliding diarthrosis/slight rotation and flexion, extension
Lumbar 5–sacrum	Between lumbar 5 body and sacral body Between inferior articular processes of lumbar 5 and articular processes of sacrum	Amphiarthrosis (symphysis)/slight movement Gliding diarthrosis/slight flexion, extension
Sacrum–hipbone	Sacroiliac	Gliding diarthrosis/slight movement
Sacrum–coccyx	Sacrococcygeal	Gliding diarthrosis that may become fused/slight movement
Coccygeal bones	—	Synarthrosis (synostosis)/no movement
Bodies of thoracic 1 to 12 and heads of ribs	Costovertebral	Gliding diarthrosis/slight movement
Transverse processes of thoracic 1 to 10	Costovertebral	Gliding diarthrosis/slight movement
Ribs and costal cartilages	—	Synarthrosis (synchondrosis)/no movement
Sternum and first costal cartilage	Sternocostal 1	Synarthrosis (synchondrosis)/no movement
Sternum and costal cartilages 2 to 7	Sternocostal 2 to 7	Gliding diarthrosis/slight movement

TEST YOUR UNDERSTANDING

1. Describe fibrous joints and list three examples.
2. Compare synchondroses with symphyses.
3. What term is a synonym for joint?

Synovial Joints

These joints allow free movement (diarthrotic) and are more complex than other types of joints. **Synovial joints** have outer layers of ligaments (**joint capsules**) and inner linings of synovial membrane that secrete synovial fluid, which lubricates these joints (**FIGURE 8-2**). Some synovial joints have shock-absorbing fibrocartilage pads called **menisci**. They may also have fluid-filled sacs (**bursae**), commonly located between tendons and underlying bony prominences

such as in the knee or elbow. The synovial fluid lubricating these joints allows for great freedom of movement. All synovial joints are freely moving diarthroses. Most joints of the body, and nearly all joints of the limbs, are synovial joints. *Fat pads* are localized adipose tissue masses that are covered by a synovial membrane layer.

The six characteristics of synovial joints are as follows:

- *Articular cartilage:* Made up of smooth hyaline cartilage covering opposing bone surfaces. Although only 1 mm (or thinner) in thickness, they absorb compression and help to keep bone ends from being crushed.
- *Articular cavity:* A potential space containing a small amount of synovial fluid.
- *Articular capsule:* This two-layered structure that encloses the joint cavity has a tough outer fibrous layer made up of dense irregular connective tissue, which is continuous with the periostea of articulating bones.

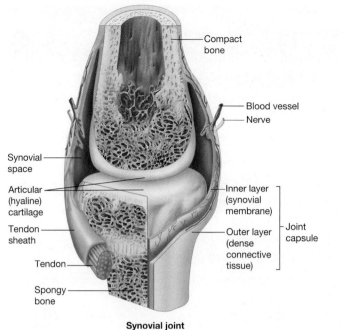

FIGURE 8-2 Synovial joint.

The capsule strengthens the joint and ensures the bones are not pulled apart. Each joint capsule's inner layer is known as the **synovial membrane**, made of loose connective tissue, that lines the fibrous layer's internal portion and covers all internal surfaces of joints that are not covered with hyaline cartilage. The synovial membrane manufactures the synovial fluid.

■ *Synovial fluid:* The slippery liquid found in all free spaces inside the joint capsule is mostly synthesized by filtration from blood in the synovial membrane capillaries. **Synovial fluid** is similar to egg whites, with a thick consistency, because of hyaluronic acid that is secreted by synovial membrane cells. When the joint is in motion, the fluid thins and becomes less viscous. Synovial fluid is also found inside articular cartilages as a slippery film. It bears weight, reducing friction between cartilages. Without it, joint surfaces would be destroyed from use. When a joint is compressed, the fluid is forced out of the cartilages. As joint pressure is relieved, it flows back into the articular cartilages quickly. This process is called *weeping lubrication*, which also provides nourishment to the cells of the joint cartilage. Synovial fluid also has phagocytic cells that patrol the joint cavity for microbes and cell debris.

■ *Reinforcing ligaments:* Band-like accessory structures that reinforce and strengthen synovial joints. They are primarily *capsular ligaments* (actually, thicker parts of the fibrous layer). They are distinct from and remain outside the capsule (*extracapsular ligaments*) or remain deep to it (*intracapsular ligaments*). The intracapsular ligaments do not actually lie within the joint cavity because they are covered with synovial membrane. The term *double-jointed* actually means a person's joint capsules and ligaments are looser, with more ability to stretch, than those of the average person.

■ *Nerves and blood vessels:* Plentiful in synovial joints, sensory nerve fibers innervate the joint capsule, whereas most of the blood vessels supply the synovial membrane. Some sensory nerve fibers detect pain, but most regulate the joint's position and stretching ability. Therefore, these fibers allow the nervous system to monitor body posture and movements. Extensive capillary beds produce the blood filtrate, which is the basis of synovial fluid.

Synovial joints sometimes have other structural components. For example, the knee and hip joints have fatty pads between the fibrous layer and the synovial membrane or bone. These add extra cushioning. Other synovial joints have fibrocartilage wedges or discs that separate articular surfaces (these *menisci*, or *articular discs*, were introduced above). They extend in from the articular capsule, dividing (or partially dividing) the synovial cavity in half. Articular discs help articulating bone ends to fit better, stabilizing the joint and lessening friction on the joint surfaces. Articular discs occur in the knees, jaw, and other areas.

The *bursae* and *tendon sheaths* are closely related to the synovial joints. They act similarly to lubricated ball bearings, reducing friction during joint activity between nearby structures. *Bursae* are flat fibrous sacs that have synovial membranes lining them. They contain a thin film of synovial fluid and are located where bones, ligaments, muscles, skin, or tendons rub together. A *tendon sheath* can be understood as lengthened bursae wrapping totally around a tendon that is subjected to friction. They are common in areas such as the wrist, where several tendons are tightly crowded inside narrow canals.

Joints must be stabilized to avoid becoming dislocated during stretching and compression. Joint stability relies on articular surface shapes, number and position of ligaments, and also on muscle tone. Articular surfaces actually play just a minor role. When they are larger and well fitting or when sockets are deep, joint stability is greatly improved. For example, the hip's ball and socket joint is very stable because of the shape of its articular surfaces.

Bones are united, and excessive or undesirable motions are prevented by the capsules and ligaments of synovial joints. Generally, the more ligaments that exist, the stronger the joint. Sometimes, excessive tension on the ligaments causes them to stretch, which is a condition that remains. Ligaments stretch approximately 6% of their length, until they break. When a joint is mostly braced by ligaments and this occurs, the joint becomes highly unstable.

Muscle tendons crossing joints are often the most important factors concerning stability. Muscle tone keeps these tendons tense. It means that the muscle, when relaxed, has low levels of contractile activity. This keeps muscles healthy and ready for stimulation. Muscle tone is vital for reinforcing areas such as the foot arches and the joints of the knees and shoulders. Articulations of the appendicular skeleton are described in **TABLE 8-3**.

TABLE 8-3

Appendicular Skeleton Articulations

Area	Articulation	Type/Movements
Sternum–clavicle	Sternoclavicular	Gliding diarthrosis/protraction, retraction, elevation, depression, slight rotation
Scapula–clavicle	Acromioclavicular	Gliding diarthrosis/slight movement
Scapula–humerus	Shoulder (glenohumeral)	Ball-and-socket diarthrosis/flexion, extension, adduction, abduction, circumduction, rotation
Humerus–ulna and humerus–radius	Elbow (humeroulnar and humeroradial)	Hinge diarthrosis/flexion, extension
Radius–ulna	Proximal radioulnar Distal radioulnar	Pivot diarthrosis/rotation Pivot diarthrosis/pronation, supination
Radius–carpals	Radiocarpal	Condylar diarthrosis/flexion, extension, adduction, abduction, circumduction
Carpal to carpal	Intercarpal	Gliding diarthrosis/slight movement
Carpal to metacarpal bone I	Carpometacarpal (thumb)	Saddle diarthrosis/flexion, extension, adduction, abduction, circumduction, opposition
Carpal to metacarpal bones II through V	Carpometacarpal	Gliding diarthrosis/slight flexion, extension, adduction, abduction
Metacarpal to phalanx	Metacarpophalangeal	Condylar diarthrosis/flexion, extension, adduction, abduction, circumduction
Phalanx/phalanx	Interphalangeal	Hinge diarthrosis/flexion, extension
Sacrum–ilium of hipbone	Sacroiliac	Gliding diarthrosis/slight movement
Hipbone–hipbone	Pubic symphysis (symphysis)	Amphiarthrosis/none
Hipbone–femur	Hip	Ball-and-socket diarthrosis/flexion, extension, adduction, abduction, circumduction, rotation
Femur–tibia	Knee	Complex, functions as hinge/flexion, extension, limited rotation
Tibia–fibula	Tibiofibular (proximal) Tibiofibular (distal)	Gliding diarthrosis/slight movement Gliding diarthrosis and amphiarthrotic syndesmosis/slight movement
Tibia and fibula with talus	Ankle (talocrural)	Hinge diarthrosis/flexion, extension (dorsiflexion, plantar flexion)
Tarsal–tarsal	Intertarsal	Gliding diarthrosis/slight movement
Tarsal–metatarsal	Tarsometatarsal	Gliding diarthrosis/slight movement
Metatarsal–phalanx	Metatarsophalangeal	Condylar diarthrosis/flexion, extension, adduction, abduction
Phalanx–phalanx	Interphalangeal	Hinge diarthrosis/flexion, extension

Types of Synovial Joints

Synovial joints are not all identical. There are six further subdivisions of synovial joints:

- *Plane (gliding) joint:* Having nonaxial movement that involves linear gliding and flat, articular surfaces. Examples include the intercarpal joints, intertarsal joints, and the joints between vertebral articular surfaces.

- *Hinge joint:* Having uniaxial movement that involves flexion and extension along a medial/lateral axis, they have cylinders and troughs. Examples include the elbow joints and interphalangeal joints.

- *Pivot joint:* Having uniaxial movement that involves rotation around a vertical axis, they have bone and ligament sleeves as well as rounded bones (axles). Examples include the proximal radioulnar joints and the atlantoaxial joint.

- *Ellipsoidal joint:* Having biaxial movement that involves adduction and abduction around an anterior/posterior axis and flexion and extension around a medial/lateral axis, with oval articular surfaces. Examples include the metacarpophalangeal (knuckle) joints and wrist joints.
- *Saddle joint:* Having biaxial movement that involves flexion and extension and adduction and abduction, saddle joints function around the same type of axis configurations as condylar joints. Articular surfaces are both concave and convex. An example is the carpometacarpal joints of the thumbs.
- *Ball-and-socket joint:* Having multiaxial movement that involves rotation, adduction, abduction, flexion, and extension. Ball-and-socket joints use vertical, anterior/posterior, and medial/lateral types of axis structures, with spherical heads in cup-like sockets. Examples include the shoulder and hip joints.

Types of synovial joints are shown in **FIGURE 8-3**.

TEST YOUR UNDERSTANDING

1. Describe the components of a synovial joint.
2. List different types of synovial joints.

Shoulder Joints

The shoulder joints are the most freely movable joints of the body, but they lack stability. They are ball-and-socket joints. The head of the humerus is large and hemispherical. It fits in the glenoid cavity of the scapula, which is shallow and small (**FIGURE 8-4**). This cavity is made slightly deeper by a fibrocartilage rim (the *glenoid labrum*). Still, it is only about one-third of the size of the humeral head, which means the shoulder joint is highly unstable. A *shoulder separation* is an

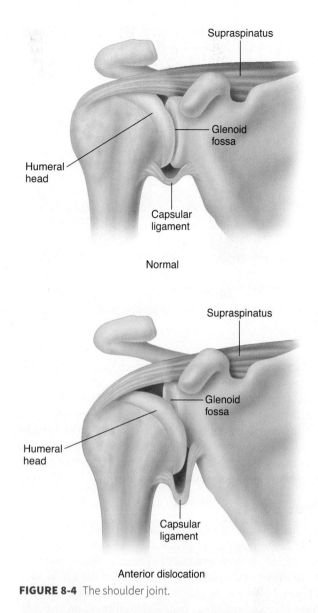

FIGURE 8-4 The shoulder joint.

injury involving partial or complete dislocation of the acromioclavicular joint.

The joint cavity is enclosed by an extremely loose, thin articular capsule. It runs from the margin of the glenoid cavity to the anatomical neck of the humerus. Only a few ligaments reinforce the shoulder joint, and these are found mostly on its anterior aspect. The superior **coracohumeral ligament** is the thickest area of the capsule. It helps to support the weight of the arm. The front of the capsule is only slightly strengthened by three **glenohumeral ligaments**. These are absent in some individuals.

Most of the stability of the shoulder joint comes from muscle tendons that cross the joint. The primary stabilizing structure is the tendon of the long head of the arm's *biceps brachii* muscle. This tendon secures the head of the humerus against the glenoid cavity. It is attached to the glenoid labrum's superior margin and travels through the shoulder joint cavity. It then continues within the intertubercular sulcus of the humerus.

Associated muscles (the subscapularis, infraspinatus, supraspinatus, and teres minor) and a total of four other

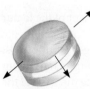

Gliding joint

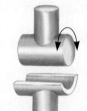

Hinge joint

Pivot joint

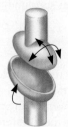

Ellipsoidal joint

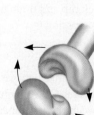

Saddle joint

Ball-and-socket joint

FIGURE 8-3 Types of synovial joints.

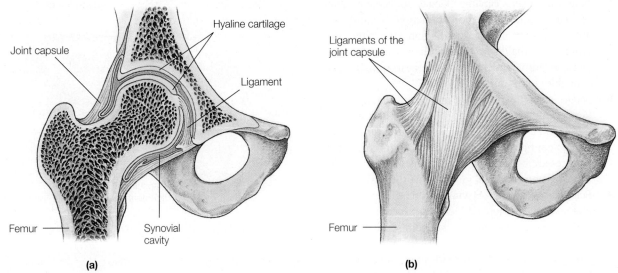

FIGURE 8-5 The hip joint, showing (A) a cross-section and (B) the ligaments of the joint capsule.

tendons comprise the **rotator cuff**, which encircles the shoulder joint. The rotator cuff blends with the articular capsule. If the arm is strongly circumducted, the rotator cuff can be stretched severely, which often occurs in athletes who pitch (such as those in baseball or softball). Instability of the shoulder joint also results in frequent dislocations. Usually, the humerus dislocates in the forward, downward direction because its reinforcements are weakest anteriorly and inferiorly.

Elbow Joints

The elbow joints allow only flexion and extension and are stable hinge joints that operate very smoothly. The radius and ulna bones both articulate inside each elbow joint with the condyles of the humerus. The hinge of the elbow joint is formed by the tight gripping of the trochlea by the trochlear notch of the ulna. Joint stabilization is provided by this structure. The articular capsule is relatively loose. It extends inferiorly from the humerus to the radius and ulna and to the **annular ligament** that surrounds the head of the radius.

The articular capsule of the elbow joint is thin both anteriorly and posteriorly. Two strong capsular ligaments restrict horizontal movements, the medial **ulnar collateral ligament** and the triangular **radial collateral ligament** on the lateral side. Several arm muscle ligaments also cross the elbow joint to make it more secure. These are the tendons of the biceps and triceps. The radius has less activity in movements of the elbow, but its head rotates inside the annular ligament during both pronation and supination of the forearm.

Hip Joints

The **hip joints** are also known as the *coxal joints*. They are ball-and-socket joints with less range than those of the shoulder. Although widely ranging movements are possible, they are limited by the deep hip sockets and strong ligaments.

Each hip joint is formed by the articulation of the femur's spherical head with the hip bone's acetabulum and its deeply cupped position (**FIGURE 8-5**). A circular rim of fibrocartilage called the **acetabular labrum** increases the depth of the acetabulum. Hip joint dislocations are rare because the articular surfaces fit tightly together. The labrum's diameter is less than that of the head of the femur, however.

Each hip joint is completely enclosed by its thick articular capsule, which extends from the rim of the acetabulum to the femur neck. The capsule is reinforced by the **iliofemoral ligament**, **pubofemoral ligament**, and **ischiofemoral ligament**. The iliofemoral ligament lies anteriorly and is very strong, with a V-shape. The pubofemoral ligament is a triangular thickening of the inferior area of the capsule. The ischiofemoral ligament spirals posteriorly. All three ligaments have an arrangement that causes a screw-like turning motion of the femur head into the acetabulum when a person stands up straight. They provide increased joint stability.

The *ligamentum teres*, which is the ligament of the femur head, is the flattened intracapsular band connecting the femur head to the acetabulum's lower edge. During most movements of the hip, it is slack. It is not important in joint stabilization but contains an artery supplying the head of the femur. When the artery is damaged, severe hip joint **arthritis** may develop. Stability of the hip joint comes from the deep socket that strongly encloses the femur head, strong capsular ligaments, thick hip and thigh muscles surrounding it, and muscle tendons crossing it.

Knee Joints

The knee joint has a single joint cavity yet is the most complex joint in the body (**FIGURE 8-6**). It is actually made up of an intermediate joint between the patella and lower femur and lateral and medial joints collectively known as the **tibiofemoral joints**. These joints lie between the femoral condyles

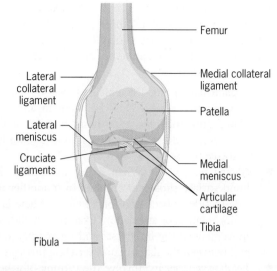

Femur

Medial collateral ligament

Lateral collateral ligament

Patella

Lateral meniscus

Cruciate ligaments

Medial meniscus

Articular cartilage

Tibia

Fibula

FIGURE 8-6 Anatomy of the knee joint.

above and the *semilunar cartilages* (C-shaped menisci) of the tibia below. The semilunar cartilages deepen the tibial articular surfaces, which are otherwise shallow. They absorb shock to the knee joint and also prevent horizontal rocking of the femur on the tibia. Unfortunately, the semilunar cartilages are often completely torn because they are only attached at their outer margins.

Flexion and extension is allowed by the hinge-like tibiofemoral joint. In actuality, it is a *bicondylar joint*, with some rotation occurring when the knee is slightly flexed or when it is extending. A fully extended knee cannot rock horizontally or rotate without difficulty because of strong ligament and menisci resistance. The patella glides across the femur's distal end during knee flexion because the femoropatellar joint is a *plane joint*.

The knee joint is the only articulation that has a cavity partially enclosed by a capsule. This capsule is thin and present only on the posterior aspects and sides of the knee. It covers most of the femoral and tibial condyles. It is absent anteriorly, and here there are three broad ligaments running from the patella to the tibia below, the *patellar, medial,* and *lateral patellar retinacula* ligaments. They merge with the articular capsule on each side. Two of them (the patellar ligament and the lateral patellar retinacula) are continuations of the tendon from the quadriceps muscle in the anterior thigh. The patellar ligament is used to test the *knee-jerk reflex.*

The knee joint's synovial cavity is also complex, with various bursae. The *subcutaneous prepatellar bursa* is an example of a bursa that is often injured by trauma to the anterior knee. The knee joint capsule is strengthened and stabilized by all three types of joint ligaments. Two of these types (capsular and extracapsular) help to prevent **hyperextension** of the knee. They are tightly stretched when the knee is extended. When the knee is extended, the extracapsular *fibular* and *tibial collateral ligaments* are crucial to prevent lateral or medial rotation. The **tibial collateral ligament**

is wide and flat, running from the femur's medial epicondyle to the tibial shaft's medial condyle. This ligament is fused to the medial meniscus. The posterior aspect of the knee joint is partially stabilized by the **oblique popliteal ligament**, which is part of the tendon of the semimembranosus muscle. It fuses with the joint capsule. The joint capsule is reinforced posteriorly by the **arcuate popliteal ligament**, which has a superior arc, from the head of the fibula over the popliteus muscle.

In the notch between the femoral condyles, the *intracapsular ligaments (cruciate ligaments)* cross each other to form an "X." They provide restraint against anterior–posterior displacement of the articular surfaces. These ligaments also secure the articulating bones during standing. They are in the joint capsule but outside the synovial cavity. Therefore, the intracapsular ligaments are nearly covered by synovial membrane and run superiorly to the femur. They are named for their tibial attachment site.

The **anterior cruciate ligament** is attached to the tibia's anterior intercondylar area and passes upward, laterally, and posteriorly to attach to the femur. Its actual point of attachment is the medial side of the femur's lateral condyle. The anterior cruciate ligament prevents the tibia from sliding forward on the femur, controlling hyperextension of the knee. It is tight during knee extension and slightly relaxed during knee flexion. The **posterior cruciate ligament** has more strength and is attached to the tibia's posterior intercondylar area. This ligament passes superiorly, medially, and anteriorly, attaching to the lateral side of the medial condyle of the femur. It prevents forward sliding of the femur or backward displacement of the tibia.

Many muscle tendons reinforce the knee capsule. Muscle strength and tone protect the knee from injury. This is especially true of the tendon of the semimembranous muscle (posteriorly) and the tendons of the quadriceps muscles in the anterior thigh.

When standing, the knees "lock in" to provide steady support. As a person rises from a sitting to a standing position, the wheel-like femoral condyles roll across the tibial condyles as the flexed leg begins to extend at the knee. The lateral femoral condyle stops rolling before the medial condyle stops. Therefore, the femur rotates medially on the tibia, followed by twisting and tightening of the collateral and cruciate ligaments of the knee. The menisci become compressed. Tension present in the ligaments makes the joint become rigid. It cannot be flexed once more until it is "unlocked," which is accomplished by the popliteus muscle. This muscle causes the ligaments to become slack and untwisted by rotating the femur laterally on the tibia.

TEST YOUR UNDERSTANDING

1. Which of the major large joints have two menisci?
2. Which ligament is used to test the knee-jerk reflex?
3. What is another name for the hip joints?

Because the knees require nonarticular factors for stability and are highly weight-bearing joints, they are often injured while playing sports. They are very vulnerable to horizontal trauma, especially when extended. The **collateral ligament** is often torn, along with the attached medial meniscus and the anterior cruciate ligament. Approximately half of all professional football players experience a serious knee injury. Most commonly, injury to the anterior cruciate ligament occurs when a hyperextended knee is excessively twisted. Repair usually requires a patellar ligament graft or another graft from the hamstring or calcaneal tendons.

Types of Joint Movements

Movements at synovial joints are produced by skeletal muscle action. In most joints, one end of a muscle is attached to a primarily immovable or fixed part and the other end of the muscle is attached to a movable part. During muscle contraction, the movable end (insertion) is pulled toward the fixed end (origin), with movement occurring at the joint. Movements are described in directional terms. These relate to the axes (lines) around which a body part moves and the body planes along which it occurs. *Nonaxial movement* involves only slipping movements, because there is no axis around which the movement can take place. *Uniaxial movement* is movement within one plane, whereas *biaxial*

movement is movement in two planes. *Multiaxial movement* is movement in or around all three planes of space and axes. Range of motion varies widely between individuals. Basically, there are three general types of movements: *angular, gliding,* and *rotation*:

- *Angular movements:* Decrease or increase the angle between two bones. This can occur in any body plane and includes extension, flexion, hyperextension, abduction, adduction, and circumduction (see below).

- *Gliding movements:* When a flat (or nearly flat) bond surface slips over or glides over another in a side-to-side or back-and-forth motion. There is no major rotation or angulation. Examples include the movement of the intertarsal and intercarpal joints and between the flat articular vertebral processes.

- *Rotation movements:* Involve the turning of a bone around its long axis. This is common at the hip and shoulder joints and is the singular movement allowed between the first two cervical vertebrae. Rotation may be directed away from the midline or toward it. Examples include the thigh's medial rotation and when the anterior surface of the femur moves toward the body's median plane. The opposite movement of medial rotation is called lateral rotation.

The following terms describe types of joint movements, with simple examples of each (as shown in **FIGURE 8-7**):

- *Flexion:* Bending parts at a joint so they come closer together. It usually occurs along the sagittal plane, decreasing the angle of the joint. Examples include bending the trunk or the knee from a straight to an angled position or bending the head forward toward the chest.

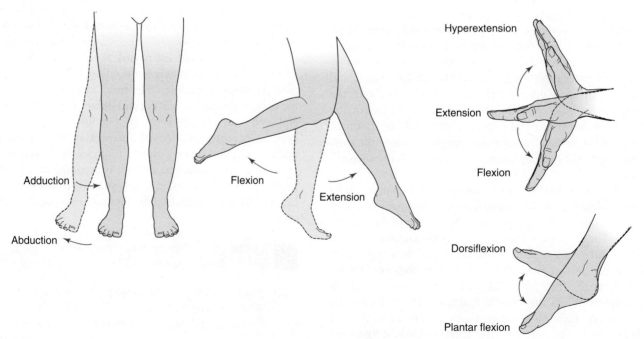

FIGURE 8-7 Types of joint movements.

- **Extension**: Straightening parts at a joint so they move farther apart. The reverse of flexion, it occurs at the same joints, also along the sagittal plane. The angle between the articulating bones is increased. This usually straightens a flexed body part, such as a limb. Examples include the straightening of a flexed elbow, neck, or knee.
- **Hyperextension**: Extending the parts at a joint beyond the normal range of motion, often resulting in injury because the anatomic position is exceeded.
- **Dorsiflexion**: Moving the ankle so the top of the foot comes closer to the shin or moving the wrist so the back of the hand comes closer to the arm (wrist extension).
- **Plantar flexion**: Moving the ankle so the foot moves farther from the shin, pointing the toes. This corresponds to wrist flexion.
- **Abduction**: Moving a part away from the midline (longitudinal axis), or median plane, of the body. An example is when the arm or thigh is raised laterally. For the toes or fingers, it means "spreading apart." However, the lateral bending of the trunk away from the body midline (in the frontal plane) is not called abduction but lateral flexion.
- **Adduction**: Moving a part toward the midline of the body. For the toes or fingers, it is moving them toward the midline of the foot or hand.

The following joint movements are shown in **FIGURE 8-8**:

- **Rotation**: Moving a part around its axis, either directed toward the midline or away from it. It is common at the hip, shoulder, and first two cervical vertebrae.

- **Circumduction**: Moving a part so its end follows a circular path, as if describing a cone in space. The distal end of a circumducting limb moves in a circle, whereas the "point" of the cone (the hip or shoulder joint) remains nearly stationary. Circumduction actually consists of the movements of flexion, then abduction, then extension, then adduction.
- **Pronation**: Turning the hand so the palm is downward, facing posteriorly. The forearm is rotated medially, moving the distal end of the radius across the ulna, forming an X between the two bones. The forearm remains in this position when a person is standing but relaxed. Pronation is not as strong a movement as supination.
- **Supination**: Turning the hand so that the palm is upward, facing anteriorly. The forearm is rotated laterally. In the anatomical position, the hand is supinated while the radius and ulnae are parallel.
- **Eversion**: Turning the foot so the plantar surface (sole) faces laterally.
- **Inversion**: Turning the foot so the plantar surface faces medially.
- **Protraction**: Moving a part forward, which is a nonangular anterior movement in the transverse plane. For example, the mandible is protracted when you stick your jaw out.
- **Retraction**: Moving a part backward, which is a nonangular posterior movement in the transverse plane. For example, the mandible is retracted when you pull your jaw back after sticking it out.
- **Elevation**: Raising a part (lifting it superiorly). When you shrug your shoulders, the scapulae are elevated.

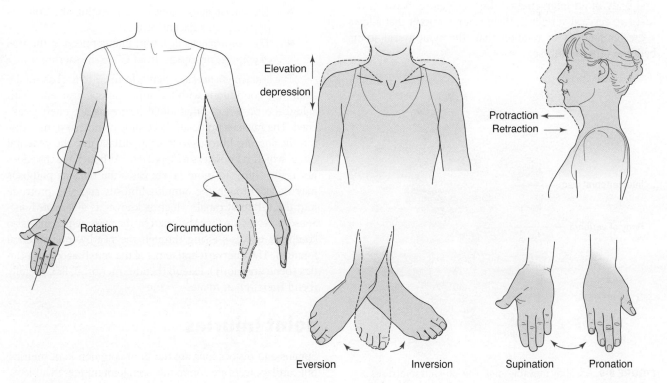

FIGURE 8-8 Joint movements.

- **Depression**: Lowering a part (moving it inferiorly). When you chew, your mandible is elevated and depressed repeatedly.
- **Opposition**: Involving the saddle joint between the trapezium and metacarpal I, the thumb performs opposition when you touch it to the tips of the other fingers on the same hand. Opposition allows us to grab a hammer or a glass of water. *Reposition* returns the thumb and fingers from opposition.

TEST YOUR UNDERSTANDING

1. Compare axial with nonaxial movements.
2. Describe angular and gliding movements.
3. Define the terms flexion, extension, and dorsiflexion.

Intervertebral Joints

Between superior and inferior articular processes of adjacent vertebrae in the spine are found **intervertebral joints** (*articulations*). These are gliding joints, allowing small movements such as flexion and rotation of the spinal column. However, only slight gliding occurs between adjacent vertebrae. Therefore, the vertebrae are separated and cushioned by *intervertebral discs*, which are pads of fibrocartilage (**FIGURE 8-9**). The bodies of the vertebrae form symphyseal joints. These joints are present between the axis and sacrum of the spine but are not present in the sacrum or coccyx. In these locations the vertebrae are fused. Also, the joints between the first and second cervical vertebrae are fused. Actually, the first cervical vertebra does not have a vertebral body or an intervertebral disc. Therefore, between the first two cervical vertebrae, there is a pivot joint that allows a greater amount of rotation than the symphyseal joints between other vertebrae.

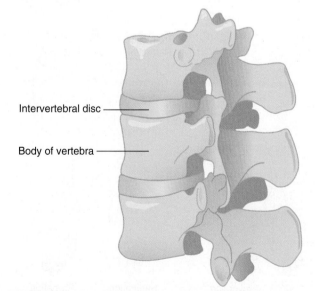

Intervertebral disc —

Body of vertebra —

FIGURE 8-9 A slightly movable joint. The intervertebral discs allow for some movement, giving the vertebral column flexibility.

Throughout most of the spine, each intervertebral disc has a tough outer layer of fibrocartilage known as the *annulus fibrosus*. Collagen fibers attach this fibrocartilage to the bodies of adjacent vertebrae. Inside the annulus fibrosis is the **nucleus pulposus**, a core that is softer, gelatinous, and more elastic. Intervertebral discs absorb shocks and have resiliency because of each nucleus pulposus. Thin *vertebral end plates* nearly cover the superior and inferior surfaces of each disc. The plates are made up of fibrocartilage and hyaline cartilage. When movement occurs, the vertebral column compresses the nucleus pulposus, displacing it in opposing directions. Gliding movements can occur while vertebral alignment remains constant.

Intervertebral discs make up nearly one-fourth of the length of the vertebral column superior to the sacrum, greatly contributing to an individual's height. However, aging causes water content of each nucleus pulposus to decrease, reducing their cushioning actions. This raises the chance of vertebral injury. The water loss results in vertebral column shortening, and the older individual actually becomes shorter over time.

Intervertebral Ligaments

The vertebrae are bound together and stabilized by many ligaments attached to their bodies. The intervertebral ligaments are as follows:

- *The anterior longitudinal ligament:* connecting anterior surfaces of adjacent vertebral bodies
- *The posterior longitudinal ligament:* connecting posterior surfaces of adjacent vertebral bodies
- *The ligamentum flavum:* connecting the laminae of adjacent vertebrae
- *The interspinous ligament:* connecting the spinous processes of adjacent vertebrae
- *The supraspinous ligament:* interconnecting the tips of spinous processes, from C7 to the sacrum

The *ligamentum nuchae* extends from C7 to the base of the skull. It is continuous with the supraspinous ligament. With aging, the posterior longitudinal ligaments are often weakened. The nucleus pulposus, becoming compressed, may distort the annulus fibrosus to force it partially into the vertebral canal, which is known as a *slipped disc*. Although the disc does not really "slip," in more severe cases the nucleus pulposus may break through the annulus fibrosus and also protrude into the vertebral canal, which is known as a *herniated disc*. Sensory nerves are then distorted by the mass, which may also compress nerves passing through the nearby intervertebral foramen. The intervertebral joints of the vertebral column can flex (bend anteriorly), extend (bend posteriorly), flex laterally (bend laterally), or rotate.

Joint Injuries

Sprains and dislocations are the most common joint injuries, but cartilage tears are commonly seen joint injuries in athletes. In a **sprain**, there is stretching or tearing of the ligaments that reinforce a joint. The most commonly sprained joint ligaments are those of the ankle, knee, and lumbar spine. Sprains are usually painful and cause the immobilization of the injured patient. When partially torn, they heal very lowly because of a lack of vascularization. However, a complete ligament tear is treated with surgery, grafting, and long-term immobilization. Ends of ligaments can be sutured together, but this is difficult to perform because of the hundreds of fibrous strands involved in each ligament. Grafting is used instead for ligaments such as the anterior cruciate ligament. In this operation, part of a muscle tendon is attached to articulating bones. For other ligaments (such as the medial collateral ligament of the knee), long-term immobilization is as effective as surgical methods.

A **dislocation** is also known as a *luxation*. It occurs when bones are forced out of alignment and usually is involved with a sprain. There is inflammation and difficulty in moving the joint. Common causes of dislocations include falling and contact sports. The most commonly dislocated joints are those of the jaw, fingers, thumbs, and shoulders. Dislocations, like fractures, must be *reduced*. This means the ends of the bones must be returned to their proper positions by a physician. Partial dislocation of a joint is called *subluxation*. Because an initial dislocation stretches a joint's capsule as well as its ligaments, repeat dislocations of the same joint often occur. The joint then has poor reinforcement because the capsule has become loose.

Tearing of cartilage causes it to break or pop because of being overstressed. The most common areas of torn cartilage occur in the knee menisci. Usually, the meniscus receives a compression and shear stress simultaneously, resulting in tearing. Cartilage usually remains torn because it cannot usually sufficiently repair itself. Loose bodies (fragments of cartilage) interfere with joint function because they cause binding or locking of the joint. Therefore, damaged cartilage is usually surgically removed via **arthroscopic surgery** (**FIGURE 8-10**). Fortunately, the patient is usually able to leave the hospital the same day as the surgery takes place. An *arthroscope* is used, which is very small, containing a miniscule lens and fiber-optic light source. The surgeon can look inside the joint to determine surgical options. Ligaments can be repaired or fragments of cartilage removed through one or several small slits. This reduces tissue damage and scarring. If only part of the meniscus is removed, mobility is not severely impaired, but the joint becomes much less stable. If the entire meniscus is removed, **osteoarthritis** usually develops in the joint earlier than normal. A meniscal transplant may be used for younger patients when cartilage is extensively damaged. Future surgeries may involve transplantation of a patient's own stem cells.

Effects of Aging on the Joints

Aging takes a heavy toll on the body's joints. Conditions such as arthritis and rheumatism are among the most prevalent complaints of elderly people. These conditions involve pain and stiffness in the joints, which may lead to immobility. Causes of arthritis include bacterial or viral infections, joint injuries, severe physical stress, and metabolic conditions.

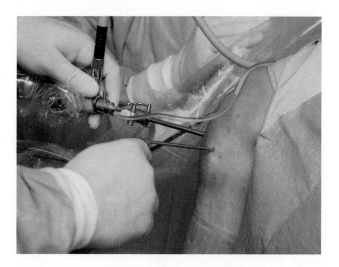

(A)

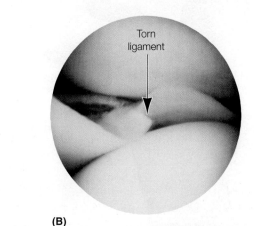

(B)

FIGURE 8-10 (A) A physician performing arthroscopic surgery. (© piotrwzk/Shutterstock, Inc.) (B) Inside view of knee joint through an arthroscope showing torn ligament. (© CNRI/Science Source)

Arthritis

Arthritis is a term that signifies more than 100 inflammatory or degenerative diseases, all of which damage the joints. Arthritis is the most common disease that results in crippling of movement in the United States, affecting one in five people. Acute arthritis usually develops from bacterial infections, whereas chronic arthritis includes the forms known as *osteoarthritis,* **rheumatoid arthritis**, and **gouty arthritis**. Rheumatoid arthritis is an autoimmune disorder that primarily affects the small joints of the hands, causing pain, stiffness, and deformity (**FIGURE 8-11**). Gouty arthritis, known also as *gout*, is caused by accumulation of uric acid and primarily affects the joints of the great toe, but can also involve the joints of the fingers, (**FIGURE 8-12**) wrists, knees, and ankles. It is much more common in men over the age of 30.

Gouty Arthritis

Gouty arthritis is a condition based on excessive, abnormal levels of uric acid deposited as needle-like urate crystals in soft tissues of joints. An inflammatory response is triggered, and

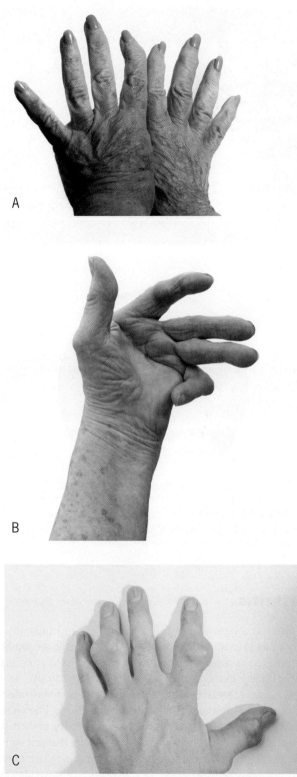

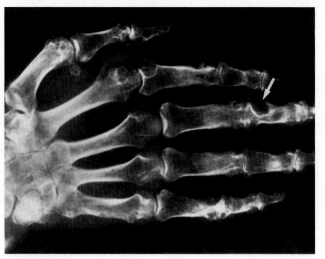

FIGURE 8-12 Radiograph of right hand of patient with gouty arthritis illustrating area of bone destruction (arrow) caused by masses of uric acid crystals. (Courtesy of Leonard V. Crowley, MD, Century College.)

If untreated, the articulating bone ends fuse to immobilize the joint. Medications include nonsteroidal anti-inflammatory drugs, colchicine, glucosteroids, and others. Dietary changes include increased water intake, avoiding alcoholic beverages, and avoiding foods such as kidneys, liver, or sardines, which are high in purine-containing nucleic acids.

Osteoarthritis

Osteoarthritis is the most common chronic form of arthritis. Degeneration of joints, via enzymatic activity, occurs due to aging in most patients (**FIGURE 8-14**). Degenerative joint disease occurs more commonly in women, usually affecting the knees and other weight-bearing joints and the distal finger joints. Nearly half of all adults develop osteoarthritis by age 85, and women are more commonly affected than men. In people with osteoarthritis, more cartilage is destroyed than can be

FIGURE 8-11 Hand changes in advanced cases of various types of arthritis. (A) Degenerative arthritis. (© Laurin Rinder/Shutterstock, Inc.) (B) Rheumatoid arthritis. (© Peterfactors/Dreamstime.com) (C) Gout. (© GIRAND/GJM/age fotostock)

extremely painful gouty arthritis occurs. Usually, the joint at the base of the great toe is first affected (**FIGURE 8-13**). Men experience gouty arthritis much more than women because of their naturally higher blood levels of uric acid. The condition may be genetically linked and often runs in families.

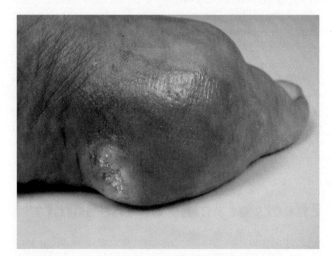

FIGURE 8-13 Gout. This is a left big toe affected by gout. The skin at the inferior of the metatarsal-phalangeal joint has broken down, and white granular material—the tophus—is extruding from the deft. The tophus is composed of urate crystals. (© GIRAND/BSIP/age fotostock)

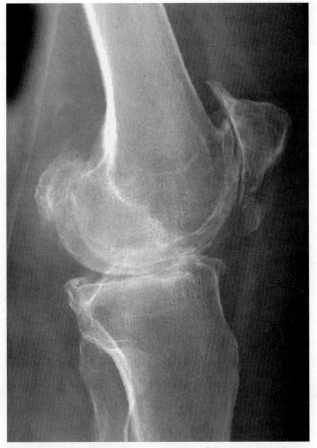

FIGURE 8-14 Degenerative joint disease of the knee, lateral x-ray. (Courtesy of Dr. Kirkland W. Davis, MD, Department of Radiology, University of Wisconsin School of Medicine and Public Health.)

normally replaced. Poorly aligned or overused joints are most likely to develop osteoarthritis. Exposed bone tissue becomes thicker over time, forming bony osteophytes (spurs). These enlarge bone ends, restricting joint movement. Affected joints may "crunch," a condition known as *crepitus*. Most commonly, the joints of the cervical or lumbar spine, fingers, knuckles, knees, and hips are affected. Osteoarthritis develops slowly, is irreversible, and causes pain, joint stiffness, and inflammation. Treatments include pain relievers, moderate activity, capsaicin, and nutritional supplements. *Continuous passive motion* helps an injured joint to repair by improving circulation of synovial fluid. This is often performed by a machine or physical therapist working with the patient.

Rheumatoid Arthritis

Rheumatoid arthritis is a chronic inflammatory disorder that usually appears between the ages of 30 and 50. It is less common than osteoarthritis and affects women three times more often than men. Initially, joint tenderness and stiffness are common. It usually manifests in the fingers, wrists, ankles, and feet, on a bilateral basis. Rheumatoid arthritis is marked by exacerbations and remissions, which may include anemia, muscle weakness, osteoporosis, and cardiovascular abnormalities. It is an autoimmune disease, in which the immune system attacks its own tissues. Although cause is not completely understood, it may be related to various

bacteria and viruses. The synovitis (synovial membrane) of an affected joint becomes inflamed first.

Lymphocytes, macrophages, and other inflammatory cells move to the joint cavity and release inflammatory chemicals. Over time, a *pannus* develops, which is a thickened, abnormal tissue that grasps to articular cartilages. The pannus erodes cartilage and bone, forming scar tissue and connecting bone ends together. When this scar tissue ossifies and the bone ends fuse, the joint becomes immobile. *Ankylosis* is the "end" condition, in which the affected areas become bent and deformed. Although ankylosis does not always develop, rheumatoid arthritis consistently results in restricted joint movement and intense pain. Treatment is aimed at disrupting the autoimmune destruction of the joints. Medications include steroidal and nonsteroidal anti-inflammatory drugs, immune suppressants, and biologic agents. Surgery may be used to replace affected joints with artificial prostheses.

Bursitis

Bursitis is inflammation of the bursae, which is often caused by trauma or friction. Examples of bursitis include conditions known as *water on the knee* and *student's elbow*. If severe, common treatments include injection of anti-inflammatory drugs into the bursae or removal of excessive fluid via needle aspiration.

Tendonitis

Tendonitis is inflammation of tendon sheaths, which is usually caused by excessive wear. This condition has similar symptoms to bursitis, which include pain and swelling. Treatment of tendonitis includes ice, rest, and anti-inflammatory drugs.

Lyme Disease

Lyme disease may also affect the joints and is caused by spirochete bacteria. It is transmitted by ticks that infest deer or mice. Lyme disease may cause joint (often knee) pain, arthritis, skin rash, flu-like symptoms, and impaired cognition. Untreated Lyme disease results in neurological and cardiovascular problems. It is very difficult to diagnose and usually requires a long course of antibiotics.

FOCUS ON PATHOLOGY

With aging, decreases in bone mass are one of the major risk factors for fractures, especially in women after menopause. This is increased by the presence of osteoporosis. Decreases in bone mass may affect the function of the joints in conditions such as osteoarthritis.

SUMMARY

Joints can be classified according to their degree of movement and by the type of tissue that binds together the bones that surround them. Joints are divided into fibrous, cartilaginous, and synovial types. Fibrous joints are tightly joined by a layer of dense connective tissue. They include sutures, syndesmoses, and gomphoses. Fibrous joints may be amphiarthrotic (having little movement, such as cartilaginous joints) or synarthrotic (immovable). Cartilaginous joints include synchondroses and symphyses. Synovial joints are covered with hyaline cartilage and are held together by a fibrous joint capsule. Synovial joints that allow free movement (diarthrotic) include ball-and-socket, hinge, condyloid, gliding, saddle, and pivot types. Synovial joints include characteristics such as articular cartilage, articular cavities, articular capsules, synovial fluid, reinforcing ligaments, nerves, and blood vessels. Both bursae and tendon sheaths are closely related to synovial joints.

Joint movements include flexion, extension, dorsiflexion, plantar flexion, hyperextension, supination, eversion, inversion, rotation, circumduction, pronation, supination, abduction, adduction, retraction, protraction, depression, and elevation. Joints must be stabilized to avoid becoming dislocated during stretching and compression. Muscle tendons crossing joints are often the most important factors concerning stability. As we age, joints may develop conditions such as arthritis or rheumatism. Many people over age 60 have osteoarthritis, which is also known as degenerative joint disease. Rheumatoid arthritis is an autoimmune disease that affects the joints. Gouty arthritis involves uric acid crystals forming in the synovial joint fluid.

KEY TERMS

Abduction
Acetabular labrum
Adduction
Amphiarthrotic
Anterior cruciate ligament
Annular ligament
Arcuate popliteal ligament
Arthritis
Arthroscopic surgery
Bursae
Bursitis
Cartilaginous joints
Circumduction
Collateral ligament
Coracohumeral ligament
Depression
Diarthrotic
Dislocation
Dorsiflexion
Elevation
Eversion
Extension

Fibrous joints
Flexion
Glenohumeral ligaments
Gomphoses
Gouty arthritis
Hip joints
Hyperextension
Iliofemoral ligament
Intervertebral joints
Inversion
Ischiofemoral ligament
Joint capsule
Joints
Lyme disease
Menisci
Nucleus pulposus
Oblique popliteal ligament
Opposition
Osteoarthritis
Plantar flexion
Posterior cruciate ligament
Pronation

Protraction
Pubofemoral ligament
Radial collateral ligament
Retraction
Rheumatoid arthritis
Rotation
Rotator cuff
Sprain
Supination
Sutures
Symphyses
Synarthrotic
Synchondroses
Syndesmoses
Synostoses
Synovial fluid
Synovial joints
Synovial membrane
Tibial collateral ligament
Tibiofemoral joints
Ulnar collateral ligament

The following learning goals correspond to the objectives at the beginning of this chapter:

1. Joints (articulations) are the junctions between bones.

2. Joints are structurally classified as fibrous, cartilaginous, and synovial joints. Joints are functionally classified as immovable (synarthrotic), slightly movable (amphiarthrotic), or freely movable (diarthrotic).

3. The structures of synovial joints include an outer layer of ligaments (joint capsules) and inner linings of synovial membrane that secrete synovial fluid. Some synovial joints have shock-absorbing fibrocartilage pads called menisci. They may also have fluid-filled sacs (bursae), commonly found between tendons and underlying bony prominences such as in the knee or elbow.

4. The six types of synovial joints are ball-and-socket, condylar or condyloid (ellipsoidal), plane (gliding), hinge, pivot, and saddle joints.

5. Common body movements include angular, gliding, and rotation movements. Angular movements decrease or increase the angle between two bones. Gliding movements include the movement of the intertarsal and intercarpal joints and between the flat articular vertebral processes. Rotation movements involve the turning of a bone around its long axis. Joint movements include flexion, extension, hyperextension, dorsiflexion, plantar flexion, abduction, adduction, rotation, circumduction, pronation, supination, eversion, inversion, protraction, retraction, elevation, depression, and opposition.

6. The most common joint injuries include sprains, dislocations, and cartilage tears. In a sprain, there is stretching or tearing of the ligaments that reinforce a joint. A dislocation is also known as a luxation and occurs when bones are forced out of alignment. They are usually involved with a sprain. Tearing of cartilage causes it to break or pop because of being over-stressed. This usually occurs in the knee menisci.

7. The common types of arthritis include osteoarthritis, which is degeneration of joints, via enzymatic activity, because of aging; rheumatoid arthritis, which is a chronic inflammatory disorder that usually appears between the ages of 30 and 50 and usually in women; and gouty arthritis, which is based on excessive, abnormal levels of uric acid deposited as needle-like urate crystals in soft tissues of joints which triggers an inflammatory response, causing extreme pain.

8. Accompanying the knee joint, there are three broad ligaments running from the patella to the tibia below: the *patellar, medial,* and *lateral patellar retinacula* ligaments. When the knee is extended, the extracapsular *fibular* and *tibial collateral ligaments* are crucial to prevent lateral or medial rotation. The posterior aspect of the knee joint is partially stabilized by the oblique popliteal ligament. The joint capsule is reinforced posteriorly by the arcuate popliteal ligament, which has a superior arc, from the head of the fibula over the popliteus muscle. The *intracapsular ligaments (cruciate ligaments)* cross each other to form an "X." The anterior cruciate ligament is attached to the tibia's anterior intercondylar area and passes upward, laterally, and posteriorly to attach to the femur. The posterior cruciate ligament has more strength and is attached to the tibia's posterior intercondylar area.

9. Gliding movements occur when a flat or nearly flat bond surface slips over or glides over another in a side-to-side or back-and-forth motion. There is no major rotation or angulation. Examples include the movement of the intertarsal and intercarpal joints and between the flat articular vertebral processes. Angular movements decrease or increase the angle between two bones. This can occur in any body plane and includes extension, flexion, hyperextension, abduction, adduction, and circumduction.

10. The causes of Lyme disease are bites from ticks that infest deer or mice and carry a specific spirochete bacterium. Lyme disease complications include joint pain, arthritis, skin rash, flu-like symptoms, and impaired cognition. If untreated, Lyme disease results in neurological and cardiovascular problems.

CRITICAL THINKING QUESTIONS

A 26-year-old professional football player injured his right knee during a game. After the team trainer examined him, he was taken off the field and directly to the emergency department. After a computed tomography, he was diagnosed with a fracture of the patella.

1. What are the three ligaments that connect the patella to the tibia?
2. If at the moment the injury occurred his knee was hyperextended and twisted, which ligament would have been damaged as well?

REVIEW QUESTIONS

1. A freely movable joint is a(n)
   A. diarthrotic joint
   B. synarthrotic joint
   C. symphysitic joint
   D. amphiarthrotic joint
2. Which of the following is an immovable joint?
   A. diarthrotic joint
   B. syndesmotic joint
   C. synarthrotic joint
   D. amphiarthrotic joint
3. The elbow joint is an example of a
   A. hinge joint
   B. pivot joint
   C. saddle joint
   D. gliding joint
4. Rotation of the forearm that causes the palm to face posteriorly is referred to as
   A. supination
   B. angulation
   C. projection
   D. pronation
5. The tibiofemoral joint functions as which of the following?
   A. gliding joint
   B. hinge joint
   C. saddle joint
   D. pivot joint
6. The amphiarthrotic articulation that limits movements between the two pubic bones is the
   A. ischial ramus
   B. pubic tubercle
   C. pubic symphysis
   D. ischial tuberosity
7. The type of synarthrosis that binds each tooth to the surrounding bony socket is a
   A. gomphosis
   B. suture
   C. symphysis
   D. synostosis

8. Extension is defined as movement that
   A. moves a limb from the midline of the body
   B. increases the angle between articulating elements
   C. moves a limb toward the midline of the body
   D. decreases the angle between articulating elements
9. The parts of the vertebral column that do not contain intervertebral discs are the
   A. first and second cervical vertebrae
   B. first thoracic and seventh cervical vertebrae
   C. first lumbar vertebrae
   D. first and second lumbar vertebrae
10. Examples of monaxial joints, which permit angular movements in a single plane, are the
    A. intervertebral joints
    B. elbow and knee joints
    C. shoulder and hip joints
    D. intercarpal and intertarsal joints
11. A movement away from the longitudinal axis of the body in the frontal plane is known as
    A. circumduction
    B. opposition
    C. adduction
    D. abduction
12. Which of the following increases the risk of fractures and is related to aging?
    A. decreases of bone mass
    B. increases of bone mass
    C. excessive degree of calcium salt deposition
    D. excessive degree of sodium and potassium in the plasma
13. Intertarsal joints are examples of
    A. ball-and-socket joints
    B. gliding joints
    C. pivot joints
    D. hinge joints

14. Which of the following are examples of saddle joints?
    A. elbow joints
    B. shoulder joints
    C. wrist joints
    D. carpometacarpal joints

15. Moving the ankle so the top of the foot comes closer to the tibial bone is called
    A. hyperextension
    B. plantar flexion
    C. dorsiflexion
    D. abduction

ESSAY QUESTIONS

1. Describe articulation.
2. Define the terms nonaxial, biaxial, and multiaxial.
3. Classify the various types of joints.
4. Discuss types of joint movements.
5. List the six characteristics of synovial joints.
6. Classify the various types of synovial joints.
7. Compare the elbow joints with the hip joints.
8. Define circumduction and pronation.
9. Describe the intervertebral ligaments.
10. Explain the effects of aging upon the joints.

Muscular System

OBJECTIVES

After studying this chapter, readers should be able to

1. Describe the structure of a skeletal muscle.
2. Compare the contraction mechanisms of skeletal muscle and cardiac fibers.
3. Describe a motor end plate and the function of a neurotransmitter.
4. Explain the relationship between cellular respiration and heat production.
5. Describe two major types of smooth muscle.
6. Distinguish between the origin and insertion of a skeletal muscle.
7. List the muscles that provide facial expressions and head movements.
8. Name the muscles of the abdominal wall and explain the action of the rectus abdominis.
9. Explain the muscles that flex and extend the thigh.
10. Describe the quadriceps femoris group and the function of the muscles it contains.

OUTLINE

Overview

Muscles are needed for many body activities, including breathing, talking, walking, and even sneezing. Important body functions performed by muscles include movement, joint stabilization, support of soft tissues, encircling digestive and urinary tract openings, posture maintenance, nutrient storage, and the generation of heat. Muscles contract by using chemical energy from nutrients. They are made up of highly specialized cells. Other actions of muscles include generating the heartbeat, distribution of heat, moving body fluids and food through the body, and providing **muscle tone**. Muscle tone does not produce active movements. Instead, it keeps muscles healthy, firm, and ready to respond to stimulation. The three types of muscle are skeletal, smooth, and **cardiac muscle**. This chapter focuses primarily on skeletal muscle. Skeletal muscle tone additionally helps to maintain posture and stabilize joints.

Skeletal Muscles

Skeletal muscles, along with other types of muscle tissue, nervous tissue, blood, and other connective tissues, make up the muscular system. Skeletal muscle attaches to bones and is the only type of muscle that is consciously controlled. It is therefore referred to as **voluntary muscle**. Skeletal muscle can, however, also be activated by reflexes. Individual skeletal muscles are separated from other muscles and held in position by layers of fibrous connective tissue known as **fascia.** Skeletal muscle controls overall body mobility. Although contractions may be rapid, skeletal muscle tires easily and requires rest after short amounts of activity.

Structure of Skeletal Muscle Fibers

A single cell that can rapidly contract in response to stimulation and relaxes when the stimulation ceases is known as a skeletal muscle fiber. These fibers are thin, elongated cylinders with rounded ends. They are very large, with a diameter ranging from 10 to 100 μm. This is up to 10 times larger than an average body cell. The length may be up to 30 cm, and skeletal muscle fibers consist of hundreds of fused embryonic cells. The cell membrane (**sarcolemma**) lies above the cytoplasm (also known as **sarcoplasm**), with many small, oval-shaped mitochondria and nuclei. The sarcoplasm is made up of many thread-like **myofibrils** arranged parallel to each other. One muscle fiber contains between several hundred and several thousand rod-like myofibrils. The sarcoplasm also contains large amounts of **glycosomes** and **myoglobin**. Myoglobin is similar to *hemoglobin*, which is the pigment that transports oxygen in the blood.

Myofibrils have thick protein filaments composed of **myosin** and thin protein filaments mostly composed of **actin** (**FIGURE 9-1**). These filaments are organized so they appear as **striations**—areas of alternating colored bands of skeletal muscle fiber. The repeating patterns of striation units that appear along each muscle fiber are referred to as **sarcomeres**, which are the functional units of skeletal muscle. Muscles are basically considered to be collections of sarcomeres. The sarcomeres contain smaller rod-like *myofilaments*. Myofilaments (which are sometimes just referred to as *filaments*) are similar to the microfilaments of cells, which contain actin or myosin. Actin and myosin are the proteins that help with motility and shape change in nearly every body cell. The collective structures that comprise myofibrils make up approximately 80% of cellular volume of muscle fibers.

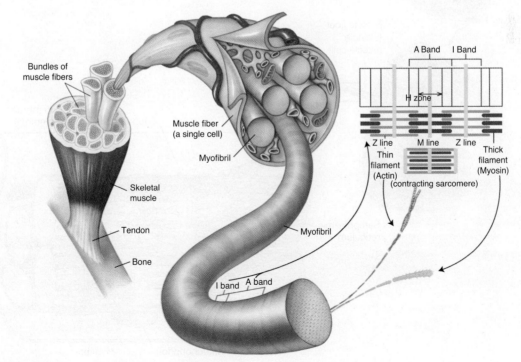

FIGURE 9-1 Details of the contractile machinery of the muscle cell.

There are two main parts of the striation pattern of skeletal **muscle fibers**, which are the longest types of muscle cells. The light bands (**I bands**) are made up of thin filaments of actin attached to round sheets known as Z lines (or **Z discs**). The Z lines or discs are made up of mostly *alpha-actinin*, a protein that anchors the thin filaments. The dark bands (**A bands**) are made up of *thick filaments* of myosin that overlap *thin filaments* of actin. The central thick filaments contain myosin and extend the entire length of the A bands. The thin filaments contain actin and extend across the I bands, part of the way into the A bands. When a muscle fiber is intact, the A bands and I bands are almost perfect in their alignment. The ability of a muscle to be stretched is known as **extensibility**.

There is a central region (**H zone**) of thick filaments, with a thickened area (the **M line**) that consists of proteins holding them in place. The H zone appears less dense because the thin filaments do not extend into it. The M line is slightly darker than the H zone because its fine protein strands hold nearby thick filaments together. The *zone of overlap* is a dark area where thin filaments lie between thick filaments. Three thick filaments surround every thin filament, and then six thin filaments surround every thick filament. Myofilaments connect to the sarcolemma and are held in an aligned pattern at the Z discs and M lines. Sarcomeres extend from one Z line to another Z line, as shown in Figure 9-1. Other proteins form the structure of myofibrils. *Elastic filaments* are composed of very large proteins known as **titins**. Each titin extends from the Z disc to thick filament, forms the core of the thick filament, and attaches to the M line. Titin binds thick filaments in place, keeping the A bands organized, and helps muscle cells to return to normal shape after being stretched. This process is called **elasticity**. **Dystrophin** is an important structural protein that links the thin filaments to the proteins of the sarcolemma. Filaments and sarcomeres are also bound by proteins such as *myomesin, nebulin,* and *C proteins*.

Inside the sarcoplasm of a muscle fiber, a network of channels surrounds each myofibril (**FIGURE 9-2**). These membranous channels form the **sarcoplasmic reticulum**, which is a smooth endoplasmic reticulum that has interconnected tubules surrounding each myofibril. Most of these tubules run longitudinally and communicate at the H zone. End sacs called *terminal cisterns* form perpendicular cross-channels at the A band–I band junctions. They occur in pairs and are larger cross-channels. The sarcoplasmic reticulum regulates intracellular levels of ionic calcium, stores calcium, and releases it when muscle fibers are stimulated to contract.

Transverse tubules (T-tubules) are other membranous channels extending inward and passing through the fiber. These tubules open to the outside of the muscle fiber and contain extracellular fluid. Each tubule lies between enlarged structures called *terminal cisternae*, near the point where actin and myosin filaments overlap. Together, the sarcoplasmic reticulum and T-tubules activate muscle contraction when stimulated. The lumen of each **T-tubule** is continuous with the extracellular space. The T-tubules form *triads,*

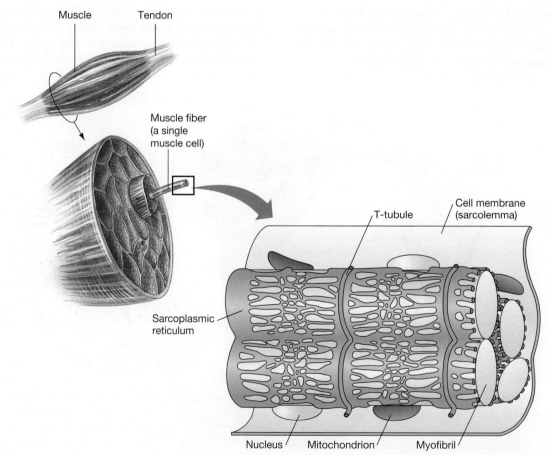

FIGURE 9-2 Location and fine structure of a muscle fiber.

which are groupings consisting of themselves in between two terminal cisterns. Ultimate control of muscle contraction is via electrical impulses initiated by nerves that travel through the sarcolemma. The continuous T-tubules conduct impulses deeply into muscle cells and all sarcomeres. This signals the release of calcium from nearby terminal cisterns. At the triads, organelles are in close contact, and integral proteins protrude into intermembrane spaces to act as voltage sensors. The proteins in this location that derive from the sarcoplasmic reticulum form gated channels. Through these channels, terminal cisterns release calcium ions.

Most skeletal muscle fibers are called *fast fibers* because they can reach peak twitch tension in 0.01 seconds, or less, after stimulation. They are large in diameter, containing large reserves of glycogen, relatively few mitochondria, and densely packed myofibrils. Muscles with fast fibers produce powerful contractions because the produced tension is proportional to the number of myofibrils, yet they fatigue quickly because adenosine triphosphate (ATP) is used in large amounts. *Slow fibers* are only about half the diameter of fast fibers, taking three times as long to reach peak tension. They can contract longer than fast fibers and are surrounded by a larger network of capillaries. They have a much higher oxygen supply to support their mitochondria. They also contain the red pigment *myoglobin*, which is similar to hemoglobin. Both pigments reversibly bind oxygen molecules. Myoglobin allows resting slow fibers to hold large oxygen reserves to be used during contractions. Slow fibers give skeletal muscles a dark red appearance because of the extensive capillaries and the large amounts of myoglobin.

Intermediate fibers look more like fast fibers, but their properties are mostly "in between" those of fast and slow fibers. They are paler because they contain low amounts of myoglobin. However, they are more resistant to fatigue than fast fibers. Muscles that have mostly fast fibers are often referred to as *white muscles*, whereas muscles that have mostly slow fibers are often referred to as *red muscles*.

Coverings of Connective Tissue

Fascia surrounds every muscle and may form cord-like tendons beyond each muscle's end. Tendon fibers may intertwine with bone fibers to attach muscles to bones. Broad sheets of fibers that may attach to bones or to the coverings of other muscles are known as **aponeuroses**.

Skeletal muscles are closely surrounded by a layer of connective tissue known as an **epimysium** (**FIGURE 9-3**). The muscle is separated into small compartments or *sheaths* by another layer known as the **perimysium**. Inside these compartments are **fascicles**, which are bundles of skeletal muscle fibers. Inside the fascicles, muscle fibers are contained within connective tissue layers. These layers form a thin covering (**endomysium**). The many layers of connective tissue that enclose and separate skeletal muscles allow a great deal of independent movement. In the endomysium are capillary networks supplying blood to the muscle fibers, *myosatellite cells* (stem cells that help repair damaged muscles), and nerve fibers controlling the muscles.

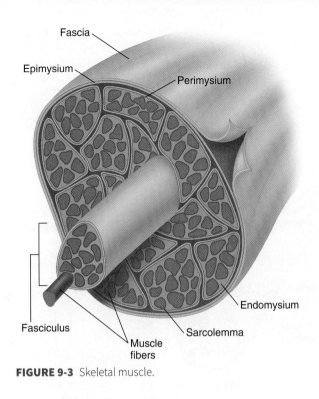

FIGURE 9-3 Skeletal muscle.

Neurological Structures

Neurons (nerve cells) conduct nerve impulses. **Motor neurons** control effectors, which include skeletal muscle. Each skeletal muscle fiber is connected in a functional manner to the axon of a motor neuron. These pass outward from the brain or spinal cord. Each functional connection is called a **synapse**. At the synapses, neurons communicate with other cells by releasing **neurotransmitters** (chemicals that enable communication). Skeletal muscle fibers usually contract when stimulated by motor neurons.

A *neuromuscular junction* is the connection between a motor neuron and a muscle fiber (**FIGURE 9-4**). A **motor end plate** is formed by specialized muscle fiber membranes and has abundant mitochondria and nuclei, with greatly folded sarcolemmas.

Motor neurons branch out and project into muscle fiber membrane recesses. Cytoplasm at these distal ends have many mitochondria and tiny synaptic vesicles that contain neurotransmitters. Upon receiving impulses, the vesicles release neurotransmitters into the synaptic cleft between the neuron and motor end plate, stimulating muscle contraction.

Motor Units

Most muscle fibers have a single motor end plate, although motor neuron axons have many branches connecting the motor neuron to various muscle fibers. When an impulse is transmitted, all connected muscle fibers contract at the same time. A **motor unit** is therefore made up of a motor neuron and the muscle fibers that it controls (innervates) (**FIGURE 9-5**).

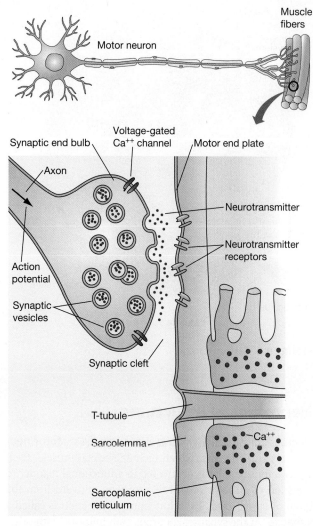

FIGURE 9-4 A synapse or neuromuscular junction.

1. Describe the basic structure of skeletal muscle fibers.
2. What is the function of a neurotransmitter?

FOCUS ON PATHOLOGY

The activities that occur at the neuromuscular junction can be affected by a variety of diseases, drugs, and toxins. A shortage of acetylcholine receptors may cause the disease known as *myasthenia gravis*, which most commonly affects the muscles of the mouth, throat, and eyelids. It also causes generalized muscle weakness. When the serum of a patient with myasthenia gravis is analyzed, there will be antibodies to acetylcholine receptors, making this disease autoimmune in nature. As it progresses, the disease destroys these receptors.

Contraction of Skeletal Muscles

Skeletal muscles contract when organelles and molecules bind myosin to actin to cause a pulling action. The myofibrils then move as the actin and myosin filaments slide, shortening the muscle fiber and pulling on its attachments. In *direct (fleshy) attachments*, the muscle's epimysium is fused to either the *periosteum* of a bone or the *perichondrium* of a cartilage. A periosteum is a specialized connective tissue covering all bones, with the potential to form bone. A perichondrium is a fibrous connective tissue layer covering all cartilage except for the articular cartilage of synovial joints. In *indirect attachments*, connective tissue wrappings of a muscle extend past the muscle in two forms: a sheet-like *aponeurosis* or a rope-like *tendon*. Indirect attachments are much more common than direct attachments. This is because they are smaller and more durable. Tendons are primarily tough collagen fibers that can withstand abrasion from bony projections that would destroy other, more delicate tissues.

Required Chemicals

Myosin molecules are made up of two protein strands with globe-shaped cross-bridges that project outward. Groups of many myosin molecules make up a myosin (thick) filament.

Actin molecules are globe-shaped with a binding site that attaches to myosin cross-bridges. Groups of many actin molecules twist in double strands (helixes) to form an actin (thin) filament, which includes the proteins known as **troponin** and **tropomyosin** (**FIGURE 9-6**).

Polypeptide strands of the rod-shaped tropomyosin protein prevent actin–myosin interaction. Tropomyosin spirals around the actin core, providing stiffening and stabilization. One subunit of the round three-polypeptide complex troponin protein molecule binds to tropomyosin, forming the troponin–tropomyosin complex. Another subunit binds to G-actin to hold the complex in position. A third subunit has a receptor binding a calcium ion. When the muscle is at rest, intracellular calcium is very low and the binding site is empty. Contractions cannot occur unless the position of the troponin–tropomyosin complex changes to expose the active sites on *filamentous actin (F-actin)*. The position change occurs when calcium ions bind to receptors on the troponin molecules. When sarcomeres shorten within a skeletal muscle fiber, a skeletal muscle contracts. This occurs because of the cross-bridges pulling on the thin filaments of F-actin. Each strand of F-actin is made up of two rows of 300 to 400 globular molecules of *G-actin*. Strands of *tropomyosin* cover the G-actin active sites and prevent actin–myosin interaction. A molecule of tropomyosin is a double-stranded protein covering seven active sites, which is bound to one molecule of troponin halfway down its length. A *troponin* molecule is made up of three globular subunits.

The **sliding filament model** or theory is so named because of the way sarcomeres shorten, with thick and thin filaments sliding past each other toward the center of the sarcomere, from both ends. If cross-bridges generate enough tension on thin filaments, shortening occurs. When the

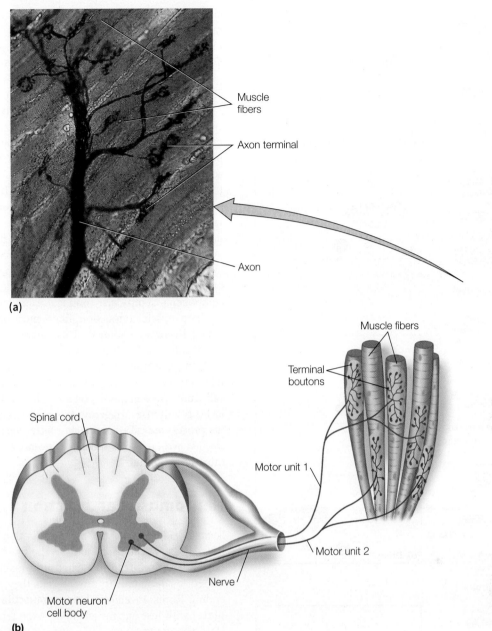

(a)

(b)

FIGURE 9-5 A motor unit is composed of a motor neuron and all the muscle fibers it innervates. (Photo: © John D. Cunningham/Visuals Unlimited)

cross-bridges become inactive, contraction stops, tension decreases, and the muscle fiber relaxes. Thin and thick filaments overlap only at the ends of A bands. Therefore, the sliding filament model states that when contraction occurs, thin filaments slide past thick filaments. Actin and myosin filaments overlap more, and myosin on thick filaments connects with myosin-binding sites on actin in the thin filaments. Sliding begins, and cross-bridge attachments form and then break several times during each contraction. They generate tension and move the thin filaments toward the center of the sarcomere. Because this occurs throughout sarcomeres in the cell at the same time, the muscle cell shortens. As thin filaments slide centrally, attached Z discs are pulled toward the M line.

Myosin filaments contain the enzyme **ATPase** in their globe-shaped portions. This enzyme catalyzes the breakdown of ATP to both adenosine diphosphate (ADP) and phosphate, releasing energy. The myosin cross-bridges assume a "cocked"

position, binding to actin to pull on the thin filament. After the pulling occurs, the cross-bridge is released from actin before the ATP splits. The cycle repeats as long as there is enough ATP for energy and muscular stimulation occurs.

To further understand, the following steps occur as a muscle cell shortens:

- I bands shorten.
- Distances between successive Z discs shorten.
- H zones (H bands) disappear.
- Contiguous A bands move closer together without changing their length.

Contraction Stimulus

The neurotransmitter that stimulates skeletal muscle to contract is **acetylcholine** (ACh). Synthesized in the cytoplasm of motor neurons, ACh is released into the synaptic

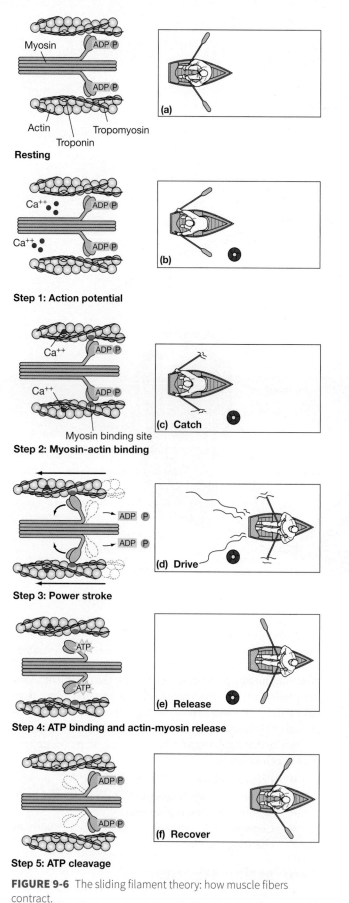

Resting

Step 1: Action potential

(a)

(b)

Step 2: Myosin-actin binding

Myosin binding site

(c) Catch

Step 3: Power stroke

(d) Drive

Step 4: ATP binding and actin-myosin release

(e) Release

Step 5: ATP cleavage

(f) Recover

FIGURE 9-6 The sliding filament theory: how muscle fibers contract.

clefts between motor neuron axons and motor end plates. It rapidly diffuses, binding to certain protein receptors in the muscle fiber membrane, increasing permeability to sodium. These charged particles stimulate a **muscle impulse** that passes in many directions over the muscle fiber membrane. This impulse eventually reaches the sarcoplasmic reticulum.

The sarcoplasmic reticulum has a high calcium ion concentration and responds by making the cisternae membranes more permeable, diffusing calcium into the sarcoplasm. Troponin and tropomyosin interact to form linkages between actin and myosin filaments. The muscular contraction also requires ATP and continues as long as ACh is released.

Muscle relaxation is caused by the decomposition of ACh via the enzyme **acetylcholinesterase**. It prevents a single nerve impulse from stimulating the muscle fiber continuously. When the stimulus ceases, calcium ions are transported back to the sarcoplasmic reticulum. The actin and myosin linkages break and the muscle relaxes. **TABLE 9-1** describes the major components of muscular contraction and relaxation.

For muscle contraction, fibers must be activated (stimulated by nerve endings). This causes a change in membrane potential. The fiber must generate an electrical current (**action potential**) in its sarcolemma, which occurs at the neuromuscular junction. This action potential is automatically moved along the sarcolemma. Intracellular calcium ion levels briefly rise, triggering the contraction. These parts of the process are called *excitation-contraction coupling*. The *contraction cycle* involves molecular events that enable skeletal muscles to contract.

Neuromuscular Junction

Somatic motor neurons are nerve cells that activate skeletal muscle fibers. They are found in the brain and spinal cord but have long, thread-like extensions (axons) that are connected inside nerves to muscle cells they serve. Each axon ending forms an elliptical **neuromuscular junction (end plate)** with just one muscle fiber. Axon terminals and muscle fibers are separated by a space called the *synaptic cleft*. Inside each axon terminal are *synaptic vesicles*, which are membranous sacs that contain ACh. Junctional folds of each sarcolemma provide large surface areas for the millions of nearby ACh receptors. Therefore, neuromuscular junctions include axon terminals, synaptic clefts, and junctional folds.

To understand more completely, the steps in which a motor neuron stimulates a skeletal muscle fiber follow:

- A nerve impulse reaches the end of an axon, and the axon terminal releases ACh into the synaptic cleft.
- ACh diffuses across the cleft, attaching to ACh receptors on the muscle fiber's sarcolemma.
- Binding of ACh triggers electrical events that generate an action potential.

The effects of ACh are quickly terminated by *acetylcholinesterase*, which breaks down ACh into its basic elements (acetic acid and choline). Therefore, continued and undesirable muscle fiber contraction, without additional nervous system stimulation, is prevented.

TABLE 9-1

Components of Muscular Contraction and Relaxation

Contraction	Relaxation
1. Nerve impulses travel down motor neuron axons.	1. Acetylcholinesterase breaks down ACh, and muscle fiber membrane is no longer stimulated.
2. Motor neuron terminals release ACh	2. Calcium ions are transported into sarcoplasmic reticulum.
3. ACh binds to ACh receptors.	3. ATP breaks links between actin and myosin without breaking down the ATP itself.
4. Sarcolemmas are stimulated; impulses travel over muscle fiber surface and deeply into fibers through transverse tubules.	4. ATP breakdown causes "cocking" of cross-bridges.
5. Impulses reach sarcoplasmic reticulum, opening calcium channels.	5. Troponin and tropomyosin inhibit interaction between myosin and actin.
6. Calcium ions diffuse into sarcoplasm, binding to troponin molecules.	6. Muscle fiber relaxes, ready to be stimulated again.
7. Tropomyosin molecules move to expose specific sites on actin.	
8. Actin and myosin link.	
9. Thin (actin) filaments are pulled to center of sarcomere by myosin cross-bridges.	

A resting sarcolemma is *polarized*, meaning there is a potential difference (voltage) across the plasma membrane, whereas the inside portion is negative compared with its outer membrane face. Action potentials occur because of a specific sequence of electrical changes. When they begin, they happen all along the sarcolemma's surface. This requires three steps: generation of an end plate potential, depolarization, and repolarization.

Energy Sources

Muscle fibers have just enough ATP for short-term contraction. ATP must be regenerated when fibers are active, using existing ATP molecules in the cells. ATP is regenerated from ADP and phosphate. **Creatine phosphate** accomplishes this with high-energy phosphate bonds. It is between four and six times more abundant in muscle fibers than ATP; however, it does not directly supply energy. It stores excess energy from the mitochondria in the phosphate bonds.

When ATP breaks down, energy from creatine phosphate is transferred to ADP molecules to convert them back into ATP. Creatine phosphate stores are exhausted rapidly when muscles are active; therefore, the muscles use cellular respiration of glucose as energy to synthesize ATP. Energy stored in creatine phosphate is eventually used to recharge ADP and convert it back to ATP. The enzyme that causes this conversion is *creatine kinase*. Muscle damage causes creatine kinase to leak across plasma membranes into the bloodstream. High blood levels of creatine kinase usually mean that serious muscle damage has occurred.

Nearly all (95%) of the ATP demands of a resting cell are provided by *aerobic metabolism*. This involves the absorption of oxygen, ADP, phosphate ions, and organic substrates such as pyruvate from surrounding cytoplasm by the mitochondria. These molecules then enter the *citric acid cycle*. Resting skeletal muscle fibers rely almost totally on aerobic metabolism of fatty acids absorbed from the circulation to generate ATP.

Oxygen Use and Debt

Oxygen is required for the breakdown of glucose in the mitochondria. Red blood cells carry oxygen, bound to **hemoglobin** molecules. Hemoglobin is the pigment that makes blood appear red. The pigment *myoglobin* is synthesized in the muscles to give skeletal muscles their reddish-brown color. Myoglobin can also combine with oxygen and temporarily store it to reduce muscular requirements for continuous blood supply during contraction.

When skeletal muscles are used for a minute or more, anaerobic respiration is required for energy. In one type of anaerobic respiration, glucose is broken down via *glycolysis* to yield pyruvic acid, which reacts by producing *lactic acid*. Lactic acid can accumulate in muscles but diffuses in the bloodstream, reaching the liver, where it is synthesized into glucose. This acid is a three-carbon molecule, which dissociates into one hydrogen ion and one negatively charged *lactate ion*. The movement of lactate to the liver and glucose back to muscle cells is called the *Cori cycle*.

When exercising strenuously, oxygen is used mostly to synthesize ATP. As lactic acid increases, an **oxygen debt**

TABLE 9-2

Changes in Muscular Metabolism

Variety of Exercise	Pathway Needed	Production of ATP	Result
Low to moderate intensity: blood flow provides enough oxygen for the cells' needs	Glycolysis, which leads to formation of pyruvic acid and aerobic respiration	For skeletal muscle, 36 ATP per glucose	Exhalation of carbon dioxide
High intensity: oxygen supply is not enough for the cells' needs	Glycolysis, which leads to formation of lactic acid	2 ATP per glucose	Accumulation of lactic acid

develops, also referred to as *excess postexercise oxygen consumption*. Oxygen debt is equivalent to the amount of oxygen that liver cells require to convert the lactic acid into glucose and the amount needed by muscle cells to restore ATP and creatine phosphate levels.

Endurance is defined as the amount of time during which a particular muscular activity can be performed without fatigue. *Anaerobic endurance* is the amount of time contraction of muscles can continue to be supported by glycolysis and the reserves of ATP and creatine phosphate. *Aerobic endurance* is the amount of time muscle contraction can continue while being supported by the activities of the mitochondria. Anaerobic endurance promotes hypertrophy, whereas aerobic endurance does not.

It may take several hours for the body to convert lactic acid back into glucose. Muscles may experience a change in their metabolic activity as exercise levels change. Increased exercise raises the muscles' capacity for glycolysis. Aerobic exercise increases the muscles' capacity for aerobic respiration. This is summarized in **TABLE 9-2**. For optimal health, you should alternate between aerobic and anaerobic exercise.

TEST YOUR UNDERSTANDING

1. Explain the basic components of muscle contraction.
2. Name the neurotransmitter that stimulates skeletal muscle fibers to contract.
3. Explain neuromuscular junctions.

Muscle Fatigue

Prolonged exercise may cause a muscle to become unable to contract. This condition is called **muscle fatigue**, and it may also occur because of interruption of muscular blood supply or occasionally a lack of ACh in the motor neuron axons. Lactic acid accumulation is the usual cause of muscular fatigue. As lactic acid lowers pH levels, muscle fibers cannot respond to stimulation. When a muscle becomes fatigued and cramps, it experiences a sustained, involuntary contraction. Although not fully understood, muscle cramps appear to be caused by changes in the extracellular fluid surrounding muscle fibers and motor neurons.

In a muscle's *recovery period*, conditions return to the normal levels present before the exertion occurred. After moderate activity, muscle fibers may need several hours to completely recover. Sustained, higher-level activity may require as much as 1 week for recovery.

FOCUS ON PATHOLOGY

Fibromyalgia is common disorder of unknown cause characterized by generalized aching; muscle, tendon, and soft tissue tenderness; muscle stiffness; fatigue; and poor sleep. Pain may worsen with fatigue, muscle strain, or overuse. Fibromyalgia is diagnosed by tests such as erythrocyte sedimentation rate, C-reactive protein, creatine kinase, and, sometimes, tests for hypothyroidism and hepatitis C because these diseases can cause general myalgia and fatigue. Fibromyalgia cannot be cured, but symptoms may be lessened by exercise, local heat, stress management, drugs that improve sleep, and analgesics.

Production of Heat

Most of the energy released in cellular respiration becomes heat. Muscle tissue generates a lot of heat because muscles form so much of the total body mass. Body temperature is partially maintained by the blood transporting heat generated by the muscle to other body tissues.

Muscle Responses

Muscle contractions can be observed by using a myogram to "see" muscle twitches. This requires electrical signals that can cause various strengths and frequencies of responses. A muscle fiber will remain unresponsive until a certain strength of stimulation (the threshold stimulus) is applied. An action potential is then generated that results in an impulse that spreads throughout the fiber, releasing calcium and activating cross-bridge binding. This causes contraction.

The contractile response of a fiber to an impulse is called a *twitch*, and it consists of a period of contraction followed

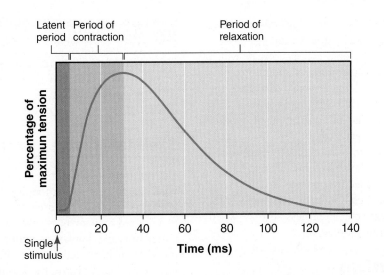

FIGURE 9-7 A myogram.

by a period of relaxation. A myogram records this pattern of events (**FIGURE 9-7**). A brief delay occurs between the stimulation time and the beginning of contraction, known as the *latent period*, which may last less than 2 msec. A myogram results from the combined twitches of muscle fibers taking part in contraction. There are two types of twitches: the fatigue-resistant slow twitch and the fatigable fast twitch. In the *contraction phase*, tension rises to a peak. This phase ends about 15 msec after stimulation. The *relaxation phase* lasts about 25 msec, and tension falls to resting levels. If stimulation occurs immediately after the relaxation phase ends, the next contraction will have a slightly higher maximum tension than the first. The increase in peak tension will continue over 30 to 50 stimulations, but after that the amount of tension will remain constant. This pattern is known as *treppe*.

The force of individual twitches combines via the process of *wave summation*. Stimulation of a muscle fiber causes it to contract and twitch. Waves of contraction add up, causing wave summation. When sustained contractions have no relaxation at all, they are referred to as either *tetanic contractions* or the condition known as *tetany* (**FIGURE 9-8**). A muscle that produces nearly peak tension during rapid contraction–relaxation cycles is described as being in *incomplete tetanus*. When the relaxation phase is eliminated by a higher stimulation frequency, *complete tetanus* occurs. High intensities of stimulation can activate many motor units (*recruitment*).

Actions of Skeletal Muscles

Skeletal muscles cause unique movements based on the type of joint they attach to and where the attachment points are. When a muscle appears to be at rest, its fibers still undergo some sustained contraction, known as muscle tone or tonus. *Isotonic contractions* involve tension rising and a change in

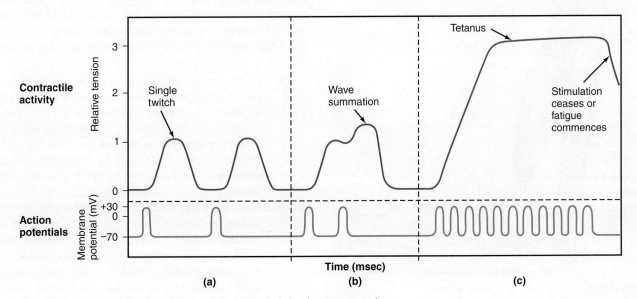

The duration of the action potentials is not drawn to scale but is exaggerated.

FIGURE 9-8 Tetany.

length of the skeletal muscle. Examples of actions involving isotonic contractions include walking and running. *Concentric contractions* are types of isotonic contractions in which muscle tension exceeds load as the muscle shortens. *Eccentric contractions* are also isotonic contractions, involving the development of peak tension that is less than the load, with the muscle lengthening because of contraction of another muscle or because of gravitational pull.

In an *isometric contraction*, tension never exceeds the load, and the muscle as a whole does not change length. Examples of isometric contractions include keeping your head up when working at a computer or carrying a baby. The involved muscles bulge, but much less so than when they are used in isotonic contractions.

Origins and Insertions

One end of a skeletal muscle usually is fastened to a relatively immovable part (**origin**) at a movable joint. The other end connects to a movable part (**insertion**) on the other side of the joint. As contraction occurs, the insertion is pulled toward the origin. There may be more than one origin or insertion, such as in the biceps brachii muscle of the arm. When this muscle contracts, the insertion being pulled toward its origin causes the forearm to flex at the elbow (**FIGURE 9-9**). Muscle contraction produces specific *actions* or *movements*.

The head of a muscle is the part closest to its origin. The term *flexion* describes a decrease in the angle of a joint, for example, a movement of the forearm that causes it to bend at the elbow. The term *extension* describes an increase in the angle of a joint, for example, a movement of the forearm that straightens the elbow.

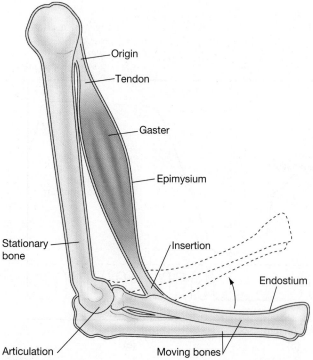

FIGURE 9-9 The parts of a muscle. The actual origin of the muscle shown is the scapula. The origin of the humerus is shown for clarity.

Skeletal Muscle Interactions

Skeletal muscles usually function in groups, with the nervous system stimulating the desired muscles to perform the intended function. A muscle that contracts to provide most of a desired movement is called a **prime mover** or **agonist**. Other muscles, known as **synergists**, work with a prime mover to make its action more effective. For example, when you bend your forearm, the agonist muscles are the biceps and the synergists are the triceps. Some synergists known as *fixators* may also assist an agonist by preventing another joint from moving to stabilize the origin of the agonist.

Other muscles act as **antagonists** to prime movers. They cause movement in the opposite direction. In the above example, the triceps are the antagonists to the biceps. Smooth body movement depends on antagonists relaxing while prime movers contract. Muscles may work opposite to each other or together to control various movements.

Manual Muscle Testing

Manual muscle testing is important for medical practitioners to determine muscular injury before treating patients with these injuries. For example, sports medicine practitioners and physical therapists use manual muscle testing on a daily basis for the diagnosis of conditions, to determine the required treatment, and to begin rehabilitation of injured muscles. These practitioners, as well as massage therapists and physical therapy assistants, must have knowledge of the locations and anatomic features of the muscles to be tested. Patients should receive a thorough explanation of what is being tested, how manual resistance will be used, what they should feel, and other information before any manual muscle tests.

There are two general tests used for gauging muscle strength:

- *Break test:* When a limb or other body part has completed its range of movement, manual resistance is applied in the direction of the "line of pull" of the involved muscle or muscles. The patient is asked to hold the part at that point and not allow the medical professional to "break" the hold with manual resistance. The break test is the most commonly used type of manual muscle test.
- *Active resistance test:* Manual resistance is applied against an actively contracting muscle or group of muscles (against the direction of movement). The medical professional gradually increases the amount of manual resistance until it reaches the ultimate level the patient can tolerate and motion ceases. This test is less often performed because it requires much skill and experience.

Resistance should be applied near the distal end of the body segment to which the muscle attaches, except when testing the hip abductors and the scapular muscles. When testing the hip abductors, resistance should be applied at the distal end of the femur, just above the knee. When testing the scapular muscles, resistance should be applied to the arm rather than on the scapula.

Muscles are graded between the numbers 0 and 5:

- *5, Normal (N):* Full range of motion or ability to maintain end-point range against maximal resistance.
- *4, Good (G):* Full range of motion against gravity or ability to tolerate strong resistance without breaking the test position but yielding to some extent at the end of its range with maximal resistance.
- *3, Fair (F):* Full range of motion against only gravity, but additional resistance, even if mild, causes the motion to break. Also, there is a Fair 1 grade that signifies a slightly greater muscle strength in some patients.
- *2, Poor (P):* Full range of motion possible only in a position that minimizes the force of gravity; this position is often described as the "horizontal plane of motion." Poor+ and Poor− grades indicate slightly greater or lesser muscle strength in some patients.
- *1, Trace activity (T):* Visual examination or palpation reveals some contractile activity in the tested muscle or muscles, but there is no movement as a result of this minimal contractile activity.
- *0, Zero/no activity (0):* Visual examination or palpation reveals no muscle activity.

Muscular Anatomy

Skeletal muscles, according to the arrangement of their fascicles, are divided into four distinct types: parallel muscles, convergent muscles, pennate muscles, and circular muscles. The pennate muscles are subdivided into *unipennate, bipennate,* and *multipennate* muscles. Most skeletal muscles are classified as *parallel muscles,* in which the fascicles are parallel to the long axes. Some are flat muscular bands with broad attachments called *aponeuroses* at each end, whereas others are thick and cylindrical, having tendons at one or both ends. When they are thick and cylindrical, they have a spindle shape with a central *body.* An example of a parallel muscle is the *biceps brachii.*

In a *convergent muscle,* the muscle fascicles extend over a broad area, converging on a single attachment site. The muscle may pull on a tendon, aponeurosis, or slender band of collagen fibers. This band is known as a *raphe.* An example of a convergent muscle is the *pectoralis major.*

In a *pennate muscle,* the fascicles create a common angle with the tendon, and muscle fibers pull at an angle. This means pennate muscles do not move tendons as far as parallel muscles do, but they have more tension because they have more muscle fibers and myofibrils. An example of a unipennate muscle is the *extensor digitorum,* of a bipennate muscle is the *rectus femoris,* and of a multipennate muscle is the *deltoid.*

In a *circular muscle* or *sphincter,* the fascicles are arranged around an opening in a concentric pattern. Muscle contractions cause a decrease in the diameter of the opening, such as the *orbicularis oris muscle* of the mouth or the *orbicularis oculi muscle* of the eye.

The skeletal muscles of the body are listed in **TABLES 9-3** to **9-19**, which are organized by body area. Muscle names

TABLE 9-3

Muscles of Facial Expression

Muscle	Action	Origin	Insertion	Innervation
Buccinator	Compresses the cheeks inward	Outer surfaces of mandible and maxilla	Orbicularis oris	Cranial nerve (VII)
Epicranius	Raises the eyebrows	Occipital bone	Muscles and skin around eye	Cranial nerve (VII)
Occipitofrontalis (frontal belly)	Raises eyebrows, wrinkles forehead	Epicranial aponeurosis	Skin of eyebrow, bridge of nose	Facial nerve (N VII)
Occipitofrontalis (occipital belly)	Tenses and retracts scalp	Occipital bone, mastoid region of temporal bones	Epicranial aponeurosis	Facial nerve (N VII)
Orbicularis oculi	Closes the eyes	Frontal and maxillary bones	Skin around eye	Cranial nerve (VII)
Orbicularis oris	Closes and protrudes the lips	Muscles near the mouth	Skin of the lips	Cranial nerve (VII)
Platysma	Draws the mouth downward	Fascia in upper chest	Lower border of mandible	Cranial nerve (VII)
Temporoparietalis	Tenses scalp, moves auricle of ear	Fascia around external ear	Epicranial aponeurosis	Facial nerve (N VII)
Zygomaticus	Raises the corners of the mouth	Zygomatic bone	Orbicularis oris	Cranial nerve (VII)

TABLE 9-4

Extrinsic Eye Muscles

Muscle	Action	Origin	Insertion	Innervation
Inferior rectus	Eye looks down	Sphenoid, around optic canal	Inferior, medial surface of eyeball	Oculomotor nerve (N III)
Medial rectus	Eye looks medially	Sphenoid, around optic canal	Medical surface of eyeball	Oculomotor nerve (N III)
Superior rectus	Eye looks up	Sphenoid, around optic canal	Superior surface of eyeball	Oculomotor nerve (N III)
Lateral rectus	Eye looks laterally	Sphenoid, around optic canal	Lateral surface of eyeball	Abducens nerve (N VI)
Inferior oblique	Eye rolls, looks up and laterally	Maxilla, at anterior portion of orbit	Inferior, lateral surface of eyeball	Oculomotor nerve (N III)
Superior oblique	Eye rolls, looks down and laterally	Sphenoid, around optic canal	Superior, lateral surface of eyeball	Trochlear nerve (N IV)

TABLE 9-5

Muscles of the Tongue, Pharynx, Larynx, and Palate

Muscle	Action	Origin	Insertion	Innervation
Tongue				
Genioglossus	Depresses and protects tongue	Medial surface of mandible, around chin	Body of tongue, hyoid bone	Hypoglossal nerve (N XII)
Hyoglossus	Depresses and retracts tongue	Body and greater horn of hyoid bone	Side of tongue	Hypoglossal nerve (N XII)
Palatoglossus	Elevates tongue, depresses soft palate	Anterior surface of soft palate	Side of tongue	Internal branch of accessory nerve (N XI)
Styloglossus	Retracts tongue, elevates side of tongue	Styloid process of temporal bone	Alongside to tip and base of tongue	Hypoglossal nerve (N XII)
Pharyngeal constrictors				
Superior constrictor	Constricts pharynx to propel bolus into esophagus	Pterygoid process of sphenoid, medial surfaces of mandible	Median raphe attached to occipital bone	Branches of pharyngeal plexus (N X)
Middle constrictor	Constricts pharynx to propel bolus into esophagus	Horns of hyoid bone	Median raphe	Branches of pharyngeal plexus (N X)
Inferior constrictor	Constricts pharynx to propel bolus into esophagus	Cricoid and thyroid cartilages of larynx	Median raphe	Branches of pharyngeal plexus (N X)
Laryngeal elevators	Elevate larynx	Range from soft palate, to cartilage around inferior portion of auditory tube, to styloid process of temporal bone	Thyroid cartilage	Branches of pharyngeal plexus (N IX and N X)
Muscles of palate				
Levator veli palatini	Elevates soft palate	Petrous area of temporal bone; tissues around auditory tube	Soft palate	Branches of pharyngeal plexus (N X)
Tensor veli palatini	Elevates soft palate	Sphenoidal spine; tissues around auditory tube	Soft palate	Trigeminal nerve (N V)

TABLE 9-6

Muscles of Mastication (Chewing)

Muscle	Action	Origin	Insertion	Innervation
Masseter	Elevates the mandible	Lower border of zygomatic arch	Lateral surface of mandible	Trigeminal nerve (V), mandibular branch
Temporalis	Elevates the mandible	Temporal bone	Coronoid process and lateral surface of mandible	Trigeminal nerve (V), mandibular branch

TABLE 9-7

Muscles That Move the Head

Muscle	Action	Origin	Insertion	Innervation
Semispinalis capitis	Extends the head, bends it to one side, and rotates the head	Processes of lower cervical and upper thoracic vertebrae	Occipital bone	Cervical spinal nerves
Splenius capitis	Rotates the head, bends it to one side, and brings it into an upright position	Spinous processes of lower cervical and upper thoracic vertebrae	Mastoid process of temporal bone	Cervical spinal nerves
Sternocleidomastoid	Pulls the head to one side, towards the chest, or raises the sternum	Anterior surface of sternum and upper surface of clavicle	Mastoid process of temporal bone	Accessory nerve (XI) and cervical spinal nerves (C_2-C_3) of cervical plexus

TABLE 9-8

Anterior Neck Muscles

Muscle	Action	Origin	Insertion	Innervation
Digastric	Depresses mandible, elevates larynx	Anterior belly from inferior surface of mandible at chin; posterior belly from mastoid region of temporal bone	Hyoid bone	Anterior: Trigeminal nerve (N V), mandibular branch; Posterior: Facial nerve (N VII)
Geniohyoid	Depresses mandible, elevates larynx, pulls hyoid bone anteriorly	Medial surface of mandible at chin	Hyoid bone	Cervical nerve C1, via hypoglossal nerve (N XII)
Mylohyoid	Elevates floor of mouth and hyoid bone, depresses mandible	Mylohyoid line of mandible	Median connective tissue band (raphe) that runs to hyoid bone	Trigeminal nerve (N V), mandibular branch
Omohyoid (superior and inferior bellies, united at central tendon anchored to clavicle and first rib)	Depresses hyoid bone and larynx	Superior border of scapula, near scapular notch	Hyoid bone	Cervical spinal nerves C_2-C_3
Sternohyoid	Depresses hyoid bone and larynx	Clavicle, manubrium	Hyoid bone	Cervical spinal nerves C_1-C_3
Sternothyroid	Depresses hyoid bone and larynx	Dorsal surface of manubrium, first costal cartilage	Thyroid cartilage of larynx	Cervical spinal nerves C_1-C_3

TABLE 9-8

Anterior Neck Muscles (continued)

Muscle	Action	Origin	Insertion	Innervation
Stylohyoid	Elevates larynx	Styloid process of temporal bone	Hyoid bone	Facial nerve (N VII)
Thyrohyoid	Elevates thyroid, depresses hyoid bone	Thyroid cartilage of larynx	Hyoid bone	Cervical spinal nerves C_1-C_2, via hypoglossal nerve (N XII)
Sternocleidomastoid	Its two bellies flex the neck; separately one side bends head toward shoulder and turns face to opposite side	Clavicular head attaches to sternal end of clavicle; sternal head attaches to manubrium	Mastoid region of skull and lateral portion of superior nuchae line	Accessory nerve (N XI) and cervical spinal nerves (C_2-C_3) of cervical plexus

TABLE 9-9

Muscles That Move the Pectoral Girdle

Muscle	Action	Origin	Insertion	Innervation
Levator scapulae	Elevates the scapula	Transverse processes of cervical vertebrae	Medial margin of scapula	Cervical nerves (C_3-C_4) and dorsal scapular nerve (C_5)
Pectoralis minor (minor means "smaller")	Pulls the scapula anteriorly and downward, or raises the ribs	Sternal ends of upper ribs	Coracoid process of scapula	Medial pectoral nerve (C_8, T_1)
Rhomboid major	Raises and adducts the scapula	Spines of upper thoracic vertebrae	Medial border of scapula	Dorsal scapular nerve (C_5)
Rhomboid minor	Adducts scapula, performs downward rotation	Spinous processes of vertebrae C_7-T_1	Vertebral border of scapula, near spine	Dorsal scapular nerve (C_5)
Serratus anterior	Pulls the scapula anteriorly and downward	Outer surfaces of upper ribs	Ventral surface of scapula	Long thoracic nerve (C_5–C_7)
Subclavius	Depresses, protracts shoulder	First rib	Clavicle (inferior border)	Nerve to subclavius (C_5–C_6)
Trapezius	Rotates the scapula, raises the arm, raises the scapula, pulls the scapula medially, and pulls the scapula and shoulder downward	Occipital bone and spines of cervical and thoracic vertebrae	Clavicle; spine and acromion process of scapula	Accessory nerve (XI) and cervical spinal nerves (C_3-C_4)

TABLE 9-10

Muscles of the Vertebral Column

Muscle	Action	Origin	Insertion	Innervation
Superficial				
Splenius cervicis	Rotates and laterally flexes the neck	Spinous processes and ligaments connecting inferior cervical and superior thoracic vertebrae	Mastoid process, occipital bone of skull, and superior cervical vertebrae	Cervical spinal nerves
Spinalis cervicis	Extends the neck	Inferior portion of ligamentum nuchae and spinous process of C_7	Spinous process of axis	Cervical spinal nerves

TABLE 9-10

Muscles of the Vertebral Column (continued)

Muscle	Action	Origin	Insertion	Innervation
Spinalis thoracis	Extends the vertebral column	Spinous processes of inferior thoracic and superior lumbar vertebrae	Spinous processes of superior thoracic vertebrae	Thoracic and lumbar spinal nerves
Longissimus capitis (longissimus means "longest")	Rotates and laterally flexes the neck	Transverse processes of inferior cervical and superior thoracic vertebrae	Mastoid process of temporal bone	Cervical and thoracic spinal nerves
Longissimus cervicis	Rotates and laterally flexes the neck	Transverse processes of superior thoracic vertebrae	Transverse processes of middle and superior cervical vertebrae	Cervical and thoracic spinal nerves
Longissimus thoracis	Extends vertebral column and produces lateral flexion	Broad aponeurosis and transverse processes of inferior thoracic and superior lumbar vertebrae; joins iliocostalis	Transverse processes of superior vertebrae and inferior surfaces of ribs	Thoracic and lumbar spinal nerves
Iliocostalis cervicis	Extends or laterally flexes neck, elevates ribs	Superior borders of vertebrosternal ribs near angles	Transverse processes of middle and inferior cervical vertebrae	Cervical and superior thoracic spinal nerves
Iliocostalis thoracis	Stabilizes thoracic vertebrae in extension	Superior borders of inferior seven ribs medial to angles	Upper ribs and transverse process of last cervical vertebra	Thoracic spinal nerves
Iliocostalis lumborum	Extends vertebral column, depresses ribs	Iliac crest, sacral crests, and spinous processes	Inferior surfaces of inferior seven ribs near angles	Inferior thoracic and lumbar spinal nerves
Deep				
Semispinalis capitis	Together, they extend the head; alone, each side extends and laterally flexes the neck	Articular processes of inferior cervical and transverse processes of superior thoracic vertebrae	Occipital bone, between nuchal lines	Cervical spinal nerves
Semispinalis cervicis	Extends vertebral column, rotates toward opposite side	Transverse processes ot T_1-T_5 or T_6	Spinous processes of C_2-C_5	Cervical spinal nerves
Semispinalis thoracis	Extends vertebral column, rotates toward opposite side	Transverse processes of T_6-T_{10}	Spinous processes of C_5-T_4	Thoracic spinal nerves
Multifidus	Extends vertebral column, rotates toward opposite side	Sacrum, transverse processes of each vertebra	Spinous processes of third or fourth more superior vertebrae	Cervical, thoracic, lumbar spinal nerves
Rotatores	Extends vertebral column, rotates toward opposite side	Transverse processes of each vertebrae	Spinous processes of adjacent, more superior vertebra	Cervical, thoracic, lumbar spinal nerves
Interspinales	Extends vertebral column	Spinous processes of each vertebra	Spinous processes of more superior vertebra	Cervical, thoracic, lumbar spinal nerves
Intertransversarii	Laterally flexes vertebral column	Transverse processes of each vertebra	Transverse processes of more superior vertebra	Cervical, thoracic, lumbar spinal nerves
Spinal flexors				
Longus capitis	Together, flex the neck; alone, each side rotates the head to that side	Transverse processes of cervical vertebrae	Base of occipital bone	Cervical spinal nerves
Longus colli	Flexes, rotates neck; limits hyperextension	Anterior surfaces of cervical and superior thoracic vertebrae	Transverse processes of superior cervical vertebrae	Cervical spinal nerves
Quadratus lumborum	Together, depress ribs; alone, each side laterally flexes vertebral column	Iliac crest, iliolumbar ligament	Last rib, transverse processes of lumbar vertebrae	Thoracic, lumbar spinal nerves

TABLE 9-11

Muscles That Move the Arm

Muscle	Action	Origin	Insertion	Innervation
Coracobrachialis	Flexes and adducts the arm	Coracoid process of scapula	Shaft of humerus	Musculocutaneous nerve (C_5-C_7)
Deltoid	Abducts the arm, extends or flexes the humerus	Acromion process, spine of scapula, and clavicle	Deltoid tuberosity of humerus	Axillary nerve (C_5-C_6)
Infraspinatus	Rotates the arm laterally	Posterior surface of scapula	Greater tubercle of humerus	Suprascapular nerve (C_5-C_6)
Latissimus dorsi	Extends and adducts the arm, rotates the humerus inwardly, pulls the shoulder downward and posteriorly	Spines of sacral, lumbar, and lower thoracic vertebrae; iliac crest; and lower ribs	Intertubercular groove of humerus	Thoracodorsal nerve (C_6-C_8)
Pectoralis major	Pulls the arm anteriorly and across the chest, rotates the humerus, and adducts the arm	Clavicle, sternum, and costal cartilages of upper ribs	Intertubercular groove of humerus	Pectoral nerves (C_5-T_1)
Subscapularis	Rotates the arm medially	Anterior surface of scapula	Lesser tubercle of humerus	Subscapular nerves (C_5-C_6)
Supraspinatus	Abducts the arm	Posterior surface of scapula	Greater tubercle of humerus	Suprascapular nerve (C_5)
Teres major (teres means "long and round")	Extends the humerus or adducts and rotates the arm medially	Lateral border of scapula	Intertubercular groove of humerus	Lower subscapular nerve (C_5 C_6)
Teres minor	Rotates the arm laterally	Lateral border of scapula	Greater tubercle of humerus	Axillary nerve (C_5-C_6)

TABLE 9-12

Muscles That Move the Forearm

Muscle	Action	Origin	Insertion	Innervation
Biceps brachii	Flexes the forearm at the elbow and rotates the hand laterally	Coracoid process and tubercle above glenoid cavity of scapula	Radial tuberosity of radius	Musculocutaneous nerve (C_5-C_6)
Brachialis	Flexes the forearm at the elbow	Anterior shaft of humerus	Coronoid process of ulna	Musculocutaneous nerve (C_5-C_6) and radial nerve (C_7-C_8)
Brachioradialis	Flexes the forearm at the elbow	Distal lateral end of humerus	Lateral surface of radius above styloid process	Radial nerve (C_5-C_6)
Pronator quadratus	Rotates the forearm medially	Anterior distal end of ulna	Anterior distal end of radius	Median nerve (C_8-T_1)
Pronator teres	Rotates the forearm medially	Medial epicondyle of humerus and coronoid process of ulna	Lateral surface of radius	Median nerve (C_6-C_7)
Supinator	Rotates the forearm laterally	Lateral epicondyle of humerus and crest of ulna	Lateral surface of radius	Deep radial nerve (C_6-C_8)
Triceps brachii				
(lateral head)	Extension at elbow	Superior, lateral margin of humerus	Olecranon of ulna	Radial nerve (C_6-C_8)
(long head)	Extension at elbow, extension and adduction at shoulder	Infraglenoid tubercle of scapula	Olecranon of ulna	Radial nerve (C_6-C_8)
(medial head)	Extension at elbow	Posterior surface of humerus inferior to radial groove	Olecranon of ulna	Radial nerve (C_6-C_8)

TABLE 9-13

Muscle	Action	Origin	Insertion	Innervation
Abductor digiti minimi	Abduction of little finger and flexion at its metacarpophalangeal joint	Pisiform	Proximal phalanx of little finger	Ulnar nerve, deep branch (C_8-T_1)
Abductor pollicis brevis	Abduction of thumb	Transverse carpal ligament, scaphoid, and trapezium	Radial side of base of proximal phalanx of thumb	Median nerve (C_6-C_7)
Abductor pollicis longus	Abduction at joints of thumb, wrist	Proximal dorsal surfaces of ulna, radius	Lateral margin of first metacarpal bone	Deep radial nerve (C_6-C_7)
Adductor pollicis	Adduction of thumb	Sides of metacarpal bones II, IV, and V	Proximal phalanx of thumb	Ulnar nerve, deep branch (C_8-T_1)
Dorsal interosseous (4)	Abduction at metacarpophalangeal joints of fingers 2 and 4; flexion at these same joints; extension at interphalangeal joints	Each originates from opposing faces of 2 metacarpal bones (I and II, II and III, III and IV, IV and V)	Bases of proximal phalanges of fingers 2 and 4	Ulnar nerve, deep branch (C_8-T_1)
Palmar interosseous (3-4), also called the *first palmar interosseous muscle*	Adduction at metacarpophalangeal joints of fingers 2, 4, and 5; flexion at these same joints; extension at interphalangeal joints	Sides of metacarpal bones II, IV, and V	Bases of proximal phalanges of fingers 2, 4, and 5	Ulnar nerve, deep branch (C_8-T_1)
Extensor carpi radialis brevis (brevis means "short")	Extends the wrist and abducts the hand	Lateral epicondyle of humerus	Base of second and third metacarpals	Radial nerve (C_6-C_7)
Extensor carpi radialis longus (longus means "long")	Extends the wrist and abducts the hand	Distal end of humerus	Base of second metacarpal	Radial nerve (C_6-C_7)
Extensor carpi ulnaris	Extends and adducts the wrist	Medial epicondyle of humerus and olecranon process	Carpal and metacarpal bones	Deep radial nerve (C_6-C_8)
Extensor digitorum	Extends the fingers	Lateral epicondyle of humerus	Posterior surface of phalanges in fingers 2 to 5	Deep radial nerve (C_6-C_8)
Extensor pollicis brevis	Extension at joints of thumb, abduction at wrist	Shaft of radius, distal to origin of adductor pollicis longus	Base of proximal phalanx of thumb	Deep radial nerve (C_6-C_7)
Extensor pollicis longus	Extension at joints of thumb, abduction at wrist	Posterior, lateral surfaces of ulna, interosseous membrane	Base of distal phalanx of thumb	Deep radial nerve (C_6-C_8)
Extensor indicis	Extension, adduction at joints of index finger	Posterior surface of ulna, interosseous membrane	Posterior surface of phalanges of index finger (2), with tendon of extensor digitorum	Deep radial nerve (C_6-C_8)
Extensor digiti minimi	Extension at joints of little finger	Via extensor tendon to lateral epicondyle of humerus, and from intermuscular septa	Posterior surface of proximal phalanx of little finger (5)	Deep radial nerve (C_6-C_8)

TABLE 9-13

Muscles That Move the Hands and Fingers (continued)

Muscle	Action	Origin	Insertion	Innervation
Flexor carpi radialis	Flexes and abducts the wrist	Medial epicondyle of humerus	Base of second and third metacarpals	Median nerve (C_6-C_7)
Flexor carpi ulnaris	Flexes and adducts the wrist	Medial epicondyle of humerus and olecranon process	Carpal and metacarpal bones	Deep radial nerve (C_6-C_8)
Flexor digitorum profundus	Flexes the distal joints of the fingers	Anterior surface of ulna	Bases of distal phalanges in fingers two to five	Palmar interosseous nerve from median nerve, and ulnar nerve (C_8-T_1)
Flexor digitorum superficialis	Flexion at proximal interphalangeal, metacarpophalangeal, wrist joints	Medial epicondyle of humerus, adjacent anterior surfaces of ulna, radius	Midlateral surfaces of middle phalanges of fingers 2–5	Median nerve (C_7-T_1)
Flexor pollicis longus	Flexion at joints of thumb	Anterior shaft of radius, interosseous membrane	Base of distal phalanx of thumb	Median nerve (C_8-T_1)
Palmaris brevis	Moves skin on medial border toward palm midline	Palmar aponeurosis	Skin of medial hand border	Ulnar nerve, superficial branch (C_8)
Palmaris longus	Flexes the wrist	Medial epicondyle of humerus	Fascia of palm	Median nerve (C_6-C_7)
Flexor digiti minimi brevis	Flexion at little finger joints	Hamate	Proximal phalanx of little finger	Ulnar nerve, deep branch (C_8-T_1)
Flexor pollicis brevis	Thumb flexion and adduction	Flexor retinaculum, capitate, trapezium, and ulnar side of first metacarpal bone	Radial and ulnar sides of proximal thumb phalanx	Branches of median and ulnar nerves
Lumbrical (4)	Flexion at metacarpophalangeal joints 2–5; extension at proximal and distal interphalangeal joints of digits 2–5	Tendons of flexor digitorum profundus	Tendons of extensor digitorum to digits 2–5	#1 and #2 by median nerve; #3 and #4 by ulnar nerve, deep branch
Opponens digiti minimi	Opposition of fifth metacarpal bone	Flexor retinaculum and trapezium	Fifth metacarpal bone	Ulnar nerve, deep branch (C_8-T_1)
Opponens pollicis	Opposition of thumb	Flexor retinaculum and trapezium	First metacarpal bone	Median nerve (C_6-C_7)

TABLE 9-14

Muscles of the Thorax and Abdominal Wall

Muscle	Action	Origin	Insertion	Innervation
Cervical Scalenes (anterior, middle, posterior)	Elevate ribs, flex neck	Transverse, costal processes of cervical vertebrae	Superior surfaces of first two ribs	Cervical spinal nerves
Thoracic Diaphragm	Contraction expands thoracic cavity, compresses abdominopelvic cavity	Xiphoid process, cartilages of ribs 4–10, anterior surfaces of lumbar vertebrae	Central tendinous sheet	Phrenic nerves (C_3-C_5)

TABLE 9-14

Muscles of the Thorax and Abdominal Wall (continued)

Muscle	Action	Origin	Insertion	Innervation
External intercostals	Elevate ribs	Inferior border of each rib	Superior border of more inferior rib	Intercostal nerves (branches of thoracic spinal nerves)
Internal intercostals	Depress ribs	Superior border of each rib	Inferior border of preceding rib	Intercostal nerves (branches of thoracic spinal nerves)
Transversus thoracis	Depress ribs	Posterior surface of sternum	Rib cartilages	Intercostal nerves (branches of thoracic spinal nerves)
Serratus posterior superior	Elevates ribs, enlarges thoracic cavity	Spinous processes of C_7-T_3, ligamentum nuchae	Superior borders of ribs 2–5 near angles	Thoracic nerves (T_1-T_4)
Serratus posterior inferior	Pulls ribs inferiorly, pulls outward also, opposing diaphragm	Aponeurosis from spinous processes of T_{10}-L_3	Inferior borders of ribs 8–12	Thoracic nerves (T_9-T_{12})
Abdominal				
External oblique (external or *externus* means "surface"; oblique means "slanted")	Tenses the abdominal wall and compresses the abdominal contents	Outer surfaces of lower ribs	Outer lip of iliac crest and linea alba	Intercostal, iliohypogastric, and ilioinguinal nerves
Internal oblique (internal or *internus* means "deeper")	Tenses the abdominal wall and compresses the abdominal contents	Crest of ilium and inguinal ligament	Cartilages of lower ribs, linea alba, and crest of pubis	Intercostal, iliohypogastric, and ilioinguinal nerves
Rectus abdominis (rectus means "straight")	Tenses the abdominal wall, compresses the abdominal contents, and flexes the vertebral column	Crest of pubis and symphysis pubis	Xiphoid process of sternum and costal cartilages	Intercostal nerves (T_7-T_{12})
Transversus abdominis (transverse means "across")	Tenses the abdominal wall and compresses the abdominal contents	Costal cartilages of lower ribs, processes of lumbar vertebrae, lip of iliac crest, and inguinal ligament	Linea alba and crest of pubis	Intercostal, iliohypogastric, and ilioinguinal nerves

TABLE 9-15

Muscles of the Pelvis

Muscle	Action	Origin	Insertion	Innervation
Bulbospongiosus	In females, it constricts the vagina; in males, it assists in the emptying of the urethra	Central tendon	Females: Pubic arch and root of clitoris Males: Urogenital diaphragm and fascia of the penis	Pudendal nerve, perineal branch (S_2-S_4)
Ischiocavernosus	Assists in the function of the bulbospongiosus	Ischial tuberosity	Pubic arch	Pudendal nerve, perineal branch (S_2-S_4)
Levator ani				
Iliococcygeus	Tenses floor of pelvis, flexes coccygeal joints, elevates and retracts anus	Ischial spine, pubis	Coccyx, median raphe	Pudendal nerve (S_2-S_4)
Pubococcygeus	Tenses floor of pelvis, flexes coccygeal joints, elevates and retracts anus	Inner margins of pubis	Coccyx, median raphe	Pudendal nerve (S_2-S_4)
External anal sphincter	Closes anal opening	Via tendon from coccyx	Encircles anal opening	Pudendal nerve, hemorrhoidal branch (S_2-S_4)

TABLE 9-15

Muscles of the Pelvis (continued)

Muscle	Action	Origin	Insertion	Innervation
Pelvic diaphragm Coccyges	Flexes coccygeal joints; tenses, supports pelvic floor	Ischial spine	Lateral, inferior borders of sacrum, coccyx	Inferior sacral nerves (S_4-S_5)
Superficial transversus perineal	Supports the pelvic viscera	Ischial tuberosity	Central tendon	Pudendal nerve, perineal branch (S_2-S_4)
Urogenital diaphragm				
Deep transverse perineal	Stabilizes central tendon of perineum	Ischial ramus	Median raphe of urogenital diaphragm	Pudendal nerve, perineal branch (S_2-S_4)
External urethral sphincter (male)	Closes urethra; compresses prostate, bulbourethral glands	Ischial and pubic rami	To median raphe at base of penis; inner fibers encircle urethra	Pudendal nerve, perineal branch (S_2-S_4)
External urethral sphincter (female)	Closes urethra; compresses vagina, greater vestibular glands	Ischial and pubic rami	To median raphe; inner fibers encircle urethra	Pudendal nerve, perineal branch (S_2-S_4)

TABLE 9-16

Muscles That Move the Thigh

Muscle	Action	Origin	Insertion	Innervation
Adductor brevis	Adduction, flexion, and medial rotation at hip	Inferior ramus of pubis	Linea aspera of femur	Obturator nerve (L_3-L_4)
Adductor longus	Adducts, flexes, and rotates the thigh laterally	Pubic bone near symphysis pubis	Posterior surface of femur	Obturator nerve (L_3-L_4)
Adductor magnus (magnus means "large")	Adducts, extends, and rotates the thigh laterally	Ischial tuberosity	Posterior surface of femur	Obturator and sciatic nerves
Gracilis	Adducts the thigh, flexes and rotates the lower limb medially	Lower edge of symphysis pubis	Medial surface of tibia	Obturator nerve (L_3-L_4)
Pectineus	Adduction, flexion, and medial rotation at hip	Superior ramus of pubis	Pectineal line inferior to femur's lesser trochanter	Femoral nerve (L_2-L_4)
Gluteus maximus (maximus means "largest")	Extends the thigh	Sacrum, coccyx, and posterior surface of ilium	Posterior surface of femur and fascia of thigh	Inferior gluteal nerve (L_5-S_2)
Gluteus medius	Abducts and rotates the thigh medially	Lateral surface of ilium	Greater trochanter of femur	Superior gluteal nerve (L_4-S_1)
Gluteus minimus (minimus means "smallest")	Abducts and rotates the thigh medially	Lateral surface of ilium	Greater trochanter of femur	Superior gluteal nerve (L_4-S_1)
Iliacus	Flexes the thigh	Iliac fossa of ilium	Lesser trochanter of femur	Femoral nerve (L_2-L_3)
Gemelli (superior and inferior)	Lateral rotation at hip	Ischial spine and tuberosity	Medial surface of greater trochanter with tendon of obturator internus	Nerves to obturator internus and quadratus femoris

TABLE 9-16

Muscles That Move the Thigh (continued)

Muscle	Action	Origin	Insertion	Innervation
Obturators (externus and internus)	Lateral rotation at hip	Lateral and medial margins of obturator foramen	Trochanteric fossa of femur (externus); medial surface of greater trochanter (internus)	Obturator nerve (externus: L_3-L_4) and special nerve from sacral plexus (internus: L_5-S_2)
Piriformis	Lateral rotation and abduction at hip	Sacrum's anterolateral surface	Femur's greater trochanter	Branches of sacral nerves (S_1-S_2)
Quadratus femoris	Lateral rotation at hip	Lateral border of ischial tuberosity	Intertrochanteric crest of femur	Special nerve from sacral plexus (L_4-S_1)
Psoas major (major means "larger")	Flexes the thigh	Lumbar intervertebral discs, bodies, and transverse processes of lumbar vertebrae	Lesser trochanter of femur	Branches of the lumbar plexus (L_2-L_3)
Tensor fasciae latae	Abducts, flexes, and rotates the thigh medially	Anterior iliac crest	Fascia of thigh	Superior gluteal nerve (L_4-S_1)

TABLE 9-17

Muscles That Move the Leg

Muscle	Action	Origin	Insertion	Innervation
Hamstring group				
Biceps femoris	Flexes the leg, extends the thigh	Ischial tuberosity and posterior surface of femur	Head of fibula and lateral condyle of tibia	Sciatic nerve; tibial portion (S_1-S_3; to long head) and common fibular branch (L_5-S_2; to short head)
Semimembranosus	Same	Ischial tuberosity	Medial condyle of tibia	Sciatic nerve (tibial portion; L_5-S_2)
Semitendinosus	Same	Ischial tuberosity	Medial surface of tibia	Sciatic nerve (tibial portion; L_5-S_2)
Quadriceps femoris group				
Rectus femoris	Extends leg at the knee	Spine of ilium and margin of acetabulum	Patella by the tendon, which continues as patellar ligament to tibial tuberosity	Femoral nerve (L_2-L_4)
Vastus intermedius	Same	Anterior and lateral surfaces of femur	Same	Femoral nerve (L_2-L_4)
Vastus lateralis	Same	Greater trochanter and posterior surface of femur	Same	Femoral nerve (L_2-L_4)
Vastus medialis	Same	Medial surface of femur	Same	Femoral nerve (L_2-L_4)
Sartorius	Flexes the leg and thigh, abducts the thigh, rotates the thigh laterally, and rotates the leg medially	Anterior superior iliac spine	Medial surface of tibia	Femoral nerve (L_2-L_3)

TABLE 9-18

Muscles of the Foot and Toes

Muscle	Action	Origin	Insertion	Innervation
Fibularis longus	Plantar flexion and eversion of the foot; also supports the arch	Lateral condyle of tibia and head and shaft of fibula	Tarsal and metatarsal bones	Superficial fibular nerve (L_4-S_1)
Fibularis brevis	Eversion of foot and extension (plantar flexion) at ankle	Midlateral margin of fibula	Base of fifth metatarsal bone	Superficial fibular nerve (L_4-S_1)
Gastrocnemius	Plantar flexion of the foot and flexion of the leg at the knee	Lateral and medial condyles of femur	Posterior surface of calcaneus	Tibial nerve (S_1-S_2)
Plantaris	Plantar flexion at ankle; flexion at knee	Lateral supracondylar ridge	Posterior calcaneus	Tibial nerve (L_4-S_1)
Soleus	Plantar flexion of the foot	Head and shaft of fibula and posterior surface of tibia	Posterior surface of calcaneus	Sciatic nerve, tibial branch (S_1-S_2)
Tibialis anterior	Dorsiflexion and inversion of the foot	Lateral condyle and lateral surface of tibia	Tarsal bone (cuneiform) and first metatarsal	Deep fibular nerve (L_4-S_1)
Tibialis posterior	Plantar flexion and inversion of the foot	Lateral condyle and posterior surface of tibia, and posterior surface of fibula	Tarsal and metatarsal bones	Sciatic nerve, tibial branch (S_1-S_2)
Flexor digitorum brevis	Flexion at proximal interphalangeal joints of toes 2–5	Calcaneus (tuberosity on inferior surface)	Sides of middle phalanges, toes 2–5	Medial plantar nerve (L_4-L_5)
Flexor hallucis brevis	Flexion at metatarsophalangeal joint, great toe	Cuboid and lateral cuneiform bones	Proximal phalanx, great toe	Medial plantar nerve (L_4-L_5)
Lumbrical (4)	Flexion at metatarsophalangeal joints; extension at proximal interphalangeal joints, toes 2–5	Flexor digitorum longus tendons	Extensor digitorum longus insertions	Medial plantar nerve (1), lateral plantar nerve (2–4)
Quadratus plantae	Flexion at joints of toes 2–5	Calcaneus (inferior, medial surfaces)	Flexor digitorum longus tendon	Lateral plantar nerve (L_4-L_5)
Extensor digitorum brevis	Extension at metatarsophalangeal joints, toes 1–4	Calcaneus (lateral and superior surfaces)	Dorsal surfaces, toes 1–4	Deep fibular nerve (L_5-S_1)
Extensor hallucis brevis	Extension of great toe	Superior surface, anterior calcaneus	Dorsal surface of base of proximal phalanx, great toe	Deep fibular nerve (L_5-S_1)
Flexor digiti minimi brevis	Flexion at metatarsophalangeal joint, toe 5	Base of metatarsal bone 5	Lateral side of proximal phalanx, toe 5	Lateral plantar nerve (S_1-S_2)
Abductor hallucis	Abduction at metatarsophalangeal joint, great toe	Calcaneus (tuberosity on inferior surface)	Medial side of proximal phalanx, great toe	Medial plantar nerve (L_4-L_5)

TABLE 9-18

Muscles of the Foot and Toes (continued)

Muscle	Action	Origin	Insertion	Innervation
Adductor hallucis	Adduction at metatarsophalangeal joint, great toe	Bases of metatarsal bones 2–4 and plantar ligaments	Proximal phalanx, great toe	Lateral plantar nerve $(S_1\text{-}S_2)$
Dorsal interosseous (4)	Abduction at metatarsophalangeal joints, toes 3 and 4	Sides of metatarsal bones	Medial, lateral sides of toe 2; lateral sides, toes 3 and 4	Lateral plantar nerve $(S_1\text{-}S_2)$
Plantar interosseous (3)	Adduction at metatarsophalangeal joints, toes 3–5	Bases and medial sides, metatarsal bones	Medial sides, toes 3–5	Lateral plantar nerve $(S_1\text{-}S_2)$
Abductor digiti minimi	Abduction at metatarsophalangeal joint, toe 5	Sides of metatarsal bones	Lateral side of phalanx, toe 5	Lateral plantar nerve $(L_4\text{-}L_5)$
Extensor digitorum longus	Dorsiflexion and eversion of the foot and extension of the toes	Lateral condyle of tibia and anterior surface of fibula	Dorsal surfaces of second and third phalanges of the four lateral toes	Deep fibular nerve $(L_4\text{-}S_1)$
Extensor hallucis longus	Extension at joints of great toe	Anterior fibula surface	Distal phalanx, superior surface, of great toe	Deep fibular nerve $(L_4\text{-}S_1)$
Flexor digitorum longus	Flexion at joints of toes 2–5	Posteromedial surface of tibia	Inferior surfaces of distal phalanges, toes 2–5	Sciatic nerve, tibial branch $(L_5\text{-}S_1)$
Flexor hallucis longus	Flexion at joints of great toe	Posterior fibula surface	Distal phalanx, inferior surface, of great toe	

often describe their sizes, shapes, locations, actions, number of attachments, or direction of fibers. **FIGURES 9-10** and **9-11** show anterior and posterior views of the superficial skeletal muscles, **FIGURE 9-12** shows the muscles of the face and anterior trunk, **FIGURE 9-13** shows the muscles of the shoulder and back, **FIGURE 9-14** shows the muscles of the anterior shoulder and arm, and **FIGURES 9-15** and **9-16** show various portions of the upper and lower leg muscles.

TABLE 9-19

Skeletal, Smooth, and Cardiac Muscle

	Skeletal	Smooth	Cardiac
Location	Skeletal muscles	Hollow viscera walls, blood vessels	Heart walls
Function	Movement of bones at joints, maintenance of posture	Viscera movement, peristalsis, vasoconstriction	Heart pumping
Striations	Present	None	Present
Nucleus	Many nuclei	Single nucleus	Single nucleus
Features	Good transverse tubule systems	No transverse tubules	Good transverse tubule systems, intercalated discs separating adjacent cells
Control	Voluntary	Involuntary	Involuntary
Contraction	Rapid contraction and relaxation	Slow contraction and relaxation, self-exciting, rhythmic	Cell network contracts as a unit, self-exciting, rhythmic

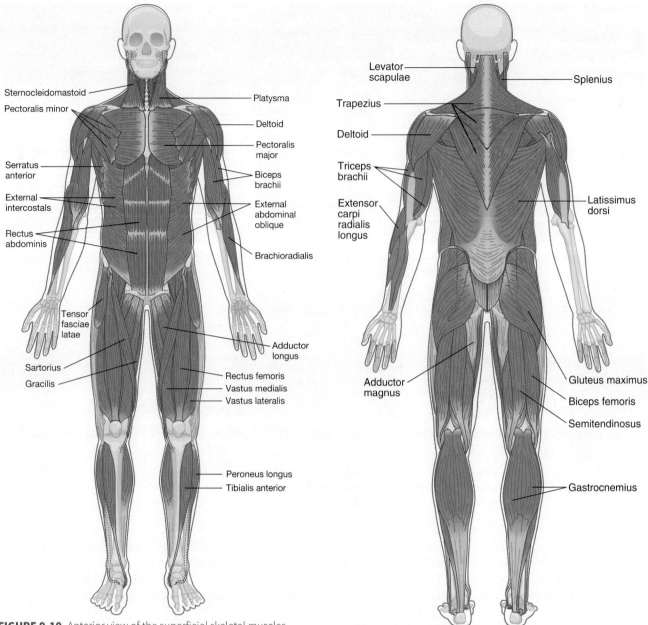

FIGURE 9-10 Anterior view of the superficial skeletal muscles.

FIGURE 9-11 Posterior view of the superficial skeletal muscles.

The diaphragm muscle is only discussed briefly here. The diaphragm is a dome-shaped muscle located below the lungs. As it moves downward, the thoracic cavity enlarges and atmospheric pressure forces air into the airways. While it is contracting and moving downward, the ribs are raised and the sternum elevates, allowing more air to enter the airways. As the diaphragm and external intercostal muscles relax after inspiration, the lungs and thoracic cage return to their original shapes. The diaphragm is pushed upward to force air inside the lungs out through the respiratory passages. The abdominal wall muscles increase pressure and force the diaphragm even higher against the lungs to squeeze additional air out of them.

FOCUS ON PATHOLOGY

Muscular *atrophy* can occur in situations where a patient is immobilized for a long time, because of a lack of use and loss of neural stimulation. Atrophied muscles degenerate and lose mass. This process begins as soon as muscles are immobilized, with up to 5% of muscle strength being lost per day.

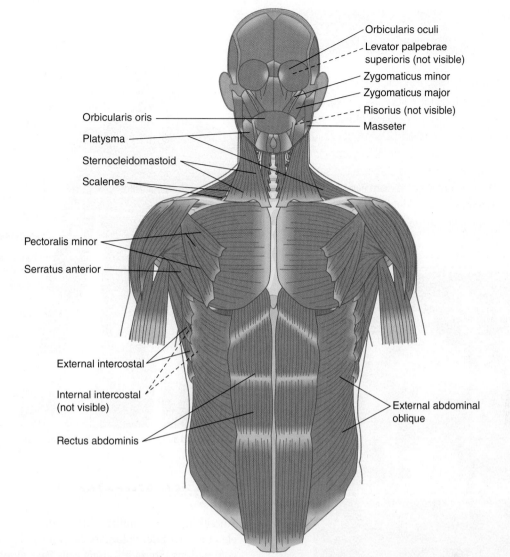

FIGURE 9-12 The muscles of the face and anterior trunk.

FOCUS ON PATHOLOGY

A disease that usually appears in childhood and destroys muscles is known as *muscular dystrophy*. At first, it causes muscles to enlarge because of fat and connective tissue deposits, but this is followed by atrophy of muscle fibers and degeneration. Eventually, all types of muscular dystrophy lead to muscle atrophy and replacement of muscle by adipose and fibrous tissues.

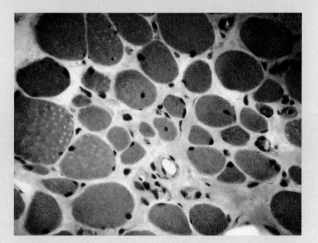

Dystrophic muscle.

Duchenne muscular dystrophy is the most common and most serious form. It is a sex-linked recessive disease that nearly always affects males, appearing between ages 2 and 7 years. It is caused by a defective gene for *dystrophin*, a cytoplasmic protein that normally helps to stabilize the sarcolemma. Affected children seldom live beyond their early twenties, usually dying of respiratory failure when the disease reaches their chest muscles.

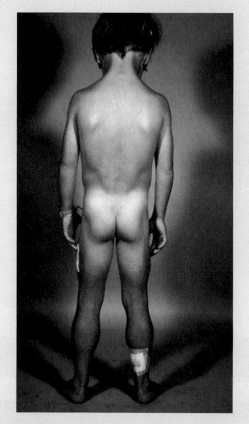

Duchenne muscular dystrophy.

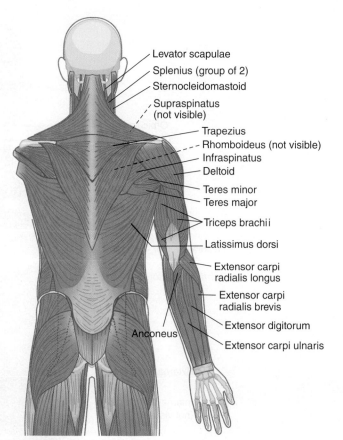

FIGURE 9-13 The muscles of the shoulder and back.

Smooth Muscles

Smooth muscle is similar, but not identical, to skeletal muscle. It is not under voluntary control and has slow, sustained contractions. Smooth muscle cells have elongated, spindle-like shapes with tapered ends, but lack striations. They have a single, centrally located nucleus and are between 5 and 10 μm in diameter. Smooth muscle fibers are between 30 and 200 μm in length, which is much smaller than skeletal muscle fibers. Their myofibrils contain actin and myosin throughout their entire lengths. Smooth muscle does not have the striations that skeletal muscle has because although smooth muscle has contractile proteins, they are poorly organized. This lack of organization means that striations cannot form. Smooth muscles' sarcoplasmic reticula

Many athletes use anabolic steroids to enhance their muscle growth, a dangerous practice because of adverse effects. These steroids are engineered variants of the male sex hormone testosterone. Pathological effects include Cushing-like bloating of the face, hair loss, acne, testicular atrophy resulting in infertility, hypercholesterolemia, and liver damage that may result in hepatic cancer. Psychological effects include depression, manic behavior, extreme rage, and delusions. The use of anabolic steroids in females may cause masculine characteristics and hirsutism.

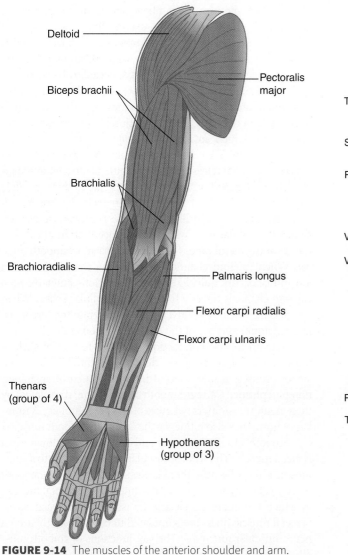

FIGURE 9-14 The muscles of the anterior shoulder and arm.

Deltoid
Biceps brachii
Brachialis
Brachioradialis
Thenars (group of 4)
Pectoralis major
Palmaris longus
Flexor carpi radialis
Flexor carpi ulnaris
Hypothenars (group of 3)

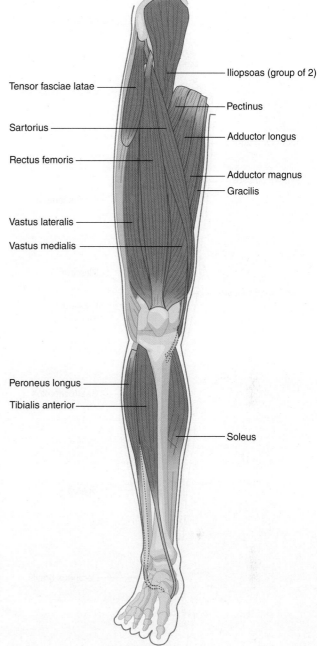

FIGURE 9-15 The superficial muscles of the anterior hip and leg.

Tensor fasciae latae
Sartorius
Rectus femoris
Vastus lateralis
Vastus medialis
Peroneus longus
Tibialis anterior
Iliopsoas (group of 2)
Pectinus
Adductor longus
Adductor magnus
Gracilis
Soleus

are not well developed. A small amount of fine endomysium is found between smooth muscle fibers. It is secreted by the smooth muscles themselves and contains blood vessels and nerves. Although smooth muscle contains both thick and thin filaments, the myosin filaments are much shorter than the actin filaments. Smooth muscle, along with skeletal and cardiac muscle, is shown in **FIGURE 9-17**.

A different type of myosin exists in smooth muscle compared with the type found in skeletal muscle. To understand further, skeletal muscle has 13 times more thin filaments than thick filaments, whereas smooth muscle only has twice as many thin filaments as thick filaments. The thin filaments of smooth muscle have no troponin complex. Also, the thick and thin filaments are arranged diagonally. There is an intermediate filament-dense body network. These intermediate filaments resist tension. *Dense bodies* are also attached to the sarcolemma, anchoring thin filaments. These dense bodies correspond to the Z discs found in skeletal muscle. In smooth muscle sarcoplasm, calcium ions interact with *calmodulin*, which is a calcium-binding protein that activates the enzyme *myosin light chain kinase*. This enables myosin heads to attach to actin. Stretched smooth muscles adapt to their

new lengths and remain able to contract on demand, a condition known as *plasticity*.

There are two types of smooth muscle: multiunit and visceral. **Multiunit smooth muscle** has separated muscle fibers and is found in the irises of the eyes and the walls of blood vessels. It contracts only when stimulated by motor nerve impulses or certain hormones. **Visceral smooth muscle** is made up of sheets of spindle-shaped cells. It is found in the walls of hollow organs such as the intestines, stomach, urinary bladder, and uterus. In these locations, it forces fluids and other substances through body channels. Smooth muscle is also found in the integumentary, respiratory, and reproductive systems. In the digestive tract, **pacesetter cells** spontaneously trigger contraction of entire sheets of muscle.

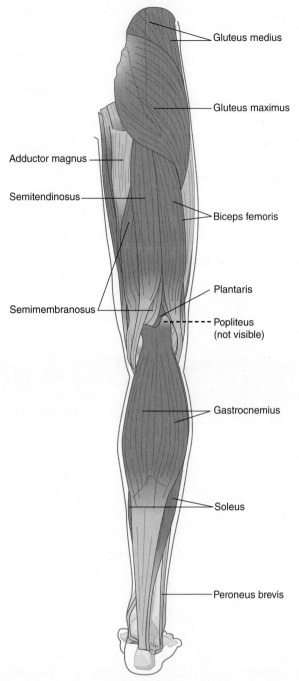

FIGURE 9-16 The superficial muscles of the posterior hip and leg.

Visceral smooth muscle fibers can stimulate each other, and adjacent fibers experience **excitability**. They display a pattern of repeated contractions known as *rhythmicity*, which is caused by self-exciting fibers. The wave-like motion of many tubular organs, known as **peristalsis**, is caused by these features of visceral smooth muscle. Peristalsis helps to move the contents of organs such as the intestines from the stomach to the outside of the body. In smooth muscles, innervating nerve fibers exist, which are part of the autonomic (involuntary) nervous system. They have many bulb-like swellings, called *varicosities*, which release neurotransmitters into a wide synaptic cleft near smooth muscle cells. These are known as *diffuse junctions*. The sarcolemma of smooth muscles has many *caveolae*, which are pouch-like infoldings. The caveolae contain some extracellular fluid with a high concentration of calcium ions near the membrane. T-tubules are absent in smooth muscle. When calcium channels open in the caveolae, calcium ion influx occurs quickly. Most of these ions enter through calcium channels directly from the extracellular space. When cytoplasmic calcium is actively transported into the sarcoplasmic reticulum and out of the cell, contraction ends.

Smooth muscle contraction is similar to that of skeletal muscle, using actin, myosin, calcium ions, and ATP; however, smooth muscle is also affected by another neurotransmitter, norepinephrine. Certain smooth muscles are stimulated by these neurotransmitters, whereas others are inhibited. A number of hormones also influence the actions of smooth muscles.

Smooth muscle contracts and relaxes more slowly than skeletal muscle. The whole muscular sheet responds to a stimulus in unison because there is electrical coupling of smooth muscle cells by *gap junctions*. This differs from skeletal muscle, in which the fibers are electrically isolated from each other. Skeletal muscle fibers are stimulated to contract by their own neuromuscular junctions. The gap junctions of smooth muscle allow the transmission of action potentials from fiber to fiber. With the correct amount of ATP, it can maintain forceful contractions for a longer period. Smooth muscles can change length without changing how taut they are.

Pacemaker cells are specific smooth muscle cells found in the stomach and small intestine. When excited, they set the pace of contraction for the entire muscle sheet. The membrane potentials of these pacemaker cells fluctuate and are self-excitatory. In the absence of external stimuli, they

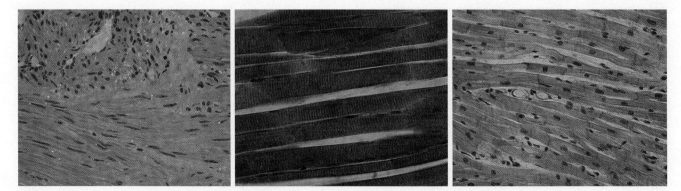

FIGURE 9-17 The three types of muscle fibers: (A) skeletal, (B) smooth, and (C) cardiac. (© Donna Beer Stolz, PhD, Center for Biologic Imaging, University of Pittsburgh Medical School.)

depolarize spontaneously. The rate and intensity of smooth muscle contraction can, however, be modified by both neural and chemical stimuli. A summary of smooth muscle contraction is as follows:

- The sliding filament mechanism occurs for the interaction of actin and myosin.
- A rise in the intracellular calcium ion level is the final trigger for contraction.
- ATP energizes the sliding process.

Smooth muscle takes approximately 30 times longer than skeletal muscle to contract and relax. However, it uses much less energy. It can maintain the same amount of contractile tension for long periods, with less than 1% of the energy expended. In small arterioles and other visceral organs, the smooth muscle regularly maintains a small amount of contraction (*smooth muscle tone*) with fatigue. Because of its low energy requirements, the aerobic pathways of smooth muscle manufacture adequate amounts of needed ATP.

Smooth muscle contraction is regulated by nerves, hormones, and local chemical changes. Neurotransmitter binding creates action potentials that are coupled with increased calcium ion concentrations in the cytosol. Certain smooth muscles respond to neural stimulation with local electrical *graded potentials* only. Other smooth muscle layers have no nerve supply. They depolarize either spontaneously or because of chemical stimuli binding to G protein–linked receptors. Some smooth muscle cells also respond to *both* neural and chemical stimuli.

Chemical factors that cause smooth muscle to contract or relax without action potentials may accomplish this by enhancing or inhibiting calcium ion entry into the sarcoplasm. These factors include histamine, certain hormones, low pH, excessive carbon dioxide, and lack of oxygen. Smooth muscle activity is altered by a direct response to these chemical stimuli. This is based on local tissue requirements and is believed to regulate smooth muscle tone. Gastrin in the stomach is an example of a chemical stimulus. It stimulates the stomach smooth muscle to contract during digestion, mixing food contents.

The *stress–relaxation response* allows hollow organs to stretch and retract slowly for large volumes of substances without causing any strong contractions (which would expel the substances). Therefore, smooth muscle can stretch more greatly and generate more tension than skeletal muscles when they are similarly stretched. Smooth muscles can generate strong *force* even when substantially stretched, in part because of their lack of sarcomeres combined with their irregular, overlapping arrangement. Smooth muscle can contract between half to twice its resting length. This is a total range of 150%. In comparison, the total length change that skeletal muscles can accomplish while retaining efficient function is only about 60%.

Although all muscle cells can increase in size (*hypertrophy*), some can also divide and increase their numbers (*hyperplasia*). An example is hyperplasia of uterine cells in response to estrogen during puberty. The uterus, at this time, grows until it reaches its adult size. When a woman becomes pregnant, high estrogen levels stimulate uterine hyperplasia so the growing fetus can be accommodated.

Myoblasts are the embryonic mesoderm cells from which most muscle tissue develops. Development occurs quickly, with the embryo experiencing skeletal muscle fiber contraction by week 7. The surfaces of developing myoblasts are initially covered with ACh receptors. Spinal nerves eventually penetrate the muscle masses. Nerve endings seek out individual myoblasts and release *agrin*, a growth factor. Agrin activates *MuSK*, a muscle kinase. This stimulates clusters of ACh receptors at new neuromuscular junctions and maintains them in each muscle fiber. The nerve endings release another chemical to eliminate receptor sites that have not been innervated or stabilized by the released agrin.

For both cardiac and smooth muscle cells, the myoblasts that produce these cells do not fuse. Instead, they develop gap junctions in the embryo very early. Within 3 weeks after fertilization, cardiac muscle is pumping blood through the embryo. Although specialized cardiac and skeletal muscle cells stop dividing very early, they remain able to lengthen and thicken during childhood and then experience hypertrophy in the adult.

Satellite cells resemble myoblasts and are associated with skeletal muscle. They aid in the repair of injured fibers. They also allow incomplete regeneration of dead skeletal muscle, but this declines during the aging process. Recent studies also show that cardiac cells do divide somewhat, yet injured cardiac muscle is mostly repaired by scar tissue. However, smooth muscles regenerate well. For example, the smooth muscle cells of blood vessels divide regularly throughout a person's lifetime.

TEST YOUR UNDERSTANDING

1. Explain the structure of smooth muscle.
2. Define diffuse junctions and gap junctions.
3. Explain the role of myoblasts in the development of muscle.
4. Describe the structure of visceral smooth muscle.
5. Besides ACh, what other neurotransmitter affects smooth muscle contraction?

Cardiac Muscle

Cardiac muscle, found only in the heart, is made up of striated cells that are connected into three-dimensional networks (Figure 9-17). The many filaments of actin and myosin in cardiac muscle resemble those of skeletal muscle. Sarcoplasmic reticula, mitochondria, and transverse tubules are also present. Less calcium is stored in cardiac muscle, however, with calcium ions being released by the larger transverse tubules into the sarcoplasm. As a result, the raised calcium sent into the extracellular fluid causes longer muscle **twitches** than in skeletal muscle.

Cross-bands at the opposite ends of cardiac muscle cells connect the ends. These cross-bands, known as *intercalated discs*, help to join cells and transmit contraction force while allowing muscle impulses to freely travel very quickly from cell to cell. Stimulation to one portion of the cardiac muscle network passes to the other parts of the network, with the entire heart contracting as one functional unit. This type of muscle is self-exciting and rhythmic, repeating contraction and relaxation to cause the heart's rhythmic contractions. Cardiac muscle contracts at a relatively stable rate, controlled by the heart's pacemaker, but increased physical activity causes neural controls to speed up the heart as needed.

The four major characteristics of cardiac muscle are summarized as follows:

- *Automaticity:* The property in which cardiac muscle tissue contracts without neural stimulation; specialized *pacemaker cells* normally determine timing of contractions.
- *Nervous system alteration:* The pace of the pacemaker cells may be altered by the nervous system, which may adjust how much tension is produced during contractions.
- *Contraction length:* Cardiac muscle cell contractions are about 10 times longer than those of skeletal muscle fibers, with longer refractory periods and little fatigue.

- *Sarcolemma properties:* Individual twitches do not undergo wave summation, and tetanic contractions are not produced. If the heart had a sustained tetanic contraction, it would not be able to pump blood.

TEST YOUR UNDERSTANDING

1. Describe the twitching of cardiac muscle.
2. Explain the actions of the intercalated discs.

Effects of Aging on the Muscular System

All muscle tissues decrease in strength and size as we age. Skeletal muscle fibers become smaller in diameter as the number of myofibrils decreases. Blood flow to active muscles does not increase as rapidly with exercise. Skeletal muscles also become less elastic as **fibrosis** occurs, which restricts movement and circulation. Tolerance for exercise decreases and overheating may become a problem as a result of exercise. The ability to recover from injuries to muscles decreases, limiting repair capabilities and causing scar tissue to form. For the elderly, exercise should be regular but not extreme to avoid damage to muscles, tendons, ligaments, bones, and joints.

SUMMARY

Skeletal muscle is voluntary striated muscle that is usually attached to bones. It has long, slender cells called muscle fibers. Cardiac muscle is involuntary striated muscle. Muscular tissue is used for movement, stability of the body, control of body passages and openings, and heat production. Muscle cells are able to carry out excitability, conductivity, contractility, extensibility, and elasticity. A skeletal muscle is composed of muscular tissue, connective tissue, nervous tissue, and blood vessels. The muscle attachment at the stationary end is called its origin, and the attachment at the moving end is called the insertion.

A muscle fiber is a long, slender cell with multiple nuclei just inside the *sarcolemma*. The *sarcoplasm* is occupied mainly by myofibrils, which are thread-like bundles of protein filaments. Each myofibril is a bundle of protein myofilaments. The thick filaments are made up mostly of myosin, and the thin filaments are made up mostly of actin. Skeletal muscle contracts only when stimulated by a somatic motor neuron. This is known as **contractility**.

Nerves and muscle fibers meet at a complex of synapses called a neuromuscular junction. Each tip of a nerve fiber ends in the synaptic knob. A narrow gap, the synaptic cleft, separates the synaptic knob from the sarcolemma. The synaptic knob contains synaptic vesicles filled with the chemical ACh. An enzyme called acetylcholinesterase, found in the synaptic cleft and as part of the sarcolemma, breaks down ACh to terminate stimulation of the muscle fiber.

Smooth muscle is similar but not identical to skeletal muscle. It is not under voluntary control and has slow, sustained contractions. Smooth muscle fibers are much smaller than skeletal muscle fibers. Smooth muscle does not have the striations that skeletal muscle has. A different type of myosin exists in smooth muscle. There are two types of smooth muscle: multiunit (found in the eyes and blood vessels) and visceral (found in hollow organs). The wave-like motion of many tubular organs, known as peristalsis, is caused by visceral smooth muscles. Smooth muscle, unlike skeletal muscle, is affected by the neurotransmitter called norepinephrine. Smooth muscle takes approximately 30 times longer than skeletal muscle to contract and relax but uses much less energy. Smooth muscle contraction is regulated by nerves, hormones, and local chemical changes.

KEY TERMS

A bands
Acetylcholine
Acetylcholinesterase
Actin
Action potential
Agonist
Antagonists
Aponeuroses
ATPase
Cardiac muscle
Contractility
Creatine phosphate
Dystrophin
Elasticity
Endomysium
Epimysium
Excitability
Extensibility
Fascia
Fascicles
Fibrosis
Glycosomes

Hemoglobin
H zone
I bands
Insertion
M line
Motor end plate
Motor neurons
Motor unit
Multiunit smooth muscle
Muscle fatigue
Muscle fibers
Muscle impulse
Muscle tone
Myoblasts
Myofibrils
Myoglobin
Myosin
Neuromuscular junction (end plate)
Neurotransmitters
Origin
Oxygen debt
Pacesetter cells

Perimysium
Peristalsis
Prime mover
Sarcolemma
Sarcomeres
Sarcoplasm
Sarcoplasmic reticulum
Sliding filament model
Striations
Synapse
Synergists
Titins
Transverse tubules
Tropomyosin
Troponin
T-tubule
Twitches
Visceral smooth muscle
Voluntary muscle
Z discs

LEARNING GOALS

The following learning goals correspond to the objectives at the beginning of this chapter:

1. Skeletal muscle fibers are thin, elongated cylinders with rounded ends. The cell membrane lies above the cytoplasm (sarcoplasm), with many small, oval-shaped mitochondria and nuclei. The sarcoplasm is made up of many thread-like myofibrils arranged in a parallel fashion. Myosin and actin filaments appear as alternating colored bands (striations). These repeating patterns are called sarcomeres. Inside the sarcoplasm, membranous channels surround each myofibril.

2. A. Skeletal muscles contract when organelles and molecules bind myosin to actin to cause a pulling action. The myofibrils then move as the actin and myosin filaments slide, shortening the muscle fiber and pulling on its attachments.

   B. Smooth, cardiac muscles contract in a similar fashion to skeletal muscles, using actin, myosin, calcium ions, and ATP; however, these muscles are also affected by the neurotransmitter norepinephrine and hormones. Smooth muscle contracts more slowly than skeletal muscle but can maintain contractions for a longer period. Smooth muscles change length without changing their tautness.

3. A motor end plate is formed by specialized muscle fiber membranes and has abundant mitochondria and nuclei, with greatly folded sarcolemmas. Neurotransmitters are contained within tiny synaptic vesicles at these distal ends. Upon receiving impulses, the vesicles release neurotransmitters into the synaptic cleft between the neuron and motor end plate, stimulating muscle contraction.

4. Most of the energy released in cellular respiration becomes heat. Muscle tissue generates a lot of heat because muscles form so much of the total body mass. Body temperature is partially maintained by the blood transporting heat generated by the muscle to other body tissues.

5. A. Multiunit smooth muscle has separated muscle fibers and is found in the irises of the eyes and the walls of blood vessels. It contracts only when stimulated by motor nerve impulses or certain hormones.

    B. Visceral smooth muscle is made up of sheets of spindle-shaped cells. It is found in the walls of hollow organs such as the intestines, stomach, urinary bladder, and uterus.

6. One end of a skeletal muscle usually is fastened to a relatively immovable part (origin) at a movable joint. The other end connects to a movable part (insertion) on the other side of the joint.

7. A. Muscles of facial expression are buccinators, epicranis, orbicularis oculi, orbicularis oris, platysma, and zygomaticus.

    B. Muscles that move the head are semispinalis capitis, splenius capitis, and sternocleidomastoid.

8. A. Muscles of the abdominal wall are external oblique, internal oblique, rectus abdominis, and transversus abdominis.

    B. The actions of the rectus abdominis are tensing the abdominal wall, compressing the abdominal contents, and flexing the vertebral column.

9. The muscles that flex the thigh are the adductor longus, gracilis, iliacus, psoas major, and tensor fasciae latae. The muscles that extend the thigh are the adductor magnus and gluteus maximus.

10. The quadriceps femoris group functions to extend the leg at the knee. It includes the rectus femoris, vastus intermedius, vastus lateralis, and vastus medialis muscles.

CRITICAL THINKING QUESTIONS

A 70-year-old man decided to go to the gym for regular workouts to build up his muscle size. After 1 year, his muscles were much stronger and more solid.

1. Describe what source of energy his muscles need to continue workouts.

2. Why will this man be unable to continue his workouts for as long as a much younger man?

3. Explain how his muscles became larger after 1 year.

REVIEW QUESTIONS

1. Which of the following terms refers to the cytoplasm of a skeletal muscle fiber?
    A. sarcomere
    B. sarcoplasm
    C. sarcosome
    D. sarcolemma

2. Which of the following is not a function of skeletal muscle?
    A. maintain body temperature
    B. maintain posture
    C. metabolize food
    D. produce movement

3. The muscle that flexes the foot is the
    A. quadriceps femoris
    B. gastrocnemius
    C. gluteus maximus
    D. gluteus medius

4. Skeletal muscles need all of the following factors to contract *except*
    A. vitamin D
    B. myosin
    C. actin
    D. calcium

5. The adductor magnus muscle is located in which portion of the body?
    A. forearm
    B. leg
    C. neck
    D. buttocks

6. The deltoid muscle can
    A. raise the arm
    B. flex the arm
    C. adduct the arm
    D. abduct the arm

7. Which of the following muscles is located in the torso?
    A. pectoralis major
    B. external oblique
    C. soleus
    D. biceps

8. What is the main muscle involved in the act of inspiration?
    A. diaphragm
    B. stomach
    C. larynx
    D. trachea

9. The cell membrane of skeletal muscle is called the
    A. sarcoplasm
    B. sarcosome
    C. sarcolemma
    D. sarcoplasmic reticulum

10. The more movable end of a muscle is the
    A. origin
    B. proximal end
    C. insertion
    D. distal end

11. Which of the following muscles can extend the arm when doing push-ups?
    A. deltoid
    B. triceps brachii
    C. biceps brachii
    D. pectoralis major

12. Cross-bridges are located on
    A. myosin molecules
    B. actin molecules
    C. troponin molecules
    D. calcium ions

13. Which of the following flexes the head?
    A. trapezius
    B. deltoid
    C. pectoralis major
    D. sternocleidomastoid

14. The sartorius muscle is located in the
    A. chest
    B. thigh
    C. abdomen
    D. foot

15. Which of the following muscles contains the calcaneal tendon?
    A. tibialis anterior
    B. vastus lateralis
    C. gastrocnemius
    D. biceps femoris

ESSAY QUESTIONS

1. What are the criteria used in naming muscles?
2. Define the terms sarcolemma, myofibrils, glycosomes, and myoglobin.
3. Define the terms I bands, A bands, Z discs, H zone, and M line.
4. Describe the decomposition of ACh and the role of ACh in muscle contraction.
5. Name three muscles used as sites for intramuscular injections.
6. Name the two muscles that flex and extend the head.
7. Why does muscle fatigue occur?
8. Define the terms prime mover, synergists, and antagonists.
9. Name two muscles of mastication.
10. Name three muscles that flex the forearm.

UNIT III

CONTROL AND COORDINATION

Hz

Neural Tissue

OBJECTIVES

After studying this chapter, readers should be able to

1. Describe the anatomical and functional divisions of the nervous system.
2. List the basic functions of the nervous system.
3. Describe the functions of astrocytes and oligodendrocytes.
4. Describe the neuron and its important structural components.
5. Describe the locations and functions of neuroglia.
6. Describe synapses and synaptic transmission.
7. Discuss the events that occur at a chemical synapse.
8. List the major types of neurotransmitters.
9. Define action potential.
10. Explain the classifications of nerve fibers.

Overview

The nervous system controls all other body systems and the communications between all body components. It is involved with actions, emotions, and thoughts. Chemical and electrical signals are used in cellular communication. They occur very rapidly, with specific goals, and responses to these signals are almost immediate. The unit upon which all nervous system activity is based is known as the neuron (nerve cell). *Neurons* require neuroglial cells (*neuroglia*), which conduct phagocytosis, fill spaces, produce components of myelin, and provide structural frameworks. There are many more neuroglial cells than neurons in the body. Neuroglia, which exist in both the central nervous system (CNS) and peripheral nervous system (PNS), can divide, whereas most neurons cannot. Neuroglia are much smaller than neurons, and their nuclei stain dark. There are approximately 10 CNS neuroglia to every one neuron. Neuroglia form approximately half the mass of the brain. Neuroglia are classified as astrocytes, ependymal cells, microglial cells, and oligodendrocytes. In the PNS, the two types of neuroglia are satellite cells and Schwann cells.

Divisions of the Nervous System

The nervous system controls all body functions, maintains homeostasis, and allows the body to respond to many varieties of changing conditions. Information is carried to the brain and spinal cord, which then stimulate the body's responses. The nervous system has millions of sensory receptors that monitor changes (**sensory input**) outside and inside of the body. The nervous system processes and interprets this information to determine how it should react (**integration**). The *effector organs* of the body are the muscles and glands, which are activated by the nervous system to respond. The responses are collectively termed **motor output**.

The **central nervous system (CNS)** consists of the brain and spinal cord, located in the dorsal body cavity. The CNS is the control center of the nervous system, integrating all of its activities. Reflexes, past happenings, and current conditions determine how it will interpret sensory input and control motor output. The **peripheral nervous system (PNS)** consists of the peripheral nerves connecting the CNS to other parts of the body (**FIGURE 10-1**). Primarily, it is made up of nerves extending from the brain and spinal cord to the rest of the body. The cranial nerves transmit impulses to and from the brain. Likewise, the spinal nerves transmit impulses to and from the spinal cord.

The CNS and PNS work together to provide sensory, integrative, and motor functions to the body. The two functional subdivisions of the PNS are the **afferent (sensory) division** and the **efferent (motor) division**. The afferent division carries impulses toward the CNS from the body's sensory receptors. *Somatic sensory fibers* transmit impulses from the joints, skeletal muscles, and skin. *Visceral sensory fibers* transmit impulses from the visceral organs of the ventral body cavity. This sensory division informs the CNS of all events happening inside and outside the body. The efferent division carries impulses from the CNS to the effector organs, activating muscles to contract and glands to secrete. They affect (cause) motor responses. The two main parts of this motor division are the **somatic nervous system** and the **autonomic nervous system** (ANS).

The somatic nervous system is made up of somatic motor fibers transmitting impulses from the CNS to the skeletal muscles. It is also called the **voluntary nervous system** because our skeletal muscles are under conscious control. However, the somatic nervous system also controls involuntary contractions, such as those involved in **reflexes**. The ANS contains visceral motor nerve fibers regulating glandular, cardiac muscle, and smooth muscle activity. In general, the ANS is not under conscious control and thus is also called the **involuntary nervous system**. The two subdivisions of the ANS are the *sympathetic* and *parasympathetic* divisions. Their actions usually oppose each other. When one division causes stimulation, the other inhibits its actions.

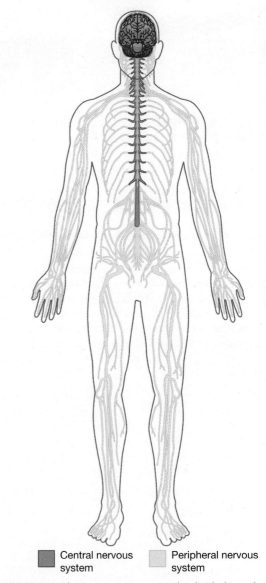

Central nervous system   Peripheral nervous system

FIGURE 10-1 The nervous system can be divided into the CNS and the PNS.

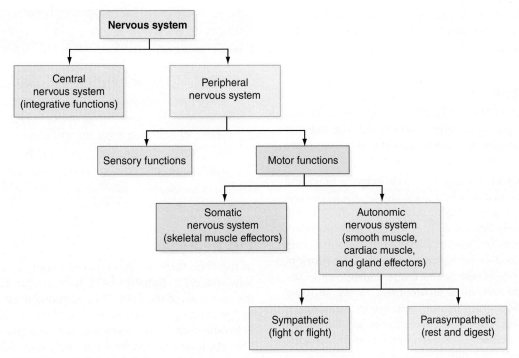

FIGURE 10-2 Major subdivisions of the nervous system.

Major subdivisions of the nervous system are summarized in **FIGURE 10-2**.

Nervous System Functions

Sensory receptors located at the ends of peripheral neurons provide the nervous system's sensory functions. They detect changes in the body's internal and external environment and relay information. These changes may involve oxygen levels, temperature, light, sound, and many other types of information. The information is converted into nerve impulses, which are integrated so they can be processed to achieve the correct reaction. Motor functions then act on the integrated information.

Response structures called **effectors** are located outside the nervous system. When stimulated by nerve impulses, these effectors, which include muscles and glands, may contract, secrete, or perform other reactive functions. Consciously controlled motor functions are handled by the somatic nervous system, which is in control of skeletal muscle. Involuntary effectors, such as the heart, various glands, and the smooth muscle in blood vessels, are controlled by the ANS. The nervous system helps maintain the body's homeostasis by using its different divisions to respond to changes that occur.

Cells of the Nervous System

Nerve tissue contains neurons and glial cells (neuroglia). Neurons are the structural units of the nervous system, whereas neuroglia support the functions of the neurons.

Neuroglia also conduct **phagocytosis**, fill spaces, produce components of **myelin**, and provide structural frameworks (**FIGURE 10-3**). There are many more neuroglial cells than neurons in the body.

Neuroglia

Neuroglia, which exist in both the CNS and PNS, can divide, whereas most neurons cannot. Most neuroglia, like neurons,

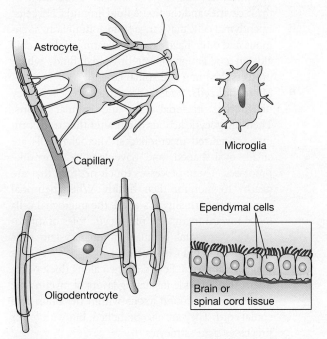

FIGURE 10-3 The four types of neuroglia cells in the CNS.

have branching processes that extend outward and a neutral cell body. Neuroglia are much smaller than neurons, and their nuclei stain dark.

CNS Neuroglia

There are approximately 10 CNS neuroglia to every one neuron. Neuroglia form approximately half the mass of the brain. Neuroglia are classified as the following types of cells:

- *Astrocytes*: Usually found between neurons and blood vessels, where they anchor these components together, astrocytes are star-shaped and delicately branched. They are the most abundant glial cells and have a variety of functions: maintain the blood–brain barrier, create the framework of the CNS, repair neural tissue damage, and control the interstitial environment. Many radiating processes grasp neurons and synaptic endings of neurons. They also cover nearby capillaries and aid in exchanges between neurons and capillaries, determining capillary permeability. Astrocytes also control migration and development of new neurons as well as the formation of synapses between neurons. They have a vital function in cleaning up leaked potassium ions and recycling released neurotransmitters. Astrocytes also respond to nerve impulses and released neurotransmitters. They are connected by gap junctions and signal each other via calcium intake as well as release of extracellular chemical messengers. They create slow intracellular calcium waves and influence neuronal functioning.
- *Ependymal cells*: These cells line central brain and spinal cord cavities, forming a permeable barrier or *ependyma* between the cerebrospinal fluid in these cavities and the tissue fluid around CNS cells. Ependymal cells may range from columnar to squamous and often have cilia. The beating of these cilia aids in circulation of cerebrospinal fluid, which protects the brain and spinal cord.
- *Microglial cells*: Found throughout the CNS, they phagocytize bacterial cells and cellular debris. Their phagocytic actions occur after they transform into specialized macrophages. Microglial cells are small, oval-shaped, and have lengthy thorn-like processes. These processes touch neurons that are nearby to monitor their health. When neuronal injury or abnormality is sensed, the microglial cells move toward them. The phagocytic roles of microglia cells are vital because immune system cells only have limited CNS access.
- *Oligodendrocytes*: Found aligned along thick nerve fibers, they provide insulating layers of myelin (the *myelin sheath*) around axons within the brain and spinal cord. They are also branched, but with fewer processes than astrocytes.

PNS Neuroglia

In the PNS, there are two types of neuroglia: satellite and Schwann cells. **Satellite cells** have similar functions to the astrocytes of the CNS. They surround neuron cell bodies, resembling satellites around a planet in outer space. **Schwann cells** (*neurolemmocytes*) are neuroglial cells in the PNS that form a myelin sheath around axons. Schwann cells do not touch one another, so there are gaps in the myelin sheath. They play a part in repairing damaged nerves in the PNS. A process called *Wallerian generation* of an axon that is distal to an injury site results in macrophages arriving to clean up debris, yet the Schwann cells themselves do not degenerate. They proliferate to form a cellular cord along the path of the original axon. In time, the damaged neuron's axon grows into the site of the injury, with the Schwann cells wrapping around the axon. Normal synaptic contacts may or may not be reestablished. This regeneration is not as common within the CNS.

Brain capillaries are formed by cells that are much more connected than the cells throughout the rest of the body. Partially due to astrocytes, this "high connectivity" forms a **blood–brain barrier** that protects the brain from many chemical substances; for example, certain antihistamines are kept from entering the brain, preventing drowsiness, a common side effect, from occurring. The actions of the Schwann cells are most similar to those of the oligodendrocytes of the CNS.

TEST YOUR UNDERSTANDING

1. Describe how the CNS integrates information.
2. Differentiate the CNS from the PNS.
3. What is the function of Schwann cells in the PNS?
4. Name the types of neuroglia that form myelin sheaths in the CNS and PNS.

Neurons

Nervous tissue consists of masses of **neurons** (nerve cells) and is highly cellular. In the CNS, the cells are densely packed and intertwined. Less than 20% of the CNS is extracellular space. Neurons are the structural and functional units of the nervous system, and each neuron has a specialized function. Billions of neurons exist in the nervous system and can function very well for a person's entire lifetime if they receive adequate nutrients. However, they are *amitotic*, losing their ability to divide, and therefore cannot be replaced if they are destroyed (in most circumstances). Neurons that can be replaced include the olfactory epithelium of the nose and certain regions of the hippocampus in the brain, which is involved in memory. Neurons are larger than other cells of the nervous system and highly specialized in their conduction of impulses. **Nerve impulses** are actually electrochemical changes transmitted by neurons to other neurons and to cells outside the nervous system. **FIGURE 10-4** shows the structure of a neuron.

Cell Bodies of Neurons

Each neuron has a rounded cell body and extensions called **dendrites** and **axons**. Dendrites, which may be numerous, receive electrochemical messages, whereas axons send out electrochemical messages. Each neuron usually has only one axon. Bundles of axons constitute nerves. The cytoplasm of an axon is called the *axoplasm*, which is surrounded by a specialized portion of the plasma membrane known as the *axolemma*. In the CNS, the axolemma may be exposed to interstitial fluid or covered by neuroglial processes. **Neuroglial cells** provide insulation, physical support, and nutrients to the neurons. Neurons require continuous, abundant oxygen and glucose supplies because they have a very high metabolic rate. Without oxygen, neurons cannot survive for more than a few minutes.

Although neurons are similar in structure, they vary greatly in size and shape. They all have a cell body or **soma**, dendrites, and an axon. The cell body, which ranges between 5 and 140 μm in diameter, is made up of a cell membrane, a granular cytoplasm or *perikaryon*, and organelles (lysosomes, a Golgi apparatus, mitochondria, and fine, thread-like **neurofibrils**). The neurofibrils are bundles of *neurofilaments*. The cytoskeleton of the perikaryon contains these, along with *neurotubules*. The well-developed Golgi apparatus forms either an arc or a circle around the nucleus. The cell body is where most biosynthesis occurs in the neuron. Therefore, it contains organelles that synthesize chemicals such as proteins. To maintain cell integrity and shape, microtubules and the neurofibrils form a structural network.

Throughout the cytoplasm are many sac-like Nissl bodies, also known as **chromatophilic substance**. These bodies are similar to the rough endoplasmic reticulum of other cells and stain darkly with commonly used dyes. Attached ribosomes synthesize protein. The center of the cell body has a large, round nucleus with a nucleolus surrounded by cytoplasm. In certain neurons, the cell body may contain pigments such as *black melanin*, a red pigment that contains iron, or a gold-brown pigment called *lipofuscin*. Most neuron cell bodies are located in the CNS and are protected by the bones of the vertebral column and skull. **Nuclei** are clusters of cell bodies in the CNS, whereas **ganglia** are clusters of cell bodies in the PNS, which lie along peripheral nerves.

Processes of Neurons

All neuron cell bodies have **processes** that extend outward. The CNS contains both neuron cell bodies and processes, whereas the PNS mostly contains just processes. In the CNS, bundles of neuron processes are called **tracts.** In the PNS, these bundles are called **nerves.** There are two types of neuron processes: *dendrites* and *axons. Dendrites* have multiple branches that act as the neuron's main receptive surfaces. The dendrites of the motor neurons are tapered, short in length, and have diffusely branched extensions. They are the primary *receptive (input) regions* of neurons, having a large surface area for receiving neuronal signals. In many parts of the brain, the finer dendrites are extremely specialized for information collection. The dendrites convey messages coming toward the cell body. These messages are usually short-distance *graded*

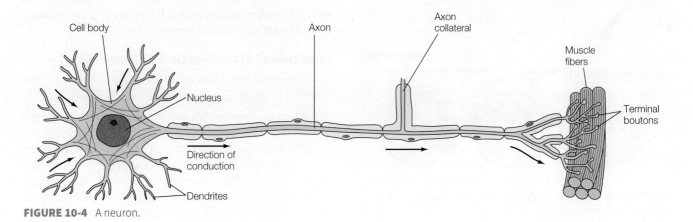

FIGURE 10-4 A neuron.

potentials instead of long-distance *action potentials*. A graded potential is also called a *local potential*. It is a change in the *transmembrane potential* that is not able to spread very far from the area that surrounds the site of stimulation.

Most neurons have a single axon arising from an elevation (the axonal hillock) on the cell body. The axonal hillock is cone-shaped, narrowing to form a slender process that retains the same diameter for the remainder of its length. Some neurons have short axons or may even lack axons. In others, axons make up almost the entire neuron length. In the skeletal muscles of the great toe, axons of motor neurons extend up to 4 feet from the lumbar region of the spine. These are the longest cells of the body, and long axons such as these are called **nerve fibers**.

Larger axons are enclosed in **myelin sheaths** that originate from Schwann cells (**FIGURE 10-5**). These cells are wound tightly around the axons. The areas of the Schwann cells containing most of the cytoplasm and nuclei are located outside the myelin sheath, comprising a **neurolemma**. Large areas of myelinated axons from oligodendrocytes are known as *internodes*, which are usually between 1 and 2 mm long. These narrow gaps between the myelin sheaths are known as **nodes of Ranvier**, which occur at regular intervals, approximately 1 mm each, along myelinated axons. The myelin sheaths are long or have a large diameter. Myelin is a whitish protein-lipoid. It occurs in segments when it forms the myelin sheath. Myelin electrically insulates fibers and protects them, increasing their transmission speed of nerve impulses.

Axon Structure

Although each neuron has only one axon, some axons have occasional branches known as **axon collaterals**, which extend at right angles in most cases. Whether an axon is branched or not, it usually has profuse branching at its end (up to approximately 10,000 branches), which are known as **terminal** branches or *telodendria*. The distal endings of these terminal branches are knob-like and are called **axon terminals**, *synaptic terminals, synaptic knobs, synaptic boutons,* or *terminal boutons*. When an impulse reaches the axon terminals, it causes neurotransmitter release into the extracellular space. This either excites or inhibits neurons (or effector cells) that are close to the axon. Axons have the same organelles as dendrites except for *rough endoplasmic reticulum* and a *Golgi apparatus*. Axons decay quickly if they are cut or experience severe damage.

FOCUS ON PATHOLOGY

Retrograde axonal transport is used by some bacterial toxins and certain viruses to reach neuron cell bodies. This mode of transport uses motor proteins, microtubules, and actin filaments. Conditions known to use this type of transport include polio, herpes simplex viruses, and rabies. The tetanus toxin also damages neurons via this transport method. Research is ongoing, in which viruses containing corrected genes or microRNA are introduced to suppress defective genes.

An axon with a myelin sheath is called *myelinated*, whereas those without myelin sheaths are called *unmyelinated*. In the CNS, dense groups of myelinated axons are white, forming the *white matter*. The white matter contains mostly fiber tracts. Those that are unmyelinated, along with neuron cell bodies, form the *gray matter* in the CNS. The gray matter contains mostly nonmyelinated fibers and nerve cell bodies.

In both the CNS and PNS, axons of the smallest diameter are nonmyelinated and are covered by long extensions from adjacent glial cells. Throughout the nervous system, myelinated fibers conduct nerve impulses more quickly than nonmyelinated fibers. Axons can regenerate when peripheral nerves become damaged, with the neurolemma playing an important role. CNS axons are myelinated by oligodendrocytes, which do not have neurolemmas. When CNS neurons are damaged, they do not usually regenerate. Collections of neural stem cells in the brain can develop new neurons or neuroglial cells. Neural stem cells are located deep within the brain and near the brain's ventricles, which contain cerebrospinal fluid.

Functional Classification of Neurons

The functional classification of neurons is based on the direction in which action potentials are conducted:

- *Sensory neurons (afferent neurons):* Carry nerve impulses from the peripheral body parts into the CNS. They may have receptor ends at the tips of the dendrites or receptor cells that are associated with the dendrites in the sensory organs or the skin. *Somatic sensory neurons* monitor the external environment, whereas *visceral sensory neurons* monitor the body's

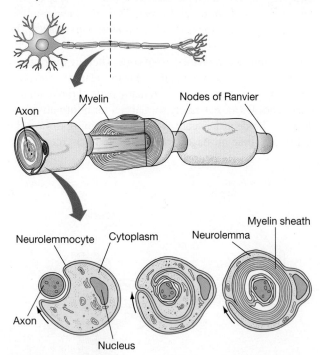

FIGURE 10-5 Larger axons are enclosed in myelin sheaths that originate from Schwann cells.

internal environment. Sensory receptors are classified as interoceptors, exteroceptors, and proprioceptors. *Interoceptors* provide sensations of deep pressure, distension, and pain and are found in the digestive, cardiovascular, respiratory, reproductive, and urinary systems. *Exteroceptors* provide perception of temperature, touch, pressure, smell, taste, equilibrium, hearing, and sight. *Proprioceptors* provide perception of skeletal muscle and joint movement and position.

- *Interneurons:* Conduct action potentials from one neuron to another within the CNS. The cell bodies of some interneurons form masses called *nuclei* in the CNS, which are similar to ganglia.
- *Motor neurons (efferent neurons):* Conduct action potentials away from the CNS, toward muscles or glands. *Somatic motor neurons* innervate skeletal muscles. Their cell bodies lie within the CNS, whereas their axons extend outward within peripheral nerves, innervating skeletal muscle fibers at the neuromuscular junctions. *Visceral motor neurons* innervate smooth and cardiac muscle, glands, and adipose tissue. The axons of these neurons that lie within the CNS innervate other visceral motor neurons in the peripheral autonomic ganglia. Visceral motor neurons that have cell bodies in these ganglia innervate and control the peripheral effectors. Axons extending from the CNS to an autonomic ganglion are known as *preganglionic fibers.* Axons that connect ganglion cells to peripheral effectors are known as *postganglionic fibers.*

Structural Classification of Neurons

Neurons are classified based on the number of processes that extend from their cell bodies. The three major structural categories of neurons are multipolar, bipolar, and unipolar:

- *Multipolar neurons:* Make up most of the neurons whose cell bodies lie within the brain or spinal cord. They have three or more processes that arise from their cell bodies, with only one process being an axon and the rest being dendrites. Multipolar neurons are the most common, and more than 99% of neurons in the human body are multipolar. They are also the most common type in the CNS.
- *Bipolar neurons:* Exist only in specialized parts of the eyes, nose, and ears. They have only two processes arising from their cell bodies. Only one process of each neuron is an axon; the other is a dendrite. Bipolar neurons are very rare in the body. They are located in certain sensory organs, such as the retinas of the eyes and in the nasal cavity.
- *Unipolar neurons:* Often aggregate in specialized ganglia located outside the brain and spinal cord. They have a single short process extending from the cell body that divides into two "T-like" branches that function more like a single axon. One branch (the more distal *peripheral process*) is associated with dendrites near a peripheral body part; the

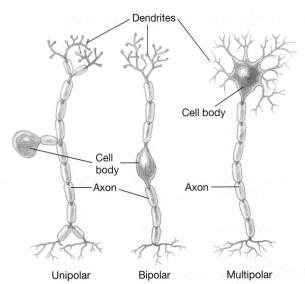

FIGURE 10-6 Structural variations in neurons.

other branch (the *central process*) enters the brain or spinal cord. Unipolar neurons originate as bipolar neurons and are more accurately described as *pseudounipolar neurons.*

Multipolar, bipolar, and unipolar neurons are shown in **FIGURE 10-6**. Classifications of neurons by function and structure are shown in **FIGURE 10-7**.

Another structural classification of neurons is termed *anaxonic*, in which the neurons are small, lacking any features that distinguish axons from dendrites. The cell processes are extremely similar in appearance. Anaxonic neurons are found in the brain and organs of the special senses and are not well understood.

TEST YOUR UNDERSTANDING

1. Describe the structures of neurons, dendrites, and axons.
2. Identify the differences between sensory and motor neurons.

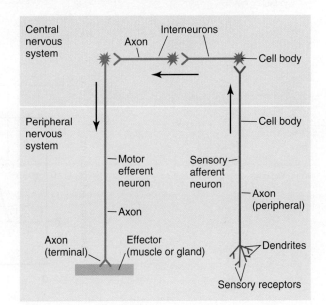

FIGURE 10-7 Classifications of neurons by function and structure.

Cell Membrane Potential

A cell membrane's surface is usually electrically charged (polarized) compared with its inner contents. This is due to unequal amounts of positive and negative ions and is important for conduction of nerve and muscle impulses. Adequate stimulation of a neuron causes generation of an electrical impulse in response. An action potential is a change in neuron membrane polarization and a return to its resting state. An action potential forms a nerve impulse propagated along an axon. The human body is electrically neutral, with the same number of positive and negative electrical charges. Some regions, however, are positively or negatively charged. Opposite charges attract each other, requiring energy to separate them. Therefore, when opposite charges come together, energy is liberated to perform cellular work.

Action Potential

The threshold potential causes permeability to suddenly change. Sodium channels open and sodium diffuses freely inward. The membrane becomes depolarized. Nearly simultaneously, potassium channels open to allow potassium to diffuse freely outward. The inside of the membrane becomes briefly hyperpolarized and then repolarized to its *resting potential*. For example, if the resting membrane potential is −70 mV and the threshold is −60 mV, a membrane potential of −62 mV will not produce an action potential. The *action potential* is defined as this rapid sequence of **depolarization**

and **repolarization**, taking only about one-thousandth of a second. Only cells with excitable membranes can generate action potentials. These cells include muscle cells and neurons. Synaptic activity produces graded potentials in postsynaptic cell plasma membranes.

The terms depolarization and **hyperpolarization** describe membrane potential changes that are related to resting membrane potential. In depolarization, the inside of the membrane becomes less negative (for example, it moves from −70 to −60 mV). In hyperpolarization, the inside of the membrane becomes more negative. Many action potentials can occur, and resting potentials can be reestablished before the concentrations of sodium and potassium significantly change. Active transport inside the membranes maintains the original concentrations on either side. Action potentials do not decay with greater distance traveled.

In skeletal muscle cells and neurons, action potential generation and transmission occur in the same way. Action potentials are usually generated only in axons, with neurons generating them only when enough stimulation occurs. Stimuli change the neuron membrane's permeability via the opening of certain voltage-gated channels on the axon. Changes in the membrane potential cause these channels to open and close is shown in **FIGURE 10-8A**. *Graded potentials* (local currents) activate them, with these currents spreading toward axons along the dendrite and cell body membranes. The method in which an *action potential* is generated is shown in **FIGURE 10-8B**.

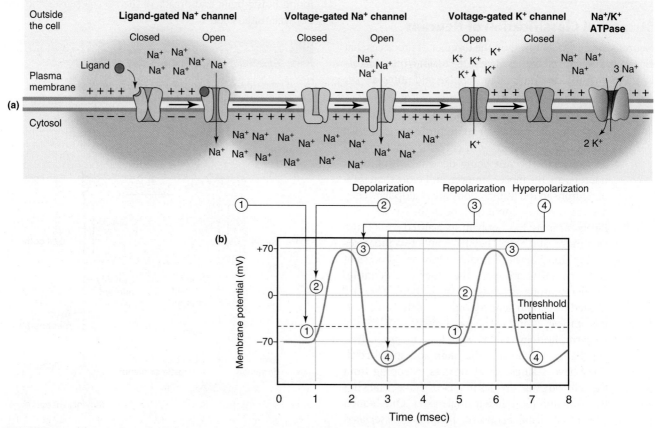

FIGURE 10-8 (A) Operation of gated channels, and (B) action potential.

Depolarization Phase

Beginning with a neuron in its polarized (resting) state, all gated sodium and potassium ion channels are closed. Leakage channels are the only ones open, and they maintain resting membrane potential. Depolarization opens sodium channels and then inactivates them. The axon membrane is first depolarized, followed by sodium channels opening and the rushing in of sodium ions into the cell. These positively charged ions depolarize the local membrane area to a greater degree, opening more sodium channels. The cell interior therefore becomes less negative on a continual basis. When threshold is reached at the stimulation site, depolarization becomes self-generating. Threshold is usually between −55 and −50 mV. Positive feedback assists the process, with depolarization being driven by ionic currents that were created by the sodium ion influx.

Repolarization Phase

In repolarization, sodium channels are inactivating, with potassium channels open. The intense rise of action potential is only about 1 msec in length, being self-limited because of the slow inactivation gates of the sodium channels closing at this time. The membrane permeability to sodium therefore reduces to resting levels. The net influx of sodium ions completely stops, meaning the action potential spike stops its rise. The slow potassium channels open, and potassium quickly leaves the cell along its electrochemical gradient. The internal negativity of the resting neuron is therefore restored (repolarization). The fast decline in sodium permeability and the increased potassium permeability aid in repolarization.

Hyperpolarization

In *hyperpolarization*, some potassium ion channels remain open, and sodium ion channels are reset. Usually, the time in which increased potassium permeability occurs lasts longer than is actually required to restore the resting state. A hyperpolarization is seen on the action potential curve, appearing as a small dip after the spike; this is the result of excessive potassium ion efflux before the closure of the potassium channels.

All-or-None Phenomenon

Action potentials are not always produced by depolarization events. For depolarization to produce an action potential, it must reach threshold values to make an axon "fire." Threshold may be the membrane potential at which potassium movement's outward current is identical to sodium movement's inward current. When the membrane has been depolarized by 15 to 20 mV from its resting value, threshold is usually reached. An action potential is therefore an **all-or-none phenomenon**, a principle occurring completely or not at all.

Refractory Periods

A neuron cannot respond to any amount of stimulus when an area of neuron membrane is generating an action potential and its voltage-gated sodium channels are opened. The **absolute refractory period** is the period from which

sodium channels open until they begin to reset to their resting state. This period results in each action potential being a unique all-or-one occurrence. It also enforces the one-way transmission of the action potential. The interval that follows the absolute refractory period is the **relative refractory period**. At this time, most sodium channels have resumed their resting state, but some potassium channels are still open, and repolarization is occurring.

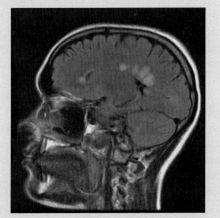
Propagation

Propagation of action potentials may occur in several different ways. In unmyelinated axons, *continuous propagation* is the method by which action potentials move. At the first segment of the axon, there is a brief change of the transmembrane potential when it becomes positive instead of negative. As sodium ions begin to move, a local current develops, spreads, and depolarizes nearby areas of the membrane. A chain reaction occurs, with the process repeating and moving the action potential forward but not backward. Backward movement is prevented by the previous axonal segment still being in its absolute refractory period. The furthest portions of the plasma membrane are eventually affected. The action potential that reaches the synaptic terminal is identical to the one that was initially generated. Continuous propagation occurs at a rate of approximately 1 meter per second, which is about 2 miles per hour. A second stimulus is needed for a second action potential to occur at the same site.

In the CNS and PNS, *saltatory propagation* moves action potentials much more quickly along axons. An action potential appearing at the first segment of a myelinated axon avoids the internodes and depolarizes the nearest node to threshold. The action potential jumps the 1- to 2-mm distance between the nodes in a large, myelinated axon. This requires less energy than continuous propagation, because there is less surface area involved and not as many sodium ions are needed to be pumped from the cytoplasm.

Ion Distribution

Because of active transport, body cells have more sodium ions outside of them and more potassium ions inside them. These cells' cytoplasm contains many negatively charged phosphate ions, sulfate ions, and proteins. Distribution of ions is determined partly by *selectively permeable channels* located in the cell membranes. Some are open, whereas others can open or close. Certain channels can allow specific ions to pass through, whereas others cannot. Potassium ions pass through cell membranes more easily than sodium ions. Therefore, potassium ions contribute greatly to membrane polarization. Membrane channels are large proteins with subunits. Their amino acid chains are distributed in a back and forth pattern across the membrane. Those known as *leakage (nongated) channels* remain open constantly. These are also called *passive channels*. *Gated channels* open and close based on certain signals. These are also called *active channels*. Every gated channel can either be closed but able to open, open (also called *activated*), or closed and unable to open (also called *inactivated*).

Chemically gated channels bind to specific chemicals to open or close. Examples include the receptors that bind acetylcholine (ACh) at neuromuscular junctions. These channels are most common on dendrites and cell bodies of neurons. *Voltage-gated channels* respond to changes in the transmembrane potential by opening or closing and are common on *excitable membranes*, which are those that can generate or conduct action potentials. These channels are common on the sarcolemma of skeletal or cardiac muscle fibers and the axons of unipolar and multipolar neurons. *Mechanically gated channels* respond to physical distortions of membrane surfaces by opening or closing. They are important in sensory receptors involving pressure, touch, or vibration.

Resting Potential

Sodium and potassium ions move from areas of high concentration to areas of low concentration, based on permeability. Because resting cell membranes are more permeable to potassium ions than sodium ions, the potassium ions diffuse out of cells more rapidly than sodium ions diffuse. More positive charges leave the cell by diffusion than enter it, making the outside of the cell membrane positive and the inside negative. This difference in charges is called a *potential difference*. In a resting nerve cell, this potential difference is called a **resting potential**. If undisturbed, the cell membrane remains polarized. Sodium and potassium continue to be actively transported, maintaining the concentrations needed for diffusion. Membrane voltage can be measured by using a *voltmeter*, with one microelectrode inserted into a neuron and the other into its extracellular fluid. Membrane voltage is approximately –70 mV. The minus sign means that the cytoplasmic (inside) portion of the membrane is negatively charged compared with the outside portion. In different types of neurons, the value of the resting membrane potential ranges from –40 to –90 mV. The resting potential only exists across the membrane, with solutions inside and outside the cell being electrically neutral. The resting potential is generated by either differences in permeability of the plasma membrane to the intracellular and extracellular fluids or differences in the *ionic composition* of these fluids.

Ionic Composition Differences

A lower concentration of sodium ions and a higher concentration of potassium ions exist in the cell cytosol, in comparison with the extracellular fluid. Anionic (negatively charged) proteins aid in balancing the positive charges of intracellular cations, which are mostly potassium ions. The positive charges of sodium and other cations are mostly balanced by chloride ions in the extracellular fluid. There are many other solutes in both fluids, including glucose and urea. Even so, potassium plays the chief role in generating the membrane potential.

Plasma Membrane Permeability Differences

When resting, the plasma membrane is not permeable to large anionic cytoplasmic proteins. It is slightly permeable to sodium but nearly 25 times more permeable to potassium. Also, it is highly permeable to chloride ions. These permeabilities are related to the leakage ion channel properties. Along their *concentration gradient*, potassium ions diffuse out of the cell very easily in comparison with how easily sodium ions can enter. The cell becomes more negatively charged inside as potassium ions flow outward. The slowly entering sodium ions cause the cell to become just slightly more positive than it would be if only potassium was flowing. Therefore, at resting potential, the cell's negative interior is based much more on the ability of potassium to diffuse outward than it is on the entrance of sodium. Via the adenosine triphosphate (ATP)-controlled *sodium-potassium pump*, three

TABLE 10-1

Nerve Impulse Events

Focus	Action
Neuron membrane	Maintains its resting potential
Threshold stimulus	Received
Sodium channels	Open in the trigger zone of the neuron
Sodium ions	Depolarize the membrane by diffusing inward
Potassium channels	Open in the membrane
Potassium ions	Repolarize the membrane by diffusing outward
Action potential	Stimulates adjacent membranes by causing a local bioelectric current
Wave of action potentials	Travels down the axon as a nerve impulse

Synapses

Nerve pathways carry nerve impulses. A **synapse** is a junction between any two communicating neurons. The actual gap between neurons is known as the **synaptic cleft**. Neurons conduct intracellular communication across these gaps (**FIGURE 10-10**). The nervous system requires impulse

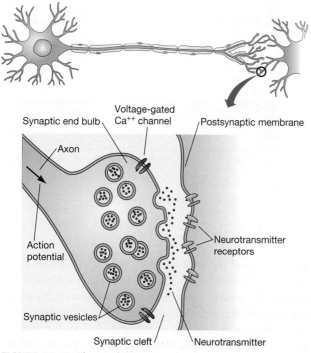

FIGURE 10-10 Chemical Synapse.

transmission through neuron chains that are functionally connected by synapses.

Axodendritic synapses are those between the axon endings of a neuron and the dendrites of other neurons. *Axosomatic synapses* are those between axon endings of one neuron and cell bodies (soma) of others. *Axoaxonal, dendrodendritic,* and *somatodendritic* synapses are less common, occurring (respectively) between axons, between dendrites, or between cell bodies and dendrites. Neurons may have between 1,000 and 10,000 axon terminals, with synapses being stimulated by an equivalent number of other neurons. Outside the CNS, postsynaptic cells may be other neurons or effector cells (gland or muscle cells).

A synapse between a neuron and a muscle cell is known as a *neuromuscular junction*. Neurons regulate or control the activities of secretory cells at *neuroglandular junctions*. Neurons also function in the *innervation* of many other types of cells, an example of which is fat cells or *adipocytes*.

A neuron carrying an impulse into a synapse is called a *presynaptic neuron*. The neuron receiving this impulse is called a *postsynaptic neuron*. The process of the impulse crossing the synaptic cleft is called *synaptic transmission*. Most neurons function as both presynaptic and postsynaptic neurons. Synaptic transmission occurs in one direction, carried by biochemicals (**neurotransmitters**).

Chemical synapses allow the release and reception of chemical neurotransmitters. *Electrical synapses* are less common than *chemical synapses*, consisting of gap junctions similar to those between certain other cells of the body. Most chemical synapses are made up of two parts: an *axon terminal* and a neurotransmitter *receptor region*. The *axon terminal* is a knob-like structure of the presynaptic neuron. The axon terminal contains many **synaptic vesicles**, which are very small membrane-bounded sacs holding thousands of neurotransmitter molecules. The neurotransmitter receptor region is located on the postsynaptic neuron's membrane. The properties of the receptors on the postsynaptic membrane determine the effect of a neurotransmitter. The neurotransmitter receptor region is usually located on the cell body or on a dendrite.

The synaptic cleft is a fluid-filled space that separates presynaptic and postsynaptic membranes. Each of these clefts is approximately one-millionth of 1 inch in width. The electrical current from the *presynaptic membrane* dissipates in each synaptic cleft. Therefore, chemical synapses prevent nerve impulses from being directly transmitted between neurons. Instead, they are transmitted through chemical events that are based on release, diffusion, and receptor binding of neurotransmitter molecules. Neurons, therefore, have *unidirectional communication* between them.

Complex *synaptic terminals* exist at each neuromuscular junction, which contain parts of the endoplasmic reticulum, mitochondria, and thousands of neurotransmitter-filled vesicles. Synaptic terminals reabsorb breakdown products of neurotransmitters, which are synthesized neurotransmitters from cell bodies, enzymes, and lysosomes. The movement of these materials is called *axoplasmic transport*, which may be slow or fast, occurring in both directions. If *anterograde*, they move from the cell body to the synaptic terminal. If moving in reverse, they are described as *retrograde*.

Information is transferred across chemical synapses beginning when an action potential arrives at an axon terminal. The voltage-gated calcium ion channels then open, allowing calcium to enter the axon terminal. This entry results in synaptic vesicles releasing neurotransmitter via exocytosis. A single nerve impulse reaching the presynaptic terminal causes up to 300 vesicles to empty into the synaptic cleft. A higher impulse frequency causes more synaptic vesicles to fuse and release their contents. This has a greater effect on postsynaptic cells. Neurotransmitter diffuses across the synaptic cleft, binding to certain receptors on the *postsynaptic membrane*. This binding opens ion channels to create graded potentials, after which the neurotransmitter's effects are terminated.

The events that occur at a cholinergic synapse, involving the release of ACh, begin with the arrival of an action potential, which depolarizes the synaptic terminal. Extracellular calcium ions enter the synaptic terminal. This triggers the exocytosis of ACh, which then binds to receptors and depolarizes the postsynaptic membrane. ACh is then removed by acetylcholinesterase. This enzyme breaks down ACh, via hydrolysis, into *acetate* and *choline*. Acetate is then absorbed and metabolized by the postsynaptic cell or by other tissues and cells. Choline is actively absorbed by the synaptic terminal so more ACh can be synthesized. This requires use of acetate that is provided by coenzyme A.

Between the arrival of the action potential at the synaptic terminal and its effect on the postsynaptic membrane, there is a *synaptic delay* of between 0.2 and 0.5 msec. During this time, an action potential is able to travel more than 7 cm (3 inches) along a myelinated axon. The less synapses involved, the shorter the total synaptic delay, meaning the faster the response. In our bodies, the fastest reflexes have only one synapse, and a sensory neuron directly controls a motor neuron. Under intense stimuli, ACh resynthesis and transport may not be able to meet the demands for the neurotransmitter. If so, *synaptic fatigue* occurs. The synapse becomes weak until ACh has been replenished.

Synaptic Transmission

The effects of neurotransmitters differ. When neurotransmitters diffuse across synaptic clefts, they react differently with specific receptor molecules located in the postsynaptic neuron membrane. Neurotransmitters may be *excitatory* or *inhibitory*. We discussed cholinergic synapses, but it important to remember that other types of synapses are also involved in synaptic transmission. For example, norepinephrine or *noradrenaline* is released at *adrenergic synapses*. Norepinephrine usually has excitatory effects that depolarize the postsynaptic membrane. The actions of adrenergic synapses are much different than those of cholinergic synapses.

Excitation and Inhibition

Excitatory neurotransmitters are those that increase postsynaptic membrane permeability to sodium ions, bringing the postsynaptic membrane closer to threshold. This may trigger nerve impulses. *Inhibitory* neurotransmitters are those that make it less probable that the threshold will be reached. They decrease the chance that a nerve impulse will occur. A single postsynaptic neuron may receive communication from thousands of neuronal synaptic knobs. The actions of the neurotransmitters sent from these knobs may be either excitatory or inhibitory. Their effects are based on which knobs are being activated. If more excitatory neurotransmitters are released, the postsynaptic neuron's threshold may be reached, triggering a nerve impulse.

Neurotransmitters

There are about 50 types of neurotransmitters, which are classified chemically and functionally. Neurons may release one or more types. The actions of neurotransmitters include effects on sleeping, anger, thinking, hunger, movement, memory, and many other functions. Synaptic transmission is commonly affected by either the enhancing or inhibiting effects of neurotransmitters, their destruction, or the blocking of receptor binding. Anything that reduces neurotransmitter activity may slow the brain's ability to communicate with the rest of the body. Usually, neurotransmitters are released at various stimulation frequencies. This helps to create more ordered synaptic transmission. Simultaneous release of two neurotransmitters from the same vesicle does still occur. Therefore, a cell can have multiple effects on its target. A summary of neurotransmitters and their actions is shown in **TABLE 10-2**.

The membrane of a synaptic knob has increased permeability to calcium ions when an action potential reaches it. Calcium ions diffuse inward and in some synaptic vesicles respond by releasing their contents into the synaptic cleft. Eventually, these vesicles separate from the membrane and reenter the cytoplasm to pick up more neurotransmitters. Neurotransmitters (such as ACh) are decomposed by specific enzymes (such as acetylcholinesterase). Others are transported back into the synaptic knobs that released them in a process known as *reuptake*. They may also be transported to neurons or neuroglial cells that are close to them. These actions prevent neurotransmitters from continually stimulating postsynaptic neurons (**TABLE 10-3**).

Neurotransmitter Chemical Classifications

ACh was the first identified neurotransmitter and is released at *neuromuscular junctions*. The neuromuscular junctions that release ACh are also known as *cholinergic synapses*. ACh is synthesized from acetic acid as *acetyl* coenzyme A and choline via the enzyme *choline aceyltransferase*. It is then transported to synaptic vesicles to be released at a later time. It is then degraded to acetic acid and choline (via the enzyme *acetylcholinesterase*). *Biogenic amines* include the *catecholamines*

TABLE 10-2

Major Neurotransmitters and Their Actions

Neurotransmitter	Action
ACh	At nicotinic ACh receptors on autonomic ganglia and in the CNS, it controls skeletal muscles, having excitatory, direct action At muscarinic ACH receptors in the CNS and on visceral effectors, it has excitatory or inhibitory functions (based on subtype of receptor) and indirect action, via second messengers Stimulates skeletal muscle contraction at neuromuscular junctions and can excite or inhibit at ANS synapses (PNS)
Amino acids	
GABA	Mostly inhibitory (CNS), having direct and indirect actions via second messengers
Glutamic acid (glutamate)	Mostly inhibitory (CNS), having mostly excitatory, direct action
Glycine	Mostly inhibitor, with direct action
Monoamines (biogenic amines)	
Dopamine	Creates a sense of well-being; deficiency is associated with Parkinson's disease (CNS) Limited ANS actions; may excite or inhibit (PNS) based on receptor type Has indirect action via second messengers
Histamine	Promotes alertness (CNS), has excitatory or inhibitory actions based on receptor type Has indirect action via second messengers
Norepinephrine	Creates a sense of well-being; deficiency may lead to depression (CNS), has excitatory or inhibitory actions based on receptor type May excite or inhibit ANS actions (PNS) Has indirect action via second messengers
Serotonin (5-HT)	Mostly inhibitory; causes sleepiness; is enhanced by selective serotonin reuptake inhibitor or selective norepinephrine reuptake inhibitor drugs (CNS) Has indirect action via second messengers but direct action at 5-HT_3 receptors
Neuropeptides	
Endorphins (including beta endorphin, dynorphin)	Mostly inhibitory, reduces pain by inhibiting substance P release (CNS) Have indirect action via second messengers
Enkephalins	Same as endorphins
Tachykinins (substance P, neurokinin A)	Excitatory; perception of pain (PNS) Have indirect action via second messengers
Cholecystokinin	Mostly excitatory; has indirect action via second messengers
Somatostatin	Mostly inhibitory; has indirect action via second messengers
Gases and lipids	
Nitric oxide	May affect memory (CNS) Either excitatory or inhibitory, has indirect action via second messengers Vasodilation (PNS)
Carbon monoxide	Either excitatory or inhibitory, has indirect action via second messengers
Endocannabinoids (anandamide, 2-arachidonoyglycerol)	Inhibitory effects, have indirect action via second messengers
Purines	
Adenosine	Mostly inhibitory, has indirect action via second messengers
ATP	Either excitatory or inhibitory based on receptor type Has direct and indirect actions via second messengers

TABLE 10-3	
Neurotransmitter Release	
Step	Event
1	Action potential passes along axons and over synaptic knobs.
2	Synaptic knobs become more permeable to calcium ions, which diffuse inward.
3	Synaptic vesicles fuse to synaptic knob membranes.
4	Synaptic vesicles release neurotransmitters into synaptic clefts.
5	Synaptic vesicles reenter axons' cytoplasm to pick up more neurotransmitters.

and *indolamines*. The catecholamines include dopamine, epinephrine, and norepinephrine. The indolamines include histamine and serotonin.

Amino acids that have identified roles as neurotransmitters include *aspartate, glutamate, gamma-aminobutyric acid (GABA),* and *glycine. Peptides* (neuropeptides) are basically amino acid chains and include a mediator of pain signals (*substance P*) and substances that reduce pain perception while under stress. These substances include the *endorphins* and *enkephalins*. Examples of endorphins include *beta endorphin* and *dynorphin*. Neuropeptides called *gut-brain peptides* are found throughout the gastrointestinal tract, produced by non-neural body tissues. These peptides include *cholecystokinin* and *somatostatin*.

Purines are chemicals that contain nitrogen, which are actually breakdown products of nucleic acids. Examples include *adenine* and *guanine*. They also include *ATP* and a part of ATP known as *adenosine*. Gases and lipids with neurotransmitter actions include *gasotransmitters* and *endocannabinoids*. Examples of gasotransmitters include nitric oxide, carbon monoxide, and hydrogen sulfide. The endocannabinoids are natural neurotransmitters that act at the same receptors as *tetrahydrocannabinol*, which is the active ingredient in marijuana. They are lipid soluble and released as needed instead of being stored in vesicles.

Neurotransmitter Functional Classifications

Functional classifications of neurotransmitters are based on their excitatory or inhibitory actions. Excitatory neurotransmitters cause depolarization, whereas inhibitory neurotransmitters cause hyperpolarization. They are also classified based on direct versus indirect actions. Those that act directly bind to and open ion channels. Those that act indirectly cause wider, longer-lasting effects via acting through intracellular second messengers (usually G protein pathways). A chemical messenger released by a neuron that affects the strength of synaptic transmission is called a *neuromodulator*. Most neuromodulators are *neuropeptides*, which are small peptide chains that are synthesized and released by synaptic terminals. They usually act by binding to receptors in the presynaptic or postsynaptic membranes, activating

cytoplasmic enzymes. *Opioids* are neuromodulators that bind to the same group of postsynaptic receptors as the drugs *opium* and *morphine*. The four classes of CNS opioids are *endorphins, enkephalins, endomorphins,* and *dynorphins*.

Overall, neuromodulators have long-term effects that usually appear slowly and trigger responses that have many steps and various involved compounds. They affect the presynaptic membrane, the postsynaptic membrane, or both. Neuromodulators also may be released alone or with a neurotransmitter. Many neurotransmitters and neuromodulators bind to receptors in the plasma membrane but require a G protein to link between first and second messengers. As a result, an enzyme called *adenylate cyclase* may be activated. It converts ATP to *cyclic adenosine monophosphate,* or *cAMP*, at the inner surface of the plasma membrane. cAMP is a second messenger that can open membrane channels, activate intracellular enzymes, or both.

Processing of Impulses

Neurons and axons within the brain and spinal cord affect impulse processing. In the CNS, neurons are organized into neuronal pools, which are groups of neurons that work together to perform a common function. These pools may have excitatory or inhibitory effects on other pools or peripheral effectors. If the net effect of an input is excitatory, a threshold may be reached, triggering an outgoing impulse. If the net effect is subthreshold (but still excitatory), an impulse is not triggered but the neuron is more excitable to incoming stimulation than previously. This state is called *facilitation*. A neuron is described as *facilitated* when its transmembrane potential shifts closer to threshold. *Presynaptic facilitation* involves activity at an axoaxonic synapse that increases the amount of neurotransmitter that is released when an action potential arrives at the synaptic terminal. The neurotransmitter *serotonin* is involved in this type of facilitation. In one form of *presynaptic inhibition*, when GABA is released, it inhibits opening of voltage-gated calcium channels in the synaptic terminal. This reduces how much neurotransmitter is released when an action potential arrives, reducing the effects of synaptic activity on the postsynaptic membrane.

Axons that originate from different areas of the nervous system but lead to the same neuron exhibit convergence, which makes it possible for impulses from different sources to have an additive effect on a neuron. If a neuron is facilitated by receiving subthreshold stimulation from an input neuron, it may reach threshold if it receives additional stimulation from a second input neuron. Therefore, a nerve impulse may travel to a particular effector to evoke a response. Convergence allows the collection of many different kinds of information as well as processing and responses by the CNS.

Impulses that leave a neuron in a neuronal pool often exhibit divergence by continuing on to several other output neurons. An impulse from one neuron may stimulate two others, which may stimulate more in a continuing process. Divergence can amplify impulses so they reach enough motor units within skeletal muscles to cause forceful contraction. Divergence can occur with motor or sensory impulses.

Graded potentials that develop in the postsynaptic membrane in response to a neurotransmitter are known as *postsynaptic potentials*. An *excitatory postsynaptic potential (EPSP)* is caused by a neurotransmitter arriving at the postsynaptic membrane, due to the opening of chemically gated membrane channels, leading to depolarization of the plasma membrane. An *inhibitory postsynaptic potential* is a graded hyperpolarization of the postsynaptic membrane. It may result from the opening of chemically gated potassium channels, during which time the neuron is described as *inhibited*. This is due to a greater than normal depolarizing stimulus required to bring the membrane potential to threshold.

Individual EPSPs have tiny effects on transmembrane potential, but when they combine through the process of *summation*, their effects become integrated. There are two types of summation: *temporal summation* and *spatial summation*. Temporal summation occurs when stimuli are added in rapid success at just one synapse that is repeatedly active. Although a typical EPSP lasts only 20 msec, with maximum stimulation, an action potential can reach the synaptic terminal every millisecond. When a second EPSP arrives before the effects of the first EPSP have disappeared, the effects combine. The degree of depolarization continually increases.

Spatial summation involves simultaneous stimuli that are applied at different locations, cumulatively affecting the transmembrane potential. Multiple synapses are active simultaneously. Each synapse moves sodium ions across the postsynaptic membrane to produce a graded potential that has localized effects. Cumulative effects occur on the initial segment.

TEST YOUR UNDERSTANDING

1. Differentiate between "excitatory" and "inhibitory" neurotransmitters.
2. What is a "neuronal pool"?

Classification of Nerve Fibers

Nerve fibers are classified by their diameter, degree of myelination, and speed of conduction. There are three primary groups of nerve fibers:

- *Group A fibers:* These mostly serve the joints, skeletal muscles, and skin and are primarily somatic sensory and motor fibers, with the largest diameter of all types of fibers and thick myelin sheaths. These fibers conduct impulses at speeds as high as 300 miles per hour.
- *Group B fibers:* Of intermediate diameter, with light myelination, group B fibers conduct impulses at speeds averaging approximately 30 miles per hour.
- *Group C fibers:* These fibers are nonmyelinated, with the smallest diameter, and cannot create saltatory conduction; they conduct impulses at 2 miles per hour or less.

Both B and C fibers include motor fibers of the ANS that serve the smaller somatic sensory fibers that transmit sensory impulses from the skin (including small touch and pain fibers), visceral sensory fibers, and those that serve the visceral organs.

FOCUS ON PATHOLOGY

Impulses can be impeded by many physical and chemical factors. If there is no sodium entry, no action potential can be generated. Therefore, agents that block the voltage-gated sodium channels, such as local anesthetics, are extremely effective. Impulse conduction is also impaired by continuous pressure and cold temperatures, which interrupt blood circulation, slowing oxygen and nutrient delivery to neuron processes. This is why a body part *goes to sleep* if it receives pressure from the rest of the body and then recovers when the pressure is removed (causing a prickly feeling that is uncomfortable).

Effects of Aging on the Nervous System

Beginning at age 30, anatomic and physiological changes begin to affect the nervous system. After age 65, there may be noticeable changes in CNS function and mental performance. As fatty deposits accumulate in the blood vessels, there is a decrease in blood flow to the brain. This can increase the chances that an affected vessel will rupture, leading to symptoms of a stroke (cerebrovascular accident).

Cerebrovascular diseases are more common in long-term smokers or when conditions such as hypertension, high cholesterol, or diabetes mellitus are present.

Verbal abilities often begin to decline at approximately age 70. If no neurologic disorders are present, intellectual performance is usually maintained until about age 80. Because the brain processes nerve impulses more slowly, performance of certain tasks and reaction times often become slower. Other disorders that affect the nervous system due to aging include depression, hypothyroidism, and degenerative brain disorders. An elderly person who exercises (both mentally and physically) often loses fewer nerve cells in the brain. Consumption of two or more drinks of alcohol every day reduces brain function.

The spine is also affected by aging, and pressure increases on the spinal cord and spinal nerve roots. This can result in decreases in sensation, strength, and balance. Peripheral nerve conduction slows because the myelin sheaths degenerate with aging. Self-repair of damaged peripheral nerve cells is also slower in older individuals.

SUMMARY

Nervous tissue includes neurons and neuroglial cells. The nervous system is divided into the CNS and PNS. Sensory functions receive stimulation from receptors concerning internal and external changes. Sensory information is used to carry out motor functions, which in turn stimulate effectors to respond. Neuroglial cells include microglial cells, oligodendrocytes, astrocytes, and ependymal cells. In the PNS, Schwann cells form myelin sheaths. A neuron consists of a cell body, dendrites, and an axon. Dendrites and cell bodies provide receptive surfaces. A single axon arises from the cell body and may be enclosed in a neurolemma and myelin sheath. Axons may have occasional branches known as axon collaterals, which usually extend in right angles. An axon with a myelin sheath is called myelinated. In the CNS, dense groups of myelinated axons form the white matter. Those that are unmyelinated, along with neuron cell bodies, form the gray matter.

Functional classifications of neurons include sensory (afferent) neurons, interneurons, and motor (efferent neurons). Structural classifications of neurons include multipolar, bipolar, and unipolar neurons. The surface of a cell membrane is usually electrically charged (polarized) compared with its inner contents. An action potential is a change in neuron membrane polarization and a return to its resting state. It is an all-or-none phenomenon, occurring completely or not at all. The absolute refractory period is the time between sodium channels opening until they begin to reset to their resting state.

Distribution of ions is determined in part by selective channels located in cell membranes. The difference in charges between the outside of the cell membrane and the inside of it in a resting cell is known as a resting potential. The cytosol of cells contains less sodium ions but more potassium ions, compared with the extracellular fluid. Potassium ions diffuse out of cells very easily in comparison with how easily sodium ions can enter. Nerve cells respond with excitability to changes in surroundings. Depolarization opens sodium channels and then inactivates them. In repolarization, sodium channels are inactivating, with potassium channels open. In hyperpolarization, some potassium ion channels remain open, and sodium ion channels are reset.

Nerve fibers are classified by their diameter, degree of myelination, and speed of conduction and are divided into group A, group B, and group C fibers. In a nerve cell membrane, an action potential causes a local bioelectric current to reach other portions of the membrane. A wave of action potentials is a nerve impulse. Impulses are conducted over the entire surface of unmyelinated axons, but there is reduced impulse conduction in myelinated axons because of the insulation provided by the myelin.

A synapse is a junction between two neurons. Presynaptic neurons carry impulses into synapses, and postsynaptic neurons respond. Axons have synaptic knobs, which secrete neurotransmitters. Neurotransmitters reaching the postsynaptic neuron membrane are either excitatory or inhibitory. ACh is released at neuromuscular junctions and is eventually degraded to acetic acid and choline via the enzyme acetylcholinesterase. The way the nervous system processes and responds to nerve impulses is based on the organization of neurons in the brain and spinal cord. The aging process affects the entire nervous system in many different ways and usually reduces function as a result of slower impulse processing abilities.

Absolute refractory period
Action potential
Afferent (sensory) division
All-or-none phenomenon
Astrocytes
Autonomic nervous system
Axon collaterals
Axons
Axon terminals
Blood–brain barrier
Central nervous system (CNS)
Chromatophilic substance
Dendrites
Depolarization
Effectors
Efferent (motor) division
Ependymal cells
Ganglia
Hyperpolarization
Integration

Involuntary nervous system
Microglial cells
Motor output
Myelin
Myelin sheaths
Nerve fibers
Nerve impulses
Nerve pathways
Nerves
Neurofibrils
Neuroglial cells
Neurolemma
Neurons
Neurotransmitters
Nodes of Ranvier
Nuclei
Oligodendrocytes
Peripheral nervous system (PNS)
Phagocytosis
Processes

Reflexes
Relative refractory period
Repolarization
Resting potential
Satellite cells
Schwann cells
Sensory input
Sensory receptors
Soma
Somatic nervous system
Synapse
Synaptic cleft
Synaptic vesicles
Terminal branches
Threshold potential
Tracts
Voluntary nervous system

LEARNING GOALS

The following learning goals correspond to the objectives at the beginning of this chapter:

1. The CNS consists of the brain and spinal cord. The PNS consists of the peripheral nerves connecting the CNS to other parts of the body. Consciously controlled motor functions are handled by the somatic nervous system. Involuntary effectors are controlled by the ANS.

2. Sensory receptors located at the ends of peripheral neurons provide the nervous system's sensory functions. They relay information in response to environmental changes. The information is converted into nerve impulses, which are then processed so motor functions can act appropriately in response. Response structures called effectors are located outside the nervous system. These include muscles and glands, which may contract, secrete, or perform other reactive functions. The somatic nervous system controls conscious motor functions and skeletal muscles. The ANS controls involuntary effectors such as the heart, certain glands, and smooth muscle in blood vessels. The nervous system maintains homeostasis.

3. Astrocytes anchor neurons and blood vessels together and aid in exchanges between neurons and capillaries, determining capillary permeability. They also control migration of new neurons as well as the formation of synapses between neurons. They have a vital function in cleaning up leaked potassium ions and recycling released neurotransmitters. Astrocytes also respond to nerve impulses and released neurotransmitters. They signal each other via calcium intake and release of extracellular chemical messengers. They create slow intracellular calcium waves and influence neuronal functioning. Oligodendrocytes provide insulating layers of myelin (the myelin sheath) around axons within the brain and spinal cord.

4. Nervous tissue consists of masses of neurons (nerve cells) and is highly cellular. Neurons are the structural and functional units of the nervous system, and each neuron has a specialized function. Billions of neurons exist in the nervous system and can function very well for a person's entire lifetime if they receive adequate nutrients. However, they are *amitotic*, losing their ability to divide. Therefore, they cannot be replaced if they are destroyed (in most circumstances). Neurons that can be replaced include the

olfactory epithelium of the nose and certain regions of the hippocampus in the brain, which is involved in memory. Neurons are larger than other cells of the nervous system and highly specialized in their conduction of impulses. Each neuron has a rounded cell body and extensions called dendrites and axons. Each neuron usually has only one axon. Neurons require continuous, abundant oxygen and glucose supplies because they have a very high metabolic rate. Without oxygen, neurons cannot survive for more than a few minutes. Although neurons are similar in structure, they vary greatly in size and shape. They all have a cell body (soma), dendrites, and an axon. The cell body is where most biosynthesis occurs in the neuron. Most neuron cell bodies are located in the CNS. All neuron cell bodies have processes that extend outward. The CNS contains both neuron cell bodies and processes, whereas the PNS mostly contains just processes. There are two types of neuron processes: dendrites and axons. Dendrites have multiple branches that act as the neuron's main receptive surfaces. The dendrites of the motor neurons are tapered, short in length, and have diffusely branched extensions. They are the primary receptive (input) regions of neurons, having a large surface area for receiving neuronal signals. Most neurons have a single axon arising from an elevation (the axonal hillock) on the cell body. Some neurons have short axons or may even lack axons. In others, axons make up almost the entire neuron length.

5. Neuroglial cells provide insulation, physical support, and nutrients to the neurons. Neuroglia include astrocytes (usually found between neurons and blood vessels), ependymal cells (cover specialized brain parts and form inner linings enclosing spaces inside the brain and spinal cord; they secrete cerebrospinal fluid), microglial cells (found through the CNS; they phagocytize bacterial cells and cellular debris), and oligodendrocytes (aligned along nerve fibers; they provide insulating layers of myelin around axons within the brain and spinal cord).

6. Synaptic transmission occurs in one direction, carried by biochemicals (neurotransmitters). When a nerve impulse reaches the synaptic knob, the synaptic vesicles release a neurotransmitter. It diffuses across the cleft to react with certain receptors on the postsynaptic neuron membrane, either exciting or inhibiting a postsynaptic cell. This depends on the combined effect of excitatory and inhibitory inputs from a single (or many) presynaptic neurons.

7. Chemical synapses allow the release and reception of chemical neurotransmitters. They are more common than electrical synapses and are usually made up of two parts: the axon terminal and a neurotransmitter receptor region. The axon terminal is a knob-like structure of the presynaptic neuron. The axon terminal contains many synaptic vesicles, which are very small membrane-bounded sacs holding thousands of neurotransmitter molecules. The neurotransmitter receptor region is located on the postsynaptic neuron's membrane. This is usually located on the cell body or on a dendrite. The synaptic cleft is a fluid-filled space that separates presynaptic and postsynaptic membranes. Each of these clefts is approximately one-millionth of 1 inch in width. The electrical current from the presynaptic membrane dissipates in each synaptic cleft. Therefore, chemical synapses prevent nerve impulses from being directly transmitted between neurons. Instead, they are transmitted through chemical events that are based on release, diffusion, and receptor binding of neurotransmitter molecules. Neurons, therefore, have unidirectional communication between them.

8. The major types of neurotransmitters are acetylcholine, amino acids (GABA and glutamic acid), monoamines (dopamine, histamine, norepinephrine, and serotonin), neuropeptides (endorphins, enkephalins, and substance P), and gases (nitric oxide).

9. An action potential is the basis for a nerve impulse. It is based on the cell membrane reaching its threshold potential and is a brief reversal of membrane potential with a change in voltage of approximately 100 mV.

10. Nerve fibers are classified by their diameter, degree of myelination, and speed of conduction. Group A fibers mostly serve the joints, skeletal muscles, and skin; they are primarily somatic sensory and motor fibers, with the largest diameter of all types of fibers and thick myelin sheaths. These fibers conduct impulses at speeds as high as 300 miles per hour. Group B fibers are of intermediate diameter, with light myelination. They conduct impulses at speeds averaging approximately 20 miles per hour. Group C fibers are nonmyelinated, with the smallest diameter, and cannot create saltatory conduction. They conduct impulses at 2 miles per hour or less.

CRITICAL THINKING QUESTIONS

A 35-year-old woman went to see her physician because of partial vision loss, lack of coordination, and the development of speech problems. She was extremely worried that she had a brain tumor. After thorough testing, it was determined that she had multiple sclerosis.

1. What happens to the axons in a person with this condition?
2. Are there any possible treatments for her condition?

REVIEW QUESTIONS

1. Which of the following is not a function of the neuroglia?
   A. phagocytosis
   B. support
   C. information processing
   D. secretion of cerebrospinal fluid

2. The brain and spinal cord comprise which of the following nervous systems?
   A. efferent
   B. afferent
   C. peripheral
   D. central

3. The neurolemma of axons in the PNS is formed by
   A. Schwann cells
   B. astrocytes
   C. microglia
   D. oligodendrocytes

4. Which of the following is the site of intracellular communication between neurons?
   A. synaptic knob
   B. synapse
   C. hillock
   D. collateral

5. Which of the following differentiates chemical synapses from electrical synapses?
   A. chemical synapses involve a neurotransmitter
   B. chemical synapses involve direct physical contact between cells
   C. chemical synapses initiate action potentials quickly
   D. chemical synapses contain special links called connexons

6. Which of the following describes membrane potential changes related to resting membrane potential?
   A. polarization
   B. hyperpolarization
   C. action potential
   D. synaptic transmission

7. Which of the following are the two major cell types in neural tissue?
   A. satellite and Schwann cells
   B. astrocytes and oligodendrocytes
   C. neurons and neuroglia
   D. ependymal cells and microglia

8. Which of the following is the responsibility of neurons?
   A. transferring information in the nervous system
   B. creating a three-dimensional framework for the CNS
   C. repair of damaged neural tissue
   D. protecting the neuroglia

9. Sensory neurons are responsible for carrying impulses
   A. from the CNS to the PNS
   B. to the PNS
   C. to the CNS
   D. away from the CNS

10. The larger the diameter of the axon, the
    A. less effect it will have on action potential propagation
    B. faster an action potential can be conducted
    C. slower an action potential will be conducted
    D. greater the number of action potentials

11. When the resting potential is –70 mV and the threshold is –60 mV, a membrane potential of –60 mV will
    A. not produce an action potential
    B. depolarize the membrane to 0 mV
    C. produce an action potential
    D. repolarize the membrane to –90 mV

12. Which of the following is the classification of neurons on the basis of their function?
    A. somatic, visceral, and autonomic
    B. central, peripheral, and autonomic
    C. multipolar, bipolar, and unipolar
    D. sensory, interneurons, and motor

13. A node along the axon represents an area where there is
    A. a section of interwoven layers of myelin and protein
    B. an absence of myelin
    C. a gap in the cell membrane
    D. a layer of fat
14. The effect of a neurotransmitter on the postsynaptic membrane depends on the
    A. width of the synaptic cleft
    B. number of synaptic vesicles
    C. nature of the neurotransmitter
    D. properties of the receptors
15. When the resting membrane potential is –70 mV, a hyperpolarized membrane is
    A. +5 mV
    B. +40 mV
    C. –65 mV
    D. –80 mV

ESSAY QUESTIONS

1. Describe how neuronal firing is determined.
2. Explain the anatomic and functional divisions of the nervous systems, with all subdivisions.
3. Describe neurotransmitter binding and the time it takes for this to occur.
4. Compare and contrast the structure of axons and dendrites.
5. Explain the differences between group A, group B, and group C fibers.
6. Describe the processes of myelination.
7. Indicate where multipolar, bipolar, and unipolar neurons are most likely to be found.
8. What are the three stages of neuron development?
9. How is the polarized membrane state maintained?
10. What events must occur in order for an action potential to be generated?

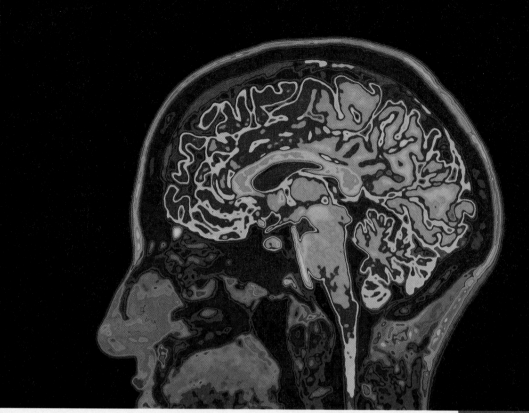

CHAPTER 11

Central Nervous System

OBJECTIVES

After studying this chapter, readers should be able to

1. Name the primary regions of the brain in adults.
2. Describe the locations of the ventricles of the brain.
3. Describe the gyri, sulci, and fissures of the brain.
4. Explain the part of the brain that is connected to pituitary gland.
5. Describe the functions of the hypothalamus and thalamus.
6. Describe the centers that control blood pressure and respiration.
7. Specify the functions of the cerebellum.
8. Explain the layers of the meninges.
9. Discuss the main structures and functions of the spinal cord.
10. Describe the effects of the aging process on the brain.

Overview

The human brain contains most of the body's neural tissue and generally weighs about 3 pounds. Brain sizes vary considerably, often in relation to body size. However, there is no relation of brain size to intelligence. The brain is divided into major structures such as the cerebrum, cerebral hemispheres, diencephalon, brain stem, and cerebellum. Higher mental functions are controlled by the cerebrum, which is the largest portion of the brain.

The spinal cord begins where nervous tissue exits the cranial cavity near the foramen magnum and extends to the lumbar section of the spine. It has nerves arising from each of its 31 segments. The spinal cord is divided into right and left halves by a deep anterior median fissure and a shallow posterior median fissure. In the central nervous system (CNS), *nuclei* are masses of gray matter. The inner core of the spinal cord is made of gray matter surrounded by white matter. Major nerve tracts are made up of long bundles of myelinated nerve fibers. A horizontal bar of gray matter in the very middle of the spinal cord surrounds its narrow *central canal* and contains cerebrospinal fluid (CSF). The spinal cord conducts nerve impulses and **spinal reflexes**, whereas reflexes processed in the brain are called *cranial reflexes*. Two-way communication flows between the brain and other body parts because of the spinal cord. Tracts carrying information to the brain are called *ascending tracts*, whereas those carrying information to the muscles and glands are called *descending tracts*.

Brain

Nearly 100 billion neurons compose the adult brain, which can be divided into the cerebrum (with two cerebral hemispheres), diencephalon, brain stem (which includes the midbrain, pons, and medulla oblongata), and cerebellum (**FIGURE 11-1**). The largest part (**cerebrum**) coordinates sensory and motor functions and higher mental functions such as memory and reasoning. The diencephalon processes additional sensory information. The nerve pathways of the brain stem connect nervous system components and regulate certain visceral activities. The cerebellum coordinates voluntary muscular movements.

The CNS is basically designed as a central cavity surrounded first by gray matter and then by white matter. The gray matter consists mostly of neuron cell bodies, whereas the white matter consists of myelinated fiber tracts. This pattern makes up most of the spinal cord. However, the brain also has extra regions of gray matter not found in the spinal cord. The cerebral hemispheres and cerebellum have an outer *cortex*, which is a layer of gray matter.

Ventricles

Interconnected cavities known as **ventricles** exist within the cerebral hemispheres and brain stem. They are continuous with the spinal cord's central canal and also contain CSF. The walls of the hollow ventricular chambers are lined by *ependymal cells*. The two large **lateral ventricles** are located inside the frontal, temporal, and occipital lobes. The third ventricle is under the **corpus callosum** in the brain's midline. The fourth ventricle is in the brain stem, and a narrow cerebral aqueduct joins it to the third ventricle.

Within each cerebral hemisphere are large C-shaped chambers known as the paired *lateral ventricles*. They demonstrate the pattern of cerebral growth and lie close together anteriorly. A thin median membrane called the **septum pellucidum** separates them. Each lateral ventricle is connected to the thin *third ventricle*, which is surrounded by the diencephalon, via a channel known as the *interventricular foramen*. The third ventricle connects to the *fourth ventricle* via the **cerebral aqueduct**, which runs through the midbrain. **FIGURE 11-2** shows the ventricles in the brain.

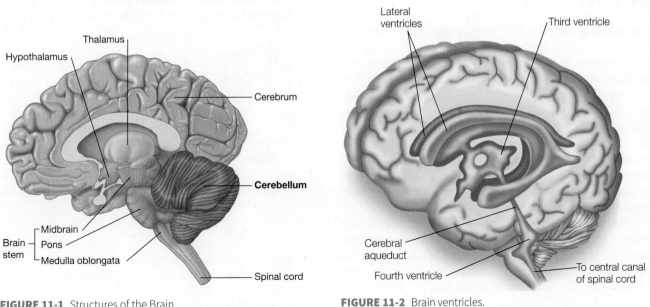

FIGURE 11-1 Structures of the Brain

FIGURE 11-2 Brain ventricles.

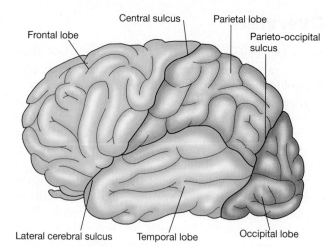

FIGURE 11-3 The lobes of the cerebrum.

TEST YOUR UNDERSTANDING

1. Describe the ventricle that is surrounded by the diencephalon.
2. Which sections of the brain have a cortex of gray matter?

Cerebral Hemispheres

The cerebrum is divided into two large **cerebral hemispheres**, one to the left and one to the right. They form the superior part of the brain and are easily visualized, making up approximately 83% of the brain's total mass. The *corpus callosum* is a deep bridge of nerve fibers that connects the hemispheres, separated by a layer of dura mater. It lies superior to the lateral ventricles, deep inside the **longitudinal fissure**. The cerebrum's surface is covered with **gyri**, which are separated by shallow or deep grooves. Each shallow groove is called a **sulcus**, and each deep groove is called a **fissure**. The fissures separate large regions of the brain. All these grooves form distinct patterns in normal brains, with the gyri and sulci being more prominent.

Several sulci divide each hemisphere into the frontal, parietal, temporal, and occipital lobes (as well as a structure called the **insula**). The insula is a brain lobe but is buried deep within the lateral sulcus, forming a portion of the brain floor. The lobes of the cerebral hemispheres refer to the skull bones they are positioned near. The cerebral hemispheres are separated by the median longitudinal fissure, whereas the *transverse cerebral fissure* separates the cerebral hemispheres from the cerebellum below them.

The three basic regions of each cerebral hemisphere are the cerebral cortex, white matter, and basal nuclei. The cerebral cortex is superficial gray matter and actually appears gray in color in fresh brain tissue. The white matter is more internal, and the basal nuclei are islands of gray matter located deep inside the white matter.

Cerebral Cortex

The **cerebral cortex,** a thin layer of gray matter comprising the outer portion of the cerebrum, is the center of the *conscious mind*. It contains about 75% of all the neuron cell bodies of the nervous system. The cerebral cortex is involved with awareness, communication, sensation, memory, understanding, and the initiation of voluntary movements. Its gray matter contains dendrites, neuron cell bodies, glia, and blood vessels. It lacks fiber tracts but contains six layers in which there are billions of neurons. The cerebral cortex is approximately 2 to 4 mm in thickness yet makes up approximately 40% of overall brain mass. Its surface area is nearly tripled by its many convolutions.

Beneath the cerebral cortex is white matter, comprising most of the cerebrum. It contains myelinated axon bundles, some of which pass from one cerebral hemisphere to the other. Others carry impulses from the cortex to nerve centers of the brain and spinal cord (**FIGURES 11-3** and **11-4**).

The lobes of the cerebral cortex are as follows:

- *Frontal lobe:* forms the anterior portion of each cerebral hemisphere
- *Parietal lobe:* lies posteriorly to the frontal lobe
- *Temporal lobe:* lies below the frontal and parietal lobes
- *Occipital lobe:* forms the posterior part of each cerebral hemisphere
- *Insula:* lies under the frontal, parietal, and temporal lobes

In most people, one side of their cerebrum acts as the **dominant hemisphere**, controlling the use and understanding of language. The left side of the cerebrum is usually responsible for activities such as speech, writing, reading, and complex intellectual functions. The nondominant hemisphere controls nonverbal functions and intuitive and emotional thoughts. The dominant hemisphere controls the motor cortex of the nondominant hemisphere.

Function

Aside from sensory and motor control, memory, and reasoning, the cerebrum also coordinates intelligence and personality. Functions overlap between regions of the cerebral cortex.

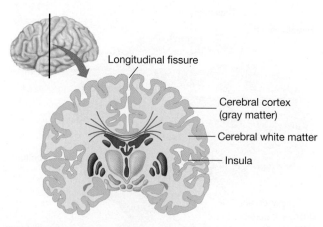

FIGURE 11-4 A coronal section through the cerebrum. The area of gray matter is greatly increased by the folding of the surface into gyri, sulci, fissures, and the insula.

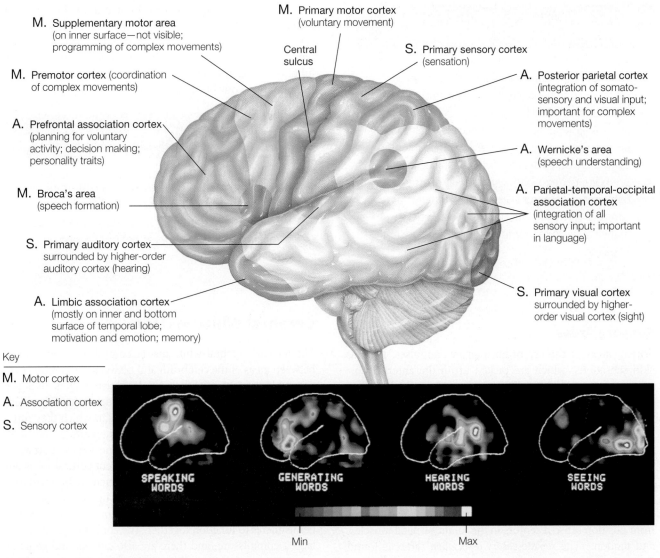

M. **Supplementary motor area**
(on inner surface—not visible;
programming of complex movements)

M. **Primary motor cortex**
(voluntary movement)

Central
sulcus

S. **Primary sensory cortex**
(sensation)

M. **Premotor cortex** (coordination
of complex movements)

A. **Posterior parietal cortex**
(integration of somato-
sensory and visual input;
important for complex
movements)

A. **Prefrontal association cortex**
(planning for voluntary
activity; decision making;
personality traits)

A. **Wernicke's area**
(speech understanding)

A. **Parietal-temporal-occipital
association cortex**
(integration of all
sensory input; important
in language)

M. **Broca's area**
(speech formation)

S. **Primary auditory cortex**
surrounded by higher-order
auditory cortex (hearing)

A. **Limbic association cortex**
(mostly on inner and bottom
surface of temporal lobe;
motivation and emotion; memory)

S. **Primary visual cortex**
surrounded by higher-
order visual cortex (sight)

Key

M. Motor cortex

A. Association cortex

S. Sensory cortex

SPEAKING WORDS   GENERATING WORDS   HEARING WORDS   SEEING WORDS

Min   Max

FIGURE 11-5 Functional regions of the cortex.

The three functional areas of the cerebral cortex are the motor, sensory, and association areas (**FIGURE 11-5**). All neurons in the cerebral cortex are *interneurons*. Each cerebral hemisphere controls the motor and sensory functions of the *contralateral* (opposite) side of the body. The hemispheres are not exactly equal in function, even though their structure is closely matched. Cortical functions are specialized, which exhibits a phenomenon known as *lateralization*. No functional area acts on its own, and conscious actions use the entire cortex in varying ways.

Motor Areas

Most of the cerebral cortex **motor areas** are located in the frontal lobes and are further defined as the *primary motor cortex, premotor cortex, Broca's area,* and *frontal eye field.* Impulses from large *pyramidal cells* in the motor areas travel through the brain stem into the spinal cord via the corticospinal tracts that form synapses with lower motor neurons. Their axons leave the spinal cord, reaching the skeletal muscle fibers.

The *primary motor cortex* is also known as the *somatic motor cortex.* It is located in the precentral gyrus of the frontal lobe of both hemispheres. The mapping of the CNS structures of the body is referred to as **somatotopy**. The *premotor cortex* lies just anterior to the precentral gyrus in the frontal lobe and helps to plan movements. **Broca's area** is found anterior to the inferior region of the premotor area and is more prevalent in the left hemisphere. It has a *motor speech area* and also becomes active just before speaking or when planning other voluntary motor activities. The *frontal eye field* is superior to Broca's area, located partly in and anterior to the premotor cortex. It controls voluntary eye movements. The central sulcus separates the primary motor areas from the somatosensory areas.

When certain local areas of the *primary motor cortex* are damaged (such as from a stroke), the muscles controlled by these areas become paralyzed. A right hemisphere lesion causes left-sided body paralysis, and vice versa. Although voluntary control is lost, muscle reflexes can still occur. If the *premotor cortex* is partially or totally destroyed, there is loss of motor skills that it normally controls. However, muscle strength and performance of discrete individual movements are not impaired.

The *gustatory (taste) cortex* is located in the insula, deep in the temporal lobe. The *visceral sensory area* controls visceral sensations and lies in the cortex of the insula, just posterior to the gustatory cortex. Its sensations include bladder fullness, stomach upset, and tightness in the lungs (such as from holding your breath).

If the *primary visual cortex* is damaged, the individual will become functionally blind. When an individual has a damaged visual association area, he or she can still see but cannot understand what is being seen.

Sensory Areas

Sensory areas of the cerebrum interpret impulses, such as skin sensations, which are picked up in the anterior portions of the parietal lobes. The posterior occipital lobes affect vision, whereas the temporal lobes affect hearing. Taste and smell receptors are located deeper within the cerebrum. Sensory fibers also cross similarly to motor fibers. Additional sensory areas include the insular and occipital lobes.

The *primary somatosensory cortex* lies in the postcentral gyrus of the parietal lobe. It is just posterior to the primary motor cortex, and its neurons receive input from the somatic sensory receptors of the skin. It also receives input from position sense receptors in the joints, skeletal muscles, and tendons. The *somatosensory association cortex* is found just posterior to the primary somatosensory cortex, is interconnected, and functions primarily to integrate temperature, pressure, and related information. The *primary visual (striate) cortex* is mostly buried in the **calcarine sulcus** of the occipital lobe but also extends to the extreme posterior occipital tip. It is the largest cortical sensory area, receiving visual information from the retinas of the eyes. The *visual association area* uses visual experiences from the past to interpret color, form, movement, and other visual stimuli.

Each *primary auditory cortex* lies in the superior margin of the temporal lobe and receives impulses from the inner ear, interpreting location, loudness, and pitch. Posteriorly, the *auditory association area* perceives sound stimuli such as speech, music, and environmental noises. The *vestibular (equilibrium) cortex* controls balance and is located in the posterior insula and the nearby parietal cortex. The *primary (olfactory) smell cortex* is present on the medial temporal lobe in the *piriform lobe* area, which is signified by its *uncus*, a hook-like structure. The olfactory cortex is part of the **rhinencephalon**, a primitive structure that includes the *orbitofrontal cortex, uncus,* and related regions on or inside the medial temporal lobe as well as the olfactory tracts and bulbs extending to the nose.

Cerebral White Matter

The internal cerebral white matter controls communication between areas of the cerebrum and between the cerebral cortex and lower centers of the CNS. Myelinated fibers, bundled into large tracts, make up most of this white matter. The fibers and tracts are classified by the directions in which they run.

Association fibers connect the various parts of the same brain hemisphere. Adjacent gyri are connected by short association fibers called *arcuate fibers*. Different cortical lobes are connected by long association fibers, which are bundled into tracts. Corresponding gray areas of both hemisphere are connected by *commissural fibers* or *commissures*, which allow the hemispheres to function together. The corpus callosum is the largest commissure, and there are also *anterior* and *posterior* commissures. *Projection fibers* enter the cerebral cortex from spinal cord or lower brain areas or descend to lower areas from the cerebral cortex. They allow motor output to leave the cerebral cortex and also sensory information to reach it. Projection fibers are different from association and commissural fibers in that they run vertically. Projection fibers at the top of the brain stem form a compact **internal capsule**, passing between the thalamus and certain basal nuclei. They then have a fan-like radiating pattern through the cerebral white matter and are therefore referred to as the **corona radiata**.

Basal Nuclei

Several masses of gray **basal nuclei** (basal ganglia) lie deep inside each cerebral hemisphere. These are the **caudate nucleus**, **globus pallidus**, and **putamen**. The basal nuclei help to control skeletal muscle activities. They filter out inappropriate responses as well as being involved in cognition and emotion. The lack of dopamine released from the basal nuclei may cause Parkinson's disease. The caudate nucleus arches superiorly over the diencephalon, joining the putamen to form the **striatum**, which has a striped appearance. The basal nuclei are linked to the *subthalamic nuclei* of the diencephalon

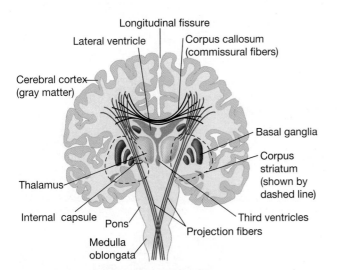

Longitudinal fissure
Lateral ventricle
Corpus callosum (commissural fibers)
Cerebral cortex (gray matter)
Basal ganglia
Corpus striatum (shown by dashed line)
Thalamus
Internal capsule
Pons
Projection fibers
Third ventricles
Medulla oblongata

FIGURE 11-6 Basal ganglia and nearby structures.

and the **substantia nigra** of the midbrain. They receive input from all of the cerebral cortex, other subcortical nuclei, and each other. The globus pallidus and substantia nigra relay information through the thalamus, reaching the premotor and prefrontal cortices. Therefore, they influence muscle movements, as controlled by the primary motor cortex. However, the basal nuclei do not directly access the motor pathways. **FIGURE 11-6** shows the basal nuclei and nearby structures.

TEST YOUR UNDERSTANDING

1. List the major divisions of the human brain.
2. Describe the functions of the cerebrum.
3. Explain the three basic regions of each cerebral hemisphere.
4. Describe the components of the basal nuclei.

Diencephalon

The **diencephalon** is mostly made up of the paired gray matter structures known as the *thalamus, hypothalamus,* and *epithalamus* and forms the central core of the forebrain. The diencephalon is surrounded by the cerebral hemispheres and itself encloses the third ventricle.

Thalamus

The superolateral walls of the third ventricle are formed by the egg-shaped, bilateral nuclei of the **thalamus**. This structure makes up 80% of the diencephalon and is found deep inside the brain. The nuclei of the thalamus are interconnected (in most individuals) by an intermediate mass known as the *interthalamic adhesion*. The thalamic nuclei are mostly named based on their location, each having functional specialties, with unique fibers connected to certain regions of the cerebral cortex.

The thalamus processes and relays all incoming and outgoing information between the cerebral cortex and the spinal cord. The thalamus mediates motor activities, sensation,

cortical arousal, learning, and memory. Related impulses are organized in groups through the internal capsule of the thalamus to the correct area of the cerebral cortex and association areas. Afferent impulses reaching the thalamus are basically recognized as either pleasant or unpleasant. Specific stimulus discrimination and localization actually occur in the cerebral cortex, not in the thalamus. Nearly all other inputs ascending to the cerebral cortex are channeled through the thalamic nuclei: inputs for memory or sensory integration projected to areas such as the **pulvinar**, lateral dorsal, or lateral posterior nuclei and inputs regulating emotional and visceral function from the hypothalamus, via the anterior nuclei. Additionally, the thalamic nuclei interpret instructions aiding in direction of motor cortical activity from the cerebellum (via the ventral lateral nuclei) and the basal nuclei (via the ventral anterior nuclei).

Hypothalamus

The **hypothalamus** is the primary visceral control center of the body. It is crucial for the homeostasis of the body, affecting nearly all body tissues. It is located below the thalamus, capping the brain stem, and forming the inferolateral walls of the third ventricle (**FIGURE 11-7**). Paired, small, and round structures bulge anteriorly from the hypothalamus. Known as **mammillary bodies**, they act as relay stations in the olfactory pathways. A stalk of hypothalamic tissue known as the **infundibulum** lies between the mammillary bodies and the optic chiasma. The infundibulum connects the **pituitary gland** to the base of the hypothalamus.

The hypothalamus controls the autonomic nervous system (ANS) and endocrine system function. It also initiates physical responses to emotions. Other regulatory functions of the hypothalamus affect body temperature, intake of food, water balance, thirst, and the sleep–wake cycle. Its control of ANS activities occur by control of brain stem and spinal cord activity. The hypothalamus is vital for the limbic system, which is the emotional part of the brain, and it acts through ANS pathways to initiate many physical expressions of emotion. The hypothalamus is also the body's thermostat, controls hormone secretion from the anterior pituitary gland, and produces the hormones antidiuretic hormone and oxytocin.

Epithalamus

The **epithalamus** is the most dorsal part of the diencephalon, forming the roof of the third ventricle. The **pineal gland** extends from its posterior border. This gland secretes the hormone **melatonin**, which helps regulate the sleep–wake cycle and also acts as an antioxidant. The caudal border of the epithalamus is formed by the *posterior commissure*.

TEST YOUR UNDERSTANDING

1. Name three major structures of the diencephalon.
2. What are the main functions of the hypothalamus?

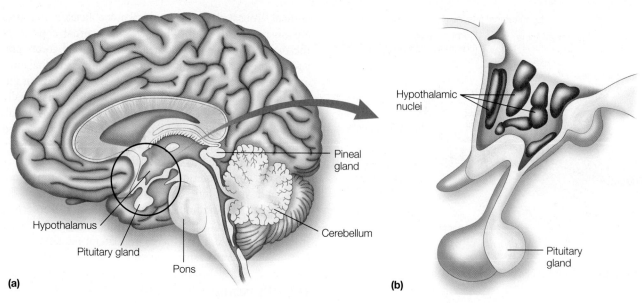

Hypothalamic nuclei

Pineal gland

Hypothalamus

Pituitary gland

Pons

Cerebellum

Pituitary gland

(a)

(b)

FIGURE 11-7 The hypothalamus.

Limbic System

On the medial aspect of each cerebral hemisphere and the diencephalon are a group of structures that comprise the **limbic system** (**FIGURE 11-8**). The upper part of the brain stem is encircled by the structures of the limbic system. An almond-shaped nucleus on the tail of the caudate nucleus, known as the **amygdaloid body,** is part of the limbic system. Other parts include the various sections of the rhinencephalon. In the diencephalon, the primary limbic structures are the *anterior thalamic nuclei* and the *hypothalamus*. Fiber tracts such as the **fornix** link all these regions. The rhinencephalon includes the cingulate gyrus, septal nuclei, the C-shaped hippocampus, the dentate gyrus, and the parahippocampal gyrus.

The emotional, feeling part of the brain constitutes the limbic system. For emotions, the critical areas are the anterior *cingulate gyrus* and the amygdaloid body, which is important for response to threats with either fear or aggression. Emotions are expressed through gestures, and frustration is resolved by the cingulate gyrus. Much of the limbic system is involved with the rhinencephalon and odors may trigger emotional reactions and memories as a result.

The limbic system can integrate and respond to many environmental stimuli because of extensive connections between it and both lower and higher brain regions. The hypothalamus relays most limbic system output. The hypothalamus processes emotional responses as well as autonomic (visceral) function; as a result, acute or prolonged emotional stress may cause visceral illnesses such as heartburn or high blood pressure. Emotion-influenced illnesses are described as *psychosomatic illnesses*. The *hippocampus* in the limbic system is responsible for storage and retrieval of new long-term memories. The amygdaloid body also functions in memory processing.

Reticular Formation

The *reticular formation* is mostly composed of white matter and extends through the core of the brain stem. A section of this formation, known as the *reticular activating system*, continually supplies impulses to the cerebral cortex to enhance its excitability (**FIGURE 11-9**). The reticular activating system also filters sensory inputs. It is inhibited by sleep centers of the hypothalamus and other regions and is affected by CNS depressants. The reticular formation also has a motor section, projecting to the spinal cord via the reticulospinal tracts.

Brain Stem

The most superior region of the **brain stem** is the *midbrain*, with descending regions including the *pons* and *medulla oblongata* (**FIGURE 11-10**). The entire brain stem only makes up about 2.5% of the total brain mass. The midbrain, pons, and medulla oblongata are each about 1 inch in length. The brain stem is organized similarly to the spinal cord, with deep gray

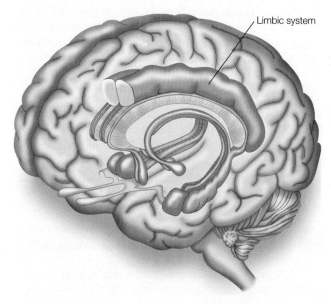

Limbic system

FIGURE 11-8 The limbic system.

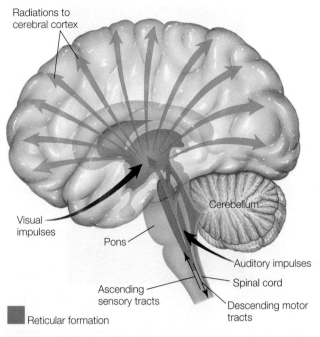

FIGURE 11-9 The reticular activating system.

matter surrounded by white matter fiber tracts. The brain stem also has nuclei of gray matter that are embedded in its white matter—this differs from the organization of the spinal cord.

Behaviors needed for survival are produced in the brain stem. These behaviors are automatic and highly controlled. The brain stem creates a pathway for fiber tracts that connect higher and lower neural centers. The brain stem nuclei are also linked to 10 pairs of the cranial nerves and are greatly involved with innervation of the head.

Midbrain

Between the diencephalon and pons is the portion of the brain stem known as the **midbrain**. It has two bulges (**cerebral peduncles**) on its ventral aspect, which support the cerebrum. Each peduncle has a *crus cerebri*, a leg-like structure containing a large corticospinal (pyramidal) motor tract that descends toward the spinal cord. Other fiber tracts, the *superior cerebellar*

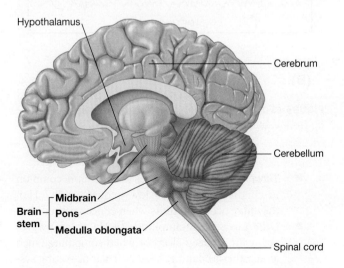

FIGURE 11-10 The brain stem consists of the medulla oblongata, pons, and midbrain.

peduncles, connect the midbrain to the cerebellum in its dorsal region. The roof of the midbrain is called the *tectum.* The cerebral aqueduct is the channel connecting the third and fourth ventricles.

In the midbrain, nuclei are also located throughout the surrounding white matter. The largest midbrain nuclei are the **corpora quadrigemina**, which create four rounded protrusions on the dorsal midbrain's surface. The *superior colliculi* are two visual *reflex centers* coordinating head and eye movements. The **inferior colliculi** relay impulses from the auditory center. The *tegmentum* is the area anterior to the cerebral aqueduct. Two pigmented nuclei are located in each side of the white matter of the midbrain: the *substantia nigra* and the **red nucleus**. The substantia nigra have a high amount of melanin pigment and appear dark in color. When dopamine-releasing neurons of the substantia nigra degenerate, Parkinson's disease results. The red nucleus has a rich blood supply and iron pigment. It is a part of the reticular formation.

Pons

Lying between the midbrain and medulla oblongata, the **pons** is a bulge in the brain stem separated dorsally from the cerebellum by the fourth ventricle. It primarily contains conduction tracts that run either longitudinally, transversely, or dorsally. The *pontine nuclei* relay information between the motor cortex and cerebellum. Three nerve pairs (the *trigeminal, abducens,* and *facial nerves*) originate from the pontine nuclei. The pons also contains ascending, descending, and transverse tracts, longitudinal tracts interconnected with other CNS structures. The middle cerebellar peduncles are connected to the *transverse fibers* that cross the anterior surface of the pons.

Medulla Oblongata

The most inferior part of the brain stem is known as the **medulla oblongata** or, more simply, the *medulla.* It joins the spinal cord smoothly, at the level of the skull's foramen magnum. Cranial nerves VIII, IX, X, and XII originate from the medulla. It plays a vital role as a center of autonomic reflexes required for homeostasis. Important functional groups of visceral *motor nuclei* are controlled by the medulla oblongata. Its *cardiovascular center* includes both the cardiac center and vasomotor center. Its respiratory centers control respiratory rhythm, rate, and depth. Various other centers of the medulla influence hiccupping, vomiting, coughing, swallowing, and sneezing. Motor nuclei send motor commands to peripheral effectors.

Cerebellum

Approximately 11% of the brain is made up by the **cerebellum**. It is the second largest portion of the brain (after the cerebrum) and appears similar to the shape of a cauliflower. It is found dorsal to the pons, medulla, and fourth ventricle. The cerebellum protrudes under the occipital lobes of the cerebral hemispheres and is separated from these lobes by the transverse cerebral fissure. The cerebellum processes inputs from the cerebral motor cortex, brain stem, and sensory receptors. It then regulates skeletal muscle movements for many different activities, such as driving a car, playing a musical instrument, or using a computer. All cerebellar activity is subconscious.

The surface of the cerebellum is highly convoluted. It has fine gyri known as **folia**, which have a folded appearance and are transversely oriented. The cerebellum is bilaterally symmetrical, with a worm-like **vermis** connecting its two hemispheres. Each cerebellar hemisphere is divided into *anterior, posterior,* and *flocculonodular lobes.* The cerebellum has its own thin outer cortex of gray matter, internalized white matter, and deep masses of gray matter. These paired masses include the **dentate nuclei**, and neurons of the cerebellum contain large **Purkinje cells**, uniquely distributing axons through the white matter to synapse with the central *cerebellar nuclei. Superior, middle,* and *inferior cerebellar peduncles* connect the cerebellum with other brain structures.

FOCUS ON PATHOLOGY

Permanent damage to the cerebellum may occur by stroke or trauma. It may also be temporarily damaged by alcohol and other drugs. A disturbance in muscular coordination called *ataxia* results. When severe, the patient will not be able to stand or sit without assistance by another person.

TEST YOUR UNDERSTANDING

1. What is the function of the limbic system?
2. What regions make up the brain stem?
3. What are the functions of the medulla oblongata?

Higher Brain Functions

Although ongoing studies continue, the human brain's higher functions are extremely difficult to truly understand. **Brain waves** are based on electrical activity, and normal brain functions involve continuous electrical activity of the neurons. Certain aspects of electrical brain activity can be recorded on an **electroencephalogram** (EEG), which involves placing electrodes on the patient's scalp. The EEG measures voltage differences between the areas of the cerebral cortex. Brain waves are the patterns of neuronal electrical activity that is recorded (**FIGURE 11-11A** and **B**). They are generated by the activity of synapses at the surface of the cortex. Every individual's brain wave patterns are unique but are grouped into four primary types:

- *Alpha waves:* Relatively regular, rhythmic, synchronous waves of low amplitude (8–13 Hz), they usually indicate calm and relaxed wakefulness.
- *Beta waves:* Rhythmic but less regular waves that have a higher frequency than alpha waves (14–30 Hz), they occur during mental alertness, such as when concentrating or looking at visual stimuli.

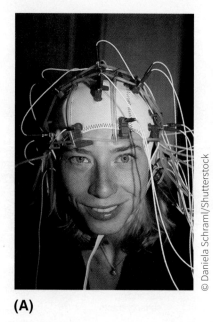

(A)

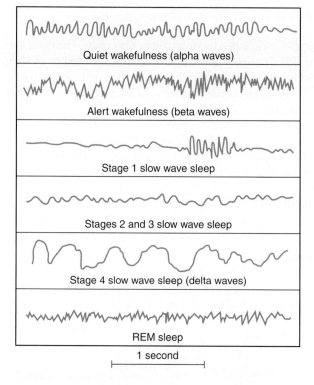

(B)

FIGURE 11-11 (A) Electrodes placed on the scalp during an EEG. (B) The four brain waves in EEGs.

- *Theta waves:* Irregular waves that are more common in children and have a low frequency (4–7 Hz), they may occur in adults when concentrating.
- *Delta waves:* High-amplitude (4 Hz or less) waves occurring in deep sleep or when something (such as anesthesia) dampens the reticular activating system; if these waves exist in a conscious adult, they indicate brain damage.

sodium ions are ejected from the cell, followed by two potassium ions being transported back in. This pump stabilizes the resting potential via maintenance of concentration gradients for both sodium and potassium.

Changes in Potential

Nerve cells respond with excitability to changes in surroundings. Some can detect specific changes such as temperature, pressure, or light from outside the body. Many neurons respond to neurotransmitters from other neurons, usually affecting the resting potential in a certain part of the nerve cell's membrane. If the resting potential decreases, it is described as being *depolarized*. The amount of change in resting potential is proportional to the amount of the stimulus. The greater the stimulus, the greater the depolarization. Sufficiently depolarized neurons cause the membrane potential to reach its **threshold potential**. When this happens, an **action potential** is reached, which is the basis for the nerve impulse. The primary method in which neurons send signals over long distances throughout the body is the generation and transmission of action potentials.

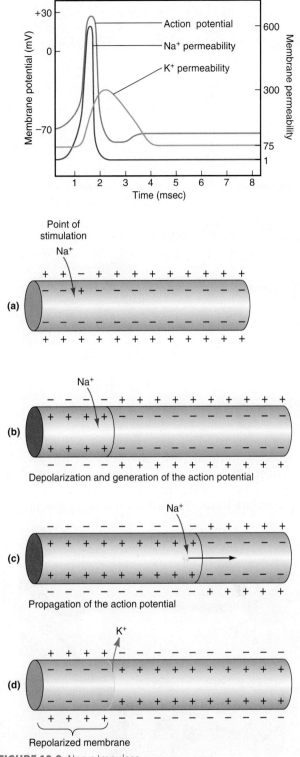

FIGURE 10-9 Nerve Impulses.

> ### TEST YOUR UNDERSTANDING
>
> 1. Explain the various phases of action potentials.
> 2. Define *resting potential* and *threshold potential*.
> 3. Explain the effects of myelination on an axon's ability to conduct action potentials.

Nerve Impulses

In a nerve cell membrane, an action potential causes a local bioelectric *current* to reach other portions of the membrane. This stimulates the adjacent membrane to its threshold level and another action potential is triggered, stimulating yet another region. These action potential waves move down to the end of the axon, constituting *nerve impulses* (**FIGURE 10-9**). **TABLE 10-1** describes the steps in the conduction of a nerve impulse. A membrane's *resistance* is defined as the level at which is restricts signal or ion movement.

Impulses are conducted over the entire surface of unmyelinated axons. Myelinated axons are insulated by their myelin content, reducing impulse conduction. The myelin sheath is interrupted by nodes of Ranvier between the Schwann cells, meaning action potentials occur at the nodes. Therefore, nerve impulses on myelinated axons appear to move from node to node. This saltatory impulse conduction is much faster than unmyelinated axon conduction. The greater the diameter of the axon, the quicker impulses are conducted. An example is the extremely fast conduction on a skeletal muscle as compared with much slower conduction on a sensory neuron.

Nerve impulses are conducted either completely or not at all, known as the *all-or-none response*. All impulses on an axon are of the same strength. If stimulation is raised, the impulses remain the same in strength but occur more rapidly. After each nerve impulse, a very brief refractory period limits the frequency of further nerve impulses. Most of the time, axons conduct impulses at the speed of 100 per second, although speeds of as high as 700 per second are possible.

Brain waves change with brain disease, aging, sensory stimuli, and the chemical balance of the body.

FOCUS ON PATHOLOGY

In the brain, electrical activity is normally synchronized between the two cerebral hemispheres. When this activity loses alignment, a *seizure* may result, which is a temporary disorder causing abnormal movements, sensations, and behaviors. Clinically, seizure disorders are called *epilepsies*. Regardless of the type of seizure disorder, there is a significant change in the pattern of electrical brain activity that can be recorded on an EEG.

Consciousness

Consciousness is defined as conscious perception of sensation, capabilities related to higher mental processing, voluntary initiation, and control of movement. Consciousness levels are graded based on alertness, drowsiness or lethargy, stupor, and coma. It involves simultaneous activity of large portions of the cerebral cortex and is superimposed on other types of neural activity (both motor control and cognition). It is holistic and completely interconnected—an example is a memory triggered by a location, an odor, a person, or other stimuli.

Sleep and Sleep Patterns

Sleep is a state of partial unconsciousness from which we may be aroused by stimulation. It is different from *coma*, from which a person cannot be aroused by stimulation. During sleep most cortical activity is depressed, but brain stem functions continue. These functions include control of heart rate, blood pressure, and respiration. The two major types of sleep are *non–rapid eye movement (NREM) sleep* and *rapid eye movement (REM) sleep*. Each of these has different patterns on an EEG. **TABLE 11-1** lists the stages of sleep.

Sleep patterns are normally based on a natural 24-hour *circadian rhythm*. The sleep cycle is controlled by the hypothalamus. Sleep occurs because of the inhibition of the brain stem's reticular activating system. The preoptic nucleus is the actual component that turns off arousal and puts the cerebral cortex to sleep. Sleep patterns usually move through the four stages of NREM sleep, into REM sleep, and then they alternate back and forth, with partial arousals occurring occasionally. After each REM episode, the individual moves toward NREM-4 again. REM sleep recurs about every 90 minutes, with each period lengthening. REM stages begin at 5 to 10 minutes' duration and eventually reach 20 to 50 minutes' duration. Longer dreams, therefore, occur toward the end of the sleep period. The individual awakes because of peptides called *orexins* that are released by hypothalamic neurons.

TABLE 11-1	
Stages of Sleep	
Stage	**Description**
NREM-1	Relaxation begins; arousal is easy; EEG shows alpha waves.
NREM-2	Arousal is more difficult; EEG is irregular with sleep spindles (short, high-amplitude bursts).
NREM-3	Sleep deepens and vital signs decline; on EEG, theta and delta waves appear.
NREM-4 (slow-wave sleep)	Arousal is very difficult; bed-wetting, nightmares, night terrors, or sleepwalking may occur; EEG is dominated by delta waves—the transition to REM sleep from this stage is marked by an abrupt change in EEG patterns, with alpha waves reappearing.
REM sleep	Most dreaming occurs; except for diaphragm and ocular muscles, the skeletal muscles are actively inhibited, which prevents acting out of dreams; more oxygen is used during REM sleep than during consciousness; in teenagers, this stage may cause sexual arousal.

Slow-wave sleep is thought to have restorative properties for the mind and body. Sleep-deprived people will spend more time in slow-wave sleep as a result, the next time they do fall asleep. Deprivation of REM sleep causes depression and moodiness, resulting in various personality disorders. Dreaming may help an individual to focus thoughts while awake. The need for sleep declines from infancy (from approximately 16 hours per day) to reach a plateau of 7.5 to 8.5 hours (in early adulthood) and then declines again in old age. Sleep patterns may change differently throughout life for every individual. Stage 4 sleep declines steadily over time

FOCUS ON PATHOLOGY

Narcolepsy is a condition in which the individual lapses into REM sleep directly from the awake state. Sleep may last approximately 15 minutes, may occur with no warning, and may be triggered by something enjoyable. Some narcoleptic individuals may experience *cataplexy* (a sudden loss of voluntary muscle control), triggered by intense emotions. Other sleep conditions include *insomnia*, a chronic inability to sleep or to sleep adequately, and *sleep apnea*, which is a temporary cessation of breathing during sleep that may cause hypoxia. Insomnia may be treated by blocking the actions of orexin, a neurotransmitter that regulates wakefulness.

and may not even occur in elderly individuals. REM sleep occupies about 50% of the sleep of infants but declines to about 25% in adults.

TEST YOUR UNDERSTANDING

1. What are the four primary types of brain wave patterns?
2. What are the two major types of sleep?
3. What are the results of REM sleep deprivation?

Language Functions

In the brain, language involves nearly all of the left association cortex, especially Broca's area and **Wernicke's area**. Lesions of Broca's area may cause difficulty speaking, writing, typing, or using sign language. Lesions of Wernicke's area may cause lack of understanding of language or the use of excessive nonsense words while speaking. Language, as controlled by the brain, also involves the basal nuclei and surrounding portions of the cerebral cortex. The right association cortex is involved in nonverbal language, or body language.

Memory Functions

Memory involves storage and retrieval of information and is required for learning, establishing behaviors, and normal conscious activity. *Short-term memory* (working memory) focuses on small pieces of information needed for a few moments and is based on approximately seven to eight groups of information. *Long-term memory* may be unlimited but is affected by changes to the body over time and declines with aging.

The transfer of information from short-term to long-term memory is influenced by your emotional state, rehearsing or repeating material, associating new information to stored information, and automatic memory (which is the unconscious memorizing of something that occurred, such as what a person was wearing).

Brain Protection

The brain is surrounded by bones, fluids, and membranes. It lies inside the skull's cranial cavity and is soft and delicate. Between the bony coverings and the soft brain tissues are layered membranes known as **meninges** that protect the brain and spinal cord (**FIGURE 11-12**). The singular term *meninx* describes just one of the meninges. Also, the CSF cushions the brain, and the **blood–brain barrier** protects it from harmful substances carried in the blood. There is also a *blood–CSF barrier*, which is formed by specialized ependymal cells surrounding the capillaries of the choroid plexus.

Meninges

There are three layers of membranes in the meninges: the **dura mater**, **arachnoid mater**, and **pia mater**. The outermost layer (dura mater) is made up of fibrous, tough, white connective tissue. It has many blood vessels and nerves and attaches to the inside of the cranial cavity; it also extends inward between the brain lobes to form protective partitions. It continues into the vertebral canal to surround the spinal cord, ending in a sac at its end. The dura mater has two layers of fibrous connective tissue. Its *periosteal layer*, which

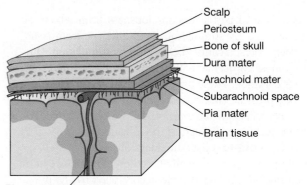

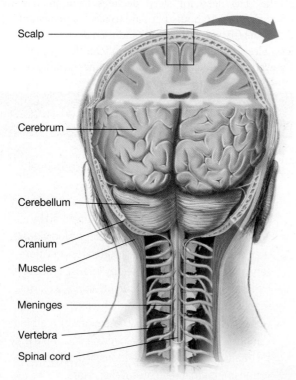

FIGURE 11-12 The CNS is protected by the meninges.

is more superficial, attaches to the periosteum (the inner surface of the skull). Around the spinal cord, there is no dural periosteal layer. The *meningeal layer* actually covers the brain, continuing caudally as the spinal dura mater in the vertebral canal. The two dural layers of the brain are fused in most areas. In certain places they separate, enclosing *dural venous sinuses*, which collect blood from the brain and channel it to the internal jugular veins in the neck.

Dural septa limit excessive brain movement and are formed from the meningeal dura mater. It contains three primary features. Its *falx cerebri* is a large fold that dips into the longitudinal fissure between the hemispheres of the cerebrum. It contains two large venous sinuses known as the *superior sagittal* and *inferior sagittal* sinuses. The *falx cerebelli* continues inferiorly from the more posterior falx cerebri, along the vermis of the cerebellum. The *tentorium cerebelli* is a nearly horizontal dural fold extending into the transverse fissure and cerebellum. It contains the *transverse sinus*.

The membrane around the spinal cord has an epidural space separating it from the vertebrae. The epidural space contains loose adipose and connective tissues, protecting the spinal cord. A thin, web-like *arachnoid mater* lies between the dura and pia maters. The *subdural space* is a narrow serous cavity that contains a fluid film.

The thin pia mater has many blood vessels and nerves that nourish the brain and spinal cord. The pia mater is closely aligned with the surfaces of these organs. It is comprised of many tiny blood vessels and delicate connective tissue. The pia mater is bound tightly to the brain and its convolutions. Small ragged bits of pia mater are briefly carried by small arteries entering the brain. There are also *spinal meninges*, which are discussed later.

FOCUS ON PATHOLOGY

The meninges, skull, other protective structures, and CSF surrounding the brain are fairly solid barriers against *cranial trauma*. More than 8 million people experience cranial trauma annually in the United States, yet only about 1 million of these people have serious brain damage as a result.

Cerebrospinal Fluid

Between the arachnoid and pia maters is a subarachnoid space containing the watery and clear **cerebrospinal fluid (CSF)**. This is similar to blood plasma but contains less protein. CSF contains more sodium, chloride, and hydrogen ions but less calcium and potassium than blood plasma. Inside the subarachnoid space are web-like extensions that function partially to bind the arachnoid mater to the pia mater. This space also contains CSF and the primary brain blood vessels. However, these blood vessels are not

protected well because the arachnoid mater is very fine and elastic. *Arachnoid villi* are knob-like projections that protrude superiorly through the dura mater into the superior sagittal sinus. They absorb CSF into the venous blood of the sinus. In adults, clusters of arachnoid villi form large *arachnoid granulations*, where CSF is actually absorbed into the venous circulation.

Small red *choroid plexuses* (specialized capillaries) secrete CSF and project into the brain ventricles. Most CSF is formed in the lateral ventricles. CSF also enters the meninges' subarachnoid space via the two *lateral apertures* and the single *median aperture* and is reabsorbed into the blood. CSF surrounds the brain and spinal cord, maintaining a stable ionic concentration and protecting CNS structures. The brain floats in CSF, which cushions it and prevents the bottom of

FOCUS ON PATHOLOGY

Hydrocephalus is a pathologic condition characterized by an abnormal accumulation of cerebrospinal fluid. The fluid is usually under increased pressure, within the cranial vault, and there is subsequent dilation of the ventricles in infants. The sutures, up until 18 months of age, are not fused. Interference with the normal flow of CSF may result from increased secretion of the fluid, or obstruction within the ventricular system. Hydrocephalus may be caused by developmental anomalies, infection, trauma, or brain tumors. It is also called *hydrocephaly*. It may be treated by draining with a ventricular shunt to the abdominal cavity.

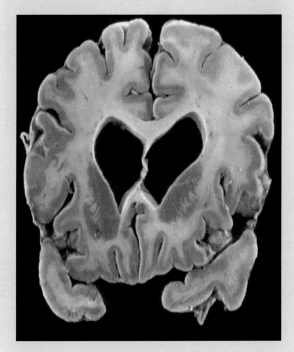

Hydrocephalus.

the brain from being crushed by its own weight. The CSF also helps to nourish the brain and may assist in carrying chemical signals concerning sleep and appetite. It also may carry hormones. The total CSF volume is about 150 mL, which is replaced every 8 hours.

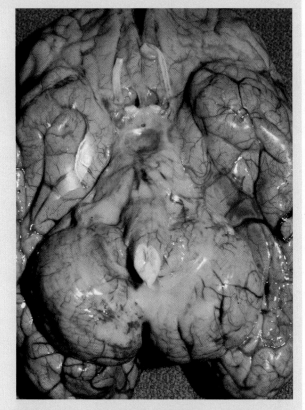
Blood-Brain Barrier

The brain requires a constant internal environment to function normally. To maintain this, the *blood–brain barrier* acts to selectively allow certain molecules to pass and to keep others from reaching the brain. The maintenance of a constant environment keeps the brain's neurons from firing uncontrollably. Before bloodborne substances can move from brain capillaries to reach neurons, three layers of the blood–brain barrier

await them: the capillary wall endothelium, a thick basal lamina surrounding every capillary's external side, and bulb-like *feet* of the astrocytes that are bound to the capillaries. These portions of astrocytes give signals to the endothelial cells and cause them to form *tight junctions*. The junctions form the actual barrier by causing a seamless pattern of endothelial cells. This capillary barrier is the least permeable of all capillary structures in the body.

The selective blood–brain barrier allows certain electrolytes, nutrients, and essential amino acids to pass through. It does not allow passage of proteins, bloodborne metabolic wastes, most drugs, and specific toxins. Also, nonessential amino acids and potassium ions are actively pumped across the capillary endothelium away from the brain. The blood–brain barrier is not effective against fatty acids, fats, carbon dioxide, oxygen, and other fat-soluble molecules that can easily diffuse through the body's plasma membranes. Therefore, bloodborne anesthetics, alcohol, and nicotine affect the brain.

The blood–brain barrier is not uniform throughout the brain and is even absent near the third and fourth ventricles. In the brain's vomiting center, bloodborne molecules can easily cross to the neural tissue, but this is part of this center's monitoring for poisons. The hypothalamus also does not have a barrier, allowing it to sample the blood's chemical composition so it can regulate many metabolic activities. In newborns and premature infants, the blood–brain barrier is not fully formed. As a result, certain toxins can enter the CNS and cause certain conditions that do not generally affect adults. Also, the blood–brain barrier can be broken down by brain injuries. When these occur, the capillary endothelial cells or their tight junctions are commonly affected.

Spinal Cord

The **spinal cord** is a thin column of nerves leading from the brain to the vertebral canal. It starts at the point where nervous tissue exits the cranial cavity near the foramen magnum and eventually tapers off to terminate near the point where the first and second lumbar are located (**FIGURE 11-13**). The spinal cord is approximately 42 cm in length and 1.8 cm in thickness. It appears as a shiny white structure, protected by bone, meninges, and CSF. The spinal cord provides two ways of communication, to and from the brain, and contains the spinal reflex centers. The spinal cord is continuous throughout its length, with slight internal structure changes. The spinal cord is divided into right and left halves by a deep anterior median fissure and a shallow posterior median sulcus. It is slightly flat from front to back.

The spinal meninges are continuous with those of the brain. In the spinal cord, the *dura mater* has a single layer and is not attached to the vertebral column. The inner surface of the dura mater contacts the outer surface of the *arachnoid mater*, which is the middle meningeal layer of the spine. An **epidural space** exists between the dura mater and vertebrae, which is padded by fat and a vein network. CSF fills the *subarachnoid space*, which lies between the arachnoid and pia mater meninges. The dural and arachnoid membranes

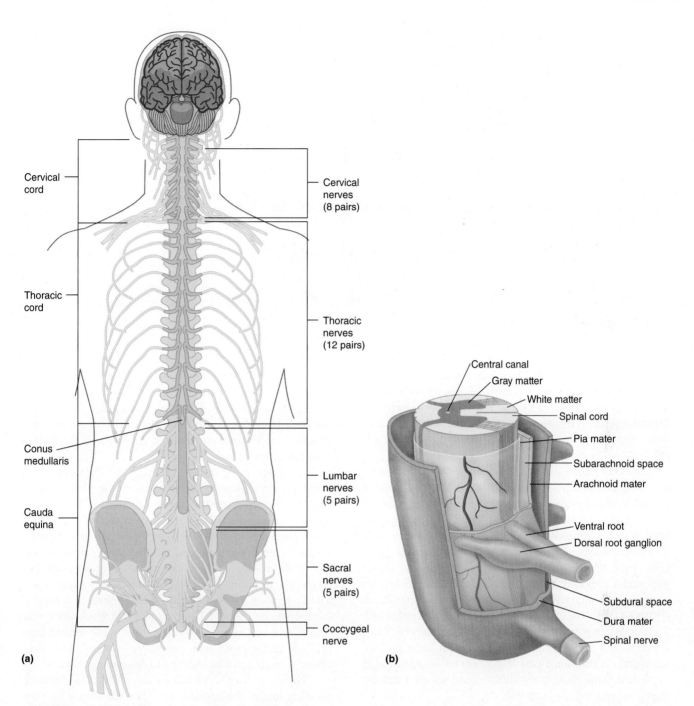

FIGURE 11-13 The spinal cord and its protective structures.

(a)

Cervical cord

Thoracic cord

Conus medullaris

Cauda equina

Cervical nerves (8 pairs)

Thoracic nerves (12 pairs)

Lumbar nerves (5 pairs)

Sacral nerves (5 pairs)

Coccygeal nerve

(b)

Central canal

Gray matter

White matter

Spinal cord

Pia mater

Subarachnoid space

Arachnoid mater

Ventral root

Dorsal root ganglion

Subdural space

Dura mater

Spinal nerve

extend inferiorly to the S_2 level, which is far below the end of the spinal cord, which ends between the L_1 and L_2 levels. The subarachnoid space inside the meningeal sac inferior to the lumbar region is an excellent spot for the removal of CSF. This procedure is called a **lumbar puncture** or *spinal tap*.

The spinal cord terminates inferiorly in a tapered, cone-shaped structure called the **conus medullaris**. A fibrous extension of the conus medullaris called the **filum terminale** extends inferiorly to the coccyx to anchor the spinal cord. Sawtooth-shaped sections of pia mater are called **denticulate ligaments** and bind the spinal cord to the dura mater meninx for its entire length. Components of

the filum terminale blend with a dense cord of collagen fibers continuous with the spinal dura mater to form the *coccygeal ligament*.

Cross-Section of the Spinal Cord

The inner core of the spinal cord is made of gray matter surrounded by white matter. Motor fibers pass out of portions of the gray matter through *spinal nerves* to skeletal muscles; however, most of the gray matter neurons are interneurons. The sensory fibers that enter the spinal cord usually end on interneurons, which receive input from the sensory neurons.

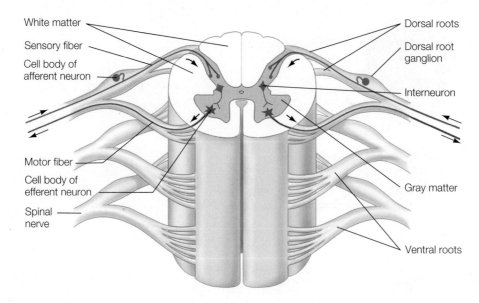

Labels on figure:
- White matter
- Sensory fiber
- Cell body of afferent neuron
- Motor fiber
- Cell body of efferent neuron
- Spinal nerve
- Dorsal roots
- Dorsal root ganglion
- Interneuron
- Gray matter
- Ventral roots

FIGURE 11-14 Cross-section of the spinal cord.

Impulses may be transmitted by the interneurons to adjacent multipolar motor neurons. The axons of these motor neurons leave in the spinal nerve's ventral root, and nerve impulses are transmitted to muscles and glands. The arrangement of these neurons enables information to enter and leave the spinal cord very quickly.

The gray matter of the spinal cord appears as a butterfly shape, also described as similar to the letter "H," within the spinal cord's white matter. Major nerve pathways called **nerve tracts** are made up of long bundles of myelinated nerve fibers. A horizontal bar of gray matter in the very middle of the spinal cord surrounds its central canal and contains CSF. This is known as the **gray commissure**. Its two dorsal gray matter projections are called the *dorsal (posterior) horns*, whereas the ventral pair are called the *ventral (anterior) horns* (**FIGURE 11-14**). They run the entire length of the spinal cord. The dorsal horns contain somatic and visceral *sensory inputs*, which receive and relay sensory information for peripheral receptors. An additional pair of gray matter columns called the *lateral horns* exist in the thoracic and superior lumbar segments (sympathetic neurons).

All neurons that have cell bodies in the gray matter of the spinal cord are multipolar. Interneurons completely make up the dorsal horns, whereas the ventral horns have mostly somatic motor neurons, with lower amounts of interneurons. The motor neurons send their axons out to the skeletal muscles, which are their effector organs, via *ventral rootlets*. These rootlets fuse together, becoming the spinal cord's **ventral roots**. Sensory and motor roots are bound together into one *spinal nerve*. This occurs distal to each dorsal root ganglion.

Cell bodies of autonomic (sympathetic division) motor neurons, which serve visceral organs, mostly make up the lateral horns. Their axons leave the spinal cord with the ventral root alongside those from the somatic motor neurons. Ventral roots serve both peripheral nervous system motor divisions because they contain somatic and autonomic efferent fibers.

The **dorsal roots** are formed by afferent fibers, which carry impulses from peripheral sensory receptors. They fan out as the *dorsal rootlets* before entering the spinal cord. Associated sensory neuron cell bodies lie in an enlarged region of each dorsal root, which is known as the **dorsal root ganglion** (*spinal ganglion*).

The white matter of the spinal cord is made up of myelinated and nonmyelinated nerve fibers. These allow communication between sections of the spinal cord and between the spinal cord and brain. The nerve fiber tracts run in three different directions. The tracts that carry information to the brain are called *ascending tracts*, and the tracts that carry information to the muscles and glands are called *descending tracts*. The ascending tracts run up to higher centers for sensory input. The descending tracts run down from the brain to the spinal cord, or inside the spinal cord to its lower levels, for motor output. The transverse tracts run across the spinal cord, from one side to the other, with commissural fibers. Most white matter is made up of ascending and descending tracts.

There are three white matter columns, called **funiculi**, on each side of the spinal cord. They are named by their positions, as the *dorsal (posterior) funiculi*, the *lateral funiculi*, and the *ventral (anterior) funiculi*. Each spinal tract contains several fiber tracts made up of axons that have similar functions and destinations. The names of the spinal tracts describe their destinations as well as origins (**FIGURE 11-15**). The anterior white columns are interconnected by the *anterior white commissure*, which is where axons cross from either side of the spinal cord. The *lateral white column* is made up by the white matter between the anterior and posterior columns on each side.

TEST YOUR UNDERSTANDING

1. List the layers of the spinal cord.
2. What are the two major functions of the spinal cord?

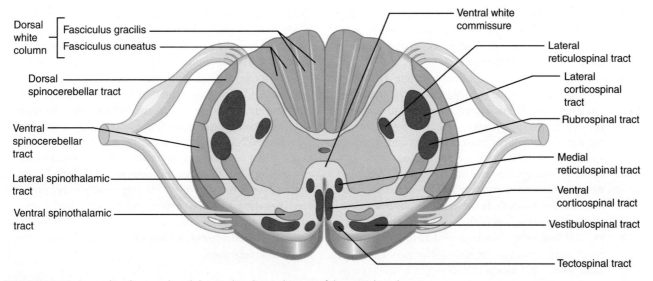

Dorsal white column
- Fasciculus gracilis
- Fasciculus cuneatus

Dorsal spinocerebellar tract

Ventral spinocerebellar tract

Lateral spinothalamic tract

Ventral spinothalamic tract

Ventral white commissure

Lateral reticulospinal tract

Lateral corticospinal tract

Rubrospinal tract

Medial reticulospinal tract

Ventral corticospinal tract

Vestibulospinal tract

Tectospinal tract

FIGURE 11-15 Ascending (sensory) and descending (motor) tracts of the spinal cord.

Spinal Neuronal Pathways

The primary spinal tracts or *fasciculi* make up *multineuron pathways* and connect the brain to the rest of the body. They contain spinal cord neurons, parts of peripheral neurons, and brain neurons. Spinal neuronal pathways are signified by *decussation, relay, somatotopy,* and *symmetry.* Most pathways cross from one side of the CNS to the other, which is described as *decussation.* Most also consist of a chain of several neurons contributing to successive pathway tracts in the relay of information. Most pathways have a precise spatial relationship among tract fibers (*somatotopy*), which resemble the body's ordered mapping. Ascending sensory tracts, for example, fibers that transmit inputs from sensory receptors in superior regions of the body, lie lateral to others that convey sensory information from inferior body regions. There is symmetry to all pathways and tracts. One member of each pair is present on either side of the brain or spinal cord.

Ascending pathways conduct sensory impulses toward the brain, and consist of three types of neurons. *First-order neurons* have cell bodies in a ganglion (either dorsal root or cranial root) and conduct impulses from the skin's cutaneous receptors and from proprioceptors to the brain stem or spinal cord. A first-order neuron synapses with a second-order neuron.

Second-order neurons have cell bodies in the spinal cord's dorsal horn or in the medullary nuclei that transmit impulses to the thalamus or cerebellum. *Third-order neurons* have cell bodies in the thalamus and send impulses to the cerebrum. There are no third-order neurons in the cerebellum.

There are three primary types of ascending pathways on each side of the spinal cord: the *dorsal column–medial lemniscal pathways, spinothalamic pathways,* and *spinocerebellar pathways.* The dorsal column–medial lemniscal pathways mediate precise transmission of inputs of certain sensory receptors, such as for discriminative touch and vibrations. The spinothalamic pathways receive signals from many sensory receptor types, making multiple synapses in the brain stem. The spinothalamic pathways transmit temperature, touch, pain, and pressure impulses. The spinocerebellar pathways transmit information about tendon or muscle stretching to the cerebellum so it can coordinate the activities of the skeletal muscles.

The descending pathways transmit impulses from the brain to the spinal cord, via direct and indirect pathways. *Upper motor neurons* are pyramidal cells of the motor cortex as well as neurons of the subcortical motor nuclei. *Lower motor neurons* are from the ventral horn and directly innervate skeletal muscles. *Direct (pyramidal) pathways* originate primarily with the pyramidal neurons in the precentral gyri and send impulses through the brain stem via large *pyramidal (corticospinal) tracts.*

The indirect pathways include all other motor pathways except the pyramidal pathways and brain stem motor nuclei. Formerly, indirect pathways were referred to as *the extrapyramidal system.* However, they are now referred to as indirect (*multineuronal*) pathways or may be individually named. Indirect pathways are most involved in maintaining balance and posture (via the axial muscles), coarse limb movements, and the following of objects in the visual field with the head, neck, and eyes. The *vestibulospinal* and *reticulospinal* tracts varying postural muscle tone to maintain balance. Flexor muscles are controlled by the *rubospinal tracts,* whereas the *superior colliculi* and *tectospinal tracts* control head movements in relation to visual stimuli.

Neuronal Pools

Throughout the CNS the interneurons are organized into a smaller amount of *neuronal pools,* which are functional groups of interconnected neurons. Neuronal pools may be scattered to involve only neurons in several brain regions or may be localized to just one certain region of the brain or spinal cord. Output of neuronal pools may stimulate or depress activities in the CNS. There are five general patterns of interaction:

- *Divergence:* The spread of information from a neuron to several other neurons or from one neuronal pool to additional neuronal pools. It allows broad distribution of specific input.
- *Convergence:* On a single postsynaptic neurons, several neurons synapse. This means the postsynaptic neuron can be affected by several patterns of activity in the presynaptic neurons. Some motor neurons can be under both conscious and subconscious control as a result of convergence.
- *Serial processing:* Information is relayed from one neuron to another or from one neuronal pool to another. An example is the relay of sensory information from one part of the brain to another.
- *Parallel processing:* When several neurons or neuronal pools process the same information at the same time. This means that divergence must occur first. Parallel processing allows many responses to occur simultaneously.
- *Reverberation:* This resembles a positive feedback loop, because collateral axon branches along the circuit extend back to the source of an impulse and stimulate presynaptic neurons again. A reverberating circuit functions until it is broken by inhibitory stimuli or synaptic fatigue and can occur in one or more neuronal pools.

TEST YOUR UNDERSTANDING

1. Describe first-order, second-order, and third-order sensory neurons.
2. Differentiate the functions of the ascending and descending spinal pathways.

Imbalances of the CNS

Brain dysfunctions are common and varied and may be caused by many different factors. This section focuses on brain trauma, cerebrovascular accidents, degenerative brain disorders, spinal cord trauma, poliomyelitis, and amyotrophic lateral sclerosis.

Brain Trauma

One of the leading causes of accidental death in the United States is head injury that results in brain trauma. In a car accident, for example, the brain is damaged by local injury at the site of the blow (the *coup* injury) and the reverse effect as the brain contacts the opposite end of the skull (the *contrecoup* injury). An alteration in brain function after a blow to the head, which is usually temporary, is called a **concussion**. Symptoms of a concussion include dizziness and loss of consciousness. Concussions, regardless of their severity, can damage the brain. If serious, the brain is bruised, resulting in permanent neurological damage. This is known as a **contusion**, which can range from the patient remaining conscious to varying lengths of loss of consciousness. If the

brain stem is contused, a coma develops that may last for hours or from which the patient will never awaken.

Brain trauma may also involve **subdural hemorrhage** or **subarachnoid hemorrhage**. These occur when blood vessels in one of these brain areas are ruptured. The patient is often lucid at first after the trauma but then develops neurological deterioration due to the hemorrhage. Accumulating blood compresses brain tissue and increases intracranial pressure. When the brain stem becomes forced inferiorly through the foramen magnum, the patient's blood pressure, respiration, and heart rate become uncontrolled. Treatment of intracranial hemorrhage is via surgery to remove the localized hematoma (blood mass) and repair vessel ruptures. Traumatic head injury may also cause swelling of the brain, called **cerebral edema**, which can aggravate a brain injury or even be fatal itself.

Cerebrovascular Accident (Stroke)

The most common nervous disorder is a **cerebrovascular accident**, which is also called a *stroke* or a *brain attack*. Strokes are the third leading cause of death in North America and occur when the brain's blood circulation is blocked, causing the death of brain tissue (**FIGURE 11-16**). Deprivation of blood to a body tissue, called **ischemia**, impairs delivery of oxygen and nutrients. Strokes are usually caused by blood clots that block cerebral arteries. The second most common cause is rupture of blood vessels in the brain, often due to hypertension (see **FIGURE 11-17**). Aneurysm is the third most common cause of stroke (**FIGURE 11-18**). Usually, the survivor of a cerebrovascular accident is paralyzed on one side of the body (*hemiplegia*).

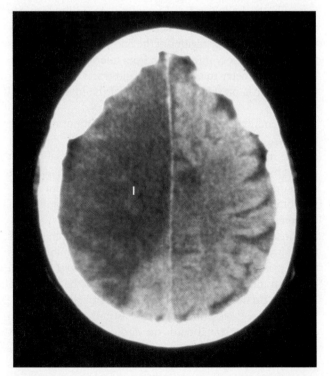

FIGURE 11-16 Computed tomography of a large hemispheric infarct. (Courtesy of Dr. Patrick Turski, Department of Radiology-MRI, University of Wisconsin School of Medicine and Public Health.)

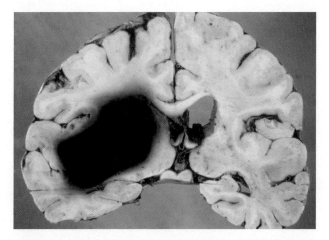

FIGURE 11-17 Large hypertensive hemorrhage in deep brain tissue.

The most critical component of a cerebrovascular accident is its long-term effect that often results in death of brain neurons. Neurons that are completely deprived of oxygen disintegrate relatively quickly, releasing an overabundance of *glutamate* (an excitatory neurotransmitter).

In strokes, glutamate acts as an *excitotoxin*, which over-excites the surrounding cells until they die. High levels of calcium ions damage mitochondria of brain cells and initiate specific protein synthesis to cause cell death via free radicals and inflammatory agents. Stroke treatments include *plasminogen activator* to dissolve blood clots and robotic surgery. New advancements include the use of stem cells to replace damaged brain neurons. Temporary episodes of reversible cerebral ischemia are known as **transient ischemic attacks**. They last between 5 and 50 minutes, causing temporary paralysis, numbness, or speech impairment.

Degeneration of the Brain

The three primary degenerative brain disorders include *Alzheimer's disease, Parkinson's disease*, and *Huntington's disease*. Alzheimer's disease is a progressive disease that eventually results in *dementia* (mental deterioration). Up to 50% of people over age 85 die because of some Alzheimer-related factor. Symptoms include disorientation, short attention span, and loss of language abilities. The brain is overcome with senile plaques that form between neurons and *neurofibrillary tangles* inside the neurons. The brain begins to shrink as its cells die (**FIGURE 11-19**). This primarily occurs in the basal forebrain and hippocampus. Glutamate excitotoxicity is also involved in the progression of Alzheimer's disease.

Parkinson's disease results from degeneration of dopamine-releasing neurons in the substantia nigra and usually begins when a person is in his or her fifties or sixties. Symptoms include "pill-rolling" hand movements, tremor of the hands at rest, a stony facial expression, slowness in movements, a shuffling gait when walking, and a forward-bending posture when walking. Although of unknown cause, Parkinson's disease may occur due to abnormalities in mitochondrial proteins and their degradation pathways. Treatments involve the medications *elodea* (*L-dopa*) and *darnel*, deep brain stimulation, gene therapy, and stem cell implantation.

Huntington's disease usually develops during middle age and is a fatal, hereditary disorder. *Huntingtin* proteins mutate and accumulate, causing death of brain tissue. The basal nuclei and cerebral cortex degenerate. Symptoms include nearly continuous jerky movements (*chorea*), which are involuntary, and eventual severe mental deterioration. Huntington's disease is usually fatal within 15 years of symptom onset. This disorder's symptoms oppose Parkinson's disease because there is over-stimulation of the motor drive instead of inhibition. Treatments include medications to block the effects of dopamine and stem cell implantation.

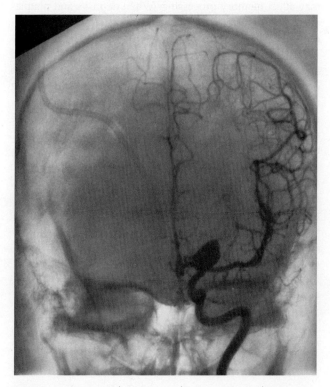

FIGURE 11-18 Carotid angiogram demonstrating radiopaque dye in a saccular aneurysm of the middle cerebral artery.

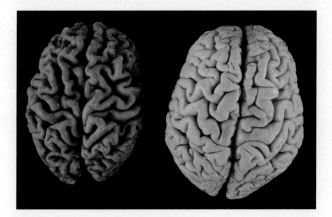

FIGURE 11-19 Atrophic brain of Alzheimer's disease (left) compared with normal brain (right).

Spinal Cord Trauma

The spinal cord is able to stretch extensively, yet direct pressure on it may cause serious loss of function. Localized damage to either the cord itself or the spinal roots causes either **paralysis** or **paresthesias**. **Flaccid paralysis** of the skeletal muscles occurs because of severe ventral root or ventral horn cell damage. Because nerve impulses do not reach the skeletal muscles, they become unable to move involuntarily or voluntarily and atrophy because of lack of stimulation. *Spastic paralysis* occurs if just the upper motor neurons of the primary motor cortex are damaged. This is because the spinal motor neurons remain intact, with spinal reflex activity continuing to irregularly stimulate the muscles. The muscles stay healthy for a longer time but lose voluntary control. They may become permanently shortened as a result.

If the spinal cord is cut in half (transected), total motor and sensory loss occurs in body regions below the site of the damage. For example, transection between the T1 and L1 levels affects both lower limbs (**paraplegia**). If transection occurs in the cervical region, all four limbs are affected (**quadriplegia**). Paralysis of one side of the body (*hemiplegia*) is usually caused by brain injury and not spinal cord injury.

Spinal shock is a collection of symptoms caused by spinal cord transection. There is a transient period of functional loss after injury and immediate depression of all reflex activity that is caudal to the lesion site. All muscles below the injury site become paralyzed and insensitive, blood pressure is reduced, and reflexes of the bowel and bladder stop. Within a few hours after injury, neural function usually returns. If this does not occur within 48 hours, paralysis is usually permanent.

Poliomyelitis

Poliomyelitis is defined as inflammation of the gray matter of the spinal cord caused by the poliovirus, which usually enters the body via water that is contaminated with feces, destroying the ventral horn motor neurons. Symptoms of poliomyelitis begin with headache, fever, muscle weakness and pain, and the loss of specific *somatic reflexes*. Paralysis eventually develops, with affected muscles experiencing atrophy. Poliomyelitis may be fatal due to cardiac arrest or paralysis of the respiratory muscles. The polio vaccines have nearly eradicated the disease worldwide.

The *poliomyelitis epidemic* of the 1940s and 1950s claimed many victims, and many survivors are today experiencing *postpolio syndrome* signified by sharp, burning muscular pain, extreme lethargy, and progressive muscle weakness and atrophy. Of unknown cause, postpolio syndrome is believed to be related to continual loss of neurons, which occurs throughout normal aging. A polio survivor may not have sufficient reserve neurons to compensate for this loss over time.

Amyotrophic Lateral Sclerosis

Amyotrophic lateral sclerosis, commonly referred to as *Lou Gehrig's disease*, is a neuromuscular condition that progressively destroys the ventral horn motor neurons and pyramidal tract fibers, causing loss of the ability to swallow, speak, and breathe. This condition is usually fatal within 5 years of onset. It is caused by a combination of genetic and environmental factors. Mutations are inherited in 10% of patients, with spontaneous mutations probably occurring in the remainder. Recent advancements have localized the mutation to genes involved in RNA processing. Excitotoxic cell death is probably involved, because of the presence of excess amounts of extracellular glutamate. The only treatment that has prolonged the lives of amyotrophic lateral sclerosis patients is the drug called *riluzole*, which interferes with glutamate signaling.

Effects of Aging on the Brain

In elderly people the brain becomes reduced in both size and weight. This is linked to a loss of cortical neurons. The synaptic organization of the brain changes as the number of dendritic branches and other structures decreases. This limits neurotransmitter production. Brain neurons accumulate abnormal intracellular deposits. Extracellular plaques may affect memory processing. When deposits and plaques exceed normal amounts caused by aging, clinical abnormalities may occur.

After young adulthood, brain neurons become damaged and die. However, only a small percentage of total brain neurons are actually lost. Continued learning throughout the life span occurs because remaining neurons can alter their synaptic connections. Aging does cause cognitive declines that may affect perception speed, spatial abilities, making decisions, reacting to occurrences, and memory loss. Cognitive declines usually only become significant when a person is in his or her seventies. Functions that do not decline with age include fluency of speech and mathematical skills. Reversible dementia may be caused by adverse effects of medications, poor nutrition, low blood pressure, hormone imbalances, dehydration, and depression. Alcoholics and athletes who experience head trauma experience greater loss of brain size and weight and at much earlier ages.

SUMMARY

The human brain controls movements, sensations, consciousness, and cognitive abilities. The adult brain is divided into the cerebrum (with cerebral hemispheres), diencephalon, brain stem, and cerebellum. The cerebral hemispheres and cerebellum contain a nuclei of gray matter surrounded by white matter and an outer gray matter cortex. Each cerebral hemisphere consists of the cerebral cortex, cerebral white matter, and basal nuclei (ganglia). The cerebral hemispheres each receive sensations from and dispatch motor impulses to the opposite side of the body. The brain contains four ventricles filled with CSF. It is covered by convolutions, gyri, sulci, and fissures.

The diencephalon includes the thalamus, hypothalamus, and epithalamus. The hypothalamus controls the ANS and part of the limbic system as well as gastrointestinal activity, body temperature, and anterior pituitary gland activity. The brain stem includes the midbrain, pons, and medulla oblongata. The cerebellum also has two hemispheres and interprets impulses from the motor cortex and sensory pathways. It coordinates motor activity in the body. The limbic system is the emotional–visceral part of the brain and also plays a role in memory.

Patterns of electrical activity in the brain are called brain waves, which can be recorded by an EEG. Brain waves include alpha, beta, theta, and delta waves. Consciousness has four basic components: alertness, drowsiness, stupor,

and coma. Sleep is a state of partial consciousness from which a person can be aroused by stimuli. The two major types of sleep are NREM and REM sleep. In most people, the left brain hemisphere controls language, whereas the right brain hemisphere controls the emotional content of language. Memory storage includes short-term and long-term memory.

The brain is protected by the meninges, CSF, and the blood–brain barrier. The meninges include the dura, arachnoid, and pia mater, which enclose the brain, spinal cord, and related blood vessels. The blood–brain barrier blocks certain molecules from entering the brain, maintaining a needed stability to the brain environment. Common brain injuries include trauma, cerebrovascular accidents (strokes), and degenerative brain disorders (Alzheimer's, Parkinson's, and Huntington's diseases).

The spinal cord is a two-way impulse conduction pathway and reflex center inside the vertebral column. The central gray matter of the spinal cord is H-shaped, and each side of its white matter has dorsal, lateral, and ventral columns known as funiculi, which each contain ascending and descending tracts. Ascending tracts are sensory, whereas descending tracts are motor. Spinal cord trauma often results in various degrees of paralysis. As we age, the CNS (primarily the brain) decreases in amount of neurons, size, and weight. Cognitive abilities may decline in specific areas or overall.

KEY TERMS

Amygdaloid body
Arachnoid mater
Basal nuclei
Blood–brain barrier
Brain stem
Brain waves
Broca's area
Calcarine sulcus
Caudate nucleus
Cerebellum
Cerebral aqueduct
Cerebral cortex
Cerebral edema
Cerebral hemispheres
Cerebral peduncles
Cerebrospinal fluid (CSF)
Cerebrovascular accident

Cerebrum
Concussion
Contusion
Conus medullaris
Corona radiata
Corpora quadrigemina
Corpus callosum
Dentate nuclei
Denticulate ligaments
Diencephalon
Dominant hemisphere
Dorsal root ganglion
Dorsal roots
Dura mater
Electroencephalogram
Epidural space
Epithalamus

Filum terminale
Fissure
Flaccid paralysis
Folia
Fornix
Funiculi
Globus pallidus
Gray commissure
Gyri
Hypothalamus
Inferior colliculi
Infundibulum
Insula
Internal capsule
Ischemia
Lateral ventricles
Limbic system

Longitudinal fissure
Lumbar puncture
Mammillary bodies
Medulla oblongata
Melatonin
Meninges
Midbrain
Motor areas
Nerve tracts
Paralysis
Paraplegia
Paresthesias
Pia mater

Pineal gland
Pituitary gland
Pons
Pulvinar
Purkinje cells
Putamen
Quadriplegia
Red nucleus
Rhinencephalon
Septum pellucidum
Somatotopy
Spinal cord
Spinal reflexes

Sulcus
Striate
Striatum
Subarachnoid hemorrhage
Subdural hemorrhage
Substantia nigra
Thalamus
Transient ischemic attacks
Ventral roots
Ventricles
Vermis
Wernicke's area

LEARNING GOALS

The following learning goals correspond to the objectives at the beginning of this chapter:

1. The adult brain is divided into the cerebrum, diencephalon, brain stem, and cerebellum. The cerebrum is divided into large left and right cerebral hemispheres, which make up most of the brain's mass. The cerebrum's surface is covered with gyri, sulci, and fissures. Several sulci divide each hemisphere into the frontal, parietal, temporal, and occipital lobes, as well as the insula, which is buried deep in the lateral sulcus. The three basic regions of each cerebral hemisphere include the cerebral cortex, white matter, and basal nuclei. The cerebral cortex is a thin layer of gray matter comprising the outer portion of the cerebrum and is the center of the conscious mind. The diencephalon is mostly made up of the paired gray matter structures known as the thalamus, hypothalamus, and epithalamus. It forms the central core of the forebrain. The diencephalon is surrounded by the cerebral hemispheres and itself encloses the third ventricle. The most superior region of the brain stem is the midbrain, with descending regions including the pons and medulla oblongata. The brain stem is organized similarly to the spinal cord, with deep gray matter that is surrounded by white matter fiber tracts. The brain stem also has nuclei of gray matter that are embedded in its white matter—this differs from the organization of the spinal cord. Behaviors that are needed for survival emanate from the brain stem. These behaviors are automatic and highly controlled. The cerebellum is the second largest portion of the brain and appears similar to the shape of a cauliflower. It is found dorsal to the pons, medulla, and fourth ventricle. The cerebellum protrudes under the occipital lobes of the cerebral hemispheres. The cerebellum process inputs from the cerebral motor cortex, brain stem, and sensory receptors. It then regulates skeletal muscle movements for many different activities.

2. Interconnected cavities known as ventricles exist within the cerebral hemispheres and brain stem. They are continuous with the spinal cord's central canal and also contain CSF. The walls of the hollow ventricular chambers are lined by ependymal cells. The two large lateral ventricles are located inside the frontal, occipital, and temporal lobes. The third ventricle is under the corpus callosum in the brain's midline. The fourth ventricle is in the brain stem, and a narrow cerebral aqueduct joins it to the third ventricle.

3. The cerebrum's surface is covered with gyri (elevated ridges or convolutions), which are separated by shallow or deep grooves. Each shallow groove is called a sulcus, and each deep groove is called a fissure. The fissures separate large regions of the brain. All these grooves form distinct patterns in normal brains, with the gyri and sulci being more prominent.

4. A stalk of hypothalamic tissue known as the infundibulum lies between the mammillary bodies and the optic chiasma. The infundibulum connects the pituitary gland to the base of the hypothalamus.

5. The hypothalamus is the primary visceral control center of the body and vital for homeostasis. Its mammillary bodies act as relay stations in the olfactory pathways. The hypothalamus also controls the ANS and endocrine system function and initiates physical responses to emotions. Other regulatory functions of the hypothalamus affect body temperature, intake of food, water balance, thirst, and sleep–wake cycles. The hypothalamus is vital for the limbic system and acts through ANS pathways to initiate many physical expressions of emotion. It is also the body's thermostat, controls hormone secretion from the anterior pituitary gland, and produces the hormones antidiuretic hormone and oxytocin. The thalamus relays information coming into the cerebral cortex. It mediates motor activities, sensation, cortical arousal, learning, and memory. Afferent impulses reaching the thalamus are basically recognized as either pleasant or unpleasant. The thalamic nuclei also interpret instructions aiding in direction of motor cortical activity from the cerebellum and the basal nuclei.

6. In the brain stem, the medulla oblongata contains a cardiovascular center, which includes both the cardiac center and vasomotor center and respiratory centers that control respiratory rhythm, rate, and depth. Therefore, the cardiovascular and respiratory centers are in control of blood pressure and respiration.

7. The cerebellum processes inputs from the cerebral motor cortex, brain stem, and sensory receptors. It then regulates skeletal muscle movements for many different activities. All cerebellar activity is subconscious.

8. The three layers of membranes in the meninges are the dura mater, arachnoid mater, and pia mater. The outermost layer (dura mater) is made up of fibrous, tough, white connective tissue. It has many blood vessels and nerves and attaches to the inside of the cranial cavity; it also extends inward between the brain lobes to form protective partitions. It has two layers of fibrous connective tissue (the periosteal and meningeal layers). A thin, web-like arachnoid mater lies between the dura and pia maters. The thin pia mater has many blood vessels and nerves that nourish the brain and spinal cord. It is closely aligned with the surfaces of these organs and is composed of many tiny blood vessels and delicate connective tissue. The pia mater is bound tightly to the brain and its convolutions.

9. The spinal cord is a thin column of nerves leading from the brain to the vertebral canal. It starts at the point where nervous tissue exits the cranial cavity near the foramen magnum and eventually tapers off to terminate near the point where the first and second lumbar are located. It is approximately 42 cm long and 1.8 cm thick. The spinal cord appears as a shiny white structure, protected by bone, meninges, and CSF. An epidural space exists between the dura mater and vertebrae, which is padded by fat and a vein network. CSF fills the subarachnoid space, which lies between the arachnoid and pia mater meninges. The spinal cord terminates inferiorly in a tapered, cone-shaped structure called the conus medullaris. A fibrous extension of the conus medullaris, called the filum terminale, extends inferiorly to the coccyx to anchor the spinal cord. Sawtooth-shaped sections of pia mater are called denticulate ligaments and bind the spinal cord to the dura mater meninx for its entire length. The spinal cord has spinal nerves that arise from each of its 31 segments, which are part of the peripheral nervous system. In the neck, the spinal cord thickens to form the cervical enlargement, which supplies nerves to the upper limbs (shoulder girdle and arms). The lumbar enlargement in the lower back supplies nerves to the lower limbs. The spinal cord is divided into right and left halves by a deep anterior median fissure and a shallow posterior median fissure. The inner core of the spinal cord is made of gray matter surrounded by white matter. Major nerve pathways called nerve tracts are made up of long bundles of myelinated nerve fibers. All neurons that have cell bodies in the gray matter are multipolar. The motor neurons send their axons out to the skeletal muscles, which are their effector organs, via ventral rootlets. These rootlets fuse together, becoming the spinal cord's ventral roots. The dorsal roots are formed by afferent fibers, which carry impulses from peripheral sensory receptors. Associated sensory neuron cell bodies lie in an enlarged region of each dorsal root, which is known as the dorsal root ganglion. The spinal cord's white matter is made up of myelinated and nonmyelinated nerve fibers. The spinal cord conducts nerve impulses and spinal reflexes, so called because

their reflex arcs pass through the spinal cord. Tracts carrying information to the brain are called ascending tracts, whereas those carrying information to the muscles and glands are called descending tracts. The ascending tracts run up to the higher centers for sensory input. The descending tracts run down from the brain to the spinal cord, or inside the spinal cord to its lower levels, for motor output.

10. In elderly people, the brain becomes reduced in both size and weight. This is linked to a loss of cortical neurons. The synaptic organization of the brain changes as the number of dendritic branches and other structures decreases. This limits neurotransmitter production. Brain neurons accumulate abnormal intracellular deposits. Extracellular plaques may affect memory processing. When deposits and plaques exceed normal amounts caused by aging, clinical abnormalities may occur. After young adulthood, brain neurons become damaged and die. However, only a small percentage of total brain neurons are actually lost. Continued learning throughout the life span occurs because remaining neurons can alter their synaptic connections. Aging does cause cognitive declines that may affect perception speed, spatial abilities, making decisions, reacting to occurrences, and memory loss. Cognitive declines usually only become significant when a person is in his or her seventies. Functions that do not decline with age include fluency of speech and mathematical skills.

CRITICAL THINKING QUESTIONS

A transcriptionist read the chart of a 62-year-old man who had a "slight tremor of both hands at rest, stony facial expression, and difficulty in initiating movement." The physician's diagnosis was Parkinson's disease.

1. Which areas of the brain have a lack of dopamine in a patient with Parkinson's disease?
2. Parkinson's disease results from degeneration of which specific neurons?

REVIEW QUESTIONS

1. Which of the following is the major region of the brain that is responsible for conscious thought processes, sensations, memory, and motor patterns?
   A. medulla
   B. cerebrum
   C. pons
   D. cerebellum

2. The brain stem consists of the
   A. diencephalon, midbrain, cerebellum, and pons
   B. cerebellum, pons, cerebrum, and medulla
   C. thalamus, hypothalamus, spinal cord, and cerebrum
   D. midbrain, pons, and medulla oblongata

3. The slender canal that connects the third ventricle with the fourth ventricle is the
   A. septum pellucidum
   B. diencephalic chamber
   C. foramen of Monro
   D. cerebral aqueduct

4. The brain is biochemically isolated from the general circulation by which of the following?
   A. choroid plexus
   B. subarachnoid space
   C. blood–brain barrier
   D. cerebrospinal fluid

5. The epithalamus is an anatomic structure of the
   A. diencephalon
   B. midbrain
   C. red nuclei
   D. cerebellum

6. The C-shaped structure in the limbic system that is responsible for storage and retrieval of new long-term memories is the
   A. cingulate gyrus
   B. corpus callosum
   C. amygdaloid body
   D. hippocampus

7. The respiratory rhythmicity centers and the cardiovascular centers are located in the
    A. pons
    B. cerebellum
    C. medulla oblongata
    D. thalamus
8. Which of the following is the center of the emotions, autonomic function, and hormone production?
    A. hippocampus
    B. hypothalamus
    C. pineal gland
    D. midbrain
9. Which of the following waves are produced in a person with a healthy brain when he or she is awake and resting, with the eyes closed?
    A. theta
    B. delta
    C. beta
    D. alpha
10. The cervical enlargement of the spinal cord supplies nerves to the
    A. shoulder girdle and arms
    B. thorax and abdomen
    C. back and lumbar region
    D. pelvis and legs
11. During a spinal tap, to withdraw CSF the needle should be inserted into the
    A. epidural space
    B. subarachnoid space
    C. subdural space
    D. arachnoid space
12. The posterior horns of the spinal cord contain
    A. somatic and visceral motor nuclei
    B. anterior and posterior columns
    C. somatic and visceral sensory nuclei
    D. ascending and descending tracts
13. The white matter of the spinal cord contains
    A. large numbers of myelinated and unmyelinated axons
    B. cell bodies of neurons and glial cells
    C. sensory and motor nuclei
    D. somatic and visceral sensory nuclei
14. The cell bodies of the associated sensory neurons are found in an enlarged region of the dorsal root called the
    A. gray commissure
    B. lateral horns
    C. dorsal root ganglion
    D. posterior funiculi
15. In cross-section, the gray matter of the spinal cord looks like the letter
    A. C
    B. W
    C. J
    D. H

ESSAY QUESTIONS

1. Explain how the cerebellum is physically connected to the brain stem.
2. Define the terms gyrus, sulcus, and fissure.
3. Describe the basal nuclei and related functions.
4. List the three parts of the diencephalon.
5. Compare the functions of the pons and medulla oblongata.
6. Describe the blood–brain barrier.
7. Compare short-term memory with long-term memory.
8. List four ways that the brain is protected.
9. Describe the spinal cord and its composition of gray and white matter.
10. Describe the layers of the meninges in the spinal cord.

Peripheral Nervous System

OBJECTIVES

After studying this chapter, readers should be able to

1. List the types of somatic and visceral sensory receptors.
2. Explain the three levels of the somatosensory system.
3. Name the 12 cranial nerves.
4. Explain reflex activity and spinal reflexes.
5. Explain dual innervation of the autonomic nervous system.
6. Describe the arrangement of sympathetic and parasympathetic neurons and ganglia.
7. Describe the relationship between preganglionic and postganglionic neurons.
8. Distinguish between the sympathetic and parasympathetic divisions of the autonomic nervous system.
9. Differentiate between cholinergic and adrenergic neurons as to the neurotransmitter secreted and the type of neuron that secretes the neurotransmitter.
10. Contrast the two types of cholinergic receptors.

Overview

The **peripheral nervous system** (PNS) consists of the peripheral nerves connecting the central nervous system (CNS) to other parts of the body. The PNS includes the cranial and spinal nerves and can be subdivided into the **somatic nervous system** (SNS) and **autonomic nervous system** (ANS). The CNS and PNS work together, providing sensory, integrative, and motor functions to the body. The PNS is made up of all neural structures that are outside the brain and spinal cord. The SNS oversees conscious activities, whereas the ANS oversees unconscious activities. The SNS consists of cranial and spinal nerve fibers connecting the CNS to the skin and skeletal muscles. The ANS includes fibers connecting the CNS to the visceral organs such as the heart, stomach, intestines, and glands. The PNS allows us to process information between our bodies and our environments. A comparison of the CNS and PNS is shown in **FIGURE 12-1.**

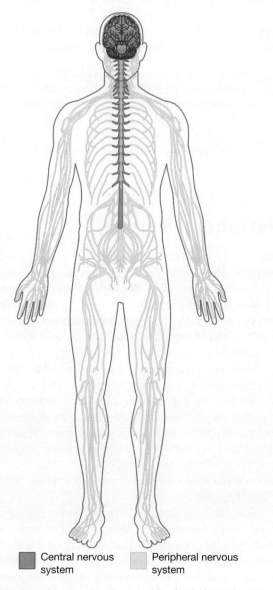

■ Central nervous system ■ Peripheral nervous system

FIGURE 12-1 The nervous system can be divided into the CNS and the PNS.

Sensory Receptors

The **sensory receptors** of the PNS are specialized to respond to **stimuli**. In most cases, a sensory receptor that is activated by enough stimuli results in graded potentials, which initiate nerve impulses along afferent fibers of the PNS. The brain can then process awareness of the stimulus (*sensation*) and interpret the meaning of the stimulus (*perception*).

Types of Sensory Receptors

Sensory receptors are classified by what stimuli they detect, their location in the body, and the complexity of their structures:

- *Chemoreceptors:* These respond to chemicals in solution, including smelled or tasted molecules, changes in blood chemistry, and changes in interstitial fluid chemistry. Chemoreceptive neurons are also found in the *carotid bodies* in the neck and the *aortic bodies* between the primary branches of the aortic arch.
- *Mechanoreceptors:* These respond to mechanical forces such as pressure, touch, stretching, and vibrations. There are three classes: *tactile receptors, baroreceptors,* and *proprioceptors.* Tactile receptors sense pressure, touch, and vibration. *Fine touch and pressure receptors* allow us to sense sources of stimulation that include exact location, shape, size, movement, and texture. *Crude touch and pressure receptors* only allow generalized sensations. Baroreceptors detect pressure changes in blood vessel walls and in areas of the urinary, reproductive, and digestive tracts. Proprioceptors sense positions of skeletal muscles and joints and tension in the ligaments and tendons.
- *Nociceptors:* These respond to stimuli that may be damaging, such as extreme heat or cold, excessive pressure, and inflammatory chemicals, resulting in pain. Various subtypes of chemoreceptors, mechanoreceptors, and thermoreceptors may be stimulated by these stimuli. Nociceptors are common in the superficial skin, around blood vessel walls, inside joint capsules, and in the periostea of bones. Painful sensations are carried on two types of fibers called *type A* and *type C* fibers. The myelinated type A fibers carry *fast pain* sensations, such as from a vaccination or a deep cut. The type C fibers carry *slow pain*, which is described as pain that feels aching or burning.
- *Photoreceptors:* These receptors respond to light, for example, the receptors in the retinas of the eyes.
- *Thermoreceptors:* These respond to temperature changes and are *free nerve endings* in the dermis, liver, skeletal muscles, and hypothalamus. Although not structurally different from each other, there are three to four more *cold receptors* to every *warm receptor*. Thermoreceptors are phasic receptors that quickly adapt to stable temperatures.

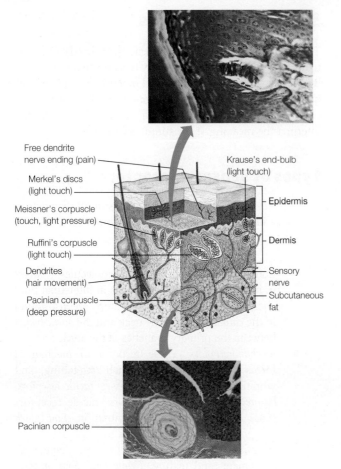

Free dendrite
nerve ending (pain)

Merkel's discs
(light touch)

Meissner's corpuscle
(touch, light pressure)

Ruffini's corpuscle
(light touch)

Dendrites
(hair movement)

Pacinian corpuscle
(deep pressure)

Krause's end-bulb
(light touch)

Epidermis

Dermis

Sensory
nerve

Subcutaneous
fat

Pacinian corpuscle

FIGURE 12-2 Three types of touch and pressure censors.
(Top photo: © Biophoto Associates/Science Source.
Bottom photo: © Donna Beer Stolz, PhD, Center for Biologic
Imaging, University of Pittsburgh Medical School.)

Classification by Receptor Structure

Most sensory receptors of the *general senses* are actually modified dendritic endings. They are located in most areas of the body and monitor the majority of different types of general sensory information (**FIGURE 12-2**). Complex *sense organs* contain the receptors for the **special senses**, which include hearing, vision, equilibrium, smell, and taste. For example, the eyes contain *sensory neurons* and non-neural cells that make up their lenses, supporting walls, and related structures.

Somatosensory System

Sensation is the awareness of environmental changes, both externally and internally. To survive, humans rely on sensation as well as how they interpret these changes (**perception**). How we respond to sensations is determined by our perceptions of them. The part of the sensory system that serves the limbs and wall of the body is known as the **somatosensory system**. Input is received from exteroceptors, interoceptors, and proprioceptors. The somatosensory system transmits information about various sensations. The sensory receptors make up the *receptor level* of this system, whereas processing in the ascending pathways makes up its *circuit level*.

The processing in the *cortical sensory areas* is called its *perceptual level*. For sensations to occur, stimuli must excite a receptor and action potentials must reach the CNS.

Sensory neurons may be called either *tonic receptors* or *phasic receptors*. Tonic receptors are always active. The rate at which action potentials are generated changes when stimulus increases or decreases. Phasic receptors are normally inactive but become active for a short period of time when a change occurs in the conditions they monitor. These receptors provide information about intensity and rates of change of a stimulus.

Adaptation is a reduced sensitivity, whereas a stimulus is consistently present. *Peripheral adaptation* occurs as levels of receptor activity change. The initial strong response subsides over time, partly because the size of the generator potential decreases gradually. This is typical of phasic receptors, and for this reason, they are also called *fast-adapting receptors*. The tonic receptors are called *slow-adapting receptors* because they show little peripheral adaptation. Pain receptors or *nociceptors* are examples of slow-adapting receptors.

Peripheral Nerves

The PNS is divided into *sensory (afferent)* and *motor (efferent)* divisions. The direction in which nerves transmit impulses also helps to classify them. **Sensory (afferent) nerves** carry impulses in one direction—toward the CNS. **Motor (efferent) nerves** carry impulses in the opposite direction—away from the CNS. **Mixed nerves** contain sensory and motor fibers and transmit impulses in both directions.

Most nerves are mixed nerves; the other two types are relatively rare. The fibers in mixed nerves are classified according to the region of the body they innervate. Therefore, they may be classified as *somatic afferent, somatic efferent, visceral afferent,* and *visceral efferent* fibers. Mixed nerves commonly carry both somatic and autonomic (visceral) nervous system fibers. The nerves of the PNS are classified as either *cranial nerves* or *spinal nerves*, based on the location in which they arise.

Ganglia are groups of neuron cell bodies that are related to peripheral nerves. *Nuclei* are groups of neuron cell bodies in the CNS. The ganglia that are associated with *afferent nerve fibers* have cell bodies of sensory neurons. These are also known as *dorsal root ganglia*. The ganglia that are associated with *efferent nerve fibers* mostly have cell bodies of autonomic motor neurons.

Because mature neurons generally do not divide, severe damage or proximity to the cell body may cause the entire neuron to die. Neurons that are regularly stimulated by the damaged neuron's axon may also die. If the cell body is still intact, however, compressed or severed axons of peripheral nerves can still regenerate. It is important to understand that the same is not generally true in the CNS, which is why brain or spinal cord damage is usually irreversible. The ability of PNS neurons to regenerate is linked to their supporting cells, which do not contain the growth-inhibiting proteins found in the oligodendrocytes of the CNS.

Cranial Nerves

There are 12 pairs of *cranial nerves*, which arise from the underside of the brain (see **FIGURE 12-3**). The first pair begin in the cerebrum and attach to the forebrain. The other 11 pairs begin in the brain stem. They all pass through the foramina of the skull. Most are mixed nerves, although the nerves for smell and vision are sensory nerves only. Sensory fibers in the cranial nerves have neuron cell bodies formed into *ganglia*. Motor neuron cell bodies are mostly located in the gray matter of the brain. The cranial nerves serve only structures of the head and neck, except the *vagus nerve*, which reaches the abdomen.

Cranial nerves are usually named based on the structures they serve or functions they provide. They are numbered using Roman numerals, beginning with the most rostral nerves and ending with the most caudal. **TABLE 12-1** lists and explains the cranial nerves in greater detail.

Spinal Nerves

There are 31 pairs of *spinal nerves* originating from the spinal cord. They are identified by their associations with adjacent vertebrae. They are mixed nerves, allowing communication back and forth between the spinal cord and the upper limbs, lower limbs, neck, and trunk. Spinal nerves have both sensory and motor fibers. Spinal nerves are grouped according to the location from which they arise. As each spinal nerve passes through the intervertebral foramen, it is grouped with

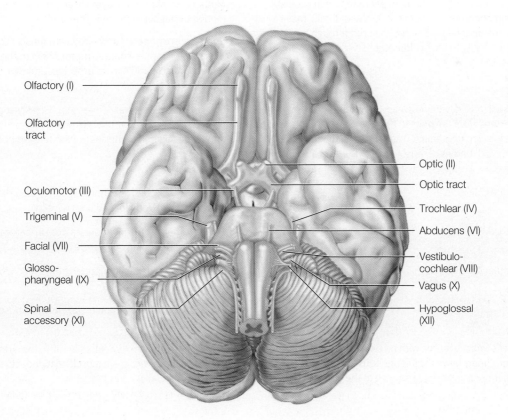

FIGURE 12-3 Cranial nerves.

TABLE 12-1

Cranial Nerves

Nerve	Function
I. Olfactory (sensory only, with no parasympathetic fibers). Olfactory nerve fibers arise from olfactory sensory neurons in olfactory epithelium of the nasal cavity, passing through the cribriform plate of the ethmoid bone. Fibers of olfactory bulb neurons extend posteriorly as the olfactory tract, running beneath the frontal lobe, entering the cerebral hemispheres, and terminating in the primary olfactory cortex. The olfactory nerve fibers attach directly to the cerebrum.	Associated with the sense of smell, they are tiny filaments that run from the nasal mucosa, synapsing with the olfactory bulbs. The olfactory bulbs and tracts are actually brain structures and not part of this nerve.
II. Optic (sensory only, with no parasympathetic fibers). Optic nerve fibers arise from the retinas. The optic nerve passes through the optic canal of each eye orbit, converging to form the optic chiasma, where fibers cross over partially, continue as optic tracts, enter the thalamus, and synapse. Thalamic fibers run as the optic radiation to the occipital (visual) cortex. The optic nerve fibers also attach directly to the cerebrum.	Associated with the sense of vision, it is actually a brain tract, because it develops as an outgrowth of the brain.
III. Oculomotor (mostly motor, contains parasympathetic fibers). Oculomotor fibers extend from the ventral midbrain, near its junction with the pons, to pass through the bony orbit via the superior orbital fissure to each eye. Certain parasympathetic cell bodies exist in the ciliary ganglia. The sensory afferents run from the same four extrinsic eye muscles to the midbrain.	*Motor fibers:* Raising eyelids (via the levator palpebrae superioris muscle), moving eyes, adjusting amount of entering light, and focusing lenses; this nerve supplies four (of the six) extrinsic muscles that move the eyeball in its orbit. These are the inferior oblique and superior, inferior, and medial rectus muscles. The parasympathetic motor fibers reach the sphincter pupillae to cause the pupil to constrict. The ciliary muscle controls lens shape. *Some sensory fibers:* Associated with muscle condition
IV. Trochlear (mostly motor, and no parasympathetic fibers). Trochlear fibers emerge from the dorsal midbrain, move around the midbrain, and enter the orbit through the superior orbital fissure, with the oculomotor nerves.	*Motor fibers:* Moving the eyes via an extrinsic eye muscle lopped through a ligament in the eye orbit. *Some sensory fibers:* Associated with muscle condition. This nerve supplies somatic motor fibers to the superior oblique muscle and carries proprioceptor fibers from this muscle.
V. Trigeminal (mixed, with no parasympathetic fibers). Trigeminal fibers extend from the pons to the face via the superior orbital fissure, forming ophthalmic, maxillary, and mandibular divisions. Cell bodies of sensory neurons are located in the large trigeminal ganglion.	The largest of all cranial nerves, supplying sensory fibers to the face and motor fibers to the muscles used for chewing. It transmits afferent impulses from touch, temperature, and pain receptors.
Ophthalmic division	*Sensory fibers:* Transmit impulses from surface of eyes, tear glands, scalp, forehead, and upper eyelids
Maxillary division	*Sensory fibers:* Transmit impulses from upper teeth, upper gum, upper lip, lining of palate, and facial skin
Mandibular division	*Sensory fibers:* Transmit impulses from skin of jaw, lower teeth, lower gum, lower lip *Motor fibers:* Transmit impulses to chewing muscles and those in the floor of the mouth
VI. Abducens (mostly motor, with no parasympathetic fibers). Abducens fibers leave the inferior pons and enter the orbit via the superior orbital fissure, running to the eye.	*Motor fibers:* Transmit impulses to move the eyes via control of the extrinsic eye muscle that abducts the eyeball (turning it laterally) *Sensory fibers:* Associated with muscle condition

TABLE 12-1

Cranial Nerves (continued)

Nerve	Function
VII. Facial (mixed, with parasympathetic fibers). Facial fibers come from the pons, just lateral to the abducens nerves, to enter the temporal bone through the internal acoustic meatus. They run through the inner ear cavity to emerge through the stylomastoid foramen and then to the lateral aspect of the face.	*Motor fibers:* Transmit impulses to facial expression muscles, tear glands, and salivary glands. They are the chief motor nerves of the face. The five major branches are the temporal, zygomatic, buccal, mandibular, and cervical branches. *Sensory fibers:* Transmit impulses associated with taste
VIII. Vestibulocochlear (mixed, with no parasympathetic fibers). Vestibulocochlear fibers arise from within the inner ear, passing through the internal acoustic meatus, entering the brain stem at the pons–medulla border. Afferent fibers from the cochlea form the cochlear division. Those from the semicircular canals and vestibule form the vestibular division.	Previously called the *auditory nerve.*
Vestibular branch: sensory nerve cell bodies are located in the vestibular ganglia.	Transmit impulses associated with equilibrium
Cochlear branch: sensory nerve cell bodies are located in the spiral ganglion within the cochlea.	Transmit impulses associated with hearing
IX. Glossopharyngeal (mixed, with parasympathetic fibers). Glossopharyngeal fibers emerge from the medulla and leave the skull via the jugular foramen, reaching the throat.	*Motor fibers:* Transmit impulses to pharynx muscles used in swallowing, and to the salivary glands. These nerves also innervate part of the tongue. *Sensory fibers:* Transmit impulses from the pharynx, tonsils, posterior tongue, and carotid arteries
X. Vagus (mixed, with parasympathetic fibers). The only cranial nerves to extend beyond the head and neck, reaching the thorax and abdomen.	*Somatic motor fibers:* Transmit impulses to muscles used for speech and swallowing *Autonomic motor fibers:* Transmit impulses to the heart, smooth muscles, and thoracic and abdominal glands *Sensory fibers:* Transmit impulses from the pharynx, larynx, esophagus, and viscera of the thorax and abdomen
XI. Accessory (mostly motor, with no parasympathetic fibers). Accessory fibers form from rootlets emerging from the spinal cord and not the brain stem. They enter the skull via the foramen magnum and exit through the jugular foramen.	They supply motor fibers to the trapezius and sternocleidomastoid muscles and convey proprioceptor impulses from the same muscles.
Cranial branch	*Motor fibers:* Transmit impulses to soft palate, pharynx, and larynx
Spinal branch	*Motor fibers:* Transmit impulses to neck and back
XII. Hypoglossal (mostly motor, with no parasympathetic fibers). Hypoglossal fibers arise by a series of roots from the medulla, exiting the skull via the hypoglossal canal.	*Motor fibers:* Transmit impulses to tongue muscles. They allow tongue movements that mix and manipulate food during chewing, and aid in swallowing and speech.

the vertebra above it. This is true for all spinal nerves except for those in the cervical area. There are 8 pairs of cervical nerves (C_1-C_8), 12 pairs of thoracic nerves (T_1-T_{12}), 5 pairs of lumbar nerves (L_1-L_5), 5 pairs of sacral nerves (S_1-S_5), and 1 pair of coccygeal nerves (Coc_1). They are identified by increased numbering moving down the spine. The lumbar, sacral, and coccygeal nerves descend past the end of the spinal cord to form

the **cauda equina** (horse's tail). Although there are eight pairs of cervical nerves, there are only seven cervical vertebrae. The first seven pairs exit the vertebral canal superior to the vertebrae for which they are named. However, C_8 emerges inferior to the seventh cervical vertebra, which is between C_7 and T_1. Below the cervical area of the spine, the spinal nerves leave the vertebral column inferior to the vertebra that has the same number.

Spinal nerves are only 1 to 2 cm in length and divide just after emerging from each foramen. Each spinal nerve divides into a small *dorsal ramus*, a larger *ventral ramus*, and an extremely small *meningeal branch*. The meningeal branch reenters the vertebral canal, innervating the meninges and blood vessels that lie inside. Each ramus is mixed, similar to the actual spinal nerve. *Rami communicantes* contain visceral (autonomic) nerve fibers that attach to the base of the ventral rami or each thoracic spinal nerve.

Spinal Nerve Innervation

From the spinal nerves, the rami and their primary branches supply all the somatic region of the body from the neck down, which consists of the skin and skeletal muscles. The posterior body trunk is supplied by the dorsal rami, and the remainder of the trunk and limbs are supplied by the thicker ventral rami. Rami differ from roots in several ways. Each root is either sensory or motor and lies medial to the spinal nerves, which they actually form. Rami carry both sensory and motor fibers and lie distal to the spinal nerves, from which they are laterally branched. All ventral rami (except for T_2-T_{12}) branch out, joining each other lateral to the vertebral column.

The main portions of the spinal nerves combine (except in the thoracic region) to form complex networks called **plexuses**. The ventral rami are the only rami that form plexuses. Recombined spinal nerve fibers innervate certain body parts, even though these fibers may originate from other spinal nerves. Each branch of a plexus formed from ventral rami contains fibers from several spinal nerves and fibers from the ventral rami, which travel to peripheral body portions via different routes. Every muscle in a specific limb receives its nerve supply from several spinal nerves, not just a single nerve. Therefore, damage to one spinal root or segment does not totally paralyze a limb muscle.

Cervical Plexuses

The **cervical plexuses** deep in the neck are formed from branches of the first four cervical nerves. Under the sternocleidomastoid muscle, a looped *cervical plexus* is formed from the ventral rami of the first four cervical nerves. Most branches of this plexus are *cutaneous nerves* supplying the skin alone. Sensory impulses are transmitted from the skin of the neck, ear region, posterior head, and shoulder. The anterior neck is innervated by other branches.

Fibers from the third, fourth, and fifth cervical nerves are combined into the right and left **phrenic nerves**, conducting motor impulses to the diaphragm. Each phrenic nerve runs inferiorly through the thorax, supplying sensory and motor fibers to the diaphragm, which is the most important muscle that causes the movements required for breathing.

FOCUS ON PATHOLOGY

Diaphragm spasms or hiccups occur when a phrenic nerve becomes irritated. If the C_3 to C_5 region of the spinal cord is crushed or otherwise destroyed or if both phrenic nerves are severed, respiratory arrest occurs because the diaphragm is paralyzed. To save the patient's life, a mechanical respirator is required, which forces air into the lungs.

Brachial Plexuses

The lower four cervical nerves and first thoracic nerve branch out to the **brachial plexuses**, found in the shoulders between the neck and armpits. They supply the skin and muscles of the arms and hands, most importantly including the musculocutaneous, median, radial, ulnar, and axillary nerves. The brachial plexuses communicate with the sympathetic trunk and are composed of the anterior branches of the lower four cervical (C_5-C_8) and first two thoracic nerves (T_1 and T_2). Sometimes, C_4 is also involved. The plexuses appear braided and allow sensory and motor axons from the spinal cord to cross and recross. The brachial plexus is a very complex structure, basically made up of ventral rami, which form trunks, then divisions, then cords. The three cords of the brachial plexus move along the axillary artery, where the main nerves of the upper limb originate. The brachial plexus ends in the axilla.

FOCUS ON PATHOLOGY

Brachial plexus injuries are common and, if severe, may cause weakness or paralysis of an entire upper limb. These injuries may occur if the shoulder receives trauma that forces the humerus to move inferiorly or when the upper limb is pulled with great force.

The *axillary nerve* branches from the posterior cord, running posteriorly to the surgical neck of the humerus. The *musculocutaneous nerve* is the major end branch of the lateral cord and runs inferiorly in the anterior arm. The *median nerve* runs down through the arm to the anterior forearm, branching off to the skin and most flexor muscles. The *ulnar nerve* branches off the medial cord of the plexus to descend along the arm's medial aspect to the elbow, behind the medial epicondyle, and along the ulna and medial forearm. The *radial nerve* is the largest branch of the brachial plexus and continues from the posterior cord. It wraps around the humerus, running anteriorly around the lateral epicondyle at the elbow, branching toward the radius and hand.

FOCUS ON PATHOLOGY

When the median nerve is injured, it is difficult to pick up a small object using the thumb and index finger. The median nerve may be compressed as a part of *carpal tunnel syndrome*. It is also injured in a suicide attempt that involves slashing of the wrist. If the radial nerve is injured, the hand cannot be extended at the wrist. It is commonly injured by sleeping with the arm extended over the edge of a bed or by using a crutch improperly.

Lumbosacral Plexuses

The **lumbosacral plexuses** are made up of the last thoracic nerve and the lumbar, sacral, and coccygeal nerves and extend into the pelvic cavity; they are associated with the skin and muscles of the lower abdominal wall, buttocks, external genitalia, thighs, legs, and feet. Their major branches include the femoral, obturator, and sciatic nerves. The anterior thoracic spinal nerves enter spaces between the ribs to become **intercostal nerves**. They supply the intercostal muscles and upper abdominal wall muscles while receiving sensory impulses from the skin of the abdomen and thorax. The lumbosacral plexuses are so named because of substantial overlap of the lumbar and sacral plexuses, with many lumbar plexus fibers combining with the sacral plexus through the *lumbosacral trunk*.

The lumbar plexuses are nervous plexuses in the lumbar region, formed by parts of the first four lumbar nerves and parts of the subcostal nerve. The nerves of the lumbar plexuses pass in front of the hip joints and mostly support the anterior thighs. Each lumbar plexus lies within the psoas major muscle, branching proximally to innervate abdominal wall muscles and the psoas muscle itself. The major branches of the lumbar plexus descend to innervate the medial and anterior thigh.

The largest terminal nerve of the lumbar plexus is the *femoral nerve*, which runs deep to the inguinal ligament. It enters the thigh, dividing into several large branches. Its motor branches innervate the quadriceps (anterior thigh muscles), which are vital to flexing the thigh and extending the knee. The cutaneous branches of the femoral nerve innervate the skin of the anterior thigh and the leg's medial surface (from knee to foot). The *obturator nerve* enters the medial thigh through the obturator foramen, innervating the adductor muscles. **TABLE 12-2** explains the branches of the lumbar plexus.

TABLE 12-2

Lumbar Plexus Nerve Branches

Ventral Rami	Lumbar Plexus Nerve
L_1	Iliohypogastric and ilioinguinal
L_1 and L_2	Genitofemoral
L_2 and L_3	Lateral femoral cutaneous
L_2-L_4	Femoral and obturator

FOCUS ON PATHOLOGY

Compression of the spinal roots of the lumbar plexus may occur because of a herniated disc, which can cause problems with walking because the femoral nerve serves the primary movers that both flex the hip and extend the knee. Compression of these roots may also cause anterior thigh pain or numbness. If the obturator nerve is also impaired, pain or numbness of the medial thigh occurs.

The *sacral plexus* lies immediately caudal to the lumbar plexus, arising from spinal nerves L_4 to S_4. It has approximately 12 named branches, half of which serve the buttocks and lower limbs. The remainder serve the structures of the pelvis and the perineum. **TABLE 12-3** summarizes the largest branches of the sacral plexus.

The *sciatic nerve* is the largest branch of the sacral plexus and is also the longest and thickest nerve in the entire body. It supplies all of each lower limb except the anteromedial thigh. The sciatic nerve is actually two nerves in a common sheath, called the *tibial* and *common fibular* nerves. The sciatic nerve moves from the pelvis, through the greater sciatic notch, deeply into the gluteus maximus muscle. It then enters the posterior thigh medial to the hip joint, with motor branches to the hamstring muscles and adductor magnus. In the hamstrings, it comprises all muscles that extend the thigh and flex the knee. Just above the knee, the tibial and common fibular nerves diverge into different directions.

The tibial nerve continues through the popliteal fossa, posterior to the knee joint, supplying the posterior compartment muscles of the leg as well as the skin of the posterior calf and sole of the foot. The common fibular nerve (also called the *common peroneal nerve*) descends to wrap around the neck of the fibula and divides into superficial and deep branches. The branches innervate the knee joint, skin of the leg (anterior and lateral), and dorsum of the foot. They also innervate the anterolateral leg, so its extensors can dorsiflex the foot.

TABLE 12-3

Sacral Plexus Nerve Branches	
Ventral Rami	**Sacral Plexus Nerve**
L_4, L_5, and S_1-S_3 (L_4-S_3) (L_4-S_2)	Sciatic nerve (Tibial, which includes sural, medial and lateral plantar, and medical calcaneal branches) (Common fibular, which includes superficial and deep branches)
L_4, L_5, and S_1	Superior gluteal
L_5-S_2	Inferior gluteal
S_1-S_3	Posterior femoral cutaneous
S_2-S_4	Pudendal

FOCUS ON PATHOLOGY

Sciatica involves intense, stabbing pain along the sciatic nerve and is a common problem. If the proximal area of the sciatic nerve is injured, the lower limb may be impaired in different ways, based on which nerve roots are affected. This type of injury may be caused by a disc herniation, a fall, or an injection into the wrong portion of the buttocks. If the nerve is transected, the leg is nearly immovable and cannot be flexed and the foot and ankle are temporarily paralyzed.

TEST YOUR UNDERSTANDING

1. Explain the most important nerve of the cervical plexus.
2. List the five primary nerves of the brachial plexus and explain their locations.
3. Differentiate between the lumbar plexus and the sacral plexus.

Peripheral Motor Endings

In the PNS, **motor endings** activate effectors via the release of neurotransmitters. Terminals of somatic motor fibers innervating voluntary muscles form complex *neuromuscular junctions* with their effector cells. The ending of each axon branch, at its target muscle fiber, splits into a cluster of *axon terminals*, branching over the sarcolemma folds of the fiber. These axon terminals contain mitochondria and synaptic vesicles that are filled with acetylcholine (ACh).

As a nerve impulse reaches the axon terminal, ACh is released, via exocytosis, diffusing across the synaptic cleft. It attaches to its receptors on the sarcolemma and the neuromuscular junction. Ligand-gated channels are opened by this ACh binding, allowing sodium and potassium ions to pass.

Because sodium enters cells more quickly than potassium is lost, the muscle cell interior becomes depolarized. This graded potential, known as the *end plate potential,* spreads to nearby areas of the membrane, causing voltage-gated sodium channels to open. An action potential results along the sarcolemma, stimulating contraction of the muscle fiber. At somatic neuromuscular junctions, the synaptic cleft is filled with a basal lamina that is rich in glycoproteins. This basal lamina is not present at other synapses. It contains acetylcholinesterase, which breaks down the ACh.

Visceral Muscle and Gland Innervation

Junctions between autonomic motor endings and their effectors are not as complex as those formed between somatic fibers and skeletal muscle cells. There is repeated branching of autonomic motor axons. Each of these forms *synapses en passant* (which means "synapses in passing") with its effector's cells. An axon serving a smooth muscle or gland has many *varicosities*, whereas an axon serving a cardiac muscle does not. Varicosities are knob-like swellings that contain mitochondria and synaptic vesicles, resembling a string of pearls. Autonomic synaptic vesicles usually contain ACh or norepinephrine (NE). Both act indirectly on their targets, using second messengers. As a result, visceral motor responds are slower than those caused by somatic motor fibers, which cause direct opening of ion channels.

TEST YOUR UNDERSTANDING

1. Explain the actions of motor endings.
2. Define the term "neuromuscular junction" and the relationship to axon terminals and the end plate potential.
3. Define the term "varicosities."

Somatic Nervous System

The SNS differs from the ANS in that it stimulates skeletal muscles, whereas the ANS innervates glands as well as cardiac and smooth muscle. Other differences are based on the physiology of the effector organs of each system. In the SNS, motor neuron cell bodies lie in the CNS, with their axons extending in spinal or cranial nerves, to reach target skeletal muscles. Somatic motor fibers are usually thick and heavy. These myelinated group A fibers conduct nerve impulses very quickly. This differs again from the ANS, which uses a two-neuron chain to reach its effectors.

Every somatic motor neuron releases ACh at its synapse with a skeletal muscle fiber. Effects are always *excitatory*. Muscle fibers contract if the stimulation reaches threshold. Both somatic and autonomic motor activities are regulated and coordinated by higher brain centers. Also, both somatic and autonomic fibers are contained in most spinal nerves and in many cranial nerves. The body's ability to adapt to most internal and external changes involves both visceral organs and skeletal muscles. A hard-working skeletal muscle requires additional glucose and oxygen, so autonomic control mechanisms increase heart rate and dilate airways.

Reflex Activity and Spinal Reflexes

A *reflex* is actually defined as a fast, automatic response to a specific stimulus. Reflex activity in the human body can be either inborn (intrinsic) or learned (acquired). Inborn reflexes are rapid and predictable motor responses to stimuli that are formed between neurons during human development. They are involuntary and subconsciously maintain body posture, help to avoid pain, and control visceral activities. For example, a response to pain is triggered by an inborn spinal reflex that operates without assistance from the brain. We may only be aware of the final outcome of one of these basic reflexes and not the process of the reflex itself. Many visceral reflexes are regulated by the brain stem and spinal cord.

A learned reflex develops over time, because of repeated reactions to stimuli. It is more complex than an inborn reflex. An example is how an older driver may access learned reflexes because of his or her experience in driving, whereas a younger driver may have yet to learn them. However, most inborn reflexes can be altered by learning and conscious effort. In a situation involving pain, the pain signals are quickly transmitted to the brain by the interneurons of the spinal cord. Withdrawing from the source of the pain involves serial processing by the spinal cord, whereas awareness of pain involves simultaneous parallel processing of the sensory stimuli.

Reflex Arc

In a **reflex arc**, sensory impulses from receptors can reach their effectors without being processed by the brain (**FIGURE 12-4**).

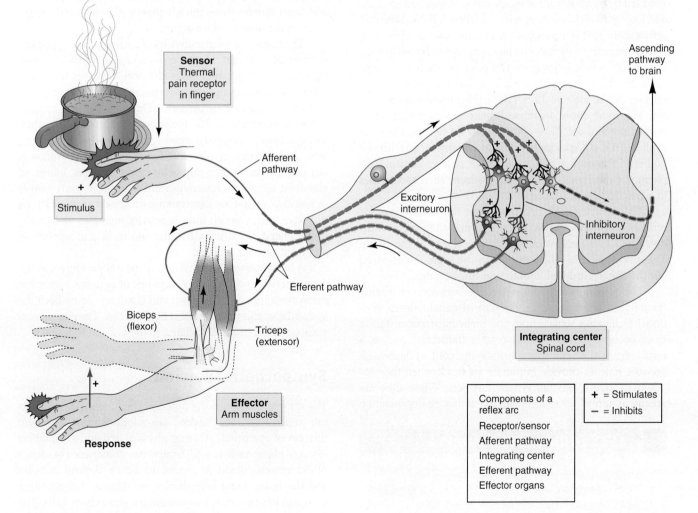

FIGURE 12-4 The functions of a reflex arc.

Some reflex arcs use interneurons and others do not. The five basic components of the reflex arc are a receptor, a sensory neuron, an integration center, a motor neuron, and an effector. A receptor is the site of the stimulus action. The sensory neuron transmits afferent impulses to the CNS. In a simple reflex arc, the integration center may be only a single synapse, located between a sensory neuron and a motor neuron, referred to as a *monosynaptic reflex*. The sensory neuron synapses directly on a motor neuron. In a more complex reflex arc, multiple synapses with chains of interneurons are involved and are referred to as *polysynaptic reflexes*. They have a longer delay between stimuli and responses than monosynaptic reflexes. The integration center for such reflexes lies within the CNS. A motor neuron conducts efferent impulses from the integration center to an effector organ, and an effector is defined as a muscle fiber or gland cell that responds to these impulses by contracting or secreting. The most complicated spinal reflexes are called *intersegmental reflex arcs*, in which many segments work together and produce coordinated motor responses that are extremely variable.

A **somatic reflex** is one that activates skeletal muscle, allowing for involuntary muscle control. Examples include *superficial*, *stretch*, and *patellar* reflexes. Sensory receptors used in stretch reflexes are *muscle spindles* that each consist of bundled *intrafusal muscle fibers*. The muscle spindle is surrounded by larger *extrafusal muscle fibers*. Somatic reflexes are also known as *deep tendon* or *myotatic* reflexes. An **autonomic reflex** is one that activates visceral effectors such as smooth or cardiac muscle or glands. An autonomic reflex is also known as a visceral reflex. In every *visceral reflex arc*, there is a receptor, a sensory neuron, and one or more interneurons. Visceral reflexes can be long or short. *Long reflexes* usually coordinate activities in an entire organ, with their actions processed by interneurons of the CNS. *Short reflexes* do not use the CNS at all but use the sensory neurons and interneurons with cell bodies in the autonomic ganglia. Short reflexes control simple motor responses, with localized effects, such as activities in a specific part of a target organ.

The spinal cord controls some common somatic reflexes, known as **spinal reflexes**, which often occur without direct involvement of the higher centers of the brain. These reflexes may still occur when the brain is destroyed but the spinal cord is still intact and functioning.

The brain is aware of most spinal reflexes and can modify them in most circumstances. For normal spinal reflexes, continual facilitating signals from the brain must occur. *Spinal shock* occurs when the spinal cord is transected, and as a result, all functions controlled by the spinal cord are depressed. Somatic reflexes provide important feedback when they are tested to assess nervous system function. When they are absent, abnormal, or exaggerated, there may be degeneration

or pathology of certain regions of the nervous system. There may be no other signs of dysfunction present.

Autonomic Nervous System

The ANS is part of the PNS. It functions autonomously (independently), without conscious effort. The ANS regulates the smooth muscles, cardiac muscles, and glands. It can respond to emotional stress and prepares the body for strenuous physical activity. Most peripheral nerve fibers lead to ganglia located outside the CNS and control visceral muscles and glands highly independent of the brain and spinal cord.

The ANS is divided into the **sympathetic** and **parasympathetic** divisions. Certain visceral organs have fibers from both divisions, controlling the activation or inhibition of their actions. The sympathetic division prepares the body for stressful or emergency situations and is part of the *fight-or-flight response*. This division can change tissue and organ activities by releasing NE at peripheral synapses and by distributing epinephrine and NE throughout the body. *Sympathetic activation*, controlled by the hypothalamus, occurs when the entire sympathetic division responds to a crisis situation. When this happens, a person feels extremely alert, energized, and euphoric; blood pressure, breathing, and heart rate increase; muscle tone is elevated; and energy reserves are mobilized for action.

The parasympathetic division functions in an opposite manner and is part of the *rest-and-digest response*. When stress occurs, the sympathetic division increases heart and breathing rates. As the stress subsides, the parasympathetic division decreases these activities. *Dual innervation* is applied so the two divisions counterbalance the effects of each other, using *cardiac, pulmonary, esophageal, celiac, inferior mesenteric*, and *hypogastric plexuses*. *Parasympathetic activation* is signified by constricted pupils for better focusing, increased glandular secretions, raised nutrient absorption, and changes in blood flow that are associated with sexual arousal. In the digestive tract, smooth muscle activity increases, defecation is stimulated, the urinary bladder contracts, and respiration and heart rate are reduced.

A little-known third division of the ANS is known as the *enteric nervous system*. It is a network of neurons and nerve networks in the digestive tract and is influenced by both the sympathetic and parasympathetic divisions. The enteric nervous system is primarily related to the visceral reflexes.

Sympathetic Division

The sympathetic division's functions include increased heart rate and respiration, reduced salivation, clammy skin, and dilation of eye pupils. During physical activity, it constricts visceral blood vessels and sometimes constricts cutaneous blood vessels. Blood is moved to active skeletal muscles and the heart. Lung bronchioles are dilated, and resulting increases in ventilation move more oxygen to body cells. The liver releases more glucose into the blood to supply energy

---

TEST YOUR UNDERSTANDING

1. Identify the five components of a reflex arc.
2. Differentiate between somatic and autonomic reflexes.
3. Explain how many spinal reflexes occur.

to the body. Simultaneously, it slows down nonessential activities such as motility in the gastrointestinal tract. The sympathetic division may be referred to as the "E division" (signifying exercise, emergency, and excitement).

Sympathetic fibers are thoracolumbar, originating in the thoracic and lumbar regions of the spinal cord (**FIGURE 12-5**). They have short *preganglionic fibers* and long *postganglionic fibers*. *Sympathetic ganglia* lie closer to the spinal cord than parasympathetic ganglia. The sympathetic division innervates more organs than the parasympathetic division, including the visceral organs of the body cavities and the visceral structures in the somatic (superficial) areas of the body. Certain glands and smooth muscle structures in the sweat glands and arrector pili muscles require autonomic innervation, served exclusively by sympathetic fibers. Sympathetic fibers also innervate the smooth muscle walls of the arteries and veins.

All preganglionic fibers arise from cell bodies of *preganglionic neurons* in spinal cord segments T_1 to L_2; hence, the *thoracolumbar division* is the alternate name for the sympathetic division. Many preganglionic sympathetic neurons exist in the spinal cord's gray matter, which form its *lateral horns*. There are no lateral horns in the sacral spinal cord regions because parasympathetic preganglionic neurons are far less abundant there when compared with the sympathetic neurons in the thoracolumbar regions. The preganglionic fibers leave the spinal cord via the ventral root, passing through a *white ramus communicans* and entering the *sympathetic trunk ganglion* to form part of the *sympathetic trunk*. The sympathetic trunks flank each side of the vertebral column and appear like strands of beads that are glistening and white. Each sympathetic trunk is also known as a *sympathetic chain*, and the sympathetic trunk ganglia are also called *paravertebral* or *chain ganglia*.

Sympathetic fibers arise only from the thoracic and lumbar spinal cord segments. There are usually 23 ganglia in each sympathetic trunk (3 cervical, 11 thoracic, 4 lumbar, 4 sacral, and 1 coccygeal). Three different things occur when a preganglionic axon reaches a trunk ganglion: The pre- and *postganglionic neurons* can either synapse at the same level, synapse at a higher or lower level, or synapse in a distant collateral ganglion. When they synapse in a distant collateral ganglion, the preganglionic fibers play a role in forming several *splanchnic nerves*. They synapse in *collateral (prevertebral) ganglia* anterior to the vertebral column. Collateral ganglia are not paired or arranged in segments and only occur in the abdomen and pelvis. However, all sympathetic ganglia are close to the spinal cord.

Parasympathetic Division

The parasympathetic division keeps energy use by the body to its lowest possible amounts. It controls digestion of food and elimination of feces and urine. For example, during digestion, blood pressure and heart rate are lowered while the gastrointestinal system is active. Also, the pupils of the eyes become constricted and the lenses are accommodated for close vision. The parasympathetic division may be referred to as the "D division" (signifying digestion,

defecation, and diuresis). Both divisions antagonize each other's effects greatly to maintain homeostasis.

Parasympathetic fibers are craniosacral, originating in the brain and sacral spinal cord. They have long preganglionic and short postganglionic fibers. Parasympathetic ganglia are mostly located in the visceral effector organs. Overall, the parasympathetic division is simpler than the sympathetic division. It is also known as the *craniosacral division* because its preganglionic fibers emerge from opposite ends of the CNS (the brain stem and sacral spinal cord). The preganglionic axons run from the CNS, nearly all the way to innervated target structures (**FIGURE 12-6**). At these points, axons synapse with postganglionic neurons of the **terminal ganglia**, lying close to, or inside, the target organs. Extremely short postganglionic axons emerge from the terminal ganglia, synapsing with nearby effector cells.

In the cranial portion of the parasympathetic nervous system, preganglionic fibers exist in the facial, oculomotor, glossopharyngeal, and vagus nerves. Cell bodies of these fibers lie in related motor cranial nerve nuclei of the brain stem. The parasympathetic fibers of the *oculomotor (III) nerves* innervate smooth muscles that cause the pupils of the eyes to constrict and the lenses to bulge, which are both used when focusing. Cell bodies of the postganglionic neurons lie in the **ciliary ganglia** inside the eye orbits.

The parasympathetic fibers of the *facial (VII) nerves* stimulate large glands located in the head. Preganglionic fibers synapse with postganglionic neurons in the *pterygopalatine ganglia*, which are just posterior to the maxillae. Preganglionic neurons stimulating salivary glands (submandibular and sublingual) synapse with postganglionic neurons in the *submandibular ganglia*.

The parasympathetic fibers of the *glossopharyngeal (IX) nerves* begin in the inferior salivary nuclei of the medulla. They synapse in the **otic ganglia**, just inferior to the foramen ovale of the skull. The entire parasympathetic innervation of the head is supplied by cranial nerves III, VII, and IX.

The two *vagus (X) nerves* make up 90% of all preganglionic parasympathetic fibers in the body. Their preganglionic axons begin primarily from the dorsal motor nuclei of the medulla. They synapse in terminal ganglia that are mostly located in the target organ walls. Branches of the vagus nerves pass to the **cardiac plexuses**, which supply fibers to the heart that slow the heart rate. Other branches supply the **pulmonary plexuses** and **esophageal plexuses**. Near the esophagus, the main trunks of the vagus nerves join fibers to form *anterior* and *posterior vagal trunks*, each with fibers from both vagus nerves. The trunk continue down to the abdominal cavity, sending fibers through the large *abdominal aortic plexus*, which is made up of the celiac, superior mesenteric, and hypogastric plexuses running along the aorta. The large abdominal aortic plexus then branches off to the abdominal viscera.

The sacral portion of the parasympathetic division serves the pelvic organs and the distal half of the large intestine. It arises from lateral gray matter neurons of spinal cord segments S_2 to S_4. Axons of these neurons continue through the ventral roots of the spinal nerves to the ventral rami. They branch to form the **pelvic splanchnic nerves** that pass

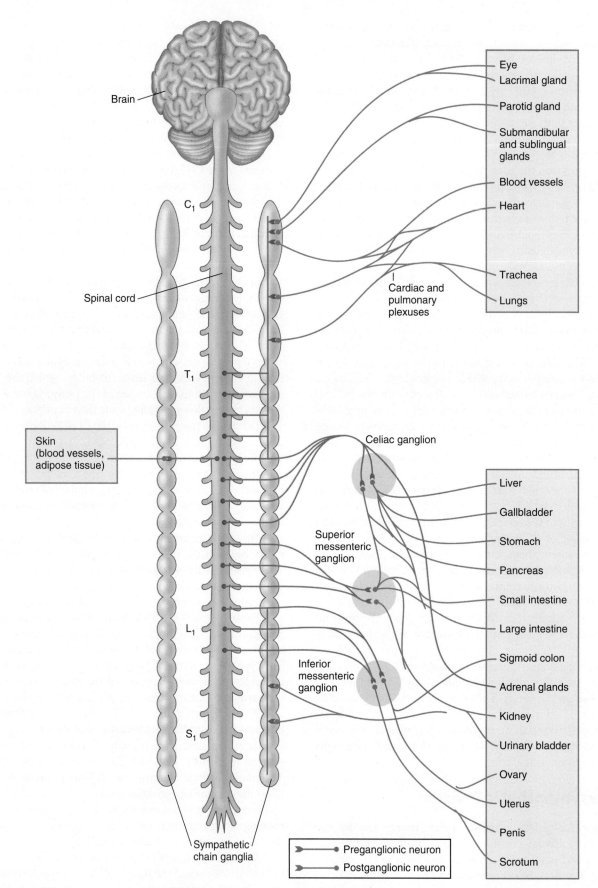

FIGURE 12-5 Sympathetic division of the ANS.

Brain

C₁

Spinal cord

T₁

Skin
(blood vessels,
adipose tissue)

L₁

S₁

Sympathetic
chain ganglia

Cardiac and
pulmonary
plexuses

Celiac ganglion

Superior
messenteric
ganglion

Inferior
messenteric
ganglion

Eye
Lacrimal gland
Parotid gland
Submandibular
and sublingual
glands
Blood vessels
Heart
Trachea
Lungs

Liver
Gallbladder
Stomach
Pancreas
Small intestine
Large intestine
Sigmoid colon
Adrenal glands
Kidney
Urinary bladder
Ovary
Uterus
Penis
Scrotum

Preganglionic neuron
Postganglionic neuron

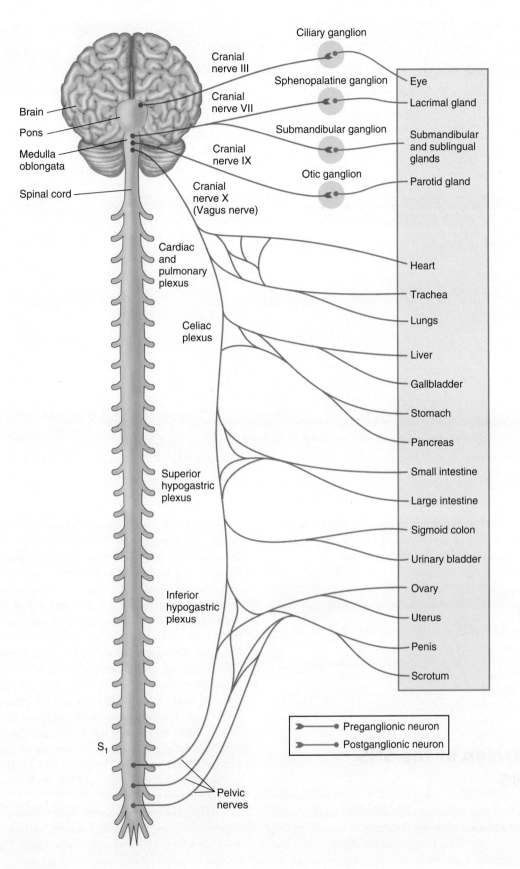

FIGURE 12-6 Parasympathetic division of the ANS.

TABLE 12-4

Differences Between the Sympathetic and Parasympathetic Divisions

Factor	Sympathetic Division	Parasympathetic Division
Functional role	Prepares body for activity (fight or flight)	Body maintenance, conservation and storage of energy (rest and digest)
Location of ganglia	Within a few centimeters of the CNS, alongside vertebral column (sympathetic trunk ganglia) and anterior to vertebral column (collateral or prevertebral ganglia)	Terminal ganglia are within the visceral organ (intramural) or near the organ served
Origin	Thoracolumbar part: lateral horns of spinal cord gray matter, segments T_1-L_2	Craniosacral part: brain stem nuclei of cranial nerves III, VII, IX, and X; spinal cord segments S_2-S_4
Degree of branching of preganglionic fibers	Extensive	Slight
Relative length of pre- and postganglionic fibers	Short preganglionic, long postganglionic	Long preganglionic, short postganglionic
Neurotransmitters	All preganglionic fibers release ACh, most postganglionic fibers release NE (adrenergic fibers); postganglionic fibers that serve sweat glands release ACh; neurotransmitter activity augmented by release of adrenal medullary hormones (epinephrine and NE)	All pre- and postganglionic fibers release ACh (cholinergic fibers)
Rami communicantes	Gray and white; the white rami contain myelinated preganglionic fibers, and the gray contain nonmyelinated postganglionic fibers	None

through the **inferior hypogastric (pelvic) plexus** in the floor of the pelvis. **TABLE 12-4** compares differences between the sympathetic and parasympathetic divisions.

Comparison of the SNS and ANS

ANS neurons are motor neurons but differ in that they contain two neurons. One neuron's cell body is located in the brain or spinal cord. The **preganglionic fiber** leaves the CNS to synapse with a second motor neuron to make a *ganglionic neuron*. The axon of the second neurons is called a **postganglionic fiber**. The *postganglionic axon* extends to the effector organ. Preganglionic axons are thin and lightly myelinated, whereas postganglionic axons are even thinner and nonmyelinated (**FIGURE 12-7**).

Autonomic motor neurons have a resting level of spontaneous activity even when there are no stimuli. This determines the *autonomic* tone, which is an important function of the ANS. By keeping a resting level of activity constant, an autonomic nerve can decrease or increase its activity, allowing for better control. Autonomic tone is important for dual innervation, but even more so when dual innervation does not occur to help balance the divisions of the body's nervous systems.

Autonomic *ganglia* are *motor ganglia* and contain the cell bodies of motor neurons. Conduction through the autonomic efferent chain is not as fast as conduction in the somatic motor system. The spinal and cranial nerves continue many pre- and postganglionic fibers throughout most of their entire length. The autonomic ganglia are sites of synapse and information transmission, from preganglionic to postganglionic neurons. The dorsal root ganglia are only part of the sensory division of the PNS, and the somatic motor division has *no ganglia at all*.

Autonomic postganglionic fibers release NE, which is secreted by most sympathetic fibers, and also release ACh, which is secreted by parasympathetic fibers. Effects are either excitatory or inhibitory, depending on the type of receptors from the target organ. The axon terminals of somatic neurons release ACh at the skeletal muscle fibers. This always has excitatory effects, causing contraction of muscle fibers. Preganglionic sympathetic and preganglionic parasympathetic fibers release ACh. However, postganglionic parasympathetic

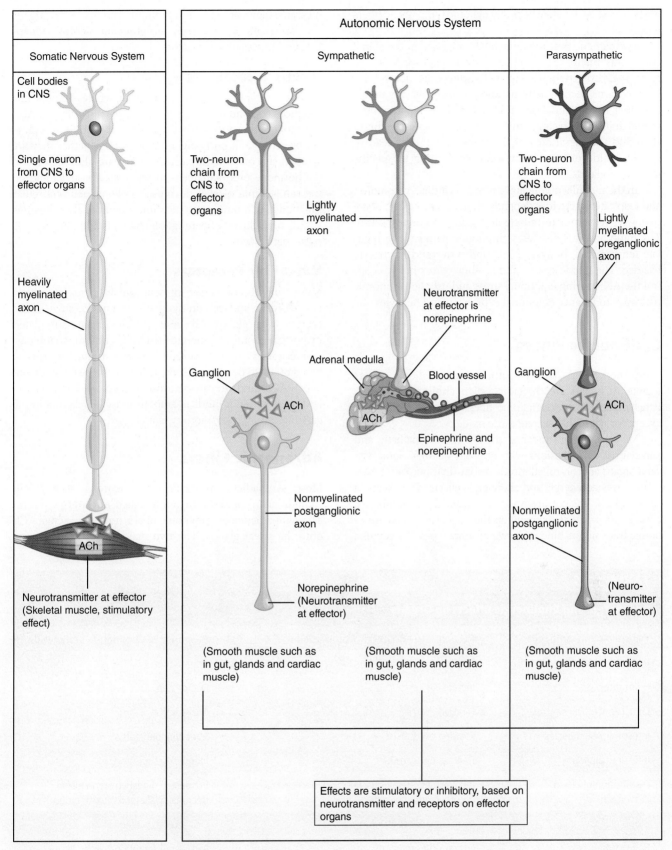

FIGURE 12-7 Neurons and neurotransmitters of the SNS and ANS.

fibers release ACh, whereas postganglionic sympathetic fibers release NE.

Sympathetic preganglionic fibers originate in the spinal cord's gray matter. These fibers leave the spinal nerves to enter the paravertebral ganglia. Preganglionic fibers form synapses with second neurons, and the axons usually return to spinal nerves and visceral effectors. In the parasympathetic division, preganglionic fibers arise from the brain stem and the sacral area of the spinal cord. They lead to ganglia inside or near the viscera, continuing to specific muscle or glands.

In the medulla oblongata, control of cardiac, vasomotor, and respiratory activities depends on using autonomic nerve pathways to stimulate muscle and gland motor responses. The hypothalamus also uses autonomic pathways to regulate temperature, hunger, thirst, and water and electrolyte balance. The limbic system and cerebral cortex help to control the ANS during emotional stress and use the autonomic pathways to balance emotional expression and behavior.

Cholinergic Fibers

Sympathetic and parasympathetic preganglionic fibers secrete ACh and are therefore called **cholinergic fibers**. Parasympathetic postganglionic fibers are also cholinergic, except for those that secrete nitric oxide.

Most organs are innervated from the sympathetic and parasympathetic divisions with opposite actions. Some visceral organs are controlled mostly by one division. **TABLE 12-5** summarizes adrenergic and cholinergic effects. The effects of ACh and NE are not always either excitatory or inhibitory, because their action depends on the related receptor. Autonomic transmitters bind with two or more types of receptors,

meaning they can activate or inhibit various body targets. The two types of cholinergic receptors are **nicotinic receptors** and **muscarinic receptors**.

Nicotinic Receptors

Nicotinic receptors respond to nicotine, whereas muscarinic receptors respond to the toxin known as *muscarine*. All ACh receptors fall into these two categories. Nicotinic receptors are present on all postganglionic neurons, whether they are sympathetic or parasympathetic. They are also present on the hormone-producing cells in the *adrenal medulla* and on the sarcolemma of skeletal muscle cells at neuromuscular junctions. ACh binding to nicotinic receptors always causes stimulation, directly opening ion channels and depolarizing postsynaptic cells.

Muscarinic Receptors

Muscarinic receptors are present on all parasympathetic target organs and certain sympathetic targets, such as the eccrine sweat glands. All these effector cells are stimulated by postganglionic cholinergic fibers. ACh binding to muscarinic receptors causes either inhibitory or stimulatory effects, based on the type of muscarinic receptor on the target organ. When ACh binds to cardiac muscle receptors, heart activity is slowed. When it binds to smooth muscle receptors in the gastrointestinal tract, motility is increased.

Adrenergic Fibers

Most sympathetic postganglionic neurons secrete NE (noradrenalin), and are therefore called **adrenergic fibers**. The sympathetic postganglionic fibers, however, secrete ACh onto the sweat glands. The two major types of adrenergic

TABLE 12-5

Adrenergic and Cholinergic Effects on Organs

Visceral Action or Effector	Response to Adrenergic Stimulation	Response to Cholinergic Stimulation
Pupils of the eyes	Dilation	Constriction
Heart rate	Increasing	Decreasing
Lung bronchioles	Dilation	Constriction
Intestinal wall muscles	Slowing peristalsis	Speeding peristalsis
Intestinal glands	Decreasing secretion	Increasing secretion
Distribution of blood	Increasing skeletal muscle blood, decreasing digestive organ blood	Increasing digestive organ blood, decreasing skeletal muscle blood
Blood glucose	Increasing concentration	Decreasing concentration
Salivary glands	Decreasing secretion	Increasing secretion
Tear glands	No action	Secretion
Gallbladder muscles	Relaxing	Contracting
Urinary bladder muscles	Relaxing	Contracting

receptors are *alpha (α) and beta (β)*. Subdivisions of these types include α_1, α_2, β_1, β_2, and β_3. One or more of these subdivisions are present on organs that respond to either NE or epinephrine, and either excitatory or inhibitory effects can occur. The determining factor is which subdivision of receptor is the denominating subdivision on the target organ. When NE binds to the β_1 receptors of cardiac muscle, for example, heart activity increases. When epinephrine binds to the β_2 receptors of bronchiole smooth muscle, it relaxes, causing the bronchiole to dilate.

TEST YOUR UNDERSTANDING

1. Define the terms "preganglionic fiber" and "postganglionic fiber."
2. Which neurotransmitters are used by the ANS?
3. Classify cholinergic and adrenergic receptors.

Drug Effects

Specific drugs can be prescribed using knowledge of how they will affect their target organs, based on cholinergic and adrenergic receptor subdivisions. *Atropine* is a drug that is often administered before surgery to dry respiratory secretions and prevent salivation. It is an anticholinergic drug that blocks the muscarinic ACh receptors. Another use for atropine is to dilate the pupils of the eyes before examination. *Neostigmine,* another anticholinergic, inhibits acetylcholinesterase, allowing ACh to accumulate in the synapses. It is used to treat myasthenia gravis, which impairs the activity of skeletal muscles because of inadequate ACh stimulation. Depression may be relieved by using drugs that prolong NE's activity upon postsynaptic membranes of the brain.

Sympathomimetic drugs mimic the effects of sympathetic activity and include many over-the-counter cold and allergy medications. They stimulate α-adrenergic receptors to constrict nasal mucosa blood vessels, which inhibits secretions. Ideally, drugs that affect just a single subdivision of receptor will be used with more frequency in the future. Fairly recently, drugs that primarily activate β_2 receptors were discovered. They can be used for asthma to dilate lung bronchioles without activating the β_1 receptors (which would increase heart rate, an unneeded effect).

Autonomic Division Interactions

Because most visceral organs receive dual innervation from the parasympathetic and sympathetic divisions, both ANS divisions are partially activated. From both subsystems, action potentials fire regularly down the axons to cause antagonism that carefully controls visceral activity. One subsystem does dominate, however, and in rare cases, there is actual cooperation between them.

Antagonism is common in the gastrointestinal system, heart, and respiratory system. The fight-or-flight syndrome involves sympathetic increases in heart rate, inhibition of digestion and elimination, and dilation of airways. The parasympathetic division then reverses these processes when the

initial stressors have ceased. It is important to understand that the sympathetic division is still the primary controller of blood pressure, even when at rest. The vascular system is almost entirely innervated by sympathetic fibers. They maintain partial constriction of blood vessels continually, which is known as *sympathetic (vasomotor) tone*. Sympathetic fibers fire more quickly when blood pressure is insufficient to maintain blood flow. The blood vessels then constrict, and blood pressure increases. If it becomes too high, sympathetic fibers fire less quickly and vessels dilate. For the occasional treatment of hypertension, *alpha-blockers* are used, which block the responses in these *vasomotor fibers*.

Inadequate blood flow to body tissues is also known as *circulatory shock*. When this occurs, or when additional blood is required for activity in the skeletal muscles, the blood vessels that serve the abdominal viscera and skin strongly constrict. This shunts blood into the overall circulation to support the skeletal muscles and vital organs.

The parasympathetic division primarily controls the heart and smooth muscle of urinary and digestive organs. *Parasympathetic tone* is maintained, which can slow down the heart and maintain normal levels of urinary and digestive activity. This can be interrupted by the sympathetic division when certain stressors occur. Medications that block parasympathetic responses speed up heart activity and cause urine and feces to be retained. Most glands are activated by parasympathetic fibers, except for sweat glands in the skin and the adrenal glands.

The external genitalia provide the primary example of cooperative ANS effects. During sexual activity, erection of the penis or clitoris is produced by parasympathetic stimulation, which dilates the blood vessels. It is understandable why anxiety can impair sexual performance, because the sympathetic division takes control. Sympathetic stimulation causes reflex contractions of the vagina and ejaculation of semen by the penis.

FOCUS ON PATHOLOGY

Autonomic neuropathy is damage to the autonomic nerves, and commonly occurs as a complication of diabetes mellitus. Other symptoms of autonomic neuropathy include sexual dysfunction in both sexes, dizziness after standing up quickly, slowed reactions of the pupils, urinary incontinence, and abnormal sweating. Strict control of blood glucose levels in diabetics is the primary method of preventing autonomic neuropathy.

Imbalances of the PNS

Because of its widespread effects, imbalances of the PNS (primarily the ANS) can cause a variety of outcomes. These include hypertension, *autonomic dysreflexia*, and

Raynaud's disease. Autonomic disorders often cause the smooth muscles to be over-controlled or under-controlled. Hypertension is commonly referred to as *high blood pressure* and may be caused by overactive sympathetic vasoconstrictor responses due to continuous stressors. It is a serious condition because it causes the heart to work harder than normal, leading to heart disease, and may harm the walls of the arteries. Treatments for hypertension may include adrenergic receptor–blocking drugs, which counteract sympathetic nervous system effects on the cardiovascular structures.

Autonomic dysreflexia occurs due to uncontrolled activation of autonomic neurons. This life-threatening disorder is common in quadriplegics and those who have spinal cord injuries above the T_6 level, within 1 year after injury. Triggers for autonomic dysreflexia include overfilling of the urinary bladder or another visceral organ or painful skin stimuli. The arterial blood pressure then becomes dangerously high and may cause a blood vessel of the brain to rupture, which precipitates a stroke. Symptoms of autonomic dysreflexia include flushing of the face, headache, cold and clammy skin below the area of the injury, and sweating above the area of the injury. This disorder's actual mechanism of action is not fully understood.

Raynaud's disease is often caused by exposure to emotional stress or cold temperatures and is an exaggerated response of vasoconstrictive activities. The patient experiences intermittent attacks, with the skin of the fingers and toes becoming pale at first and eventually cyanotic and painful. The disease may be an uncomfortable condition or can cause severe constriction of the blood vessels, leading to ischemia and gangrene (death of tissue). Adrenergic blockers and other vasodilators are often used for treatment. If the disease is extremely severe, preganglionic sympathetic fibers that serve the affected regions are surgically severed (*sympathectomy*).

Dilation of the involved vessels can then occur, and adequate blood flow to the region is reestablished.

Effects of Aging on the PNS

The effects of aging reduce the efficiency of PNS function. There are structural changes in certain preganglionic axon terminals. These terminals become clogged with neurofilaments. Common symptoms of ANS dysfunction include constipation (because of reduced gastrointestinal tract motility) and both drying and infection of the eyes (because of a reduced ability to form tears). Other effects of aging on the PNS include *orthostatic hypotension*, which is defined as low blood pressure after changes in position such as standing up quickly. This occurs because pressure receptors become less responsive to changes in blood pressure. The cardiovascular centers become less able to maintain healthy blood pressure. Most of these effects can be controlled by implementing changes in lifestyle or using artificial aids. Older adults are advised to change position slowly, to allow the sympathetic nervous system to adjust the blood pressure. *Artificial tears* are eye drops used to alleviate dry eyes and resultant conditions.

SUMMARY

The PNS consists of peripheral nerves, which connect the CNS to the rest of the body. It is divided into the SNS and ANS. Peripheral sensory receptors are specialized to respond to stimuli. They include chemoreceptors, mechanoreceptors, nociceptors, photoreceptors, and thermoreceptors. Complex sense organs contain the receptors for the special senses, which include hearing, vision, equilibrium, smell, and taste. The somatosensory system serves the limbs and wall of the body. Sensory (afferent) nerves carry impulses toward the CNS, whereas motor (efferent) nerves carry impulses away from the CNS.

There are 12 pairs of cranial nerves and 31 pairs of spinal nerves. The main portions of the spinal nerves mostly combine to form complex networks called plexuses. Peripheral motor endings activate effectors via the release of neurotransmitters. The SNS stimulates skeletal muscles, whereas the ANS innervates glands, cardiac muscle, and smooth muscle. Reflexes are either inborn (intrinsic) or learned (acquired). A reflex arc is formed by five components: a receptor, a sensory neuron, an integration center, a motor neuron, and an effector.

The ANS is divided into the sympathetic and parasympathetic divisions. The sympathetic division signifies exercise, emergency, and excitement and uses fibers that originate in the thoracic and lumbar regions of the spine. The parasympathetic division signifies digestion, defecation, and diuresis and uses fibers that originate in the brain and sacral spinal cord. Preganglionic fibers leave the CNS to synapse with second motor neurons to make ganglionic neurons. Axons of second neurons are called postganglionic fibers. Sympathetic and parasympathetic preganglionic fibers secrete ACh and are therefore called cholinergic fibers.

The two types of cholinergic receptors are nicotinic and muscarinic receptors. Most sympathetic postganglionic neurons secrete NE (noradrenalin) and are therefore called adrenergic fibers. Imbalances of the PNS (mostly the ANS) include hypertension, autonomic dysreflexia, and Raynaud's disease. Common symptoms of ANS dysfunction due to aging include constipation, drying and infection of the eyes, and orthostatic hypotension.

KEY TERMS

Adrenergic fibers
Autonomic nervous system
Autonomic reflex
Brachial plexuses
Cardiac plexuses
Cauda equina
Cervical plexuses
Cholinergic fibers
Ciliary ganglia
Dorsal root
Esophageal plexuses
Ganglia
Inferior hypogastric (pelvic) plexus
Intercostal nerves
Lumbosacral plexuses

Mixed nerves
Motor (efferent) nerves
Motor endings
Muscarinic receptors
Nicotinic receptors
Otic ganglia
Parasympathetic
Pelvic splanchnic nerves
Perception
Peripheral nervous system
Phrenic nerves
Plexuses
Postganglionic fiber
Preganglionic fiber
Pulmonary plexuses

Reflex arc
Sensation
Sensory (afferent) nerves
Sensory receptors
Somatic nervous system
Somatic reflex
Somatosensory system
Special senses
Spinal reflexes
Stimuli
Sympathetic
Terminal ganglia
Ventral root

The following learning goals correspond to the objectives at the beginning of this chapter:

1. The types of somatic and visceral sensory receptors include chemoreceptors, which respond to chemicals in solution, including smelled or tasted molecules, changes in blood chemistry, and changes in interstitial fluid chemistry; mechanoreceptors, which respond to mechanical forces such as pressure, touch, stretching, and vibrations; nociceptors, which respond to stimuli that may be damaging, resulting in pain (stimuli include extreme heat or cold, excessive pressure, and inflammatory chemicals; various subtypes of chemoreceptors, mechanoreceptors, and thermoreceptors may be stimulated by these stimuli); photoreceptors, which respond to light, such as the receptors in the retinas of the eyes; and thermoreceptors, which respond to temperature changes.

2. The somatosensory system is the part of the sensory system that serves the wall of the body and the limbs. It has three primary levels of neural integration: the receptor level, which consists of sensory receptors; the circuit level, in which processing occurs in ascending pathways; and the perceptual levels, in which processing occurs in cortical sensory levels.

3. The 12 cranial nerves are as follows: I, olfactory; II, optic; III, oculomotor; IV, trochlear; V, trigeminal; VI, abducens; VII, facial; VIII, vestibulocochlear; IX, glossopharyngeal; X, vagus; XI, accessory; and XII, hypoglossal.

4. Reflexes can be either inborn (intrinsic) or learned (acquired). Inborn reflexes are rapid, predictable motor responses to stimuli. Learned reflexes develop from repetition over time. The five essential components of a reflex arc are a receptor, a sensory neuron, an integration center, a motor neuron, and an effector. Reflexes are functionally classified as somatic or autonomic (visceral). Somatic reflexes activate skeletal muscle, whereas autonomic reflexes activate visceral effectors, which include smooth or cardiac muscle or glands. Spinal reflexes are somatic reflexes controlled by the spinal cord, often without direct involvement of higher brain centers. The brain can intercede on spinal reflexes due to continuous monitoring. Spinal shock may occur if the spinal cord is transected. Tests of somatic reflexes are used to assess nervous system functioning.

5. Dual innervation of the autonomic nervous system helps to balance the sympathetic and parasympathetic divisions. Via dual innervation, the divisions counterbalance each other, keeping the systems of the body functioning normally. Both divisions generally cause opposite effects on the same visceral organs. Cooperative dual innervations involve the fibers of both systems working together to produce a response. Dual innervations may also be antagonistic or complementary.

6. In the sympathetic division, all preganglionic fibers arise from cell bodies of preganglionic neurons in the spinal cord, from the level of T_1 down to L_2; hence, another name is the "thoracolumbar division." The many preganglionic sympathetic neurons in the spinal cord gray matter form the lateral horns, which are just posterolateral to the ventral horns that contain the somatic motor neurons. After leaving the spinal cord via the ventral root, preganglionic sympathetic fibers pass through a white ramus communicans to enter an adjoining sympathetic trunk ganglion that forms part of the sympathetic trunk. The sympathetic trunks consist of the sympathetic ganglia and fibers that run from one ganglion to another. Sympathetic fibers arise only from the thoracic and lumbar spinal cord segments. Once a preganglionic axon reaches a trunk ganglion, it can either synapse at the same level, synapse at a higher or lower level, or synapse in a distant collateral ganglion. In the parasympathetic division, also called the craniosacral division, preganglionic fibers emerge from opposite ends of the CNS (the brain stem and sacral spinal cord). Preganglionic axons extend from the CNS to nearly reach the structures they innervate. The axons then synapse with postganglionic neurons in the terminal ganglia. Short postganglionic axons emerge from the terminal ganglia to synapse with nearby effector cells.

7. In the ANS, preganglionic neurons are the cell bodies of the first neurons and are found in the brain or spinal cord. Their axons synapse with second motor neurons, also known as postganglionic or ganglionic neurons. Their cell bodies are in autonomic ganglia outside the CNS. Their axons extend to effector organs. Preganglionic axons are thin and lightly myelinated. Postganglionic axons are thinner and nonmyelinated. Conduction through the autonomic efferent chain is therefore slower than conduction in the somatic motor system. Much of the length of pre- and postganglionic fibers are within the spinal and cranial nerves. Autonomic ganglia are motor ganglia that are sites of synapse and information transmission from preganglionic to postganglionic neurons.

8. The sympathetic and parasympathetic divisions of the PNS have many differences. The sympathetic division mobilizes the body during activity, whereas the parasympathetic division promotes maintenance functions and conserves energy. Often, one division stimulates reactions while the other inhibits them. The sympathetic division can be thought of as the "E" division because it is in charge of emergencies, excitement, and exercise. The parasympathetic division can be thought of as the "D" division because it is in charge of digestion, defecation, and diuresis. The two divisions maintain a dynamic antagonism so they can balance homeostasis. Sympathetic fibers are thoracolumbar in origination, whereas parasympathetic fibers are craniosacral. The sympathetic division has short preganglionic fibers and long postganglionic fibers, which is the opposite of the parasympathetic division. Sympathetic ganglia lie close to the spinal cord, whereas most parasympathetic ganglia are located in the visceral effector organs.

9. Cholinergic neurons and their resultant fibers release ACh. Adrenergic neurons and their fibers release NE. In the ANS, ACh is secreted by somatic motor neurons as well as all ANS preganglionic axons and all parasympathetic postganglionic axons at synapses with their effectors. Most sympathetic postganglionic axons release NE and are therefore "adrenergic fibers," except for sympathetic postganglionic fibers, which secrete ACh onto sweat glands. The action of either neurotransmitter depends on the receptor to which it binds. Each binds with two or more types of receptors, exerting different effects (activation or inhibition) at different targets.

10. The two types of cholinergic receptors, which bind ACh, are named for drugs that bind to them, mimicking the effects of ACh. Nicotinic receptors respond to nicotine. Muscarinic receptors can be activated by muscarine, a poison that comes from mushrooms. Nicotinic receptors are found on the sarcolemma of skeletal muscle cells, at neuromuscular junctions, sympathetic and parasympathetic postganglionic neurons, and the cells of the adrenal medulla that produce hormones. ACh binding to these receptors is always stimulatory. Muscarinic receptors exist on all effector cells that are stimulated by postganglionic cholinergic fibers. These includes all parasympathetic target organs and some sympathetic targets, such as eccrine sweat glands. ACh binding can be either inhibitory or stimulatory, based on the subclass of receptor.

CRITICAL THINKING QUESTIONS

An Iraq war veteran went to see his physician. During a conversation with the receptionist, he got very angry about his bill and couldn't be calmed down. The physician asked him to come back into the examination room for a private discussion. After a while, the physician was able to calm the veteran down.

1. In this scenario, which part of the ANS system released neurotransmitters that contributed to his stress?
2. List the other effects of this part of the ANS in a condition such as this.

1. Which of the following neurotransmitters is released by cholinergic synapses?
   A. serotonin
   B. acetylcholine
   C. norepinephrine
   D. adrenaline

2. Adrenergic fibers release which of the following neurotransmitters?
   A. dopamine
   B. acetylcholine
   C. norepinephrine
   D. serotonin

3. Which of the following cranial nerves attach directly to the cerebrum?
   A. olfactory nerves
   B. trigeminal nerves
   C. oculomotor nerves
   D. trochlear nerves

4. The brachial plexuses are composed of the anterior branches of which of the following cervical nerves?
   A. C_1 to C_3
   B. C_3 to C_6
   C. C_5 to C_8
   D. C_6 to C_7

5. Motor fibers of which cranial nerves transmit impulses to pharynx muscles, the salivary glands, and part of the tongue?
   A. facial
   B. glossopharyngeal
   C. abducens
   D. accessory

6. Nociceptors are sensory receptors for
   A. pain
   B. temperature
   C. physical distortion
   D. chemical concentration

7. The somatic nervous system initiates somatic motor commands that direct the
   A. contractions of smooth and cardiac muscles
   B. control of skeletal muscles
   C. stimulation of the autonomic nervous system
   D. activities of fat cells and glands

8. Adrenergic stimulation is able to do which of the following?
   A. accelerate heart rate
   B. decrease force of cardiac contractions
   C. decrease diameter of respiratory passageways
   D. increase salivation

9. The cranial nerve with a cervical origin in the spinal cord is the
   A. optic nerve
   B. hypoglossal nerve
   C. accessory nerve
   D. abducens nerve

10. A major nerve of the lumbar plexus is the
    A. sciatic nerve
    B. tibial nerve
    C. ilioinguinal nerve
    D. vagus nerve

11. Nerves that carry impulses from the CNS are only
    A. motor nerves
    B. mixed nerves
    C. afferent nerves
    D. efferent nerves

12. The sciatic nerve is composed of which two nerves?
    A. tibial and common fibular
    B. common fibular and tibial
    C. posterior femoral cutaneous and tibial
    D. pudendal and fibular

13. Which of the following cranial nerves only has sensory fibers?
    A. facial
    B. trigeminal
    C. oculomotor
    D. olfactory

14. A fracture of the ethmoid bone may result in damage to which cranial nerve?
    A. vagus
    B. optic
    C. olfactory
    D. accessory

15. If the dorsal root of a spinal nerve were cut, which of the following may result?
    A. complete loss of sensation
    B. complete loss of involuntary and voluntary movement
    C. complete loss of voluntary movement
    D. loss of neither sensation nor movement but only of autonomic control

1. Explain the relationship of the peripheral nervous system to the central nervous system.
2. Describe the function and components of the peripheral nervous system.
3. Define sensation and perception.
4. Describe the composition of a spinal nerve.
5. Compare and describe the autonomic nervous system and somatic nervous system.
6. Describe the subdivisions of the autonomic nervous system.
7. Explain preganglionic and postganglionic components of the autonomic nervous system and their secretions.
8. Describe the meaning and importance of sympathetic tone and parasympathetic tone.
9. In the elderly, explain manifestations of decreased autonomic nervous system efficiency that are commonly seen.
10. Identify the effects of sympathetic and parasympathetic activation of the sweat glands, pupils of the eyes, and the penis.

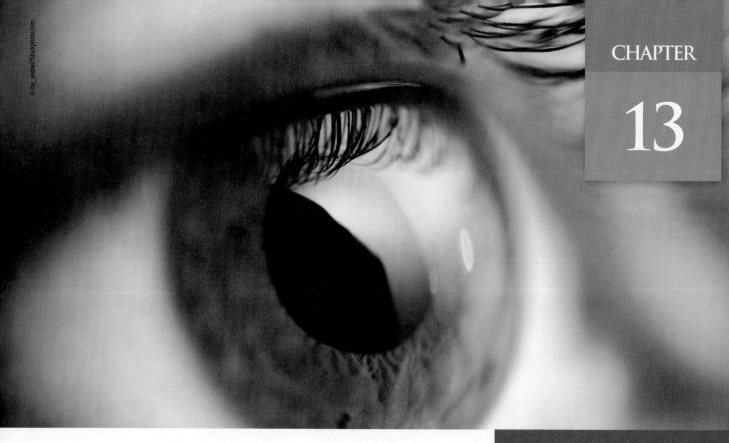

The Senses

OBJECTIVES

After studying this chapter, readers should be able to

1. Describe the sensory organs of taste.
2. Name five kinds of general receptors.
3. Name the five primary taste sensations.
4. Explain the mechanism for the sense of smell.
5. Describe sensory adaptation.
6. Identify the accessory structures of the eye.
7. Describe how refraction occurs within the eye.
8. Describe the structures of the middle and inner ear.
9. Distinguish between static and dynamic equilibrium.
10. Describe the parts of the inner ear and their roles in equilibrium.

Overview

The central nervous system (CNS) processes and interprets nerve impulses from sensory receptors that detect environmental changes. Feelings and sensations are the body's responses to these nerve impulses. The general, or *somatic* senses are pressure, temperature, pain, and touch. General sense receptors are found in the skin and deeper tissues. The general senses involve relatively simple receptors. Receptors that function in the special senses are much more complex than those functioning in the general senses. The special senses are smell, taste, hearing, equilibrium, and sight.

Types of Receptors

Sensory receptors are diverse but sensitive to certain types of environmental changes. These receptors send information to the brain as sensations. The brain interprets sensations as perceptions. There are five types of sensory receptors:

- **Chemoreceptors:** Stimulated by changes in chemical concentrations
- **Pain receptors** (*nociceptors*)*:* Stimulated by tissue damage
- **Thermoreceptors:** Stimulated by temperature changes
- **Mechanoreceptors:** Stimulated by pressure or movement changes
- **Photoreceptors:** Stimulated by light energy

When the brain becomes aware of sensory impulses, a sensation occurs. When the brain interprets the impulses, a perception occurs. Each type of sensation depends on which area of the brain receives the nerve impulse. Certain receptors, such as those measuring blood oxygen, do not trigger sensations. When a sensation is formed, the brain's cerebral cortex causes it to seem to come from the stimulated receptors in a process called *projection*. Therefore, the ears actually only "seem" to hear and the eyes "seem" to see.

The brain prioritizes sensory information to control its inflow. **Sensory adaptation** is the ability to ignore unimportant stimuli. It can result from receptors that become unresponsive (known as *peripheral adaptation*) or from CNS inhibition along sensory pathways of the cerebral cortex (known as *central adaptation*).

TEST YOUR UNDERSTANDING

1. List the various types of receptors.
2. Explain the terms *sensation* and *perception*.

General Senses

The general senses, touch, pressure, temperature, and pain, are spread throughout the body via muscle, joint, skin, and visceral receptors. Touch and pressure senses are derived from the following three types of receptors:

- *Free nerve endings:* Common in epithelial tissues, with free ends extending between epithelial cells; they control the sensation of itching.
- *Meissner's (tactile) corpuscles:* Oval yet flattened connective tissue cells inside connective sheaths, with two or more fibers branching into each corpuscle to end in small knobs; located in hairless skin (fingertips, lips, palms, soles, external genitalia, and nipples), they respond to objects that lightly touch the skin.
- *Pacinian (lamellated) corpuscles:* Relatively large structures of connective tissue, common in deeper dermal and subcutaneous tissues as well as tendons and ligaments; they respond to heavy pressure.

Temperature is sensed via *warm receptors* and *cold receptors*. Warm receptors are most sensitive to temperatures above 77°F (25°C), becoming unresponsive to temperatures above 113°F (45°C). At this temperature pain receptors are stimulated to produce a burning sensation. Cold receptors are most sensitive to temperatures between 50°F (10°C) and 68°F (20°C) to produce a freezing sensation. These receptors work rapidly, and sensation begins to fade away after approximately 1 minute of continuous stimulation.

Free nerve endings sense pain throughout the skin and internal tissues (except the brain). Pain receptors are stimulated by tissue damage but adapt to improving conditions poorly. They may send pain impulses persistently to the CNS regardless of whether tissue damage is continuing, making pain persist. Pain is triggered by releases of certain chemicals and deficiency of oxygen-rich blood (a condition known as *ischemia*) or the stimulation of certain mechanoreceptors.

Pain receptors in the visceral organs act differently from those located in surface tissues. When visceral tissues are stimulated on a widespread basis, strong pain sensations can follow. This type of pain appears to be caused by mechanoreceptor stimulation, decreased oxygenated blood flow, or accumulation of pain-stimulating chemicals. Visceral pain may seem to be coming from a different area of the body from the one actually being stimulated. This is known as **referred pain**. Heart pain, for example, may appear to be occurring in the shoulder or upper left arm.

Referred pain may arise from different areas, including the skin and viscera. Heart pain impulses travel through the same nerve pathways as do skin pain impulses, such as those from the skin of the left shoulder and upper left arm. A heart attack may therefore fool the cerebral cortex into interpreting pain impulses as if they are coming from the shoulder or arm instead.

Acute pain fibers are thin, myelinated nerve fibers that conduct nerve impulses rapidly and mostly produce sharp pain. Acute pain is usually sensed as coming from the skin. *Chronic pain fibers* are thin, unmyelinated nerve fibers that conduct impulses more slowly and mostly produce dull, aching pain. Chronic pain is usually sensed as coming from deeper within the body. Pain stimulation often causes both types of sensations—a sharp pain followed by a dull ache.

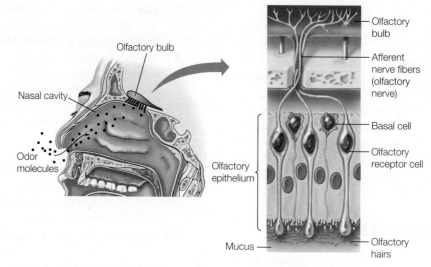

FIGURE 13-1 Location and structure of the olfactory epithelium.

The aching pain is often more intense, worsening as time passes, and can cause prolonged suffering.

The cranial nerves sense pain impulses originating from the head. All other pain impulses travel through the spinal nerves. The spinal cord's neurons process pain impulses in its gray matter to transmit them to the brain. Other neurons conduct impulses to the thalamus, hypothalamus, and cerebral cortex. Pain awareness occurs when pain impulses reach the thalamus; however, it is the cerebral cortex that controls the body's response to pain. The midbrain, pons, and medulla oblongata regulate how pain impulses move from the spinal cord. Biochemicals are released to block pain signals by inhibiting presynaptic nerve fibers in the spinal cord.

The posterior horn of the spinal cord releases **enkephalins** to suppress pain impulses of various severities. Enkephalins bind to the same receptor sites on neuronal membranes as the drug morphine. **Serotonin** is also released, which helps by stimulating further enkephalin release. **Endorphins** also have pain suppression actions and are found in the pituitary gland. Both enkephalins and endorphins are released in response to extreme pain.

TEST YOUR UNDERSTANDING

1. Differentiate between acute and chronic pain.
2. Define the term *referred pain*.

Special Senses

Although the general receptors of the sensory neurons are distributed widely throughout the body, the special sensory receptors are distinct receptor cells. They are located in the head region and are highly localized. The special senses of smell, taste, hearing, equilibrium, and sight require large, complex sensory organs, including the olfactory organs, taste buds, ears, and eyes.

Sense of Smell

The upper nasal cavity contains smell (olfactory) receptors. The sense of smell works closely with the sense of taste. The **olfactory organs** are yellow-brown masses of pseudostratified epithelium covering the upper part of the nasal cavity, the superior nasal conchae, and part of the nasal septum. Bipolar neurons surrounded by column-like epithelial cells are called *olfactory receptor cells* (**FIGURE 13-1**) or *olfactory sensory neurons*. The dendrites of these neurons are covered at the distal end by hair-like and mostly stationary cilia, which greatly increase the receptive surface area. Mucus from the *olfactory glands* helps to capture and dissolve airborne odorants. The sensory neurons are surrounded and cushioned by supporting cells that are columnar in arrangement. Short **olfactory stem cells** lie at the base of the olfactory epithelium. Unlike many other sensory neurons, those involved in olfaction are often damaged, with a life span of only 30 to 60 days. They are replaced when olfactory stem cells in the olfactory epithelium differentiate. *Odorant molecules* stimulate varieties of olfactory receptor proteins to differentiate between odors. These molecules must partially condensate from gases to fluids before receptors can detect them. The receptors of both smell and taste are *chemoreceptors*. These two senses complement each other, responding to different groups of chemicals.

Olfactory receptor cell fibers synapse with neurons located in the enlarged **olfactory bulbs**, which lie on either side of the ethmoid bone. These bulbs analyze impulses, which are transmitted along the olfactory tracts to the limbic system. Most smells are interpreted in the olfactory cortex within the temporal lobes of the brain and at the lower frontal lobes in front of the hypothalamus. Filaments of the olfactory nerves synapse with *mitral cells*, which are actually second-order sensory neurons. This occurs in complex *olfactory glomeruli*. Activation of the mitral cells causes impulses to flow from the olfactory bulbs through the olfactory tracts. Odors are consciously interpreted and identified to the part of the frontal lobes just above the orbit, and only some of this information reaches the thalamus. Another pathway reaches the hypothalamus, amygdala, and other limbic system regions. Emotional responses, to smells such as gas or smoke, may be elicited there, triggering the fight-or-flight response. Salivation and digestive tract actions are stimulated by appetizing odors. Protective choking or sneezing reflexes may occur if an unpleasant odor is detected.

Olfactory stimulation occurs as biochemical pathways are activated, allowing an influx of sodium ions, triggering an action potential. There are several hundred types of olfactory receptor cells. They can bind to several types of odorant molecules, and vice versa. Because the olfactory organs are high up in the nasal cavity, faint odors may be difficult to perceive. The sense of smell is more intense with a new odor at first, fading over time. Because the olfactory epithelium is located high up in the nasal cavity, it is not as efficient in detecting certain odors as it is in other animals. Sniffing the air pulls more odorant molecules across this epithelium, intensifying olfaction.

A single odor may be made up of hundreds of chemicals. Unlike the sense of taste, the sense of smell is not easily classified in regard to how it works. Our olfactory sensory neurons are stimulated by different combinations of olfactory qualities, which together can allow us to distinguish approximately 10,000 odors. In the human nose about 400 "olfactory genes" are active, with each gene encoding a unique receptor protein. Each protein is believed to respond to one or more odors, with each odor binding to several different types of receptors. Only one type of receptor protein, however, belongs to each receptor cell. Nasal cavities also contain temperature and pain receptors that are affected by irritants. Sharp, cooling, or spicy irritants create impulses from these receptors, which reach the CNS through trigeminal nerve afferent fibers. To smell a certain odorant, it must be in a gaseous state (volatile) as it enters the nasal cavity. It must also dissolve in the fluid that coats the olfactory epithelium.

FOCUS ON PATHOLOGY

The sense of smell may be reduced because of many different factors, including nasal congestion, colds, allergies, viral illnesses, aging, nasal polyps, nasal septal deformities, nasal or brain tumors, Alzheimer's dementia, endocrine disorders, head trauma (especially to the ethmoid bone), nervous disorders, and nutritional disorders.

Sense of Taste

The special organs of taste, the **taste buds**, number over 10,000. Most are found on the surface of the tongue, with tiny elevations called **papillae** (**FIGURE 13-2**). Taste buds are found on the tops of mushroom-shaped **fungiform papillae**, scattered over the surface of the tongue, as well as in the epithelium of the large and round **circumvallate papillae** and the side walls of the **foliate papillae**, which are also called *filiform papillae*. The circumvallate papillae are the least numerous yet largest of the various types of papillae. Between 7 and 12 circumvallate papillae form an inverted V shape on the posterior tongue.

In addition, about 1,000 taste buds are found in the roof of the mouth and the throat walls. Each taste bud has up to 150 taste cells (gustatory epithelial cells), which are replaced every 3 days. The spherical, flask-shaped taste buds have openings called *taste pores* and tiny projections called **taste hairs**. The taste hairs are the sensitive parts of the taste receptor cells. Stimulation triggers an impulse on a nearby nerve fiber, traveling to the brain. There are three

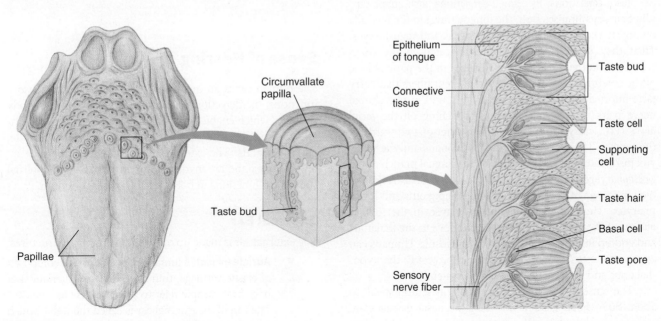

FIGURE 13-2 The taste buds of the tongue.

or more types of gustatory epithelial cells, which may either form synapses with sensory dendrites and release serotonin or lack synaptic vesicles and release adenosine triphosphate as a neurotransmitter. The taste buds also have *basal epithelial cells.*

Chemicals must dissolve in the saliva, diffuse into taste pores, and contact gustatory hairs before they can be tasted. A food chemical is known as a *tastant.* When a tastant binds to receptors in a gustatory epithelial cell membrane, a graded depolarizing potential is induced, causing neurotransmitter release. Although taste cells in taste buds are similar in appearance, there are five types:

- Those that sense *sweetness* (such as sugar)
- Those that sense *sourness* (such as lemons)
- Those that sense *saltiness* (such as table salt)
- Those that sense *bitterness* (such as caffeine)
- Those that sense *umami* or *deliciousness* (responding to specific amino acids and related chemicals such as monosodium glutamate, or MSG)

Other sensations that may be sensed are *alkaline* and *metallic* sensations, and it is widely believed that humans can take long-chain fatty acids from lipids. This may explain why foods containing fats are so popular. Additionally, there are *water receptors* located mostly in the pharynx. Their sensory output is processed in the hypothalamus and affects water balance, regulation of blood volume, and antidiuretic hormone secretion.

Flavors are tasted because of combinations of the primary sensations. The sense of smell also influences the flavors that are tasted. Although taste cells are spread over the tongue, they are, in general, concentrated in the following areas of the tongue:

- *Tip of the tongue:* sweetness
- *Sides of the tongue:* sourness
- *Front and sides:* saltiness
- *Back of the tongue:* bitterness and umami

Taste sensations, like smell sensations, also adapt rapidly. Sensory impulses from the tongue travel to the medulla oblongata via the facial, glossopharyngeal, and vagus nerves. Then they move to the thalamus (located in the diencephalon) and gustatory cortex (located in the parietal lobe of the cerebrum). Mostly, however, afferent fibers that carry taste information from the tongue are found in two cranial nerve pairs. The *chorda tympani,* branching off the *facial nerve (VII),* carry impulses from the anterior two-thirds of the tongue. The posterior third of the tongue and the pharynx just behind this are serviced by the lingual branch of the *glossopharyngeal nerve (IX).* The *vagus nerve (X)* is responsible for carrying taste impulses from the epiglottis and lower pharynx. The afferent taste fibers synapse in the *solitary nucleus* of the medulla. Impulses then move to the thalamus and end up in the *gustatory cortex* of the insula. Humans can appreciate tastes because of fibers that project to the hypothalamus and structures of the limbic system.

The sense of taste is actually mostly based on smell, to about 80%. Food lacks taste when the nasal passages are congested. Without smell, the sense of taste would be very inefficient, and much of what we enjoy from various flavors could no longer be appreciated. The sense of taste is intensified by food temperatures and textures. Thermoreceptors, mechanoreceptors, and nociceptors in the mouth are involved here. An example is a spicy pepper that becomes more pleasurable because, in addition to its taste, it excites pain receptors in the mouth.

Taste sensitivity among individual people differs widely. A variety of inherited conditions influences your taste sensitivity, such as the compound known as *phenylthiourea or phenylthiocarbamide.* Approximately 70% of people throughout the world perceive this substance as bitter, whereas others cannot taste it at all. It does not occur in food, but related chemicals do, mostly in certain Asian or Australian fruits.

TEST YOUR UNDERSTANDING

1. Name the five primary taste sensations.
2. Describe which types of receptors are used in the senses of smell and taste.

FOCUS ON PATHOLOGY

The sense of taste may be impaired due to a variety of reasons. Often, impairment of the sense of smell also results in impaired taste sensation. Causes of impaired taste include advanced age, Bell's palsy, colds, influenza, nasal infection, nasal polyps, sinusitis, pharyngitis, strep throat, salivary gland infections, ear surgery, heavy smoking, trauma, mouth dryness, certain medications, gingivitis, and deficiencies of vitamin B_{12} or zinc.

Sense of Hearing

The human ear is an organ that serves two special sensory functions: the detection of sound and the detection of body position, which enables us to maintain balance. The ear consists of three separate portions: the external (outer), middle, and inner parts. The external and middle ear structures are less complex and are involved only in hearing. The internal (inner) ear functions in both hearing and equilibrium.

External Ear

The external ear is made up of the following three structures:

- **Auricle** (*pinna*): A funnel-shaped structure composed of elastic cartilage, thin skin, and small amounts of hair; most people refer to this structure as "the ear." The rim of the external ear is called the **helix**, which is slightly thicker and has a fleshy *lobule* (earlobe)

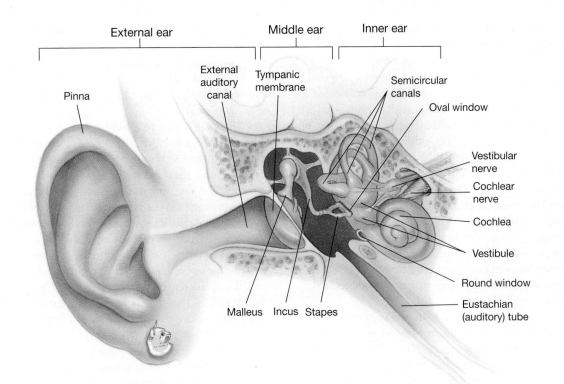

External ear | Middle ear | Inner ear

Pinna

External auditory canal

Tympanic membrane

Semicircular canals

Oval window

Vestibular nerve

Cochlear nerve

Cochlea

Vestibule

Round window

Eustachian (auditory) tube

Malleus Incus Stapes

FIGURE 13-3 The ear.

that dangles because of a lack of supporting cartilage. The auricle functions to funnel sound waves to the external acoustic meatus.

- **External acoustic meatus** (*external auditory canal*): An S-shaped tube leading through the temporal bone for approximately 2.5 cm, extending from the auricle to the eardrum. It is framed in elastic cartilage near the auricula, but its remainder is inside the temporal bone. Skin bearing hairs, sebaceous glands, and modified apocrine sweat glands (**ceruminous glands**) lines the entire canal. The ceruminous glands secrete **cerumen**, a yellow-brown waxy substance commonly referred to as *earwax*. Cerumen helps to trap foreign particles and repel insects from entering the ear. Normally, cerumen dries and falls out of the external acoustic meatus, providing a natural cleaning function. It is moved out because of the effects of jaw movements during talking, eating, and other functions. However, in certain people cerumen may become compacted if it builds up excessively, requiring medical intervention.
- **Eardrum** (*tympanic membrane*): A semitransparent membrane covered by thin skin on the outside and mucous membrane on the inside that actually moves back and forth in response to sound waves; it is the boundary between the outer and middle ear. The eardrum itself is thin, translucent, and covered on its external face by skin. It is a connective tissue membrane, which is covered internally by mucosa. The eardrum appears as a flat cone, with

its apex protruding medially into the middle ear. Its shape is maintained by one of the **auditory ossicles** (the malleus). Sound waves, collected by the auricle and directed through the external acoustic meatus, cause the eardrum to vibrate, transferring sound energy to the tiny middle ear bones, making them also vibrate. These collective vibrations reproduce the vibrations of the source of the sound waves.

FIGURE 13-3 shows the major parts of the ear.

Middle Ear

The middle ear (**tympanic cavity**) inside the petrous portion of the temporal bone is filled with air and contains the *auditory ossicles* (the *malleus, incus,* and *stapes*). These bones are attached to the tympanic cavity wall by ligaments and bridge the eardrum and inner ear to transmit vibrations. They are very small in size, with all three collectively smaller than a penny. The hammer-shaped malleus, attached to the eardrum at three points, vibrates along with it. Vibrations are passed to the anvil-shaped incus and then the stirrup-shaped stapes, which is held to an opening (the **oval window**) by ligaments. Vibration of the stapes moves fluid within the inner ear to stimulate hearing receptors.

The middle ear is lined with mucus. The superior oval window and the inferior **round window** are found in the bony wall that flanks this region. The tympanic cavity arches superiorly upward as the *epitympanic recess*, which forms the roof of the middle ear cavity. The *mastoid antrum* is a canal in its posterior wall and allows it to communicate with *mastoid air cells* in the mastoid process.

The ossicles also amplify the force of vibrations, concentrating the force, with pressure inside the inner ear much higher than the outer ear. Each middle ear is connected to the throat via the **auditory tube** (Eustachian tube), which conducts air and helps to maintain equal air pressure on both sides of the eardrum. The auditory tube is clinically known as the *pharyngotympanic tube*. It runs obliquely down to the middle ear cavity, linking it with the nasopharynx and mucosa of the middle ear. The auditory tube is normally flat and closed but opens briefly with yawning or swallowing, which equalizes pressure in the middle ear cavity with external ear pressure. If altitude changes, air pressure outside the eardrum increases, pushing it inward and impairing hearing. When air pressure equalizes, the membrane moves back into normal position, producing a popping sound, reducing normal hearing.

The ossicles are associated with two very small skeletal muscles, known as the *tensor tympani* and the *stapedius*. The tensor tympani emerge from the wall of the auditory tube, inserting on the malleus. The stapedius links the posterior wall of the middle ear to the stapes. Loud sounds cause these muscles to contract in a reflex action, limiting ossicle vibration and reducing damage to hearing receptors.

FOCUS ON PATHOLOGY

Middle ear inflammation (*otitis media*) often follows a sore throat, especially in children. This is because their auditory tubes are shorter than those of adults and are more horizontal. Otitis media is the most common cause of childhood hearing loss. Its acute, infectious form causes the eardrum to bulge with inflammation and redden. Antibiotics are typically used for treatment. If excessive fluid or pus has accumulated, the eardrum may need to be lanced in a procedure called an emergency *myringotomy*, quickly relieving ear pressure. A small tube is then implanted in the eardrum to drain pus out into the external ear. The tube falls out on its own within a year of placement.

Internal Ear

The internal ear is complex, with chambers and tubes forming the **bony labyrinth** (**FIGURE 13-4**). The *bony labyrinth* is an osseous canal deep inside the temporal bone, and the **membranous labyrinth** lies beneath it. Both structures contain **perilymph** fluid, and another fluid (**endolymph**) is also found in the membranous labyrinth. Inside the labyrinth structures are three **semicircular canals**, which aid

in equilibrium, and a **cochlea**, which functions in hearing. The bony cochlea is curved, resembling a snail's shell. The upper compartment of the cochlea (the scala vestibuli) leads from the oval window to the apex of the cochlear spiral. The lower compartment (the scala tympani) extends to the *round window*.

The egg-shaped **vestibule** is found in the central portion of the bony labyrinth, posterior to the cochlea and anterior to the semicircular canals. It flanks the middle ear medially, and the oval window is in its lateral wall. Two membranous sacs, the **saccule** and **utricle**, are suspended in the perilymph of the vestibule. They are joined by a small duct, and the smaller saccule is continuous with the membranous labyrinth. It extends anteriorly into the cochlea as the *cochlear duct*. The larger utricle is continuous with the anterior, posterior, and lateral *semicircular ducts* that extend into the semicircular canals posteriorly. Equilibrium receptor regions of the saccule and utricle are called **maculae**. They respond to gravity and transmit impulses concerning changes in head position.

Together, the semicircular canals and vestibule are known as the *vestibular complex*. The *semicircular canals* are found lateral and posterior to the vestibule. Each canal makes up about two-thirds of a circle. Their cavities project from the posterior section of the vestibule, creating an anterior, posterior, and lateral semicircular canal in each internal ear. In a vertical plane the anterior and posterior canals are oriented at right angles to each other. The lateral canal is placed horizontally. Through each semicircular canal there is a membranous *semicircular duct* communicating with the utricle anteriorly. Each duct has an enlarged swelling at the end called an **ampulla**. Each ampulla contains an equilibrium receptor region (**crista ampullaris**) that responds to rotational movements of the head.

The *cochlea* is a snail-shaped, spiral, and conical chamber that is very small—only about as large as a split pea. The cochlea links the anterior vestibule, coiling about 2½ times around the bony, pillar-like *modiolus*. The membranous cochlear duct runs through its center and contains the organ of Corti (*spiral organ*), the site of cochlear hair cells. Threaded through the modiolus is the *osseous spiral lamina*. Along with the cochlear duct, this divides the cavity of the cochlea into the *scalae*. The duct is separated from the *scala vestibuli* by Reissner's (vestibular) membrane and from the *scala tympani* by a *basilar membrane* (**FIGURE 13-5**). The cochlear duct ends at the cochlear apex. The scala vestibuli lies superior to the cochlear duct. It continues on from the vestibule and meets the oval window. The cochlear duct is also known as the *scala media*. The scala tympani, which are inferior to the cochlear duct, terminate at the round window.

The scala media is filled with endolymph, whereas the scala vestibuli and scala tympani contain perilymph. These scalae are continuous with each other at the **helicotrema**, which is another name for the cochlear apex. The *vestibular membrane* makes up the roof of the cochlear duct and separates the scala media from the scala vestibuli. The *stria vascularis* (external wall of the cochlear duct) is made up of heavily

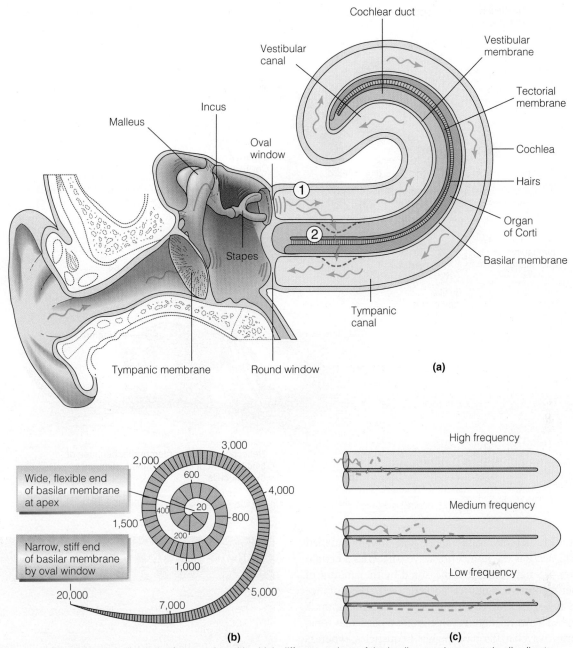

The numbers indicate the frequencies with which different regions of the basilar membrane maximally vibrate.

FIGURE 13-4 The inner ear.

vascularized mucosa, from which endolymph is secreted. The osseous spiral lamina and *basilar membrane* make up the floor of the cochlear duct. The basilar membrane is fibrous and supports the spiral organ. The basilar membrane is thick but narrow near the oval window yet becomes thinner and wider near the cochlear apex. From the spiral organ, through the modiolus, the cochlear nerve runs onward, eventually to the brain. It is a division of the vestibulocochlear nerve (VIII).

Cochlear hair cells possess large stereocilia on their superficial surfaces and serve as receptors for sound. Above the hair cells is the *tectorial membrane*, which is attached to the cochlea's bony shelf. Neurotransmitters are released to stimulate sensory nerve fibers and transmit impulses along the vestibulocochlear nerve to the auditory cortex in the brain's temporal lobe. Younger people can normally hear sound frequencies ranging from 20 to 20,000 vibrations per second. Most older people hear a smaller range of frequencies because of the aging process. The cerebrum interprets auditory impulses on both sides of the brain. **TABLE 13-1** lists the steps involved in the sense of hearing.

Sound is actually a pressure disturbance made up of varying areas of low and high pressure produced by a vibrating object and duplicated by various types of molecules. It depends on elasticity of various structures. *Sound waves* are series of pressures that radiate in many directions. They are also called *sound cycles*. A sound wave may be illustrated as an S-shaped curve, which is also known as a *sine wave*.

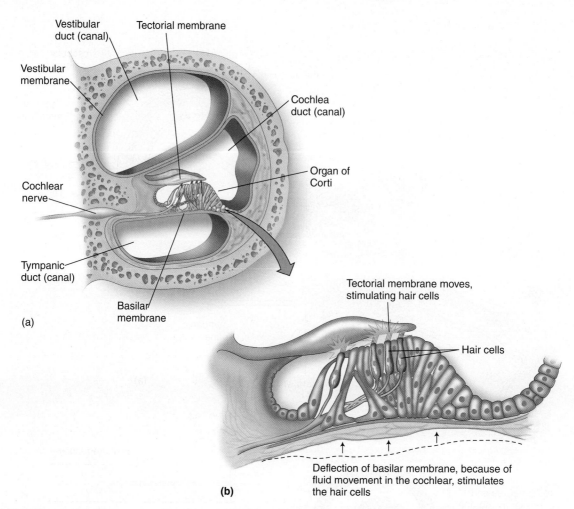

Vestibular duct (canal)

Tectorial membrane

Vestibular membrane

Cochlea duct (canal)

Cochlear nerve

Organ of Corti

Tympanic duct (canal)

Basilar membrane

(a)

Tectorial membrane moves, stimulating hair cells

Hair cells

Deflection of basilar membrane, because of fluid movement in the cochlear, stimulates the hair cells

(b)

FIGURE 13-5 The cochlea. The cross-section of the cochlea (A) and the spiral organ and tectorial membrane (B).

It contains crests (compressed areas) and troughs (rarefied areas). *Frequency* is the number of waves that pass a certain point over a certain time. It is measured by the amount of cycles per second via a unit called *hertz (Hz)*. The distance between two crests or two troughs is called the sound's *wavelength*. The wavelength is constant for a particular tone, and shorter wavelengths have higher frequencies, whereas longer wavelengths have lower frequencies.

Humans perceive various sound frequencies as *pitch* differences. Higher frequencies have higher pitches, and vice versa. Most sounds are mixtures of several frequencies, and this characteristic is called the *quality* of a sound, which provides richness and complexity. The height of a sine wave's crests is referred to as *amplitude* and signifies the intensity of the sound. *Loudness* is a term referring to how our ears interpret amplitude.

TEST YOUR UNDERSTANDING

1. Name the three tiny bones needed for the sense of hearing.
2. What is the function of the Eustachian tube?
3. Describe the semicircular canals.
4. Define the basilar membrane and its role in hearing function.

FOCUS ON PATHOLOGY

Tinnitus is a condition in which the ears experience ringing or clicking sounds without any auditory stimuli. It is usually a symptom of other conditions such as cochlear nerve degeneration or inflammation of the middle or internal ears or may be an adverse effect of aspirin or other medications.

FOCUS ON PATHOLOGY

Hearing loss commonly occurs with aging, which is called **presbycusis**. Heredity and chronic exposure to loud noises are the primary factors that contribute to hearing loss over time. Other factors include earwax blockage, inner ear damage, infections, and a ruptured tympanic membrane.

TABLE 13-1

How the Ears Hear

Action	Area of Ear
Sound waves enter.	Acoustic meatus
Waves of changing pressures cause reproduction of vibration from the sound wave source.	Eardrum
Vibrations are amplified and transmitted to the end of the stapes.	Auditory ossicles
Movement of stapes transmits vibrations to perilymph in the scala vestibuli.	Stapes at the oval window
Vibrations pass through and enter endolymph of the cochlear duct.	Vestibular membrane
Different frequencies of vibration stimulate different sets of receptor cells.	Endolymph
As depolarization occurs, cell membranes become more permeable to calcium ions.	Receptor cells
Inward diffusion of calcium ions causes release of neurotransmitter.	Vesicles at base of receptor cells
Neurotransmitter stimulates ends of those sensory neurons that are nearby.	Nearby sensory neurons
Sensory impulses are triggered.	Fibers of the cochlear branch of the vestibulocochlear nerve, the axons of which enter the medulla oblongata to synapse at the *cochlear nucleus*; the cell bodies of bipolar sensory neurons monitoring impulses are located in the *spiral ganglion* of the bony cochlea
Sensory impulses are interpreted by the CNS.	Auditory cortex of temporal lobe

FOCUS ON PATHOLOGY

Deafness actually is defined as any amount of hearing loss. It is classified as either *conduction deafness* or *sensorineural deafness*. Conduction deafness may be caused by compacted earwax, a ruptured (perforated) eardrum, otitis media, or *otosclerosis* of the ossicles. Otosclerosis is described as "hardening of the ear" caused by overgrowth of bony tissue. The base of the stapes becomes fused to the oval window, or the ossicles become joined together. The skull bones then conduct sound to the affected ear, altering its ability to hear normally. Otosclerosis requires surgical correction. Sensorineural deafness is caused by damage to any neural structures, including the cochlear hair cells and auditory cortical cells. As hair cells are gradually lost over time, this type of deafness may develop, although hair cells can also be destroyed in earlier life by explosive sounds or prolonged high-level sound exposure. Sensorineural deafness can also be due to degeneration of the cochlear nerve, a stroke, or an auditory complex tumor. Hair cells do not regenerate, but new medical advances such as cochlear implants may help people with this type of deafness. A recess is drilled into the temporal bone and the implant placed, which converts sound energy into electrical signals.

Both loudness and amplitude are measured in *decibels (dB)*, which are logarithmic units. Decibels of very quiet sounds begin at 0 dB, which is barely audible, up to the loudest sound possible to hear without extreme pain (120 dB). Every 10 dB signify an increase in sound intensity (amplitude) of 10 times. Severe hearing loss may occur with prolonged or frequent exposure to sounds louder than 90 dB.

Sense of Equilibrium

The sense of equilibrium consists of **static equilibrium** and **dynamic equilibrium**. In static equilibrium the position of the head is sensed while the head and body are still, maintaining stability. The organs of static equilibrium are located in the *vestibule*. The *vestibular apparatus* contains the equilibrium receptors in the semicircular canals and vestibule. The receptors in the vestibule are related to static equilibrium. Those in the semicircular canals are related to dynamic equilibrium.

In the labyrinth of the vestibule both the utricle and saccule have a tiny, flat *macula*, with many sensory *hair cells*, which respond to linear acceleration. These hair cells are surrounded by *supporting cells* and are embedded in an overlying **otolith membrane**. This consists of a mass of jelly-like material containing tiny stones made of calcium carbonate crystals called *statoconia*. These stones are known as *otoliths*, which are very dense and increase the weight of the membrane as well as its resistance to changes in motion.

When the head is upright, the hairs project upward into the gelatinous material. When the head bends forward, backward, or to one side, the hairs bend to signal nerve fibers. Nerve impulses travel into the CNS via the vestibulocochlear nerve, and the brain controls the skeletal muscles to maintain balance. In the utricle, the macula is horizontal, with the hairs remaining vertical while the head is upright. Therefore, the utricular maculae respond well to acceleration in the horizontal plane and the tilting of the head to the side. This is because vertical movements do not displace the horizontal otolith membrane. The situation is different in the saccule, because the macula is almost vertical and the hairs protrude horizontally through the otolith membrane. Therefore, this area responds best to vertical movements. A thin passage called the *endolymphatic duct* is continuous, with the narrow endolymphatic duct connecting the utricle and saccule. The endolymphatic duct ends in a closed cavity known as the *endolymphatic sac*. **FIGURE 13-6** shows how the maculae respond to changes in head position.

Fibers of the *vestibular nerve* synapse with these hair cells. The endings of these fibers are coiled around their bases. The vestibular nerve is another division of the vestibulocochlear nerve. Nearby *superior* and *inferior vestibular ganglia* contain cell bodies of the sensory neurons.

In dynamic equilibrium, when the head and body move or rotate, the motion is detected, aiding in balance. The organs of dynamic equilibrium are the three semicircular canals in the labyrinth. Each crista ampullaris is bound to a gelatinous mass known as the *cupula*, into which its sensory hair cells extend. The strands of the cupula radiate out and contact the "hairs" of the hair cells. The base of each hair cell is encircled by dendrites of vestibular nerve fibers. The free surface of every hair cell supports up to 100 long *stereocilia*, which resemble long microvilli. Every hair cell in the vestibule also has a single large cilium known as a *kinocilium*. The cristae are excited by acceleration and deceleration movements of the head and are mostly stimulated by rotational movements. Each crista has both supporting and hair cells that are similar to those of the cochlea and maculae. **FIGURE 13-7** shows the crista ampullaris within the ampulla.

When the head or body turns rapidly, the hair cells of the crista ampullaris are stimulated, but the fluid inside the canals remains stationary. The hair cells within the cupula are bent, sending signals to the brain. The cerebellum can predict consequences of rapid body movements and trigger the skeletal muscles to maintain balance. Additionally, mechanoreceptors associated with the neck joints communicate with the brain about position changes, and the eyes assist in maintaining balance. During rotation of the head and immediately after this movement, a condition known as *vestibular nystagmus* occurs, in which the eyes make a series of odd movements linked to impulses that are transmitted from the semicircular canals of the ears, because of movement of the endolymph. Vestibular nystagmus often occurs with the condition known as *vertigo*, which is a balance disorder similar to dizziness.

TEST YOUR UNDERSTANDING

1. Differentiate between static equilibrium and dynamic equilibrium.
2. Where are sensory hair cells located in the inner ear? Explain their functions.

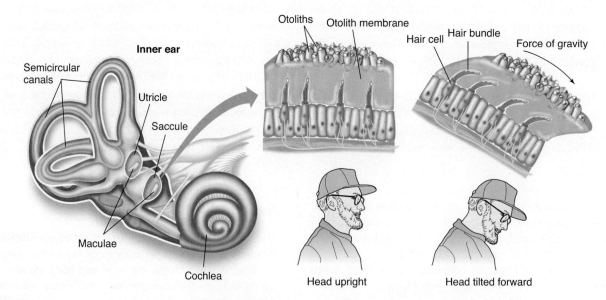

FIGURE 13-6 How the maculae respond to changes in the head position.

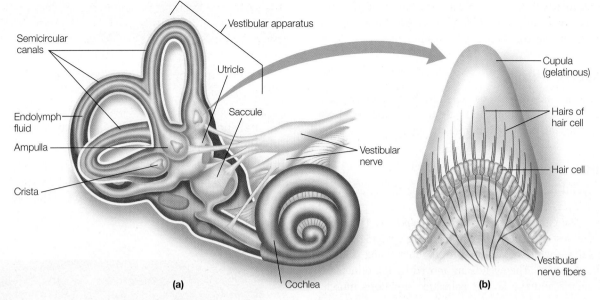

FIGURE 13-7 The crista ampullaris is located within the ampulla of each semicircular canal.

FOCUS ON PATHOLOGY

Impaired equilibrium may be linked to viral or bacterial ear infections, head injuries, and blood circulation disorders affecting the inner ear or brain. Aging and certain medications may also be related. Sometimes, impaired equilibrium is linked to low blood pressure, arthritis, or eye muscle imbalance.

FOCUS ON PATHOLOGY

Problems with equilibrium are completely reflexive and are often unpleasant. They include dizziness, loss of balance, and nausea. Sometimes nystagmus occurs even without rotational stimulus. *Motion sickness* is linked to a "mismatching" of sensory input, such as when you are inside a cabin on a ship. The cabin appears stationary, but the ship may be rocking to various degrees because of ocean waves. The confusion in stimuli often leads to motion sickness. Other signs that motion sickness is developing include pallor, excessive salivation, profuse sweating, and deep, rapid breathing. The condition is treated by either removing the stimuli or with over-the-counter antimotion drugs. However, these are most effective when taken before the stimuli occur.

FOCUS ON PATHOLOGY

All three parts of the internal ear may be affected by *Meniere's syndrome*, which causes chronic vertigo, nausea, and vomiting. Even standing up becomes almost impossible in this syndrome because of severe disturbances to equilibrium. Dizziness may last for at least 30 minutes or up to 24 hours. Hearing is often also impaired or lost, and a loud form of tinnitus is common. Meniere's syndrome may be caused by excessive endolymph, leading to distortion of the membranous labyrinth. Another cause may be rupture of various membranes, in which endolymph and perilymph become mixed. The condition may also be linked to excessive salt in the diet, caffeine, alcohol, or stress. Severe cases require drainage of excess endolymph, or when hearing loss becomes complete, surgical removal of the entire labyrinth. When mild, antimotion drugs, diuretics, and a low-salt diet may be effective in decreasing endolymph volume.

Sense of Sight

The sense of sight (vision) is our dominant sense, with approximately 70% of all sensory receptors found in the eyes, which are the organs of sight. Almost half of the cerebral cortex of the brain is used to some degree for visual processing. The eyes work along with accessory organs, including the eyelids, eyebrows, conjunctiva, lacrimal apparatus, and extrinsic muscles. All these organs are housed within the orbital cavity (or orbit) of the skull. Each orbit also contains blood vessels, fat, connective tissues, and nerves.

Eyebrows

The *eyebrows* consist of coarse, short hairs overlying the supraorbital skull margins and help to shade the eyes from light and to trap perspiration from the forehead.

Eyelids

Each **eyelid** has skin, muscle, connective tissue, and conjunctiva layers that collectively protect the anterior portion of the eye. The clinical term for eyelid is *palpebrae*. The eyelid is the thinnest portion of skin on the body, covering the lid's outer surface while being fused to its inner lining near the margin of the lid. The eyelids are moved by the orbicularis oculi muscle and the levator palpebrae superioris muscle. They are separated by the *palpebral fissure* yet are connected at the *medial canthus* and the *lateral canthus*. Internally, the eyelids are supported by *tarsal plates*, which are made of thin connective tissue. The tarsal plates also function to anchor the eyelid muscles. The orbicularis muscle encircles the eye, and its contraction causes the eye to close. In each eye the upper eyelid is more mobile than the lower eyelid, mostly because of the levator palpebrae superioris muscle, because it raises the upper eyelid to open the eye. The functions of the eyelids include protection as well as blinking, a reflex action that normally occurs every 3 to 7 seconds. Blinking causes secretions from the accessory structures to spread across the surface of the eyeball, which moistens it. These secretions include mucus, oil, and saline solution.

The *eyelashes* are hairs that project from the free margin of each eyelid. Eyelash follicles are innervated by many hair follicle receptors (nerve endings). Reflex blinking is therefore triggered by anything that touches the eyelashes, including the wind, an insect, and various particles. Within the tarsal plates are *tarsal glands*, which have ducts that open at the edge of the eyelid, slightly posterior to the eyelashes. The tarsal glands are modified sebaceous glands and produce an oily secretion that has two functions: preventing the eyelids from sticking together and lubricating both the eye and the eyelid. At the medial canthus of the eyelids, the *lacrimal caruncle* contains glands that produce *rheum*, the gritty substance that is often present when we awaken. Commonly, rheum is known as "sleep."

FOCUS ON PATHOLOGY

When a tarsal gland becomes infected, it causes a *chalazion* to develop, which is an ugly-looking cyst. When a smaller gland of the eye becomes inflamed, this is known as a *sty* or *stye*.

FOCUS ON PATHOLOGY

Inflammation of the conjunctiva is known as *conjunctivitis*. When caused by allergens, conjunctivitis is not contagious. However, the viral and bacterial forms are highly contagious. Signs and symptoms include pink or red color of the sclera, swelling of the conjunctiva, discharge of tears or pus, itchy or scratchy eyes, burning, photophobia, and crusting of the eyelids or eyelashes. Conjunctivitis is also known as *pink eye*.

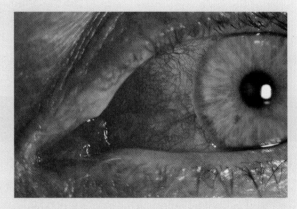

Conjunctivitis. (Courtesy of John T. Halgren, M.D./University of Nebraska Medical Center.)

Conjunctiva

The **conjunctiva**, also known as the *palpebral conjunctiva*, is a clear mucous membrane lining the inner eyelids. It folds back, covering the anterior eyeball surface (except for the central cornea). In the area where it folds back, it is described as the *bulbar* or *ocular conjunctiva*. The area where the palpebral conjunctiva becomes continuous with the bulbar conjunctiva is called the *fornix*. The primary function of the conjunctiva is to produce mucus that lubricates the eyes and prevents drying.

Lacrimal Apparatus

The lacrimal apparatus contains the **lacrimal gland**, which secretes tears. It also has a series of ducts carrying tears into the nasal cavity (**FIGURE 13-8**). The lacrimal gland actually lies in the orbit over the eye's lateral end and can be seen through the conjunctiva when the eyelid is everted. The diluted saline solution released by the lacrimal gland is known as *lacrimal secretion*, or collectively as *tears*. Tears are actually secreted continuously, exiting through tubules flowing downward and medially across the eye. Tears moisten and lubricate the eye and eyelid linings and contain the hormone *lysozyme*, which is antibacterial. Tears also contain mucus and antibodies. Collectively, the components of tears

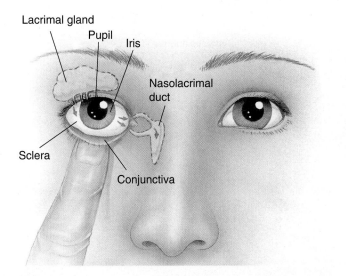

FIGURE 13-8 The lacrimal gland, lacrimal sac, and nasolacrimal duct.

clean and protect the surface of the eye while they lubricate and moist it. Blinking of the eye causes tears to spread down and across the eye to the *medial commissure*. Here, through the two tiny *lacrimal puncta*, they enter the paired *lacrimal canaliculi*. The lacrimal puncta appear as two tiny red dots on each eyelid's medial margin. The tears then drain from the lacrimal canaliculi into the *lacrimal sac* and *nasolacrimal duct*. This duct empties into the nasal cavity at the *inferior nasal meatus*.

Extrinsic Eye Muscles

The six **extrinsic muscles** move the eye in many directions, with each strap-like muscle associated with one primary action. The extrinsic muscles originate from the walls of the eye orbit. They insert into the eyeball's outer surface, allowing the eye to follow moving objects. These muscles also hold it within the orbit and help to maintain the eyeball's shape. The extrinsic muscles are shown in **FIGURE 13-9**. **TABLE 13-2** lists the functions of the extrinsic and eyelid muscles.

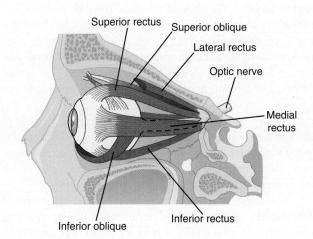

FIGURE 13-9 The six extrinsic muscles of the eye.

TABLE 13-2		
Extrinsic and Eyelid Muscle Functions		
Muscle	**Function**	**Control Nerve**
Eyelid muscles		
Orbicularis oculi	Closes the eye	Facial nerve (VII)
Levator palpebrae superioris	Opens the eye	Oculomotor nerve (III)
Extrinsic muscles		
Superior rectus	Rotates the eye upward, toward midline	Oculomotor nerve (III)
Inferior rectus	Rotates the eye downward, toward midline	Oculomotor nerve (III)
Medial rectus	Rotates the eye toward midline	Oculomotor nerve (III)
Lateral rectus	Rotates the eye away from midline	Abducens nerve (VI)
Superior oblique	Rotates the eye downward, away from midline	Trochlear nerve (IV)
Inferior oblique	Rotates the eye upward, away from midline	Oculomotor nerve (III)

Originating from the *common tendinous (annular) ring* are four *rectus muscles*. The common tendinous ring is found at the back of the eye orbit, and the rectus muscles connect it to their insertion points on the eyeball. Each rectus muscle is named for its location and the movements it controls: *superior, inferior, lateral,* and *medial*. The *superior oblique muscle* originates with the rectus muscles and lies along the medial wall of the eye orbit. However, it soon makes a nearly 90-degree (right-angle) turn to pass through the **trochlea**, a loop of fibrocartilage on the superolateral eyeball.

From the medial orbit surface, the *inferior oblique muscle* originates to run laterally and obliquely. It inserts on the inferolateral eye surface. The two oblique muscles assist the four rectus muscles in providing even more defined eye movements. The lateral rectus and superior oblique muscles are innervated by, respectively, the *abducens* and *trochlear* nerves. However, all of the extrinsic eye muscles are served by the *oculomotor* nerves.

Anatomy of the Eyeball

The eye is hollow, spherical, and about 2.5 cm (1 inch) in diameter. Also referred to as the *eyeball*, it is slightly irregular in shape. It has three distinct layers—the outer, middle,

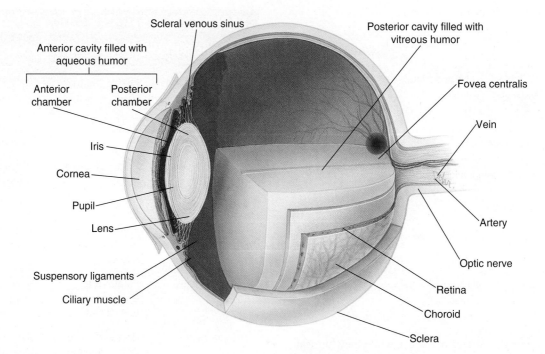

FIGURE 13-10 The eye.

and inner layers. The internal cavity of the eye is filled with *humors*, which are fluids that help to maintain its shape. **FIGURE 13-10** shows a transverse section of the right eye, with all three layers.

FOCUS ON PATHOLOGY

Strabismus is a condition in which the affected eye rotates medially or laterally. It may be caused by congenital weakness of the external eye muscles. The eyes may then attempt to compensate by focusing on objects in an alternating manner. Some individuals are only able to focus the controllable eye. When this occurs, the brain stops processing input from the deviant eye, which eventually becomes functionally blind. Eye exercises may be used to strengthen the external eye muscles, or a patch may be placed over the stronger eye so the weaker eye must be used. When these methods are not effective, surgery is indicated.

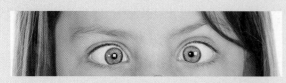

Strabismus. (© Justin Paget/Shutterstock, Inc.)

FOCUS ON PATHOLOGY

Diplopia is commonly known as "double vision." It may be caused by weakness or paralysis of specific extrinsic muscles or neurological disorders or as a result of acute alcohol intoxication. The affected individual sees two images instead of one because he or she cannot normally focus the images of the same area of the visual field from each eye. In diplopia, movements of the external muscles of both eyes are not in perfect coordination.

Outer Layer The fibrous, anterior layer or *tunic* bulges forward to form the transparent **cornea** (the "window of the eye"), which helps to focus entering light rays and is continuous along its circumference with the white **sclera**. The border between the cornea and sclera is called the *corneal limbus*. The sclera is opaque, protective, and the attachment for the extrinsic muscles. It is pierced at the back by the **optic nerve** and certain blood vessels. The visible portion of the eye is only one-sixth of its anterior surface. The remaining parts of the eye are enclosed in the walls of the bony orbit and cushioned by a layer of *orbital fat*. This layer of the eye is made up of dense, avascular connective tissue.

The sclera makes up most of the outer layer and is described as "glistening." The cornea is completely clear and controls much of the refractory power of the eye, on a constantly occurring basis. It has many pain receptors and other nerve endings. Touching the cornea causes reflexive blinking and tearing. It is the part of the eye that is primarily exposed and often damaged. Even so, it can regenerate and repair itself to a large degree. The cornea lacks blood vessels and cannot be affected by the immune system activities. Therefore, it can be transplanted between humans with nearly no risk of being rejected by the recipient.

Middle Layer   The vascular tunic or *uvea* includes the **choroid coat**, **ciliary body**, and **iris**. The choroid coat is joined to the sclera and has many pigment-producing melanocytes. It is therefore dark brown in color and rich in blood vessels. The choroid coat is also referred to simply as the *choroid* and forms the posterior five-sixths of the middle layer. Blood vessels of the choroid supply nutrients to all layers of the eye. The choroid helps to absorb light and prevent it from scattering and reflecting. The ciliary body develops anteriorly from the choroid and forms a thick internal ring around the front of the eye, with radiating folds (ciliary processes) and bundles of smooth ciliary muscles. The ciliary processes secrete the fluid that fills the *anterior cavity* of the eyeball. The ciliary body extends posteriorly to the *ora serrata*, which is the serrated anterior edge of the thick, inner portion of the eye's inner layer.

Many *suspensory ligaments* hold the transparent, biconvex **lens** in position behind the iris and pupil; the lens adjusts its shape to focus, a phenomenon called **accommodation**. In accommodation, the refractory power of the lens is increased. *Lens fibers* are the cells in the interior of the lens that have lost their nuclei and other organelles. The lens is supported vertically by the **ciliary zonule** and divides the eyeball into *anterior* and *posterior* segments. The body of the lens is formed by transparent, folded proteins known as *crystallins,* which are also present in the lens fibers.

The suspensory ligaments pull to adjust the lens and help it to focus, controlled by the ciliary muscles. Contraction of the ciliary muscles is regulated by the parasympathetic fibers of the oculomotor nerves. When the lens is no longer stretched, its elastic fibers recoil and bulge. This provides a shorter focal length, so an object close to the retina can be seen more clearly. The lens is actually enclosed by a thin, elastic capsule and is avascular, like the cornea. The lens enlarges throughout life because new fibers are continually being added. It becomes less elastic, more convex, and more dense. This gradually reduces its ability to focus light properly.

The iris is a thin diaphragm that appears as the visible colored portion of the eye, lying between the cornea and lens. The iris is continuous with the ciliary body posteriorly and contains two smooth muscle layers with groups of sticky elastic fibers that randomly form patterns during gestation. The muscle fibers of the iris allow it to reflexively change shape, varying pupil size. The iris actually contains only brown pigment, even though the irises of different individuals appear in different colors. Darker eyes simply contain more pigment. A newborn baby usually has blue or gray iris color because the iris pigment is not fully developed.

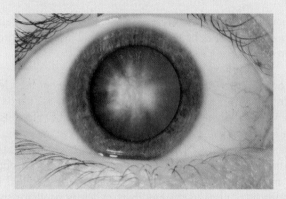
The iris divides the anterior cavity into an *anterior chamber* and a *posterior chamber.* The anterior chamber can be better understood as being "between the cornea and the iris." The posterior chamber can be better understood as being "between the iris and the lens." A clear, watery fluid called the **aqueous humor** is secreted by the epithelium on the inner surface of the ciliary body. All the anterior segment is filled with aqueous humor, which is similar to blood plasma in composition. The aqueous humor circulates from the posterior chamber through the **pupil** into the anterior chamber, and vice versa, at a rate of 1 to 2 μL per minute. When aqueous humor leaves the anterior chamber, it filters through connective tissue fibers near the base of the iris to enter the *scleral venous sinus* or *canal of Schlemm.* This is a passageway extend around the eye, at the level of the corneal limbus. Collecting channels then bring the aqueous humor to veins in the sclera. In general, this movement is at the same pace as the rate of generation at the ciliary processes. Therefore, aqueous humor is recycled a few hours after it has formed.

The *intraocular pressure* of the eye can be measured in the anterior chamber, because the fluid pushes against the inner corneal surface. This is usually done by *applanation*

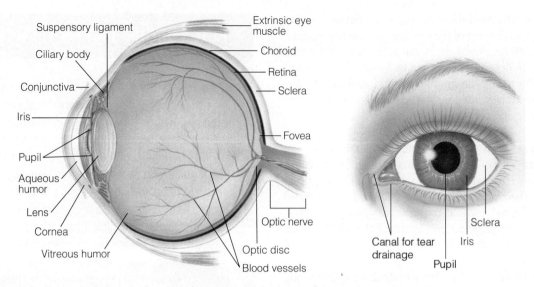

FIGURE 13-11 (A) The lens and ciliary body viewed from behind. (B) Dilation of the pupil.

tonometry, which involves a small, flattened disk being placed on the anesthetized cornea. Normal intraocular pressure is between 12 and 21 mm Hg.

The pupil is the round central opening of the iris and allows light to enter the eye. When the pupil contracts, less light enters, controlling the amount of light the eye needs to see in specific conditions. Close vision or bright light causes the circular *sphincter pupillae* muscles to contract, which constricts the pupil. Distant vision or dim light causes the radial *dilator pupillae* muscles to contract, dilating the pupil so more light can enter. Pupillary dilation is controlled by sympathetic nervous system fibers, whereas papillary constriction is controlled by parasympathetic nervous system fibers. The pupils commonly dilate because of an interesting sight, fear, or when we are trying to solve a problem. Pupil constriction often occurs because of unpleasant sights or boredom. **FIGURE 13-11A** and **B** shows the lens and ciliary body viewed from behind and the dilation of the pupil. **FIGURE 13-12** shows how accommodation works.

Inner Layer   The nervous tunic, which consists of the **retina**, contains approximately 130 million visual receptor cells called *photoreceptors*. These cells convert light energy, in a process called *transduction*. Light actually passes through the structures of the eye in this order: cornea, aqueous humor, lens, vitreous humor, and then through the entire neural layer of the retina. The retina also contains other neurons that process light responses and glial cells (glia). The retina has a complex structure of distinct layers, with a central depression (the **fovea centralis**) in the portion of the retina that produces the sharpest vision and a yellowish spot (the *macula lutea*). The fovea centralis is only 0.4 mm in depth. The **optic disc** is the point where nerve fibers leave the retina and join the *optic nerve*, in the posterior wall (*fundus*). This area is not strengthened by the sclera. Because the optic disc area lacks receptor cells, it is referred to as the *blind spot*. Light focused on the optic disc cannot be seen. The *posterior cavity* is filled with a clear, jelly-like fluid called **vitreous humor**, which along with collagenous fibers makes

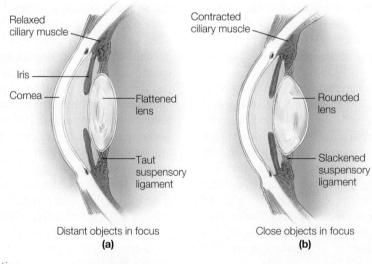

FIGURE 13-12 Accommodation.

up the *vitreous body* of the eye, giving it support and shape. The vitreous humor contains large amounts of water, contributes to *intraocular pressure* by helping to counteract the forces of the extrinsic eye muscles, supports the posterior lens surface, holds the neural retinal layer against the pigmented layer, and transmits light. The vitreous humor forms in the human embryo and lasts throughout life. Unlike the aqueous humor, the vitreous humor does not form or drain continually and is not always in motion. **FIGURE 13-13** shows the layers of the retina and how light waves enter. In total, only a small portion of the eye is involved in photoreception.

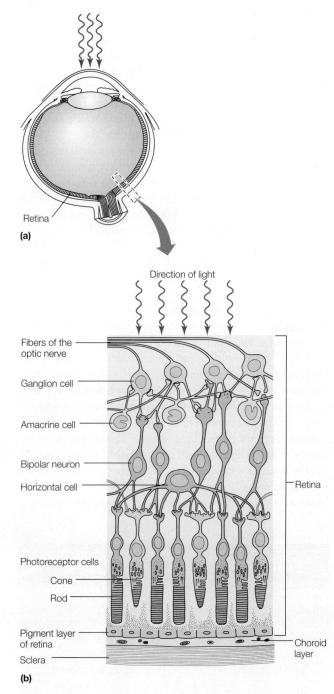

FIGURE 13-13 The retina: (a) gross section through the wall of the eye, and (b) arrangement of the cellular components of the retina.

FOCUS ON PATHOLOGY

Scotomas are abnormal blind spots in the field of vision at areas other than the optic disc. These permanent abnormalities remain in the same part of the visual field and are caused by optic nerve compression, photoreceptor damage, or damage to the center part of the visual pathway. Floaters, or small spots that drift across the visual field, are usually temporary and caused by cellular debris or blood cells in the vitreous body.

FOCUS ON PATHOLOGY

Prolonged period of reading can result in eyestrain because the eye muscles become tired. They tire because of the need for nearly continuous accommodation, papillary constriction, and convergence.

TEST YOUR UNDERSTANDING

1. List the six extrinsic muscles of the eyes.
2. What is the purpose of accommodation?

Light waves enter the eye, focusing the image of the object on the retina. When light waves bend to focus, the phenomenon is called **refraction**. It occurs when light waves pass at oblique angles from one optical density medium to a different one. Because the lens has a convex surface, it causes light waves to converge (**FIGURE 13-14**). The lens differs from the cornea in

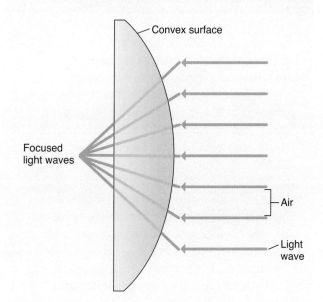

FIGURE 13-14 A lens allows light waves to be focused in the eye.

that its high elasticity allows it to change shape and bend light actively instead of on a constant basis, allowing fine focusing to occur. Most refraction occurs when light reaches the corneal tissues, but additional refraction occurs when the light passes from the aqueous humor into the lens. This additional refraction is required to focus light rays from an object toward a *focal point*, which is a certain point of intersection on the retina. The *focal distance* of the lens is the distance between its center and the focal point. Focal distance is determined by the distance of the object from the lens and the shape of the lens. The closer an object is to the lens, the greater the focal distance. The more round the lens is in shape, the more refraction occurs.

The neural layer of the retina contains the rods and cones. Rods have long, thin projections and provide black and white vision. Rods are hundreds of times more sensitive to light than cones, providing vision in dim light, without color. Cones have short, blunt projections and provide color vision. Cones provide sharper images, whereas rods provide more general outlines of objects. In the fovea centralis the ratio of ganglion cells and cones is approximately 1:1. Ganglion cells that monitor cones are called *P cells*. They provide information about color, fine detail, and edges of objects in bright light.

Up to 1,000 rods may conduct information via bipolar cells to just one ganglion cell. The larger ganglion cells that monitor information from the rods are called *M cells*. These are less numerous than the P cells found in the cones. In dim light, M cells function to provide information about object shapes as well as motion and shadows. Certain ganglion cells known as *on-center neurons* are inhibited by light striking the edges of their receptive field but are excited by light that arrives in the center of their sensory field. *Off-center neurons* function in the opposite way. Together, on-center and off-center neurons help to improve detection of the edges of objects in the visual field.

FOCUS ON PATHOLOGY

Normal vision is referred to as 20/20, which means you should be able to clearly see objects 20 feet away that most normal people can also see at that distance. If you have 20/30 vision, this means you must be 20 feet away from an object to see it clearly that a person with normal vision could see clearly at 30 feet. Once *visual acuity* falls below 20/200, even if contact lenses or glasses are used, the person is considered to be *legally blind*. Most of these individuals are over the age of 65. The term *blindness* actually means a total absence of vision because of eye or optic pathway damage. Conditions that may lead to blindness include diabetes mellitus, cataracts, corneal scarring, glaucoma, retinal detachment, and even hereditary factors.

Each eye receives a slightly different visual image. This is because the fovea of each eye is 2 to 3 inches, or 5 to 7.5 cm, apart. The view of the opposite side is blocked by the nose and eye socket. By comparing the relative positions of objects within the images seen by each eye, *depth perception* is achieved. Depth perception is defined as the interpretation of three-dimensional relationships among viewed objects. Visual images from both eyes overlap as we look straight ahead. Visual information of the left eye's field of vision reaches the visual cortex of the right occipital lobe, and vice versa.

Lateral to the blind spot of each eye is an oval region known as the **macula lutea** (yellow spot). In its center is the fovea centralis, which is the size of the head of a pin. The foveae have enough cone density for detailed color vision. Focusing directly on an object causes its image to fall on the fovea centralis. If an imaginary line were drawn from the object's center through the center of the eye lens to the fovea, this would establish the eye's *visual axis*. Both rods and cones are located in the deep portion of the retina near a layer of pigmented epithelium. The epithelial pigment helps to keep light from reflecting off of surfaces inside the eye. Visual receptors are only stimulated when light reaches them. The rods and cones synapse with approximately 6 million neurons that are known as *bipolar cells*. These cells then synapse inside layers of *ganglion cells* near the posterior cavity of the eye. A *horizontal cell network* continues across the outer retina between photoreceptors and bipolar cells. Where the bipolar cells synapse with ganglion cells, there is a layer of *amacrine cells*, which are involved in cellular communications and alter the retina's sensitivity. **FIGURE 13-15** shows the structures of rods and cones.

Rods and cones contain light-sensitive pigments. **Rhodopsin** is a light-sensitive biochemical in rods that is also known as *visual purple*. In the presence of light, rhodopsin breaks down into a clear protein called *opsin* and a yellowish pigment called *retinal* or *retinine*, which is made from *vitamin A*. The light-sensitive proteins in cones are made of retinal and three different opsin proteins. The three types of cones each contain one of three visual pigments, erythrolabe (sensitive mostly to red light waves), chlorolabe (sensitive mostly to green light waves), or cyanolabe (sensitive mostly to blue light waves). Therefore, the three types of cones are referred to as *red cones*, *green cones*, and *blue cones*. Color blindness occurs when certain cone pigments are lacking.

FOCUS ON PATHOLOGY

Color blindness is a condition that is more common in males than in females. It is caused by a congenital lack of one or several cone pigments and is an inherited X-linked condition. Most often, *red-green color blindness* occurs, in which these colors are seen as being the same.

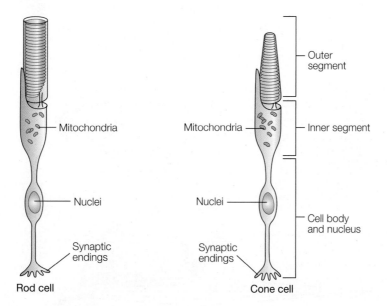

FIGURE 13-15 Rods and cones.

The process of photoreception involves photons striking the retinal portions of rhodopsin molecules in the membranes of photoreceptor discs. Opsin is then activated, which in turn activates transducin, a G protein. This activates phosphodiesterase, an enzyme that breaks down cyclic guanosine monophosphate. As cyclic guanosine monophosphate levels decline, gated sodium channels close. The dark current is reduced, and the rate of release of neurotransmitter declines. Each adjacent bipolar cell then senses that the photoreceptor has absorbed a photon.

Visual nerve pathways begin as axons of the retinal neurons and leave the eyes to form optic nerves. They then form the X-shaped optic chiasma with crossed fibers. The fibers from the nasal half of the left eye and temporal half of the right eye form the right optic tract, and fibers from the nasal half of the right eye and temporal half of the left eye form the left optic tract. Most fibers enter the thalamus and synapse in its lateral geniculate body, where visual impulses enter nerve pathways called *optic radiations*, leading to the visual cortex of the occipital lobe.

After you spend 30 minutes or more in the dark, nearly all visual pigments become fully receptive to stimulation, which is known as the *dark-adapted state*. The visual system is very sensitive at this time, with a single road hyperpolarizing in response to a single photon of light. If only seven rods absorb photons at one time, you experience a "flash" of light. Turning the room lights on at first seems excessively bright, but over a few minutes sensitivity to light decreases as *bleaching* occurs. This is soon balanced by the speed at which the visual pigments reform, which is called the *light-adapted state*.

In the brain stem, visual processing is integrated with movements of the head and neck. This affects how other brain stem nuclei function. The *pineal gland*, along with the *suprachiasmatic nucleus*, uses visual information to establish the *circadian rhythm*. This rhythm is the daily patterns of visceral activity that occurs because of the day–night cycle. This important cycle affects endocrine function, metabolism, blood pressure, digestion, the sleep–wake cycle, and many behavioral processes.

TEST YOUR UNDERSTANDING

1. Name the structures required to see color.
2. Explain light refraction.

FOCUS ON PATHOLOGY

The leading causes of vision and impairment include age-related eye diseases such as macular degeneration, cataracts, and glaucoma. Vision loss may also be caused by eye injury and birth defects.

Focusing Light on the Retina

Light is focused on the retina's photoreceptors because of the actions of the cornea and lens. The cornea differs from the lens in that it cannot be adjusted to focus on objects that are up close. The flexibility of the lens is controlled by the ciliary body muscles, which are attached via the suspensory ligament. **FIGURE 13-16** illustrates the refraction of light by the cornea and lens. The lens becomes thicker yet shorter and more curved to focus on a nearby object. This process is called *accommodation*. When a nearby object is viewed, the eyes actually turn inward to converge, which focuses the image on each fovea. *Convergence* occurs so much during our daily lives that it can cause straining of the extrinsic eye muscles. Eyestrain and headaches commonly result.

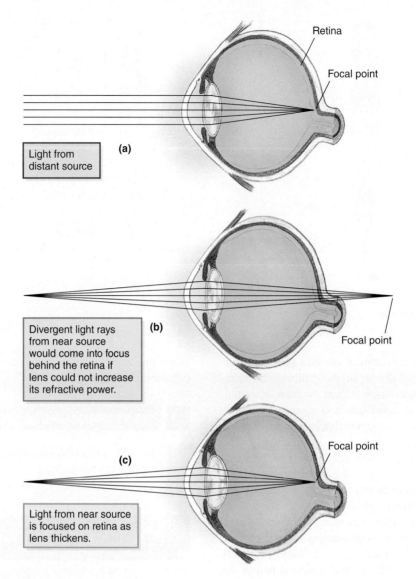

Retina

Focal point

Light from distant source

(a)

Divergent light rays from near source would come into focus behind the retina if lens could not increase its refractive power.

(b)

Focal point

Focal point

(c)

Light from near source is focused on retina as lens thickens.

FIGURE 13-16 Refraction of light by the cornea and lens.

FOCUS ON PATHOLOGY

Astigmatism is a condition in which the amount of curvature in the cornea or lens of the eye varies from one axis to another. Minor astigmatism is very common, and many people are not even aware they have the condition. As it becomes more serious, light passing through the cornea and lens is refracted improperly, causing distortion of visual images. Treatments include glasses, contact lenses, corneal modification procedures, and laser surgery.

Effects of Aging on the Senses

Aging affects each of the senses in varying ways. The eyes begin to lose the ability to see clearly up close or to focus when not in bright light. The tissues of the eyes may become

FOCUS ON PATHOLOGY

Night blindness is a condition wherein the function of the rods of the eyes is impaired. Also known as *nyctalopia*, it may make it very dangerous to drive a car at night because of the oncoming lights of other vehicles. Night blindness may be caused by nearsightedness, glaucoma, cataracts, diabetes, retinitis pigmentosa, or vitamin A deficiency. *Retinitis pigmentosa* is actually a group of inherited retinopathies that are the most common inherited visual abnormalities. In these retinopathies, visual receptors deteriorate over time, leading to blindness. The visual pigments of the membrane photoreceptors discs become mutated.

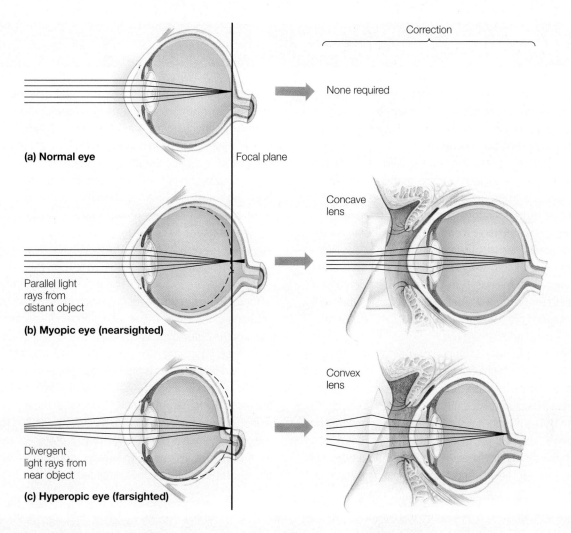

Correction

None required

(a) Normal eye

Focal plane

Concave
lens

Parallel light
rays from
distant object

(b) Myopic eye (nearsighted)

Convex
lens

Divergent
light rays from
near object

(c) Hyperopic eye (farsighted)

FIGURE 13-17 Common visual problems.

drier and the skin around the eyes may sag. The iris loses flexibility and cataracts may form slowly over time. Pressure changes in the eyes can lead to glaucoma. Macular degeneration destroys sharp, central vision. **FIGURE 13-17** illustrates common visual problems.

Hearing loss progresses with age and affects men more than women. The ear canals become thinner, earwax production changes, and the ability to perceive certain ranges of frequencies becomes difficult or even impossible. The eardrums thicken, and loss of hair cells in the ear brings about hearing difficulties. Causes of hair cell loss include nerve damage, trauma, loud noises, and certain medications. Aging also affects our balance and coordination and the perception of smells and tastes.

SUMMARY

Sensory receptors sense change in their surroundings and include chemoreceptors, nociceptors, thermoreceptors, mechanoreceptors, and photoreceptors. Each type of receptor is most sensitive to a distinct type of stimulus. Sensations are feelings resulting from sensory stimulation. General senses are associated with receptors in the skin, muscles, joints, and viscera. The general senses include touch, pressure, temperature, and pain. Special senses have receptors within large, complex sensory organs of the head. The special senses are smell, taste, hearing, equilibrium, and sight. Olfactory organs consist of receptors and supporting cells in the nasal cavity. Taste receptors consist of taste cells and supporting cells. The five basic types of taste sensations are sweetness, sourness, saltiness, bitterness, and umami (deliciousness).

The outer, middle, and inner ear work together to receive vibrations, which are perceived as sounds. The outer ear consists of the auricle (pinna), external acoustic meatus (external auditory canal), and eardrum (tympanic membrane). The middle ear (tympanic cavity) contains the auditory ossicles (malleus, incus, and stapes) and is connected to the throat via the auditory (Eustachian) tube. The complex inner ear is also important to establish the sense of equilibrium. It contains chambers and tubes that form its bony labyrinth, which lies above a membranous labyrinth. The semicircular canals aid in equilibrium, whereas the cochlea functions in hearing. The sense of equilibrium consists of static and dynamic equilibrium. In static equilibrium, the position of the head is sensed while the head and body are still. In dynamic equilibrium, motion is detected when the head and body move or rotate, aiding in balance.

The sense of sight (vision) is the dominant sense. The eye has three distinct layers. The outer layer is fibrous and anterior in position, bulging forward to form the transparent cornea. The cornea and lens of each eye refract light waves to focus an image on the retina, which transmits visual perceptions to the brain. The white-colored sclera makes up most of the outer layer. The middle layer of the eye, called the uvea, is vascular and includes the choroid coat, ciliary body, and iris. The lens is held in position by many suspensory ligaments behind the iris and pupil. The inner layer of the eye is the nervous layer and consists of the retina and its millions of photoreceptors. When light waves bend to focus, the phenomenon is called refraction. Photoreceptors known as rods provide vision in dim light, without color. Other photoreceptors called cones provide color vision.

KEY TERMS

Accommodation
Ampulla
Aqueous humor
Auditory ossicles
Auditory tube
Auricle
Bony labyrinth
Cerumen
Ceruminous glands
Chemoreceptors
Choroid coat
Ciliary body
Ciliary zonule
Circumvallate papillae
Cochlea
Conjunctiva
Cornea
Crista ampullaris
Dynamic equilibrium
Eardrum

Endolymph
Endorphins
Enkephalins
External acoustic meatus
Extrinsic muscles
Eyelid
Foliate papillae
Fovea centralis
Fungiform papillae
Helicotrema
Helix
Iris
Lacrimal gland
Lens
Macula lutea
Maculae
Mechanoreceptors
Membranous labyrinth
Olfactory bulbs
Olfactory organs

Olfactory stem cells
Optic disc
Optic nerve
Otolith membrane
Oval window
Pain receptors
Papillae
Perilymph
Photoreceptors
Presbycusis
Pupil
Referred pain
Refraction
Retina
Rhodopsin
Round window
Saccule
Sclera
Semicircular canals
Sensory adaptation

Serotonin
Static equilibrium
Taste buds
Taste hairs

Thermoreceptors
Trochlea
Tympanic cavity
Utricle

Vestibule
Vitreous humor

LEARNING GOALS

The following learning goals correspond to the objectives at the beginning of this chapter:

1. The sensory organs of taste include over 10,000 taste buds, each of which has up to 150 taste cells. Taste pores have tiny projections called taste hairs, which are the sensitive parts of the taste receptor cells. Stimulation triggers an impulse on a nearby nerve fiber, traveling to the brain.

2. The five kinds of general receptors are chemoreceptors, pain receptors, thermoreceptors, mechanoreceptors, and photoreceptors.

3. The five primary taste sensations are sweetness, sourness, saltiness, bitterness, and umami (deliciousness).

4. The mechanism for the sense of smell concerns olfactory receptors, which work with the sense of taste as well. The olfactory organs are masses of epithelium covering the upper part of the nasal cavity, superior nasal conchae, and part of the nasal septum. Olfactory receptor cells have hair-like cilia, which help to differentiate among odors. Odorant molecules must partially condensate from gases to fluids before receptors can detect them. Impulses are analyzed by olfactory bulbs and interpreted in the olfactory complex of the brain.

5. Sensory adaptation is the ability to ignore unimportant stimuli. It can result from receptors that become unresponsive or CNS inhibition along sensory pathways of the cerebral cortex.

6. The accessory structures of the eye include the eyelids, lacrimal apparatus, and extrinsic muscles, all housed within the orbital cavity (orbit) of the skull.

7. The eye refracts light by bending light waves in order to focus. Light waves enter the eye, focusing the image of the object on the retina. Refraction occurs when light waves pass at oblique angles from one optical density medium to a different one. Because the lens has a convex surface, it causes light waves to converge.

8. The middle ear structures include the auditory ossicles (malleus, incus, and stapes), ligaments, and oval window. The inner ear structures include the osseous labyrinth, membranous labyrinth, three semicircular canals, the cochlea, round window, and organ of Corti.

9. Static equilibrium concerns the maintenance of stability when the position of the head is sensed while the head and body are still. Dynamic equilibrium concerns the maintenance of stability when the head and body move or rotate.

10. The parts of the inner ear that also function in equilibrium include the vestibule and its two expanded chambers (the utricle and saccule), with a tiny macula containing many sensory hair cells. When the head is upright, the hairs project upward into a gelatinous material. When the head bends forward, backward, or to one side, the hairs bend to signal nerve fibers. The organs of dynamic equilibrium are the three semicircular canals in the labyrinth. A swelling called an ampulla houses sensory organs, each known as a crista ampullaris. Hair cells within a cupula are bent to signal the brain.

CRITICAL THINKING QUESTIONS

A 69-year-old man went to his physician complaining about recurring dizziness and tinnitus in both ears. He also described a feeling of ear pressure. He characterized the dizziness as lasting sometimes less than an hour and sometimes the entire day.

1. Related to his condition, which structures of the ears may be involved in these symptoms?
2. What are the probable causes of this man's condition?

REVIEW QUESTIONS

1. Which of the following sensory receptors are the pain receptors?
   A. mechanoreceptors
   B. chemoreceptors
   C. thermoreceptors
   D. nociceptors

2. The general senses
   A. involve receptors that are relatively simple
   B. do not conduct action potentials
   C. have receptors only in the brain and spinal cord
   D. involve little input from the brain

3. Gustatory receptors are located
   A. in the nose
   B. on the surface of the tongue
   C. on the skin
   D. in the ear

4. How many types of taste sensations exist?
   A. 2
   B. 5
   C. 6
   D. 8

5. The lining of the visible outer surface of the eye is the
   A. iris
   B. cornea
   C. anterior chamber
   D. conjunctiva

6. The pigmented portion of the eye is the
   A. cornea
   B. iris
   C. pupil
   D. conjunctiva

7. The greatest amount of refraction occurs when light passes from the air into the
   A. cornea
   B. iris
   C. lens
   D. vitreous humor

8. The external auditory canal ends at the
   A. cochlea
   B. oval window
   C. tympanic membrane
   D. vestibule

9. The senses of equilibrium and hearing are provided by receptors located in the
   A. oval window
   B. inner ear
   C. middle ear
   D. outer ear

10. The thick, gel-like fluid that helps support the structure of the eyeball is the
    A. perilymph
    B. aqueous humor
    C. vitreous humor
    D. endolymph

11. Which of the following is not one of the primary taste sensations?
    A. sour
    B. spicy
    C. sweet
    D. salty

12. Sound waves are converted into mechanical movements by the
    A. round window
    B. oval window
    C. tympanic membrane
    D. organ of Corti

13. The hair cells of the utricle and saccule are clustered in the
    A. maculae
    B. cristae
    C. ampullae
    D. oval window

14. Cones are responsible for
    A. low light vision
    B. color vision
    C. night vision
    D. none of the above

15. The iris is a part of the
    A. nervous tunic
    B. fibrous tunic
    C. vascular tunic
    D. muscle tissue

ESSAY QUESTIONS

1. Describe the three types of receptors that function in the sense of touch.
2. Name the five primary taste receptors and the cranial nerves that serve the sense of taste.
3. Where are the locations of the olfactory sensory neurons?
4. Describe the structures of the external ear.
5. Define the bony labyrinth and the membranous labyrinth.
6. Compare perilymph and endolymph and their functions.
7. Describe the role of the vestibule, semicircular canals, and cochlea.
8. How do the rods and cones differ functionally?
9. Where is the fovea centralis, and why is it important?
10. Why can humans see so many colors when there are only three types of cones?

Endocrine System

OBJECTIVES

After studying this chapter, readers should be able to

1. List the hormones released from the anterior and posterior lobes of the pituitary gland.
2. Discuss from where the various types of hormones are derived.
3. Describe the location of the thyroid gland and identify the hormones produced by this gland.
4. Explain the functions of parathyroid hormones.
5. Describe the location, structure, and general functions of the adrenal glands.
6. Identify the hormones produced by the adrenal cortex and medulla.
7. Identify the hormones produced by the pancreas, and specify the functions of those hormones.
8. Describe the functions of the hormones produced by the kidneys, heart, and thymus.
9. Identify the hormones produced by the testes and ovaries.
10. Describe the hormones of special importance to normal growth.

OUTLINE

Overview

The endocrine system works along with the nervous system to regulate the functions of the human body to maintain homeostasis. However, the endocrine system works much more slowly than the nervous system, which can cause responses to occur within milliseconds. The *endocrine system* and its widely scattered glands secrete **hormones** that diffuse from the interstitial fluid into the bloodstream. The hormones, which are chemical messengers, act on **target cells**, regulating their metabolic functions. Hormones affect most body cells, regulating growth and development, balance of blood components, body defenses, cellular metabolism, energy balance, and even reproduction. Hormones are considered "long-distance" chemical signals.

However, there are also "short-distance" chemical signals: the paracrines and autocrines. **Paracrine** secretions are those that affect only neighboring cells. An example of paracrine actions is when somatostatin from certain pancreatic cells stops insulin release by other pancreatic cells. **Autocrine** secretions are those that affect the secreting cell only. An example of these chemicals are specific prostaglandins that are released by smooth muscle cells and cause contraction of these cells. *Exocrine glands* are those that secrete nonhormonal substances outside the body through ducts and include the sweat and salivary glands. The endocrine system controls body processes for long periods of time.

Endocrine System

The endocrine system, like the nervous system, uses chemical signals that bind to receptor molecules. Similarities and differences between the two systems are summarized in **TABLE 14-1**. The glandular cells of the endocrine system release hormones into the bloodstream, carrying messenger molecules throughout the body. Endocrine glands are ductless glands. They help regulate metabolism, controlling chemical reactions, transporting substances, regulating water and electrolyte balances, and aiding in reproduction, growth, and development. Endocrine glands release hormones into the surrounding tissue fluid. These glands usually have a large amount of both vascular and lymphatic drainage of their hormones.

The major endocrine glands include the pituitary gland, thyroid gland, parathyroid glands, adrenal glands, pancreas, pineal gland, thymus gland, and reproductive glands (**FIGURE 14-1**). The endocrine functions of the *hypothalamus* include the production and release of hormones, so it is considered to be a **neuroendocrine organ**. Also, several organs may secrete hormones, including the stomach, small intestine, kidneys, and heart. These are discussed in detail later in this chapter.

Actions of Hormones

Most hormones are either steroids or steroid-like substances, which are made from cholesterol, or nonsteroidal, including amines, glycoproteins, peptides, or proteins made from amino acids. Even low concentrations of hormones can stimulate target cell changes. The type of target cell influences the precise response that occurs. For example, epinephrine stimulates certain smooth muscle cells to contract but does not cause other types of cells to contract. **FIGURE 14-2** shows three classes of hormones, and **TABLE 14-2** lists various types of hormones.

Steroid hormones, which are synthesized from cholesterol, are insoluble in water but soluble in lipids, which are also known as *fats*. Therefore, they can easily diffuse into nearly any cell in the body, because lipids make up most cell membranes. Only gonadal and adrenocortical hormones are steroids. **FIGURE 14-3** depicts the following steps involved in a steroid hormone entering a target cell:

1. The steroid hormone diffuses through the cell membrane.
2. It binds to a specific protein molecule, which is its receptor.
3. The resulting complex binds inside the nucleus to certain parts of the target cell's DNA, activating transcription of specific genes into messenger RNA (mRNA) molecules.
4. These mRNA molecules leave the nucleus and enter the cytoplasm.
5. The mRNA molecules are associated with ribosomes, directing the synthesis of certain proteins.

TABLE 14-1

Endocrine System and Nervous System

Location or Action	Endocrine System	Nervous System
Cells	Glandular epithelium	Neurons
Chemical signal	Hormone	Neurotransmitter
Duration of action	Brief, or lasting for days even if secretion stops	Very brief, unless there is continued neuronal activity
Specificity of response	Receptors on target cell	Receptors on postsynaptic cell
Speed of onset	Seconds, minutes, or hours	Seconds

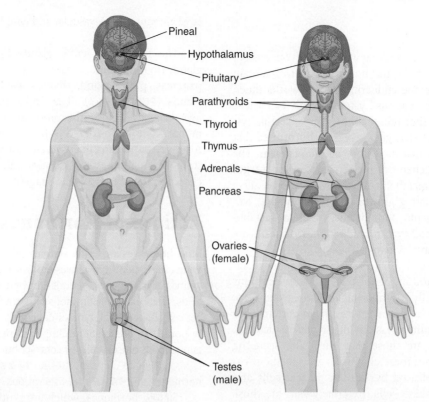

FIGURE 14-1 The organs of the endocrine system and the endocrine glands.

However, most hormones are amino acid based and not steroid based. Molecular sizes of these hormones range from simple amino acid derivatives to peptides to proteins. The nonsteroidal hormones usually bind receptors in target cell membranes by uniting with the binding site of their receptor. The activity site of a hormone is where it exerts its effects. Receptor binding can alter enzyme function and membrane transport mechanisms. The *first messenger* is the hormone that triggers this chain of biochemical activity. *Second messengers* are biochemicals in the cell that cause changes in response to the hormone's binding. Signal transduction describes the entire process of direct chemical communication from outside cells to inside them. **Cyclic adenosine monophosphate (cAMP)** is the second messenger associated with one group of hormones. **FIGURE 14-4** shows how it works, following the steps listed below:

1. A hormone binds its receptor.
2. The resulting complex activates a *G protein*.

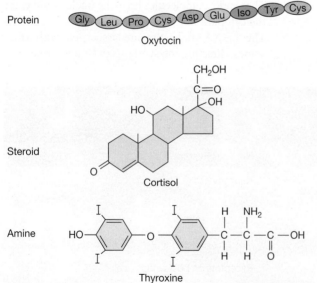

FIGURE 14-2 Three chemical classes of hormones.

TABLE 14-2		
Types of Hormones		
Type	Examples	Derived From
Steroids	Aldosterone, cortisol, estrogen, testosterone	Cholesterol
Amines	Epinephrine, norepinephrine	Amino acids
Glycoproteins	FSH, LH, TSH	Carbohydrates and proteins
Peptides	ADH, oxytocin, thyrotropin-releasing hormone	Amino acids
Proteins	GH, PTH, PRL	Amino acids

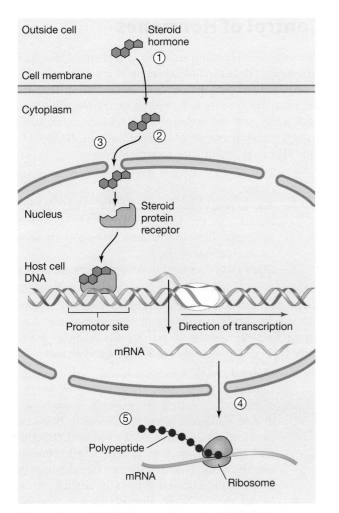

3. This activates the enzyme *adenylate cyclase*, which is a membrane protein.
4. This catalyzes the circularization of adenosine triphosphate into cAMP.
5. This activates enzymes called protein kinases to cause phosphorylation, altering the shapes of and activating substrate molecules. *Protein kinase C*, when activated, results in phosphorylation of calcium channel proteins. This open channels, allows extracellular calcium ions to enter the cells, and begins a positive feedback loop. This rapidly elevates intracellular calcium ion concentrations.
6. The calcium ions act as messengers, usually in combination with the intracellular protein **calmodulin**. Certain cytoplasmic enzymes are activated, resulting in stimulatory effects occurring when epinephrine or norepinephrine activates α_1 receptors. The activation of calmodulin is also used in response to oxytocin and to certain regulatory hormones from the hypothalamus.

Hormones act on their receptors in one of two general ways. The steroid and thyroid hormones, which are lipid soluble, act on receptors inside the cell, directly activating genes. The amino acid–based hormones, except thyroid hormone, are water soluble and act on receptors in the plasma membrane. These receptors are usually coupled to one or more intracellular second messengers by regulatory molecules known as *G proteins*. The intracellular second messengers mediate the response of the target cell.

Cellular processes are then altered by these steps to cause the hormone's effects, based on the kinds of protein substrate molecules present. The enzyme *phosphodiesterase* then inactivates the cAMP quickly. Because of this, a target

FIGURE 14-3 Five steps involved in a steroid hormone entering a target cell.

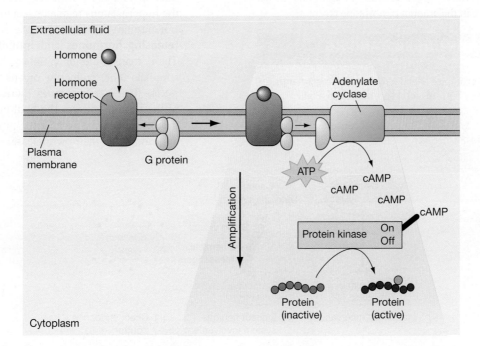

FIGURE 14-4 Cyclic adenosine monophosphate (also known as cyclic AMP or cAMP).

cell's continuing response requires a continuing signal from hormone molecules that bind the target cell's membrane receptors. Other second messengers include *diacylglycerol* and *inositol triphosphate*.

A third group of hormones, the **eicosanoids**, include *leukotrienes* and *prostaglandins*. These substances are biologically active lipids manufactured from arachidonic acid. Nearly all cell membranes release them. *Leukotrienes* release signals that regulate inflammation and certain allergic reactions.

Prostaglandins are lipids made from arachidonic acid in cell membranes of the kidneys, heart, liver, lungs, pancreas, brain, reproductive organs, and thymus. They usually act more locally than hormones and are very potent in small quantities. They are made just before release and are rapidly inactivated. They often have diverse or opposite effects. Prostaglandins stimulate hormone secretions and influence sodium and water movements in the kidneys, helping to regulate blood pressure. They increase uterine contractions during the birthing process and also have effects on blood clotting, inflammation, and pain.

A cell must have specific receptor proteins on its plasma membrane or interior, to which the hormone can bind, to respond to the hormone. For example, the receptors for adrenocorticotropic hormone (ACTH) are usually found on specific cells of the adrenal cortex. Oppositely, thyroxine receptors are found in almost all body cells because thyroxine is the main hormone that stimulates cellular metabolism. Target cell activation also depends on three additional factors: the blood levels of the hormone, the amount of receptors for that hormone on or in target cells, and the strength or *affinity* of how the hormone and receptor are bound. Hormones also influence the amount of receptors that respond to other hormones. An example is progesterone, which antagonizes the actions of estrogen by *down-regulating* estrogen receptors in the uterus. Conversely, estrogen enhances the same cells' ability to respond to progesterone by causing them to produce more progesterone receptors. The process of *up-regulation* involves the absence of a hormone, which triggers an increase in the amount of hormone receptors.

TEST YOUR UNDERSTANDING

1. List several examples of endocrine and exocrine glands.
2. What are the effects of steroid hormones on a cell?
3. Describe target cells.
4. Describe the types of hormones that consist entirely of lipid-soluble hormones.

Control of Hormones

Increasing or decreasing secretion of a hormone results in increased or decreased blood levels of the hormone. This is because hormones are continually excreted in the urine and broken down mostly by liver enzymes. **Negative feedback** is the mechanism that controls hormone secretion. It is triggered by an internal or external stimulus. **FIGURE 14-5** shows the steps of hormone secretion:

1. The nervous system directly stimulates certain glands.
2. The hypothalamus regulates the release of hormones from the anterior pituitary gland, with its proximity allowing constant communication about the internal environment.
3. Other glands respond directly to internal changes.

As hormone levels rise, negative feedback inhibits the system and secretion decreases. As blood levels of hormones decrease, the system starts up again. Hormones in the bloodstream fluctuate resultantly but remain relatively stable. Three types of stimuli trigger endocrine gland actions:

- *Humoral stimuli:* Changing blood levels of certain vital ions and nutrients. They are the simplest type of endocrine controls. An example is when parathyroid gland cells or *chief cells* monitor blood calcium and secrete *parathyroid hormone* (PTH) when they detect lower than normal levels. Humoral stimuli are also linked to release of insulin from the pancreas and aldosterone from the adrenal cortex.
- *Neural stimuli:* Nerve fiber stimulation. The best example is how the sympathetic nervous system responds to stress by stimulating the adrenal medulla to release norepinephrine and epinephrine.
- *Hormonal stimuli:* Hormone release due to the production of other hormones. An example is when the hypothalamus regulates secretion of most anterior pituitary hormones via the actions of its own **releasing hormones** and **inhibiting hormones**. Then, many anterior pituitary hormones act to stimulate other endocrine organs to cause them to release their own hormones. Increasing blood levels of the hormones from the final target glands then inhibit the release of anterior pituitary hormones and, therefore, their own release.

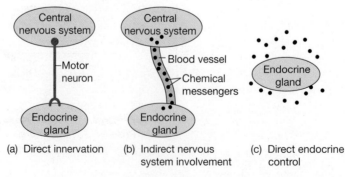

(a) Direct innervation   (b) Indirect nervous system involvement   (c) Direct endocrine control

FIGURE 14-5 The steps of hormone secretion.

Remember that multiple hormones may act on the same target cells at the same time, often with unpredictable reactions. There are three basic types of hormone interaction:

- *Permissiveness:* One hormone is not able to exert its full effects without the presence of another hormone. An example is when reproductive system hormones require the presence of thyroid hormone to develop reproductive structures at their normal times in the life span. If the thyroid hormone is lacking, reproductive development is delayed.
- *Synergism:* One hormone produces the same effects as another hormone at the target cell, amplifying their combined effects. An example is when glucagon from the pancreas, along with epinephrine, signals the liver to release glucose into the blood.
- *Antagonism:* One hormone opposes another hormone's actions. An example is when insulin is antagonized by glucagon. Insulin lowers blood glucose levels while glucagon raises them, an opposite effect.

Hormones may also produce complimentary yet different effects in certain organs and tissues that are described as *integrative effects.*

Pituitary Gland

The *pituitary gland,* also known as the *hypophysis* (**FIGURE 14-6**), is located at the base of the brain, attached to the hypothalamus, superiorly, by a stalk called the **infundibulum**. The pituitary is about 1 cm in diameter. It lies in the sella turcica of the sphenoid bone and secretes a number of different hormones. The description of the pituitary gland's appearance is that of a "pea on a stalk." Arterial blood is delivered to the pituitary gland via hypophyseal branches of the internal carotid arteries. Veins leaving the gland drain into the dural sinuses.

The *anterior pituitary* and *posterior pituitary* lobes have differing functions. The anterior pituitary gland is also called the *adenohypophysis* and is composed of glandular tissue. It manufactures and releases a variety of hormones. The anterior lobe has three regions:

- *Pars distalis:* The largest, most anterior part of the pituitary gland.
- *Pars tuberalis:* The extension that wraps around the adjacent area of the infundibulum.
- *Pars intermedia:* The slender and narrow band that borders the posterior lobe of the pituitary gland; this section may secrete two types of *melanocyte-stimulating hormone,* which is also known as *melanotropin.* It stimulates the melanocytes of the skin to increase production of melanin, and release of melanocyte-stimulating hormone is inhibited by dopamine.

Releasing hormones from the hypothalamus control the anterior pituitary's secretion and travel in the hypothalamus's capillary network. These *fenestrated* capillaries contain structures that resemble *pores* and form the **hypophyseal portal veins**, passing along the pituitary stalk to the capillary network of the anterior pituitary (**FIGURE 14-7**). The hypothalamus releases substances that are carried directly to the anterior pituitary via the blood. Releasing actions of the anterior pituitary are mostly stimulatory, although some have inhibitory effects. The primary and secondary capillary plexuses, along with the hypophyseal portal veins, are the structures that comprise the *hypophyseal portal system.* Via this system, the releasing and inhibiting hormones from the ventral hypothalamus circulate to the anterior pituitary and regulate its hormone secretion. Releasing hormones stimulate synthesis and secretion of one or several hormones at the anterior lobe, while inhibiting hormones prevent this from occurring.

Anterior Pituitary Hormones

The anterior pituitary consists of dense, collagenous connective tissue (**FIGURE 14-6**), and is known as the "master endocrine gland." Its numerous hormones, which are all proteins, regulate the activity of other endocrine glands. It has six types of secretory cells: growth hormone (GH), prolactin (PRL), thyroid-stimulating hormone (TSH), ACTH, follicle-stimulating hormone (FSH), and luteinizing hormone (LH).

An appropriate chemical stimulus from the hypothalamus causes the anterior pituitary to release one or more of its hormones. Each target cell is able to distinguish its received messages and respond so it secretes the correct hormone, regulated by the specific *releasing hormones.* Hormone release is likewise shut off, according to specific *inhibiting hormones.* The *tropic hormones,* also called *tropins,* regulate the secretory actions of other endocrine glands. These include TSH, ACTH, FSH, and LH. Except for GH, all the anterior pituitary hormones affect their target cells via a cAMP second-messenger system.

Growth Hormone

Growth hormone (GH) is produced by *somatotropic cells* of the anterior pituitary and is also called *somatotropin.* It stimulates cells to grow and divide more frequently and enhances the movement of amino acids to stimulate growth. This hormone has both direct metabolic and growth-promoting actions. It mobilizes fats for transport to cells, which increase blood levels of fatty acids to be used for fuel. GH decreases rates of glucose uptake and metabolism to conserve glucose. It encourages liver breakdown of glycogen so glucose can be released to the blood. Therefore, GH is said to have *glucose-sparing* actions and *anti-insulin effects.* It also increases amino acid uptake into the cells so these acids can be incorporated into proteins. The hypothalamus, as well as the patient's nutritional state, influences GH secretion via growth hormone-releasing hormone and growth hormone release-inhibiting hormone. More GH is released when protein is deficient and blood glucose is low. Also, *ghrelin,* known as the "hunger hormone," also stimulates

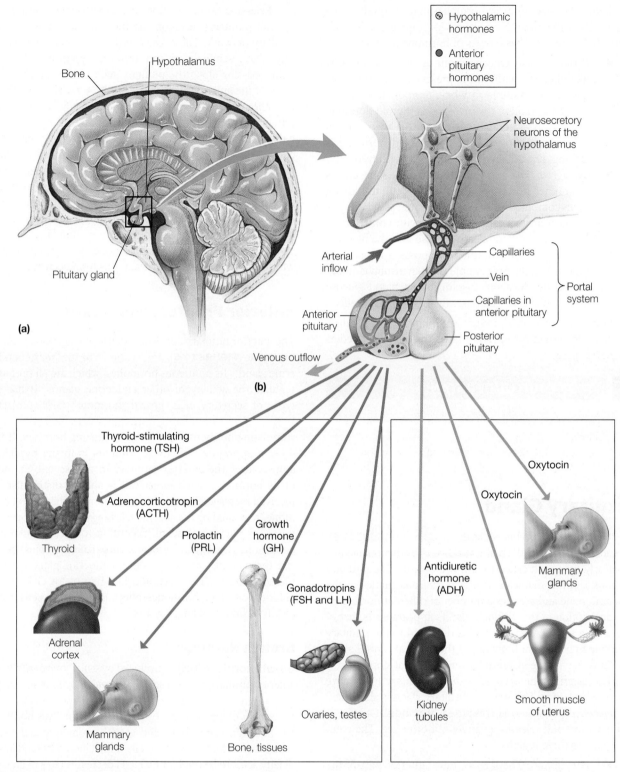

FIGURE 14-6 The pituitary gland.

the release of GH. GH secretion undergoes a diurnal cycle (**FIGURE 14-8**) in that during sleep and strenuous exercise, blood levels of GH are at their highest. As we age, GH secretion declines gradually.

GH uses various growth-promoting proteins known as *insulin-like growth factors (IGFs)*, which allow it to have indirect growth-enhancing effects. IGFs are produced by tissues such as the liver, bone, and skeletal muscle in response to GH. In the liver, IGFs act as hormones, but those produced by other tissues act locally as *paracrines*. The actions required for growth, as stimulated by IGFs, are as follows:

- Uptake of blood nutrients for incorporation into proteins and DNA, which allows growth by cell division.

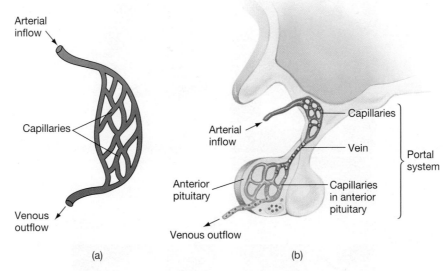

Arterial
inflow

Capillaries

Venous
outflow

(a)

Arterial
inflow

Anterior
pituitary

Venous outflow

Capillaries

Vein

Capillaries
in anterior
pituitary

Portal
system

(b)

FIGURE 14-7 Compare the typical vascular arrangement (A) to the portal system (B).

■ Collagen formation and bone matrix deposition. The major targets of GH are bone and skeletal muscle. Long bone growth occurs via epiphyseal plate stimulation. Muscle mass increases by stimulation of skeletal muscles.

FOCUS ON PATHOLOGY

Structural abnormalities can occur because of hypersecretion or hyposecretion of GH. In children hypersecretion causes **gigantism**, because GH targets the active epiphyseal plates. The child, over time, can reach a height of up to 8 feet, with mostly normal body proportions. Hyposecretion of GH in children slows the growth of long bones, which is known as **pituitary dwarfism**. If the epiphyseal plates have already closed, excessive GH causes **acromegaly**, in which the bones of the hands, feet, and face continue to grow, whereas the other bones usually do not.

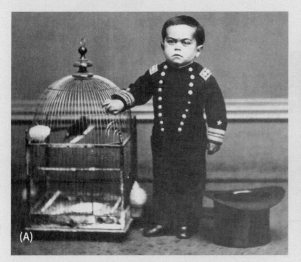

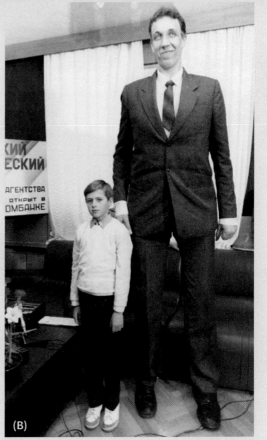

(A) Pituitary dwarf. (B) Pituitary giant. (© NYPL/Science Source © AP Images)

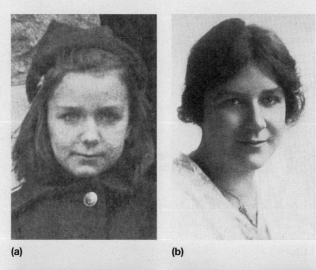

(a)   (b)

(c)   (d)

Acromegaly. There is no sign of the disorder at age 9 (A) or age 16 (B). Symptoms are evident at age 33 (C) and age 52 (D). (Reproduced from Am. J. Med., vol. 20, Mendelhoff, A. I., and Smith, D. E., Acromegaly, diabetes, hypermetabolism, proeinuria and heart failure, pp. 133-144. © 1956, with permission from Elsevier.)

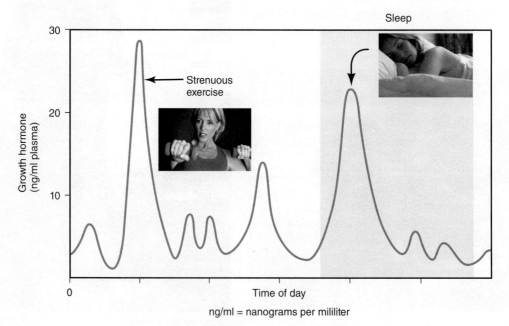

ng/ml = nanograms per mililiter

FIGURE 14-8 Growth hormone secretion in an adult. (Left photo: © LiquidLibrary; Right photo: © Photos.com)

Prolactin

Prolactin (PRL) is a protein hormone that controls milk production in women after they give birth. In males, it may also help to maintain sperm production. Elevated levels of PRL can interrupt sexual function in both females and males. The secretion of PRL is regulated by a *neuroendocrine reflex*, a reflex involving both the endocrine and nervous systems (**FIGURE 14-9**). During the breastfeeding process, sensory fibers in the breast are stimulated, sending nerve impulses to the hypothalamus. The hypothalamus responds by secreting PRL-releasing hormone, causing PRL release. The PRL-inhibiting hormone is *dopamine*. Lower PRL-inhibiting hormone secretion causes increased PRL release. There are many PRL-releasing factors, one of which is thyroid-releasing hormone. In women, estrogen stimulates PRL release, which is part of the cause of breast tenderness before menstruation.

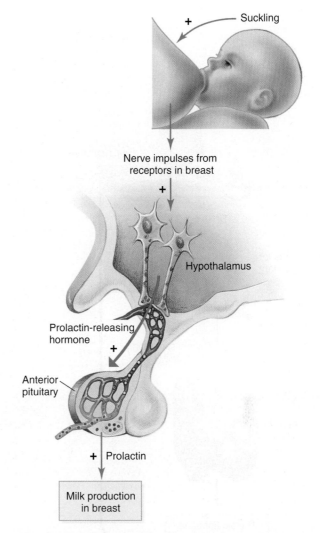

FIGURE 14-9 Neuroendocrine reflex and prolactin secretion.

FOCUS ON PATHOLOGY

Hypersecretion of PRL is a more common occurrence than hyposecretion. The most common abnormality caused by anterior pituitary tumors is hyperprolactinemia, signified by lack of menses, inappropriate lactation, and infertility in women. If it occurs in men, it causes impotence.

Thyroid-Stimulating Hormone

Thyroid-stimulating hormone (TSH) controls the thyroid, and TSH secretion is regulated by the hypothalamus via thyroid-releasing hormone. Receptors in the hypothalamus control levels of circulating thyroxine. When these levels are low, receptors signal the hypothalamus to release thyroid-stimulating hormone releasing hormone. As thyroxine levels increase, TSH releasing hormone secretion declines (**FIGURE 14-10**) in a process called negative feedback control of TSH secretion. The secretion of TSH releasing hormone is also stimulated by cold and stress. TSH is also known as *thyrotropin*.

Adrenocorticotropic Hormone

Adrenocorticotropic hormone (ACTH) controls hormone secretion from the cortex of the adrenal gland, partly via *corticotropin-releasing hormone (CRH)* from the hypothalamus. Stress may also increase ACTH secretion. Negative feedback controls the secretion of ACTH (**FIGURE 14-11**). ACTH is also known as *corticotropin*, because it is secreted by the *corticotropic cells*. It stimulates the release of corticosteroid hormones from the adrenal cortex, of which glucocorticoids are most important, because they play a role in resisting stressors. Every day, the release of ACTH occurs in a rhythm,

wherein levels are highest in the morning, just before we awake. As levels of glucocorticoids rise, CRH secretion is blocked, as is ACTH release. However, normal ACTH rhythm can be altered by factors such as fever, all types of stressors, and hypoglycemia.

Gonadotropins

Follicle-stimulating hormone (FSH) and **luteinizing hormone (LH)** are *gonadotropins*, affecting the reproductive organs or *gonads*. In males these are the *testes* and in females, the *ovaries*. In males LH regulates testosterone production, and in females it triggers ovulation and regulates ovarian hormone synthesis. Gonadotropins become more active during puberty, prompted by hypothalamic release of *gonadotropin-releasing hormone (GRH)*.

Posterior Pituitary and Hypothalamic Hormones

The posterior pituitary differs from the anterior pituitary in that it is made up of mostly nerve fibers and neuroglial cells

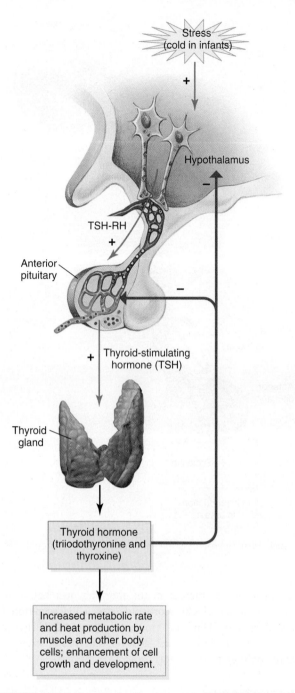

FIGURE 14-10 Negative feedback control of TSH secretion.

(**FIGURE 14-12**). The hypothalamic neurons are located in supraoptic or paraventricular nuclei, synthesizing oxytocin and antidiuretic hormone (ADH). These *neurohormones* received from the hypothalamus actually function as a storage area for hormones instead of a manufacturing area. Along with the infundibulum, the posterior lobe of the pituitary gland makes up the **neurohypophysis**. This term is often used to describe just the posterior lobe itself, but this is incorrect. The posterior lobe is actually part of the brain and is formed by a down growth of hypothalamic tissue. Its neural connection with the hypothalamus is via a nerve bundle called the *hypothalamic-hypophyseal tract,* which runs through the infundibulum. The hypothalamic-hypophyseal tract is formed by neurons in the *supraoptic* and *paraventricular nuclei* of the hypothalamus.

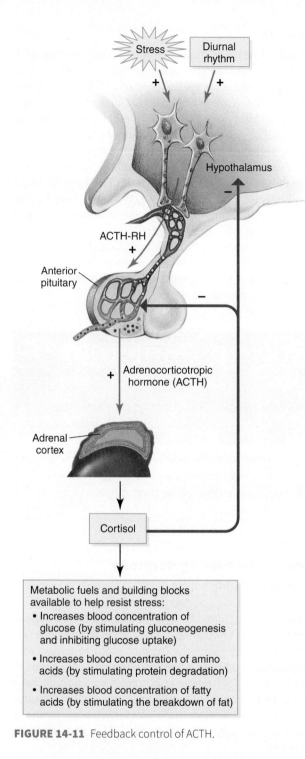

FIGURE 14-11 Feedback control of ACTH.

Specialized *supraoptic* and *paraventricular* neurons of the hypothalamus produce, respectively, the posterior pituitary's hormones, **antidiuretic hormone** and **oxytocin**. ADH is also called *vasopressin*. Nerve impulses from the hypothalamus release these hormones into the blood. A *diuretic* is a chemical that increases urine production, whereas an *antidiuretic* decreases urine formation (**FIGURE 14-13**).

Antidiuretic Hormone

ADH regulates the water concentration of body fluids by reducing water excretion by the kidneys. It acts to prevent both water overload and dehydration from occurring.

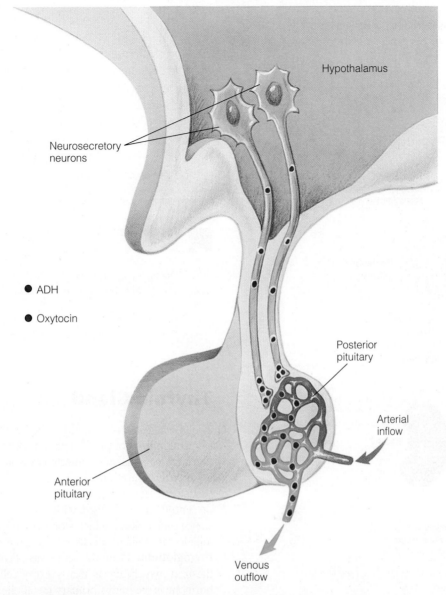

Hypothalamus

Neurosecretory neurons

● ADH

● Oxytocin

Posterior pituitary

Arterial inflow

Anterior pituitary

Venous outflow

FIGURE 14-12 The posterior pituitary.

Decreased levels of ADH causes polyuria and diabetes insipidus.

Osmoreceptors sense increases in osmotic pressure due to dehydration and use ADH to signal the kidneys to produce less urine. If too much water is in the body, ADH release is inhibited and urine production increases. ADH targets kidney tubules, via cAMP, and the tubules then reabsorb more water from the forming urine, returning it to the bloodstream. Therefore, less urine is produced and solute concentrations of the blood decline. This triggers the osmoreceptors to stop depolarizing, which nearly stops the release of ADH. Other triggers for ADH release include low blood pressure, pain, morphine, barbiturates, and nicotine. Alcohol intake inhibits ADH secretion and increases urine output, as does consuming high amounts of water. An alcoholic hangover is signified by dehydration, including intense thirst and dry mouth. Oppositely, diuretics antagonize ADH effects, removing water from the body. They are used for certain types of hypertension and edema, such as in congestive heart failure. In severe blood loss conditions, extremely high amounts of ADH are released, causing vasoconstriction mostly of visceral blood vessels. The blood pressure then rises. This response uses different ADH receptors on vascular smooth muscle; hence, the alternate name of ADH is *vasopressin*.

Oxytocin

Oxytocin stimulates uterine contractions during childbirth and milk letdown, which is the ejection of milk from the breast glands soon after suckling begins. Oxytocin receptors peak in number near the end of pregnancy, and the hormone's stimulatory effects are most effective on uterine smooth muscle. Oxytocin release, at this time, is triggered by afferent impulses that reach the hypothalamus. When blood levels of oxytocin rise, uterine contractions increase

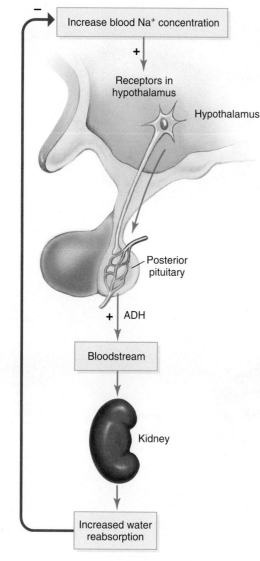

FIGURE 14-13 Role of ADH in regulating fluid levels.

until expulsion of the fetus occurs. In the brain oxytocin acts as a neurotransmitter and is involved in affection and sexual behaviors as well as promoting trust, nurturing behaviors, and the bonding of two individuals as a "couple." **TABLE 14-3** discusses the pituitary gland hormones in greater detail.

FOCUS ON PATHOLOGY

Diabetes insipidus is a condition related to ADH deficiency in which the patient experiences intense thirst and excessive urine output. It is not related to insulin deficiency. Diabetes insipidus may be caused by trauma to the hypothalamus or posterior pituitary gland. It may become life threatening if the patient is

unconscious or comatose. Oppositely, hypersecretion of ADH may be caused by meningitis in children and by neurosurgery, cancer, hypothalamic injury, general anesthesia, or certain drugs in adults. This leads to *syndrome of inappropriate ADH secretion*, signified by fluid retention, headache, disorientation, weight gain, brain edema, and decreased blood solute concentrations. It is treated with fluid restriction and careful blood sodium monitoring.

TEST YOUR UNDERSTANDING

1. Define the term *gonadotropin*.
2. List the effects of ACTH and PRL.
3. List the hormones stored in the posterior lobe of the pituitary gland.
4. Describe the physiology of vasopressin and oxytocin.

Thyroid Gland

The *thyroid gland* is located just below the larynx, on either side and in front of the trachea (**FIGURE 14-14**). It consists of two large *lobes* that are connected by a broad *isthmus*, forming a "butterfly" shape, and is covered by a capsule of connective tissue with secretory parts called *follicles*. The thyroid's *lumen* or central cavity is filled with a clear, amber-colored substance called *colloid*, which stores hormones produced by the follicles. Its follicular cells produce the glycoprotein called **thyroglobulin**. From this substance, *thyroid hormone* is synthesized, which affects nearly every cell in the body. This hormone is the body's primary metabolic hormone, containing **thyroxine,** which is also known as *tetraiodothyronine* or T_4, and **triiodothyronine** or T_3. The number of each of these iodine-containing amine hormones indicates the number of atoms of iodine. T_3 is five times as potent as T_4. The thyroid hormones regulate metabolism of carbohydrates, lipids, and proteins, determining the body's basal metabolic rate. Thyroid hormones are required for growth, development, and maturation of the nervous system. Thyroxine is the major hormone of the thyroid follicles. Most triiodothyronine forms at target tissues because of thyroxine. Most molecules of the thyroid hormones attach to *thyroid-binding globulins* upon entering the bloodstream. In the circulation, most remaining molecules attach to *transthyretin*, which is also called *thyroid-binding prealbumin*, or to albumin itself.

Thyroid hormones enter target cells, binding to intracellular receptors in the cell's nucleus. They control transcription of mRNA needed for protein synthesis. The many effects of thyroid hormones include increase of basal metabolic rate, increase of body heat production or *the calorigenic effect*, regulation of tissue growth and development, and maintenance of blood pressure.

TABLE 14-3

Pituitary Gland Hormones

Hormone	Source	Action
Anterior Lobe		
GH	GH releasing hormone and GH release-inhibiting hormone from the hypothalamus	Increases size and division rate of body cells, enhances amino acid movement across membranes
PRL	PRL release-inhibiting hormone and PRL-releasing factor from the hypothalamus	Sustains milk production after birth
TSH	Thyroid-releasing hormone from the hypothalamus	Controls thyroid gland hormone secretion
ACTH	Corticotropin-releasing hormone (CRH) from the hypothalamus	Controls adrenal cortex hormone secretion
FSH	Gonadotropin-releasing hormone (GRH) from the hypothalamus	Develops egg-containing follicles in females and also stimulates secretion of estrogen; stimulates production of sperm cells in males
LH	GRH from the hypothalamus	Promotes sex hormone secretion; aids in release of female egg cells
Posterior Lobe		
ADH	Hypothalamus in response to changes in water concentration in body fluids	Causes conservation of water in kidneys; in high concentrations increases blood pressure
Oxytocin	Hypothalamus in response to stretching of uterine and vaginal walls and stimulation of breasts	Contracts uterine wall muscles; contracts milk-secreting gland muscles

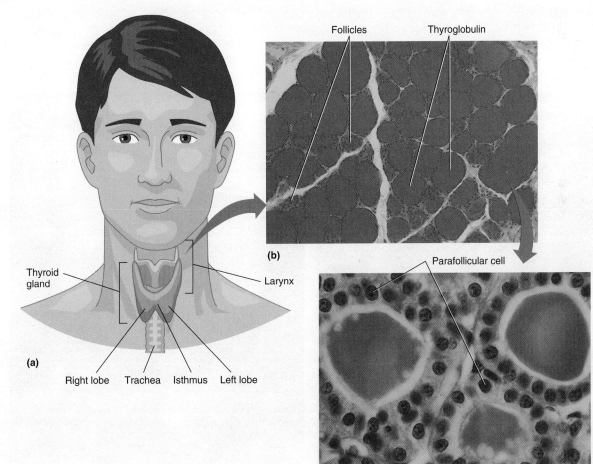

FIGURE 14-14 The thyroid gland. (A) Thyroid gland in the neck. (B) Thyroid follicles produce thyroid hormones. (C) Enlargement showing calcitonin-producing cells known as parafollicular cells. (Top photo: © Dr. Robert Calentine/Visuals Unlimited; Bottom photo: © Dr. David Phillips/Visuals Unlimited)

Iodine salts or *iodides* are needed by the follicular cells to secrete thyroid hormones. Thyroid hormone secretion is controlled by the hypothalamus and pituitary gland. **Calcitonin** is another hormone secreted by the thyroid, although it is produced by its parafollicular cells, also known as *C cells*, rather than the follicular cells. These cells lie in the follicular epithelium, protruding into the connective tissue surrounding the thyroid follicles. Calcitonin is a polypeptide hormone that regulates concentrations of blood calcium and phosphate ions, and its release is controlled by blood concentration of calcium ions. Calcitonin inhibits osteoclast activity, which inhibits bone resorption and release of calcium from the bone matrix. It also stimulates calcium uptake and incorporation into the bone matrix. **TABLE 14-4** discusses the actions of thyroid hormones.

Parathyroid Glands

The *parathyroid glands* are located on the posterior thyroid gland surface (**FIGURE 14-14**). There are usually four parathyroid glands—one superior and one inferior gland on each of the thyroid gland's two lobes. They are covered in thin connective tissue capsules and appear yellowish-brown.

Parathyroid hormone (PTH) is secreted by the cells of the parathyroid glands. Also called *parathormone*, it increases blood calcium concentration and decreases blood phosphate ion concentration to affect the bones, intestines, and kidneys. The most important hormone that controls blood calcium levels, PTH stimulates reabsorption of bone while causing kidney conservation of blood calcium and excretion of more phosphate ions in urine. It stimulates absorption of calcium

FOCUS ON PATHOLOGY

Severe metabolic disturbances can occur because of thyroid gland overactivity or underactivity. *Myxedema* describes a severe hypothyroid syndrome in adults signified by chills, low metabolism, constipation, eye puffiness, thickening and drying of the skin, edema, lethargy, and mental sluggishness. If myxedema is caused by a lack of iodine, a *goiter*, which is an enlarged and protruding thyroid gland, develops. Severe hypothyroidism in an infant is called *cretinism*, signified by mental retardation, body disproportion, and thickened tongue and neck. *Graves' disease* is the most common type of hyperthyroidism and causes elevated metabolism, heartbeat abnormalities, sweating, weight loss, nervousness, and protrusion of the eyeballs.

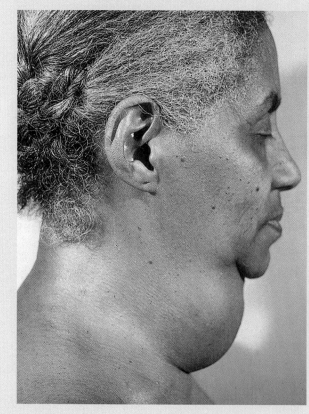

Goiter. (© Ken Greer/Visuals Unlimited)

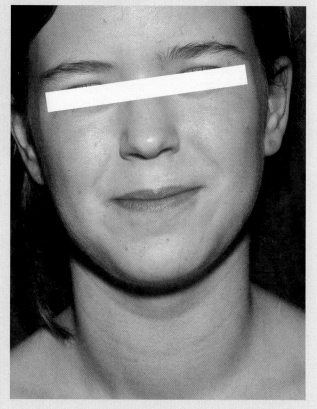

Graves' disease. (Courtesy of Leonard V. Crowley, MD, Century College.)

TABLE 14-4

Thyroid Gland Hormones

Hormone	Source	Action
Thyroxine (T$_4$)	TSH from anterior pituitary	Increases energy release from carbohydrates; increases protein synthesis; accelerates growth; stimulates nervous system activity
Triiodothyronine (T$_3$)	TSH from anterior pituitary	Same as T$_4$ but five times more potent
Calcitonin	Blood calcium concentration	Lowers blood calcium and phosphate ion concentrations by inhibiting calcium and phosphate ion release from bones, and by increasing kidney excretion of these ions

from food in the intestines. PTH secretion is regulated by negative feedback between the parathyroid glands and the blood calcium concentration. More PTH is secreted as blood calcium concentration drops, and vice versa. PTH is important, along with calcitonin, for stable blood calcium concentration.

FOCUS ON PATHOLOGY

Hypoparathyroidism is usually caused by parathyroid gland trauma or removal of the gland during thyroid surgery. It may also be caused by extended deficiency of dietary magnesium, resulting in hypocalcemia. Symptoms include tingling, tetany, convulsions, and possible respiratory paralysis and death. *Hyperparathyroidism* is a rare condition, usually caused by a parathyroid gland tumor. The bones soften and become deformed due to fibrous connective tissue replacing their mineral salts. A severe form is known as *osteitis fibrosa cystica*, which causes bone weakening and spontaneous fracture. Resulting hypercalcemia is primarily signified by nervous system depression, abnormal reflexes, weak skeletal muscles, and kidney stones.

Calcitonin decreases above-normal blood calcium concentrations, whereas PTH increases below-normal blood calcium concentrations.

Adrenal Glands

The pyramid-shaped *adrenal glands* sit on top of each kidney like caps and are embedded in the adipose tissue enclosing each kidney (**FIGURE 14-15**). The adrenal glands are also known as the *suprarenal glands* because of their position.

The adrenal glands have a central *adrenal medulla* and an outer *adrenal cortex*, each secreting different hormones. The adrenal medulla is closely connected with the sympathetic division of the autonomic nervous system and appears more like a mass of nervous tissue than a gland. The adrenal cortex consists of layers of cells, including an outer zone or *zona glomerulosa*, a middle zone or *zona fasciculate*, and an inner zone or *zona reticularis*. It is derived from the embryonic mesoderm. Both the adrenal medulla and cortex are well supplied with blood vessels.

Adrenal Medulla

The adrenal medulla secretes **epinephrine** or *adrenaline* and **norepinephrine** or *noradrenaline*. Epinephrine makes up 80% of adrenal medulla secretions, the rest being norepinephrine. These hormones aid in coping with stressors and participate

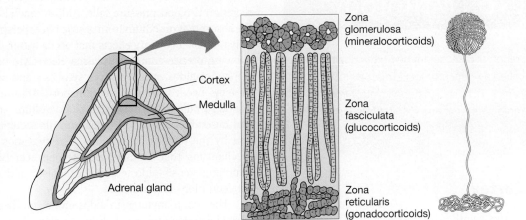

FIGURE 14-15 The adrenal gland.

TABLE 14-5

Adrenal Medullary Hormones

Affected Part or Function	Epinephrine	Norepinephrine
Heart	Increases rate and force of contraction	Increases rate and force of contraction
Blood vessels	Dilates skeletal muscle vessels, decreasing blood flow resistance	Increases skeletal muscle blood flow because of constriction of blood vessels in skin and viscera
Systemic blood pressure	Increases somewhat because of increased cardiac output	Increases greatly because of vasoconstriction
Airways	Dilates	Dilates slightly
Reticular brain formation	Activates	Little effect
Liver	Promotes glycogen-to-glucose breakdown; increases blood sugar concentration	Little effect on blood sugar concentration
Metabolic rate	Increases	Increases

in the fight-or-flight response. Epinephrine is stronger in its stimulation of bronchial dilation, metabolic activities, and increased blood flow to the heart and skeletal muscles. It is used clinically as a bronchodilator and heart stimulant. Norepinephrine more greatly influences blood pressure and peripheral vasoconstriction.

One group of chemicals produced in nervous tissue, called *catecholamines,* regulate many different functions, including thought processes, hormone secretions, blood pressure, and heart rate. The most common catecholamines are epinephrine, norepinephrine, dopamine, and serotonin. The adrenal medulla is a modified sympathetic ganglion.

The adrenal medulla's secretions have long-lasting effects. They increase heart rate, cardiac muscle contraction force, breathing rate, and blood glucose level, while elevating blood pressure and decreasing digestive activity. In response to stress, the hypothalamus releases impulses to control the adrenal medulla. These impulses prepare the body for the "fight-or-flight response." **TABLE 14-5** discusses adrenal medullary hormones and their effects.

FOCUS ON PATHOLOGY

Hypersecretion of catecholamines, often due to a tumor called a *pheochromocytoma,* produces hyperglycemia, increased metabolic rate, hypertension, rapid heartbeat and palpitations, extreme nervousness, and sweating.

Adrenal Cortex

The adrenal cortex synthesizes more than 30 **corticosteroids**. This synthesis begins with cholesterol, using a variety of intermediate substances in relation to the hormone being made. Steroid hormones are not stored in cells, and their rate of release is based on their rate of synthesis. Some of these hormones are vital for survival, especially aldosterone, cortisol, and some sex hormones.

Mineralocorticoids

Mineralocorticoids mainly function in the regulation of mineral salt or electrolyte concentrations in the extracellular fluids, mostly regulating sodium and potassium. The regulation of sodium is connected to the regulation of potassium, hydrogen, bicarbonate, and chloride. The regulation by mineralocorticoids of sodium and potassium is vital for overall homeostasis. Aldosterone accounts for more than 95% of the mineralocorticoids produced.

The outer adrenal cortex or *zona glomerulosa* synthesizes **aldosterone**, a mineralocorticoid that helps regulate mineral electrolyte concentrations. Aldosterone helps the kidneys to balance sodium and potassium and stimulates water retention via the process of osmosis. If blood sodium decreases or blood potassium increases, the adrenal cortex secretes aldosterone. The kidneys also stimulate aldosterone secretion if blood pressure falls. Aldosterone also enhances the absorption of sodium from gastric juice, perspiration, and saliva. It has regulatory effects that occur within 20 minutes, allowing precise control of plasma electrolyte balance. The activity of aldosterone involves synthesis and activation of proteins needed for sodium transport. Aldosterone secretion is stimulated by decreased blood volume and pressure and raised blood levels of potassium. Its secretion is inhibited by the opposite conditions. The two most important mechanisms that regulate aldosterone secretion are the renin-angiotensin-aldosterone mechanism and the plasma concentrations of potassium.

The renin-angiotensin-aldosterone mechanism regulates aldosterone release, helping to control blood volume, blood pressure, and the reabsorption of sodium and water by the kidneys. When blood pressure or volume falls, certain cells of the *juxtaglomerular complex* of the kidneys are excited, which respond by releasing *renin* into the blood. The renin cleaves off part of the plasma protein known as **angiotensinogen**. This causes an enzymatic cascade to occur, forming *angiotensin II*. This substance stimulates cells of the glomerulosa to release aldosterone. All the effects of this mechanism ultimately raise blood pressure.

The cells of the zona glomerulosa in the adrenal cortex are directly influenced by fluctuating blood levels of potassium. When increased, potassium stimulates aldosterone release, and the opposite is also true. ACTH normally has very little effect on aldosterone release. However, when stressors are prevalent, the hypothalamus secretes more CRH. ACTH rises in the blood, increasing aldosterone secretion slightly. This helps to deliver nutrients and respiratory gases in an attempt to cope with the stressors.

Atrial natriuretic peptide is a hormone from the heart that is secreted when blood pressure rises. It regulates blood pressure and sodium–water balance and greatly inhibits the renin-angiotensin-aldosterone mechanism. Renin and aldosterone secretion are blocked, and atrial natriuretic peptide also inhibits other mechanisms that enhance sodium and water reabsorption. Overall, it decreases blood pressure by allowing sodium and water to leave the body in the urine.

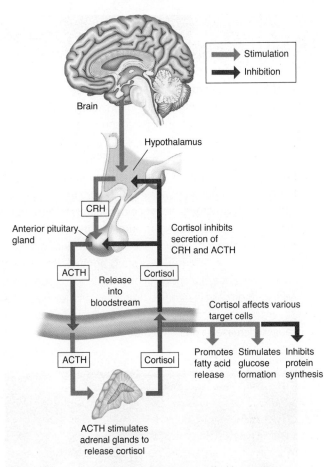

FIGURE 14-16 Cortisol secretion is controlled by negative feedback. (Adapted from Shier, D. N., Butler, J. L., and Lewis, R. Hole's Essentials of Human Anatomy & Physiology, Tenth edition. McGraw-Hill Higher Education, 2009.)

FOCUS ON PATHOLOGY

Aldosteronism is hypersecretion of aldosterone and is usually caused by adrenal tumors. The two major types of problems that result are hypertension and edema because of excessive sodium and water retention and increased excretion of potassium ions. When this second problem is extreme, the neurons become nonresponsive and muscles weaken until they eventually become paralyzed.

Glucocorticoids

In general, the *glucocorticoids* help us to resist stressors and influence energy metabolism. **Cortisol** is a glucocorticoid produced in the middle adrenal cortex or *zona fasiculata* that also influences protein and fat metabolism. It inhibits protein synthesis, promotes fatty acid release, and stimulates the liver to synthesize glucose from non-carbohydrates. Cortisol, which is also known as *hydrocortisone*, helps balance blood glucose and is controlled by negative feedback. ACTH stimulates the adrenal cortex to release cortisol, and stress plays an important part in triggering cortisol release. **FIGURE 14-16** shows how negative feedback regulates cortisol secretion. Other glucocorticoid hormones include *cortisone* and *corticosterone*, but

these are relatively insignificant compared with cortisol. Acute stress interrupts normal cortisol rhythm, resulting in increased ACTH blood levels. Cortisol responds to stress by causing a large rise in blood glucose, amino acids, and fatty acids. Its metabolic effect known as *gluconeogenesis* is defined as the formation of glucose from fats and proteins. Cortisol, in an attempt to conserve glucose for the brain, mobilizes fatty acids from adipose tissue so they can be used for energy. Stored proteins are broken down, vasoconstriction is enhanced, and nutrients are dispersed to the cells more quickly than normal. Excessive cortisol, however, causes anti-inflammatory and anti-immune effects to a large degree. When excessive, cortisol depresses cartilage formation, bone formation, and the immune system. It disrupts normal cardiovascular, gastrointestinal, and neural function and inhibits inflammation via the decrease in release of inflammatory chemicals.

Gonadocorticoids

The inner adrenal cortex or *zona reticularis* produces sex hormones. In males, these are known as **adrenal androgens**, which can be converted to female *estrogens* in the adipose

Cushing's syndrome is caused by excessive glucocorticoid release. If caused by an ACTH-releasing pituitary tumor, an ACTH-releasing malignancy, or an adrenal cortex tumor, it is called *Cushing's disease*. However, it is usually caused by administration of glucocorticoid drugs. Cushing's syndrome is indicated by persistently elevated blood glucose, sodium and water retention, muscle protein and bone protein loss, hypertension, and edema. The patient often develops a swollen, "moon-shaped" face, fat redistribution to the abdomen and posterior neck, poor wound healing, and easy bruising. In the posterior neck fat distribution is commonly referred to as a "buffalo hump." Infections may become very severe before the recognized symptoms develop. Over time, muscle weakening and spontaneous fractures often occur. The only treatment is to remove the tumor or discontinue the drug. The major hyposecretory disorder of the adrenal cortex is known as **Addison's disease**. It results from atrophy or destruction of both adrenal glands, which leads to a deficiency of all the steroid hormones. Usually, Addison's disease is caused by an autoimmune disorder. Less often, adrenal destruction may result from tuberculosis, histoplasmosis, or metastatic cancer. Because of glucocorticoid deficiency, blood glucose levels may decline and hypoglycemia may develop. Addison's disease is signified by weight loss, lowered plasma glucose and sodium, and increased blood potassium. Severe hypotension and dehydration often occur, and therapy is with corticosteroid replacements. It also commonly causes increased skin pigmentation that accompanies the rise in ACTH secretion.

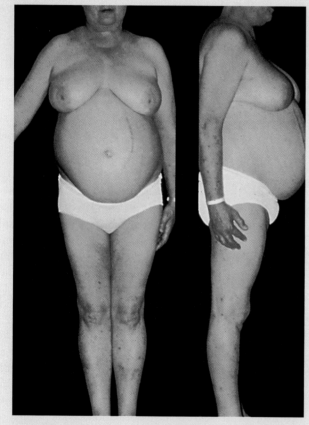

Cushing syndrome. (Courtesy of Leonard V. Crowley, MD, Century College.)

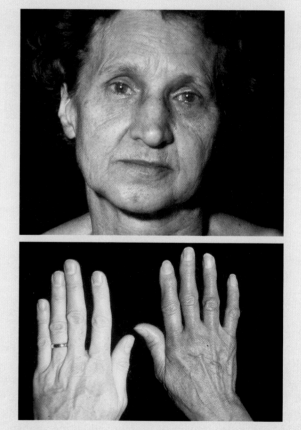

Addison's disease. (Courtesy of Leonard V. Crowley, MD, Century College.)

tissue, liver, and skin. These hormones may supplement sex hormones from the gonads and stimulate early reproductive organ development. Adrenal sex hormones are also called **gonadocorticoids**. The amount of these hormones produced by the adrenal cortex is insignificant compared with the amounts produced during late puberty and adulthood by the gonads. Their release is linked to ACTH. **TABLE 14-6** discusses the adrenal cortex hormones.

Hypersecretion of gonadocorticoids causes *masculinization,* or *adrenogenital syndrome.* In prepubertal males and in females this may cause dramatic developments. In males, maturity of the reproductive organs and appearance of secondary sex characteristics is early, with a much-heightened sex drive. In females, a beard may develop, and body hair distribution appears masculine. The clitoris may grow large enough to resemble a small penis.

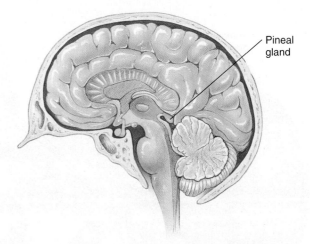

FIGURE 14-17 The pineal gland. (© Jones & Bartlett Learning)

TEST YOUR UNDERSTANDING

1. What are the names of the hormones released from the adrenal glands?
2. Explain the effects of aldosterone in the kidneys.
3. Which pituitary hormone stimulates the adrenal cortex?

Pineal Gland

The small, cone-shaped *pineal gland* is located deep in the cerebral hemispheres and is attached to the thalamus near the upper part of the third ventricle (**FIGURE 14-17**). It secretes the hormone **melatonin** in response to light conditions in the external environment, from its *pinealocytes,* which are arranged in tight cords and clusters. Between the pinealocytes, in adults calcium salts are contained in dense particles. The calcium salts are radiopaque, and therefore the pineal gland is used as an aid in determining the orientation of the brain when x-rays are taken. When it is dark, nerve impulses from the eyes decrease and the secretion of melatonin increases. Melatonin is an amine hormone derived from serotonin.

Melatonin functions as a biologic clock and can help to regulate the **circadian rhythms,** which are associated with environmental day and night cycles and help the body to

distinguish day from night. Melatonin is not fully understood but appears to inhibit gonadotropin secretion, to help regulate the female reproductive cycle, and to control the onset of puberty. In children, melatonin may inhibit early sexual maturation. The *biologic clock* of humans is the *suprachiasmatic nucleus* of the hypothalamus. Its large amount of melatonin receptors react to bright light, altering the biologic clock. Therefore, altered melatonin levels may result in variations of appetite, body temperature, and sleep habits.

Other Glands, Organs, or Tissues

Other organs in the body produce hormones, but their main functions are not to produce these hormones. These structures include the thymus, reproductive organs, digestive glands, pancreas, heart, kidneys, adipose tissue, skeleton, and skin.

Thymus

The *thymus,* located deep inside the mediastinum posterior to the sternum, between the lungs, is larger in children than in adults. It shrinks with age and is important in early immunity. The lobulated thymus secretes hormones called **thymosins,**

TABLE 14-6

Adrenal Cortex Hormones

Hormone	Factor or Area	Action
Aldosterone	Body fluid electrolyte concentrations	Helps to regulate extracellular electrolyte concentrations by conserving sodium and excreting potassium
Cortisol	CRH from the hypothalamus and ACTH from the anterior pituitary	Decreases protein synthesis, increases fatty acid release, and stimulates glucose synthesis from noncarbohydrates
Adrenal androgens	Inner zone of the adrenal cortex	Supplement sex hormones from gonads; may be converted to estrogens in females

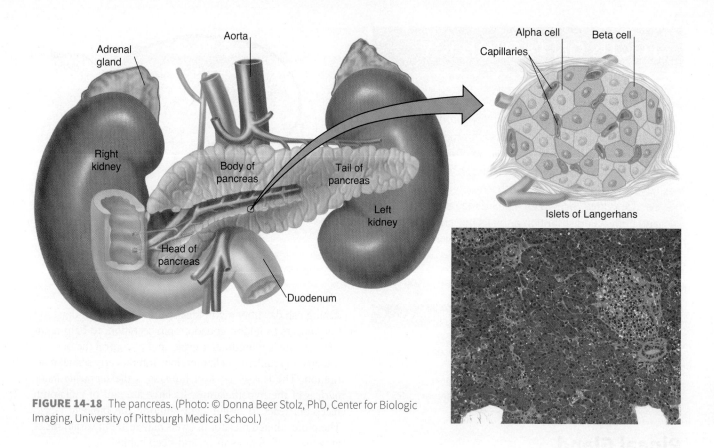

Adrenal gland
Aorta
Right kidney
Body of pancreas
Tail of pancreas
Left kidney
Head of pancreas
Duodenum

Alpha cell   Beta cell
Capillaries
Islets of Langerhans

FIGURE 14-18 The pancreas. (Photo: © Donna Beer Stolz, PhD, Center for Biologic Imaging, University of Pittsburgh Medical School.)

affecting production and differentiation of lymphocytes, as well as *thymulin* and *thymopoietins*. Although considered hormones, these substances primarily act locally as paracrines. By the time of old age, the thymus has changed to a structure made of adipose and fibrous connective tissues.

Reproductive Organs

The reproductive organs important for hormone secretion include the ovaries, which produce *estrogens* and *progesterone*; the testes, which produce *testosterone* in their *interstitial cells*; and the **placenta**, which produces estrogens, progesterone, and *gonadotropins*. The placenta is a temporary endocrine organ that sustains the fetus during pregnancy and secretes steroid and protein hormones that regulate pregnancy. Gonadotropins regulate the release of gonadal hormones. Estrogens help the reproductive organs to mature and cause the appearance of the secondary sex characteristics of females at the time of puberty. Along with progesterone, estrogens promote the menstrual cycle and breast development. In males at puberty, testosterone initiates maturation of reproductive organs and appearance of secondary sex characteristics as well as sex drive. It is also required for normal production of sperm and to maintain reproductive organs in adult males.

Digestive Glands

The digestive glands that secrete hormones are found in the linings of the stomach and small intestine. For example, the stomach secretes **gastrin** and **ghrelin**. The duodenum releases **secretin**, **cholecystokinin**, and **incretins**.

Pancreas

The *pancreas* functions as two things: an exocrine gland secreting digestive juice and an endocrine gland releasing hormones. It is an elongated, slightly flattened organ posterior to the stomach, behind the parietal peritoneum. It is joined to the duodenum of the small intestine, transporting digestive juice into the intestine (**FIGURE 14-18**).

The endocrine part of the pancreas consists of groups of cells called *pancreatic islets,* or *islets of Langerhans.* Of these cells, *alpha cells* secrete the hormone glucagon and *beta cells* secrete the hormone insulin. *Delta cells* produce a peptide hormone that is identical to *GH-inhibiting hormone.* It suppresses release of glucagon and insulin and slows food absorption and enzyme secretion in the digestive tract. *F cells* produce *pancreatic polypeptide*, a hormone that inhibits gallbladder contractions while regulating pancreatic enzyme production. **Glucagon**, a 29-amino-acid polypeptide, stimulates the liver to break down glycogen in the process known as *glycogenolysis* and to convert certain noncarbohydrates, including amino acids, into glucose in the process called *gluconeogenesis*. This raises the blood sugar concentration much more effectively than epinephrine is able to do. Glucagon secretion is regulated by negative feedback and prevents hypoglycemia from occurring when glucose concentration is relatively low. Glucagon is so powerful that just one molecule can trigger the release of 100 million glucose molecules into the bloodstream. Humoral stimuli cause the alpha cells to secrete glucagon, although stimulation from the sympathetic nervous system and rising amino acid levels also play a role. The release of glucagon is suppressed by insulin, somatostatin, and rising blood glucose levels.

Insulin, a 51-amino-acid protein, works in a manner opposite of glucagon by stimulating the liver to form glycogen from glucose and inhibiting conversion of noncarbohydrates into glucose. It consists of two amino acid chains that are linked by disulfide or -S-S- bonds and is synthesized as part of *proinsulin*, a larger polypeptide chain. Insulin decreases blood glucose concentration, promotes amino acid transport into cells, increases protein synthesis, and stimulates adipose cells to make and store fat. Insulin secretion is also controlled by negative feedback, and insulin prevents high blood glucose concentrations by promoting glycogen formation. Insulin secretion decreases as glucose concentrations fall. Just after we eat, insulin lowers blood glucose levels and also influences protein and fat metabolism. Insulin enhances membrane transport of glucose into, primarily, fat and muscle cells, inhibits glycogen breakdown into glucose, and inhibits conversion of fats or amino acids to glucose.

Because the brain, kidneys, and liver have easy access to blood glucose, no matter what the insulin level currently is, insulin is not required for glucose entry into these organs. In the brain it plays roles in feeding behaviors, learning, memory, and neuronal development. Insulin and glucagon function together to maintain stable blood glucose concentration, even though the amount of carbohydrates ingested by a person may vary widely. Nerve cells are partially sensitive to blood glucose concentration changes. Such changes can alter brain functions.

Heart

The atria of the heart secretes atrial natriuretic peptide, which stimulates urinary sodium excretion. This peptide decreases sodium in the extracellular fluid, reducing blood pressure and volume.

Kidneys

The kidneys secrete **erythropoietin**, which is a red blood cell GH. Erythropoietin is a glycoprotein hormone that causes the bone marrow to increase production of red blood cells. They also release **renin**, initiating the renin-angiotensin-aldosterone mechanism of aldosterone release.

Adipose Tissue

The adipose cells release **leptin**, and hormone-producing cells exist in the walls of the stomach, small intestine, kidneys, and even the heart. Leptin functions to inform the body how much stored fat is present that may be used for energy. Blood levels of leptin are higher when there is more stored fat. It helps to control appetite and stimulate increased expenditure of energy. Two other adipose cell hormones play different roles. **Resistin** is an insulin antagonist, whereas **adiponectin** enhances the sensitivity to insulin. In the gastrointestinal tract, *enteroendocrine cells* secrete hormones such as *gastrin, ghrelin, secretin,* and *cholecystokinin* and are found throughout the gastrointestinal mucosa.

Skeleton

The bones, via their osteoblasts, secrete **osteocalcin**, which causes pancreatic beta cells to divide, secreting more insulin. Osteocalcin restricts fat storage by the adipocytes and triggers *adiponectin* release, improving handling of glucose and reducing body fat.

Skin

In the skin, *cholecalciferol*, which is an inactive form of vitamin D$_3$, is produced because of ultraviolet radiation exposure. Eventually, cholecalciferol becomes fully activated by the kidneys, forming *calcitriol*, which is required to regulate how

FOCUS ON PATHOLOGY

Hyposecretion or hypoactivity of insulin causes *diabetes mellitus*. Type 1 diabetes mellitus develops when insulin is absent. Type 2 diabetes mellitus develops when the effects of insulin are deficient. After a meal both types cause blood glucose levels to remain elevated because glucose is unable to enter most tissue cells. Excess glucose is lost from the body in the urine in the process known as *glycosuria*. In severe cases, blood levels of fatty acids and their metabolites, such as acetone and acetoacetic acid, are dramatically raised. Fatty acid metabolites, which are also called *ketones* or *ketone bodies,* accumulate in the blood, and blood pH drops. This results in *ketoacidosis*, with ketone bodies spilling into the urine, which is known as *ketonuria*. Ketoacidosis may be life threatening if it is severe, disrupting heart activity and oxygen transport and leading to severe nervous system depression and coma. The three cardinal signs of diabetes mellitus are *polyuria*, leading to dehydration; *polydipsia* or excessive thirst; and *polyphagia* or excessive hunger and food consumption. *Hyperinsulism* causes low blood glucose levels, which is known as *hypoglycemia*, and causes anxiety, nervousness, tremors, and weakness. It is usually caused by an insulin overdose and is treated by ingestion of glucose.

TABLE 14-7

Hormones from Other Organs

Origination	Hormone
Thymus	Thymulin, thymopoietins, thymosins
Reproductive organs	Estrogens and progesterone (ovaries), testosterone (testes), estrogens/progesterone/gonadotropin (placenta)
Gastrointestinal tract mucosa	Gastrin and ghrelin (stomach), secretin and cholecystokinin (duodenum of the small intestine), incretins (glucose-dependent insulinotropic peptide and glucagon-like peptide 1) from the duodenum and other gut regions
Heart (atria)	Atrial natriuretic peptide
Kidneys	Erythropoietin
Adipose tissue	Leptin, resistin, adiponectin
Skeleton	Osteocalcin
Skin (epidermal cells)	Cholecalciferol (provitamin D_3)

intestinal cells absorb calcium from the diet. Without calcitriol the bones soften and weaken. Osteocalcin is also involved in regulating the mineralization of the bones and teeth. **TABLE 14-7** illustrates the hormones produced by other organs.

Stress

Homeostasis ensures survival. When danger is sensed, the hypothalamus triggers physiologic responses, which include increased sympathetic activity and increased secretion of adrenal and other hormones. A factor stimulating this type of response is a stressor, and the condition it produces is *stress*. Many stresses are opposed by specific homeostatic changes. For example, when body temperature declines, it leads to shivering and changes in the pattern of blood flow. This can restore normal body temperature.

The body also has a general response to stress that occurs while other, more specific responses are under way. When exposure to a wide variety of stress-causing factors occurs, it produces the same general pattern of hormonal and physiologic changes. These responses are part of the general adaptation syndrome that is also known as the *stress response*.

Physical factors and psychological factors both can produce stress. Physical factors include temperature changes, decreased oxygen concentration, infections, injuries, prolonged exercises, and loud sounds. Physiological factors include real or imagined dangers, personal loss, and unpleasant social situations. Psychological stressors also include anger, fear, anxiety, depression, grief, and guilt. Positive stimuli can also be stressful in certain situations.

The hypothalamus controls the stress response, as part of the *general adaptation syndrome*. Reactions occur in either the immediate "alarm" stage or the longer term "resistance" stage. The hypothalamus first prepares the body for the fight-or-flight syndrome by raising blood glucose, glycerol, and fatty acids and by increasing heart rate, blood pressure, and breathing rate. It dilates the air passages, moves blood from the skin and digestive organs to the skeletal muscles, and increases epinephrine secretion from the adrenal medulla (**FIGURE 14-19**).

The resistance response involves the release of CRH to stimulate the secretion of ACTH, which stimulates cortisol secretion. This increases blood amino acids, release of fatty acids, and glucose formation. The body is being prepared for physical action to alleviate the stress. Energy sources are mobilized and blood volume is increased, which is important during bleeding or heavy sweating.

TEST YOUR UNDERSTANDING

1. What hormones are secreted by the placenta, thymus gland, and stomach?
2. List the hormones produced from the adipose tissue, skin, heart, and skeleton.

Effects of Aging on the Endocrine System

The endocrine system is one of the systems least affected by aging. The levels of TSH, ADH, PTH, thyroid hormones, PRL, and glucocorticoids remain relatively constant throughout life. However, the major exception to this is the decline in reproductive hormone production. Some endocrine tissues also are not as responsive to stimulation during later life. GH and insulin are not secreted in nearly the same amounts after eating carbohydrates as they were earlier in life. The effects of these hormonal changes include reduced bone density and muscle mass. Peripheral tissues also may become less responsive to certain hormones such as ADH and glucocorticoids.

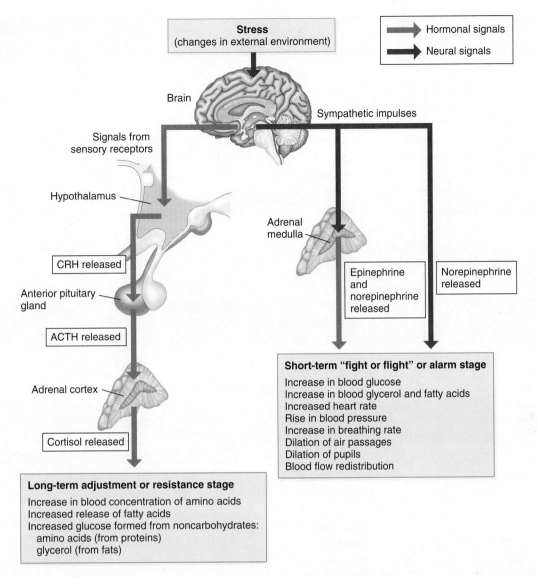

Stress
(changes in external environment)

→ Hormonal signals
→ Neural signals

Brain

Sympathetic impulses

Signals from
sensory receptors

Hypothalamus

Adrenal
medulla

CRH released

Epinephrine
and
norepinephrine
released

Norepinephrine
released

Anterior pituitary
gland

ACTH released

Adrenal cortex

Short-term "fight or flight" or alarm stage
Increase in blood glucose
Increase in blood glycerol and fatty acids
Increased heart rate
Rise in blood pressure
Increase in breathing rate
Dilation of air passages
Dilation of pupils
Blood flow redistribution

Cortisol released

Long-term adjustment or resistance stage
Increase in blood concentration of amino acids
Increased release of fatty acids
Increased glucose formed from noncarbohydrates:
  amino acids (from proteins)
  glycerol (from fats)

FIGURE 14-19 Stress response.

SUMMARY

The endocrine and nervous systems maintain homeostasis. The endocrine system is a network of glands that secrete hormones. These hormones, which are quite potent, travel through the bloodstream to affect the functioning of target cells. The nervous and endocrine systems both exert very precise effects. Hormones include steroids, amines, peptides, proteins, and glycoproteins. Steroid hormones enter target cells and bind receptors, forming complexes in the nuclei. Nonsteroid hormones bind receptors in target cell membranes. The concentration of each hormone in the body fluids is regulated.

The pituitary gland has an anterior lobe and a posterior lobe. Its secretions are mostly controlled by the hypothalamus. The anterior pituitary gland secretes GH, PRL, TSH, ACTH, FSH, and LH. The posterior pituitary gland secretes ADH

and oxytocin. The thyroid gland in the neck consists of two lobes and secretes thyroxine and triiodothyronine. The parathyroid glands, on the posterior thyroid gland, secrete PTH.

The adrenal glands, located atop the kidneys, consist of a medulla and a cortex, each with differing functions. The medulla secretes epinephrine and norepinephrine, and the cortex secretes aldosterone, cortisol, and sex hormones. The pancreas secretes digestive juices as well as hormones and is vital for normal balancing of glucagon and insulin. Other endocrine glands include the pineal gland, thymus, ovaries, testes, digestive glands, and hormone-producing organs. The pineal gland is located deep in the cerebral hemispheres and secretes the hormone melatonin. The thymus is located deep inside the mediastinum posterior to the sternum, shrinks with aging, and is important in early immunity. The ovaries secrete estrogens and progesterone, whereas the testes secrete the testosterone. The digestive glands secrete gastrin, ghrelin, secretin, cholecystokinin, and incretins.

Hormone-producing organs include the heart, kidneys, and skin. The adipose tissue and skeleton also secrete hormones. The heart's atria secretes atrial natriuretic peptide, which stimulates urinary sodium excretion. The kidneys secrete erythropoietin, a red blood cell GH. The skin secretes cholecalciferol, an inactive form of vitamin D_3. The adipose tissue cells release leptin,

resistin, and adiponectin. The bones, via their osteoblasts, secrete osteocalcin, which functions in insulin secretion.

Stress occurs when the body responds to stressors that threaten homeostasis. Stress responses include increased sympathetic nervous system action and increased adrenal hormone secretion. Physical factors and psychological factors both can produce stress. The hypothalamus controls the stress response, also known as general adaptation syndrome. The resistance response involves the release of CRH to stimulate the secretion of ACTH, which stimulates cortisol secretion. This prepares the body for physical action to alleviate the stress.

KEY TERMS

Acromegaly	Erythropoietin	Neurohypophysis
Adiponectin	Follicle-stimulating hormone (FSH)	Norepinephrine
Addison's disease	Gastrin	Osteocalcin
Adrenal androgens	Ghrelin	Oxytocin
Adrenocorticotropic hormone (ACTH)	Gigantism	Paracrine
Aldosterone	Glucagon	Parathyroid hormone (PTH)
Angiotensinogen	Gonadocorticoids	Pituitary dwarfism
Antidiuretic hormone	Growth hormone (GH)	Placenta
Autocrine	Hormones	Prolactin (PRL)
Calcitonin	Hypophyseal portal veins	Prostaglandins
Calmodulin	Incretins	Releasing hormones
Cholecystokinin	Infundibulum	Renin
Circadian rhythms	Inhibiting hormones	Resistin
Corticosteroids	Insulin	Secretin
Cortisol	Leptin	Target cells
Cushing's syndrome	Luteinizing hormone (LH)	Thymosins
Cyclic adenosine monophosphate (cAMP)	Melatonin	Thyroglobulin
	Mineralocorticoids	Thyroid-stimulating hormone (TSH)
Eicosanoids	Negative feedback	Thyroxine
Epinephrine	Neuroendocrine organ	Triiodothyronine

LEARNING GOALS

The following learning goals correspond to the objectives at the beginning of this chapter:

1. The anterior pituitary gland secretes growth hormone, prolactin, thyroid-stimulating hormone, adrenocorticotropic hormone, follicle-stimulating hormone, and luteinizing hormone. The posterior pituitary gland secretes antidiuretic hormone and oxytocin.

2. Steroids are derived from cholesterol. Amines, peptides, and proteins are derived from amino acids. Glycoproteins are derived from both carbohydrates and proteins.

3. The thyroid gland is located just below the larynx, on either side and in front of the trachea. The thyroid

gland produces thyroxine or T_4 and triiodothyronine or T_3, as well as calcitonin.

4. PTH increases blood calcium concentration and decreases blood phosphate ion concentration to affect the bones, intestines, and kidneys. It stimulates reabsorption of bone while causing kidney conservation of blood calcium and excretion of more phosphate ions in urine. It also stimulates absorption of calcium from food in the intestines. Along with calcitonin, PTH is important for stable blood calcium concentration because it increases blood calcium concentrations.

5. The adrenal glands sit on top of each kidney like caps and are embedded in the adipose tissue enclosing each kidney. They have a central adrenal medulla and an outer adrenal cortex. The medulla is closely connected with the autonomic nervous system. It increases heart rate, cardiac muscle contraction force, breathing rate, and blood glucose level, while elevating blood pressure and decreasing digestive activity. This prepares the body for the fight-or-flight response.

6. The adrenal medulla produces norepinephrine and norepinephrine. The adrenal cortex produces more than 30 steroids, as well as hormones such as aldosterone, cortisol, and some sex hormones.

7. The pancreas produces the hormones glucagon and insulin. Glucagon stimulates the liver to break down glycogen and convert certain noncarbohydrates, including amino acids, into glucose. This raises the blood sugar concentration very effectively. Glucagon secretion prevents hypoglycemia from occurring when glucose concentration is relatively low. Insulin works in a manner opposite of glucagon. It decreases blood glucose concentration, promotes amino acid transport into cells, increases protein synthesis, and stimulates adipose cells to make and store fat. Insulin secretion decreases as glucose concentrations fall.

8. The kidneys secrete erythropoietin, which is a red blood cell GH. The heart secretes atrial natriuretic peptide, which stimulates urinary sodium excretion. The thymus is important in early immunity, secreting hormones called thymosins, affecting production and differentiation of lymphocytes.

9. The testes produce testosterone. The ovaries produce estrogen and progesterone.

10. Normal growth requires growth hormone, which is stimulated by growth hormone-releasing hormone. Thyroid hormones are also required for growth and include thyroxine or T_4 and triiodothyronine or T_3.

CRITICAL THINKING QUESTIONS

A 45-year-old woman had hypertension, a moon-shaped face, and a "buffalo hump" on her back. Her physician diagnosed her with Cushing's syndrome.

1. Dysfunction of which endocrine glands can produce these symptoms?

2. Name six hormones from the anterior pituitary gland, and five major substances secreted from the adrenal glands.

REVIEW QUESTIONS

1. Which of the following statements is true about the hormone oxytocin?
    A. It is responsible for milk production in the mammary glands.
    B. It regulates blood pressure.
    C. It promotes uterine contractions.
    D. It controls the ovarian cycle.

2. Which of the following pituitary hormones controls the release of glucocorticoids from the adrenal cortex?

    A. LH
    B. GH
    C. TSH
    D. ACTH

3. Which of the following hormones may cause blood sugar levels to fall?
    A. glucagon
    B. insulin
    C. aldosterone
    D. cortisol

4. Which of the following hormones is released by the adrenal cortex?
    A. epinephrine
    B. aldosterone
    C. norepinephrine
    D. insulin
5. The placenta secretes
    A. progesterone
    B. cortisone
    C. aldosterone
    D. testosterone
6. Calcitonin is secreted from the
    A. heart
    B. liver
    C. pituitary gland
    D. thyroid gland
7. Growth hormone is also called
    A. melanotropin
    B. somatotropin
    C. adrenocorticotropin
    D. gonadotropin
8. Parathyroid hormone does all the following, *except*
    A. increase urine formation
    B. inhibit osteoblast activity
    C. stimulate osteoclast activity
    D. increase reabsorption of calcium in the kidneys
9. Diabetes insipidus is caused by decreased levels of which hormone?
    A. glucagon
    B. prolactin
    C. vasopressin
    D. cortisol
10. The zona glomerulosa of the adrenal cortex produces
    A. epinephrine
    B. norepinephrine
    C. glucocorticoids
    D. mineralocorticoids
11. The posterior pituitary gland secretes
    A. TSH
    B. LH
    C. ADH
    D. ACTH
12. Hormones known as catecholamines are
    A. steroids
    B. lipids
    C. peptides
    D. derivatives of amino acids
13. The hypothalamus controls secretions of the anterior pituitary by
    A. releasing and inhibiting hormones
    B. direct neural stimulation
    C. direct mechanical control
    D. altering ion concentrations in the anterior pituitary
14. All the following hormones are produced by the adenohypophysis, *except*
    A. LH
    B. GH
    C. ADH
    D. TSH
15. The pituitary hormone that triggers the release of thyroid hormone from the thyroid gland is
    A. FSH
    B. GH
    C. TSH
    D. LH

ESSAY QUESTIONS

1. Define "hormone."
2. Describe the locations of the pineal gland, adrenal glands, parathyroid glands, and pituitary gland.
3. List the hormones that are stored in the posterior lobe of the pituitary gland.
4. Name the hormones secreted from the adipose tissue and the skeleton.
5. List the major hormones that are released from the adrenal cortex.
6. Describe the mechanism of the renin-angiotensin-aldosterone system.
7. Explain the roles of insulin and glucagon on glucose in the blood.
8. Describe how prolactin and oxytocin affect the female reproductive system.
9. Define and compare diabetes insipidus with diabetes mellitus.
10. Name two endocrine glands that are important in the body's response to stress.

UNIT IV

TRANSPORT

Blood

OBJECTIVES

After studying this chapter, readers should be able to

1. Describe the important components of the blood.
2. Specify the composition of plasma.
3. List three types of plasma proteins.
4. List the characteristics of the functions of red blood cells.
5. Describe the functions of hemoglobin.
6. Categorize the various white blood cells on the basis of their structures and functions.
7. Describe the function and production of platelets.
8. Distinguish between granulocytes and agranulocytes.
9. Discuss mechanisms that control blood loss after an injury.
10. Explain the importance of blood typing and the basis for ABO and Rh incompatibilities.

Overview

The *cardiovascular system* consists of the heart, blood, and blood vessels. Blood is pumped by the heart through a closed circuit of blood vessels to the body tissues, returning back to the heart. This chapter focuses on the structure and functions of the blood. The blood's functions include transportation, protection by fighting foreign invaders, and clotting to prevent bleeding. The blood is also involved in acid-base balance, fluid and electrolyte balance, and the regulation of body temperature.

Blood Components

The *blood* is made up of cells, fragments of cells, and dissolved biochemicals containing nutrients, oxygen, hormones, and wastes (**FIGURE 15-1**). It helps to distribute body heat and maintain stable interstitial fluid. Blood is actually a connective tissue with its cells suspended in a liquid, the extracellular matrix. It is heavier and thicker than water, is the only fluid tissue in the body, and is a *homogenous liquid*. This means it has a similar composition throughout. Blood contains formed elements such as red blood cells (*RBCs*), white blood cells (*WBCs*), and platelets. Of these, only the leukocytes or *WBCs* are complete cells, containing nuclei and organelles. Most of the formed elements exist in the bloodstream for only a few hours or days before they are replaced by new cells. Also, most of them do not divide and are replaced by stem cells that continuously divide in the red bone marrow. The liquid portion of blood is called **plasma**.

Blood Functions

The various components of the blood function in distribution, regulation, and protection. These are broken down by function as follows:

- *Distribution:* Delivery of oxygen from the lungs, delivery of nutrients from the gastrointestinal tract to all cells in the body, transport of hormones from endocrine organs to target organs, and transport of metabolic waste products from cells to various elimination sites; these include the kidneys, for disposal of nitrogenous wastes in the urine, and the lungs, for the elimination of carbon dioxide.

- *Regulation:* Maintenance of proper fluid volume in the circulatory system; proteins in the blood prevent excessive fluid loss from the bloodstream into tissue spaces; therefore, fluid volume remains in the blood vessels, supporting efficient blood circulation throughout the body; maintenance of body temperature by absorption and distribution of body heat, as well as to the skin surfaces for heat loss; maintenance of normal pH in body tissues, with proteins and other bloodborne solutes becoming buffers, preventing serious changes in blood pH; the blood also is a reservoir for bicarbonate ions, which are the body's *alkaline reserve*.

- *Protection:* Prevention of infection, via the actions of antibodies, complement proteins, and WBCs; this protects the body against bacteria, viruses, and other foreign agents; prevention of blood loss via the actions of platelets and plasma proteins, which begin clot formation and slow or stop blood loss.

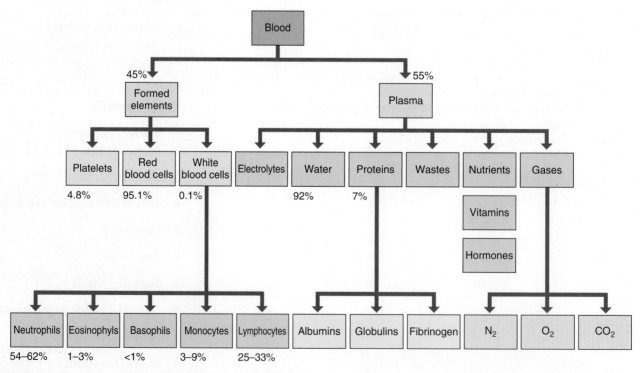

FIGURE 15-1 Blood composition.

TABLE 15-1

Plasma Proteins

Protein	Origin	% of Total	Function
Albumins	Liver	60	Help maintain colloid osmotic pressure
Globulins		36	
Alpha	Liver		Transport lipids and fat-soluble vitamins
Beta	Liver		Transport lipids and fat-soluble vitamins
Gamma	Lymphatic tissues		Constitute a type of antibody
Fibrinogen	Liver	4	Plays key roles in blood coagulation

Plasma

Plasma suspends the cells and platelets of the blood. It is a clear, straw-colored liquid made up of 92% water, with organic and inorganic biochemicals. In many respects the composition of plasma resembles interstitial fluid. Concentrations of major plasma ions are similar to those of the interstitial fluid, differing greatly from the concentrations inside cells. This is because water, ions, and over 100 small solutes are continuously exchanged between plasma and interstitial fluid across the walls of capillaries. Normally, the capillaries deliver more liquid and solutes to tissues than they remove from them. Plasma helps to transport gases, hormones, nutrients, and vitamins while helping to regulate fluid and electrolyte balance as well as pH levels. Electrolytes such as sodium and chloride are the most prevalent of the solutes in the plasma. **Plasma proteins** are heavier than electrolytes and are not typically used as energy sources, remaining in the blood and interstitial fluids. By weight alone, the plasma proteins are the most abundant of the plasma solutes, making up approximately 8% of plasma weight. The liver synthesizes and releases more than 90% of the plasma proteins, including all albumins, fibrinogen, and most globulins. The plasma also contains products of cell activity and wastes.

Albumins are the smallest of the plasma proteins but make up around 60% of these proteins by weight. They are made in the liver and play an important role in the plasma's osmotic pressure, transporting smaller molecules such as hormones and ions. Plasma proteins are too large to move through capillary walls, so they create an osmotic pressure to hold water in the capillaries, which is known as *colloid osmotic pressure*. This helps regulate water movement between blood and tissues, to aid in controlling blood volume and blood pressure. Therefore, albumins act as important blood buffers.

Globulins, which include alpha, beta, and gamma globulins, make up around 36% of the plasma proteins. **Fibrinogen**, which makes up around 4% of the plasma proteins, is important for blood coagulation. Under certain conditions fibrinogen molecules interact to form large, insoluble strands of **fibrin**. This substance provides the basic framework for a blood clot. Fibrinogen is made in the liver and is the largest,

in size, of the plasma proteins. **TABLE 15-1** summarizes albumin, globulin, and fibrinogen.

Oxygen and carbon dioxide are the most important blood gases, with nitrogen also contained in the plasma. Plasma nutrients include amino acids, nucleotides, lipids, and simple sugars absorbed from the digestive tract. Glucose is transported in the plasma from the small intestine to the liver.

In the liver, glucose is stored as glycogen or converted to fat. The concentration of glucose in the blood is represented in milligrams per deciliter (mg/dL). When the blood concentration of glucose drops, the potentially dangerous situation called *hypoglycemia* occurs. When glucose is elevated, it is called hyperglycemia, which can lead to diabetes (**TABLE 15-2**). Plasma carries amino acids to the liver to manufacture proteins or to be used for energy. Plasma lipids include triglycerides, cholesterol, and phospholipids.

TABLE 15-2

Blood Glucose Levels

Level	Description	Resulting Conditions
Less than 70 mg/dL	Hypoglycemia	Can be potentially fatal; symptoms include lethargy, impaired mental functioning, irritability, and loss of consciousness
Between 70 and 110 mg/dL	Normal	Levels are usually lower in the morning and rise after meals
Between 110 and 125 mg/dL	Borderline hyperglycemia	Does not result in diabetes mellitus
126 mg/dL or greater	Hyperglycemia	If persistent, can result in diabetes mellitus, which can cause eye, kidney, and nerve damage

Lipids are not water soluble, but the plasma is mostly made of water. Hence, lipids join with proteins to form *lipoproteins*, which the plasma can carry.

Nonprotein nitrogenous substances have nitrogen atoms but are not proteins. In the plasma these include amino acids, urea, and uric acid. Blood plasma also contains many electrolytes, which include potassium, calcium, sodium, magnesium, chloride, phosphate, bicarbonate, and sulfate ions. The most abundant types are sodium and chloride ions. All plasma constituents are regulated so their blood concentrations remain mostly stable.

TEST YOUR UNDERSTANDING

1. Which plasma protein plays a key role in blood coagulation?
2. What are the functions of globulins?
3. Define the terms *albumins, fibrinogen,* and *fibrin*.

FOCUS ON PATHOLOGY

Clotting disorders are a group of conditions in which there is an increased tendency for excessive clotting. Each year, more than 600,000 people in the United States die from abnormal blood clots. Thrombosis is a very common medical problem, and approximately 2 million Americans experience a deep vein thrombosis every year. Nearly half of these patients experience long-term health consequences.

Formed Elements

Red blood cells make up about 45% of blood volume, which is known as the **hematocrit**. WBCs and platelets make up less than 1%. The remainder is plasma, which appears as a clear, straw-colored liquid. Plasma contains water, amino acids, carbohydrates, lipids, proteins, hormones, electrolytes, vitamins, and cellular wastes. An average adult has approximately 5 liters or approximately 5.3 quarts of blood in his or her body.

All formed elements arise from the hematocytoblasts, which are also called *hematopoietic stem cells*, which are undifferentiated precursor cells in the red bone marrow. Different modes of maturation of formed elements exist. Once a cell becomes committed to a certain blood cell pathway, it is unable to change. Membrane surface receptors appear, which signal the cell's commitment to one blood cell pathway. The receptors respond to specific growth factors or hormones. These assist the cell in becoming even more specialized. In a healthy male adult the normal hematocrit value is 47%, plus or minus 5%. In a healthy female adult,

it is 42%, plus or minus 5%. Less than 1% of blood volume consists of platelets and leukocytes. Most of the remaining 55% of whole blood is made up by the plasma (**FIGURE 15-2**). The components that make up whole blood can be separated or *fractionated* to be clinically analyzed.

Red Blood Cells

Red blood cells (erythrocytes) have a biconcave shape, meaning they are basically round, with a center that is depressed in comparison with their edges. This shape helps them to transport gases by increasing the surface area of the cell, allowing more diffusion. This shape also ensures the cell membrane is nearer to the **hemoglobin**, which carries oxygen, inside the cell. Erythrocytes, when mature, are bound by a plasma membrane. Red blood cells are about one-third hemoglobin, a protein that gives them their red color. Therefore, hemoglobin is the major protein in red blood cells. **FIGURE 15-3** shows the various types of blood cells.

The formation of erythrocytes, called *erythropoiesis*, occurs only in the red bone marrow or the *myeloid tissue,* which is tissue that performs *hematopoiesis*. Erythrocytes have nuclei that are shed as they mature, allowing more room for hemoglobin. Lacking nuclei, mature RBCs cannot synthesize proteins or divide to form more cells. They produce adenosine triphosphate through glycolysis because they do not have mitochondria and use none of the oxygen carried in their hemoglobin. Erythrocytes also have nearly no organelles and contain mostly antioxidant enzymes and structural proteins. The structural proteins allow them to change shape and return to their original shape afterward. A network of proteins, primarily one called *spectrin*, is attached to the cytoplasm of red blood cell plasma membranes. This maintains the biconcave shape. Spectrin forms a net that allows RBCs to bend, turn, and become more concave as needed to move through tiny capillaries. For example, in lung capillaries RBCs pick up oxygen and release it to tissue cells through other body capillaries. They also move approximately 20% of the carbon dioxide from tissue cells back to the lungs. Red blood cells are highly efficient in these tasks because they generate adenosine triphosphate via anaerobic mechanisms and do not have mitochondria. This means they do not consume any of the oxygen they carry. Oxygen is picked up from the alveoli by the red blood cells, and it binds with hemoglobin. The RBCs carry oxygen to the tissue cells.

Hemoglobin

Hemoglobin is responsible for the ability of the cells to transport oxygen and carbon dioxide, and most oxygen carried in the blood is bound to hemoglobin. When hemoglobin easily and reversibly binds with oxygen, oxyhemoglobin is formed. *Oxyhemoglobin* is bright red and has a three-dimensional structure. When oxygen is released, deoxyhemoglobin is formed. *Deoxyhemoglobin* is darker red, and blood rich in deoxyhemoglobin may appear bluish when seen through blood vessels. Deoxyhemoglobin is also known as *reduced hemoglobin*.

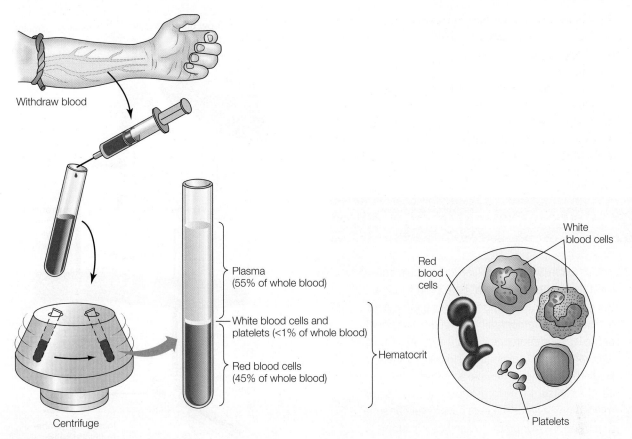

FIGURE 15-2 The composition of whole blood.

Erythrocytes 98%

Leukocytes 2%

Erythromyeloid lineage

• Granular leukocytes

  Neutrophils 45–74% of leukocytes

  Basophils <1% of leukocytes

  Eosinophils 1–5% of leukocytes

• Monocytes 3–11% of leukocytes

Lymphoid lineage 20–47% of leukocytes

• T cells

• B cells

FIGURE 15-3 Various blood cells.

Approximately 20% of the carbon dioxide that is transported by the blood is combined with hemoglobin. However, the carbon dioxide binds to the amino acids of the globin portion of hemoglobin instead of the *heme* portion. This forms *carbaminohemoglobin*, and the process occurs more easily when the hemoglobin is dissociated from oxygen. This is known as its *reduced state*. The loading of carbon dioxide occurs in the tissues, with transport occurring from the tissues to the lungs, where it is eliminated from the body.

Mature RBCs contain an adult-type of hemoglobin called HbA. In an embryo or fetus, a different form of hemoglobin, known as *fetal hemoglobin* or *HbF*, is contained in the RBCs. This binds oxygen more readily than adult hemoglobin. Therefore, a developing fetus can "steal" oxygen from the mother's bloodstream via the placenta. Fetal hemoglobin begins to convert to adult hemoglobin shortly before birth and continues over the next year.

The way hemoglobin is contained in the RBCs prevents two major occurrences. The hemoglobin does not break into fragments and therefore does not leak out of the bloodstream through the walls of the capillaries. Also, the hemoglobin is prevented from increased blood viscosity and raising osmotic pressure. The viscosity of the blood is mostly determined by the erythrocytes. When the number of RBCs exceeds the normal range, blood flows more slowly because it has become more viscous. Oppositely, blood thins and flows more quickly when the RBC count drops below the normal range.

A red blood cell count is the number of RBCs in a microliter of blood. Normal ranges are as follows:

- *Adult males:* 4.7 million to 6.1 million cells per microliter
- *Adult females:* 4.2 million to 5.4 million cells per microliter

Increased numbers of circulating RBCs increase the blood's oxygen-carrying capacity, which can affect health positively. RBC counts are taken to diagnose many diseases and evaluate their courses.

FOCUS ON PATHOLOGY

Thalassemia is a genetic disorder in which deficient production of alpha or beta globulin affects the rate of synthesis of normal *hemoglobin A*. As a result, more *hemoglobin F* or *fetal hemoglobin*, or the less common *hemoglobin A2*, is increased to compensate. Thalassemia is most prevalent in Mediterranean countries, parts of Africa, and in Southeast Asia. In the form known as *thalassemia major*, homozygous patients have severe anemia that develops in infancy, causing death during childhood or adolescence. In this form, increased destruction of immature erythrocytes in the bone marrow causes decreased production of RBCs.

Erythropoiesis

In humans, RBCs are mostly developed in spaces within bones that are filled with red bone marrow. RBCs usually live for 120 days, with replacement cells created to maintain a relatively stable RBC count. The rate of RBC formation is controlled by negative feedback via the hormone **erythropoietin**. It is released by the kidneys and liver in response to prolonged oxygen deficiency (**FIGURE 15-4**).

The formation of all types of blood cells is known as *hematopoiesis* and occurs in the red bone marrow. In this bone marrow, there is a soft network of reticular connective tissue. This tissue borders *blood sinusoids*, which are wide blood capillaries. The network contains immature blood cells, fat cells, macrophages, and *reticular cells*. The reticular cells secrete the connective tissue fibers. In an adult, red bone marrow is mostly found in the axial skeleton bones and girdles and in the proximal epiphyses of the femur and humerus.

Production of RBCs continues at a heightened rate until the amount of them in the blood circulation is enough to supply oxygen to the body tissues. The stages of formation of RBCs and other types of blood cells from *hemocytoblasts* are shown in **FIGURE 15-5**. These stages have been individually named by hematologists. Approximately 1 ounce of new blood is created every day. This ounce of blood contains approximately 100 billion new cells.

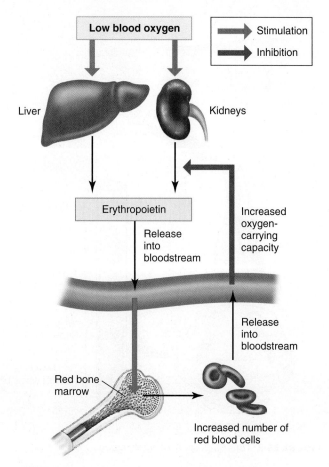

FIGURE 15-4 The rate of RBC formation is controlled by negative feedback via the hormone erythropoietin. It is released by the kidneys and liver in response to prolonged oxygen deficiency. (Adapted from Shier, D. N., Butler, J. L., and Lewis, R. Hole's Essentials of Human Anatomy & Physiology, Tenth edition. McGraw-Hill Higher Education, 2009.)

The stages of RBC maturation are described briefly, as follows:

- Hemocytoblasts or *multipotent stem cells*, in the red bone marrow, produce *myeloid stem cells*; myeloid stem cell division creates *progenitor cells*, from which all formed elements derive, except for lymphocytes.
- The myeloid stem cells divide, producing RBCs and several types of WBCs.
- *Lymphoid stem cells* divide to produce various types of lymphocytes.
- Cells that will become RBCs initially differentiate into *proerythroblasts*.
- These cells then mature through several *erythroblast* stages, actively synthesizing hemoglobin.
- After approximately 4 days, the erythroblasts are then called *normoblasts* and shed their nuclei to become *reticulocytes*; the reticulocytes contain 80% of the hemoglobin of a mature RBC and are immature cells found in the peripheral blood.
- Hemoglobin synthesis continues for up to 3 more days; the cytoplasm of these cells still contains RNA.

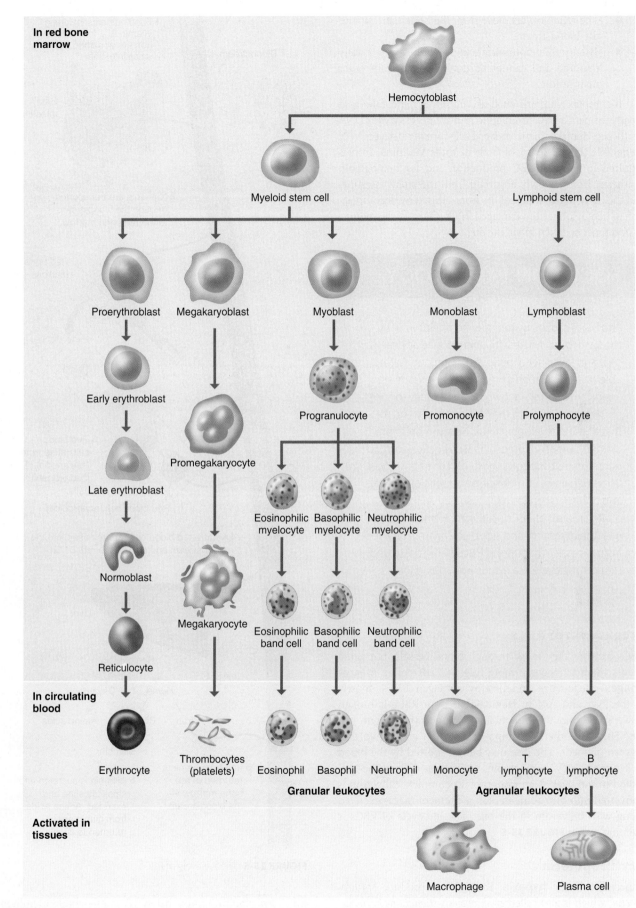

FIGURE 15-5 The stages of formation of the blood cells from hemocytoblasts. (Adapted from Shier, D. N., Butler, J. L., and Lewis, R. Hole's Essentials of Human Anatomy & Physiology, Tenth edition. McGraw-Hill Higher Education, 2009.)

- The reticulocytes move from the bone marrow into the bloodstream.
- Twenty-four hours later, the reticulocytes are fully matured and cannot be distinguished from other mature RBCs.

B-complex vitamins such as vitamin B_{12} and folic acid greatly influence RBC production and are necessary for DNA synthesis. Hematopoietic or *blood cell–forming* tissue is very vulnerable to deficiency of both of these vitamins. Iron is required for normal RBC production and for hemoglobin synthesis. Iron is slowly absorbed from the small intestine, and the body reuses much of the iron released by decomposition of hemoglobin from damaged RBCs. Only small amounts of iron must be taken in via the diet.

FOCUS ON PATHOLOGY

Anemia is caused by too little hemoglobin or by too few RBCs. People with anemia may appear pale and lack energy because their blood is not able to carry enough oxygen. Iron-rich foods are important for pregnant women especially to supply enough oxygen to their blood supply and to that of their developing fetus. Because pregnant women's blood volume increases because of fluid retention that supports the fetus, their hematocrit levels decrease. Iron-deficiency, pernicious, renal, and aplastic anemias are caused by an inadequate amount of RBCs produced. Hemolytic anemia, thalassemias, and sickle-cell anemia develop from excessive amounts of RBCs being destroyed. Hemorrhagic anemia results from blood loss.

Breakdown of RBCs

RBCs bend as they move through blood vessels, but aging causes them to become more fragile. Cells called **macrophages** phagocytize and destroy damaged RBCs, mostly in the liver and spleen. Hemoglobin from RBCs is broken down into *heme*, which contains iron, and the protein *globin*. The heme then decomposes into iron and **biliverdin**, a green pigment. The iron may be transported by the blood to synthesize new hemoglobin, with about 80% of the iron stored in the liver as an iron–protein complex. Biliverdin is converted into **bilirubin**, an orange pigment that is excreted along with biliverdin in the bile. The life cycle of RBCs is summarized in **FIGURE 15-6**.

Erythropoietin

Especially during **hypoxia**, the kidneys produce *erythropoietin*, which is also called *erythropoiesis-stimulating hormone*. Erythropoietin stimulates production of erythroblasts from bone marrow. Therefore, bone marrow can increase the rate of

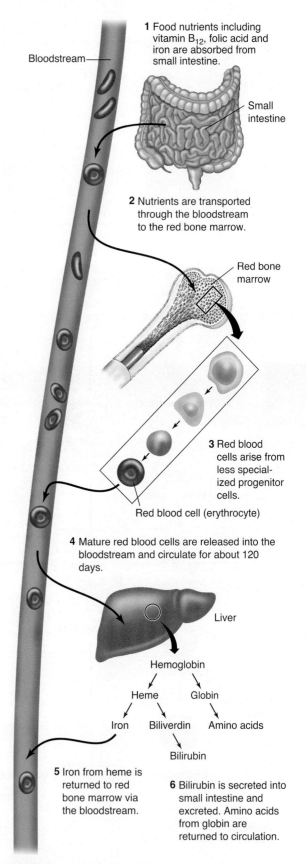

1 Food nutrients including vitamin B_{12}, folic acid and iron are absorbed from small intestine.

Bloodstream

Small intestine

2 Nutrients are transported through the bloodstream to the red bone marrow.

Red bone marrow

3 Red blood cells arise from less specialized progenitor cells.

Red blood cell (erythrocyte)

4 Mature red blood cells are released into the bloodstream and circulate for about 120 days.

Liver

Hemoglobin

Heme   Globin

Iron   Biliverdin   Amino acids

Bilirubin

5 Iron from heme is returned to red bone marrow via the bloodstream.

6 Bilirubin is secreted into small intestine and excreted. Amino acids from globin are returned to circulation.

FIGURE 15-6 The life cycle of RBCs.

RBC formation by approximately 10 times—about 30 million cells per second. This process aids the patient during recovery from a severe loss of blood.

Erythropoietin is actually a glycoprotein hormone. There is a small amount of erythropoietin in the blood consistently, which sustains a basal rate of RBC production. The kidneys are important for erythropoietin production, and the liver produces lesser quantities. If certain kidney cells are deficient in oxygen, enzymes that are oxygen-sensitive cannot function normally. *Hypoxia-inducible factor* is an intracellular signaling molecule that accumulates as a result, increasing the synthesis and release of erythropoietin. This condition may be caused by iron deficiency, in which there is insufficient hemoglobin in each RBC; high altitudes or pneumonia, which cause reduced availability of oxygen; excessive destruction of RBCs; or hemorrhage, which results in reduced numbers of RBCs. Oppositely, erythropoietin production is depressed by excessive oxygen or excessive erythrocytes in the bloodstream. In the bloodstream, erythropoietin stimulates red bone marrow cells that are already committed to forming erythrocytes, causing them to mature more quickly.

FOCUS ON PATHOLOGY

Self-injection of erythropoietin is becoming more prevalent today among athletes, with potentially deadly results. Although injection may raise hematocrit from normal levels up to 65%, extreme physical activity can cause blood concentration, because of dehydration. The blood becomes thick and sticky, which can lead to clotting, heart failure, and stroke.

Testosterone also enhances production of erythropoietin in the kidneys. Female sex hormones do not do this. Therefore, testosterone may account somewhat for higher hemoglobin levels and RBC counts in males. RBC production may also be heightened by many different chemicals released by leukocytes, platelets, and some reticular cells.

Iron

Amino acids, lipids, and carbohydrates are required for erythropoiesis to occur. Hemoglobin synthesis requires iron, which is available in the diet. The cells of the intestines accurately control iron absorption into the bloodstream as a result of changing amounts of iron that are stored in the body. Hemoglobin contains approximately 65% of the body's supply of iron, which is about 4,000 mg. The liver and spleen store most of the rest of body iron, with small amounts also stored in the bone marrow. Iron is stored inside cells as protein–iron complexes called *ferritin* and *hemosiderin*, because free iron ions are toxic to the body. Iron is loosely bound to a transport protein called *transferrin* in the blood. Erythrocytes that are developing take up iron as required to form hemoglobin. Every day we lose small amounts of iron via

the feces, perspiration, and urine. Men lose approximately 0.9 mg per day, and women lose approximately 1.7 mg per day. Menstruation is the reason for additional average daily loss of iron in women.

When a blood sample is spun in a centrifuge, the heavier formed elements sink, whereas the plasma rises. A thin, whitish-colored layer called the *buffy coat* is present at the point where the RBCs joint the plasma. This layer is made up of leukocytes and platelets.

As erythrocytes age they become less flexible and more fragile and rigid. The hemoglobin degenerates, with these RBCs fragmenting and becoming trapped in the smaller vessels, mostly those of the spleen. They are engulfed and destroyed by macrophages, with the heme portion of their hemoglobin being split from the globin portion. The iron core is saved and bound to ferritin or hemosiderin for future use. The remainder of the heme group is degraded, becoming *bilirubin*, the yellow pigment that is released to the blood. Bilirubin is bound to albumin to be transported and then picked up by the liver, which secretes it in the bile into the intestine. There, it is metabolized to become *urobilinogen*. Most of it then leaves the body via the feces as the brown pigment known as *stercobilin*. The globin portion of the hemoglobin is transformed into amino acids and released to the blood circulation.

TEST YOUR UNDERSTANDING

1. Describe the function of hemoglobin.
2. Explain how RBCs produce adenosine triphosphate.
3. Which hormone is required for the formation of erythrocytes?

FOCUS ON PATHOLOGY

Polycythemia is an abnormal excess of RBCs, which increases blood viscosity until the blood flows much too slowly. This condition also increases the amounts of hematocrit and hemoglobin. *Primary polycythemia* is caused by inherent problems in the process of RBC production. *Secondary polycythemia* usually occurs because of other factors or underlying conditions that promote RBC production.

White Blood Cells

Leukocytes, also known as **white blood cells**, protect the body against disease. They develop from hemocytoblasts in the red bone marrow in response to hormones. These hormones are either **interleukins** or **colony-stimulating factors (CSFs)**. Interleukins are classified with different numbers, such as IL-3, whereas most of the CSFs are named for the type of cells they stimulate, such as granulocyte CSF, or G-CSF. WBCs are transported to sites of infection, and may then leave the bloodstream.

The four primary characteristics of circulating WBCs are as follows:

- *All WBCs are able to migrate out of the bloodstream:* When they contact and stick to the vessel walls, the process is known as *margination;* when they later interact with endothelial cells to become activated and squeeze between the cells to enter surrounding tissue, the process is known as *emigration* or *diapedesis.*
- *All WBCs can use amoeboid movement:* This is a gliding motion related to the flow of cytoplasm into thin cellular processes extending in the direction of movement; as a result, WBCs move through endothelial linings into peripheral tissues.
- *All WBCs are attracted to certain chemical stimuli:* This is known as *positive chemotaxis* and moves WBCs to invading pathogens, other active WBCs, and damaged tissues.
- *Phagocytosis is conducted by neutrophils, eosinophils, and monocytes:* Sometimes, neutrophils and eosinophils are called *microphages* to distinguish them from the larger *macrophages* that exist in connective tissues; macrophages are monocytes that have become actively phagocytic after moving out of the bloodstream

Usually, five types of WBCs are found in circulating blood, differing in size, cytoplasm nature, nucleus shape, and staining characteristics. Leukocytes with granular cytoplasm are called **granulocytes**; those without are called **agranulocytes**. Most granulocytes, including eosinophils, basophils, and neutrophils, are about two times as large as a RBC. Like RBCs, granulocytes develop in the red bone marrow but only live about 12 hours. To various degrees, all granulocytes are phagocytes. Agranulocytes include lymphocytes and monocytes, which lack visible cytoplasmic granules. Their nuclei are usually kidney shaped or spherical. The process of lymphocyte production is known as *lymphopoiesis.*

FOCUS ON PATHOLOGY

Infectious mononucleosis is highly contagious, caused by the Epstein-Barr virus, and usually affects young children. It is signified by excessive amounts of mostly atypical agranulocytes. Symptoms include body aches, tiredness, low-grade fever, and chronic sore throat. Although incurable, the patient is advised to rest and let the condition resolve on its own. This usually takes a few weeks.

Neutrophils

Neutrophils have small granules that appear light purple in neutral stain. Older neutrophils are sometimes called *segs* and have lobed nuclei in three to six segments connected by thin chromatin strands. Because of the structure of the nucleus, a neutrophil may be referred to as *polymorphonuclear,* or simply as a *poly.* Younger neutrophils have C-shaped nuclei and are called *bands* (**FIGURE 15-5**). Neutrophils make up 50% to 70% of the leukocytes in most adults. Neutrophils are highly mobile and, because of this, are usually the first type of WBC to arrive at an injury site. They are very active cells, attacking and digesting bacteria. An acute bacterial infection causes the numbers of neutrophils to greatly increase. They are active phagocytes that are chemically attracted to areas of inflammation and primarily target bacteria and also certain fungi. The process of this attraction is called a *respiratory burst,* in which the cells metabolize oxygen. This creates strong oxidizing substances such as hydrogen peroxide and bleach, which kill the invaders. When granules containing defensins merge with a phagosome containing a microbe, defensin-mediated lysis occurs. Spearlike structures are formed by the *defensins,* which make holes in the membranes of the ingested pathogens. Neutrophils are approximately twice as large as erythrocytes. The process of reducing the number of granules in cytoplasm via interaction with defensins is known as *degranulation.*

Most neutrophils have a short life span, surviving in the bloodstream for only about 10 hours. When they actively engulf debris or pathogens, they may last for only up to 30 minutes. Each neutrophil dies after engulfing between 1 and 2 dozen bacteria. As a neutrophil breaks down, it releases chemicals that attract other neutrophils to the site. A mixture of dead neutrophils and cellular debris forms *pus,* which is associated with infected wounds. The production of WBCs is known as *leukopoiesis.* It is stimulated by the interleukins and *CSFs.*

There are four types of colony-stimulating factors, identified by their targets:

- *M-CSF:* stimulates monocyte production
- *G-CSF:* stimulates granulocyte production; these include basophils, eosinophils, and neutrophils
- *GM-CSF:* stimulates production of granulocytes and monocytes
- *Multi-CSF:* speeds up production of granulocytes, monocytes, platelets, and RBCs

Eosinophils

Eosinophils have coarse, same-sized granules that appear dark red in the acidic eosin stain (**FIGURE 15-5**). Because the granules also stain with other acid types, they are sometimes called *acidophils.* Their nuclei usually have just two lobes, which is called *bilobed,* and they make up only 2% to 4% of circulating leukocytes. The eosinophil granules resemble lysosomes and are filled with a specific type of digestive enzymes. Eosinophils are similar in size to neutrophils. Eosinophils are particularly effective against multicellular parasites, such as parasitic flukes, including flatworms and tapeworms, and roundworms, including hookworms and pinworms, which are too big to engulf. The number of circulating eosinophils increases dramatically during a parasitic infection. Eosinophils also increase in number during an allergic reaction and asthmatic conditions.

Basophils

Basophils are similar to neutrophils or eosinophils. However, they are more irregular and become deep blue or purple in basic stain (**FIGURE 15-5**). Basophils usually account for less than 1% of circulating leukocytes. They migrate to sites of injury and cross the capillary endothelium to accumulate in the damaged tissues, where they release the inflammatory chemical *histamine*, which dilates blood vessels. Histamine also attracts other WBCs to areas of inflammation. Therefore, *antihistamines* work by opposing this effect. Basophils also release *heparin*, a compound that prevents blood clotting. Stimulated basophils release these chemicals into the interstitial fluids. These chemicals enhance the local inflammation initiated by **mast cells**. Although the same compounds are released by mast cells in damaged connective tissues, both mast cells and basophils originate differently from each other. The cytoplasm of basophils holds histamine-containing granules that are large and coarse. These granules have an affinity for basic types of dye. The nuclei of basophils are usually "S" or "U" shaped and have either one or two visible constrictions. The nuclei of mast cells are more oval in shape instead of being lobed. Both mast cells and basophils bind to immunoglobulin E, which is the antibody that causes histamine release.

Monocytes

Monocytes are the largest type of blood cells, up to three times as large as RBCs (**FIGURE 15-5**). Their average diameter is 18 μm. They have nuclei that may be either kidney-shaped, lobed, oval, or round. Their cytoplasm is abundant and pale-blue in color, whereas their "U" shaped or kidney shaped nuclei stain dark purple. Monocytes usually make up 3% to 8% of circulating leukocytes and live for either weeks or months. A single monocyte remains in the circulation for only about 24 hours before it enters the peripheral tissues. There it becomes a *tissue macrophage*. Macrophages are aggressive phagocytes that are very important in the defense against viruses, chronic infections such as tuberculosis, and certain intracellular bacterial parasites. They often attempt to engulf items as large as themselves. When they are involved in phagocytosis, they release chemicals that attract and stimulate neutrophils, monocytes, and other phagocytic cells.

Lymphocytes

Lymphocytes are usually only a little larger than RBCs, with large, round nuclei inside a thin cytoplasm rim (**FIGURE 15-5**). Lymphocytes make up between 20% and 30% of circulating leukocytes and may live for years. They continuously migrate from the bloodstream, through the peripheral tissues, and back to the bloodstream. Circulating lymphocytes represent a very small fraction of all lymphocytes. At any particular moment most of the body's lymphocytes are

in other connective tissues and organs of the lymphatic system. Their nuclei stain dark purple and appear so large they take up nearly all of the cell volume. Lymphocytes are named because of their close association with the lymph nodes, spleen, and other lymphoid tissues.

The circulating blood contains two functional classes of lymphocytes:

- **B cells** or B lymphocytes are responsible for humoral immunity, which is a specific defense mechanism that involves the production of antibodies. Activated B cells differentiate into **plasma cells**, which are specialized to secrete antibodies.
- **T cells** or T lymphocytes are responsible for cell-mediated immunity and activate B cells. They act directly against tumor cells and virus-infected cells.

WBCs protect the body in a variety of ways. Some leukocytes phagocytize bacterial cells; others create proteins called *antibodies* that disable or destroy foreign particles. *Diapedesis* is the process of leukocytes squeezing between cells of the blood vessel walls to leave the circulation. They can then move through interstitial spaces, self-propelled, via *amoeboid motion*.

Normally, there are 4,800 to 10,800 WBCs in a microliter of human blood. This is called a *white blood cell count*, abbreviated as either *WBCC* or *WCC*. WBC counts are of interest to determine patients' clinical conditions.

Percentages of the types of leukocytes in a blood sample are listed in a *differential WBC count*, which is useful to determine more exactly the type of condition. Bacterial infections usually cause neutrophil counts to increase, whereas certain parasitic infections cause the number of eosinophils to increase. AIDS causes certain types of lymphocyte counts to drop sharply.

FOCUS ON PATHOLOGY

Leukemia refers to various cancerous conditions that involve overproduction of abnormal WBCs. These cells are descendants of just one cell that remains unspecialized. They proliferate greatly and impair the function of normal red bone marrow. The red bone marrow becomes filled with cancerous leukocytes, and immature WBCs proliferate in the bloodstream. Severe anemia and bleeding develop as the other types of blood cells are crowded out, and additional symptoms include bone pain, fever, and weight loss. The large amounts of leukocytes are not functional, and the body defenses are weakened greatly. Leukemia usually causes death from an overwhelming infection and internal bleeding.

■ **TEST YOUR UNDERSTANDING**

1. Explain the five types of WBCs.
2. Which type of WBCs are the most active phagocytes?
3. Explain the term *white blood cell count*.
4. Which type of WBCs turns into a macrophage in the tissues?

Platelets

Platelets in nonmammalian vertebrates are nucleated cells called **thrombocytes**. They are incomplete cells arising from extremely large red bone marrow cells called **megakaryocytes** that have become fragmented. Megakaryocytes, which are up to 60 μm in diameter, develop from hemocytoblasts because of the hormone **thrombopoietin**. Plasma membranes from each megakaryocyte fragment seal quickly around their cytoplasm to form a platelet. The formation of platelets is known as *thrombocytopoiesis*. Platelets lack nuclei and are approximately one-fourth of the size of a lymphocyte and less than one-half the size of an erythrocyte. In actual size, platelets measure between 2 and 4 μm in diameter. They live for about 10 days and are capable of amoeboid movement. Usually, platelet counts range from 150,000 to 400,000 per μL. They can circulate freely and are inactivated during this activity by prostacyclin and nitric oxide from endothelial cells of the blood vessels. Approximately one-third of the body's platelets are held in the spleen and other vascular organs instead of in the bloodstream. These reserves are mobilized during a circulatory crisis such as severe bleeding. The function of platelets is primarily to block injuries to damaged blood vessels and to start forming blood clots. They accomplish this by sticking to the damaged site and forming a temporary plug to seal the broken area. The characteristics of RBCs, WBCs, and platelets are listed in **TABLE 15-3**.

When a blood smear is performed, each platelet's outer region stains blue, whereas the inner area has granules that stain purple. The granules contain many chemicals used for clotting, including enzymes, adenosine diphosphate, platelet-derived growth factor, calcium ions, and serotonin.

■ **TEST YOUR UNDERSTANDING**

1. Name the three major types of blood cells.
2. Explain how platelets participate in the clotting process.

Hemostasis

The stoppage of bleeding is known as **hemostasis**. When blood vessels are damaged, this vital process helps to limit or prevent blood loss. It involves several steps, including

TABLE 15-3

Characteristics of Blood Cells and Platelets

Type	Function	Amount	Description
RBCs (erythrocytes)	Transport carbon dioxide and oxygen	4.2 million to 6.2 million per microliter	Biconcave discs with no nucleus, about one-third hemoglobin
WBCs (leukocytes)	Destroy parasites and pathogens and remove worn cells	5,000–10,000 per microliter	
Granulocytes			About twice the size of RBCs, with cytoplasmic granules
Neutrophils	Phagocytize small particles	54–62% of WBCs	Nuclei have 2–5 lobes; granules stain light purple
Eosinophils	Help control allergic reactions and inflammation and kill parasites	1–3% of WBCs	Bilobed nuclei; granules stain dark red
Basophils	Release histamine and heparin	Less than 1% of WBCs	Bilobed nuclei; granules stain blue
Agranulocytes			No cytoplasmic granules
Monocytes	Phagocytize large particles	3–9% of WBCs	2–3 times larger than RBCs; varied nuclei shape
Lymphocytes	Provide immunity	25–33% of WBCs	Only slightly larger than RBCs, with very large nuclei
Platelets (thrombocytes)	Help control blood loss from broken vessels and begin clotting process	130,000–360,000 per microliter	Cytoplasmic fragments

blood vessel spasms, the formation of a platelet plug, and coagulation of the blood. The process of hemostasis is quick and localized, involving a variety of *clotting factors* from the plasma, along with substances released by platelets and injured tissue cells. The three steps of hemostasis are vasospasm or *vascular spasm*, platelet plug formation, and *coagulation* (blood clotting). After hemostasis, the clot retracts and eventually dissolves to be replaced by fibrous tissue that prevents any additional blood loss.

Vasospasm

When a smaller blood vessel is cut or broken, smooth muscles in its walls contract, which is known as **vasospasm**, and loss of blood slows nearly immediately. A vasospasm has the potential to completely close the ends of a severed vessel. The vascular spasm lasts for approximately 30 minutes and is also known as the *vascular phase of hemostasis*. The endothelial cells contract to expose the basement membrane to the bloodstream. Chemical factors and local hormones begin to be released by the endothelial cells. Also released are *endothelins*, which are peptide hormones that stimulate smooth muscle contraction and promote vascular spasms. They also stimulate endothelial cell division, smooth muscle cell division, and fibroblast division to accelerate repair of damaged tissue.

Platelet Plug Formation

In the *platelet phase,* a platelet plug forms because of *platelet aggregation*, and blood begins coagulating (**FIGURE 15-7**). Platelets release **serotonin** to contract smooth muscles in blood vessels, reducing blood loss. In *platelet adhesion*, the platelets stick to rough surfaces and connective tissue collagen under the endothelial blood vessel lining. They also stick to each other to form a platelet plug in the area of the blood vessel injury. Larger breaks may require a blood clot to stop bleeding. The growth of the platelet plug is limited by several important factors:

- The endothelial cells release a prostaglandin known as *prostacyclin*, which inhibits platelet aggregation.
- WBCs entering the area release inhibitory compounds.
- Adenosine diphosphate near the platelet plug is broken down by circulating plasma enzymes.
- Compounds such as serotonin inhibit platelet plug formation once they are present in high quantities.
- The development of a blood clot strengthens the platelet plug but isolates the platelet plug from the general circulation.

Coagulation

The formation of a blood clot is known as **coagulation**. The *coagulation phase* requires many biochemicals known as *clotting factors* or *procoagulants*. Some clotting factors promote coagulation, whereas others inhibit it, so a delicate balance between these two types is achieved to address the specific injured tissue. Many present proteins or *proenzymes* control vital reactions in the clotting response. Calcium ions and *vitamin K* are very important for nearly all of the coagulation process. Adequate amounts of vitamin K must be present in the liver for it to synthesize prothrombin and other clotting factors.

The most important event in coagulation is the conversion of the plasma protein fibrinogen into the insoluble threads of the protein called *fibrin*. The first step is the release of tissue thromboplastin, which results in the production of prothrombin activator. **FIGURE 15-8** describes the blood-clotting cascade.

The three pathways to the activation of the clotting system are the *extrinsic pathway,* the *intrinsic pathway,* and the *common pathway.* When damaged endothelial cells or peripheral tissues release *Factor III* or *tissue factor*, the extrinsic pathway begins. Tissue factor combines with calcium ions and *Factor VII*, forming an enzyme complex that is able to activate *Factor X*, which is the first stage of the common pathway. The *intrinsic pathway* starts with activation of proenzymes, primarily *Factor XII*, exposed to collagen fibers at the site of injury. A platelet factor known as *PF-3* assists the process. Other factors speed up the reactions in this pathway, and eventually, activated *Factor VIII* and *Factor IX* combine, forming an enzyme complex that can activate *Factor X*. The common pathway begins as the enzyme *prothrombinase* is formed.

Prothrombin is an alpha globulin made in the liver on a continual basis and is always present in the blood plasma. Prothrombinase converts prothrombin into **thrombin**, which causes fibrinogen to be cut into sections of fibrin. This fibrin then joins to form long threads. The threads stick to surfaces of damaged blood vessels to create a mesh that traps blood cells and platelets. The result is a blood clot. A clear, yellowish liquid remains after formation of the clot. This liquid is called **serum** and is plasma minus its clotting factors.

More prothrombinase becomes present if tissue damage is more severe. Continual clotting occurs to stop greater damage. Positive feedback is used to stimulate more clotting action based on the original clotting action. However, this continual process can only work for a short time because it interrupts the stability of the body's internal environment. Excess thrombin is normally carried away to avoid the formation of a massive blood clot. As a result, blood coagulation usually occurs in blood that is not moving or only moving slowly. Clotting stops where a clot contacts the circulating blood.

Blood clots in ruptured vessels are invaded by fibroblasts to produce fibrous connective tissue that helps seal blood vessel breaks. Clots that form in tissues as a result of blood leakage are called hematomas, which disappear over time. This process requires the plasma protein plasminogen to be converted to plasmin, an enzyme that digests threads of fibrin and other proteins involved in clotting. Although plasmin may dissolve entire clots, those that fill large blood vessels usually are not removed naturally.

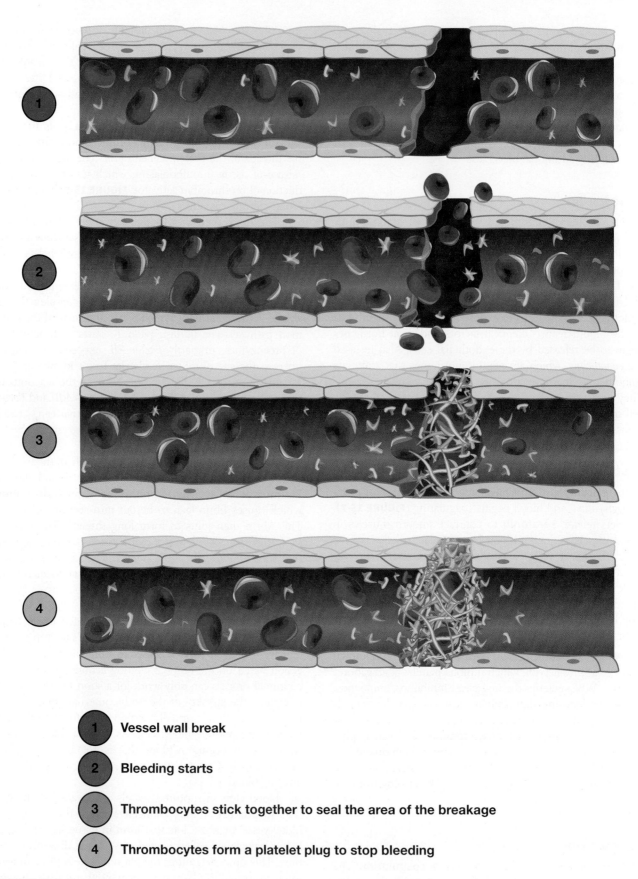

1. **Vessel wall break**

2. **Bleeding starts**

3. **Thrombocytes stick together to seal the area of the breakage**

4. **Thrombocytes form a platelet plug to stop bleeding**

FIGURE 15-7 Platelet plug.

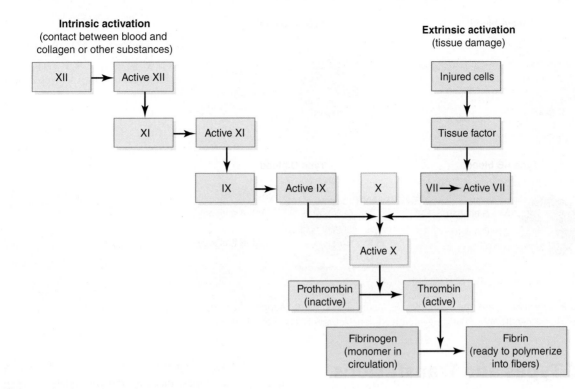

Intrinsic activation
(contact between blood and collagen or other substances)

XII → Active XII

XI → Active XI

IX → Active IX

Extrinsic activation
(tissue damage)

Injured cells

Tissue factor

VII → Active VII

X

Active X

Prothrombin (inactive) → Thrombin (active)

Fibrinogen (monomer in circulation) → Fibrin (ready to polymerize into fibers)

FIGURE 15-8 The clotting cascade.

FOCUS ON PATHOLOGY

A **thrombus** is a clot that forms abnormally in a vessel. An **embolus** is a clot that dislodges or fragments to be carried away in the blood flow. Emboli usually move until they reach narrow vessels, which they may block. When a blood clot forms in a vital organ's vessels, it kills the tissues served by the vessel, which is known as *infarction*, a potentially fatal occurrence. If this occurs in the heart, it is known as *coronary thrombosis*. If it occurs in the brain, it is known as *cerebral thrombosis*. *Pulmonary embolism* describes a clot blocking a vessel supplying the lungs. In *atherosclerosis*, the endothelial linings of blood vessels change because of fatty deposits that accumulate.

Substances that Control Coagulation

Certain substances deactivate or remove clotting factors as well as other stimulatory agents from the blood to control coagulation. Examples of these substances include *plasma anticoagulants* such as *antithrombin III*; *heparin*, which is released by basophils and mast cells; *aspirin*; *thrombomodulin*, which is released by endothelial cells, binds to thrombin, and converts it to an enzyme that activates *protein C*, which inactivates

clotting factors and helps to form *plasmin*; *prostacyclin*, which inhibits platelet aggregation and opposes thrombin and adenosine diphosphate; *alpha-2-macroglobulin*, which inhibits thrombin; and *C1 inactivator*, which inhibits several intrinsic clotting factors.

Retraction of the Clot

Syneresis is also known as *clot retraction*, in which the torn edges of a damaged vessel are pulled closer together. This reduces bleeding and stabilizes the site of injury. It also reduces the size of the area of damage, so that fibrocytes, endothelial cells, and smooth muscle cells can continue the repair process.

Fibrinolysis

Over time, the clot dissolves as *fibrinolysis* starts by activation of plasminogen by thrombin as well as *tissue plasminogen activator*. This activator is released by damaged tissues at the injury site. Plasminogen then leads to production of *plasmin*, the enzyme that begins digestion of the fibrin strands and erosion of the clot.

TEST YOUR UNDERSTANDING

1. What is the difference between a thrombus and an embolus?
2. List the major steps involved in blood clot formation.
3. Define the terms *hemostasis, vasospasm,* and *prothrombin.*

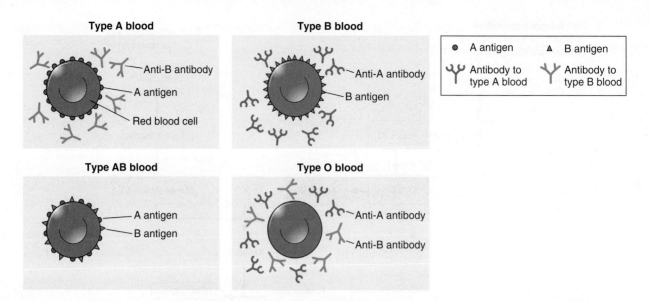

FIGURE 15-9 Various antigens and antibodies distinguish blood types. (Adapted from Shier, D. N., Butler, J. L., and Lewis, R. Hole's Essentials of Human Anatomy & Physiology, Tenth edition. McGraw-Hill Higher Education, 2009.)

Blood Types and Transfusions

Blood consists of different types, not all of which are *compatible*. Safe blood transfusions of whole blood depend on matching the blood types of both donors and recipients. The clumping of RBCs after a transfusion reaction is called **agglutination**. This involves RBC surface molecules called **antigens** or *agglutinogens* that react with **antibodies** or *agglutinins* from the plasma. There are at least 50 kinds of *surface antigens* on RBC membranes. Three surface antigens are of particular importance: A, B, and Rh or "D" antigens. They can produce serious transfusion reactions, including antigens of the ABO group and those of the Rh group.

Classifications are determined by the presence or absence of specific surface antigens in RBC cell membranes are called *blood types*. The ABO blood group is based on the presence or lack of the major protein antigens A and B on RBC membranes. Erythrocytes may have one of the following four antigen combinations:

- *Antigen A only:* type A blood
- *Antigen B only:* type B blood
- *Both antigen A and B:* type AB blood, the least common type
- *Neither antigen A or B:* type O blood, the most common type

Blood types are inherited. Antibodies related to each type of antigen are produced between 2 and 8 months after birth. For example, if antigen A is absent, the antibody called *anti-A* is produced. Therefore, people with type A blood, meaning that antigen A is present but antigen B is absent, have *anti-B* antibody. The opposite is true for people with type B blood. Those with type AB blood have neither of the two antibodies. People with type O blood have both antibodies (**FIGURE 15-9**). The anti-A and anti-B antibodies are very large and cannot cross the placenta. This means that a pregnant woman and her fetus may have different blood types,

and agglutination in the fetus cannot occur. **TABLE 15-4** summarizes blood types, antigens, and antibodies.

Antibodies of a certain type react with antigens of the same type and cause clumping of RBCs, so these combinations must be avoided. For example, a person with type A or *anti-B* blood must not receive blood of either type B or type AB to avoid clumping. A person with type B or *anti-A* blood must not receive type A or type AB blood. A person with type O or *anti-A and anti-B* blood must not receive type A, B, or AB blood. Because type AB blood lacks both anti-A and anti-B antibodies, those with type AB blood can receive transfusions from any other type. Because of this, type AB individuals are called *universal recipients*.

Rapid transfusion must be avoided, however, because agglutination can still occur because of certain antibodies in the blood being transfused. It is therefore always best to transfer blood from the same type into the person requiring the transfusion (**TABLE 15-5**). Note the permissible donor types listed in Table 15-5 should be used only in extreme emergencies. *Cross-match testing* involves exposing donor RBCs to samples of a recipient's plasma under careful control to reveal significant cross-reactions involving surface antigens

TABLE 15-4

ABO Blood Group Antigens and Antibodies

Blood Type	Antigen Present	Antibody Present
A	A	Anti-B
B	B	Anti-A
AB	Both A and B	Neither anti-A nor anti-B
O	Neither A or B	Both anti-A and anti-B

TABLE 15-5

Blood Transfusion Rules

Recipient's Blood Type	Preferred Donor Type	Permissible Donor Type
A	A	O
B	B	O
AB	AB	A, B, and O
O	O	No alternate types

other than the A, B, or Rh antigens. Lost blood can also be replaced with synthetic blood substitutes because these do not contain surface antigens.

FIGURE 15-10 illustrates the concepts of agglutination. Because type O blood lacks antigens A and B, it can be transfused, in extreme emergencies, into people with any other type. Because of this, people with type O blood are called *universal donors*. Type O blood still should be given slowly to people of other blood types so it will be diluted by the recipient's blood volume, minimizing chances of an adverse reaction.

For blood typing, blood is drawn from a vein, and the blood sample is mixed with antibodies against type A and B blood. It is checked to see whether the blood cells *agglutinate* or not. When they agglutinate, the blood has reacted with one of the antibodies. The next step is called *back typing*. The blood serum is mixed with blood that is known to be either type A or type B, which accurately determines the blood type. Also, Rh typing is performed with a similar method of testing.

Rh Blood Group

The *Rh blood group* got its name from the rhesus monkey, because it was in this type of monkey the blood group was first studied. There are several Rh antigens or *factors* in humans, the most prevalent of which is antigen D. If present on the RBC membranes, the blood is called *Rh-positive*. If not, it is called *Rh-negative*. Only 15% of the U.S. population is Rh-negative. The presence or absence of Rh antigen is inherited, but the antibodies that react with it, which are

called *anti-Rh antibodies*, are not spontaneous. They form only in Rh-negative people because of specific stimulation.

A similar condition can occur when an Rh-negative woman is pregnant with an Rh-positive fetus (**FIGURE 15-11**). Although the pregnancy may be normal, at birth or miscarriage the placental membranes tear, allowing some of the fetal Rh-positive RBCs to enter the mother's circulation. This may stimulate her tissues to begin producing anti-Rh antibodies. If she becomes pregnant a second time and the fetus is Rh-positive, these antibodies or *hemolysins* cross the placental membrane to destroy the fetal RBCs. The fetus develops erythroblastosis fetalis, which is also called *hemolytic disease of the fetus and newborn*. Although extremely rare because of the careful management of Rh status, erythroblastosis fetalis may cause the death of the fetus or infant. Signs of this condition in an infant include anemia, enlarged liver or spleen, generalized swelling, and newborn *jaundice*, which is yellowing of the skin and eyes due to liver or bile duct abnormalities resulting in high levels of circulating bilirubin.

FOCUS ON PATHOLOGY

An Rh-negative person receiving Rh-positive blood will begin producing anti-Rh antibodies. The first transfusion usually causes no serious problems, but after that the Rh-negative person has become *sensitized* to Rh-positive blood. A second transfusion, even months later, usually causes the donated RBCs to agglutinate. When RBCs agglutinate and hemolyze, the reaction is called a *cross-reaction*.

TEST YOUR UNDERSTANDING

1. Which blood type is the universal recipient, and which blood type is the universal donor? Why?
2. Explain the Rh blood group and name the condition it may cause in a fetus.
3. Define the terms *agglutination, antigens,* and *antibodies.*

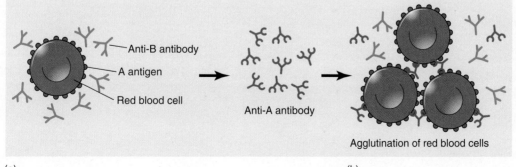

(a) (b)

FIGURE 15-10 Agglutination. (Adapted from Shier, D. N., Butler, J. L., and Lewis, R. Hole's Essentials of Human Anatomy & Physiology, Tenth edition. McGraw-Hill Higher Education, 2009.)

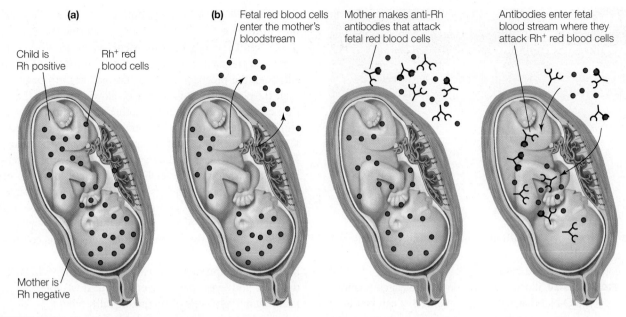

(a)

Child is Rh positive

Rh⁺ red blood cells

Mother is Rh negative

(b) Fetal red blood cells enter the mother's bloodstream

Mother makes anti-Rh antibodies that attack fetal red blood cells

Antibodies enter fetal blood stream where they attack Rh⁺ red blood cells

FIGURE 15-11 The Rh factor and pregnancy.

Diagnostic Blood Tests

Various changes in the blood can reveal many different health conditions. The presence of **leukocytosis** signifies infections. When infections are severe, the hematocrit will have a buffy coat that is larger than normal. Diabetics regularly test their own blood to control their blood sugar levels and make smart dietary choices. Lipidemia causes the blood to have a yellowish tint, whereas anemia causes the blood to appear pale, with a low hematocrit. The size and shape of erythrocytes under the microscope may indicate pernicious or iron-deficiency anemias.

An effective diagnostic testing method is the *differential WBC count*. This test determines relative proportions of various types of leukocytes. For example, if eosinophils are high, the patient may have significant allergies or even a parasitic infection. The state of a person's hemostasis can be gauged via the *prothrombin time* test, which determines the ability of normal clotting to occur. If *thrombocytopenia* is suspected, the *platelet count* is taken. If platelet counts exceed 1 million per microliter, *thrombocytosis* is present. For routine physical examinations and before hospitalization, a *complete blood count* (CBC) and a computerized *sequential multiple analysis test* (SMAC) are performed. The CBC includes counts of the formed elements, hematocrit, hemoglobin content, and RBC size. The second test, also known as the *SMAC, chemistry panel*, and *comprehensive metabolic panel*, measures electrolytes, glucose, and various markers that signify kidney and liver conditions. Together, the CBC and SMAC give an accurate and comprehensive view of a person's overall health.

Effects of Aging on the Blood

Aging can cause a variety of changes to the blood, including decreased hematocrit levels, increased risk of thrombi, and pooling of blood in the legs. A thrombus is a stationary blood clot that can detach, pass through the heart, and lodge in a small artery. This usually occurs in the lungs, causing a pulmonary embolism. When blood pools in the legs, it is usually because the valves of the leg veins are no longer working normally.

SUMMARY

Blood is a type of connective tissue. It consists of RBCs, WBCs, and platelets suspended in a liquid plasma, called the extracellular matrix. The RBCs, WBCs, and platelets are collectively described as formed elements, but the blood also contains a liquid portion that transports these elements. The RBCs or *erythrocytes* are mostly developed in the red bone marrow. They are primarily involved in the supply of oxygen and nutrients to the body tissues. The WBCs or *leukocytes* protect the body against disease. Of the leukocytes, B cells are responsible for humoral immunity, and T cells are responsible for cell-mediated immunity. The platelets are vital for blood coagulation. Plasma suspends the cells and platelets of the blood.

Blood transports substances between body cells and the external environment. Blood plasma transports gases and nutrients, helps maintain stable pH, and helps regulate fluid and electrolyte balance. Hemostasis is the stoppage of bleeding and involves the steps of blood vessel spasm, platelet plug formation, and blood coagulation. It helps to maintain a stable internal environment.

Blood can be typed on the basis of cell surface antigens. The ABO blood group concerns the presence or absence of antigens A and B. The Rh blood group concerns the Rh antigen, which is present on the RBC membranes of Rh-positive blood, but is negative in Rh-negative blood.

KEY TERMS

Agglutination
Agranulocytes
Albumins
Antibodies
Antigens
Basophils
B cells
Bilirubin
Biliverdin
Coagulation
Colony-stimulating factors (CSFs)
Embolus
Eosinophils
Erythropoietin
Fibrin
Fibrinogen

Globulins
Granulocytes
Hematocrit
Hemoglobin
Hemostasis
Hypoxia
Interleukins
Leukocytes
Leukocytosis
Lymphocytes
Macrophages
Mast cells
Megakaryocytes
Monocytes
Neutrophils
Nonprotein nitrogenous substances

Plasma
Plasma cells
Plasma proteins
Platelets
Prothrombin
Red blood cells (erythrocytes)
Serotonin
Serum
T cells
Thrombin
Thrombocytes
Thrombopoietin
Thrombus
Vasospasm
White blood cells (leukocytes)

The following learning goals correspond to the objectives at the beginning of this chapter:

1. The blood is made up of cells, fragments of cells, and dissolved biochemicals containing nutrients, oxygen, hormones, and wastes. RBCs transport gases, WBCs fight disease, and platelets aid in clotting. RBCs, WBCs, and platelets are collectively called formed elements; the liquid portion of the blood is called plasma.

2. Plasma is a clear, straw-colored liquid containing water, amino acids, carbohydrates, lipids, proteins, hormones, electrolytes, vitamins, and cellular wastes.

3. Plasma proteins include albumins, the smallest type, making up around 60% of plasma proteins by weight; globulins, making up around 36% of the total; and fibrinogen, the largest type, making up around 4% of the total.

4. RBCs have a biconcave shape that helps them transport gases by increasing the surface area of the cell, allowing more diffusion. The hemoglobin portion of an RBC carries oxygen. They produce adenosine triphosphate through glycolysis. RBC formation is controlled by negative feedback via the hormone erythropoietin. RBCs are vital in supplying the body tissues with oxygen.

5. Hemoglobin carries oxygen inside RBCs and makes up about one-third of each RBC. Hemoglobin gives RBCs their red color and binds with oxygen to form oxyhemoglobin, which is bright red. When oxygen is released, deoxyhemoglobin is formed, which is a darker red color. RBCs have nuclei that are shed as they mature, allowing more room for hemoglobin. None of the oxygen carried in hemoglobin is used by an RBC. Iron is required for normal RBC production and for hemoglobin synthesis. Anemia is caused by too little hemoglobin or by too few RBCs. Hemoglobin is broken down into heme and globin, with the heme then decomposing into iron and biliverdin.

6. The five types of WBCs in circulating blood are as follows:
    A. *Neutrophils:* Have small granules; older neutrophils or *segs* have lobed nuclei, whereas younger neutrophils or *bands* have C-shaped nuclei. Neutrophils phagocytize small particles.
    B. *Eosinophils:* Have bilobed nuclei; eosinophils help control allergic reactions and inflammation, and kill parasites.
    C. *Basophils:* Similar to eosinophils, but with irregular granules; basophils release histamine and heparin.
    D. *Monocytes:* Types of basophils without granules; monocytes phagocytize large particles.
    E. *Lymphocytes:* Types of basophils without granules; lymphocytes provide immunity.

7. Platelets or *thrombocytes* are incomplete cells arising from megakaryocytes that have become fragmented. They lack nuclei and are less than half the size of RBCs. Their function is primarily to block injuries to damaged blood vessels and to start forming clots.

8. Granulocytes are leukocytes with granular cytoplasm. Agranulocytes are leukocytes without granular cytoplasm.

9. The stoppage of bleeding is known as hemostasis. When a small blood vessel is cut or broken, smooth muscles in its wall contract, which is called *vasospasm*, and loss of blood slows nearly immediately. After about 30 minutes, a platelet plug forms and blood begins coagulating. Platelets release serotonin to contract smooth muscles in blood vessels, reducing blood loss. Larger breaks may require a blood clot to stop bleeding. The formation of a blood clot is known as coagulation, requiring biochemicals known as clotting factors. The most important event in coagulation is the conversion of the plasma protein fibrinogen into the insoluble threads of the protein called fibrin.

10.
    A. Blood typing is important because safe blood transfusions of whole blood depend on matching the blood types of both donors and recipients. If done incorrectly, a transfusion reaction called agglutination, which is the clumping of RBCs, may occur.
    B. Type A blood has antigen A only, type B blood has antigen B only, type AB blood has both antigens A and B, and type O blood has neither antigen A nor B. These antigens influence the type of antibodies they produce. Combinations of incompatible blood types must be avoided because of potential agglutination. It is always best to transfer blood from the same type into a person requiring a transfusion. Type A people can receive A or O blood; type B people can receive B or O blood; type AB people can receive A, B, or O blood; and type O people can receive only O blood.
    C. If the Rh antigen called antigen D is present on a person's RBC membranes, their blood is called Rh-positive. If not, it is Rh-negative.

An Rh-negative person receiving Rh-positive blood begins producing anti-Rh antibodies. Although an initial transfusion of this type causes no serious problems, a second transfusion usually causes the donated RBCs to agglutinate. A similar condition can occur when an Rh-negative woman is pregnant with an Rh-positive fetus. The fetus is in danger of developing erythroblastosis fetalis when the mother's body tries to destroy the fetal RBCs.

CRITICAL THINKING QUESTIONS

A 25-year-old woman was pregnant and undernourished. Her blood was also Rh-negative. The physician advised her to take some iron supplements.

1. Why is iron so important for pregnant women to have in their diet?

2. If the fetus was Rh positive, what are the potential consequences?

REVIEW QUESTIONS

1. Which of the following terms means "the process of RBC production"?
    A. erythropoiesis
    B. erythrocytosis
    C. erythropenia
    D. hemocytosis

2. Immature RBCs are found in peripheral blood samples and are referred to as
    A. myeloblasts
    B. erythroblasts
    C. reticulocytes
    D. normoblasts

3. The formed elements of the blood are called
    A. clotting proteins
    B. lipoproteins
    C. albumins
    D. blood cells

4. Which of the following are the most abundant proteins in blood plasma?
    A. fibrinogens
    B. albumins
    C. lipoproteins
    D. globulins

5. Which of the following WBCs produce antibodies?
    A. monocytes
    B. lymphocytes
    C. eosinophils
    D. basophils

6. Platelets are formed from cells in the bone marrow known as
    A. megakaryocytes
    B. erythroblasts
    C. lymphoblasts
    D. myeloblasts

7. Which of the following vitamins is needed for the formation of clotting factors?
    A. vitamin A
    B. vitamin D
    C. vitamin K
    D. vitamin E

8. Thrombocytes are
    A. small cells that lack a nucleus
    B. small cells with many-lobed nuclei
    C. fragments of large megakaryocytes
    D. large cells with prominent nuclei

9. Which of the following WBCs release histamine and heparin?
    A. basophils
    B. monocytes
    C. neutrophils
    D. eosinophils

10. Erythrocytes are formed in
    A. the spleen
    B. red bone marrow
    C. yellow bone marrow
    D. the liver

11. Which of the following hormones regulates production of RBCs?
    A. erythropoietin
    B. thymosin
    C. epinephrine
    D. somatotropin

12. Which of the following is the major protein in a RBC?
    A. myoglobin
    B. fibrinogen
    C. albumin
    D. hemoglobin

13. Older erythrocytes are broken down by the
    A. kidneys
    B. lungs
    C. spleen
    D. pancreas

14. Allergies stimulate an increased _____ count.
    A. erythrocyte
    B. eosinophil
    C. monocyte
    D. neutrophil

15. People in which of the following blood groups are known as universal recipients?
    A. group O
    B. group A
    C. group B
    D. group AB

ESSAY QUESTIONS

1. Describe blood functions.
2. Define plasma and formed elements.
3. Discuss hemoglobin structure.
4. Describe erythropoiesis and hormonal controls.
5. Describe general structural and functional characteristics of leukocytes.
6. Classify granulocytes and agranulocytes.
7. Define thrombopoietin and megakaryocytes.
8. Discuss hemostasis.
9. Describe whole blood transfusions.
10. Classify human blood groups and Rh blood groups.

The Heart

OBJECTIVES

After studying this chapter, readers should be able to

1. Describe the size of the heart and its location in the thorax.
2. Identify the layers of the heart wall and the function of each.
3. Identify the four chambers of the heart, and list its associated great vessels.
4. Name the four heart valves, and describe the locations and functions of each.
5. Describe the vascular supply to the heart.
6. Identify the electrical events associated with a normal electrocardiogram tracing.
7. Draw a diagram of a normal electrocardiogram.
8. Define cardiac output, and describe the factors that influence this variable.
9. Describe normal heart sounds and define murmurs.
10. Explain the role of the autonomic nervous system in controlling cardiac output.

Overview

The human heart pumps blood through the blood vessels. In the capillaries, nutrients, electrolytes, dissolved gases, and waste products are exchanged between the blood and surrounding tissues. The heart performs an amazing amount of work over a person's lifetime, beating an average of 70 to 80 times per minute. An adult heart pumps about 4,000 gallons of blood every day. By the time a person reaches the age of 70, the heart will have contracted about 2.5 billion times.

Heart rate is affected by emotions and physical stressors. The heart is made up of two pumps. Its right side receives blood that is low in oxygen from the body tissues. It pumps this blood to the lungs to collect oxygen and drop off carbon dioxide. The heart's left side receives oxygenated blood from the lungs. It pumps this blood to the body to supply the tissues with nutrients and oxygen. The receiving chambers of the heart are its right and left **atria**. The pumping chambers of the heart are its right and left **ventricles**. The heart requires approximately 1/20th of the body's blood supply even though it makes up only about 1/200th of the weight of the body. The left ventricle is the portion that receives the most blood.

Blood Circulation

The heart consists of two pumps located side by side, which supply blood to the *pulmonary circuit* and *systemic circuit*. Blood enters the pulmonary circuit from the right ventricle through the pulmonary trunk, which extends upward posteriorly from the heart. It divides into right and left pulmonary *arteries*, which enter the right and left lungs, respectively. Repeated divisions connect to arterioles and capillary networks associated with the walls of the alveoli, where gas is exchanged between blood and air. The pulmonary *capillaries* lead to venules and then *veins*. Four **pulmonary veins**, two from each lung, return blood to the left atrium, completing the vascular loop of the pulmonary circuit. Capillaries are also called *exchange vessels* because their thin walls allow the exchange of dissolved gases, nutrients, and waste products between surrounding tissues and the blood.

The systemic circuit involves the movement of freshly oxygenated blood from the left atrium to the left ventricle and then into the **aorta** and its branches, leading to all body tissues. Eventually, it makes its way to the companion vein system that returns blood to the right atrium. **FIGURE 16-1** shows the pulmonary and systemic circuits.

Structures of the Heart

The heart lies inside the thoracic cavity, resting on the diaphragm (**FIGURE 16-2**). It is hollow and cone-shaped, varying in size. The heart is within the **mediastinum**, which is the medial cavity of the thorax, in between the lungs. Its posterior border is near the vertebral column, and its anterior border is near the sternum. It is not situated in the exact center of the thorax, and approximately two-thirds of the heart lies to the left of the midsternal line. It is partially obscured, laterally, by the lungs.

The average adult heart is about 14 cm (5 inches) long by 9 cm (3.5 inches) wide and weighs approximately 300 g. The **base** of the heart is actually the upper portion, where it is attached to several large blood vessels. This wide portion of the heart lies beneath the second rib. The distal end of the heart extends downward, to the left, ending in a blunt point called the *apex*, which is even with the fifth intercostal space. The apex points toward the left hip. Just below the left nipple, between the fifth and sixth ribs, the *apical impulse* can easily be felt. This is caused by the apex touching the chest wall.

Coverings of the Heart

The heart and proximal ends of the large blood vessels are enclosed within the double-walled **pericardium**, which is a serous membrane that surrounds the heart. It has an outer, fibrous *parietal* layer and an inner *visceral* layer. The *fibrous pericardium* is made of dense connective tissue attached to the central diaphragm, posterior sternum, vertebral column, and large blood vessels connected to the heart. Deeper inside lies the *serous pericardium*, which is thin and slippery. It consists of two layers of serous membrane that enclose heart. The *parietal layer* lines the inner surface of the fibrous pericardium. An inner, double-layered *visceral pericardium* or *epicardium* covers the heart as well. At the base of the heart the visceral pericardium folds back to become the *parietal pericardium*. Between the parietal and visceral layers is the pericardial cavity, containing between 15 and 50 mL of lubricating *serous fluid* that reduces friction between the pericardial membranes as the heart moves within them. This fluid is also known as *pericardial fluid*.

FOCUS ON PATHOLOGY

When *pericarditis* develops, the pericardium makes the serous membranes become rough. The heart then rubs against the *pericardial sac* as it beats, and a "creaking" sound can be heard with a *stethoscope* that is clinically described as *pericardial friction rub*. The patient experiences a deep pain in the sternum, and adhesions may develop over time. If this occurs, the visceral and parietal pericardia stick together, affecting normal heart function. In severe pericarditis, great quantities of fluid move into the pericardial cavity, compressing the heart. This condition is known as *cardiac tamponade*, commonly called "heart plug." Treatment involves insertion of a syringe into the pericardial cavity to drain off the excessive amounts of fluid.

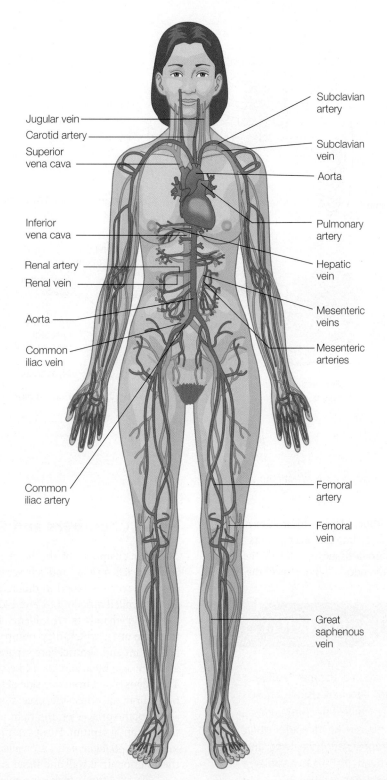

FIGURE 16-1 The blood pathway (pulmonary and systemic circulation).

Heart Layers

The three layers composing the wall of the heart are the outer epicardium, middle myocardium, and inner endocardium (**FIGURE 16-3**). The **epicardium** protects the heart by reducing friction and is the visceral portion of the *pericardium* on the surface of the heart. It consists of connective tissue and some deep adipose tissue. The thick *myocardium* is made mostly of cardiac muscle tissue that is organized in planes and richly supplied by blood capillaries, lymph capillaries, and nerve fibers. It pumps blood out of the chambers of the heart. The **endocardium** is made up of squamous epithelium and connective tissue with many elastic and collagenous fibers. It also contains blood vessels and specialized cardiac muscle

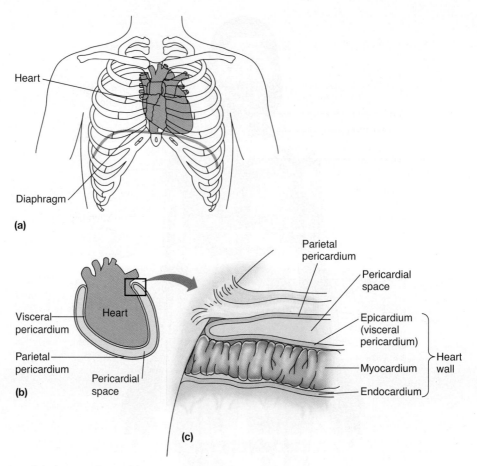

FIGURE 16-2 Location of the heart in the mediastinum.

fibers known as **Purkinje fibers**. The endocardium rests on the inner myocardial surface, lining the chambers of the heart and covering the fibrous tissue that forms the heart valves. It is continuous with endothelial linings of the heart's blood vessels.

Heart Chambers and Great Vessels

The four chambers of the heart are the *right atrium*, *right ventricle*, *left atrium*, and *left ventricle* (**FIGURE 16-4**). Each chamber receives blood in different ways. The upper chambers are called *atria* and receive blood returning to the heart. The lower chambers are called *ventricles* and receive blood from the atria, which they pump out into the arteries. The left atrium and ventricle are separated from the right atrium and ventricle by a solid wall-like structure called a **septum**. This keeps blood from one side of the heart from mixing with blood from the other side, except in a developing fetus. There are smooth surfaces on the right atrium's posterior wall and the interatrial septum. However, prominent ridges of muscles known as *pectinate muscles* or *musculi pectinati* are found on the anterior atrial wall and inner surface of the auricle.

The left atrium makes up most of the *base* of the heart. Four *pulmonary veins* enter the left atrium, carrying blood from the lungs. The pulmonary veins are most easily seen in a posterior view of the heart. The blood passes from the left atrium into the left ventricle through the *left atrioventricular (A-V) valve* or **mitral valve**, which prevents it from flowing back into the left atrium from the ventricle. Like the **tricuspid valve**, the **papillary muscles** and **chordae tendineae** prevent the mitral valve's cusps from swinging back into the left atrium when the ventricle contracts. The mitral valve closes passively, directing blood through the large artery known as the *aorta*.

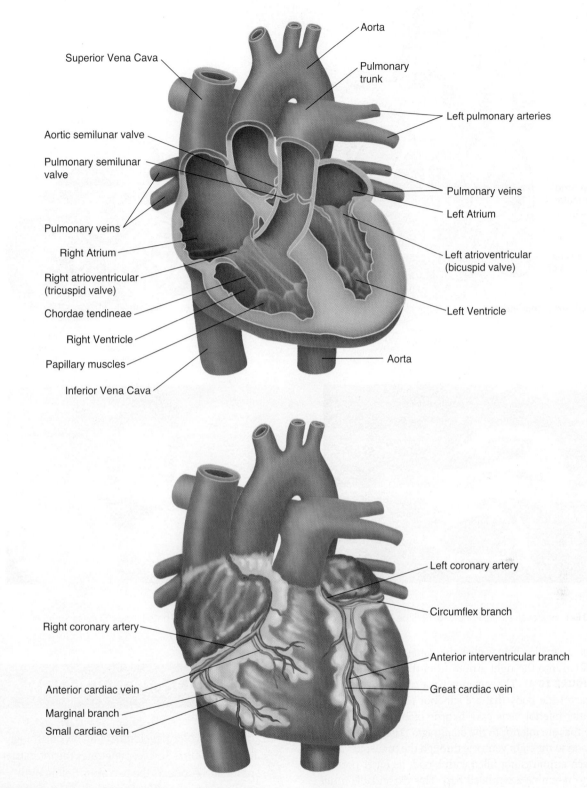

FIGURE 16-3 Anatomy of the heart.

The left ventricle forms most of the apex and inferoposterior area of the heart. The left ventricle is thicker because it must force blood through the *aorta* to all body parts, which have a much higher resistance to blood flow. The cavity of the left ventricle is almost circular. The area where the septum separates the right and left ventricles is marked on the heart's surface by the *anterior interventricular sulcus*. This groove cradles the anterior interventricular artery and continues to become the *posterior interventricular sulcus*. This sulcus is visible on the posteroinferior surface of the heart.

The right atrium receives blood from two large veins called the **superior vena cava** and the **inferior vena cava**

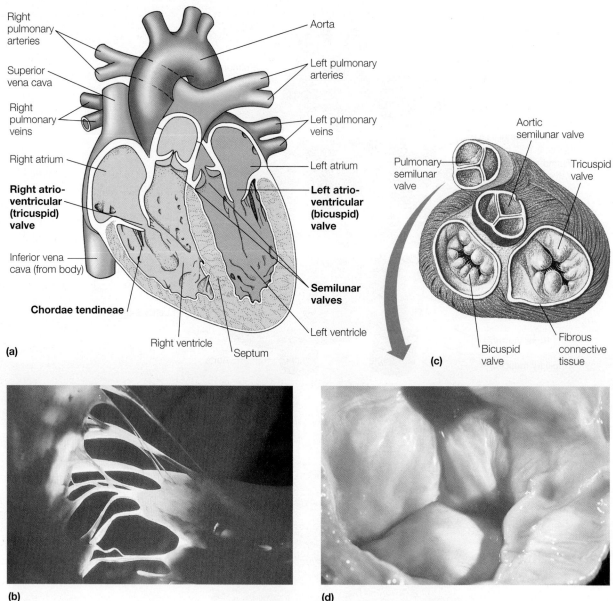

(a)

- Right pulmonary arteries
- Superior vena cava
- Right pulmonary veins
- Right atrium
- **Right atrio-ventricular (tricuspid) valve**
- Inferior vena cava (from body)
- **Chordae tendineae**
- Aorta
- Left pulmonary arteries
- Left pulmonary veins
- Left atrium
- **Left atrio-ventricular (bicuspid) valve**
- **Semilunar valves**
- Left ventricle
- Septum
- Right ventricle

(c)

- Pulmonary semilunar valve
- Aortic semilunar valve
- Tricuspid valve
- Bicuspid valve
- Fibrous connective tissue

(b)

(d)

FIGURE 16-4 Heart valves. (Left photo: © Phillipe Plailly/Science Source; Right photo: © Science Photo Library/Science Source)

and from a smaller vein called the *coronary sinus,* which drains blood into the right atrium from the heart's myocardium (**FIGURE 16-4**). The superior vena cava returns blood from areas of the body that are superior to the diaphragm, whereas the inferior vena cava returns blood from areas of the body that are inferior to the diaphragm. The right atrium sends blood to the right ventricle through the tricuspid valve. When each atrium is not filled with blood, its outer portion deflates to resemble a wrinkled flap. This expandable *atrial appendage* is also called an *auricle*.

The right ventricle forms most of the anterior surface of the heart. Its muscular wall is about three times thinner than that of the left ventricle, because it only pumps blood to the lungs, which have a low resistance to blood flow. The inner surface of the right ventricle contains a series of muscular ridges called *trabeculae carnae*. The cavity of the right ventricle is flatter than that of the left ventricle, with a crescent shape and partially enclosing the left ventricle. As the right ventricle contracts, its blood increases in pressure to passively close the tricuspid valve. Therefore, this blood can only exit through the *pulmonary trunk*, which divides into the left and right pulmonary arteries that supply the lungs. At the trunk's base is a **pulmonary valve** that allows blood to leave the right ventricle while preventing backflow into the ventricular chamber. The pulmonary valve contains three cusps. Before the pulmonary valve, the superior end of the right ventricle becomes tapered, forming a cone-shaped pouch called the *conus arteriosus*.

Heart Valves

The blood flow through the heart is in one direction because of the actions of the heart valves. The four heart valves open and close because of pressure differences in each chamber. The four heart valves are the two *A-V valves* and the two semilunar valves.

A-V Valves

The tricuspid valve and bicuspid or *mitral valve* are known as *A-V valves* because they lie between the atria and ventricles. They prevent backflow or *regurgitation* of blood from the ventricles to the atria while the ventricles contract. The *tricuspid valve*, also known as the *right A-V valve*, has three flexible projections called *cusps* and lies between the right atrium and ventricle. The cusps are actually flaps of endothelium that are reinforced by cores of connective tissue. This valve allows blood to move from the right atrium into the right ventricle while preventing backflow. The cusps of the tricuspid valve are attached to strong fibers called *chordae tendineae*, which originate from small *papillary muscles* that project inward from the ventricle walls. These muscles contract as the ventricle contracts. When the tricuspid valve closes, the papillary muscles pull on the chordae tendineae to prevent the cusps from swinging back into the atrium.

The *mitral valve* is located between the left atrium and left ventricle. It is also called the *bicuspid valve* because it has two cusps. When the left atrium is filled with oxygenated blood, it pushes the mitral valve open, sending the blood into the left ventricle. **FIGURE 16-4** shows various views of the heart valves.

Semilunar Valves

The pulmonary and aortic valves have half-moon shapes and are therefore referred to as *semilunar valves*. The pulmonary and aortic valves prevent backflow of blood from the aorta

and pulmonary trunk back into their associated ventricles. They respond to pressure differences, similar to the A-V valves. The semilunar valves are forced open, causing their cusps to flatten against the artery walls as blood moves past them. This occurs when the ventricles contract, increasing intraventricular pressure above the pressure in the aorta and pulmonary trunk. When the ventricles are relaxed, the blood can then flow back toward the heart, filling the cusps and closing the valves.

At the base of the aorta is the *aortic valve*, which has three cusps. This valve opens to allow blood to leave the left ventricle during contraction and flow into the *ascending aorta*. Blood then flows through the *aortic arch* and into the *descending aorta*. When the left ventricle relaxes, the valve closes to prevent blood from backing up into the ventricle. The *pulmonary valve* is located in the right ventricle and opens to the pulmonary trunk to send deoxygenated blood to the lungs. Near each cusp of the aortic valve are sac-like structures called *aortic sinuses*, which prevent the cusps from sticking to the aortic wall as the valve opens. **TABLE 16-1** summarizes the various heart valves.

Connective tissue arranged in "rings" surrounds the proximal ends of the pulmonary trunk and aorta, providing firm attachments for heart valves and muscle fibers. They prevent the outlets of the atria and ventricles from dilating during contraction. These rings, as well as other dense connective tissue masses, form the heart's "skeleton."

TABLE 16-1		
Heart Valves		
Heart Valve	**Location**	**Action**
Tricuspid valve	Between the right atrium and right ventricle	During ventricular contraction, it prevents blood from moving from the right ventricle into the right atrium.
Pulmonary valve	At the entrance to the pulmonary trunk	During ventricular relaxation, it prevents blood from moving from the pulmonary trunk into the right ventricle.
Mitral (bicuspid) valve	Between the left atrium and left ventricle	During ventricular contraction, it prevents blood from moving from the left ventricle into the left atrium.
Aortic valve	At the entrance to the aorta	During ventricular relaxation, it prevents blood from moving from the aorta into the left ventricle.

Even if the valves of the heart leak blood to a certain degree, the heart can continue to function. When the valves are severely deformed, cardiac function is seriously impaired. An insufficient heart valve is described as "incompetent" and causes the heart to pump the same blood again and again because of improper valve closure and backflow of blood. The term *carditis* and its various forms describe inflammation of the heart, which is often linked to *rheumatic fever*. Often, because of scar tissue caused by *endocarditis* or due to calcium salt deposits, valve flaps stiffen. This condition is known as *valvular stenosis*, a form of *valvular heart disease*. The heart must contract with abnormally intense force, increasing its workload and weakening it severely over time. Most often, it is the mitral valve that becomes faulty. However, this can be replaced with a mechanical valve or one from a cow or pig heart. The replacement valve must be treated with chemicals to prevent rejection. Another option is to use a cryopreserved valve from a human cadaver. The term "cryopreserved" is defined as *specially frozen*. Today, tissue engineering is allowing heart valves to be "grown" from a patient's own cells, using a biodegradable scaffold.

TEST YOUR UNDERSTANDING

1. Identify the locations of the A-V and semilunar valves.
2. Explain the location and functions of the mitral valve.
3. Discuss the components that make up the "skeleton" of the heart.

FOCUS ON PATHOLOGY

When coronary blockage is prolonged, the condition becomes much more serious. Myocardial cells begin to die, and the result may be a *myocardial infarction* or *heart attack*. Most dead heart tissue is replaced with scar tissue, which does not contract. This is because most adult heart tissue is *amitotic*, meaning it is able to divide but not replicate. The extent and location of heart damage determine whether the patient can survive the heart attack. Because the left ventricle is the systemic pump, damage to this ventricle is more serious than to

the right ventricle. Risk factors for myocardial infarction include atherosclerosis, increased blood cholesterol, hypertension, use of tobacco, diabetes mellitus, and family history.

Various tests are available to rule out a myocardial infarction, such as electrocardiogram, clinical assessment, and blood tests. The blood is tested to detect increases in cardiac troponins, which are sensitive and highly specific markers for dying heart cells. Either cardiac troponin I or cardiac troponin T are biomarkers unique to the heart. Unfortunately, these tests take 3 to 4 hours after a myocardial infarction occurs to reveal its diagnosis. Other substances that show changes in their levels, in relation to myocardial infarction, include creatine kinase, myoglobin, and natriuretic peptides.

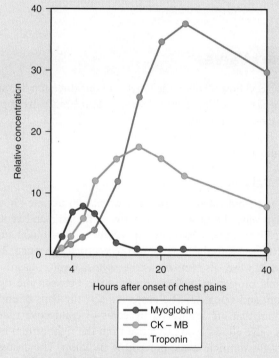

Cardiac enzyme elevations after a myocardial infarction.

Heart Circulation

The heart is nourished via the *coronary circulation*. This is the shortest circulation in the entire body and the functional blood supply of the heart. It is important to remember that blood flows through the heart in only one direction, controlled by the four heart valves. The valves open and close as a result of differences in pressure on their two sides.

Coronary Arteries

The first two aortic branches are called the right and left **coronary arteries**. They supply blood to the heart tissues, with openings lying just beyond the **aortic valve**. The coronary arteries deliver blood when the heart is relaxed and have less function while the ventricles are contracting because they are compressed by the **myocardium**.

Both of these coronary arteries enclose the heart in the *coronary sulcus* and provide the arterial supply of the coronary circulation. The *left coronary artery* runs toward the left side of the heart, whereas the *right coronary artery* runs toward the right side. The left coronary artery is divided into the *anterior interventricular artery* and the *circumflex artery*. The anterior interventricular artery is also known as the *left anterior descending artery*. It supplies blood to the anterior walls of both ventricles and to the interventricular septum. This artery follows the *anterior interventricular sulcus*. The circumflex artery supplies the posterior walls of the left ventricle and the left atrium.

Coronary artery branches supply many capillaries in the myocardium. These arteries have smaller branches with connections called **anastomoses** between vessels that provide alternate blood pathways. Known as *collateral circulation*, these pathways may supply oxygen and nutrients to the myocardium when blockage of a coronary artery occurs. The *right coronary artery* is divided into the *right marginal artery* and the *posterior interventricular artery*. The right marginal artery serves the myocardium of the heart's lateral right side. There also may be more than one marginal artery. The posterior interventricular artery supplies the posterior ventricular walls and runs to the heart **apex**. It merges or *anastomoses* near the apex of the heart with the *anterior interventricular artery*.

Coronary Veins

The **coronary veins** are basically located along the same paths as the coronary arteries. They join to form the enlarged **coronary sinus**, emptying into the right atrium. On the posterior aspect of the heart, the coronary sinus can easily be seen. It empties into the *great cardiac vein, middle cardiac vein,* and *small cardiac vein*. Also, several *anterior cardiac veins* empty into the right atrium's anterior portion. The *posterior cardiac vein* also empties into the great cardiac vein or coronary sinus.

Heart Contraction

Some *cardiac muscle cells* are self-excitable, whereas each skeletal muscle fiber requires stimulation by a nerve ending to contract. Certain cardiac muscle cells are interconnected by *intercalated discs*, at which point interlocking membranes of nearby cells are linked by gap junctions and held together by desmosomes. The intercalated discs transfer the force of contractions from cell to cell and propagate action potentials.

There are three major differences between the ways in which cardiac muscle and skeletal muscle contract. First, self-excitable cardiac muscle cells can also initiate the depolarization of the rest of the heart, spontaneously and with rhythm. This property is known as **automaticity** or *autorhythmicity*. Second, cardiac muscle has a property in which either all heart fibers contract as a unit or not at all. This is coordinated because all cardiac muscle cells are electrically linked together into one contractile unit by gap junctions. As a result, the wave of depolarization moves across the heart's cells via ion passage along the gap junctions. All this differs from skeletal muscle, in which impulses do not spread from cell to cell. Contraction of muscle fibers occurs from individual stimulation by nerve fibers. Contraction is usually with just some of the motor units being activated. Third, in cardiac muscle cells, the absolute refractory period lasts over 200 milliseconds (ms), which is almost as long as the contraction. This normally prevents tetanic contractions from occurring, which would stop the heart from pumping. In skeletal muscle cells, contractions last only 15 to 100 ms and have brief refractory periods of 1 to 2 ms. The *absolute refractory period* is the period of no excitation, in which sodium ion channels remain open or are inactivated. As a result of the long refractory period, cardiac muscle cannot exhibit tetany.

Energy Requirements

Cardiac muscle needs much more oxygen for energy metabolism than skeletal muscle and also has more mitochondria. The heart needs aerobic respiration primarily. Therefore, without oxygen, cardiac muscle cannot operate very well for very long. Skeletal muscle differs in that it can contract for a long time via anaerobic respiration and restore oxygen and fuel reserves via excessive oxygen consumption after exercise.

Glucose, fatty acids, and other fuel molecules are used by cardiac and skeletal muscle. However, because it is more adaptable, cardiac muscle easily changes metabolic pathways so it can use whatever nutrients are available. Such nutrients include lactic acid, which is generated by skeletal muscle activity. Therefore, a lack of oxygen is much more dangerous to the myocardium than any lack of nutrients.

Functions of the Heart

The heart chambers are coordinated so their actions are effective. The atria contract, which is called atrial **systole,** as the ventricles relax, which is called ventricular **diastole**. Likewise, ventricles contract, in ventricular systole, as atria relax, in atrial diastole. Then, a brief period of relaxation of both atria and ventricles occurs. This complete series of events makes up a heartbeat, also called a **cardiac cycle**. During ventricular systole's early stages, the ventricles contract isometrically and are described as being in *isovolumetric contraction*, meaning all the valves of the heart are closed, ventricular volume does not change, and ventricular pressure rises. Once pressure has exceeded the pressure in the arterial trunks, the semilunar valves open. Blood flows into the pulmonary and aortic trunks, which is the beginning of *ventricular ejection*. Each ventricle ejects between 70 and 80 mL of blood, which is the heart's *stroke volume*. At rest, this amount is about 60% of the end-diastolic volume. This ejection fraction varies with demands placed on the heart. At the end of ventricular systole, pressures in the ventricles fall quickly. The amount of blood remaining in each ventricle when the semilunar valve closes is called the *end-systolic volume*, which is about 50 mL, or 40% of the end-diastolic volume. During ventricular diastole, while the heart valves are closed and the ventricular myocardium relaxes, blood cannot flow into the ventricles. This is because ventricular pressures are still higher than atrial pressures, known as *isovolumetric relaxation*. The duration of ventricular diastole, which depends totally on heart rate, is called ventricular *filling time*.

Conduction System

Strands and clumps of specialized cardiac muscle contain only a few myofibrils and are located throughout the heart. These areas initiate and distribute impulses through the myocardium, comprising the **cardiac conduction system,** which coordinates the cardiac cycle (**FIGURE 16-5**). This system is also known as the *conducting system* or *nodal system* and includes the *sinoatrial (S-A) node, atrioventricular (A-V) node,* and *conducting cells*, which are found in *intermodal pathways* that distribute contractile stimuli to atrial muscle cells.

Depolarization and contraction of cardiac muscle are intrinsic and do not depend on the nervous system. The heart can continue to beat in rhythm even when all nerve connections are severed. However, a normal healthy heart has many autonomic nerve fibers able to alter its rhythm. Noncontractile cardiac cells are specialized to initiate and then distribute impulses in the heart, keeping its depolarization and contraction orderly and in sequence.

A stable resting membrane potential is maintained in uninsulated contractile cardiac cells. However, the *cardiac pacemaker cells* have an unstable resting potential. These *autorhythmic* cells continuously depolarize and move slowly toward threshold. Their spontaneously changing membrane potentials are called *prepotentials*, or *pacemaker potentials*. These potentials initiate action potentials, which spread through the heart and trigger contractions. In pacemaker cells, the three parts of an action potential are *pacemaker potential, depolarization,* and *repolarization*. Cardiac pacemaker cells exist in the S-A node, A-V node, atrioventricular (A-V) bundle, right and left bundle branches, and Purkinje fibers. Impulses pass across the heart in this order, beginning with the S-A node and ending with the Purkinje fibers.

S-A Node

The **sinoatrial node** (**S-A node**) is a small crescent-shaped mass of specialized tissue just beneath the epicardium, in the right atrium. It is located near the opening of the *superior vena cava*, with fibers continuous with those of the atrial syncytium. The S-A node's cells can reach threshold on their own, initiating impulses through the myocardium, stimulating contraction of cardiac muscle fibers. Its rhythmic activity occurs 70 to 80 times per minute in a normal adult. Because it generates the heart's rhythmic contractions, it is often referred to as the **pacemaker**. No other part of the conduction system has a faster depolarization rate than the S-A node. The path of a cardiac impulse travels from the S-A node into the atrial syncytium. The atria begin to contract almost simultaneously. The characteristic

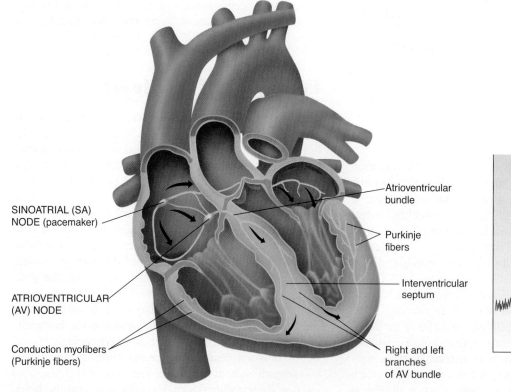

SINOATRIAL (SA)
NODE (pacemaker)

ATRIOVENTRICULAR
(AV) NODE

Conduction myofibers
(Purkinje fibers)

Atrioventricular
bundle

Purkinje
fibers

Interventricular
septum

Right and left
branches
of AV bundle

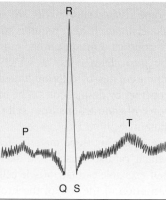

FIGURE 16-5 Conduction system with the tracing of an ECG.

rhythm of the S-A node is called the *sinus rhythm*, which determines heart rate.

A-V Node

The impulse passes along junctional fibers of the conduction system to a mass of specialized tissue called the **atrioventricular node** (**A-V node**), located in the inferior *interatrial septum*, beneath the *endocardium*. The A-V node provides the only normal conduction pathway between the atrial and ventricular syncytia. Impulses are slightly delayed for 0.1 second because of the small diameter of the junctional fibers. The atria therefore have more time to contract and empty all their blood into the ventricles before ventricular contraction occurs. Impulse conduction is slower in the A-V node than in other parts of the conduction system.

A-V Bundle

When the cardiac impulse reaches the distal A-V node, it passes into a large **A-V bundle**, or *bundle of His*, entering the upper part of the *interventricular septum*. The atria and ventricles are not connected by gap junctions even though they meet each other. The only electrical connection between them is the A-V bundle.

Right and Left Bundle Branches

The A-V bundle soon splits into the *right and left bundle branches*. These branches move along the interventricular septum toward the apex of the heart.

Purkinje Fibers

Nearly halfway down the septum, the right and left bundle branches spread into enlarged *Purkinje fibers*, extending into the papillary muscles. The fibers consist of long strands of barrel-shaped cells with only a few myofibrils, which continue to the heart's apex, curving around the ventricles and passing over their lateral walls. They complete the pathway through the interventricular septum. The Purkinje fibers have numerous small branches that become continuous with cardiac muscle fibers and irregular whorls. Superiorly, the Purkinje fibers turn into the ventricular walls. Purkinje fiber stimulation causes the ventricular walls to contract in a twisting motion to force blood into the aorta and pulmonary trunk. The Purkinje fibers are also referred to as the *subendocardial conducting network*.

TEST YOUR UNDERSTANDING

1. Explain the major differences between cardiac and skeletal muscle fibers.
2. Describe aerobic respiration and its effects on the heart.
3. Identify the locations of cardiac pacemaker cells.
4. Why is it important for impulses from the atria to be delayed at the A-V node before they pass into the ventricles?

Electrocardiogram

An **electrocardiogram** (**ECG**) is used to record electrical changes in the myocardium during the cardiac cycle, using a machine known as an *electrocardiograph*. As action potentials stimulate cardiac muscle fiber contraction, a specific pattern appears—it is not the same as individual action potentials. Because body fluids conduct electrical currents, these electrical changes can be detected on the body's surface. Nodes are placed on the skin and connected by wires to the electrocardiograph. Typically, 12 leads or *electrodes* are used that respond to weak electrical changes by moving a pen or stylus on a moving strip of paper. The movements correspond to myocardial electrical changes. The regular movement of the paper allows the distance between the pen movements to record the time between phases of the cardiac cycle.

Three of the electrodes are bipolar leads. They measure voltage differences between both arms or between one arm and one leg. Nine of the electrodes are unipolar leads. The total of 12 leads provide a complete picture of the electrical activity of the heart.

A normal electrocardiographic pattern includes several waves or *deflections* during each cardiac cycle. In between, muscle fibers remain polarized, and the pen does not move except for indicating the baseline reading. As the S-A node triggers an impulse, the atrial fibers depolarize to produce a recordable electrical change. The first pen movement produces a P wave that shows the depolarization of the atrial fibers leading to atrial contraction. The P wave lasts about 0.08 seconds.

As the impulse reaches ventricular fibers, they quickly depolarize, showing a greater electrical change because of the thicker ventricular walls. When the change ends, the resulting mark is called the QRS complex, consisting of a Q wave, R wave, and S wave that correspond to the depolarization of ventricular fibers before ventricular contraction. The QRS complex has an intricate shape because there is a constant change in the paths of depolarization waves through the ventricular walls. The QRS complex also takes about 0.08 seconds.

As the ventricles repolarize, a T wave is produced and recorded. Atrial repolarization is missing from the pattern because atrial fibers repolarize at the same time the ventricular fibers are depolarizing. The T wave lasts about 0.16 seconds. Because repolarization is slower than depolarization, the T wave appears more spread out, with a lower amplitude height than the QRS complex. It is often obscured by the larger QRS wave being recorded simultaneously.

Electrocardiographic patterns are used to assess the heart's conduction of impulses. The P-Q interval is the time period between the P wave and the QRS complex and can indicate impulse transmission times between the S-A node and A-V node to indicate ischemia or other conditions that affect the A-V conduction pathways. Damage to the A-V bundle can extend the QRS complex, showing a different recording on an ECG. The P-Q interval takes about 0.16 seconds and is also referred to as the P-R interval if the Q portion is not visible. The P-R interval includes atrial depolarization, contraction, and the passage of the depolarization wave through the remainder of the conduction system.

The S-T segment occurs when the action potentials of the ventricular myocytes are in their plateau phases. At this tie, all the ventricular myocardium is depolarized. The Q-T interval lasts about 0.38 seconds. It is the period from the start of ventricular depolarization through ventricular repolarization.

FOCUS ON PATHOLOGY

Deflection waves are usually consistent in a healthy heart. Abnormal ECG findings may indicate heart disease or damage and conduction system problems. Examples include a prolonged Q-T interval, which involves abnormal repolarization, increasing chances of ventricular **arrhythmias**; an enlarged R wave, involving enlarged ventricles; and elevation or depression of the S-T segment, involving cardiac ischemia.

Speed of Conduction

From the time the S-A node generates an impulse until depolarization of the final ventricular muscle cells takes only 220 ms in a healthy heart. After the ventricular depolarization wave, ventricular contraction is nearly immediate. The motion of contraction starts at the heart apex, moves toward the atria, and follows the excitation wave's direction through the ventricle walls. Some contained blood is ejected superiorly into the large arteries that leave the ventricles.

Various speeds of spontaneous depolarization also exist. The heart normally beats 75 times per minute because of the actions of the S-A node. If the S-A node was not there, the A-V node would depolarize approximately 50 times per minute. If the A-V node was not providing input, the A-V bundle and remainder of the conduction system would depolarize only approximately 30 times per minute, even though their conduction speed is extremely rapid.

Without the conduction system, cardiac impulses would travel very slowly. Instead of moving several meters per second in most areas, they would move only 0.3 to 0.5 meters per second. This would reduce the effectiveness of the heart's pumping action because it would allow certain muscle fibers to contract a long time before others.

Parasympathetic and Sympathetic Innervation

When the body requires more blood, such as during exercise, the heart rate increases to pump more blood to the body. Parasympathetic fibers that innervate the heart arise from neurons in the medulla oblongata of the brain. Many of these fibers branch out to the S-A and A-V nodes. Nerve impulses reach nerve fiber endings, secreting acetylcholine, decreasing S-A and A-V node activity, and decreasing heart rate.

The *cardioacceleratory center* of the medulla oblongata projects to sympathetic preganglionic neurons in levels T1 to T5 of the spinal cord. These neurons synapse with postganglionic neurons located in the cervical and upper thoracic sympathetic trunk. Postganglionic fibers then run through the cardiac plexus to the heart, innervating the S-A and A-V nodes as well as the heart muscle and coronary arteries. The *cardioinhibitory center* sends impulses to the parasympathetic dorsal vagus nucleus, also in the medulla oblongata. This sends inhibitory impulses to the heart via vagus nerve branches.

Continual parasympathetic fiber activity can increase or decrease heart rate, working in opposing fashion. Increased parasympathetic impulses slow heart rate while decreased parasympathetic impulses raise heart rate. Sympathetic fibers reach the heart structures and nodes, and their ends secrete norepinephrine in response to nerve impulses that increase myocardial contraction rates and forces. Basically, the sympathetic nervous system is described as "accelerating" heart rate, whereas the parasympathetic nervous system is described as "decelerating" heart rate.

Effects of the sympathetic and parasympathetic nerve fibers are balanced by baroreceptor reflexes that involve the brain's cardiac control center. Sensory impulses are received and relayed between the brain and heart. Baroreceptors detect changes in blood pressure. Cerebral or hypothalamic impulses also influence the cardiac control center, as do temperature changes and certain ions.

Ions

The most important ions that influence heart action are potassium and calcium. Excess extracellular potassium ions or *hyperkalemia* decrease contraction rates and forces, whereas deficient extracellular potassium ions or *hypokalemia* may cause a potentially life-threatening abnormal heart rhythm or *arrhythmia*. Excess extracellular calcium ions, a condition called *hypercalcemia*, can cause the heart to contract for an abnormally long time, whereas deficient extracellular calcium ions, known as *hypocalcemia*, depress heart action.

TEST YOUR UNDERSTANDING

1. Describe how an ECG records electrical heart activities.
2. Define what is occurring during the P-R interval, QRS complex, and the T wave on an ECG.
3. Contrast the cardioacceleratory and cardioinhibitory centers.

Heart Sounds

A heartbeat makes a characteristic double thumping sound when heard through a stethoscope, because of vibrations of the heart tissues related to the valves closing. The first thumping sound occurs during ventricular contraction when the A-V valves close and indicates when ventricular pressure rises above atrial pressure. This is the beginning of ventricular *systole*. The first sound is usually the loudest, longest, and most resonant heart sound. The second sound occurs during ventricular relaxation when the pulmonary and aortic or *semilunar* valves close. This is the beginning of ventricular relaxation or *diastole*, and the sound is shorter and sharper than the first. The two heart sounds are often described as "lub-dup," "pause," "lub-dup," "pause," and so on.

The mitral valve closes just before the tricuspid valve. Also, the aortic semilunar valve usually closes just before the pulmonary valve. Auscultating the four specific regions of the thorax distinguishes each individual valve sound. The four points are not directly superficial to the valves because the sounds take various paths to reach the chest wall. However, these points help to define the four corners of a normal heart. By understanding a normal heart's location and size, one can more easily recognize a disease and/or enlarged heart.

The four points of auscultation used to hear each individual valve sound are as follows:

- *Aortic valve:* second intercostal space at the right sternal margin
- *Pulmonary valve:* second intercostal space at the left sternal margin
- *Mitral valve:* over the heart apex, in the fifth intercostal space, in line with the middle of the clavicle
- *Tricuspid valve:* usually heard in the right sternal margin of the fifth intercostal space

FOCUS ON PATHOLOGY

Abnormal heart sounds are called *heart murmurs* and are generated when blood strikes obstruction and can be heard with a stethoscope. Even though the heart may be totally healthy, heart murmurs are somewhat common in young children and some elderly people, likely due to thinness of their heart walls and because they may vibrate more than in the average adult. Most heart murmurs indicate valve problems. If insufficient or incompetent, a "swishing" sound can be heard when the blood flows back or is regurgitated through a valve that remains partially opened when it should have closed. A *stenotic* aortic valve causes a high-pitched sound or a click to occur when the valve should be wide open but is not. Stenosis causes heart valves to be unable to open completely, restricting blood flow through them.

Cardiac Cycle

One *cardiac cycle* causes pressure in the heart chambers to rise and fall and valves to open and close. Early during diastole, pressure in the ventricles is low, causing the A-V valves to open and the ventricles to fill with blood. Nearly 70% of returning blood enters the ventricles before contraction.

As the atria contract, the remaining 30% is pushed into the ventricles. As the ventricles contract, ventricular pressure rises. When it exceeds atrial pressure, the A-V valves close and papillary muscles contract, preventing the cusps of the A-V valves from bulging into the atria excessively. During ventricular contraction, the A-V valves are closed and atrial pressure is low. Blood flows into the atria while the ventricles are contracting, so the atria are prepared for the next cardiac cycle.

As ventricular pressure exceeds pulmonary trunk and aorta pressure, the pulmonary and aortic valves open. Blood is ejected from the ventricles into these arteries, and ventricular pressure drops. When it is lower than in the aorta and pulmonary trunk, the semilunar valves close. When ventricular pressure is lower than atrial pressure, the A-V valves open and the ventricles begin to refill.

Cardiac muscle fibers are similar in function to skeletal muscle fibers but are connected in branched networks. If any part of the network is stimulated, impulses are sent throughout the heart, and it contracts as a single unit. A **functional syncytium** is a mass of merging cells that function as a unit. There are two of these structures in the heart, one in the atrial walls and one in the ventricular walls. A small area of the right atrial floor is the only part of the heart's muscle fibers not separated by the fibrous *cardiac skeleton*. Here, the atrial syncytium and the ventricular syncytium are connected by cardiac conduction system fibers.

Cardiac Output

Heart action determines the amount of blood entering the arterial system with each ventricular contraction. **Stroke volume** is defined as the volume of blood discharged from the ventricle with each contraction. An average adult male's stroke volume is relatively constant, at about 70 mL. The movements and forces that are generated during contractions of the heart are referred to as *cardiodynamics*. The **cardiac output** is defined as the volume discharged from the ventricle per minute. It is calculated by multiplying the *stroke volume* by the heart rate, in beats per minute. So, if the stroke volume is 70 mL and heart rate is 75 beats per minute, the cardiac output is 5,250 mL per minute. Blood pressure varies with cardiac output and increases or decreases based on similar changes in stroke volume or heart rate. If the heart is seriously weakened or blood volume decreases greatly, stroke volume declines, and cardiac output is maintained by increasing contractility and heart rate.

The average adult cardiac output is calculated as follows:

$$CO = HR \times SV = \frac{75 \text{ beats}}{\text{Minute}} \times \frac{70 \text{ ml per beat}}{\text{Beat}}$$
$$= \frac{5,250 \text{ mL}}{\text{Minute}} = \frac{5.25 \text{ L}}{\text{Minute}}$$

Cardiac output increases when stroke volume increases, when the heart beats faster, or both. It decreases when one or both of these factors decrease.

Remember that stroke volume represents the difference between end-diastolic volume and end-systolic volume. *End-diastolic volume* is the amount of blood that collects in a ventricle during diastole. *End-systolic volume* is the amount of blood that remains in a ventricle after it has already contracted. End-diastolic volume is normally 120 mL, and end-systolic volume is normally 50 mL. Therefore, the difference between them is 120 mL minus 50 mL, which equals 70 mL.

Preload

The three most important things to remember about the regulation of stroke volume are preload, contractility, and afterload. *Preload* is the degree the heart muscle can stretch just before contraction. Preload controls stroke volume, and in normal conditions the higher the preload, the higher the stroke volume. The relationship between the preload and stroke volume is called the *Frank-Starling law of the heart*. Resting cardiac cells are usually shorter than their optimal length, so stretching can cause significant increases in contractile force. The most important factor concerning preload is *venous return*, which is the amount of blood returning to the heart and distending its ventricles. The *atrial reflex* or *Bainbridge reflex* concerns adjustments made to heart rate as a response to increases in venous return.

Contractility

Contractility is the contractile strength achieved at a certain muscle length. Extrinsic factors increasing contractility of the heart muscle can also enhance stroke volume. Greater contractility results in more blood being ejected from the heart, which increases stroke volume and lowers end-systolic volume. Contractility is increased when sympathetic stimulation is increased. Various substances also affect contractility. *Positive inotropic agents* are substances that increase contractility and include epinephrine, glucagon, thyroxine, digitalis, and extracellular calcium ions. *Negative inotropic agents* decrease contractility and include excessive hydrogen ions, increased extracellular potassium levels, and calcium channel blockers.

Afterload

Afterload is the back pressure exerted by the arterial blood on the aortic and pulmonary valves. The ventricles must overcome this pressure to eject blood. This pressure is about 80 mm Hg in the aorta and about 10 mm Hg in the pulmonary trunk. When a person is healthy, afterload is relatively constant, but in hypertensive people, afterload reduces the ventricles' ability to eject blood. As a result, the heart retains more blood after systole, which increases end-systolic volume and decreases stroke volume.

Cardiac reserve is the difference between the resting and maximal cardiac output. It is usually four to five times the resting cardiac output in a nonathletic person. This resting output is 20 to 25 liters per minute. However, in a trained athlete, cardiac output may reach seven times the resting cardiac output, which is 35 liters per minute.

Regulation of Heart Rate

Stroke volume is fairly consistent in a healthy heart and cardiovascular system. Regulation of heart rate includes homeostatic mechanisms such as autonomic, chemical, hormonal, and other forms of regulation.

Autonomic Regulation

The most important extrinsic controls on heart rate occur because of the autonomic nervous system. Anxiety, exercise, or fright activate the sympathetic nervous system, and related nerve fibers release norepinephrine at their cardiac synapses. This binds to β_1-adrenergic receptors in the heart, and threshold can be reached faster. Therefore, the S-A node fires more quickly, and the heart beats faster. Sympathetic stimulation also speeds relaxation by enhancing contractility. It accomplishes this by enhancing calcium ion movements in contractile cells.

A ventricular contractile cell's resting potential of –90 mV is similar to that of a resting skeletal muscle's resting potential of –85 mV. Once the membrane of a ventricular muscle cell reaches threshold, or about –75 mV, an action potential begins. The action potential then proceeds in three steps, the first of which is *rapid depolarization*, using *fast sodium channels*. The next step is *plateau*, which involves *slow calcium channels*. As these channels begin closing, the third step, *repolarization,* occurs as *slow potassium channels* begin opening.

When resting, both divisions of the autonomic nervous system repeatedly send impulses to the S-A node, with mostly inhibitory effects. The heart is described as having *vagal tone*, with the heart rate usually slower than if it was not innervated by vagal nerves. If the vagal nerves were cut, there would be a fast increase in its rate of approximately 25 beats per minute. This shows the 100 beats per minute inherent rate of the S-A node. When various types of sensory input activate either autonomic division strongly, the other division is inhibited temporarily. Most of this sensory input comes from *baroreceptors*, which respond to systemic blood pressure changes.

Chemical Regulation

Heart rate is also influenced by many chemicals, especially when they are present in very high or very low amounts. Hormones and ions are implicated here. Hormones include epinephrine and thyroxine. During sympathetic activation, epinephrine is liberated by the adrenal medulla. This hormone produces equivalent cardiac effects to those from norepinephrine when it is released by the sympathetic nerves. The heart rate and contractility are both enhanced. Thyroxine from the thyroid gland increases production of body heat as well as metabolic rate. In large amounts, the heart rate increases and remains sustained. Thyroxine acts directly on the heart while enhancing effects of both epinephrine and norepinephrine. Intracellular and extracellular ions, in normal levels, also maintain normal heart function. When plasma electrolytes are out of balance, the heart may be affected to a severe degree.

The heart is depressed by *hypocalcemia* and increases its rate and contractility as a result of *hypercalcemia*. However, this effect is limited. Extremely high calcium ion levels interfere with heart function and may cause potentially fatal arrhythmias. *Hypokalemia* or *hyperkalemia* occurs in a variety of conditions and is extremely dangerous. Excessive potassium depolarizes the heart's resting potential, potentially causing **heart block** and cardiac arrest. Very low potassium may cause the heart to beat weakly and arrhythmically, which can also threaten life.

Other Types of Regulation

Heart rate is also influenced by age, body temperature, exercise, and gender. The resting heart rate of infants is highest, at 140 to 160 beats per minute, but gradually declines throughout life. Women have an average heart rate that is higher than men's. In women, this is 72 to 80 beats per minute and in men, 64 to 72 beats per minute. Via the sympathetic nervous system, exercise raises the heart rate and increases systemic blood pressure. In a physically fit adult, resting heart rate is usually much lower than in people who are out of shape. By enhancing the metabolic rate of cardiac cells, heat increases heart rate. For example, a high fever often makes you feel as if your heart is pounding rapidly. This is similar to the effects of extreme exercise, because the

muscles are generating large amounts of heat. Oppositely, the heart rate is directly decreased by cold temperatures.

1. What causes the sounds of the heart?
2. What is a cardiac cycle?
3. Name the factors that affect cardiac output.
4. Differentiate between autonomic, chemical, and hormonal regulation of heart rate.
5. What are common causes of tachycardia?

Congenital heart defects are found in more than 30,000 infants in the United States every year, making them the most common type of birth defect. The most common defects involve either mixing of oxygen-depleted blood with oxygenated blood or narrowed blood vessels or heart valves, which greatly increase the heart's workload. Examples include *septal defects, patent ductus arteriosus, coarctation of the aorta,* and *tetralogy of Fallot.*

Effects of Aging on the Cardiovascular System

Aging changes the heart and the blood vessels. The heart may experience a reduction in maximum output, changes to the nodal and conducting cells, reduction of elasticity of its fibers, progressive atherosclerosis that can restrict circulation through the heart, and the replacement of damaged cardiac muscle with scar tissue. Other age-related changes that affect the heart include valve thickening and stenosis and declines in cardiac reserve. Stiffening or *stenosis* of heart valves usually affects the mitral valve, resulting in heart murmurs. An older heart is less able to respond to the need for increased cardiac output that is both sudden and prolonged. Maximum heart rate declines because sympathetic innervation becomes less efficient. Cardiac muscle cell death results in more fibrous tissue, stiffening the heart. It then fills less efficiently, and stroke volume is reduced. Fibrosis may also affect the nodes of the heart, which increases likelihood of arrhythmias and other conduction problems. Atherosclerosis is intensified by stress, smoking, and inactivity. Serious results include coronary artery occlusion, hypertensive heart disease, heart attack, and stroke. Diet also contributes significantly to atherosclerosis. Physicians advise that Americans reduce their consumption of salt, cholesterol, and animal fat.

Extreme, repeated variances in heart rate usually indicates cardiovascular disease. **Tachycardia** is a heart rate of more than 100 beats per minute and is commonly caused by elevated body temperature, certain drugs, heart disease, or stress. Sometimes, tachycardia results in **fibrillation**. **Bradycardia** is a heart rate of less than 60 beats per minute commonly caused by certain drugs, low body temperature, or parasympathetic nervous activation. Although bradycardia is a desired result of endurance training, in people with low physical activity, it may be caused by extremely poor blood circulation and can be an indicator of brain edema after trauma to the head.

SUMMARY

The cardiovascular system consists of the heart and blood vessels. It provides oxygen and nutrients to tissues while removing wastes. The heart is located within the *mediastinum*, resting on the diaphragm. The pulmonary circuit consists of vessels that carry blood from the right ventricle to the lungs and back to the left atrium. The systemic circuit consists of vessels that lead from the left ventricle to the body cells and back to the heart, including the aorta and its branches. The aorta is the largest artery in the body, with respect to diameter.

The wall of the heart has three layers: epicardium, myocardium, and endocardium. The heart is divided into two atria and two ventricles. Blood low in oxygen and high in carbon dioxide enters the right side of the heart and is pumped into the pulmonary circulation. After oxygenation in the lungs and some removal of carbon dioxide, it returns to the left side of the heart. The left ventricle pumps blood out of the heart to the rest of the body.

The cardiac cycle consists of the atria contracting while the ventricles relax, and vice versa. Electrical activity of the cardiac cycle can be recorded via an ECG. The cardiac cycle consists of the P wave, QRS complex, and T wave. Blood vessels form a closed circuit of tubes that carry blood from the heart to the body cells and back again. Blood pressure is the force that blood exerts against the insides of blood vessels.

KEY TERMS

Anastomoses
Aorta
Aortic valve
Apex
Arrhythmias
Atria
Atrioventricular node
   (A-V node)
Automaticity
A-V bundle
Base
Bradycardia
Cardiac conduction system
Cardiac cycle
Cardiac output

Chordae tendineae
Coronary arteries
Coronary sinus
Coronary veins
Diastole
Electrocardiogram (ECG)
Endocardium
Epicardium
Fibrillation
Functional syncytium
Heart block
Inferior vena cava
Mediastinum
Mitral valve
Myocardium

Pacemaker
Papillary muscles
Pericardium
Pulmonary valve
Pulmonary veins
Purkinje fibers
Septum
Sinoatrial node
   (S-A node)
Stroke volume
Superior vena cava
Systole
Tachycardia
Tricuspid valve
Ventricles

The following learning goals correspond to the objectives at the beginning of this chapter:

1. The human heart is hollow and cone-shaped, varying in size. An average adult has a heart that is about 14 cm or 5 inches long, by 9 cm or 3.5 inches wide, and weighs approximately 300 g. The heart lies inside the thoracic cavity, resting on the diaphragm. It is within the mediastinum, which is the medial cavity of the thorax, in between the lungs. Its posterior border is near the vertebral column, and its anterior border is near the sternum. It is not situated in the exact center of the thorax, and approximately two-thirds of the heart lies to the left of the midsternal line. It is partially obscured, laterally, by the lungs.

2. The heart wall is made up of the outer epicardium, middle myocardium, and inner endocardium. The epicardium protects the heart by reducing friction. The thick myocardium pumps blood out of the chambers of the heart. The endocardium has many elastic and collagenous fibers and contains blood vessels as well as the Purkinje fibers. It lines the chambers of the heart and covers the fibrous tissue that forms the heart valves. It is continuous with the endothelial linings of the heart's blood vessels.

3. The four chambers of the heart are the right atrium, left atrium, right ventricle, and left ventricle. The right atrium receives blood from two large veins called the superior vena cava and the inferior vena cava and from a smaller vein, the coronary sinus, that drains blood into the right atrium from the heart's myocardium. Four pulmonary veins enter the left atrium, supplying it with blood from the lungs. The right ventricle sends blood to the pulmonary trunk and pulmonary arteries. The left ventricle sends blood into the aorta and its branches, which are the right and left coronary arteries.

4. The four heart valves are the two A-V valves and the two semilunar valves. The A-V valves consist of the tricuspid and bicuspid or mitral valves. The semilunar valves consist of the aortic and pulmonary valves. The A-V valves lie between the atria and ventricles, with the tricuspid valve lying between the right atrium and right ventricle and the bicuspid or mitral valve lying between the left atrium and left ventricle. The semilunar valves lie between the ventricles and the large arteries that emerge from them. Their names explain their locations. The aortic valve lies between the left ventricle and the aorta, whereas the pulmonary valve lies between the right ventricle and the pulmonary trunk and arteries.

5. The first two aortic branches are called the right and left coronary arteries. They supply blood to the heart tissues, with openings lying just beyond the aortic valve. The coronary arteries deliver blood when the heart is relaxed and have less function while the ventricles are contracting because they are compressed by the myocardium. Both coronary arteries enclose the heart in the coronary sulcus and provide the arterial supply of the *coronary circulation*. The anterior interventricular artery is also known as the left anterior descending artery. It supplies blood to the anterior walls of both ventricles and to the interventricular septum. The circumflex artery supplies the posterior walls of the left ventricle and the left atrium. Coronary artery branches supply many capillaries in the myocardium. These arteries have smaller branches with connections called *anastomoses* between vessels providing alternate blood pathways, which is known as collateral circulation. The coronary veins join to form the enlarged coronary sinus, emptying into the right atrium. The coronary sinus empties into the great cardiac vein, middle cardiac vein, and small cardiac vein. Also, several anterior cardiac veins empty into the right atrium's anterior portion.

6. An ECG normally reveals the following electrical events:
   - *P wave:* shows depolarization of atrial fibers leading to atrial contraction
   - *QRS complex:* corresponds to the depolarization of ventricular fibers before ventricular contraction
   - *T wave:* depicts the repolarization of ventricles

7. A diagram of a normal ECG should show a P wave, QRS complex, T wave, and U wave.

8. Cardiac output is defined as the volume discharged from the ventricle per minute. It is calculated by multiplying the stroke volume by the heart rate, in beats per minute. The factors that influence cardiac output include increases or decreases in stroke volume or heart rate.

9. A heartbeat makes a characteristic double thumping sound when heard through a stethoscope. The first thumping sound occurs during ventricular contraction when the A-V valves close. It is usually the loudest, longest, and most resonant heart sound. The second sound occurs during ventricular relaxation when the pulmonary and aortic or *semilunar* valves close. It is

shorter and sharper than the first sound. The two heart sounds are often described as "lub-dup," "pause," "lub-dup," "pause," and so on. Abnormal heart sounds are called heart murmurs. They are generated when blood strikes obstruction and can be heard with a stethoscope. Heart murmurs are somewhat common in young children and some elderly people. Most heart murmurs indicate valve problems. If insufficient or incompetent, there is a "swishing" sound when the blood flow back or is regurgitate through a valve that remains partially opened when it should have closed.

10. Anxiety, exercise, or fright activate the sympathetic part of the autonomic nervous system and related nerve fibers release norepinephrine at their cardiac synapses. This binds to β_1-adrenergic receptors in the

heart, and threshold can be reached faster. Therefore, the S-A node fires more quickly, and the heart beats faster. Sympathetic stimulation also speeds relaxation by enhancing contractility. It accomplishes this by enhancing calcium ion movements in contractile cells. When resting, both autonomic nervous system divisions repeatedly send impulses to the S-A node, with mostly inhibitory effects. The heart is described as having vagal tone, with the heart rate usually slower than if it was not innervated by vagal nerves. When various types of sensory input activate either autonomic nervous system division strongly, the other division is inhibited. Most of this sensory input comes from baroreceptors, which respond to systemic blood pressure changes.

CRITICAL THINKING QUESTIONS

A 56-year-old man went to his physician for a routine physical examination. The physician took an ECG, which was normal. Forty-eight hours later the man experienced angina pectoris and was taken to the emergency room. This time, the patient was admitted to the intensive care unit, where

he was diagnosed as having had a myocardial infarction of the left ventricle.

1. What are the risk factors for myocardial infarction?
2. In the intensive care unit, what tests would be performed to rule out a myocardial infarction?

REVIEW QUESTIONS

1. Blood returning to the heart from the systemic circuit first enters the
   A. left atrium
   B. left ventricle
   C. right atrium
   D. right ventricle
2. Blood leaving the left ventricle enters the
   A. pulmonary trunk
   B. pulmonary artery
   C. inferior vena cava
   D. aorta
3. The right ventricle pumps blood to the
   A. systemic circuit
   B. lungs
   C. left atrium
   D. right atrium

4. The visceral pericardium is the same as the
   A. epicardium
   B. endocardium
   C. myocardium
   D. parietal pericardium
5. The mitral valve is located between the
   A. right atrium and right ventricle
   B. left atrium and left ventricle
   C. left ventricle and aorta
   D. right ventricle and pulmonary trunk
6. Depolarization of the ventricles is represented on an electrocardiogram by the
   A. P wave
   B. T wave
   C. PR complex
   D. QRS complex

7. The function of an atrium is to
   A. pump blood to the lungs
   B. pump blood into the systemic circuit
   C. pump blood to the heart muscle
   D. collect blood

8. The pacemaker cells of the heart are located in the
   A. S-A node
   B. A-V node
   C. left ventricle
   D. left atrium

9. The T wave on an ECG tracing represents
   A. ventricular depolarization
   B. atrial repolarization
   C. ventricular repolarization
   D. atrial depolarization

10. Each of the following factors increases cardiac output, *except*
    A. increased parasympathetic stimulation
    B. increased sympathetic stimulation
    C. increased venous return
    D. increased heart rate

11. Blood leaves the right ventricle by passing through the
    A. mitral valve
    B. pulmonary valve
    C. tricuspid valve
    D. aortic valve

12. As a result of the long refractory period, cardiac muscle cannot exhibit
    A. fatigue
    B. tonus
    C. tetany
    D. recruitment

13. All the following conditions can increase heart rate, *except*
    A. increased levels of epinephrine in the interstitial fluid surrounding the myocardium
    B. increased permeability of the myocardial membrane to sodium ions
    C. increased sympathetic stimulation of nodal fibers
    D. increased parasympathetic stimulation of nodal fibers

14. The property of heart muscle to contract in the absence of neural or hormonal regulation is called
    A. bradycardia
    B. automaticity
    C. systole
    D. arrhythmia

15. If the membranes of the cardiac muscle cells in the S-A node become more permeable to potassium ions, the
    A. heart rate will decrease
    B. stroke volume will increase
    C. membranes will depolarize
    D. heart rate will increase

ESSAY QUESTIONS

1. Describe the location and position of the heart in the body.
2. Describe three layers of the heart wall.
3. Locate and discuss the heart valves.
4. Describe the heart chambers and associated great vessels.
5. Describe coronary circulation.
6. Discuss the conduction system of the heart.
7. Describe electrocardiography.
8. Describe normal heart sounds, and explain how heart murmurs differ.
9. Define cardiac output and stroke volume.
10. Describe the autonomic nervous system's regulation of heart rate.

Vascular System

OBJECTIVES

After studying this chapter, readers should be able to

1. Distinguish the structures and functions of various blood vessels.
2. Explain the difference between pulmonary and systemic vessels.
3. Define blood flow, blood pressure, and resistance.
4. Describe the effects of the sympathetic and parasympathetic nervous systems on the blood vessels.
5. Describe the factors that influence blood pressure and explain how blood pressure is regulated.
6. List the major arteries that supply the head and abdomen.
7. Identify the main arteries and veins of the lower limbs.
8. List the major veins that carry blood away from the lower limbs.
9. Describe the hepatic portal system.
10. Define pulse pressure and list locations on the body surface where the pulse can be detected.

Overview

Blood moves on a continual basis through the heart, **arteries** and their smaller branches, **capillaries**, the smaller vein branches, and then the **veins** themselves, returning back to the heart. The blood vessels constrict, relax, and pulsate as they conduct blood and other substances to the body tissues. They form a closed delivery system, beginning and ending with the heart. The **systemic circuit** has a long pathway through all of the body and is powered by the left ventricle. Along this circuit, there is about five times more resistance to **blood flow** than in the **pulmonary circuit**. All body tissues require circulation to survive. Although the two heart ventricles have uneven workloads, equal volumes of blood are pumped to the pulmonary and systemic circuits simultaneously. The pulmonary circuit is a short, low-pressure circulation. It is served by the right ventricle of the heart (**FIGURE 17-1**).

The five general classes of blood vessels in the cardiovascular system are the arteries, **arterioles**, capillaries, **venules**, and veins. In total, the blood vessels of an average human adult, if stretched out, are about 60,000 miles in length. *Arteries* are very strong elastic vessels that are able to carry blood away from the heart under high pressure. They subdivide into thinner tubes that give rise to branched, finer arterioles. In the systemic circuit, the arteries carry only oxygenated blood, whereas the veins carry only deoxygenated blood. In the pulmonary circuit, the reverse is true. The only blood vessels that closely contact tissue cells and serve the needs of the cells are the capillaries. The extremely thin capillary walls allow most exchanges that occur between blood and tissue cells. When oxygenated blood leaves the alveolar capillaries, it enters venules that eventually unite, forming larger blood vessels that transport blood to the *pulmonary veins*. The pulmonary circuit is completed by the four pulmonary veins, two from each lung, that empty into the left atrium to complete the pulmonary circuit.

Blood Vessel Structure

An artery's wall consists of three distinct layers and a blood-containing space known as the **lumen**. The innermost **tunica intima** is made up of a layer of simple squamous epithelium known as the **endothelium**. It rests on a connective tissue membrane with many elastic, collagenous fibers. The endothelium helps prevent blood clotting and may also help in regulating blood flow. It releases nitric oxide to relax smooth muscle of the vessel. In arteries, the outer margin has a thick layer of elastic fibers known as the *internal elastic membrane*.

The middle **tunica media** makes up most of an arterial wall, including smooth muscle fibers arranged mostly in circles and a thick elastic connective tissue layer. The smooth muscle fiber activity is controlled by many chemicals and the autonomic nervous system's sympathetic *vasomotor nerve fibers*. The tunica media is separated from the next layer, the tunica externa, by a thin band of fibers known as the *external elastic membrane*.

The outer **tunica externa,** also known as the *tunica adventitia*, is thinner, made mostly of connective tissue with irregular fibers. It is attached to the surrounding tissues (**FIGURE 17-2**) and contains many lymphatic vessels and nerve fibers. The tunica externa of larger blood vessels contains many tiny blood vessels, which comprise a system known as the **vasa vasorum**. This system nourishes the outer tissues of blood vessel walls. The luminal inner portions of vessels obtain nutrients directly from the blood.

In arteries and arterioles, **vasomotor fibers** receive impulses to contract and reduce blood vessel diameter, a process known as **vasoconstriction**. When inhibited, the muscle fibers relax and the vessel's diameter increases in a process known as **vasodilation**. Changes in artery and arteriole diameters greatly affect blood flow and pressure.

Arterial System

The arterial system consists of the aorta and the left and right pulmonary arteries. The aorta sends oxygenated blood to the various body systems, whereas the pulmonary arteries carry deoxygenated blood to the lungs. Arteries are grouped based

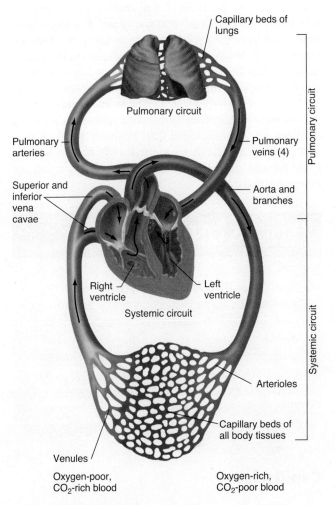

Capillary beds of lungs

Pulmonary circuit

Pulmonary arteries

Pulmonary veins (4)

Superior and inferior vena cavae

Aorta and branches

Right ventricle

Left ventricle

Systemic circuit

Arterioles

Capillary beds of all body tissues

Venules

Oxygen-poor, CO_2-rich blood

Oxygen-rich, CO_2-poor blood

Pulmonary circuit

Systemic circuit

FIGURE 17-1 The blood pathway includes two circuits. The right ventricle supplies the pulmonary circuit, and the left ventricle supplies the systemic circuit.

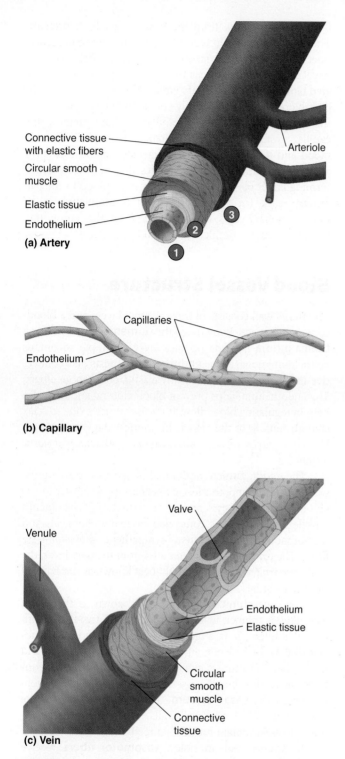

(a) Artery

Connective tissue with elastic fibers
Circular smooth muscle
Elastic tissue
Endothelium
Arteriole

Capillaries
Endothelium

(b) Capillary

Venule
Valve
Endothelium
Elastic tissue
Circular smooth muscle
Connective tissue

(c) Vein

FIGURE 17-2 Blood vessels. (A) The wall of an artery, (B) the wall of a capillary, and (c) the wall of a vein.

on whether they are elastic or muscular. Smaller arteries are called arterioles.

Elastic Arteries

Elastic arteries are located near the heart and have thick walls. They include the aorta and its primary branches. They are the arteries of largest diameter in the body and the most elastic.

The elastic arteries range between 2.5 and 1 cm in diameter, with large lumens. The size of their lumens causes them to be low-resistance pathways for blood as it moves from the heart to the medium-sized arteries. Elastic arteries are also known as *conducting arteries*.

There is more *elastin* in the elastic arteries than in the other types of arteries. Elastin is found in all three tunics, with the tunica media being the most elastic. In the tunica media, the elastin has holes and is found between layers of smooth muscle cells. When atherosclerosis and similar conditions cause the blood vessels to lose elasticity, the blood flows through with more difficulty, raising the **blood pressure**.

Muscular Arteries

The smaller, distal **muscular arteries**, also known as *distributing arteries*, deliver blood to body organs. They have the thickest tunica media of all blood vessels, in proportion to their size. The tunica media of muscular arteries, in comparison with elastic arteries, have relatively more smooth muscle and less elastic tissue. Because of this, they have more vasoconstrictive actions but are less able to stretch.

Arterioles

The arterioles are the smallest of all arteries. The diameter of their lumens is between 0.3 mm and 10 μm. The largest arterioles have three tunics, whereas the smallest arterioles are basically a single layer of smooth muscle cells circled around an endothelial lining. The tunica media of larger arterioles is mostly made up of smooth muscle, with a small amount of elastic fibers in various areas. The smaller arterioles lead directly into the capillary beds. With *resistance* describing the force that opposes blood flow, arterioles are also called *resistance vessels* because more pressure is needed to push blood through them than arteries. This is because they are more constricted.

FOCUS ON PATHOLOGY

An *aneurysm* may result when local arterial pressure exceeds the capacity of the elastic components of arterial tunics. An aneurysm is a bulge in a weakened artery wall, which may result in a serious hemorrhage. Ruptured aneurysms are most dangerous in the brain, leading to strokes, or in the aorta, which can cause the death of the patient within only a few minutes.

Capillaries

The smallest-diameter blood vessels are capillaries, which connect the smallest arterioles to the smallest venules. The walls of capillaries are also composed of endothelium and

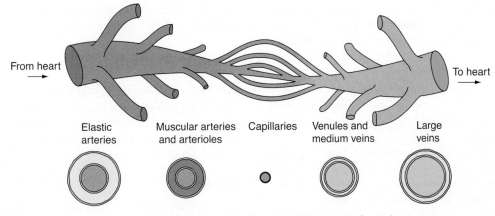

From heart →
To heart →

Elastic arteries | Muscular arteries and arterioles | Capillaries | Venules and medium veins | Large veins

FIGURE 17-3 The composition and diameter of our blood vessel walls varies with the type of vessel.

form the semipermeable layer through which substances in blood are exchanged with substances in tissue fluids surrounding cells of the body (**FIGURE 17-3**). The capillaries are microscopic blood vessels with extremely thin walls. Their walls contain a thin tunica intima and nothing else. Sometimes, a single endothelial cell makes up the entire circumference of the wall of the capillary.

In *continuous capillaries,* the endothelium forms a complete lining. Most of the body is supplied with continuous capillaries. Most capillaries average 1 mm in length with an average lumen diameter of 8 to 10 μm, causing red blood cells to move through them one at a time. Although most tissues have many capillaries, tendons and ligaments are examples of tissues that only have a small amount. These tissues get their nutrients from the blood vessels of adjacent connective tissues. In the eye, the cornea and lens lack vessels, receiving nutrients from the aqueous humor.

In *fenestrated capillaries,* window-like pores penetrate the endothelial lining, which allow rapid exchange of solutes and water between the interstitial fluid and plasma. An example of these capillaries is the *choroid plexus* of the brain. *Sinusoidal capillaries* or *sinusoids* are similar to fenestrated capillaries but are more irregular in shape, with a flattened appearance. They allow free exchange of solutes and water, including plasma proteins, between interstitial fluid and blood.

Capillary walls have thin slits where endothelial cells overlap. These slits have various sizes, affecting permeability. Capillaries of muscles have smaller openings than those of the glands, kidneys, and small intestine. Tissues with higher metabolic rates, such as muscles, have many more capillaries than those with slower metabolic rates, such as cartilage.

Some capillaries pass directly from arterioles to venules, whereas others have highly branched networks (**FIGURE 17-4**). Precapillary sphincters control blood distribution through capillaries. Based on the demands of cells, these sphincters constrict or relax so blood can follow specific pathways to meet tissue cellular requirements. Gases, metabolic byproducts, and nutrients are exchanged between capillaries and the tissue fluid surrounding body cells. Capillary walls allow diffusion of blood with high levels of oxygen and nutrients and also allow high levels of

carbon dioxide and other wastes to move from the tissues into the capillaries.

Plasma proteins usually cannot move through the capillary walls because of their large size, so they remain in the blood. Blood pressure generated when capillary walls contract provides force for filtration via hydrostatic pressure. Blood pressure is strongest when blood leaves the heart and

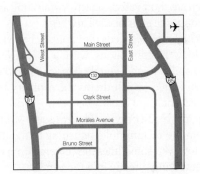

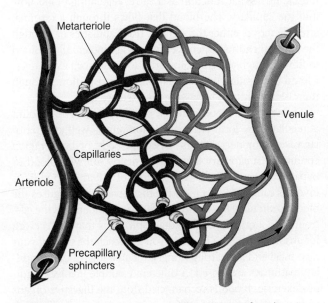

Metarteriole

Venule

Capillaries

Arteriole

Precapillary sphincters

FIGURE 17-4 Just as we travel on different types of roads, our vasculature consists of several different types of vessels.

weaker as the distance from the heart increases because of friction known as **peripheral resistance** between the blood and the vessel walls. Therefore, blood pressure is highest in the arteries, less so in the arterioles, and lowest in the capillaries. Filtration occurs mostly at the arteriolar ends of capillaries because the pressure is higher than at the venular ends. Plasma proteins trapped in capillaries create an osmotic pressure that pulls water into the capillaries, known as *colloid osmotic pressure*.

Capillary blood pressure favors filtration, whereas plasma colloid osmotic pressure favors reabsorption. At the venular ends of capillaries, blood pressure is decreased because of resistance so reabsorption can occur. The capillaries of the body provide direct access to most cells and are perfectly located and formed to easily exchange gases, hormones, nutrients, and other components between the interstitial fluid and blood.

Capillaries form interwoven networks that are referred to as *capillary beds* or *capillary plexuses*. The term *microcirculation* is used to describe blood flow through the capillary beds, which lie between the arterioles and the venules. The two types of vessels in capillary beds, which exist in most areas of the body, include *true capillaries*, which are the actual exchange vessels, and *vascular shunts*, also called *metarterioles* or *precapillary arterioles*, which are short vessels directly connecting arterioles and venules at opposite ends of capillary beds.

A *terminal arteriole* feeds the capillary bed via the metarteriole, which is continuous with a *thoroughfare channel* between a capillary and a venule. This channel then joins the *postcapillary venule*, which drains the capillary bed. In each capillary bed, there are usually between 10 and 100 capillaries, varying per organ or type of body tissue. Most often, they branch from the metarteriole, returning to the thoroughfare channel. However, sometimes they emerge from the terminal arteriole, emptying directly into the venule.

A *precapillary sphincter* surrounds each true capillary's root at the metarteriole. This sphincter is a cuff of smooth muscle fibers that function as a valve, regulating blood flow into the capillary. The blood that flows through a terminal arteriole moves either through the true capillaries or through the vascular shunts. Open precapillary sphincters allow blood to flow through the true capillaries for tissue cell exchanges. Closed precapillary sphincters cause blood to flow through the vascular shunts, bypassing the tissue cells.

How much blood enters a capillary bed? The amount is regulated by local chemical conditions as well as arteriolar vasomotor nerve fibers. Based on body or body region conditions, a capillary bed may be nearly full with blood or bypassed almost totally. An example of differing conditions involves eating. After a meal the digestive process causes the blood to circulate freely through the true capillaries of the gastrointestinal organs so breakdown products may be received for absorption by the body. As you approach the time of your next meal and are getting hungry, the majority of these capillary pathways are closed. A different example involves vigorous exercise. Blood is rechanneled from the digestive organs to the skeletal muscles, where it is needed more. Vigorous exercise after a meal "confuses" the body's management of

blood to the capillaries and may end up causing abdominal problems such as cramping or indigestion.

Venous System

Venules are microscopic vessels that link capillaries to *veins*, which carry blood back to the atria. Vein walls are similar but not identical to arteries but have poorly developed middle layers. Because they have thinner walls and are less elastic than arteries, their lumens have a greater diameter.

Venules

The capillaries join to form venules. These vessels range between 8 and 100 μm in diameter, with the smallest or *postcapillary* venules made up only of endothelium, surrounded by pericytes or *contractile cells*. The larger venules have a thin tunica externa and one to two layers of smooth muscle cells making up their tunica media. Venules combine to form veins.

Veins

Many veins have flap-like valves projecting inward from their linings. These valves often have two structures that close if blood begins to back up in the vein. They aid in returning blood to the heart, opening if blood flow is toward the heart and closing if it reverses.

Veins mostly have three tunics, but these have thinner walls and larger lumens then the arteries to which they correspond. In a vein the tunica media has little smooth muscle or elastin. Even in larger veins the tunica media is relatively thin, with the heaviest wall layer being the tunica externa. As a result, veins can contain large amounts of blood. They are also called *blood reservoirs* and *capacitance vessels*. Veins can hold nearly 65% of the blood supply of the body at any given moment but are usually only partially filled (**FIGURE 17-5**). Veins are usually in no danger of bursting because their blood pressure is relatively low. Veins have specialized structures that help them to return blood to the heart at the same rate it was pumped into the circulation via the arteries. These structures include their larger lumens, through which blood passes with little resistance.

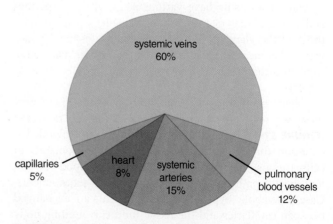

FIGURE 17-5 Relative proportion of blood volume in the cardiovascular system.

TABLE 17-1

Characteristics of Blood Vessels

Type of Vessel	Vessel Wall	Actions
Artery	Three-layered thick wall (endothelial lining, middle smooth muscle and elastic connective tissue layer, and outer connective tissue layer)	Carries relatively high pressure blood from the heart to the arterioles
Arteriole	Three-layered thinner wall (smaller arterioles have an endothelial lining, some smooth muscle tissue, and a small amount of connective tissue)	Helps control blood flow from arteries to capillaries by vasoconstricting or vasodilating
Capillary	One layer of squamous epithelium	Has a membrane allowing nutrients, gases, and wastes to be exchanged between blood and tissue fluid
Venule	Thinner wall than arterioles, with less smooth muscle and elastic connective tissue	Connects capillaries to veins
Vein	Thinner wall than arteries but similar layers; poorly developed middle layer; some have flap-like valves	Carries relatively low pressure blood from venules to the heart; valves prevent blood backflow; veins serve as blood reservoirs

Veins also act as reservoirs for blood in certain conditions, such as during arterial hemorrhage. Resulting venous constrictions help to maintain blood pressure by returning more blood to the heart, ensuring an almost normal blood flow even when up to one-fourth of the **blood volume** is lost. **TABLE 17-1** summarizes the blood vessel characteristics.

Venous Valves

The valves of veins prevent blood from flowing backward. **Venous valves** form from folds of the tunica intima (**FIGURE 17-6**). In appearance, they are similar to the heart's semilunar valves and have similar functions. More venous

FOCUS ON PATHOLOGY

When the valves of a vein become incompetent, they start to leak. They become dilated and tortuous, forming bluish bulges called **varicose veins**. This condition affects the lower limbs predominantly in more than 15% of adults. Conditions that lead to varicose veins include heredity, prolonged standing in one position, pregnancy, and obesity. Pregnancy and obesity exert downward pressure on blood vessels in the groin, and blood flow returning to the heart becomes restricted. Therefore, blood collects in the lower limbs, weakening the valves over time and stretching the walls of the veins. The veins that are most susceptible to this condition are the superficial veins, because they have little support from nearby tissues. Varicose veins are also caused by elevated blood pressure. Straining to have a bowel movement or to give birth raises intra-abdominal pressure, causing varicosities in the anal veins known as *hemorrhoids*.

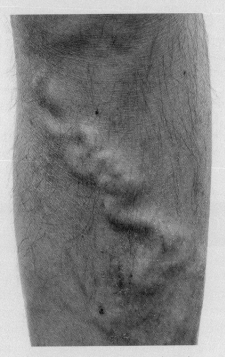

Varicose veins (© Audie/Shutterstock, Inc.)

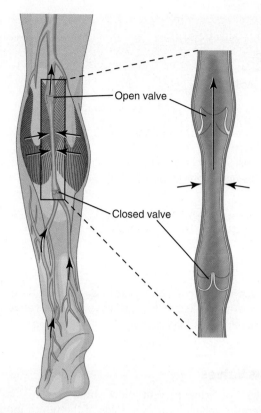

FIGURE 17-6 Valves in veins.

valves exist in the limb veins. Here, gravity opposes upward blood flow. In the abdominal and thoracic body cavities, the veins mostly do not contain valves.

Vascular Anastomoses

Vascular anastomoses are interconnections formed by blood vessels. *Arterial anastomoses* form by the merging of arteries that supply the same body tissues. Such anastomoses provide *collateral channels* so blood can reach these tissues. For example, if an artery is blocked by a clot or cut, a collateral channel may be able to provide required blood to the region.

Arterial anastomoses develop around joints in areas where blood flow through a channel may be slowed or stopped by active movement. These anastomoses also commonly occur in the brain, heart, and abdominal organs. The arteries of the kidneys, retina, and spleen usually do not anastomose or have little collateral circulation. Blood flow interruption to these areas usually causes cellular death.

Blood Circulation

The blood must continue to circulate to sustain life. The heart acts as the circulation pump, and the arteries are pressurized reservoirs and channels. The arterioles control distribution of blood via resistance, the capillaries provide sites for exchange, and the venules and veins collect blood, acting as reservoirs and conducts. It is essential to define three related terms: *blood flow, blood pressure,* and *resistance:*

- *Blood flow:* The amount or *volume* of blood that flows through blood vessels, organs, or the systemic circulation, in milliliters per minute (mL/min). Throughout the body, blood flow is equivalent to cardiac output. When resting, this is relatively constant, yet in certain body organs, blood flow may be different from others because of individual requirements.
- *Blood pressure:* Defined as the force that blood exerts against the inner walls of blood vessels. It most commonly refers to pressure in arteries supplied by the aortic branches, even though it actually occurs throughout the vascular system. Blood flow is generated by the heart's pumping action, and blood pressure results from resistance opposing blood flow. Blood pressure is expressed in millimeters of mercury (mm Hg). *A blood pressure of 120 mm Hg is the same as a column of mercury that is 120 mm in height.*
- *Resistance:* The friction between blood and blood vessel walls. Blood pressure must overcome this force for the blood to continue flowing. Factors that alter peripheral resistance therefore change blood pressure. **Viscosity** is defined as the ease with which

FOCUS ON PATHOLOGY

The legs are the most common locations in which blood clots form in the veins. The most common causes of blood clots or *thrombosis* include cancer, inherited tendency for blood clotting, pregnancy, contraceptive use, and prolonged immobility. Blood clots may develop in veins that are just under the skin or deep within a limb. When superficial, a blood clot commonly appears as a red streak along the vein and is often inflamed. Deep vein thrombosis causes symptoms in only half of all affected patients. When symptoms are present, they may include leg swelling, pressure, and/or fullness. The clot itself can cause inflammation, warmth, redness, and tenderness.

a fluid's molecules flow past one another. The higher the viscosity, the greater the resistance to flowing. Blood viscosity is increased by blood cells and plasma proteins. The greater the resistance, the more force needed to move the blood. Blood pressure rises as blood viscosity increases, and vice versa. Conditions such as excessive numbers of red blood cells, which is known as *polycythemia*, can cause both blood viscosity and resistance to increase. Some anemias, which cause low red blood cell counts, reduce viscosity and peripheral resistance.

Total blood vessel length and resistance are interrelated. There is more resistance over a longer vessel length in comparison with a shorter vessel length. As an infant grows into a child and then an adult, blood vessels lengthen. Therefore, the individual's blood pressure and peripheral resistance increase with growth. In healthy people blood viscosity and vessel length are basically constant because they are relatively unchanging once adulthood is reached. Blood vessel diameter changes often, however, and this does change peripheral resistance.

Relationship Between Flow, Pressure, and Resistance

Blood pressure is calculated by multiplying cardiac output by peripheral resistance. Normal arterial pressure is maintained by regulating these two factors. Ideally, the volume of blood discharged from the heart should be equal to the volume entering the atria and ventricles. Fiber length and force of contraction are interrelated, because of the stretching of the cardiac muscle cell just before contraction. Known as the *Frank-Starling law of the heart*, it is important during exercise when greater amounts of blood return to the heart from the veins.

Peripheral resistance also controls blood pressure. Changes in the diameters of arterioles regulate peripheral resistance. The **vasomotor center** of the medulla oblongata controls peripheral resistance. When arterial blood pressure increases suddenly, baroreceptors in the aorta and carotid arteries alert the vasomotor center, which vasodilates the vessels to decrease peripheral resistance. Carbon dioxide, oxygen, and hydrogen ions also influence peripheral resistance by affecting precapillary sphincters and smooth arteriole wall muscle.

Blood Pressure

Blood pressure is the pressure exerted by the blood's circulating volume on the walls of the arteries, veins, and heart chambers. It is regulated by the body's homeostatic mechanisms, involving blood volume, the lumens of arteries and arterioles, and the force of cardiac contraction. The *systemic blood pressure* is at its highest level in the aorta, declining along the blood pathways, until it is at 0 mm Hg in the right atrium. The largest drop in blood pressure occurs in the

arterioles, which have the most resistance to blood flow. The pressure gradient continues, even though it is small, allowing blood to flow all the way back to the heart.

Arterial Blood Pressure

Arterial blood pressure rises and falls according to cardiac cycle phases. The maximum pressure during ventricular contraction is called the **systolic pressure**, averaging 120 mm Hg in a healthy adult. **FIGURE 17-7** shows changes in blood pressure as distance from the left ventricle increases. The lowest pressure that remains in the arteries before the next ventricular contraction is called the **diastolic pressure**, which averages between 70 and 80 mm Hg in a healthy adult. Therefore, *systole* refers to periods of contraction, whereas *diastole* refers to periods of relaxation. The cardiac cycle includes atrial systole and diastole, followed by ventricular systole and diastole. An electrocardiogram illustrates all these mechanical events. The cardiac cycle is signified by continual pressure and blood volume changes within the heart.

In diastole the aortic valve closes. Blood cannot flow back into the heart. There is a recoiling of the walls of the aorta and other elastic arteries. There is enough pressure maintained so the blood can flow into the smaller vessels. Aortic pressure drops to its lowest level at this time, which is described as the diastolic pressure. The difference between the systolic and diastolic pressures is known as **pulse pressure**. During systole, it is felt in an artery as a throbbing pulsation. This is due to ventricular contraction, which forces blood into the elastic arteries, expanding them. Pulse pressure is temporarily raised by increased stroke volume and quicker blood ejection because of increased contractility from the heart.

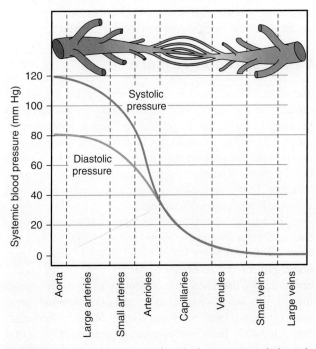

FIGURE 17-7 Blood pressure in the circulatory system. (Adapted from Shier, D.N., Butler, J.L., and Lewis, R. Hole's Essentials of Human Anatomy & Physiology, Tenth Edition. McGraw Hill Higher Education, 2009.)

Pulse pressure is chronically increased by atherosclerosis. This is because of the loss of elasticity in the elastic arteries.

Arterial blood pressure is measured with a device called a *sphygmomanometer* or blood pressure cuff. Its results are reported as a fraction of the systolic pressure over the diastolic pressure. The upper or *first* number indicates the arterial systolic pressure in mm Hg, and the lower or *second* number indicates the arterial diastolic pressure, also in mm Hg. A millimeter of mercury is a unit of pressure equal to 0.001316 of normal atmospheric pressure. This means a blood pressure of 120/80 displaces 120 mm of Hg on a sphygmomanometer, showing the systolic pressure, and also displaces 80 mm of Hg on the same device, showing diastolic pressure. *Mean arterial pressure* is used to report a single blood pressure value. To calculate it, the diastolic pressure is added to one-third of the pulse pressure.

The artery walls are distended as blood surges into them from the ventricles, but they recoil almost immediately. This expansion and recoiling can be felt as a pulse in an artery near the surface of the skin. Most commonly, the radial artery is used to take a person's pulse, although the carotid, brachial, and femoral arteries also can be used. Arterial blood pressure depends on heart rate, stroke volume, blood volume, peripheral resistance, and blood viscosity. The recoiling of arteries to their original dimensions is known as *elastic rebound*.

Capillary Blood Pressure

In the capillaries blood pressure drops off to only approximately 35 mm Hg, with the ends of capillary beds having only 17 mm Hg of pressure. This is important because the capillaries are fragile and easily ruptured. They are also extremely permeable, and low capillary pressures can cause filtrate to be forced out of the bloodstream into the interstitial space.

Venous Blood Pressure

The venous blood pressure is steady and regular. It does not pulsate with the ventricular contractions like the arterial blood pressure. In the veins, the pressure gradient is only approximately 15 mm Hg. Consider that from the aorta to the ends of the arterioles, the pressure is approximately 60 mm Hg. Venous blood pressure is usually too low to cause venous return to be adequate. Therefore, the *muscular pump*, *respiratory pump*, and *sympathetic venoconstriction* are used.

The *muscular pump* uses skeletal muscle activity to contract and relax around the veins, moving blood toward the heart. Each vein valve keeps blood that has passed from flowing backward. As pressure changes in the body's ventral cavity during breathing, the *respiratory pump* moves blood toward the heart. Inhalation increases abdominal pressure, squeezing local veins and forcing blood to the heart. Simultaneously, the chest pressure decreases. The internal and external thoracic veins then expand and increase blood entry into the right atrium. The volume of blood in the veins is then reduced by *sympathetic venoconstriction*. Sympathetic control causes the smooth muscle layer around the veins to constrict, reducing venous volume. Blood is therefore pushed toward the heart. Together, the muscular pump, respiratory pump, and sympathetic venoconstriction increase venous return and stroke volume.

Total Peripheral Resistance

The difference in pressure over the entire systemic circuit is sometimes called *circulatory pressure*. This is approximately 100 mm Hg. *Total peripheral resistance* is defined as the resistance of the entire cardiovascular system. For circulation to occur, the circulatory pressure must overcome the total peripheral resistance. The relatively high pressure of the arterioles is mostly reflected by the large pressure gradient of the arterial network, which is about 65 mm Hg. Total peripheral resistance combines vascular resistance, blood viscosity, and turbulence. *Vascular resistance* is defined as forces that oppose blood flow in the blood vessels. It is the most important component of total peripheral resistance and involves vessel length and diameter. *Viscosity*, or the resistance to blood flow caused by interactions among molecules and suspended materials, is the second component. *Turbulence* is defined as changes that increase resistance and slow blood flow, including irregular surfaces, high flow rates, and sudden changes in the diameters of blood vessels.

Net Filtration Pressure

The *net filtration pressure* is the difference between the net osmotic pressure and the net hydrostatic pressure. At arterial ends of capillaries, this is usually 10 mm Hg. This positive value shows that fluid usually moves out of capillaries, into the interstitial fluid. This means that filtration is occurring. However, at the venous ends of capillaries, the net filtration pressure is usually –7 mm Hg. This negative value shows that fluid usually moves into the capillaries, meaning that reabsorption is occurring. Whenever net filtration pressure is zero, hydrostatic and osmotic forces are equal. Therefore, the transition between filtration and reabsorption occurs where capillary hydrostatic pressure is 25 mm Hg.

Tissue Perfusion

Blood flow through tissues is also known as *tissue perfusion*. This occurs by homeostatic regulation of cardiovascular activities so that needs for oxygen and nutrients are met. The factors affecting tissue perfusion are cardiac output, peripheral resistance, and blood pressure. Cardiovascular regulation ensures that blood flow changes occur at appropriate times in areas of the body that require it without significantly changing blood pressure and flow to the vital organs.

The three mechanisms that are involved include autoregulation, neural mechanisms, and endocrine mechanisms. *Autoregulation* involves local factors that alter blood flow inside capillary beds, with precapillary sphincters opening and closing because of chemical changes in interstitial fluids. *Neural mechanisms* occur in response to arterial pressure changes or blood gas level changes in certain areas. *Endocrine mechanisms* involve hormones that enhance short-term changes and that also balance long-term changes in cardiovascular activities.

Dilation of precapillary sphincters are promoted by *vasodilators*. At the tissue level, *local vasodilators* help to speed up blood flow through their tissues of origin. Local vasodilators include acids from tissue cells, such as lactic acid; increased carbon dioxide or decreased tissue oxygen levels; increased concentrations of hydrogen or potassium ions in interstitial fluid; endothelial cells releasing nitric oxide; elevations in local temperature; and release of chemicals, such as nitric oxide or histamine during local inflammation. Also, *local vasoconstrictors*, such as thromboxanes, prostaglandins, and endothelins, stimulate precapillary sphincters to constrict. Together, local vasodilators and vasoconstrictors balance blood flow in single capillary beds. Higher concentrations of these factors affect arterioles as well.

Blood Volume

Blood volume is defined as the sum of formed elements and plasma volumes in the vascular system. Blood volume varies with age, body size, and gender. Most adults have approximately 5 liters of blood, which makes up 8% of the body's weight in kilograms. This is only slightly more than 1 gallon of blood. Blood pressure and volume are usually directly proportional. Any changes in volume can initially alter pressure. When measures are taken to restore normal blood volume, normal blood pressure can be reestablished. Fluid balance fluctuations may also affect blood volume. The entire blood supply pumps through each side of the heart about once per minute.

TEST YOUR UNDERSTANDING

1. Explain blood pressure and how it is calculated.
2. Contrast systolic and diastolic blood pressure.
3. Describe the differences between arterial and venous blood pressure.

Neural Controls of Blood Vessels

Most neural controls of blood vessels operate because of reflex arcs, which involve baroreceptors and related afferent fibers. The reflexes are controlled by the cardiovascular center of the medulla in the brain. Their output travels thorough autonomic fibers to the heart and vascular smooth muscle. The neural control mechanism is sometimes influenced by input from chemoreceptors and higher brain centers.

Sympathetic efferents known as *vasomotor fibers* are used to transmit highly steady impulses from the *vasomotor center*, which controls blood vessel diameter. Vasomotor fibers emerge from the T1 through the L2 levels of the spinal cord and innervate the smooth muscle of primarily arterioles but also of other blood vessels. This means the arterioles are nearly always slightly contracted. This is known as **vasomotor tone**, which is different between various body organs. For example, vasomotor impulses are more frequent in the skin and digestive viscera arterioles but less frequent in the skeletal muscles. As a result, they have more constriction than in the skeletal muscles. Generalized vasoconstriction and increased blood pressure results from any increase in sympathetic activity. Vascular muscle can relax slightly because of decreased sympathetic activity. This allows blood pressure to reduce to basal levels. There are three ways that cardiovascular center activity is modified:

- From baroreceptors, which respond to arterial pressure changes and stretching
- From chemoreceptors, which respond to changes in carbon dioxide, hydrogen, and oxygen levels in the blood
- From the higher brain centers

Baroreceptor Reflexes

Baroreceptors are activated by increased arterial blood pressure and are located in the **carotid sinuses**, which provide the brain's major blood supply; in the **aortic arch**; and in the walls of most large neck and thoracic arteries. Stretching causes the baroreceptors to send impulses quickly to the cardiovascular center. This inhibits the cardioacceleratory and vasomotor centers while stimulating the cardioinhibitor center. Blood pressure decreases as a result of these actions. Baroreceptors are also found in the *aortic sinuses* of the *ascending aorta* of the heart and wall of the right atrium. *Atrial baroreceptors* monitor blood pressure at the venae cavae and right atrium, which constitute the end of the systemic circuit. The *atrial reflex* responds to stretching of the wall of the right atrium.

The circulation is buffered from acute changes in blood pressure by the quick responses of the baroreceptors. Primarily in the head, blood pressure falls as we stand up after lying down. The blood supply to the brain is protected by the baroreceptors and their actions in the *carotid sinus reflex*. The baroreceptors that are activated in the *aortic reflex* help balance blood pressure in the overall systemic circuit. Sustained pressure changes, such as chronic hypertension, usually override the effects of baroreceptors. The baroreceptors become adapted to monitor pressure changes at the new, higher "set point."

Chemoreceptor Reflexes

Chemoreceptors in the *aortic arch* and large neck arteries send impulses to the cardioacceleratory center, increasing cardiac output. They also send impulses to the vasomotor center, causing reflex vasoconstriction. Chemoreceptors act with *chemoreceptor reflexes* when carbon dioxide levels rise, pH falls, or blood oxygen levels drop quickly. The resultant blood pressure increase causes blood to return to the heart and lungs more quickly. The *carotid* and *aortic* bodies close to the baroreceptors of the carotid sinuses and aortic arch are the most important chemoreceptors. They play a greater role in regulating respiratory rate, however, than blood pressure.

High Brain Center Influences

The brain stem's medulla oblongata integrates reflexes that maintain blood pressure. The cerebral cortex and hypothalamus have the ability to change arterial pressure by using relays to the centers of the medulla oblongata. The fight-or-flight response is an example. It is controlled by the hypothalamus, with large effects on blood pressure. Redistribution of blood flow and other cardiovascular responses is also regulated by the hypothalamus. Examples of this redistribution include during body temperature changes and exercise.

Hormonal Controls

Hormonal controls help to control blood pressure in short-term peripheral resistance changes as well as long-term blood volume changes. Local chemicals known as *paracrines* help to bring adequate blood flow to serve certain tissues' metabolic needs. Rarely, large releases of paracrines can affect blood pressure. Short-term hormonal controls involve antidiuretic hormone (ADH), angiotensin II, atrial natriuretic peptide (ANP), and the hormones of the adrenal medulla.

- *ADH:* Also called **vasopressin**, ADH is produced by the hypothalamus. It stimulates the kidneys to conserve water. Although not usually important for regulation of blood pressure on a short-term basis, if blood pressure falls to extremely low levels, its release is greatly increased. Severe hemorrhage is an example of a situation that triggers this release. ADH then helps to restore arterial blood pressure via extensive vasoconstriction.
- *Angiotensin II:* This hormone is generated by the enzymatic actions of *renin*. The kidneys release renin when blood pressure or volume is low. **Angiotensin II** stimulates extensive vasoconstriction, causing a fast rise in systemic blood pressure. Its other effects include stimulation of the release of ADH and aldosterone. These hormones enhance blood volume for the long-term regulation of blood pressure.
- *ANP:* Produced by the atria of the heart, ANP helps to reduce blood pressure and volume. It acts by antagonizing aldosterone, causing the kidneys to excrete more water and sodium. This reduces blood volume and also results in generalized vasodilation.
- *Adrenal medulla hormones:* These include epinephrine and norepinephrine, which are released by the adrenal gland during times of stress. In the blood these hormones increase cardiac output and promote generalized vasoconstriction, enhancing the sympathetic response. Generally, sympathetic stimulation, which releases epinephrine, causes vasoconstriction and therefore increased blood pressure. However, the parasympathetic nervous system has the opposite effect and generally causes vasodilation and decreased blood pressure.

Renal Controls

Long-term control of blood pressure involves the kidneys. This alters blood volume instead of peripheral resistance and cardiac output. There are two mechanisms: direct and indirect.

Direct Renal Mechanism

The direct renal mechanism changes blood volume without using hormones. The rate of fluid filtering from the bloodstream to the kidney tubules becomes faster when either blood pressure or blood volume rises. When this occurs, more fluid leaves the body in urine because the kidneys cannot reabsorb the filtrate quickly enough. Therefore, both blood pressure and volume become lowered. When they are low, water is conserved. It is returned to the bloodstream, and blood pressure increases.

Indirect Renal Mechanism

The indirect renal mechanism uses the renin-angiotensin-aldosterone mechanism. *Renin* is an enzyme that is released by certain kidney cells into the blood when arterial blood pressure declines. It causes enzymatic claving of *angiotensinogen*, which is a plasma protein manufactured by the liver. Renin converts angiotensinogen to *angiotensin I*. Then, *angiotensin-converting enzyme* converts angiotensin I to *angiotensin II*. The activity of angiotensin-converting enzyme is linked with the capillary endothelium primarily in the lungs but also in other body tissues.

There are four ways in which angiotensin II stabilizes extracellular fluid volume and arterial blood pressure:

- Angiotensin II stimulates the adrenal cortex to secrete *aldosterone*. This hormone enhances renal absorption of sodium. Sodium moves into the bloodstream, followed by water, conserving blood volume. Angiotensin II also directly stimulates the kidneys' reabsorption of sodium.
- Angiotensin II causes the posterior pituitary to release ADH. This promotes additional water reabsorption by the kidneys.
- Angiotensin II increases the thirst sensation via activation of the hypothalamic thirst center. Water consumption therefore increases, restoring blood volume and blood pressure.
- Angiotensin II is a very potent vasoconstrictor. It increases peripheral resistance, which increases blood pressure.

Homeostatic Imbalances

Homeostatic imbalances in blood pressure involve hypertension and hypotension. **Hypertension** is chronically elevated blood pressure, defined as a sustained increase in either systolic pressure or diastolic pressure. In hypertension, systolic pressure is usually above 140 mm Hg and diastolic pressure is usually above 90 mm Hg. Chronic hypertension is common and dangerous because the heart must pump harder against greater resistance, causing the myocardium to enlarge. Nearly 90% of hypertensive patients have *primary* or *essential* *hypertension*, which has no identified, underlying cause. Primary hypertension may be linked to heredity, diet, obesity, age, diabetes mellitus, stress, and smoking. It can usually be controlled but cannot be cured. *Secondary hypertension* is from an identifiable condition such as kidney disease, renal artery obstruction, hyperthyroidism, or Cushing's syndrome.

Hypotension, defined as blood pressure below 90/ 60 mm Hg, is often linked simply to old age. It is usually only dangerous if it leads to dizziness or fainting and, when acute, is an important sign of circulatory shock. *Orthostatic hypotension* is a temporary blood pressure drop, which causes dizziness, when a person stands up suddenly after sitting or lying down. It is most common in the elderly. *Chronic hypotension* may be linked to a more serious disorder such as Addison's disease, hypothyroidism, or severe malnutrition.

FOCUS ON PATHOLOGY

Circulatory shock is defined as a condition in which blood does not circulate normally and the blood vessels are not sufficiently filled. Tissues do not receive adequate blood flow and the condition leads to cellular death and organ damage. The three major forms are hypovolemic, vascular, and cardiogenic shock. *Hypovolemic shock*, the most common form, is caused by extensive blood or fluid loss, often due to extensive burns, acute hemorrhage, severe vomiting, or severe diarrhea. Fluid volume must be replaced as quickly as possible. *Vascular shock* is caused by extreme vasodilation, often due to anaphylactic shock, failure of autonomic nervous system regulation, and septicemia. It may also be linked to extensive sunbathing. *Cardiogenic shock* occurs when the heart cannot pump enough blood to maintain adequate circulation. It is usually caused by damage to the myocardium, such as from multiple heart attacks.

TEST YOUR UNDERSTANDING

1. Describe baroreceptor reflexes that control blood pressure changes.
2. Explain the location of chemoreceptors and their roles.
3. Describe how ADH and aldosterone regulate blood pressure.

Blood Vessel Pathways and Divisions

The blood vessel pathways make up the vascular system, which is divided into the systemic and pulmonary circulation systems. Each of these two systems has its own unique arteries, capillaries, and veins. The systemic circulation is much larger than the pulmonary circulation (**FIGURE 17-8**) and receives blood from the heart via just one systemic artery: the aorta. This differs from the pulmonary circulation, in which the heart receives returning blood via two terminal veins: the superior and inferior venae cavae. The only exception is the blood coming from the myocardium that is collected by the cardiac veins. It reenters the right atrium through the coronary sinus. The three major differences between systemic blood vessels are as follows:

- *The arteries are deep, whereas the veins are either deep or superficial:* The deep veins run similarly to the course of the arteries. Names of both the systemic arteries and the systemic deep veins are similar. Because there are superficial systemic veins but no such arteries, their names do not correspond to those of any arteries.
- *Veins have more interconnections than arteries:* Therefore, many veins are made up by two vessels with similar names and are more difficult to follow than arteries.
- *Unique drainage systems exist in the brain and digestive system:* Blood draining from the brain goes into the large dural venous sinuses instead of typical veins. Blood draining from the digestive system enters the *hepatic portal system*, moving through the liver, and then reentering the general systemic circulation.

Aorta and Its Branches

The **aorta** is the body's largest artery and emerges from the left ventricle of the heart. Its walls are approximately 2 mm in thickness, and its internal diameter is 2.5 cm. Backflow of blood during diastole is prevented by the aortic valve, at the base of the aorta. An *aortic sinus* opposes each cusp of the aortic valve. Each aortic sinus contains baroreceptors required for reflex regulation of blood pressure. The aorta consists of four portions: the ascending aorta, aortic arch, descending aorta, and abdominal aorta.

- The first portion of the aorta is the *ascending aorta*. It runs posteriorly and to the right of the pulmonary trunk for a short length of only 5 cm before it curves to the left as the aortic arch. The *right and left coronary arteries* are the only branches of the ascending aorta. They supply the myocardium with blood.
- The *aortic arch* curves across the superior surface of the heart and is deep to the sternum. It begins at the sternal angle, at the T4 level. The aortic arch connects the ascending aorta with the descending aorta. Three arteries originate along the aortic arch that deliver blood to the head, neck, shoulders, and upper limbs:
  - The **brachiocephalic trunk**: Superior, under the right sternoclavicular joint, it branches after a short distance into the *right common carotid artery* and *right subclavian artery*. The brachiocephalic trunk

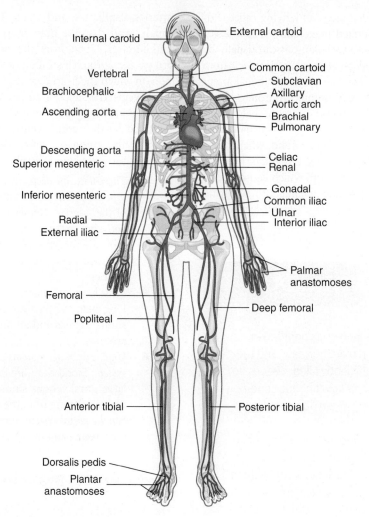

Internal carotid

External cartoid

Vertebral

Brachiocephalic

Ascending aorta

Common cartoid
Subclavian
Axillary
Aortic arch
Brachial
Pulmonary

Descending aorta
Superior mesenteric

Celiac
Renal

Inferior mesenteric

Gonadal
Common iliac
Ulnar
Interior iliac

Radial
External iliac

Palmar anastomoses

Femoral

Deep femoral

Popliteal

Anterior tibial

Posterior tibial

Dorsalis pedis
Plantar anastomoses

FIGURE 17-8 Overview of the arteries.

is also known as the *innominate artery*. There are three primary branches from each subclavian artery before it leaves the thoracic cavity: the *internal thoracic artery, vertebral artery,* and *thyrocervical trunk.*

- *The left common carotid artery*
- *The left subclavian artery*

■ The descending aorta is continuous with the aortic arch. It runs along the anterior spine. The diaphragm divides the descending aorta into a superior thoracic aorta, from T5 to T12, and an inferior abdominal aorta. The branches of the thoracic aorta are the bronchial, pericardial, esophageal, mediastinal, and intercostal arteries.

■ The abdominal aorta, beginning immediately inferior to the diaphragm, is a continuation of the thoracic aorta. It delivers blood to the abdominopelvic organs and structures, running to the L4 level. Its major branches to the visceral organs are not paired. The branches arise on the anterior surface of the abdominal aorta, extending into the

mesenteries. The *inferior phrenic arteries* supply the inferior diaphragm surface and inferior esophagus. The *adrenal arteries*, which originate on either side of the aorta, near the bottom of the superior mesenteric artery, supply the adrenal glands. The *renal arteries* arise just inferior to the superior mesenteric artery, traveling posterior to the peritoneal lining to reach the adrenal glands and kidneys. The *gonadal arteries* begin between the mesenteric arteries and are called the *testicular arteries* in males and the *ovarian arteries* in females. The small *lumbar arteries* arise on the aorta's posterior surface to supply the spinal cord, vertebrae, and abdominal wall. Unpaired branches in the abdomen include the *celiac trunk* and the superior and inferior mesenteric arteries. The celiac trunk supplies blood to the liver, stomach, and spleen. The superior mesenteric artery arises approximately 2.5 cm inferior to the celiac trunk and supplies the arteries of the pancreas, small intestine, and right and middle parts of the large intestine. The inferior mesenteric artery

TABLE 17-2

Major Branches of the Aorta

Branch	Area of Aorta	Main Regions or Organs Supplied
Right and left coronary arteries	Ascending aorta	Heart
Brachiocephalic artery	Arch of the aorta	Right upper limb and right side of head
Left common carotid artery		Left side of head
Left subclavian artery		Left upper limb
Descending aorta	Thoracic aorta	
Bronchial artery		Bronchi
Pericardial artery		Pericardium
Esophageal artery		Esophagus
Mediastinal artery		Mediastinum
Posterior intercostal artery		Thoracic wall
Descending aorta	Abdominal aorta	
Celiac artery		Upper digestive tract organs
Phrenic artery		Diaphragm
Superior mesenteric artery		Small and large intestines
Suprarenal artery		Adrenal gland
Renal artery		Kidney
Gonadal artery		Ovaries or testes
Inferior mesenteric artery		Lower large intestine
Lumbar artery		Abdominal wall (posterior)
Middle sacral artery		Sacrum and coccyx
Common iliac artery		Lower abdominal wall, pelvic organs, lower limbs

supplies blood to the terminal portions of the colon, which include the left large intestine, sigmoid colon, and rectum. The abdominal aorta divides into the right and left common iliac arteries.

TABLE 17-2 summarizes the major branches of the aorta.

Head and Neck Arteries

The head and neck are supplied by four paired arteries: the common carotid arteries plus three branches from each subclavian artery, the *vertebral arteries, thyrocervical trunks,* and *costocervical trunks.* The common carotid arteries have the largest blood distribution, with each being divided into two primary branches: the internal and external carotid arteries. A slight dilation of the internal carotid artery, known as the carotid sinus, is located at the division point. In the carotid sinus are baroreceptors that help to control blood pressure. Chemoreceptors involved in the control of respiration are nearby and are known as the **carotid bodies**. Pressure applied to the neck, near the carotid sinuses, can cause unconsciousness because this increases blood pressure, leading to vasodilation and impaired blood delivery to the brain.

Common Carotid Arteries The right common carotid artery arises from the brachiocephalic trunk, whereas the left common carotid artery is the second branch of the aortic

arch (**FIGURE 17-9**). Both arteries ascend through the lateral neck. In some elderly people the common carotid artery can be atherosclerotic, which is a major factor for stroke. Sometimes, physicians perform a *carotid angiogram* to confirm stenosis or occlusion of the carotid artery (**FIGURE 17-10**).

At the level of the Adam's apple, they divide into their primary branches: the external and internal carotid arteries. Most of the head, except for the brain and orbits, is supplied by the external carotid arteries. Each of these arteries runs superiorly. Its branches include

- *Superior thyroid artery:* supplying the thyroid gland and larynx
- *Lingual artery:* supplying the tongue
- *Facial artery:* supplying the skin and anterior face muscles
- *Occipital artery:* supplying the posterior scalp

Each of the *external carotid arteries* ends when they split into a superficial temporal artery and a maxillary artery. The *superficial temporal artery* supplies most of the scalp as well as the parotid salivary gland. The *maxillary artery* supplies both jaws, teeth, nasal cavity, and muscles used for chewing. The middle meningeal artery is a branch of the maxillary artery that enters the skull through the foramen spinosum. It supplies the inner parietal bone surface, squamous section of the temporal bone, and the dura mater underneath.

The orbits and more than 80% of the cerebrum are supplied by the larger *internal carotid arteries.* They run

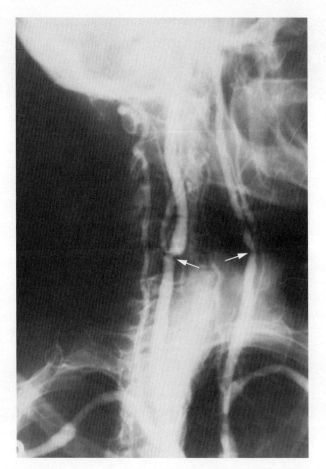

FIGURE 17-9 Carotid artery angiogram.

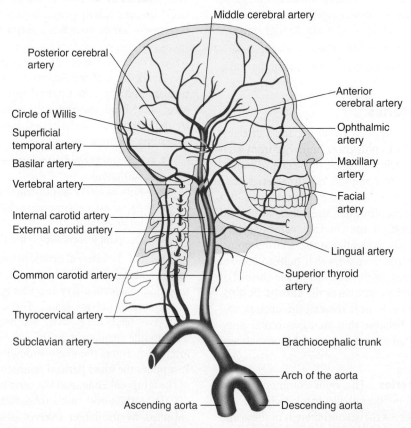

Middle cerebral artery

Posterior cerebral artery

Anterior cerebral artery

Circle of Willis

Ophthalmic artery

Superficial temporal artery

Basilar artery

Maxillary artery

Vertebral artery

Facial artery

Internal carotid artery

External carotid artery

Lingual artery

Common carotid artery

Superior thyroid artery

Thyrocervical artery

Subclavian artery

Brachiocephalic trunk

Arch of the aorta

Ascending aorta

Descending aorta

FIGURE 17-10 Common carotid artery.

TABLE 17-3

Major Branches of the Carotid Arteries

Branch	Carotid Artery	Main Regions or Organs Supplied
Superior thyroid artery	External	Larynx and thyroid gland
Lingual artery		Salivary glands and tongue
Facial artery		Chin, lips, nose, palate, and pharynx
Occipital artery		Meninges, neck muscles, and posterior scalp
Posterior auricular artery		Ear and lateral scalp
Maxillary artery		Cheeks, eyelids, jaw, and teeth
Superficial temporal artery		Parotid salivary gland and surface of face and scalp
Ophthalmic artery	Internal	Eyes and eye muscles
Anterior choroid artery		Brain and choroid plexus
Anterior cerebral artery		Frontal and parietal lobes of brain

deeply, entering the skull through the temporal bones' carotid canals. In the cranium, each of them branches into a primary *ophthalmic artery* and then into the *anterior* and *middle cerebral arteries*. The eyes, forehead, nose, and orbits are supplied by the *ophthalmic arteries*. The medial surface of the frontal and parietal lobes of the cerebral hemisphere are supplied by each *anterior cerebral artery*. This also anastomoses with its paired opposing artery via a short *anterior communicating artery*. The *middle cerebral arteries* supply the lateral sections of the frontal, parietal, and temporal lobes. These arteries run in the lateral sulci of each cerebral hemisphere. **TABLE 17-3** summarizes the major branches of the carotid arteries.

Vertebral Arteries   At the root of the neck, the *vertebral arteries* emerge from the subclavian arteries, continuing through the foramina in the transverse processes of the cervical vertebrae. They enter the skull via the foramen magnum, branching to the vertebrae, cervical spinal cord, and various deep neck structures. In the cranium, the *basilar artery* is formed by the joining of the left and right vertebral arteries. The basilar artery ascends along the brain stem's anterior aspect and branches to the cerebellum, pons, and inner ear. It also divides, at the pons–midbrain border, into two *posterior cerebral arteries*. These arteries supply the inferior sections of the temporal lobes and the occipital lobes.

The posterior cerebral arteries are connected by the *posterior communicating arteries* to the middle cerebral arteries, anteriorly. There are two posterior and single anterior communicating arteries that continue the arterial anastomosis known as the **cerebral arterial circle**, which is also called the *circle of Willis*. The circle of Willis encircles the optic chiasma and pituitary gland. It joins the anterior and posterior blood supplies of the brain and balances blood pressure in these areas. It also provides alternative routes for blood to be able to reach the brain should occlusion of a vertebral or carotid artery occur.

Thyrocervical and Costocervical Trunks   The *thyrocervical trunk* and *costocervical trunk* are short vessels emerging from the subclavian artery, lateral to the vertebral arteries on both sides. The thyrocervical trunk primarily supplies the thyroid gland, parts of the cervical vertebrae and spinal cord, and certain scapular muscles. The costocervical trunk supplies muscles of the deep neck and the superior intercostal muscles.

Upper Limb and Thoracic Arteries

The subclavian arteries branch to supply all portions of the upper limbs (**FIGURE 17-11**). First, they branch off to the neck but then run laterally to enter the axilla by moving between the clavicle and first rib on each side. At this point they are renamed the *axillary arteries*. The wall of the thorax is supplied by vessels from either the thoracic aorta or from subclavian artery branches. Small branches of the thoracic aorta supply most of the blood to the visceral thoracic organs.

Axillary Artery   Each axillary artery branches to the axilla, chest wall, and shoulder girdle. These axillary branches include the *thoracoacromial, lateral thoracic, subscapular artery,* and the *anterior and posterior circumflex humeral arteries*. The thoracoacromial artery supplies the pectoral region and deltoid muscle. The lateral *thoracic artery* supplies the breast and lateral chest wall. The subscapular artery supplies the dorsal thorax wall, the scapula, and a portion of the latissimus dorsi muscle. The anterior and posterior circumflex humeral arteries help to supply the deltoid muscle and shoulder joint. The axillary artery becomes the brachial artery as it emerges from the axilla.

Brachial Artery   The *brachial artery* supplies the anterior flexor arm muscles. A major branch is the *deep artery of the arm*, which serves the posterior triceps brachii muscle. Near the elbow, the brachial artery branches to contribute to an anastomosis that serves the elbow joint and connect it to the forearm arteries. Crossing the anterior midline aspect of the elbow, it provides the brachial pulse, which is easily palpated. Just beyond the elbow, it branches to form the radial and ulnar arteries.

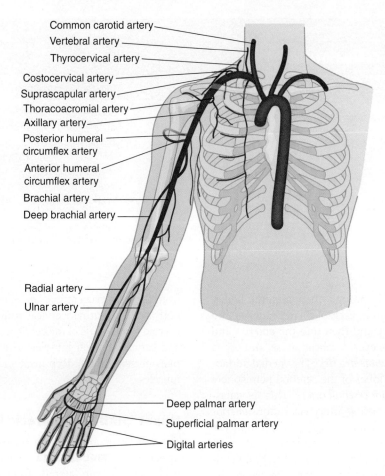

Common carotid artery
Vertebral artery
Thyrocervical artery
Costocervical artery
Suprascapular artery
Thoracoacromial artery
Axillary artery
Posterior humeral circumflex artery
Anterior humeral circumflex artery
Brachial artery
Deep brachial artery

Radial artery
Ulnar artery

Deep palmar artery
Superficial palmar artery
Digital arteries

FIGURE 17-11 Upper limb and thoracic arteries.

Radial Artery   The *radial artery* proceeds from the cubital fossa's median line, reaching the styloid process of the radius. It supplies the lateral forearm, wrist, thumb, and index finger muscles. At the thumb's root it provides the radial pulse.

Ulnar Artery   The *ulnar artery* the medial aspects of the forearm and index finger as well as the third, fourth, and fifth fingers. It gives off a short proximal branch known as the *common interosseous artery*, running between the radius and ulna, serving the forearm's deep flexors and extensors. At the wrist both the ulnar and radial arteries fuse, forming the *superficial* and *deep palmar arches*.

Palmar Arches   The superficial and deep *palmar arches* are formed by branches of the radial and ulnar arteries that anastomose in the palm. Blood supply to the fingers arises from the palmar arches, becoming the *metacarpal arteries* and *digital arteries*.

Internal Thoracic Arteries   The thoracic wall is supplied by the *internal thoracic arteries* as well as the *posterior intercostal arteries* and *superior phrenic arteries*. Formerly known as the *internal mammary arteries*, the internal thoracic arteries emerge from the subclavian arteries. They supply blood to most of the thoracic wall. Each descends lateral to the sternum, branching to form the *anterior intercostal arteries* and supplying the intercostal spaces anteriorly. Superficial branches are also sent to the skin, mammary glands, anterior abdominal wall, and diaphragm.

Posterior Intercostal Arteries   The costocervical trunk branches to form the posterior two pairs of *posterior intercostal arteries*. Nine additional pairs arise from the thoracic aorta, anastomosing anteriorly with the anterior intercostal arteries. A pair of *subcostal arteries* arises from the thoracic aorta, inferior to the 12th rib. The posterior intercostal arteries supply the deep muscles of the back, the posterior intercostal spaces, the vertebrae, and the spinal cord. The intercostal muscles are supplied by both the posterior and anterior intercostal arteries.

Superior Phrenic Arteries   The posterior superior diaphragm surface is served by either one or more paired *superior phrenic arteries*.

Thoracic Viscera Arteries   The arteries of the thoracic viscera include the pericardial, bronchial, esophageal, and mediastinal arteries. The tiny *pericardial arteries* supply the posterior pericardium. The two left and one right *bronchial*

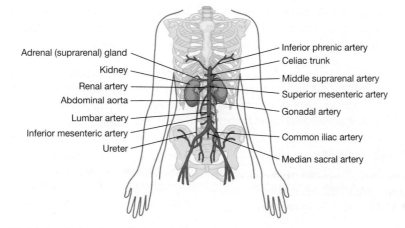

Adrenal (suprarenal) gland
Kidney
Renal artery
Abdominal aorta
Lumbar artery
Inferior mesenteric artery
Ureter

Inferior phrenic artery
Celiac trunk
Middle suprarenal artery
Superior mesenteric artery
Gonadal artery
Common iliac artery
Median sacral artery

FIGURE 17-12 Branches of the abdominal aorta.

arteries supply oxygenated blood to the bronchi, lungs, and pleurae. Four or five *esophageal arteries* supply the esophagus. The posterior mediastinum is served by the many small *mediastinal arteries*.

Abdominal Arteries

The *abdominal aorta* branches to form the abdominal arteries. Nearly half of all arterial flow moves through these vessels during rest. All of them are paired vessels except for the celiac trunk, median sacral artery, and the superior and inferior mesenteric arteries (**FIGURE 17-12**). The abdominal arteries supply the abdominal wall, diaphragm, and visceral organs inside the abdominopelvic cavity and include the *inferior phrenic arteries, celiac trunk, superior mesenteric artery, suprarenal arteries, renal arteries, gonadal arteries, inferior mesenteric artery, lumbar arteries, median sacral artery,* and *common iliac arteries*.

Inferior Phrenic Arteries   The *inferior phrenic arteries* serve the inferior diaphragm surface, emerging from the aorta just inferior to the diaphragm at the T12 level.

Celiac Trunk   The *celiac trunk* consists of large, unpaired arteries from the abdominal aorta. This divides soon after emerging into the *common hepatic, splenic,* and *left gastric* arteries. The common hepatic artery branches to the stomach, pancreas, and duodenum. At the point where the *gastroduodenal artery* branches, the common hepatic artery becomes the *hepatic artery proper*. This splits into the left and right branches serving the liver. The *splenic artery* branches to the pancreas and stomach as it passes deep to the stomach, terminating at the spleen. Part of the stomach and the inferior esophagus are supplied by the *left gastric artery*. The *right gastroepiploic artery* branches from the gastroduodenal artery, whereas the *left gastroepiploic artery* branches from the splenic artery. Both serve the stomach's greater curvature. The *right gastric artery* supplies the stomach's lesser curvature. It may emerge from either the hepatic artery proper or the common hepatic artery.

Superior Mesenteric Artery   The *superior mesenteric artery* is large and unpaired, emerging from the abdominal aorta just below the celiac trunk and the L1 level. Running deep to the pancreas, it enters the mesentery, featuring many anastomosing branches serving almost all the small intestine, through the *intestinal arteries*. It also serves the appendix, cecum, and ascending colon via the *ileocolic* and *right colic arteries*. Additionally, the superior mesenteric artery services part of the transverse colon via the *middle colic artery*.

Suprarenal Arteries   Emerging from the abdominal aorta, the *middle suprarenal arteries* flank the origin of the superior mesenteric artery. The adrenal or suprarenal glands above the kidneys are supplied with blood from these arteries. Two sets of branches, the *superior suprarenal branches*, from the inferior phrenic arteries, and the *inferior suprarenal branches*, from the renal arteries, also supply the adrenal glands.

Renal Arteries   The right and left *renal arteries* are short in length but wide. They emerge from the lateral aortic surfaces just below the superior mesenteric artery between the L1 and L2 levels. Each renal artery serves the kidney on its side.

Gonadal Arteries   The two *gonadal arteries* have different names in either gender. In women they are known as the *ovarian arteries*, whereas in men they are known as the *testicular arteries*. The ovarian arteries serve part of the uterine tubes and the ovaries. They are much shorter than the testicular arteries, which descend to enter the scrotum and serve the testes.

Inferior Mesenteric Artery   The final major branch of the abdominal aorta is the single *inferior mesenteric artery*. It emerges from the anterior aorta at the L3 level. It supplies the distal large intestine, from the mid transverse colon to the mid rectum. The inferior mesenteric artery accomplishes this through its *left colic, sigmoidal,* and *superior rectal branches*. There are looped anastomoses between the superior and inferior mesenteric arteries, which help to move blood to the digestive viscera when there is trauma to one of these arteries.

Lumbar Arteries   Four pairs of *lumbar arteries* arise from the posterolateral aortic surface in the lumbar area. They supply the posterior wall of the abdomen.

Median Sacral Artery The single *median sacral artery* emerges from the posterior abdominal aorta's surface at its terminus. This artery is very small and delivers blood to the sacrum and coccyx.

Common Iliac Arteries The aorta splits into the right and left *common iliac arteries* at the L4 level. They deliver blood to the pelvic organs, lower abdominal wall, and lower limbs.

Pelvic and Lower Limb Arteries

The *common iliac arteries* are divided into two major branches at the level of the sacroiliac joints: the internal and external iliac arteries (**FIGURE 17-13**). Blood is distributed by the internal iliac arteries primarily to the pelvic region. The external iliac arteries mostly supply the lower limbs but also branch to the abdominal wall.

Internal Iliac Arteries The two *internal iliac arteries* carry blood to the pelvic walls, bladder, rectum, and specific organs in either gender. In females these organs are the uterus and vagina, whereas in males they are the prostate and ductus deferens. The internal iliac arteries also use the *superior and inferior gluteal arteries* to serve the gluteal muscles, the *obturator artery* to serve the adductor muscles of the medial thigh, and the *internal pudendal artery* to serve the external genitalia and perineum.

External Iliac Arteries The *external iliac arteries* supply the lower limbs, branching also to the anterior abdominal wall. They pass under the inguinal ligaments, enter the thigh, and eventually become the femoral arteries.

Femoral Arteries Each *femoral artery* passes down the anteromedial thigh to branch to the thigh muscles. Of the deep branches, the largest is called the *deep artery of the thigh* or *deep femoral artery*. It is the primary supplier of blood to the hamstrings, adductors, and quadriceps of the thigh. Proximal branches from the deep femoral artery are known as the *lateral and medial circumflex femoral arteries*. They encircle the neck of the femur, with the medial circumflex artery being the primary vessel to the head of the femur. When torn, the bone tissue in the head of the femur dies. From the lateral circumflex artery, a long descending branch supplies the vastus lateralis muscle. The femoral artery passes, near the knee, posteriorly through a gap in the adductor magnus muscle called the *adductor hiatus*. The femoral artery then enters the popliteal fossa, where it is then known as the popliteal artery.

Popliteal Artery The *popliteal artery* is on the posterior side of the leg, contributing blood to an arterial anastomosis to supply the knee area. It then splits into the anterior and posterior tibial arteries.

Anterior Tibial Artery The *anterior tibial artery* courses through the anterior leg compartment, supplying the extensor muscles. It becomes the *dorsalis pedis artery* at the ankle, supplying the ankle and the dorsum of the foot. Another branch, the *arcuate artery*, links the *dorsal metatarsal arteries* to the metatarsus of the foot. The dorsalis pedis' superficial portion ends as it penetrates the sole, forming the medial *plantar arch*. This artery provides the *pedal pulse*, which can be felt to assess blood supply to the leg.

Posterior Tibial Artery The large *posterior tibial artery* moves through the posteromedial leg to supply the flexor muscles. It gives off a large branch proximally, known as the *fibular* or *peroneal artery*. This artery supplies the lateral fibularis muscles. At the medial side of the foot, the artery divides into *lateral and medial plantar arteries*. These serve the plantar foot surface. The lateral end of the plantar arch is formed by the lateral plantar artery. From the plantar arch arise the *plantar metatarsal arteries* and *digital arteries* to the toes.

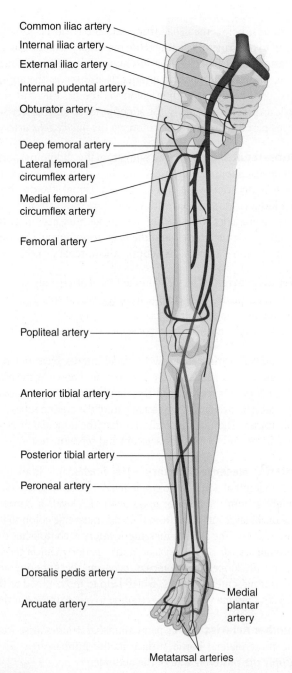

Common iliac artery
Internal iliac artery
External iliac artery
Internal pudental artery
Obturator artery
Deep femoral artery
Lateral femoral circumflex artery
Medial femoral circumflex artery
Femoral artery
Popliteal artery
Anterior tibial artery
Posterior tibial artery
Peroneal artery
Dorsalis pedis artery
Arcuate artery
Medial plantar artery
Metatarsal arteries

FIGURE 17-13 Pelvic and lower limb arteries.

1. Name the largest diameter artery in the body, and describe its location.
2. Which arteries supply the larynx, tongue, meninges, and teeth with blood?
3. What is the circle of Willis?
4. Why would compression of the common carotid arteries cause a person to lose consciousness?

FOCUS ON PATHOLOGY

Arteriosclerosis describes several blood circulation disorders involving the cardiovascular system. It is commonly known as "hardening of the arteries." It occurs over many years as vessels become hard, brittle, thickened and lose elasticity. Arteriosclerosis occurs because of calcium deposition in artery walls and generally leads to increased blood pressure or *hypertension*. It can also cause nodules in the arterial walls, ultimately blocking arteries completely. Arteriosclerosis is commonly linked to diabetes, obesity, and smoking.

Veins and Their Branches

Three major veins return blood from the body to the right atrium: the **coronary sinus**, **superior vena cava**, and **inferior vena cava**. The coronary sinus returns deoxygenated blood from the walls of the heart. The superior vena cava returns blood from the head, neck, thorax, and upper limbs. The inferior vena cava returns blood from the abdomen, pelvis, and lower limbs (**FIGURE 17-14**).

The three major types of veins are the superficial veins, deep veins, and sinuses. Most superficial veins are larger than the deep veins, but in the head and trunk the opposite is true. Venous sinuses are mostly found in the cranial cavity and the heart. The cardiac veins transport blood from the wall of the heart, returning it via the coronary sinus to the right atrium.

Large veins have all three tunica layers. They include the superior and inferior venae cavae and their tributaries inside the thoracic and abdominopelvic cavities. A thick tunica externa, made of elastic and collagen fibers, surrounds a thin tunica media. The *medium-sized veins* are similar in size to the muscular arteries, ranging in internal diameter between 2 and 9 mm. Their thickest layer is the tunica externa, with the tunica media being thin and having few smooth muscle cells in relation to other veins.

Head and Neck Veins

From the head and neck, three pairs of veins collect most of the draining blood: the **external jugular veins**, *internal jugular veins*, and *vertebral veins* (**FIGURE 17-15**). The more superficial external jugular veins drain blood mostly from the posterior head and neck, emptying into the subclavian veins. The larger, deeper internal jugular veins drain blood from the cranial cavity and the anterior head, neck, and face. The vertebral veins empty into the **brachiocephalic vein**. Most extracranial veins have the same names as their related extracranial arteries. However, their locations and connections are different.

The *dural venous sinuses* are interconnected, enlarged chambers between the layers of the dura mater. It is here that most veins of the brain drain blood. In the falx cerebri, which is located down between the cerebral hemispheres, are found the *superior and inferior sagittal sinuses*. Most *inferior cerebral veins* converge to form the *great cerebral vein*. Posteriorly, the inferior sagittal sinus drains into the *straight sinus*. Then, the superior sagittal and straight sinuses drain into the *transverse sinuses*. These sinuses are located inside shallow grooves on the occipital bone's internal surface. They drain into the *sigmoid sinuses*, which are S-shaped. The sinuses then become the *internal jugular veins* when they leave the skull via the jugular foramen. The *cavernous sinuses* receive blood from the *ophthalmic veins* of the orbits and facial veins. These sinuses flank the sphenoid body and drain the nose and upper lip region. On the way to the face and orbits, the internal carotid artery; cranial nerves III, IV, and VI; and part of cranial nerve V run through the cavernous sinus.

External Jugular Veins Superficial scalp and face structures supplied by the external carotid arteries are drained by the left and right *external jugular veins*. They anastomose often, and an amount of superficial drainage from them also enters into the internal jugular veins. The external jugular veins descend through the lateral neck, passing obliquely over the sternocleidomastoid muscles. They finally empty into the subclavian veins. The superficial head and neck veins converge to form the *temporal, facial,* and *maxillary veins*. The temporal and maxillary veins drain into the *external jugular vein*.

Vertebral Veins The *vertebral veins* are not similar to the vertebral arteries in that they do not serve most areas of the brain. They drain the spinal cord, cervical vertebrae, and some of the neck's small muscles. They are located inferiorly through the cervical vertebrae's transverse foramina. The vertebral veins join the brachiocephalic veins at the root of the neck.

Internal Jugular Veins Most of the blood draining from the brain is received by the two *internal jugular veins*, the largest paired veins that drain the head and neck, emerging from the dural venous sinuses. The internal jugular veins exit the skull through the *jugular foramina* and descend through the neck beside the internal carotid arteries. Further downward, they receive blood from certain deep face and neck veins that are branches of the *facial and superficial temporal veins*. On either side of the base of the neck, each internal jugular vein joins its subclavian vein, forming a brachiocephalic vein. Then, as previously described, the two brachiocephalic veins join and form the superior vena cava.

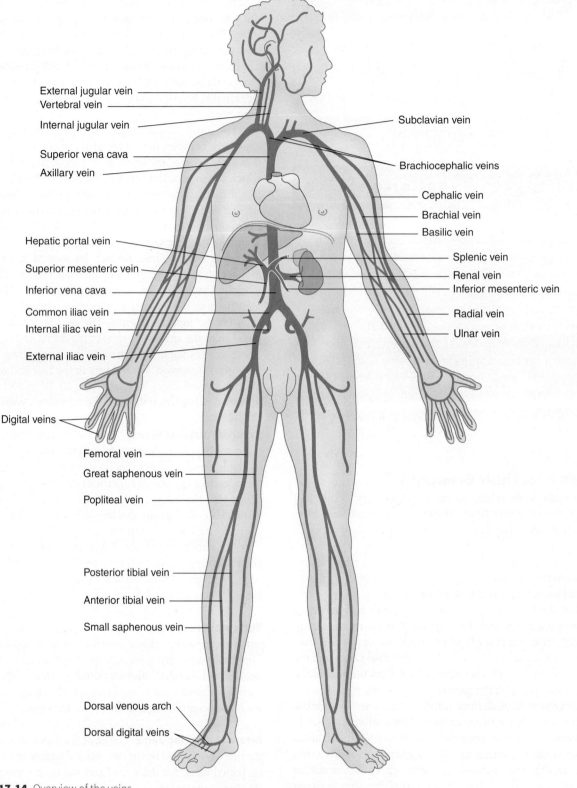

External jugular vein
Vertebral vein
Internal jugular vein
Superior vena cava
Axillary vein
Hepatic portal vein
Superior mesenteric vein
Inferior vena cava
Common iliac vein
Internal iliac vein
External iliac vein
Digital veins
Femoral vein
Great saphenous vein
Popliteal vein
Posterior tibial vein
Anterior tibial vein
Small saphenous vein
Dorsal venous arch
Dorsal digital veins

Subclavian vein
Brachiocephalic veins
Cephalic vein
Brachial vein
Basilic vein
Splenic vein
Renal vein
Inferior mesenteric vein
Radial vein
Ulnar vein

FIGURE 17-14 Overview of the veins.

Upper Limb and Thoracic Veins

As previously described, the deep upper limb veins follow their related arteries' paths and therefore have the same names. Most are paired veins flanking their related artery, except for the largest veins. Because the superficial upper limb veins are larger than the deep veins, they can be easily seen

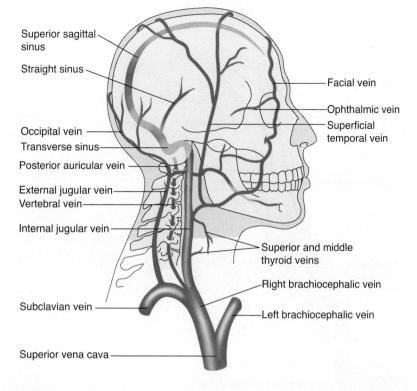

FIGURE 17-15 Head and neck veins.

Labels in figure:
- Superior sagittal sinus
- Straight sinus
- Occipital vein
- Transverse sinus
- Posterior auricular vein
- External jugular vein
- Vertebral vein
- Internal jugular vein
- Subclavian vein
- Superior vena cava
- Facial vein
- Ophthalmic vein
- Superficial temporal vein
- Superior and middle thyroid veins
- Right brachiocephalic vein
- Left brachiocephalic vein

beneath the skin. The subclavian vein drains blood from the cephalic and axillary veins. The axillary vein receives blood from the basilic and brachial veins. The communication between the cephalic and basilic veins in the elbow creates the median cubital vein. For drawing blood or administering medications, the median cubital vein is commonly used. It crosses the anterior elbow.

Deep Upper Limb Veins   The radial and ulnar veins are the most distal deep veins of the upper limbs. From the hand, the *deep and superficial venous palmar arches* empty into the *radial and ulnar veins* of the forearm. Then they join, forming the *brachial vein* of the arm. At the axilla, the brachial vein becomes the *axillary vein*. Then, at the level of the first rib, it becomes the *subclavian vein*.

Superficial Upper Limb Veins   The *dorsal venous network* begins the superficial veins of the upper limbs. It is a plexus of superficial veins located in the dorsum of the hand. The *digital veins* empty into the *superficial* and *deep palmar veins* of the hand, which join to form the *palmar venous arches*. The dorsal venous network drains into two major superficial veins in the distal forearm, the *cephalic and basilic veins*, which have many anastomoses as they continue upward. As it continues in this manner, the *cephalic vein* encircles the radius and continues to the shoulder by moving up the lateral superficial aspect of the arm. At the shoulder, the cephalic vein moves into the groove between the deltoid and pectoralis muscles. Here, it joins the axillary vein. **FIGURE 17-16** shows the upper limb and thoracic veins.

The *basilic vein* continues along the forearm's posteromedial aspect, crossing the elbow, and joining the brachial vein in the axilla to form the axillary vein. The *medial cubital vein* connects the basilic and cephalic veins at the anterior aspect of the elbow. The *median antebrachial vein*, between the radial and ulnar veins, usually ends at the elbow as it enters either the basilic or cephalic vein. The *radial* and *ulnar veins* arise from the deep palmar veins of the hand.

Azygos Vein   The *azygos vein* is located against the right side of the vertebral column. It begins in the abdomen, via the *right ascending lumbar vein*. This vein drains most of the right abdominal cavity wall. The azygos vein also begins from the *right posterior intercostal veins*, except for the first of these. These veins drain the muscles of the chest. At the T4 level, the azygos vein arches over the great vessels that supply the right lung. The azygos vein empties into the superior vena cava. Other veins that drain the abdomen include the lumbar, gonadal, hepatic, renal, adrenal, and phrenic veins.

Hemiazygos Vein   The *hemiazygos vein* ascends on the vertebral column's left side, emerging from the *left ascending lumbar vein* and the 9th to 11th *posterior intercostal veins*. The hemiazygos vein is similar to the inferior portion of the azygos vein on the right side. It passes in front of the vertebral column at about the midthorax level, joining the azygos vein. Both the azygos and hemiazygos veins also collect blood from the esophageal veins as well as smaller veins that drain other structures of the mediastinum.

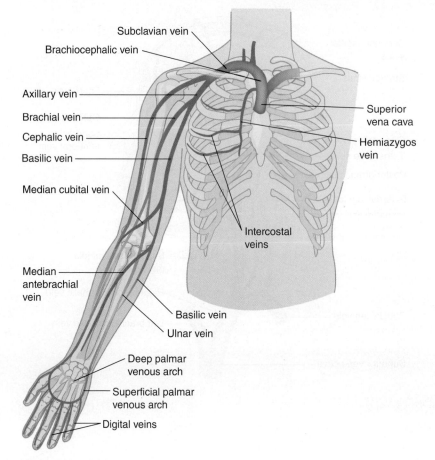

FIGURE 17-16 Upper limb and thoracic veins.

Accessory Hemiazygos Vein   Venous drainage of the left, middle thorax is completed by the *accessory hemiazygos vein*, a superior continuance of the hemiazygos vein that receives blood from the fourth to eight posterior intercostal veins. The accessory hemiazygos vein then crosses to the right and empties into the azygos vein. It receives deoxygenated systemic blood from the bronchial veins, which is the same as what the azygos vein receives.

TEST YOUR UNDERSTANDING

1.   Explain the branches of the subclavian veins.
2.   Define the medical cubital vein and its origination.
3.   Explain the junctions of the brachial vein.

Hepatic Portal System

The pathway of blood flow from the gastrointestinal tract and spleen to the liver via the portal vein and its tributaries is called the *hepatic portal circulation*. The **hepatic portal system** is made up of a series of vessels and contains two distinct capillary beds lying between the arterial supply and the final venous drainage. In this system the initial capillary beds are found in the stomach and intestines. They drain into vessels of the hepatic portal vein, and the blood is then carried to a second capillary bed inside the liver. The *hepatic portal vein* is short, starting at the L2 level. A group

of vessels from the stomach and pancreas contributes to the hepatic portal system. However, there are three major vessels: the superior mesenteric vein, splenic vein, and inferior mesenteric vein.

The *superior mesenteric vein* drains all the small intestine, the ascending and transverse regions of the large intestine, and the stomach. The *splenic vein* collects blood from parts of the stomach and pancreas as well as all of the spleen. It joins the superior mesenteric vein, forming the hepatic portal vein. The *inferior mesenteric vein* drains the distal large intestine and rectum. It joins the splenic vein just prior to its uniting with the superior mesenteric vein (**FIGURE 17-17**). The hepatic portal vein receives blood from the left and right *gastric veins* of the stomach and from the *cystic vein* of the gallbladder.

FOCUS ON PATHOLOGY

Portal hypertension is an increased venous pressure in the portal circulation caused by compression or occlusion in the portal or hepatic vascular system. It results in large collateral veins, splenomegaly, ascites, and esophageal varices. Portal hypertension is often associated with cirrhosis of the liver.

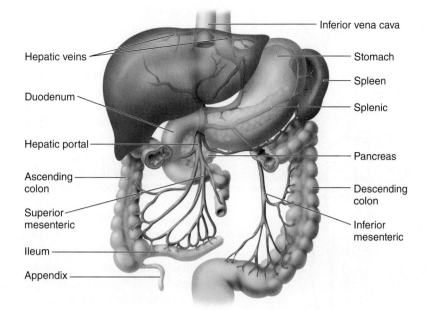

FIGURE 17-17 Veins that drain the abdominal viscera.

Pelvic and Lower Limb Veins

Most of the pelvic and lower limb veins also have the same names as their accompanying arteries. Veins that drain blood from the lower limbs are also subdivided, similar to those of the upper limbs, into deep and superficial groups (**FIGURE 17-18**). Many of these veins are double. The two *superficial saphenous veins* are where varicosities often occur, because they are not supported very well by surrounding tissues. In coronary bypass operations the great saphenous vein is often excised and used as a replacement blood vessel. The *gonadal veins* drain the ovaries in females and testicles in males.

Deep Veins   The *posterior tibial vein* ascends deep in the calf muscle after it forms via the union of the *medial and lateral plantar veins*. The posterior tibial vein receives blood from the *fibular* or *peroneal vein*. The superior continuation of the *dorsalis pedis vein* of the foot is the *anterior tibial vein*. It unites, at the knee, with the *posterior tibial vein*, forming the *popliteal vein* across the back of the knee. The popliteal vein emerges from the knee to become the *femoral vein*; draining the deep thigh structures. The femoral vein receives blood from the great saphenous, deep femoral, and femoral circumflex veins. As it enters the pelvis, the femoral vein becomes the *external iliac vein*. In the pelvis this vein joins the *internal iliac vein*, becoming the *common iliac vein*. The internal iliac veins are arranged very similar to the arrangement of the internal iliac arteries.

Superficial Veins   From the *dorsal venous arch* of the foot, the *great and small saphenous veins* emerge, anastomosing often with each other as well as the nearby deep veins. The longest vein in the body is the *great saphenous vein*. It runs from the foot to the femoral vein, distal to the inguinal ligament. It travels superiorly along the medial aspect of the leg

to the thigh. The *small saphenous vein* runs from the foot to the knee. It is located along the lateral aspect of the foot, moving through the deep fascia of the calf muscles. The small saphenous vein drains the calf muscles and empties into the popliteal vein.

TEST YOUR UNDERSTANDING

1. Which veins return blood to the right atrium?
2. What is the name of the vein that carries blood from the stomach, intestines, pancreas, and spleen through to the liver?
3. Describe the hepatic portal system.
4. Compare the structures and functions of the superior vena cava with the great saphenous vein.
5. Define cavernous sinuses and sigmoid sinuses.
6. Describe the brachiocephalic veins and from which parts of the body they receive blood.

Effects of Aging on the Vascular System

In the blood vessels aging causes atherosclerosis, which can lead to an *aneurysm* and resultant stroke, myocardial infarction, or hemorrhaging. The depositing of calcium salts can weaken the vessel walls to increase risk of stroke or myocardial infarction. Atherosclerotic plaques can also cause the formation of thrombi. Atherosclerosis usually begins to cause problems in middle or old age.

Between ages 25 and 45 men begin to have higher rates of developing atherosclerosis because they lack the amounts of estrogen to protect the blood vessels, which women have. Estrogen reduces resistance to blood flow as well as the risk of developing atherosclerosis in several ways: enhanced

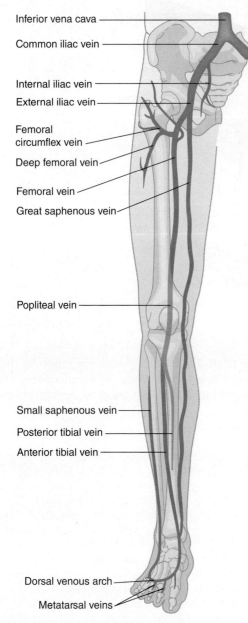

Inferior vena cava
Common iliac vein
Internal iliac vein
External iliac vein
Femoral circumflex vein
Deep femoral vein
Femoral vein
Great saphenous vein
Popliteal vein
Small saphenous vein
Posterior tibial vein
Anterior tibial vein
Dorsal venous arch
Metatarsal veins

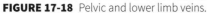

FIGURE 17-18 Pelvic and lower limb veins.

production of nitric oxide, blocking of voltage-gated calcium ion channels, and inhibition of the release of *endothelin,* a protein that constricts blood vessels and raises blood pressure.

Estrogen also causes the liver to produce enzymes that increase catabolism of low-density lipoproteins and the production of high-density lipoproteins. However, estrogen production begins to decline starting at age 45, and women then have closer rates of developing atherosclerosis to men of the same age. By age 65, men and women have the same risk for developing cardiovascular disease.

Congenital vascular problems, unlike congenital heart problems, are rare. However, aging causes *venous valves* to weaken and purple *varicose veins* to appear. Signs of reduced circulation include cramping of muscles and tingling in the digits. Blood pressure also changes with age. With normal, healthy adults under age 40, average blood pressure is 120/80 mm Hg. After this age, hypertension occurrence is much more common, along with heart attacks, renal failure, strokes, and vascular disease. Other factors that result in vascular disease over our lifetimes include high-protein and high-lipid diets, empty calorie snacks, high stress levels, lack of aerobic exercise, smoking, and high alcohol intake. Cardiovascular disease can be prevented by regular aerobic exercise, healthy diet, avoiding smoking, and only using alcohol in moderation.

FOCUS ON PATHOLOGY

Cerebrovascular accidents or *strokes* occur when the brain's vascular blood supply is interrupted. Most strokes occur in the *middle cerebral artery,* which is a primary branch of the cerebral arterial circle. If the stroke blocks this artery on the left side of the brain, aphasia develops, and both sensory and motor paralysis occur on the right side of the body. If the stroke occurs on the right side instead, the paralysis is on the left side of the body, and the individual has reduced hand–eye coordination and inability to interpret spatial relationships. Strokes that affect the lower brain stem are usually fatal.

SUMMARY

The vascular system of the human body is made up of the systemic and pulmonary circuits. The five general classes of blood vessels include the arteries, arterioles, capillaries, venules, and veins. The walls of arteries consist of three distinct layers and a blood-containing space known as the lumen. In arteries and arterioles, vasomotor fibers receive impulses to contract and reduce blood vessel diameter, which is called vasoconstriction. When inhibited the muscle fibers relax, and the vessel's diameter increases, which is called vasodilation. The arterial system consists of the aorta and pulmonary arteries.

The smallest diameter blood vessels are capillaries, which connect the smallest arterioles to the smallest venules. Venules are microscopic vessels that link capillaries to veins, which carry blood back to the atria. Vein walls are similar but not identical to arteries but have poorly developed middle layers. Many veins have flap-like valves projecting inward from their linings, preventing blood from flowing backward. Veins often act as blood reservoirs. Vascular anastomoses are interconnections formed by blood vessels.

The blood must continue to circulate to sustain life, with the heart acting as the circulation pump. Blood pressure is calculated by multiplying cardiac output by peripheral resistance. It is the pressure exerted by the blood's circulating volume on the walls of the arteries, veins, and heart chambers. The maximum pressure during ventricular contraction is called the systolic pressure. The lowest pressure that remains in the arteries before the next ventricular contraction is called the diastolic pressure. The venous blood pressure is steady and regular and does not pulsate with ventricular contractions like the arterial blood pressure. Blood volume is the sum of formed elements and plasma volumes in the vascular system.

Most neural controls of blood vessels operate because of reflex arcs, which involve baroreceptors and related afferent fibers. Baroreceptors are activated by increased arterial pressure. Chemoreceptors in the aortic arch and large neck arteries send impulses to the cardioacceleratory center to increase cardiac output. The brain stem's medulla oblongata integrates reflexes that maintain blood pressure. Short-term hormonal controls involve ADH, angiotensin II, ANP, and the hormones of the adrenal medulla. Long-term control of blood pressure involves the kidneys. Homeostatic imbalances in blood pressure involve hypertension and hypotension.

Arteries are deep, whereas veins are either deep or superficial. Veins have more interconnections than arteries. The aorta is the body's largest artery and emerges from the left ventricle of the heart. It consists of four portions: the ascending aorta, aortic arch, descending aorta, and abdominal aorta. The head and neck are supplied by four paired arteries: the common carotid arteries plus three branches from each subclavian artery. The subclavian arteries branch to supply all portions of the upper limbs. The abdominal aorta branches to form the abdominal arteries. The common iliac arteries are divided into the internal and external iliac arteries.

Three major veins return blood from the body to the right atrium: the coronary sinus, superior vena cava, and inferior vena cava. From the head and neck three pairs of veins collect most of the draining blood: the external jugular veins, internal jugular veins, and vertebral veins. The deep upper limb veins and most of the pelvic and lower limb veins follow their related arteries' paths and therefore have the same names. The pathway of blood flow from the gastrointestinal tract and spleen to the liver via the portal vein and its tributaries is called the hepatic portal circulation. Aging causes atherosclerosis in the blood vessels. Venous valves weaken and purple varicose veins appear. Hypertension is common, along with heart attacks, renal failure, strokes, and vascular disease.

KEY TERMS

Angiotensin II	Blood pressure	Cerebral arterial circle
Aorta	Blood volume	Chemoreceptors
Aortic arch	Brachiocephalic trunk	Circulatory shock
Arteries	Brachiocephalic vein	Coronary sinus
Arterioles	Capillaries	Diastolic pressure
Baroreceptors	Carotid bodies	Elastic arteries
Blood flow	Carotid sinuses	Endothelium

External jugular veins	Superior vena cava	Vasodilation
Hepatic portal system	Systemic circuit	Vasomotor center
Hypertension	Systolic pressure	Vasomotor fibers
Hypotension	Tunica intima	Vasomotor tone
Inferior vena cava	Tunica externa	Vasopressin
Lumen	Tunica media	Veins
Muscular arteries	Varicose veins	Venous valves
Peripheral resistance	Vasa vasorum	Venules
Pulmonary circuit	Vascular anastomoses	Viscosity
Pulse pressure	Vasoconstriction	

LEARNING GOALS

The following learning goals correspond to the objectives at the beginning of this chapter:

1. Arteries have three layers and a blood-containing space known as the lumen. In the systemic circuit the arteries carry only oxygenated blood, whereas the veins carry only deoxygenated blood. In the pulmonary circuit the reverse is true. Arteries are grouped based on whether they are elastic or muscular. Smaller arteries are called arterioles, which bring blood to the capillaries. The smallest diameter blood vessels are the capillaries, which connect the smallest arterioles to the smallest venules. The capillaries are microscopic blood vessels with extremely thin walls. Venules are microscopic vessels that link capillaries to veins, which carry blood back to the atria. Vein walls are similar to artery walls but have poorly developed middle layers. Their lumens have a greater diameter than those of arteries. Veins often have flap-like valves that help to return blood to the heart and prevent backflow of blood. Veins mostly have three tunics.

2. The systemic circuit has a long pathway through all of the body and is powered by the left ventricle. Along this circuit, there is about five times more resistance to blood flow than in the pulmonary circuit. The systemic circuit is served by the left ventricle of the heart. Equal volumes of blood are pumped to the pulmonary and systemic circuits simultaneously. The pulmonary circuit is a short, low-pressure circulation. It is served by the right ventricle of the heart. In the systemic circuit the arteries carry only oxygenated blood, whereas the veins carry only deoxygenated blood. In the pulmonary circuit, the reverse is true.

3. Blood flow is the amount or volume of blood that flows through blood vessels, organs, or the systemic circulation, in millimeters per minute (mL/min). Blood pressure is the force that blood exerts against the inner walls of blood vessels. Resistance is the friction between blood and blood vessel walls.

4. Generally, sympathetic stimulation, which releases epinephrine, causes vasoconstriction and therefore increased blood pressure. However, the parasympathetic nervous system has the opposite effect and generally causes vasodilation and decreased blood pressure.

5. The factors that influence blood pressure include homeostatic mechanisms such as cardiac output, peripheral resistance, blood pressure, and lumen size of the arteries and arterioles. Blood pressure is regulated by the regulation of cardiac output with peripheral resistance. Changes in the diameters of arterioles regulate peripheral resistance, which is controlled by the vasomotor center of the medulla oblongata. Peripheral resistance is also influenced by carbon dioxide, oxygen, and hydrogen ions. Arterial blood pressure rises and falls according to cardiac cycle phases. The control of blood vessel size, and therefore blood pressure, is also related to neural activities via reflex arcs, baroreceptors, related afferent fibers, chemoreceptors, high brain center influences, hormonal controls, and renal controls.

6. The major arteries that supply the head are the common carotid arteries plus three branches from each subclavian artery, which include the vertebral arteries, thyrocervical trunks, and costocervical trunks. The major arteries that supply the abdomen are the abdominal aorta branches, which form the abdominal arteries. All these arteries are paired vessels except for the celiac trunk, median sacral artery, and superior and inferior mesenteric arteries. The abdominal arteries also include the inferior phrenic arteries, suprarenal arteries, renal arteries, gonadal arteries, lumbar arteries, and common iliac arteries.

7. The main arteries and veins of the lower limbs include the common iliac artery, femoral artery, popliteal artery, tibial artery, common iliac vein, femoral vein, popliteal vein, and saphenous vein.

8. The major veins that carry blood away from the lower limbs are named similar to the lower limb arteries and are the femoral veins, great saphenous veins, popliteal veins, posterior tibial veins, anterior tibial veins, small saphenous veins, dorsal venous arches, and dorsal digital veins.

9. The hepatic portal system is made up of a series of vessels. The pathway of blood flow from the gastrointestinal tract and spleen to the liver via the portal vein and its tributaries is called the hepatic portal circulation. The hepatic portal system contains two distinct capillary beds lying between the arterial supply and the final venous drainage. These initial capillary beds are in the stomach and intestines and drain into the hepatic portal veins vessels. The three major vessels of the hepatic portal system are the superior mesenteric vein, splenic vein, and inferior mesenteric vein.

10. The difference between the systolic and diastolic pressures is known as pulse pressure. During systole, it is felt in an artery as a throbbing pulsation. This is due to ventricular contraction, which forces blood into the elastic arteries, expanding them. Pulse pressure is temporarily raised by increased stroke volume and quicker blood ejection because of increased contractility from the heart. Pulse pressure can be detected most easily at the locations of the radial, carotid, brachial, and femoral arteries.

CRITICAL THINKING QUESTIONS

A 63-year-old woman was brought to the emergency department. Her blood pressure was 80/50, and her pulse was 120 per minute. Physical examination revealed splenomegaly and ascites. Her husband told the physician she has smoked two packs of cigarettes per day and consumed alcohol heavily for the past 20 years.

1. Explain which of her veins may have had varices, resulting in rupture and internal bleeding.
2. Explain the hepatic portal system and its relation to this patient's condition.

REVIEW QUESTIONS

1. The left and right pulmonary arteries carry blood to the
    A. brain
    B. liver
    C. lungs
    D. kidneys
2. Deoxygenated blood from the cranial cavity returns to the heart via veins called the
    A. internal jugular veins
    B. brachial veins
    C. great saphenous veins
    D. azygos veins

3. Branches off of the aortic arch include the
    A. brachial and right axillary arteries
    B. right and left subclavian arteries
    C. left common carotid artery and brachiocephalic trunk
    D. right subclavian and right common carotid arteries
4. Nutrients from the digestive tract enter the
    A. hepatic vein
    B. hepatic portal vein
    C. inferior vena cava
    D. azygos vein

5. The longest vein in the human body is the
   A. inferior vena cava
   B. superior vena cava
   C. saphenous vein
   D. femoral vein

6. Which of the following is *not* related to the way blood moves forward through the veins?
   A. valves in the veins prevent the backflow of blood
   B. contractions of skeletal muscles
   C. contraction and relaxation pumping of the smooth muscle in the wall of the vein
   D. pressure in the veins is lower than in the arteries

7. Each of the following changes results in increased blood flow to a tissue, *except*
   A. increased vessel diameter
   B. relaxation of precapillary sphincters
   C. increased blood pressure
   D. increased blood volume

8. At the carotid sinus,
   A. the internal carotid arteries fuse with the vertebral arteries
   B. the external carotid artery forms the internal carotid
   C. the common carotid artery forms internal and external branches
   D. the aorta gives rise to the common carotid arteries

9. The external iliac artery branches to form which of the following arteries?
   A. radial and ulnar
   B. femoral and tibial
   C. tibial and popliteal
   D. femoral and deep femoral

10. The radial and ulnar veins fuse to form which of the following veins?
    A. basilic
    B. axillary
    C. brachial
    D. azygos

11. Which of the following layers of a vessel contain collagen fibers with scattered bands of elastic fibers?
    A. tunica media
    B. tunica externa
    C. tunica intima
    D. internal elastic membrane

12. The smallest arterial branches are the
    A. venules
    B. capillaries
    C. arteries
    D. arterioles

13. The inferior vena cava is classified as a(n)
    A. large vein
    B. venous valve
    C. arteriovenule
    D. venule

14. Blood pressure is determined by measuring the
    A. force of contraction of the right ventricle
    B. degree of turbulence in a closed vessel
    C. force exerted by blood in a vessel against air in a closed cuff
    D. size of the pulse

15. Blood flow through a capillary is regulated by the
    A. capillary plexus
    B. precapillary sphincter
    C. vasa vasorum
    D. arterial anastomosis

ESSAY QUESTIONS

1. Describe the structure of capillaries and their functions.
2. Distinguish the anatomy of arteries and veins.
3. Define peripheral resistance, blood flow, blood viscosity, and blood pressure.
4. List three main branches that arise on the anterior surface of the abdominal aorta.
5. Describe the common factors linked to arteriosclerosis.
6. Describe the hepatic portal system and its major veins.
7. Compare and describe arterial, capillary, and venous blood pressure.
8. Describe the risk factors for primary hypertension.
9. Describe neural and chemical effects exerted on the blood vessels.
10. Describe the location of the celiac trunk and its branches.

CHAPTER 18

Lymphatic System and Immunity

OBJECTIVES

After studying this chapter, the reader should be able to

1. Define immunity and explain its relationship to the lymphatic system.
2. Identify the major components of the lymphatic system.
3. Describe the structure of lymphoid tissues, vessels, and organs.
4. Describe the major functions of the lymphatic system.
5. Describe a lymph node and its functions.
6. Explain the difference between nonspecific and specific defenses.
7. Explain the role of lymphocytes in the immune response.
8. Explain the roles of the thymus and spleen.
9. Identify the body's three lines of defense against pathogens.
10. Distinguish between humoral and cellular immunity.

OUTLINE

Overview

Similarly to the cardiovascular system, the *lymphatic system* transports fluids through a network of vessels. The primary functions of the lymphatic system are the production, maintenance, and distribution of *lymphocytes*. Another major function is to transport excess fluid out of interstitial spaces in tissues and return it to the bloodstream (**FIGURE 18-1**), which may be up to 3 liters of fluid per day. Without the lymphatic system, fluid would accumulate in tissue spaces. The production of lymphocytes is called *lymphopoiesis*.

The biochemicals and cells of the lymphatic system attack "foreign" particles in the body, allowing the destruction of infectious microorganisms and viruses, toxins, and cancer cells. Many organs and body systems work together to maintain life and proper health. The lymphatic system is vital in this capacity, responsible for defending the body against environmental hazards, such as various pathogens, and internal threats, such as cancer cells.

The lymphatic system is the structural basis of our immune system. Lymphoid organs and tissues contain lymphocytes and phagocytic cells. Together, these play essential roles in how the body defends itself and resists disease. Our immune system is divided into two parts: the *innate* or *nonspecific* and *adaptive* or *specific* defense systems. The innate defense system protects the body continuously and quickly from foreign substances. The skin and mucous membranes comprise the *first line of defense* against pathogens. When either of these is compromised, the *second line of defense* uses phagocytes, antimicrobial proteins, and various other cells that attack invaders. **Inflammation** is the most important feature of the second line of defense. The adaptive or specific defense system provides a *third line of defense* and focuses on *certain* foreign substances. It acts much slower than the innate or nonspecific defense system. The term *specificity* refers to the activation of needed lymphocytes and production of antibodies to achieve targeted effects.

Effective immune function protects the body from a wide variety of potentially harmful substances and agents, such as cancer cells, infectious microorganisms, and transplanted tissue. This is accomplished by direct cellular attack and by indirect release of protective antibodies and chemicals that mobilize its protective agents. Our immune systems must be ready to handle any antigen whenever it is confronted. This *versatility* occurs partially from the many types of lymphocytes in the body and from the structural variability of synthesized antibodies.

Organization of the Lymphatic System

Lymphatic capillaries form tiny tubes called **lymphatic pathways**, which merge to form larger vessels, eventually uniting with veins in the thorax. Microscopic **lymphatic capillaries** extend into interstitial spaces in complex networks (**FIGURE 18-2**). The walls of lymphatic capillaries consists of a single layer of squamous epithelium that allows tissue fluid to enter. The fluid inside these capillaries is called **lymph**. Lymphatic capillaries are found in loose connective tissues between tissue cells and blood capillaries but are not found in bones, bone marrow, teeth, and all of the central nervous system. In the central nervous system, excess tissue fluid drains into the cerebrospinal fluid.

Proteins easily enter lymphatic capillaries but cannot enter blood capillaries. Inflammation of tissues cause lymphatic capillaries to develop openings through which larger particles can pass. These particles may include cancer cells, cell debris, and pathogens. The pathogens can then use the lymphatics to travel elsewhere in the body. However, because lymph moves through the lymph nodes, the particles are usually removed and "evaluated" by the immune system cells.

Lacteals are special lymphatic capillaries located in the small intestine's lining that absorb digested fats and carry them to the venous circulation. The name "lacteal" comes from the appearance of the lymph, which resembles milk. It is actually fatty lymph, known as **chyle**, that drains from the intestinal mucosa villi, which are finger-like in appearance.

Similar to veins but with thinner walls, **lymphatic vessels** have valves preventing backflow of lymph. Therefore, lymph moves through them in only one direction: toward the heart. Larger vessels lead to specialized organs known

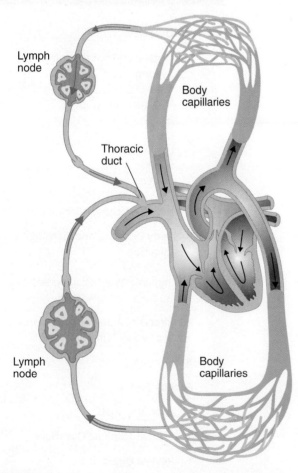

FIGURE 18-1 The lymphatic system transports fluids through a network of vessels.

Lymph node

Body capillaries

Thoracic duct

Lymph node

Body capillaries

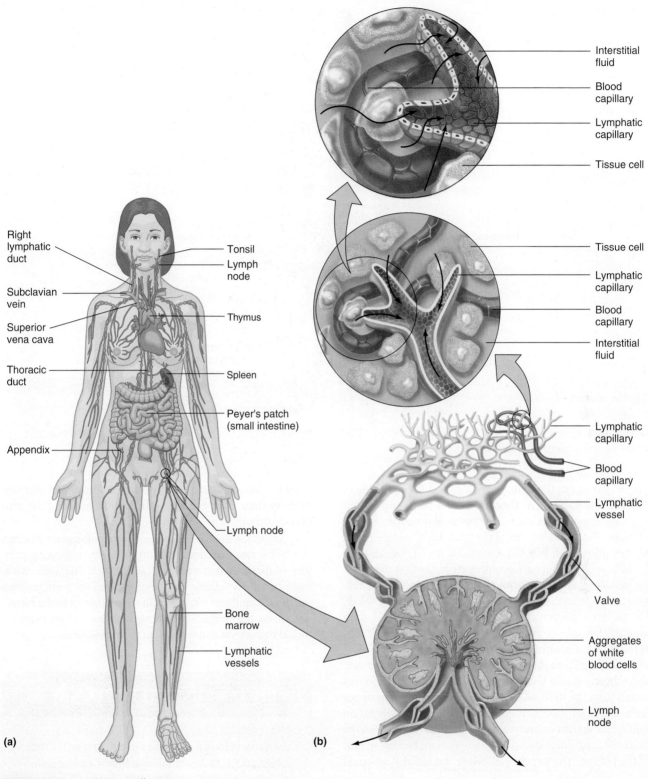

Right lymphatic duct

Subclavian vein

Superior vena cava

Thoracic duct

Appendix

Tonsil

Lymph node

Thymus

Spleen

Peyer's patch (small intestine)

Lymph node

Bone marrow

Lymphatic vessels

(a)

(b)

Interstitial fluid

Blood capillary

Lymphatic capillary

Tissue cell

Tissue cell

Lymphatic capillary

Blood capillary

Interstitial fluid

Lymphatic capillary

Blood capillary

Lymphatic vessel

Valve

Aggregates of white blood cells

Lymph node

FIGURE 18-2 Lymphatic capillaries.

as **lymph nodes** and then continue on to form larger lymphatic trunks. Similar to veins, the *collecting lymphatic vessels* have three tunics but with thinner walls. The vessels also have more internal valves and experience anastomoses more frequently. Basically, skin lymphatics are routed alongside superficial veins, but in the trunk and digestive viscera the deeper lymphatic vessels are found alongside the deep

arteries. The exact locations of lymphatic vessels are more varied among different people than the distribution of the veins.

The major **lymphatic trunks** of the body are the paired *lumbar trunks, bronchomediastinal trunks, subclavian trunks, jugular trunks,* and the single *intestinal trunk.* The lymph from lymphatic vessels drains as they join one of two **collecting ducts**. **FIGURE 18-3** depicts the right lymphatic duct and

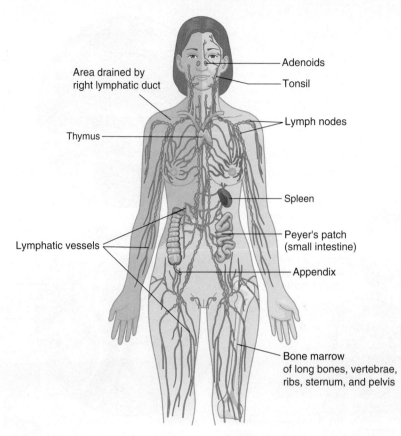

Area drained by right lymphatic duct

Adenoids

Tonsil

Lymph nodes

Thymus

Spleen

Lymphatic vessels

Peyer's patch (small intestine)

Appendix

Bone marrow of long bones, vertebrae, ribs, sternum, and pelvis

FIGURE 18-3 Lymphatic pathways. The right lymphatic duct drains lymph from the upper right side of the body, and the thoracic duct drains lymph from the rest of the body.

lymph drainage of the right upper limb and the right side of the head and thorax. The **thoracic duct** is larger and longer, receiving lymph from the lower limbs, abdominal regions, left upper limb, and left side of the head, neck, and thorax. It empties into the left subclavian vein near the left jugular vein.

The thoracic duct arises anteriorly to the first two lumbar vertebrae as the **cisterna chyli**, an enlarged sac. It collects lymph from the lumbar trunks and the intestinal trunk. The superior portion of the thoracic duct receives lymph from the left side of the head, left upper limb, and left side of the thorax. On either side of the body, each terminal duct empties lymph into the veins where the internal jugular vein and subclavian vein join. The **right lymphatic duct** receives lymph from the right side of the head and neck, right upper limb, and right thorax. It empties into the right subclavian vein near the right jugular vein. Lymph then moves from the two collecting ducts into the venous system, becoming part of the plasma. This occurs just before the blood is returned to the right atrium.

Tissue Fluid and Lymph Formation

Lymph is basically the same as tissue fluid but is referred to as lymph once it has entered a lymphatic capillary. Tissue fluid is made up of water and dissolved substances from the blood capillaries. It is very similar to blood plasma, containing gases, hormones, and nutrients. However, it lacks plasma proteins because their size does not permit them to

leave the blood capillaries. Plasma colloid osmotic pressure helps to draw fluid back into the capillaries using the process of osmosis.

Lymph forms because filtration from blood plasma occurs at a higher rate than does reabsorption. The hydrostatic pressure of tissue fluid is increased, inducing tissue fluid movement into the lymphatic capillaries. Most of the small proteins the blood capillaries filtered earlier are returned to the bloodstream via the lymph. Lymph also carries foreign particles, including bacteria and viruses, to the lymph nodes.

FOCUS ON PATHOLOGY

Lymphangitis is a condition in which the pathway of associated superficial lymphatics can be seen through the skin as red lines. These lines are tender to the touch, causing discomfort. It occurs because severe inflammation of lymphatic vessels causes the related vessels of the vasa vasorum to become congested with blood. Like larger blood vessels, larger lymphatics receive their nutrient blood supply from branches of the vasa vasorum.

Movement of Lymph

The movement of lymph is influenced by muscular activity because the lymphatic system has no organ that "pumps" lymph throughout its vessels. Lymph itself is under low hydrostatic pressure, and it moves similarly to how blood moves through the veins. Without contraction of skeletal muscles, smooth muscle contraction in the larger lymphatic trunks, and breathing-related pressure changes, lymph may not flow easily. Skeletal muscles, for example, compress lymphatic vessels to move the lymph inside, with valves preventing any backflow. Breathing creates a relatively low thoracic cavity pressure during inhalation, aiding lymph circulation. The diaphragm increases abdominal cavity pressure, squeezing lymph out of abdominal vessels and into thoracic vessels. Increased passive movements or physical activity cause lymph to flow more quickly. This balances the increased rate of fluid loss from the blood. Therefore, if a part of the body has a serious infection, immobilization results in decreased flow of inflammatory material out of it.

The continuous movement of lymph stabilizes fluid volume in the body's interstitial spaces. When tissue fluid accumulates in the interstitial spaces, known as *edema*, it is because of an interference with lymph movement. Edema commonly occurs after surgery when lymphatic tissue is removed, such as when a breast tumor is removed. In this example, axillary lymph nodes may be removed as part of the surgery to prevent cancer cells from being transported via nearby lymphatic vessels. This can obstruct upper limb draining, resulting in edema.

FOCUS ON PATHOLOGY

Severe localized edema known as *lymphedema* occurs when something prevents the normal return of lymph to the blood. Examples of causes of lymphedema include removal of lymphatics as part of cancer surgery or the blockage of lymphatics by tumors. In most cases other vessels in the area grow to reestablish drainage of lymph.

TEST YOUR UNDERSTANDING

1. Identify the major components of the lymphatic system.
2. Differentiate between tissue fluid and lymph and include sources of both.
3. Describe from which parts of the body the left and right lymphatic ducts receive lymph.
4. Detail how lymph actually forms.
5. Explain the movement of lymph.

Lymphoid Cells

The primary cells of the lymphatic system are lymphocytes. Lymphocytes are vital for the body's ability to resist or overcome diseases and infections and include T lymphocytes and B lymphocytes. *Plasma cells* are a type of B lymphocytes that produce antibodies. Normal lymphocyte populations are mostly maintained by the red bone marrow. One type of lymphoid stem cell remains in the red bone marrow, whereas the other type migrates to the thymus gland. In the red bone marrow lymphoid stem cells divide, producing immature B cells and natural killer (NK) cells. The development of B cells involves close contact with large *stromal cells* inside the bone marrow.

Besides the lymphocytes, lymphoid cells include **macrophages**, *dendritic cells,* and *reticular cells.* Macrophages are vital for protection of the body and for immune response. They phagocytize foreign substances and assist in the activation of T cells or T lymphocytes. Spiked cells called **dendritic cells** capture antigens and transport them to lymph nodes. **Reticular cells** are similar to fibroblasts and produce **stroma**, which is a reticular fiber network that supports other lymphoid cell types. Macrophages are widely distributed throughout the connective tissues and lymphoid organs. They often present antigens to T cells for them to be activated. Some effector T cells release chemicals that activate macrophages, which are killer cells that both secrete bactericidal chemicals and actively phagocytize invaders.

B cells may activate when encountering an antigen whose shape fits the B cell's antigen receptor shape, dividing repeatedly and expanding its *clone*. However, B cells usually require T cells to activate. T cells that encounter B cells bound to identical foreign antigens release cytokines that stimulate the B cells. The cytokines attract macrophages and leukocytes. Some of the B cell's clones differentiate into more *memory* cells. These memory B cells respond quickly to reexposure to specific antigens. Other B-cell clones differentiate into antibody-secreting plasma cells, which can combine with their corresponding foreign antigens and react against them (**FIGURE 18-4**). B cells can produce between 10 million and 1 billion varieties of antibodies, each specific to an antigen. When the B cells are prepared to undergo activation, they are described as being *sensitized.*

Lymphoid Tissues

In the immune system, **lymphoid tissue** is very important for two major reasons. It contains lymphocytes and provides a place for them to proliferate, and it gives lymphocytes and macrophages excellent areas to conduct their surveillance of various particles. Lymphoid tissue is mostly made up of loose, *reticular connective tissue*. Except for the thymus, all lymphoid organs consist mostly of this tissue. The macrophages are found on the reticular connective tissue fiber network. Many lymphocytes slip through the postcapillary venule walls of this network and occupy its spaces for a short period of time. Lymphocytes can reach

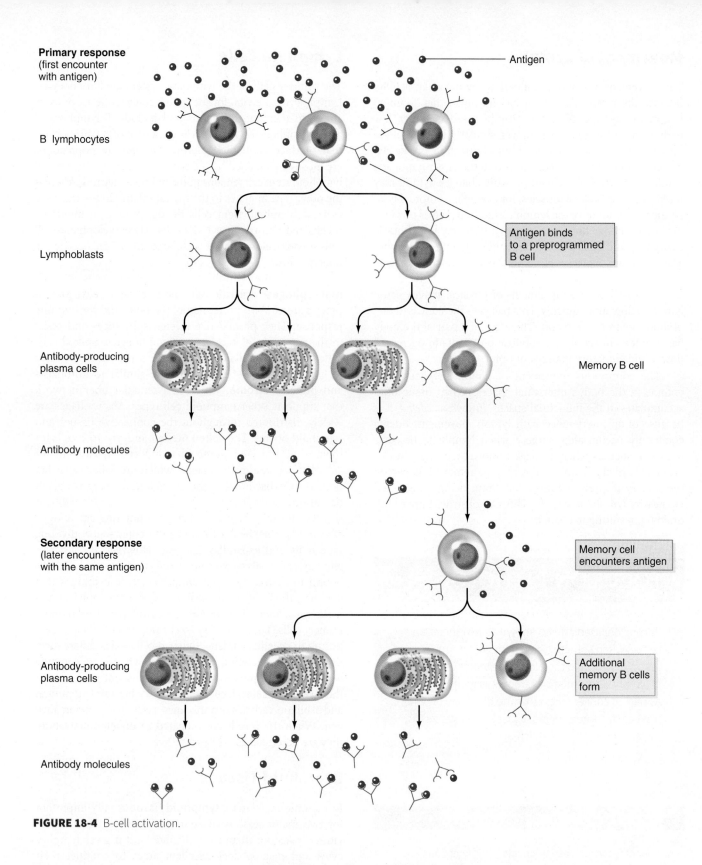

Primary response
(first encounter
with antigen)

Antigen

B lymphocytes

Antigen binds
to a preprogrammed
B cell

Lymphoblasts

Antibody-producing
plasma cells

Memory B cell

Antibody molecules

Secondary response
(later encounters
with the same antigen)

Memory cell
encounters antigen

Antibody-producing
plasma cells

Additional
memory B cells
form

Antibody molecules

FIGURE 18-4 B-cell activation.

sites of damage or infection quickly because of their regular cycling between lymphoid tissues, circulatory vessels, and loose connective body tissues. You should remember that the *primary lymphoid organs* are only the thymus and bone marrow. All other lymphoid organs are called *secondary lymphoid organs.*

The *mucosa-associated lymphoid tissue* protects the epithelia of the respiratory, digestive, urinary, and reproductive systems. *Aggregated lymphoid nodules* or *Peyer's patches* are clustered lymphoid nodules lying deep to the intestinal epithelial lining. The appendix and tonsils are also examples of mucosa-associated lymphoid tissue.

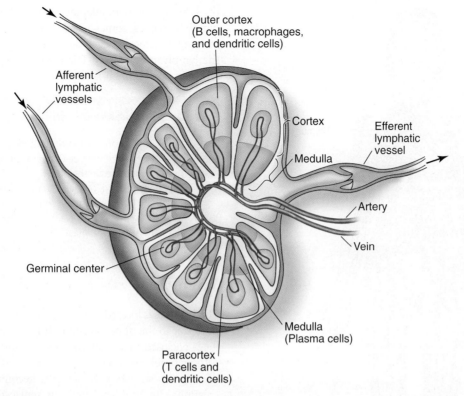

FIGURE 18-5 Lymph nodes.

Lymph Nodes

Lymph nodes are actually *lymph glands*. Totaling in the hundreds, they are found along the lymphatic pathways and contain many lymphocytes and macrophages that fight invading microorganisms. Although they vary in size and shape, they are generally bean-shaped and less than 2.5 cm in length (**FIGURE 18-5**). An indented region of each node, called the **hilum**, is where blood vessels and nerves are attached. In general, lymph nodes are hidden inside connective tissue structures called *capsules*. Large clusters are found near the surface of the body in the axillary, cervical, and inguinal regions. In these locations, lymphatic vessels merge and form the lymphatic trunks.

Each lymph node is enclosed and subdivided by a dense, fibrous capsule. Strands called *trabeculae* divide each node into compartments. A lymph node's internal framework or stroma consists of reticular fibers, which support the lymphocytes that continually change inside it. The **cortex** and **medulla** of a lymph node are distinct. Tightly packed follicles are contained in the superficial area of the cortex. Inside are areas where B cells germinate and divide. Follicles are almost totally surrounded by dendritic cells. The follicles touch the *deeper cortex* or *paracortical area*, which mostly contains transitional T cells. These T cells circulate between the blood, lymph, and lymph nodes, continually surveilling particles. The medulla of each lymph node contains plasma cells and B cells organized into long *medullary cords*.

Both types of lymphocytes that exist are contained in the *medullary cords*, which are inward extension from the cortical lymphoid tissue. The *lymph sinuses* are found throughout each lymph node. Many macrophages on the reticular fibers phagocytize foreign matter in lymph that flows through the sinuses.

The functional units of a lymph node are the **lymph nodules** or follicles, which consist of B cells and macrophages located in the node's cortex. Lymph nodules occur either alone or in groups. The tonsils are partially encapsulated lymph nodules, and groups of nodules called *Peyer's patches* are found in the lining of the small intestine. **Lymph sinuses** are spaces inside a node that comprise complex channels through which lymph moves. There are more macrophages in the lymph sinuses than in any other parts of a node.

Lymph nodes are grouped along larger lymphatic vessels but do not exist in the central nervous system (**FIGURE 18-6**). Lymph nodes have two main functions: filter potentially harmful particles from the lymph before it is returned to the bloodstream and monitor body fluids. Immune surveillance occurs via the action of the lymphocytes and macrophages. Lymphocytes are produced in the lymph nodes and red bone marrow. They attack viruses, bacteria, and parasitic cells. Macrophages engulf and destroy cellular debris, damaged cells, and foreign substances.

Lymph Node Circulation

A variety of *afferent lymphatic vessels* conducts lymph through the convex side of each lymph node. The lymph moves through a large *subcapsular sinus* into many smaller sinuses crossing the cortex and entering the *medullary sinuses*. It eventually leaves the lymph node at its *hilum* though *efferent lymphatic vessels*. There are more afferent vessels supplying

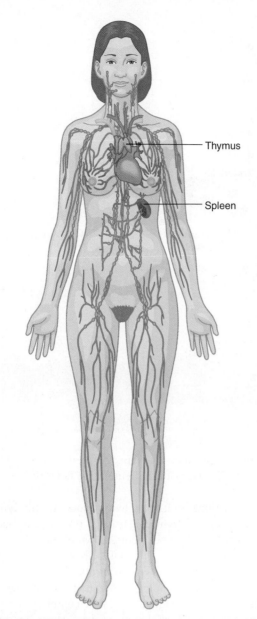

FIGURE 18-6 Lymphatic vessels.

the lymph node than efferent vessels draining it. Therefore, lymph becomes somewhat stagnant. During this slowed movement, macrophages and lymphocytes can "examine" the lymph more closely. The lymph passes through several lymph nodes before it is totally cleansed.

TEST YOUR UNDERSTANDING

1. Describe the general functions of the lymph nodes.
2. Describe the general size of the lymph nodes and their primary locations in the body.
3. Explain lymphoid follicles and the lymphocytes that dominate in their germinal centers.
4. Why do lymph nodes have more afferent lymphatics than efferent lymphatics?

Thymus

The **thymus** is located in the thorax, anterior to the aorta and posterior to the upper sternum. It is soft and consists of two lobes enclosed in a connective tissue capsule (**FIGURE 18-7**). Although relatively large in infancy and early childhood, the thymus shrinks after puberty, becoming much smaller in adults. Its lymphatic tissue is replaced during the later years of life by adipose and connective tissues. The thymus is highly active during the first year of life. It continues to produce **immunocompetent** cells throughout life, but this production declines with aging.

The thymus is divided into lobules by inward-extending connective tissues or *septa*. Each lobule has a dense outer *cortex* and a central *medulla* that is paler in color. The lobules contain large amounts of lymphocytes, including primarily inactive thymocytes. Some thymocytes mature into T lymphocytes, which leave the thymus after 3 weeks and provide immunity in the body. Thymosins are secreted by the thymus's reticular epithelial cells and cause T lymphocytes to mature. In the medulla, these cells form *thymic corpuscles*, also called *Hassall's corpuscles*. In the cortex of the thymus, lymphocytes are densely packed during their rapid division. Lesser numbers of macrophages are scattered throughout this area.

The thymus is different from other lymphoid organs in three major ways. First, it lacks B cells and therefore has no follicles. Second, the thymus does not directly fight antigens, unlike every other lymphoid organ. It is simply a place where T-lymphocyte precursors can mature and be isolated from foreign antigens so they are not prematurely activated. A *blood–thymus barrier* stops bloodborne antigens from entering the thymus. Third, its stroma consists of epithelial cells and not reticular fibers. These cells create the chemical and physical environment needed for T-lymphocyte maturation.

Spleen

The **spleen** is located in the upper left abdominal cavity, inferior to the diaphragm and posterior and lateral to the stomach. It is the body's largest lymphatic organ, resembling

FOCUS ON PATHOLOGY

Large numbers of bacteria or other potential pathogens can overwhelm a lymph node. When this happens, the lymph node becomes swollen, inflamed, and tender to the touch. Infected lymph nodes are called *buboes*. A lymph node may also develop into a secondary cancer site. This often occurs when metastasis of cancer cells occurs into lymphatic vessels. However, lymph nodes infiltrated by cancer cells are usually not painful and only feel swollen. This helps in the identification of cancerous lymph nodes rather than infected ones. Chronic or excessive lymph node enlargement is known as *lymphadenopathy*.

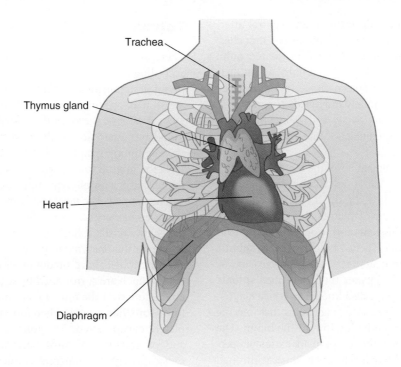

FIGURE 18-7 The thymus.

a large, subdivided lymph node. The spleen is about as large as an adult's fist and is attached to the stomach's lateral border by a broad band of mesentery known as the *gastrosplenic ligament*. The spleen is a soft organ that contains the largest amount of lymphatic tissue and lymphoid nodules in an adult's body. It differs from lymph nodes in that its venous sinuses are filled with blood, not lymph. The two types of tissues inside the splenic lobules (**FIGURE 18-8**) are white and red pulp.

■ *White pulp* is located throughout the spleen in small "islands," made up of splenic nodules containing many proliferating lymphocytes. Immune function occurs in the white pulp, which is primarily made up of lymphocytes suspended on reticular fibers.

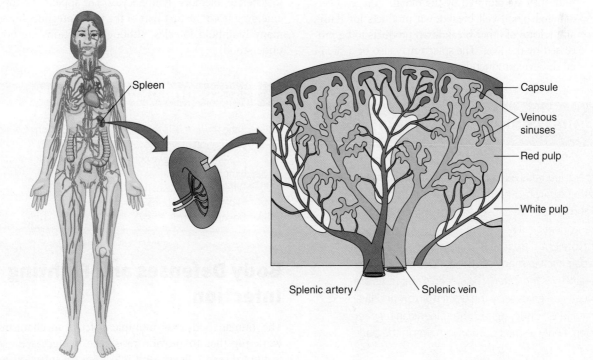

FIGURE 18-8 The structures of the spleen.

Clusters of white pulp form around central arteries, which are the small splenic artery branches, making them appear as "islands" in the red pulp. The names "white pulp" and "red pulp" reflect their appearance in fresh spleen tissue, not how they stain to be microscopically examined. The *trabecular arteries* branch extensively, and white pulp surrounds their finer branches. Capillaries move blood into the *red pulp*.

■ *Red pulp* fills the remainder of the lobules. Basically, all splenic tissue that is not white pulp is considered to make up the red pulp. It contains many red blood cells and macrophages. In the red pulp, bloodborne pathogens and worn out red blood cells are destroyed. The red pulp consists of **splenic cords**, which are areas of reticular connective tissue. The splenic cords separate the blood-filled **splenic sinusoids**, which are also known as *venous sinuses*. The sinusoids empty into small veins that join the *trabecular veins*, continuing toward the hilum. The blood capillaries of the red pulp are extremely permeable, and red blood cells easily squeeze through the capillary walls to enter the venous sinuses. Older red blood cells may be damaged during this process and so are engulfed by macrophages inside the splenic sinuses. Via the action of macrophages and lymphocytes, the spleen filters blood similarly to the way that lymph nodes filter lymph. The large splenic artery and vein serve the spleen, entering and exiting its hilum on the concave anterior surface. Immune surveillance and response occur to a great degree in the spleen, but its cleansing of blood may be its most important function. Other functions of the spleen include storage of blood platelets and monocytes until they are required by the blood, storage of certain red blood cell breakdown products for reuse, and release of other breakdown products to be processed by the liver. The spleen may also be a site of erythrocyte production in the unborn fetus.

FOCUS ON PATHOLOGY

The spleen has a very thin capsule and may be rather easily ruptured by severe infections or direct trauma. Rupture causes blood to spill into the peritoneal cavity. Although *splenectomy* was once the preferred treatment, the spleen can actually repair itself in many circumstances. When splenectomy is indicated, the spleen's functions are mostly taken over by the bone marrow and liver. In children under age 12 the spleen can regenerate even if only a small portion remains in the body.

Tonsils

There are a variety of different **tonsils**, which are named according to their location. The tonsils create a ring of lymphoid tissue surrounding the entrance to the pharynx. They are seen as swellings of the mucosa. The two **palatine tonsils** are largest, the ones that usually get infected, and are found on either side of the posterior end of the oral cavity. The lumpy lymphoid follicles at the base of the tongue form the **lingual tonsil**. The **pharyngeal tonsil** is located in the posterior nasopharynx and is referred to as the *adenoids* when enlarged. The *tubal tonsils* are very small and surround the openings of the auditory tubes at the pharynx. Collectively, the tonsils collect and remove a variety of pathogens that enter the pharynx, in inhaled air, or in food.

The tonsils have predominant germinal centers in follicles, which are surrounded by scattered lymphocytes. The epithelium over the tonsils continues deeply inside them to form **tonsillar crypts**. Therefore, the tonsils are not completely encapsulated. The tonsillar crypts collect bacteria and other particles. Most bacteria are destroyed as they move through the mucosal epithelium into the lymphoid tissue of the tonsils. This procedure causes many immune cells to be produced that remember the various trapped pathogens.

Peyer's Patches and Appendix

Peyer's patches, also known as the *aggregated lymphoid nodules*, are found in the walls of the distal small intestine (ileum). They are large, clustered lymphoid follicles that resemble the tonsils. Along with the **appendix**, **Peyer's patches** are located extremely well for the destruction of bacteria and also to generate "memory" lymphocytes. The appendix is tube-like, emerging from the first part of the large intestine. It contains many lymphoid follicles, although its actions are not fully understood.

TEST YOUR UNDERSTANDING

1. If the thymus fails to produce thymic hormones, which population of lymphocytes will be affected?
2. Explain which organ contains the largest amount of lymphatic tissue.
3. Differentiate between white pulp and red pulp.
4. Explain the functions of the tonsils.
5. Define the terms *Peyer's patches* and *appendix*.

Body Defenses and Fighting Infection

The human body has multiple defense mechanisms that work together to provide resistance, which is the ability to fight disease, illness, and infection. An infection may be caused by the presence and multiplication of a disease-causing agent or **pathogen**, which can be a virus, bacterium, fungus, or protozoan. Body defenses can be divided into two general categories: innate or nonspecific and adaptive or specific defenses. **Innate (nonspecific) defense** defends against many different types of pathogens. This type of defense, which is present at birth, includes **mechanical barriers**, **chemical barriers**, NK cells, inflammation, **phagocytosis**, fever, and species resistance.

Specific defenses are more precise and target specific pathogens to provide **adaptive (specific) defense** or **immunity**. In this type of defense, specialized lymphocytes recognize foreign molecules and act against them. Both innate and adaptive defense mechanisms work together to fight infection. Innate defenses act more rapidly than adaptive defenses. Specific defenses depend on the activity of lymphocytes.

Innate (Nonspecific) Defenses

Our innate or nonspecific defenses prevent or limit microorganisms and other environmental hazards from approaching, entering, or spreading. These defenses are often able to prevent infection by destroying pathogens, without needing the help of any other defenses. Sometimes, however, the adaptive immune system is needed to assist the nonspecific defenses. Nonspecific defenses are the first line of defense and include intact skin and mucosae. When pathogens penetrate the skin or mucosae, the second line of defense is activated. This relies on internal defenses, including antimicrobial proteins and phagocytes. *Inflammation* is the most important process in the second line of defense. The nonspecific defenses are classified as mechanical barriers, which cover body surfaces, and chemical substances, which are involved with invading pathogens.

Mechanical Barriers

Also known as *physical barriers*, mechanical barriers include the skin and the mucous membranes that line the respiratory system, digestive system, urinary system basement membranes, and reproductive passageways. They protect against certain infectious agents. The body's hair, sweat, and mucus also act as mechanical barriers. The mechanical barriers of immunity are ready to act when we are born. The skin's keratinized epithelial membrane stops most microorganisms on the skin from penetrating it. Keratin itself resists many weak bases and acids as well as toxins and bacterial enzymes. Inside the body, the mucous membranes function in much the same capacity.

Chemical Barriers

Provided by enzymes and other chemical substances in body fluids, these include pepsin and hydrochloric acid in the stomach; tears; **lysozyme** in tears, saliva, breast milk, and mucus; salt in perspiration; interferons; mucin; *defensins*; certain lipids in sebum; *dermicidin*; and complement. Interferons and complement proteins are the most important antimicrobial proteins in the body:

- **Interferons** are hormone-like peptides that bind to uninfected cells and stimulate them to make protective proteins. Interferons are secreted by infected cells and diffuse to nearby cells, stimulating protein synthesis that interferes with viral replication. Interferons block viral RNA from synthesizing proteins and also degrade the viral RNA itself. *Interferon-α* and *-β* also activate NK cells. *Interferon-γ*, also known as *immune interferon*, is secreted by lymphocytes. It activates macrophages and has wide ranging immune mobilization effects.

- *Acid mantle* components inhibit bacterial growth. These consist of the acidity of the skin, stomach secretions, and vagina.

- *Enzymes* such as *lysozyme* destroy bacteria. Lysozyme is found in the respiratory mucus, lacrimal fluid of the eye, and saliva. In the stomach, protein-digesting enzymes kill a variety of different microorganisms.

- *Mucin* is a substance that forms mucus when dissolved in water. This mucus is thick and sticky, lining the passageway of the digestive and respiratory systems. It functions to trap a variety of microorganisms. The mucin of the saliva is different in that it traps microorganisms but washes them from the mouth to the stomach, where they are digested.

- *Defensins* are broad-spectrum antimicrobial peptides secreted from the skin and mucous membranes. They are produced in much higher quantities when surface barriers are breached and inflammation develops. They help to control colonization by bacteria and fungi in different ways, including disruption of the membranes of these microorganisms.

- *Dermicidin* found in eccrine sweat is toxic to bacteria, similar to the effects of certain lipids in the body's sebum.

- *Complement* is a group of proteins in plasma and other body fluids that interact to cause inflammation and phagocytic activities. Plasma contains at least 20 special complement or *C* proteins that comprise the complement system, including proteins C1 through C9; factors called B, D, and P; and also several proteins that have a regulatory effect. The term *complement* refers to the way this system "complements" the action of antibodies. The complement proteins interact in chain reactions or *cascades* that are similar to those of the clotting system. Activated complement also acts by lysing and killing certain cells and bacteria. There are additional chemical barriers in the respiratory tract mucosae. When microorganisms make it past the chemical barriers, the internal innate defenses begin to combat them. Interferons are not *virus-specific*, and those produced against a certain virus protect against other viruses as well. The interferons are a group of immune modulating proteins with slightly different effects. They also play an indirect role in fighting cancer.

Fever

Fever is the elevation of body temperature that reduces iron in the blood, which inhibits bacterial and fungal reproduction; fever also causes increased phagocytosis by macrophages. Fever is a systemic response to invading microorganisms. Exposure of leukocytes and macrophages to foreign substances causes the release of *pyrogens*, which cause the hypothalamus to raise the body temperature. As a result of fever, the spleen and liver keep iron and zinc away from the rest of the body somewhat so they cannot be used to support bacterial growth. Cells are repaired more quickly because fever increases their metabolic rate. Active macrophages release a cytokine that is called *endogenous pyrogen* or *interleukin-1*.

Inflammation

Inflammation is a tissue response to injury or infection that may include four *cardinal signs*: redness, swelling, heat, and pain. Infected cells attract white blood cells, which engulf them. *Impaired function* is a fifth occurrence that many experts consider to be the fifth cardinal sign of inflammation. When functions such as movement become impaired, the injured area may be temporarily forced to rest so it can heal. Masses of leukocytes, bacterial cells, and damaged tissue may form a thick fluid called **pus**. The body may react to inflammation by forming a network of fibrin threads where the infection is centered. This closes off the infected area to inhibit the spread of pathogens. *An inflammatory response* is triggered when mast cells release histamine, serotonin, and heparin. The inflammatory response is a tissue-level reaction and is therefore related to the tissues and integumentary system. The inflammatory response helps to dispose of pathogens and cell debris, triggers the adaptive immune system to act, and prepares the body to repair damaged tissues.

Inflammatory chemicals may be released by injured tissue cells, stressed tissue cells, and immune cells. They can also be formed by *mast cells*. The strong inflammatory chemical known as *histamine* is released by mast cells. Macrophages are able to recognize invaders and trigger a chemical response by using surface membrane or *toll-like* receptors. Additionally, inflammatory chemicals such as *kinins, prostaglandins,* and *complement* help to dilate localized arterioles and cause additional leakage from localized capillaries. They may cause leukocytes to be attracted to an injured area for additional inflammatory actions.

The redness and heat of inflammation are caused by vasodilation. Local *hyperemia* occurs when local arterioles dilate, which means that there is congestion in the area with blood. Fluid containing clotting factors and antibodies, known as *exudate*, leaks from the blood into the tissue spaces, causing local swelling or *edema*. This condition increases pain by pressing on nearby nerve endings. Bacterial toxins that are released also contribute to pain. Released prostaglandins and kinins contribute to sensitizing effects, and pain relief by aspirin or other anti-inflammatory drugs is based on the inhibition of prostaglandin synthesis.

Phagocytosis

Injured tissues attract neutrophils and monocytes, which engulf and digest particles such as pathogens and cell debris; monocytes influence the development of macrophages that attach to blood and lymphatic vessels. Neutrophils, along with eosinophils, are termed *microphages* because of their smaller size. Together, these various phagocytic cells make up the **mononuclear phagocytic system** to remove foreign particles from the lymph and blood. Neutrophils are the most abundant and begin to engulf invaders when they find infectious material in the body tissues. *Macrophages* are larger in size, mostly derived from monocytes, and provide most phagocytic activities. Both free and fixed types of macrophages exist, which are similar in structure and function. The free macrophages search tissue spaces for invaders or cellular debris. Fixed macrophages live permanently inside certain organs, such as the liver's *stellate macrophages*. All the various phagocytes are collectively called the *monocyte macrophage system* or *reticuloendothelial system*.

NK Cells

Natural killer (NK) cells patrol the blood and lymph as part of **immunologic surveillance**. They are able to lyse and kill both cancer and viral cells before activation of the adaptive immune system. They are part of the cells known as *large granular leukocytes* and have wider actions against pathogens than the lymphocytes of the adaptive immune system. They detect generalized abnormalities, such as when cell-surface proteins known as major histocompatibility complex (MHC) are lacking. However, they are not phagocytic and kill by contacting target cells directly, in the same way as cytotoxic T cells kill. Cytotoxic T cells secrete a poisonous *lymphotoxin* that kills target cells. The inflammatory response is increased by strong chemicals secreted by NK cells. NK cells recognize abnormal cells, adhere to them, and use their Golgi apparatus to produce *perforins*, which are proteins that diffuse to the target cell. The perforins create holes or pores in the target cell's membrane, resulting in lysis of the abnormal cell. NK cells attack cancer cells and those infected with viruses. The plasma membranes of cancer cells contain *tumor-specific antigens*, which the NK cells use to find them. Some cancer cells can destroy NK cells, via a process of either avoiding their detection or neutralizing body defenses. This process is called *immunological escape*.

Species Resistance

A final form of innate, nonspecific defense is **species resistance**. For example, a human may be resistant to certain diseases that affect other species of animals. A pathogen effective against a dog, for example, may be unable to survive in a human. In reverse, humans can be infected with measles, gonorrhea, mumps, and syphilis, none of which affects other animal species.

Pus, which is a mixture of pathogens, neutrophils, and broken-down tissue cells, may accumulate in wounds that have become severely infected. Collagen fibers may form, creating a pustular sac and forming an abscess. Before healing may occur, an abscess may require surgical drainage. Certain bacteria resist digestion by macrophages and instead remain safe inside them. An example is tuberculosis bacilli, which are therefore highly resistant to prescription antibiotics. *Infectious granulomas*, which are tumor-like growths, then form. They have a central area of infected macrophages that is surrounded by noninfected macrophages and a fibrous capsule on the outside. Pathogens may remain in granulomas for years without causing symptoms, only to emerge when the immune system is weakened.

Immunity (Specific) Defenses

Immunity, or *adaptive specific defenses*, also known as the *third line of defense*, is defined as resistance to specific pathogens or their toxins and metabolic byproducts. Adaptive immune responses are carried out by lymphocytes and macrophages that recognize and remember certain foreign molecules. As a fetus develops, cells learn to recognize proteins and large molecules as being "self." The lymphatic system, as it develops, responds to "nonself" or foreign antigens and not, if the system is normal, the "self" antigens. Immunity is therefore "triggered" by initial exposures to antigens. After exposure, it can effectively protect the body. When immunity is disabled or fails to protect the body, serious diseases such as AIDS or cancer can develop. The actions of the adaptive immune system greatly increase the inflammatory response. Most complement activation also occurs because of this system.

Complement activation involves the *classical pathway* and the *alternative pathway*. The classical pathway is the fastest and most effective pathway, beginning with binding of complement protein C1 to an antibody, already attached to its specific antigen, which may be a bacterial cell wall. When antibody molecules are absent, the *alternative* or *properdin pathway* activates the complement system. This slow, less effective pathway begins when *properdin* or *factor P*, *factor B*, and *factor D* interact in the plasma. These are all various types of complement proteins. This interaction may be triggered by exposure to foreign materials. The alternative pathway also ends, like the classical pathway, with conversion of inactive C3 protein into activated C3b protein. The activation of complement results in formation of pores, increased phagocytosis, and release of histamine.

Antigens

Antigens include proteins, polysaccharides, glycoproteins, and glycolipids that are commonly found on cell surfaces. Antigens can mobilize adaptive defenses and cause an immune response. All adaptive immune responses ultimately target antigens, which are usually large and complex molecules not normally present in the body. Antigens may be natural or synthetic in nature and *complete* or *incomplete*. *Complete antigens* have both immunogenicity and reactivity. **Immunogenicity** is the ability to stimulate certain lymphocytes to multiply. **Reactivity** is the ability to react with activated lymphocytes and antibodies that are released via immunogenic reactions. Proteins are the strongest types of antigens. Microorganisms and grains of pollen are immunogenic because their surfaces hold many different types of foreign macromolecules.

A small molecule, or *incomplete antigen*, which cannot stimulate an immune response by itself, is known as a **hapten**. It is found in certain drugs such as penicillin, in dust particles, animal dander, poison ivy, detergents, cosmetics, and in various household and industrial chemicals. Haptens usually combine with larger, more complex molecules to elicit an immune response.

Before birth, red bone marrow releases lymphocyte precursors, about half of which reach the thymus. They specialize into *T lymphocytes or T cells*, which later make up between 70% and 80% of circulated blood lymphocytes. T lymphocytes do not produce antibodies and make up the cellular component of adaptive immunity. Other T cells exist in lymphatic organs, particularly in lymph nodes, the white pulp of the spleen, and the thoracic duct. Others remain in the red bone marrow, eventually differentiating into *B lymphocytes or B cells*. They are distributed by the blood and make up between 20% and 30% of the circulating lymphocytes. B cells are abundant in the lymph nodes, bone marrow, intestinal lining, and spleen. B lymphocytes control humoral immunity and do not activate naive T cells. They present antigens to *helper T cells*, which in turn help to activate the B cells. Cell surface proteins that identify cells as "self" include various glycoproteins known as *MHC proteins*. The genes of the MHC code for these glycoproteins. Because there are millions of possible combinations, any two people, except identical twins, are unlikely to have the same MHC proteins.

Humoral Immune Response

The humoral immune response involves B lymphocytes. This response is provoked when a B cell encounters its antigen. In the humoral immune response, antibodies specific for that antigen are manufactured.

Activation of B Cells

An antigen encountered by a B cell provokes the *humoral immune response*. As a result, antibodies that are specific for that antigen develop. A naive, immunocompetent B lymphocyte becomes *activated* when its surface receptors are bound to matching antigens. Cross-linking occurs of the adjacent receptors. Most cloned cells differentiate into **plasma cells**. The plasma cells are humoral response *effector cells* that secrete antibodies. They secrete antibodies at a rate of approximately 2,000 molecules every second. This activity continues for between 4 and 5 days before each plasma cell dies. The secreted antibodies have the identical antigen-binding properties as the receptor molecules of the parent B lymphocyte's surface. These secreted antibodies circulate in blood or lymph. **Memory cells** develop from any clone cells that do not become plasma cells. If these cells encounter the same antigen later, they can cause a humoral response almost immediately (**FIGURE 18-9**).

Immunological Memory

A *primary immune response* is constituted by activation of B cells or T cells after they first encounter the antigens for which they are specialized to react. This usually occurs within 3 to 6 days. Over nearly this same period of time, B cells specific for that antigen proliferate into approximately 12 generations. Plasma antibody levels increase after a mobilization period to reach their peak within about 10 days and then decline. Plasma cells release antibodies into the lymph, followed by IgG. The antibodies are transported to the blood and throughout the body to help destroy antigen-bearing agents. This continues for several weeks.

Some of the B cells then remain as memory cells so if the identical antigen is reencountered, clones of these memory cells enlarge and send IgG to the antigen. These memory B cells, along with memory T cells, produce a *secondary immune response*. After a primary immune response, detectable concentrations of antibodies appear in the blood plasma, usually 5 to 10 days after exposure to antigens, and a secondary immune response can then occur within 1 to 2 days. Memory cells live much longer than newly formed antibodies, which live between a few months and a few years. Secondary immune responses occur faster, with more effectiveness, than primary immune responses. They also last longer. The memory cells are "ready for action" because they were previously alerted to antigens. Therefore, these cells provide *immunological memory*.

Memory T_C cells are produced in the same way as cytotoxic T cells. They do not differentiate any more after an antigen triggers an immune response. When the antigen appears again, however, memory T cells immediately differentiate into cytotoxic T cells, which a fast and deadly response. *Memory helper T cells* are produced along with active helper T cells when the helper T cells that have CD4 T markers are activated and then divide.

Active Humoral Immunity *Active humoral immunity* is signified by antibodies produced by B cells after encountering antigens. Active humoral immunity is acquired either *naturally* or *artificially*. Examples of natural means of acquiring active humoral immunity include development of bacterial or viral infections, whereas examples of artificial means of acquiring active humoral immunity include **vaccines**. Most vaccines contain dead or *attenuated* pathogens or components of them. The term "attenuated" means the pathogens are extremely weakened but still alive. There are two major benefits of vaccines: they do not cause most of the uncomfortable signs and symptoms that normally occur during the primary response, and their weakened antigens provide immunogenic, reactive functional determinants of antigens. During the primary response, the level of antibody activity in the plasma, or *antibody titer*, does not peak until 1 to 2 weeks after the initial exposure. **TABLE 18-1** explains the various types of acquired immunity.

Booster shots are vaccines that can intensify the immune response when the same antigen is encountered at a later time. Diseases that have been eradicated, nearly eradicated, or extremely weakened by vaccines include smallpox, measles, polio, and whooping cough. In the United States, unfortunately, immunization of adults seems to be of less importance to many people than immunization of children. Even so, vaccines have greatly reduced serious outcomes from hepatitis B, influenza, pneumonia, and tetanus.

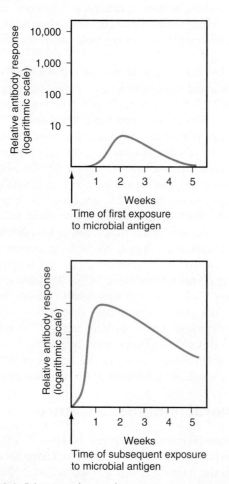

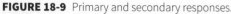

FIGURE 18-9 Primary and secondary responses.

TABLE 18-1

Types of Acquired Immunity

Type	Exposure	Outcome
Artificially acquired active immunity	Exposure to vaccine containing weakened or killed pathogens or their components	Immune response is stimulated without severe disease symptoms
Artificially acquired passive immunity	Injection of gamma globulin containing antibodies	Short-term immunity without an immune response
Naturally acquired active immunity	Exposure to live pathogens	Immune response is stimulated with disease symptoms
Naturally acquired passive immunity	Antibodies passed from mother who has active immunity to her fetus or to newborn via breast milk from mother who has active immunity	Short-term immunity for newborn without an immune response

Passive Humoral Immunity *Passive humoral immunity* is different from active humoral immunity in two major ways: the amount of protection it provides and its antibody source. In passive humoral immunity, antibodies are introduced into the body. Therefore, antigens do not challenge B lymphocytes. No immunologic memory occurs, and the introduced antibodies eventually degrade, ending their protection. When a fetus or infant is affected by antibodies from the mother's placenta or milk, passive immunity is transferred *naturally*. The baby is protected from all antigens to which the mother was previously exposed for several months after he or she is born.

An example of the *artificial* transference of passive humoral immunity is when exogenous antibodies such as *gamma globulin* are administered. These may be collected from the plasma of an immune donor. Examples of the use of exogenous antibodies include the prevention of botulism, hepatitis A, rabies, and as an antivenom to poisonous snakebites or antitoxin to tetanus. These diseases have the ability to be rapidly fatal. Therefore, because active immunity takes too long to occur, artificial passive humoral immunity can save the lives of people who contract them. Antibodies used in this type of immunity have short-lived effects of only 2 to 3 weeks but provide immediate protection.

TEST YOUR UNDERSTANDING

1. Explain how active humoral immunity may be acquired.
2. Describe how vaccines protect children against various common illnesses.
3. Describe how active and passive immunity differ.

Antibodies

B cells divide and differentiate into plasma cells, producing **antibodies** or *immunoglobulins* that react to destroy antigens or antigen-containing particles. This is called the **humoral immune response**. There are millions of different types of T and B cells. Each variety originates from a single early cell to form a **clone** of cells identical to the original cell. Each variety

has a certain antigen receptor responding to only a specific antigen. **TABLE 18-2** compares characteristics of T and B cells. Humoral immunity is also called *antibody-mediated immunity*. Its name comes from the antibodies that are present in the body fluids, which used to be referred to as the body's "humors." Antibodies are produced by lymphocytes and circulate in the blood and lymph, where they mostly bind to *extracellular targets* such as free viruses, bacteria, and bacterial toxins.

Antibodies, also known as *immunoglobulins or Igs,* make up the **gamma globulin** portion of blood proteins. These proteins are secreted as a response to an antigen by the plasma cells. Antibodies bind specifically with that antigen. They are formed as a response to many different antigens.

Each antibody has four looped polypeptide chains connected by sulfur-to-sulfur or disulfide bonds. The chains form a molecule known as an **antibody monomer**. This monomer

TABLE 18-2

Comparison of T and B Cells (Lymphocytes)

T Cells	B Cells
Originate in red bone marrow	Originate in red bone marrow
Differentiate in the thymus (a primary lymphoid organ)	Differentiate in red bone marrow (also a primary lymphoid organ)
Primarily located in lymphatic tissues	Primarily located in lymphatic tissues
Make up 70%–80% of circulating lymphocytes	Make up 20%–30% of circulating lymphocytes
Provide cellular immune response	Provide humoral immune response
Interact directly with antigens or antigen-bearing agents to destroy them	Interact indirectly to produce antibodies that destroy antigens or antigen-bearing agents

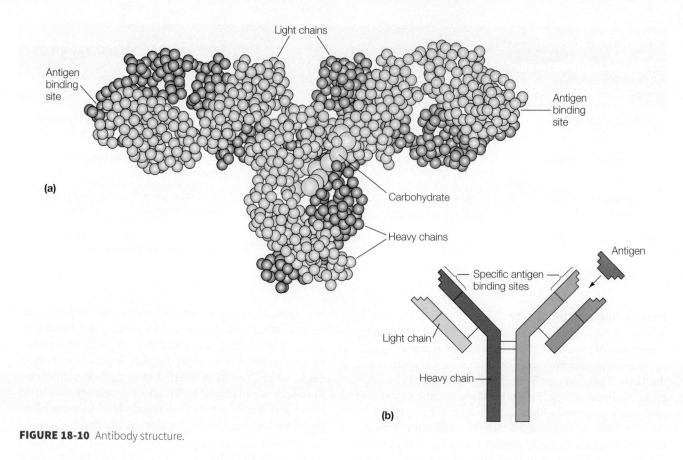

FIGURE 18-10 Antibody structure.

has two halves that are identical. Overall, the antibody monomer is shaped like a "Y" or a "T" (**FIGURE 18-10**). The two *heavy or H chains* of a monomer are identical to each other. The other two *light or L chains* are only half as long as each H chain but are also identical to each other. Near their middles, the heavy chains have a *hinge region* that is flexible. On each chain the loops are made up of disulfide bonds. These bonds cause the intervening parts of the polypeptide chains to "loop out."

At the other end of each chain, there is a **variable (V) region** at one end and a **constant (C) region** at the other. Extremely different V regions exist in antibodies that respond to different regions. However, their C regions are nearly the same, or identical, in all antibodies of the same class. The V regions of the heavy and light chains make up an **antigen-binding site** that has a shape fitting a certain antigenic determinant. As a result, in each monomer arm, each antibody monomer has two of these antigen-binding regions.

The *stem* of the antibody monomer is formed by two C regions, which determine the class of antibody. They also have common functions in all antibodies. The C regions are the *effector regions* of the antibody. They determine the body's cells and chemicals to which the antibody may bind. They also determine how the antibody class eliminates antigens. Some antibodies circulate in the blood, whereas others are found mostly in body secretions. Others fix complement, and still others can cross the barrier of the placenta. Many other functions exist.

Antibodies commonly attack antigens directly, activate complement, or stimulate *inflammation*. They combine with antigens, causing clumping or *agglutination* or forming insoluble substances, which is known as *precipitation*. Phagocytosis then can occur more easily. Sometimes antibodies neutralize the toxic effects of antigens. Complement activation is generally more important in protecting against infection than direct antibody attack, however. Antigens that are close together may result in antibodies binding to antigenic determinant sites on two separate antigens. The antibodies can then link many antigens together, creating a three-dimensional *immune complex*.

When certain antibodies combine with antigens, they trigger many reactions that lead to the activation of the complement proteins. Effects include coating the antigen–antibody complexes or **opsonization**, attracting macrophages and neutrophils in a process called **chemotaxis**, making the complexes more susceptible to phagocytosis, clumping antigen-bearing cells, rupturing foreign cell membranes via lysis, and altering viral molecular structures to make them harmless. In all types of macrophages, phagocytosis begins with *adhesion*, which is the attachment of a phagocyte to its target.

Immunoglobulin Groups   The major five groups of immunoglobulins are IgM, IgA, IgD, IgG, and IgE. These groups are defined according to the basis of the C regions in the heavy chains. **TABLE 18-3** explains each class of immunoglobulins. Compared with the others, IgM in the blood plasma is much larger. It is made up of five *monomers* or Y-shaped units that are linked, forming a *pentamer*, which has five parts. A monomer with one part, or a *dimer* with two parts, may be formed by IgA. The other immunoglobulins all are monomers, with similar Y-shaped structures.

TABLE 18-3

Immunoglobulin Groups

Immunoglobulin	Actions	Description
IgM (pentamer)	The first Ig secreted by plasma cells during primary response; it fixes and activates complement.	IgM in plasma usually indicates current pathogen infection; the monomer form acts as an antigen receptor on B-cell surfaces; the pentamer form circulates in plasma; it has many antigen-binding sites and is a strong agglutinating agent.
IgA (dimer)	The dimer form is known as *secretory IgA*, which is found in saliva, sweat, intestinal secretions, and milk; it helps to stop pathogens from attaching to epithelial cell surfaces, such as those of the epidermis and mucous membranes.	The monomer form is found in only limited amounts in plasma.
IgD (monomer)	It functions as a B-cell antigen receptor (similar to IgM).	Located on B-cell surfaces.
IgG (monomer)	Found in highest numbers of all groups in the plasma; it makes up 75%–85% of circulating antibodies; it is the primary antibody of both secondary and late primary responses and fixes as well as activates complement.	Protects against bacteria, toxins, and viruses in the blood and lymph; it crosses the placenta to confer passive immunity from mother to fetus.
IgE (monomer)	The stem ends of IgE bind to basophils or mast cells; antigens bind to its receptor end, triggering release of histamine and other chemicals that mediate allergic reactions and inflammation.	It is secreted by plasma cells in the skin, gastrointestinal mucosae, respiratory mucosae, and tonsils; is only found in trace amounts in plasma; its levels increase during chronic parasitic infections of the gastrointestinal tract or during severe allergic attacks.

TEST YOUR UNDERSTANDING

1. Describe the common effects of antibodies.
2. Contrast the basic differences between T cells and B cells.
3. Explain the five immunoglobulin groups.

Cell-Mediated Immunity

T cells attach to foreign, antigen-bearing cells such as bacterial cells and interact with direct cell-to-cell contact. This is known as **cellular immune response** or cell-mediated immunity. T cells, along with some macrophages, also synthesize polypeptides called *cytokines* that enhance responses to antigens. *Interleukin-1* and *interleukin-2* stimulate synthesis of cytokines from other T cells. Other cytokines, called *colony-stimulating factors*, stimulate leukocyte production in red bone marrow, activate macrophages, and cause B cells to grow. In the cellular immune response, lymphocytes themselves defend the body. The targets of cell-mediated immunity are cancer cells, cells of foreign grafts, and tissue cells infected with viruses or parasites. Lymphocytes either directly kill infected cells or cause their death by releasing their chemicals that enhance inflammation or activate other lymphocytes or macrophages. Both B and T lymphocytes acquire immunocompetence and *self-tolerance* in different locations in the body.

Certain activated T cells kill body cells that are infected by bacteria or viruses directly. They also may directly kill cells that are cancerous or abnormal and cells from foreign tissues that have been transplanted or infused. Different T cells release chemicals that regulate the immune response. T cells that mediate cellular immunity are much more complicated in function and classification that B cells. The two primary types of T cells are identified by *cell differentiation glycoproteins* known as CD4 or CD8. Both are surface receptors that are different from T cell antigen receptors and help with interactions between other cells and T cells. Activation of naive CD4 and CD8 cells causes them to differentiate into three types of *effector cells*, called *helper T cells, cytotoxic T cells,* or *regulatory T cells*. Activated CD4 and CD8 cells can also become *memory T cells*. All T cells have a *CD3 receptor complex* in the plasma membranes that eventually activates them to recognize antigens.

Antigen-Presenting Cells Before it can respond to an antigen, a lymphocyte must be activated. T cells are activated by the presence of processed antigen fragments attached to the surface of an **antigen-presenting cell**, also called an *accessory cell*, which may be macrophages, B cells, or other types of cells. Antigen-presenting cells have important auxiliary functions in regard to antigens and respond to them differently than lymphocytes do. When a macrophage phagocytizes a bacterium and digests it in its lysosomes, T-cell activation begins. Some bacterial antigens then move to the surface of the macrophage.

They are displayed near certain protein molecules that make up the *MHC*. MHC antigens help T cells recognize foreign antigens. Helper T cells contact displayed foreign antigens. If the antigen combines with the helper T cell's antigen receptors, it becomes activated and stimulates a B cell to produce antibodies specific for the displayed antigen. The membrane glycoproteins formed as part of the MHC are known as *MHC proteins* or *human leukocyte antigens*.

Class I MHC proteins are found in the plasma membrane of every nucleated cell. Their activation eventually results in destruction of abnormal cells, which is a significant component why donated organs are often rejected. *Class II MHC proteins* are only found in plasma membranes of antigen-presenting cells and lymphocytes. Phagocytic antigen-presenting cells break down and engulf foreign antigens or pathogens. This *antigen processing* creates antigen fragments, which become bound to class II MHC proteins and then inserted into the plasma membrane. The class II MHC proteins only appear in the plasma membrane when the cell is processing antigens. **TABLE 18-4** summarizes B cell and T cell antibody production activities.

TABLE 18-4

Antibody Production by B and T Cells

B Cell	T Cell
Antigen-bearing agents enter tissues.	Antigen-bearing agents enter tissues.
An antigen that fits antigen receptors is encountered.	An accessory cell phagocytizes the antigen-bearing agent and lysosomes digest the agent.
Activation occurs, and the B cell proliferates, enlarging its clone.	Antigens are displayed on the membrane of the accessory cell.
Further differentiation occurs as B cells become plasma cells.	A helper T cell activates when it encounters a displayed antigen fitting its antigen receptors.
Plasma cells synthesize and secrete antibodies with molecular structure similar to that of activated B-cell antigen receptors.	The activated helper T cell releases cytokines when encountering a B cell that has combined with an identical antigen-bearing agent.
Antibodies combine with antigen-bearing agents to help destroy them.	Cytokines stimulate B-cell proliferation.
	Some newly formed B cells give rise to cells differentiating into antibody-secreting plasma cells.
	Antibodies combine with antigen-bearing agents to help destroy them.

TEST YOUR UNDERSTANDING

1. Explain the actions of lymphocytes in cell-mediated immunity.
2. Differentiate between the ways that lymphocytes and antigen-presenting cells respond to antigens.
3. Explain the primary functions of helper T cells.

Imbalance of Immune System Homeostasis

The production or function of immune cells or specific molecules may be impaired. A congenital or acquired condition that causes this to occur is termed an *immunodeficiency*. Complement and antibodies may both be impaired. *AIDS* is the most devastating condition affecting the immune system because it interferes with the actions of the helper T cells. AIDS was first identified in the United States in 1981, primarily among homosexual men and intravenous drug users. It is signified by night sweats, severe weight loss, frequent opportunistic infections, swollen lymph nodes, a rare pneumonia called *pneumocystis pneumonia*, and *Kaposi's sarcoma*, a cancer affecting blood vessels that causes purple-colored lesions on the skin. In many cases, AIDS results in total debilitation, with death caused by overwhelming infections or cancer.

FOCUS ON PATHOLOGY

Severe combined immunodeficiency disease or *SCID* is a condition in which an individual is born unable to develop cell-mediated or antibody-mediated immunity. Normal B cells and T cells are absent, and lymphocyte counts are low. Infants with SCID often die from even mild infections because they have no immune response. Treatments for SCID include total isolation from potential pathogens, bone marrow transplantation from a close relative or other compatible donor, and new gene-splicing therapies.

Autoimmune Conditions   Sometimes, the immune system can no longer distinguish between "self" and "foreign" antigens. The body then produces **autoantibodies** and cytotoxic T cells that destroy the "self" tissues. This condition, called **autoimmunity**, may lead to a disease state called *autoimmune disease*. An autoimmune disease of one type or another affects approximately 5% of adults in the United States, two-thirds of them female. **TABLE 18-5** explains the most important autoimmune diseases.

Autoimmune diseases are treated with agents such as *corticosteroids*, which suppress the entire immune system. Today, treatments aim at only specific immune responses. There are many possible "targets" for these treatments because of the immune system's complexity. Commonly, there are

TABLE 18-5

Autoimmune Diseases

Disease	Description
Rheumatoid arthritis	Causes systematic joint destruction
Systemic lupus erythematosus	A systemic disease mostly affecting the heart, kidneys, lungs, and skin
Glomerulonephritis	Damages the filtration membrane of the kidneys, severely impairing renal function
Multiple sclerosis	Destroys the myelin of the brain and spinal cord's white matter
Type 1 diabetes mellitus (insulin-dependent)	Destroys pancreatic beta cells, causing an insulin deficit and an inability to use carbohydrates
Myasthenia gravis	Impairs communication between nerves and skeletal muscles
Graves' disease	Causes the thyroid gland to produce excessive thyroxine, and results in anterior protrusion of the eyeballs

two major therapies. One blocks cytokine actions by using antibodies that oppose them or their receptors, and the other blocks costimulatory molecules needed to activate effector cells. Newly investigated therapies involve "restarting" self-tolerance by either activating regulatory T cells, using vaccines to induce self-tolerance, or directing antibodies to destroy self-reactive immune cells. This is all difficult to achieve because the selective blocking of autoimmune responses often also blocks responses required to fight infection.

Hypersensitivities

When the immune system damages tissues while fighting off threats such as animal dander or pollen, *hypersensitivities* develop. Hypersensitivities are classified by how long they persist and if they involve T cells or antibodies. *Delayed hypersensitivities* are related to T-cell activity. *Immediate* and *subacute hypersensitivities* are caused by antibody-associated reactions. *Immediate hypersensitivities* are also called *acute or type I hypersensitivities*. Commonly, people refer to this type as *allergies*.

Type I Hypersensitivities When an immune response occurs because of a nonharmful substance, it is called an *allergic response*. Immune and allergic responses *sensitize* the lymphocytes, and the antibodies produced may combine with antigens. Allergic reactions can damage tissues, however, whereas normal immune responses cannot. **Allergens** are a type of antigens that trigger allergic responses, which begin within seconds after contact.

A fairly rare type I hypersensitivity is *anaphylactic shock*, which is systemic. It is usually caused by an allergen directly entering the blood and circulating quickly through the body. The most frequent causes of anaphylactic shock include injection of foreign substances such as penicillins, which act as *haptens*; bee stings; and spider bites. Prompt administration of *antihistamines* can block actions of histamine and prevent many signs and symptoms of immediate hypersensitivity. Popular antihistamines include the over-the-counter drug *diphenhydramine hydrochloride (Benadryl®)*. Severe anaphylaxis is treated with injectable antihistamines, epinephrine, and corticosteroids.

Type II Hypersensitivities Both the type II and type III hypersensitivities are classified as "subacute." They are also caused by antibodies but not the same one as in the type I hypersensitivities. They have a slower onset and a longer reaction. They usually occur within 1 to 3 hours after antigen exposure and last for between 10 and 15 hours.

Type II hypersensitivities are related to IgG and are also called *cytotoxic reactions*. They occur when antibodies bind to antigens on certain body cells. Cytotoxic reactions stimulate phagocytosis and complement-mediated lysis of cellular antigens. These reactions may occur after transfusion of blood that was not matched correctly, which results in complement lysing the transfused blood cells.

Type III Hypersensitivities Type III hypersensitivities are known as *immune-complex hypersensitivities*. They are related to IgM and occur when antigens are distributed throughout the body or blood, with the many formed insoluble antigen–antibody complexes unable to be cleared from a certain area. Often, this is linked to an autoimmune disease or a persistent infection. Intense inflammation results, including complement-mediated cell lysis and death via the actions of neutrophils. This severely damages local tissues, which is known as *necrosis*. Examples of immune-complex hypersensitivities include glomerulonephritis caused by systemic lupus erythematosus and *farmer's lung* caused by inhalation of moldy hay.

Type IV Hypersensitivities Type IV hypersensitivities are also called *delayed hypersensitivities* and are linked to T cells. They develop over 1 to 3 days, with inflammation and tissue damage occurring because of cytokine-activated macrophages or cytotoxic T cells. Examples include *allergic contact dermatitis*, often caused by contact with poison ivy, nickel and other metals, cosmetics, and deodorants. Also, type IV hypersensitivities are used when testing the skin for tuberculosis. After introduction of tubercle antigens, a person who has been sensitized to these antigens develops a small, hard lesion that lasts for days. This constitutes a positive result, and tuberculosis is diagnosed.

Tissue Rejection Reaction Another type of reaction concerns transplantation and tissue rejection. When a body part is transplanted from one person to another, the receiving patient's immune system may recognize the transplanted part as foreign and attempt to destroy its tissues, causing a *tissue rejection reaction*. The greater the difference between the antigens on cell surface molecules of the donor and recipient, the greater and more rapid the rejection reaction. Therefore, donor and recipient tissues must be matched to minimize these reactions. Immunosuppressive drugs are used to reduce tissue rejection. Although they reduce the immune response by suppressing antibody and T-cell formation, they weaken the recipient's immune system. Frequently, transplant patients survive the transplant but die from an infection caused by a weakened immune system.

Effects of Aging on the Lymphatic System and Immunity

The lymphatic system becomes less effective at fighting disease as we age, resulting in lowered immunity. T cells weaken, and fewer of them can respond to infections. As the thymus shrinks with age, there are lower circulating levels of thymic hormones. The number of helper T cells is reduced, B cells are less responsive, and antibody levels do not rise after exposure to antigens with the same speed they used to. Viral and bacterial infections are able to proliferate more. This is why vaccinations for diseases such as influenza and pneumococcal pneumonia are recommended for elderly patients. With decreased immunity, tumor cells are not eliminated as effectively, and cancer rates increase with age.

SUMMARY

The lymphatic system is related very closely to the cardiovascular system. It transports excess tissue fluid to the bloodstream. It also absorbs fats and helps to defend against disease-causing agents. Lymphoid cells consist of the T and B lymphocytes, plasma cells, macrophages, dendritic cells, and reticular cells. Lymphoid tissue dominates nearly all lymphoid organs and is mostly composed of reticular connective tissue. Lymph returns protein molecules to the bloodstream and transports foreign particles to lymph nodes. Along with the lymph nodes, the thymus and spleen are the predominant organs of the lymphatic system, along with tonsils, Peyer's patches, and appendix.

Tissue fluid originates from blood plasma. Lymph forms from interstitial fluid and is called *lymph* when it enters the lymphatic vessels. Lymph moves toward the heart via the lymphatic capillaries and lacteals, collecting lymphatic vessels, and lymphatic trunks. The lymphatic trunks lead to two collecting ducts—the thoracic duct and the right lymphatic duct. The body has defenses that protect it against infection: innate, nonspecific defenses and adaptive, specific defenses. The adaptive specific defenses are also known as *immunity*. T cells and B cells reside in lymphatic tissues and organs and are vital for the body's self-protection. Lymphocytes originate in red bone marrow and are released into the blood. Antibodies are gamma globulin proteins called immunoglobulins and include five major types: IgG, IgA, IgM, IgD, and IgE. Naturally acquired immunity arises as a result of natural events, whereas artificially acquired immunity is caused by a medical procedure. Active immunity lasts much longer than passive immunity. The presence of allergens in the body can produce various types of allergies that the body may respond to either immediately or in a delayed manner. Another type of body reaction concerns rejection of transplanted tissue.

KEY TERMS

Adaptive (specific) defense
Allergens
Antibodies
Antibody monomer
Antigen-binding site
Antigen-presenting cell
Antigens

Appendix
Autoantibodies
Autoimmunity
Cellular immune response
Chemical barriers
Chemotaxis
Chyle

Cisterna chyli
Clone
Collecting ducts
Complement
Constant (C) region
Cortex
Dendritic cells

Gamma globulin
Hapten
Hilum
Humoral immune response
Immunity
Immunocompetent
Immunogenicity
Immunologic surveillance
Inflammation
Innate (nonspecific) defense
Interferons
Lacteals
Lingual tonsil
Lymph
Lymph nodes
Lymph nodules
Lymph sinuses

Lymphatic capillaries
Lymphatic pathways
Lymphatic trunks
Lymphatic vessels
Lymphoid tissue
Lysozyme
Macrophages
Mechanical barriers
Medulla
Memory cells
Mononuclear phagocytic system
Natural killer (NK) cells
Opsonization
Palatine tonsils
Pathogen
Peyer's patches
Phagocytosis

Pharyngeal tonsil
Plasma cells
Pus
Reactivity
Reticular cells
Right lymphatic duct
Species resistance
Spleen
Splenic cords
Splenic sinusoids
Stroma
Thoracic duct
Thymus
Tonsillar crypts
Tonsils
Vaccine
Variable (V) region

LEARNING GOALS

The following learning goals correspond to the objectives at the beginning of this chapter:

1. Immunity is also known as adaptive specific defense; it targets specific pathogens via specialized lymphocytes that recognize foreign particles. Immunity is aided by the lymphatic system, which contains B cells and T cells. The lymphatic system transports fluids through a network of vessels, out of interstitial spaces, and returns it to the bloodstream. Its biochemicals and cells attack "foreign" particles to destroy microorganisms, viruses, toxins, and cancer cells. A normally functioning immune system keeps persistent infections, allergies, autoimmune disorders, and cancers from developing.

2. The lymphatic system is made of many vessels, including lymphatic pathways, capillaries, trunks, and collecting ducts. It transports a fluid called lymph, which is filtered in a variety of ways. Lymph nodes are structures important in filtering the lymph, and the spleen is important in filtering the blood. The thoracic duct drains lymph mostly from the left side of the body and the right lymphatic duct drains lymph mostly from the right side of the body.

3. Lymphoid tissues and organs are composed primarily of squamous epithelium, which allows tissue fluid to enter. Lymphatic vessels are similar to veins but have thinner walls and valves that prevent the backflow of lymph.

4. The lymphatic system transports lymph and other fluids so interstitial fluid does not accumulate in tissue spaces. It also absorbs digested fats and sends them to the venous circulation. It coordinates the destruction of infectious microorganisms of many types, as well as toxins and cancer cells. Lymphocytes and macrophages are used to engulf and destroy them.

5. Lymph nodes are actually lymph glands found along the lymphatic pathways, containing lymphocytes and macrophages. They are usually bean-shaped and less than 2.5 cm in length. The functional units of a lymph node are the lymph nodules or follicles, such as the tonsils. Lymph nodes filter potentially harmful particles from the lymph before it is returned to the bloodstream and also monitor body fluids in immune surveillance.

6. Nonspecific, innate defense defends against many different types of pathogens and includes mechanical barriers, chemical barriers, NK cells, inflammation, phagocytosis, fever, and species resistance. Nonspecific defense acts more rapidly than specific defense. Specific, adaptive defense, also known as immunity, is more precise and targets specific pathogens. Specialized lymphocytes recognize foreign particles and act against them.

7. Lymphocytes are important in the immune response because, along with macrophages, they fight invading microorganisms. They assist the lymph nodes in immune surveillance by helping to filter harmful products from the lymph and body fluids. Lymphocytes are produced in the lymph nodes and in red bone marrow and attack viruses, bacteria, and parasitic cells.

8. The thymus is important in early immunity and shrinks after puberty. It contains large amounts of lymphocytes, some of which mature into T cells. The spleen is filled with blood instead of lymph and contains many red blood cells, lymphocytes, and macrophages. It filters blood similar to the way that lymph nodes filter lymph.

9.
   A. The first line of defense consists of mechanical barriers: the skin, mucous membranes, hair, sweat, and mucus.
   B. The second line of defense includes chemical barriers, fever, inflammation, NK cells, phagocytosis, and species resistance.
   C. The third line of defense is immunity, which is also known as a specific defense. It is defined as resistance to specific pathogens or their toxins and metabolic byproducts.

10. Humoral immunity involves the humoral immune response. In this type of response, B cells divide and differentiate into plasma cells, producing antibodies or immunoglobulins, which react to destroy antigens or antigen-containing particles. Cellular immunity or cell-mediated immunity involves the cellular immune response. In this type of response, T cells attach to foreign, antigen-bearing cells such as bacterial cells, and interact with direct cell-to-cell contact.

CRITICAL THINKING QUESTIONS

Scott is 6 months old. He has been admitted three times for various types of infectious diseases. The physician has diagnosed him with an underdeveloped thymus.

1. What is the role of the thymus in the immune system?
2. Why will this child have numerous infectious diseases?

REVIEW QUESTIONS

1. Which of the following cells produce antibodies?
   A. mast cells
   B. monocytes
   C. plasma cells
   D. neutrophils

2. Which of the following organs lack(s) lymphocytes?
   A. spleen
   B. thymus gland
   C. lymph nodes
   D. brain

3. The largest collection of lymphatic tissue in the adult body is located in the
   A. spleen
   B. tonsils
   C. thymus
   D. liver

4. Which of the following is the first line of cellular defense against pathogens?
   A. plasma cells
   B. lymphocytes
   C. phagocytes
   D. mast cells

5. Which of the following is the primary function of the lymphatic system?
   A. production, maintenance, and distribution of plasma proteins
   B. production, maintenance, and distribution of lymphocytes
   C. transportation of hormones
   D. circulation of nutrients

6. Which of the following are responsible for cellular immunity?
   A. plasma cells
   B. T lymphocytes
   C. B lymphocytes
   D. macrophages

7. Immunoglobulins that attach to mast cells and basophils and are involved in allergic reactions are abbreviated as which of the following?
   A. IgE
   B. IgG
   C. IgM
   D. IgA

8. T lymphocytes must mature in which of the following organs before they can stimulate B lymphocytes?
   A. bones
   B. liver
   C. thymus
   D. spleen

9. Lymphatic vessels commonly occur in association with
   A. blood vessels
   B. peripheral nerves
   C. motor nerve endings
   D. sensory nerve endings

10. Portions of the spleen that contain the largest numbers of lymphocytes are known as
    A. red pulp
    B. white pulp
    C. adenoids
    D. lymph nodes

11. Which type of immunoglobulin is composed of five single molecules found together?
    A. IgG
    B. IgD
    C. IgM
    D. IgA

12. Lacteals are special lymphatic capillaries located in which of the following organs?
    A. right lymphatic duct
    B. hilum of the spleen
    C. lymph nodes
    D. small intestine

13. Peyer's patches are found in the
    A. red pulp of the spleen
    B. lining of the small intestine
    C. lobules of the thymus
    D. tonsils

14. Which of the following is not a physical barrier to infection?
    A. basement membranes
    B. epithelium
    C. body hair
    D. complement

15. During a primary immune response, which of the following immunoglobulins first appears in the lymph?
    A. IgG
    B. IgA
    C. IgM
    D. IgE

1. Describe the major lymphatic trunks.
2. Describe the anatomy of the lymph nodes and their major functions.
3. Discuss the role of the thymus in the immune system.
4. Describe the structure of the spleen and its functions.
5. Describe the functions of the tonsils in the pharynx.
6. Describe the physical barriers of the body.
7. Define immunological surveillance, NK cells, and phagocytosis.
8. Describe immunity and antigens.
9. Describe the major immunoglobulins.
10. Compare humoral immunity with cell-mediated immunity.

ENVIRONMENTAL EXCHANGE

Respiratory System

OBJECTIVES

After studying this chapter, the reader should be able to

1. Describe the primary functions of the respiratory system.
2. Identify the organs of the upper respiratory system and describe their functions.
3. Discuss the structure of the airway outside the lungs.
4. Describe the functional anatomy of the alveoli.
5. Define and compare the processes of external respiration and internal respiration.
6. Describe the major steps involved in external respiration.
7. Explain the important structures of the respiratory membrane.
8. Describe how oxygen is picked up, transported, and released in the blood.
9. Describe the factors that influence the respiration rate.
10. Identify the four distinct respiratory volumes.

Overview

The functions of the **respiratory system** include the intake of oxygen and the removal of carbon dioxide. Cells need oxygen to break down nutrients to release energy and produce adenosine triphosphate. Carbon dioxide results from this process, and it must be excreted. The respiratory system includes tubes that filter incoming air while transporting it into and out of the lungs. Gases are exchanged in microscopic air sacs. Respiratory organs entrap incoming air particles, control temperature and water content in the air, produce vocal sounds, regulate blood pH, and are essential for the sense of smell.

Respiration is the process of gas exchange between the atmosphere and cells. Four major events are involved in respiration, with the first two handled by the respiratory system and the last two handled by the cardiovascular or *circulatory* system:

- Movement of air into and out of the lungs, called pulmonary ventilation or *breathing*, involving inward movement or *inspiration* and outward movement or *expiration*, in which gases are changed and refreshed continuously.
- Gas exchange between air in the lungs and the blood, or *external respiration*; oxygen diffuses from the lungs to the blood, whereas carbon dioxide diffuses from the blood to the lungs.
- Gas transport in blood between the lungs and body cells, accomplished by the cardiovascular system, using blood as the transporting fluid; oxygen is transported from the lungs to the body's tissue cells, whereas carbon dioxide is transported from the tissue cells to the lungs.
- Gas exchange between the blood and the cells, or *internal respiration*; oxygen diffuses from the blood to the body's tissue cells, whereas carbon dioxide diffuses from the tissue cells to the blood.

All four processes must occur for the respiratory system to obtain oxygen and eliminate carbon dioxide. Both systems are closely linked, and if either fails, the cells of the body die from lack of oxygen. The process of using oxygen and carbon dioxide at the cellular level is called *cellular respiration*. It is the basis of all chemical reactions in the body that produce energy. Cellular respiration is a circulatory function, not a respiratory function.

Organization of the Respiratory System

The upper respiratory tract includes the nose, nasal cavity, paranasal sinuses, and pharynx. The lower respiratory tract includes the larynx, trachea, and lungs. The lungs contain the bronchi, bronchioles, and *alveoli*. **FIGURE 19-1** shows the structures of the respiratory system.

Nose and Paranasal Sinuses

The only externally visible part of the respiratory system is the *nose*. It has a variety of functions, such as providing an airway so respiration can occur, conditioning incoming air, filtering and cleaning the air, functioning as a resonating chamber for speaking, and containing the smell or *olfactory* receptors. The conditioning of incoming air consists of *moistening* and *warming*.

Nasal Cavity

The **nasal cavity** is a hollow space located behind the nose divided into right and left portions by the **nasal septum.** This structure is made up of the vomer bone and the perpendicular plate of the ethmoid bone posteriorly and septal cartilage anteriorly. Posteriorly, the nasal cavity is continuous with the nasal portion of the pharynx, via the *posterior nasal apertures*, which are funnel-like structures also known as *choanae*.

The roof of the nasal cavity comprises the skull's ethmoid and sphenoid bones. Its floor is made up of the *palate*, a structure that separates it from the oral cavity below. Anteriorly, the palate is supported by processes of the maxillary bones and the palatine bones. This area is called the *hard palate*. There is also a *soft palate*, which is the unsupported posterior section.

Most of the nasal cavity is lined with *respiratory mucosa*, which is pseudostratified ciliated epithelium containing many scattered, mucus-secreting **goblet cells**. This epithelium includes a network of blood vessels and rests on a lamina propria, which has a rich supply of seromucous *nasal glands*. Every day, these glands secrete approximately 1 liter of mucus, which contains the antibacterial enzyme known as *lysozyme*. The filtration mechanisms that prevent contamination of the respiratory system are referred to as the *respiratory defense system*.

As air passes through from the nostrils and over the mucosal surfaces, heat from the blood in these underlying capillary plexuses warms the air to more closely match the body's temperature. Incoming air is also moistened from water evaporation out of the mucous lining. The lysozyme-containing mucus, pushed by the cilia of the epithelial lining, entraps dust and other small particles and carries them toward the pharynx. The lysozyme attacks and chemically destroys bacteria. The respiratory mucosa cells also secrete *defensins*, which function as natural antibiotics. The defensins kill invading microorganisms. The respiratory mucosa has ciliated cells that create a slight current, moving the contaminated mucus posteriorly, toward the throat. Once swallowed, the mucus and its contained microorganisms are destroyed by the gastric juice of the stomach.

There is a rich supply of sensory nerve endings in the nasal mucosa. When they contact irritating dust, pollen, and other particles, the *sneeze reflex* is triggered. When we sneeze, air is forced outward violently, which effectively expels irritants.

The bones and bone processes that project in a curved shape from the nasal cavity's lateral walls, dividing it into passages, are called the **nasal conchae** (**FIGURE 19-2**).

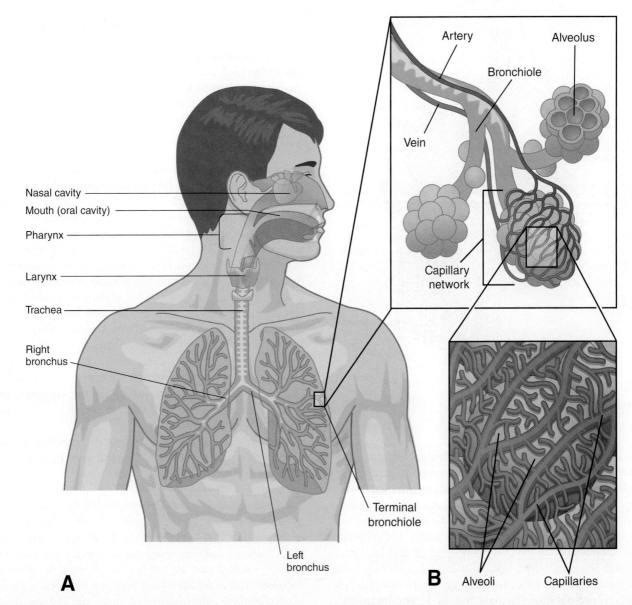

FIGURE 19-1 The respiratory system. (A) The air-conducting portion and the gas-exchange portion of the human respiratory system. The inset shows a higher magnification of the alveoli where oxygen and carbon dioxide exchange occurs. (B) A scanning electron micrograph of the alveoli, showing the rich capillary network surrounding them. (© Dr. David Phillips/Science Source)

These include the *superior, middle,* and *inferior nasal conchae.* Together, they increase the mucosal surface area that is exposed to air as well as the air turbulence in the nasal cavity.

Paranasal Sinuses

The **paranasal sinuses** are a ring of air-filled spaces inside the skull bones that open into the nasal cavity. Located inside the maxillary, frontal, ethmoid, and sphenoid bones of the skull, they are lined with mucous membranes that are continuous with the lining of the nasal cavity. These sinuses reduce the skull's weight and resonate, affecting the quality of the voice. They also help to warm and moisten the incoming air. Mucus produced by the paranasal sinuses eventually flows to the nasal cavity. When you blow your nose, a suctioning effect is created that helps to drain the sinuses.

Pharynx

The funnel-shaped **pharynx,** commonly called the throat, is behind the oral cavity and connects the nasal cavity to the larynx. The pharynx extends for about 13 cm, or 5 inches, from the base of the skull to the level of the sixth cervical vertebra. Food travels from the oral cavity through the pharynx to the esophagus. Also, air passes through the nasal cavity through the pharynx into the larynx. The pharynx helps to produce the sounds of speech (**FIGURE 19-2**).

Posterior to the nasal cavity is the **nasopharynx,** which also lies inferior to the sphenoid bone but superior to the soft palate's level. The nasopharynx is a passageway for air only, because it is located above the mouth. It is continuous with the nasal cavity via the posterior nasal apertures and is lined with pseudostratified ciliated epithelium, which assists

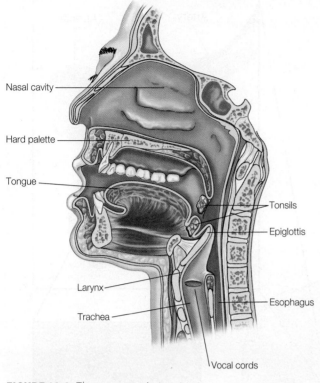

FIGURE 19-2 The upper respiratory tract.

Labels: Nasal cavity, Hard palette, Tongue, Tonsils, Epiglottis, Larynx, Esophagus, Trachea, Vocal cords

lies directly posterior to the epiglottis. The laryngopharynx extends to the larynx, at which point respiratory and digestive paths separate. The esophagus is the tube-like structure that allows food and fluids to pass to the stomach. Air enters the larynx anteriorly. When we swallow, passage of air temporarily stops so food can pass.

Larynx

An enlargement in the airway above the trachea and below the pharynx is called the **larynx**, commonly called the *voice box*. The larynx is about 5 cm, or 2 inches, in length, extending from the level of the third to the sixth cervical vertebra. It attaches to the hyoid bone superiorly, opening into the laryngopharynx, and is continuous with the trachea inferiorly.

The larynx controls how air and food are passed into their proper channels. It also functions to produce a person's voice. It conducts air into and out of the trachea while preventing foreign objects from entering and houses the vocal chords. The larynx is made up of muscles and nine cartilages that are bound by elastic tissues, consisting of ligaments and membranes. The cartilages include the **thyroid cartilage**, **cricoid cartilage**, and **epiglottic cartilage** (**FIGURE 19-3**). All the laryngeal cartilages, except for the epiglottis, are *hyaline* cartilages. These cartilages are bound to each other by intrinsic ligaments.

Two cartilage plates fuse to form the large *thyroid cartilage*, which resembles a shield in shape. At its midline, a *laryngeal prominence* exists, which is externally visible. This is commonly known as the *Adam's apple*. In males this is usually larger, and its growth is stimulated by male sex hormones during puberty. The thyroid cartilage makes up most of the anterior and lateral surface of the larynx. The ring-shaped *cricoid cartilage* is inferior to the thyroid cartilage and is located above the trachea, to which it is inferiorly anchored. Part of the lateral and posterior laryngeal walls are formed by three pairs of *arytenoid, cuneiform,* and *corniculate cartilages*. The pyramid-shaped arytenoid cartilages are most important, because they anchor the vocal folds.

the efforts of the nasal mucosa to transport mucus. The **pharyngeal tonsil**, also called the *adenoids*, is located very high up on the posterior wall of the nasopharynx. This tonsil traps pathogens from the incoming air and destroys them.

The **oropharynx** is continuous with the oral cavity via an archway known as the *isthmus of the fauces*. The oropharynx lies posterior to the oral cavity. Both air and food pass through the oropharynx because it extends inferiorly from the level of the soft palate to the epiglottis. The oropharynx contains two **palatine tonsils** as well as the **lingual tonsil**.

The **laryngopharynx** also allows air and food to pass and is also lined with a stratified squamous epithelium and

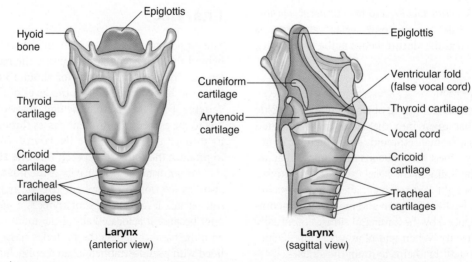

Labels (anterior view): Hyoid bone, Epiglottis, Thyroid cartilage, Cricoid cartilage, Tracheal cartilages

Labels (sagittal view): Epiglottis, Cuneiform cartilage, Arytenoid cartilage, Ventricular fold (false vocal cord), Thyroid cartilage, Vocal cord, Cricoid cartilage, Tracheal cartilages

Larynx (anterior view)

Larynx (sagittal view)

FIGURE 19-3 The larynx.

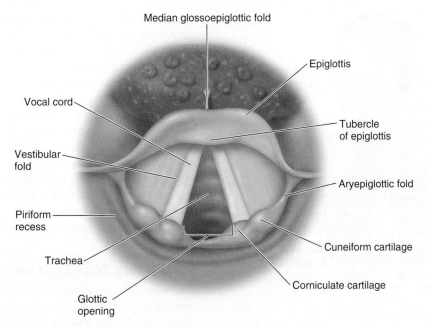

Median glossoepiglottic fold

Epiglottis

Vocal cord

Tubercle
of epiglottis

Vestibular
fold

Aryepiglottic fold

Piriform
recess

Cuneiform cartilage

Trachea

Corniculate cartilage

Glottic
opening

FIGURE 19-4 The vocal cords as viewed from above with the glottis opened.

The flap-like structure that actually allows the larynx to "control" whether air or food passes is the **epiglottis**. It is actually the ninth cartilage of the larynx and extends from the tongue's posterior aspect to where it is anchored, on the anterior rim of the thyroid cartilage. When swallowing, the larynx rises and the epiglottis presses downward, partially covering the opening into the larynx to help prevent foods and liquids from entering the air passages. The epiglottis is spoon-shaped, highly elastic, and nearly covered by a mucosa that contains taste buds.

During breathing, the larynx is wide open and the free edge of the epiglottis projects upward. Anything besides air that enters triggers the cough reflex so the substance can be expelled. However, the cough reflex does not work when a person is unconscious. Liquids should therefore never be given to an unconscious person.

Under the laryngeal mucosa, on each side, are the highly elastic *vocal ligaments* that attach the arytenoid cartilages to the thyroid cartilage. They form horizontal vocal folds inside the larynx extend inward and are divided into upper and lower folds. The upper folds are called *false vocal cords* or *vestibular folds* because they do not create sounds (**FIGURE 19-4**); they help close the airway during swallowing. The lower vocal folds are called *true vocal cords* because they actually create sounds when air is forced between them, causing them to vibrate from side to side. In appearance, the true vocal cords are pearly white in color, because they lack blood vessels. Using the tongue and lips to change the shape of the pharynx and oral cavity transforms sound waves into words. The contraction or relaxation of the vocal cords alters their tension, controlling the pitch they emit. Increasing tension raises pitch, whereas decreasing tension lowers pitch. The loudness of a sound is controlled by the force of air passing through the vocal cords. During breathing, the **glottis** is a triangular slit between the vocal cords. When food or liquid is swallowed, the glottis closes to prevent it from entering the trachea.

Trachea

The **trachea** or *windpipe* is a cylindrical tube about 2 cm in diameter. It is extremely mobile and flexible, with a length of approximately 10 to 12 cm, or 4 inches (**FIGURE 19-5**). The trachea extends downward from the larynx, anterior to the esophagus into the mediastinum of the thoracic cavity, where it splits into right and left bronchi. The trachea has layers known as the *mucosa, submucosa,* and *adventitia,* as well as a hyaline cartilage layer. The ciliated mucosa, like nearby structures, contains goblet cells in a pseudostratified epithelium. It moves trapped particles up into the pharynx where they can be swallowed along with mucus. The submucosa is a connective tissue layer that contains seromucous glands, which help to produce sheets of mucus. The adventitia is the outermost layer of connective tissue, encasing the hyaline cartilage rings of the trachea.

Inside the trachea are about 20 pieces of hyaline cartilage, each shaped like the letter "c." Their open ends are toward the spine. These rings of cartilage prevent the trachea from collapsing. The soft tissue near the back of each ring allows the esophagus to expand as food moves toward the stomach. The open posterior parts of these rings of cartilage are connected by smooth muscles in the *trachealis,* as well as by soft connective tissues. When the trachealis muscle contracts, the diameter of the trachea increases, and expired air is caused to rush upward with great force from the lungs. This helps to expel mucus when coughing, at speeds of approximately 100 miles per hour. A cartilage structure called the *carina* projects posteriorly from the final tracheal cartilage. This is the point where the trachea branches into the two primary bronchi.

Bronchi and Subdivisions

Branched airways leading from the trachea to the alveoli make up the **bronchial tree**. These branches begin with the

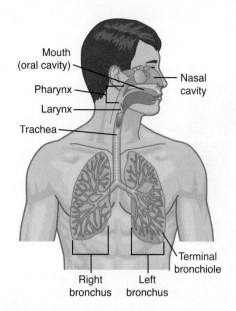

Mouth (oral cavity)

Nasal cavity

Pharynx

Larynx

Trachea

Terminal bronchiole

Right bronchus

Left bronchus

FIGURE 19-5 The structures of the trachea.

right and left **primary bronchi**, near the level of the fifth thoracic vertebra. Each primary bronchus divides into a secondary bronchus, then into tertiary bronchi, and even finer tubes. The right bronchus or *bronchus dexter* is wider, shorter, and more vertical than the left bronchus or *bronchus sinister*. The right bronchus branches off to the upper lobe of the right lung. This branch is called the eparterial branch because it arises above the right pulmonary artery. It then passed below the artery at the hyparterial branch and divides into two branches for the middle and lower lobes. The left bronchus has no eparterial branch because there is no third lobe in the left lung.

Bronchioles are smaller tubes that continue to divide and include terminal bronchioles, respiratory bronchioles, and thin **alveolar ducts**. These ducts lead to outpouchings called **alveolar sacs**, which lead to microscopic **alveoli** or *air sacs* inside capillary networks (**FIGURE 19-5**).

Bronchi have less cartilage than the trachea, and bronchioles have no cartilage. Smaller and smaller respiratory tubes have smooth muscle instead of cartilage. The alveoli provide a large surface of epithelial cells that allow easy exchange of gases. Oxygen diffuses from the alveoli into the capillaries, and carbon dioxide diffuses from the blood into the alveoli.

Conducting Zone Structures

The structures of the *conducting zone* include all respiratory passageways except for those that make up the respiratory zone. The conducting zone structures are relatively rigid, and the organs within function to clean, humidify, and warm the incoming air. Therefore, when this air reaches the lungs, it contains less dust, bacteria, and other irritants than when it entered the nose and has become warm and damp.

The trachea divides into the *right main bronchi* and the *left main bronchi*, also known as *primary bronchi*. Both are found at the level of T_7 when a person is standing. The bronchi run obliquely in the mediastinum. They then move downward

into the hilum, or medial depression, of the lungs. The left main bronchus is thinner, longer, and less vertical than the right main bronchus. It is more common for a foreign object to be inhaled and stuck in the right main bronchus because of its size, shape, and position.

Within the lungs, each main bronchus is divided into secondary or *lobar* bronchi. There are three on the right and two on the left, each one of them supplying a single lung lobe. There are three lobes in the right lung and only two in the left lung. The lobar bronchi then further divide into tertiary or *segmental* bronchi and so forth, into smaller and smaller bronchi. The term *bronchioles* refers to bronchial passages that are smaller than 1 mm in diameter. The smallest are called *terminal bronchioles*, which are less than 0.5 mm in diameter.

Respiratory Zone Structures

The *respiratory zone* is where actual gas exchange occurs. It is made up of microscopic structures, which include the respiratory bronchioles, alveolar ducts, and alveoli. The alveoli are thin-walled air sacs. The respiratory zone starts at the point of the terminal bronchioles feeding into the *respiratory bronchioles* inside the lungs. Scattered alveoli protrude from the respiratory bronchioles, which also lead into twisting and turning *alveolar ducts*. The walls of the alveolar ducts are completely made up of diffuse rings of connective tissue fibers, alveoli, and smooth muscle cells. The ducts lead to *alveolar sacs* or *alveolar saccules*, which are terminal clusters of alveoli.

The alveoli are not the same as the alveolar sacs. The alveoli are the actual sites of gas exchange. The alveolar sacs resemble bunches of grapes, with the alveoli being the individual grape-like structures. There are approximately 300 million alveoli in the lungs, all of them filled with gas. They make up most of the body's lung volume, creating a huge surface area for gas exchange.

In each alveolus the walls are mostly made up of one layer of squamous epithelial cells, also called *type I alveolar cells*. These are surrounded by a thin respiratory basement membrane. The alveolar walls are 15 times thinner than one sheet of paper. There are also scattered, cuboidal *type II alveolar cells*. These secrete *surfactant*, which coats the alveolar surfaces that are exposed to gas. The type II cells also secrete many antimicrobial proteins, needed for innate immunity (**FIGURE 19-6**).

Lungs and Pleurae

The paired **lungs** are located in the thoracic cavity and consist of soft, spongy, cone-shaped tissue. The right and left lungs are separated medially by the mediastinum and are enclosed by the thoracic cage and **diaphragm**. The mediastinum contains the heart, major blood vessels, bronchi, esophagus, and various organs. Air is inhaled by the active contraction of the respiratory muscles, including the diaphragm. Each lung occupies most of the available thoracic space on its side and is suspended by a bronchus and large blood vessels that enter on the lung's medial surface. The collective term for

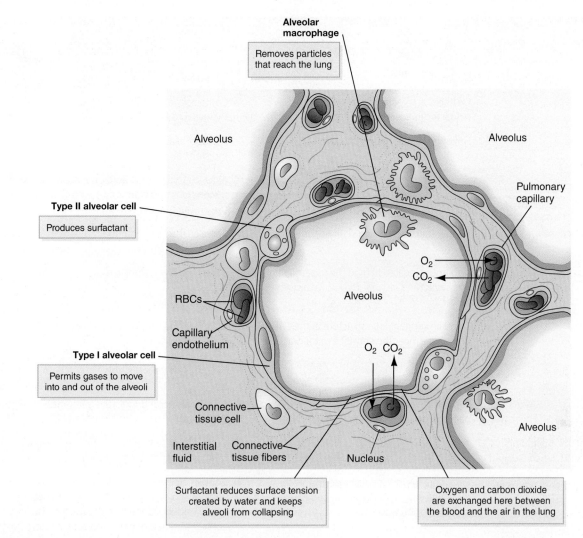

Alveolar macrophage
Removes particles that reach the lung

Alveolus

Alveolus

Pulmonary capillary

Type II alveolar cell
Produces surfactant

O_2
CO_2

Alveolus

RBCs

Capillary endothelium

Type I alveolar cell
Permits gases to move into and out of the alveoli

O_2 CO_2

Connective tissue cell

Alveolus

Interstitial fluid

Connective tissue fibers

Nucleus

Surfactant reduces surface tension created by water and keeps alveoli from collapsing

Oxygen and carbon dioxide are exchanged here between the blood and the air in the lung

FIGURE 19-6 The alveolar macrophage.

each lung's vascular and bronchial attachments is the *root*. Just below the clavicle bone on each site is the lung's narrow superior tip or *apex*. The *base* of the lung is the concave inferior surface that rests on the diaphragm muscle. Each lung's mediastinal surface has an indentation known as the *hilum*. Pulmonary and systemic blood vessels and bronchi, lymphatic vessels, and nerves enter and leave the lung at this point.

The lungs are not symmetrical. The three-lobed right lung is larger because the two-lobed left lung's space has to accommodate the heart as well. The left lung has a *cardiac notch*, which is a concavity in its medial aspect that accommodates the heart. Each lung lobe is supplied by a major branch of the bronchial tree and is connected to blood and lymphatic vessels. In the right lung, the superior and middle lobes are separated by the *horizontal fissure*, and the middle and inferior lobes are separated by an inferior *oblique fissure*. In the left lung, the fissure separating the superior and inferior lobes is also called the *oblique fissure*.

Each lung contains air passages, alveoli, blood vessels, connective tissues, lymphatic vessels, and nerves. **TABLE 19-1** lists the parts of the respiratory system. At the lung surface, resembling hexagons, are the lung *lobules*, the smallest

subdivisions of the lungs that can be seen without a microscope, which are less than 1 inch in size. Each lobule is served by a large bronchiole and its branches. Smoking or regularly inhaling pollution causes the connective tissue between the lobules to turn black, as they collect carbon.

Most of the lungs contain air spaces, with the remainder, called the *stroma*, which is primarily elastic connective tissue. This makes the lungs very soft, spongy, and light. They collectively weigh slightly more than 1 kg, or 2.2 pounds. Their elasticity makes the ability to breathe easier. The elastic components of the lungs recoil when the muscles of inhalation relax. The action of the diaphragm and rib cage returning to their normal positions is called *elastic rebound*.

The lungs have two types of circulation, pulmonary and bronchial, which are very different. The *pulmonary arteries* deliver systemic venous blood that is deoxygenated. These arteries are located anterior to the main bronchi. They are highly branched, similar to the bronchi, and eventually bring blood to the *pulmonary capillary networks* that surround the alveoli. Freshly oxygenated blood from the respiratory zone is brought by the *pulmonary veins* from the lungs to the heart. These veins flow to the hilum with corresponding bronchi as well as in the connective tissue septa between the

TABLE 19-1

Respiratory System

Structure	Description	Function
Nose	Centered above the mouth and inside and below the space between the eyes	Contains the nostrils, which provide entrances to the nasal cavity
Nasal cavity	Hollow space behind the nose	Transports air to the pharynx; filters, warms, and moistens air
Oral cavity	The mouth cavity, containing the teeth, tongue, salivary glands, etc.	Allows passage of air and food; transports air to the pharynx and warms and moistens it; aids in the production of vocal sounds
Paranasal sinuses	Hollow spaces in certain skull bones	Serve as resonant chambers; also help to reduce the weight of the skull
Pharynx	A chamber located behind the nasal cavity, oral cavity, and larynx; also known as the throat	Transports air to the larynx
Epiglottis	Flap-like cartilaginous structure at the back of the tongue, near the entrance to the trachea	Covers the opening to the trachea when swallowing occurs
Larynx	Enlargement at top of trachea; commonly known as the voice box; houses the vocal cords	Produces sounds; transports air to the trachea; helps to filter, warm, and moisten incoming air
Trachea	Tubular structure in the neck through which air passes	Warms, filters, and moistens air; transports air to the lungs
Bronchial tree (including bronchi and bronchioles)	Tubes that branch outward, connecting the trachea to the alveoli	Conducts air from trachea to alveoli, with a mucous lining that filters incoming air
Lungs	Pair of organs in the chest responsible for providing oxygen to the blood and for exhaling carbon dioxide waste	Contain air passages, alveoli (the area where alcohol and carbon dioxide exchange occurs), blood vessels, connective tissues, lymphatic vessels, and nerves of the lower respiratory tract

bronchopulmonary structures. When a pulmonary artery is blocked by any type of embolus, including blood clots, air bubbles, or fat masses, a *pulmonary embolism* occurs. This can cause alveolar collapse, respiratory failure, congestive heart failure, and death.

Although the pulmonary circuit has a high-volume circulation, the pressure inside is low. All the blood in the body passes through the lungs approximately one time per minute. Therefore, the endothelium of lung capillaries is a perfect place for enzymes that affect materials in the blood. These enzymes include *angiotensin-converting enzyme*, which activates a vital blood pressure hormone, and enzymes that inactivate various prostaglandins.

Different from the pulmonary circulation, the *bronchial arteries* bring oxygenated systemic blood to the lung tissues. They arise from the aorta, entering the lungs at the hilum. These arteries move along the bronchi as they become branched and provide blood that is highly pressurized but low in volume. They do not bring this blood to the alveoli. Some systemic venous blood from the lungs is drained by the small bronchial veins. However, there are many anastomoses between the pulmonary and bronchial circulations. Therefore, most venous blood that returns to the heart does so through the pulmonary veins.

Parasympathetic and sympathetic motor fibers, along with visceral sensory fibers, innervate the lungs. The visceral sensory fibers enter each lung through the *pulmonary plexus*, which is located on each lung root, and run along the bronchial tubes and lung blood vessels. The parasympathetic motor fibers constrict the air tubes, known as *bronchoconstriction*, whereas the sympathetic fibers cause them to dilate, known as *bronchodilation*. Excessive parasympathetic stimulation, which occurs in *asthma*, may almost totally prevent airflow along terminal bronchioles.

The **visceral pleura** consists of a layer of serous membrane attached to each lung surface that folds back to become the **parietal pleura**. The parietal pleura forms part of the mediastinum and lines the inner thoracic cavity (**FIGURE 19-7**). It also forms the superior face of the diaphragm. The slit-like potential space between the visceral and parietal pleurae is called the **pleural cavity**. It contains a thin film of serous fluid or *pleural fluid* that reduces friction as the pleurae move against each other during breathing. The visceral pleura covers the external lung surfaces and lines their fissures. The *pleurae* are relatively thin, even though they have two layers. Although they can slide across each other with ease, their separation is highly resisted by the surface tension of the pleural fluid.

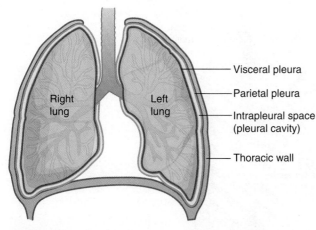

Visceral pleura
Parietal pleura
Intrapleural space (pleural cavity)
Thoracic wall

Right lung

Left lung

FIGURE 19-7 The lungs reside in the pleural cavities, subdivisions of the thoracic cavity. They are lined with a serous membrane called the pleura. The intrapleural space is located between the visceral and parietal pleura.

FOCUS ON PATHOLOGY

Inflammation of the pleurae is known as *pleurisy*. This condition is often caused by pneumonia and results in a roughening of the pleurae, friction, and stabbing pains every time a breath is taken. Over time, excessive amounts of pleural fluid may be produced, which can somewhat relieve the pain but may increase pressure on the lungs and make breathing more difficult. Other fluids may collect in the pleural cavity. These include blood from damaged vessels and blood filtrate, which is watery and leaks from lung capillaries due to left-sided heart failure. When fluid accumulates in the pleural cavity, it is generally referred to as *pleural effusion*.

TEST YOUR UNDERSTANDING

1. List the lobes of each lung.
2. Describe the differences between the left and right bronchial trees.
3. Discuss how the vocal chords produce the sounds used in speech.
4. Explain how the alveoli participate in gas exchange.
5. Differentiate between pulmonary and bronchial circulation.

Mechanics of Breathing

Breathing is also known as *pulmonary ventilation* or *respiration*. It consists of ventilation, which is the movement of air from outside of the body into and out of the bronchial tree and alveoli. Inhalation is also known as **inspiration**, and exhalation is also known as **expiration**.

During normal inspiration, when inside pressure decreases, atmospheric pressure pushes outside air into the airways. Phrenic nerve impulses stimulate the diaphragm to contract, moving downward. The thoracic cavity then enlarges, internal pressure falls, and atmospheric pressure forces air into the airways (**FIGURE 19-8A** and **B**).

As the diaphragm contracts, the external or *inspiratory* intercostal muscles between the ribs are stimulated to contract. The ribs raise and the sternum elevates, enlarging the thoracic cavity further. The lungs expand in response to these movements as well as those of the pleural membranes. When the external intercostal muscles move the thoracic wall upward and outward, the parietal pleura also moves, as does the visceral pleura. The lungs then expand in all directions.

In the alveoli, there is an opposing effect. The attraction of water molecules creates **surface tension** that makes it difficult for the alveoli to inflate. The mixture of lipids and proteins that is known as **surfactant** is synthesized, reducing the tendency of the alveoli to collapse and easing inflation of the alveoli. When a deeper breath is required, muscles contract more forcefully than usual, and other muscles help pull the thoracic cage further upward and outward, decreasing internal pressure.

Expiration occurs because of the elastic recoil of tissues and surface tension. As the diaphragm lowers, it compresses the abdominal organs below it. The elastic tissues cause the lungs and thoracic cage to return to their original shapes, and the abdominal organs move back into their previous shapes to push the diaphragm upward. Surface tension decreases the diameters of the alveoli, increasing alveolar air pressure. Air inside the lungs is forced out, meaning that normal resting expiration is a passive process. If more forceful exhalation is required, the posterior internal or *expiratory* intercostal muscles contract. This pulls the ribs and sternum downward and inward to increase the pressure in the lungs. The abdominal wall muscles squeeze the abdominal organs inward, forcing the diaphragm even higher against the lungs.

Pressure Relationships in the Thoracic Cavity

The force that moves air into the lungs is atmospheric pressure, and respiratory pressures are always expressed in relation to this pressure. Atmospheric pressure is defined as the pressure exerted by the gases, which comprise the *air* that surrounds us. At sea level, normal air pressure is equal to 760 mm Hg. It is exerted on every surface in contact with the air. The pressure on the inside of the lungs and alveoli is almost equal to outside air pressure. Atmospheric pressure may also be expressed in atmospheric units, which means that 760 mm Hg equals 1 atmospheric unit.

A region of the world is lower than atmospheric pressure when there is a negative respiratory pressure. For example, a respiratory pressure of –2 mm Hg means the pressure is lower than atmospheric pressure by 2 mm Hg. So, 760 mm Hg minus 2 mm Hg leaves 758 mm Hg, which is described as the *absolute pressure* of the given region. A zero respiratory pressure is equal to atmospheric pressure. A positive respiratory pressure is higher than atmospheric pressure.

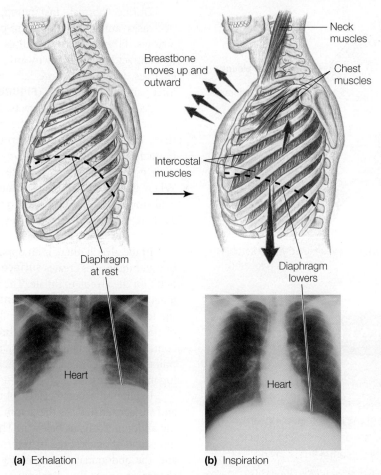

FIGURE 19-8 (A) Expiration and (B) inspiration. (Photos: © SIU/Visuals Unlimited.)

Intrapulmonary pressure is also known as *intra-alveolar pressure*, abbreviated as "P_{pul}," and defined as the pressure inside the alveoli. Intrapulmonary pressure increases and decreases during normal breathing but always becomes equalized with atmospheric pressure eventually. The pressure inside the pleural cavity is known as *intrapleural pressure*, abbreviated as "P_{ip}," and also increases and decreases during normal breathing. However, intrapleural pressure is always approximately 4 mm Hg lower than intrapulmonary pressure. It is therefore described as always *negative* to the intrapulmonary pressure.

This occurs because there are opposing forces in the thorax. Two forces pull the visceral pleura of the lungs away from the parietal pleura of the wall of the thorax, causing the lungs to collapse: the natural tendency of the lungs to recoil and the surface tension of the alveolar fluid. Because the lungs are highly elastic, they always form the smallest size they possibly can form. The molecules of the fluid that lines the alveoli are attracted to each other. This causes surface tension, which continually draws the alveoli to their smallest possible dimensions. The natural elasticity of the chest wall opposes these lung-collapsing forces. The forces of the chest wall pull the thorax outward, enlarging the lungs.

To have a negative intrapleural pressure, the amount of pleural fluid in the pleural cavity needs to remain as little as possible. On a continuous basis, pleural fluid is pumped out of the pleural cavity, entering the lymphatics. Otherwise, it would accumulate in the intrapleural space and produce a positive pressure in the pleural cavity. The negative pressure in the intrapleural space and the snug joining of the lungs to the wall of the thorax are extremely critical. If a condition equalizes intrapleural pressure with either intrapulmonary or atmospheric pressure, immediate lung collapse occurs. The difference between the intrapulmonary and intrapleural pressures is called the *transpulmonary pressure*. This pressure keeps the air spaces in the lungs open, keeping them from collapsing.

Pulmonary Ventilation

Pulmonary ventilation is a mechanical process that consists of inspiration and expiration. It is based on volume changes in the thoracic cavity. You should remember the following:

- *Volume changes always lead to pressure changes.*
- *Pressure changes lead to flow of gases, to equalize pressure.*

The relationship between pressure and volume of a gas is explained by *Boyle's law*, which states that at a constant temperature, the pressure of a gas changes inversely with its volume:

$$P_1 V_1 = P_2 V_2$$

FOCUS ON PATHOLOGY

Pneumothorax is the presence of air in the pleural cavity. It can be reversed by drawing the air out of the intrapleural space via chest tubes. The pleurae can then heal, the lung can reinflate, and normal respiratory function can return. One lung can collapse without affecting the other because they are each inside their own cavity. Lung collapse is known as *atelectasis*. It may follow pneumonia, which often leads to plugging of a bronchiole. The associated alveoli then absorb all of the contained air and collapse. Other causes of atelectasis include chest wounds or visceral pleura rupture that cause air to enter the pleural cavity. Then, air from the respiratory tract can enter the pleural cavity.

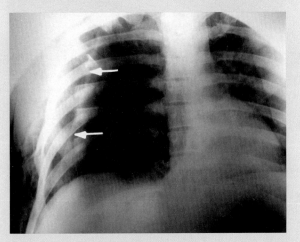

Pneumothorax. (Courtesy of Leonard V. Crowley, MD, Century College.)

FOCUS ON PATHOLOGY

Pneumonia is a lung infection classified as *lobar pneumonia,* which affects only specific areas of the lungs; *bronchopneumonia,* which is mostly located in the bronchi; and *pneumonitis* or *interstitial pneumonia,* which affects the alveolar walls. Lobar pneumonia is commonly caused by *Streptococcus pneumonia.* It may be diagnosed by chest x-ray and by classic symptoms of respiratory distress, fever, and leukocytosis. Bronchopneumonia is caused by obstruction of small bronchi by foreign objects, mucus, aspirated gastric contents, or neoplasm.

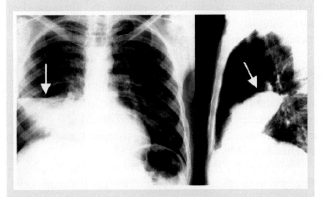

Lobar pneumonia. (Courtesy of Laura Vasquez.)

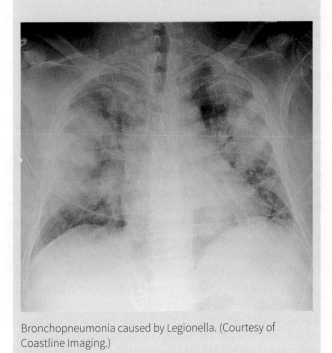

Bronchopneumonia caused by Legionella. (Courtesy of Coastline Imaging.)

where *P* is the pressure of the gas, *V* is its volume, and 1 and 2 indicate the initial condition and the resulting condition, respectively.

Gases always fill their containers, so the size of a container influences the space between gas molecules. A larger container will cause gas molecules to be farther apart and, therefore, pressure to be lower. Reducing container volume brings the gas molecules closer and increases the pressure. This is a simple way to understand how gases work inside our lungs.

TEST YOUR UNDERSTANDING

1. Describe the force that controls pulmonary ventilation.
2. During inspiration, explain how intrapulmonary pressure decreases.
3. Identify the actions of the diaphragm and intercostal muscles in inspiration.

Airway Resistance

Friction is the primary nonelastic source of resistance to gas flow. Also referred to as "drag," it occurs in the respiratory passageways. Gas flow is related to pressure and resistance. Equivalent factors determine gas flow in the respiratory system and blood flow in the cardiovascular system. Usually, tiny differences in pressure produce significant changes in gas flow volume. During normal, quiet breathing, the average pressure gradient is 2 mm Hg or less. This small amount is able to move 500 mL of air, with each breath, in and out of the lungs!

Alveolar Surface Tension

Surface tension is a state of tension at a liquid's surface that is produced by unequal attraction. At the boundary of a gas and a liquid, the liquid molecules are attracted to each other more strongly than they are attracted to the gas molecules. Surface tension pulls liquid molecules closer together. It lessens their contact with the gas molecules, because they are not similar. Surface tension also resists forces that tend to increase the liquid's surface area.

Water is an example of a liquid with very high surface tension. It is made up of highly polar molecules. Water makes up a major percentage of the liquid film coating the walls of the alveoli. As a result, it helps to reduce the alveoli to their smallest possible size. However, if this film was only made of water, the alveoli would collapse between every breath taken. Why does it not collapse?

Surfactant is a mix of lipids and proteins that resembles a detergent in its effects. It is produced by type II alveolar cells. Surfactant makes water molecules become less cohesive. This reduces the surface tension of the alveolar fluid. As a result, lower amounts of energy are needed to expand the lungs and keep the alveoli from collapsing. The type II alveolar cells are stimulated to secrete more surfactant by breaths that are deeper than normal.

Respiratory Volumes

There are four distinct **respiratory volumes** that can be measured by using *spirometry*, which is also known as *pulmonary function testing*. Spirometry is used to measure the functional capacity of the lungs (**FIGURE 19-9**). **TABLE 19-2** shows average values of respiratory volumes for men and women of normal weight at about 21 years of age. As previously discussed, about 500 mL of air move in and out of the lungs with each breath during normal, quiet breathing. This is known as **tidal volume**. However, between 2,100 and 3,200 mL of air can be inspired forcibly beyond the tidal volume. This is known as the **inspiratory reserve volume**.

The amount of air that can be expelled from the lungs after a normal tidal volume expiration is between 1,000 and 1,200 mL. This is known as the **expiratory reserve volume**. However, after the most strenuous expiration of air, there are still about 1,200 mL remaining in the lungs. Called the **residual volume**, it helps to prevent lung collapse and keep the alveoli open, which is also referred to as being *patent*.

FOCUS ON PATHOLOGY

Bronchiectasis occurs when bronchial walls in the lung are weakened because of severe inflammation or other factors, resulting in dilation of the affected bronchi. In children who have pertussis, bronchiectasis may be a complication. The condition may be a complication of cystic fibrosis or chronic obstructive pulmonary disease. Bronchiectasis is diagnosed by a *bronchogram*.

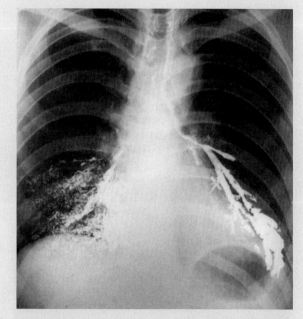

Bronchiectasis. (Courtesy of Leonard V. Crowley, MD, Century College.)

TEST YOUR UNDERSTANDING

1. Explain airway resistance and the factors involved.
2. Describe how surfactant keeps the alveoli from collapsing.
3. Differentiate respiratory volumes from respiratory capacities.

Respiratory Capacities

Respiratory capacities, as well as respiratory volumes, are useful for diagnosing problems with pulmonary ventilation. On average, adult females have smaller bodies and lung volumes than do adult males, which is why there are gender-related differences regarding respiratory volumes and capacities (**TABLE 19-3**).

Respiratory capacities include inspiratory, functional residual, vital, and total lung capacities. Two or more lung volumes always make up the respiratory capacities (**FIGURE 19-10**). The **inspiratory capacity** is the total air that can be inspired after one normal tidal volume expiration. Therefore, tidal volume plus inspiratory reserve volume equals inspiratory capacity.

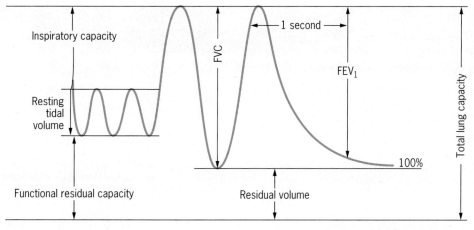

FIGURE 19-9 Pulmonary function test.

Functional residual capacity is the air that remains in the lungs after one normal tidal volume expiration. Therefore, residual volume plus expiratory reserve volume equals functional residual capacity. **Vital capacity** is the total amount of exchangeable air and is made up of the total volume, inspiratory reserve volume, and expiratory reserve volume. **Total lung capacity** is the total of all lung volumes added together.

Dead Space

A certain amount of inspired air does not contribute to alveolar gas exchange but fills the conducting respiratory passageways. *Anatomic dead space* is made up of the volume of these conducting conduits. The dead space is approximately 150 mL. For example, only 350 mL of air are used in alveolar ventilation, out of a tidal volume of 500 mL. In conditions of alveolar collapse or mucous obstruction, gas exchange may stop. Then, the *alveolar dead space* is added to the anatomic dead space, comprising a volume that is not used, known as the *total dead space*.

TEST YOUR UNDERSTANDING

1. Explain how total lung capacity is calculated.
2. Describe the importance of surfactant.
3. Explain the diaphragm's function in respiration.

Testing Pulmonary Function

Originally, a **spirometer** was used to test pulmonary function. Today, a small electronic measuring device is used instead, into which the patient blows air. Electronic spirometry is used for evaluating lost respiratory function and for studying respiratory disease progression. Although not diagnostic, it can distinguish between *obstructive* and *restrictive* diseases of the pulmonary region. Obstructive pulmonary diseases, such as chronic bronchitis, involve increased airway resistance. The lungs hyperinflate, increasing total lung capacity, functional residual capacity, and residual volume. Restrictive diseases involve a reduction in total lung capacity. Because lung expansion is limited, there are decreases in vital capacity, total lung capacity, functional residual capacity, and residual volume.

The rate at which gas moves in and out of the lungs is expressed in *forced vital capacity* (FVC) and *forced expiratory volume* (FEV). FVC measures how much gas is expelled after taking a deep breath and forcefully, maximally, and rapidly exhaling. FEV determines how much air is expelled during certain time intervals of the FVC test. FEV_1 is the volume exhaled during the first second. Healthy people can exhale approximately 80% of their FVC in 1 second. Obstructive pulmonary diseases cause an individual to be unable to exhale anywhere near this percentage. In restrictive diseases, even though there is reduced FVC, the patient can exhale 80% or higher in 1 second.

TABLE 19-2

Respiratory Volumes in Average Adults

Respiratory Volumes	Average Adult Males	Average Adult Females	Comments
Tidal volume	500 mL	500 mL	Under resting conditions, the air inhaled or exhaled with each breath
Inspiratory reserve volume	3,100 mL	1,900 mL	Air that can be forcibly inhaled after normal tidal volume inspiration
Expiratory reserve volume	1,200 mL	700 mL	Air that can be forcibly exhaled after normal tidal volume expiration
Residual volume	1,200 mL	1,100 mL	Air remaining in lungs after forced expiration

TABLE 19-3

Respiratory Capacities in Average Adults

Respiratory Capacities	Average Adult Males	Average Adult Females	Comments
Total lung capacity	6,000 mL	4,200 mL	Maximum air contained in lungs after maximum inspiratory effort (TV + IRV + ERV + RV)
Vital capacity	4,800 mL	3,100 mL	Maximum air that can be expired after maximum inspiratory effort (TV + IRV + ERV)
Inspiratory capacity	3,600 mL	2,400 mL	Maximum air that can be inspired after normal tidal volume expiration (TV + IRV)
Functional residual capacity	2,400 mL	1,800 mL	Air remaining in lungs after normal tidal volume expiration (ERV + RV)

TV, tidal volume; IRV, inspiratory reserve volume; ERV, expiratory reserve volume; RV, residual volume.

Alveolar Ventilation

The total amount of gas flowing into or out of the respiratory tract, in 1 minute, is called the *minute ventilation*. In a healthy individual during normal, quiet breathing, this is approximately 500 mL per breath. At 12 breaths per minute, this is about 6 liters of air. The minute ventilation may increase to 200 L/min during vigorous exercise. These values help to assess respiratory efficiency.

A better indicator is the **alveolar ventilation rate**, because it includes the air in the dead space. It measures the flow of gases into and out of the alveoli during a certain interval of time. The alveolar ventilation rate is calculated by multiplying the frequency of breaths per minute by the tidal volume minus the dead space, both in milliliters of air per breath. The alveolar ventilation rate is based on millimeters of air per minute.

Gas Exchange

The alveoli in the lungs carry on the exchange of gases between air and the blood. The alveoli are microscopic air sacs clustered around the distal ends of the narrowest

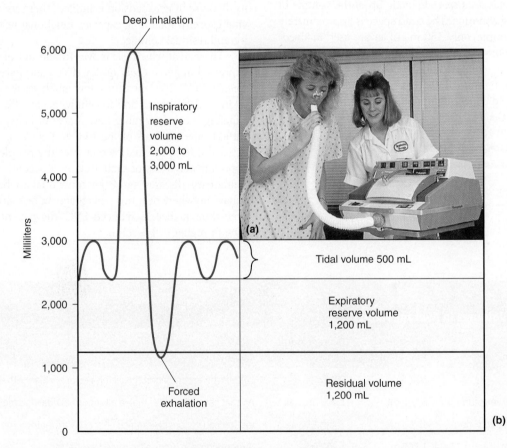

FIGURE 19-10 Respiratory volumes and capacities. (Photo: © SIU/Visuals Unlimited.)

respiratory tubes called the *alveolar ducts*. Each alveolus consists of a tiny space inside a thin wall, separating it from adjacent alveoli. The inner lining is made up of simple squamous epithelium. Dense networks of capillaries are found near each alveolus. At least two thicknesses of epithelial cells and a fused basement membrane layer separate the air in an alveolus from the blood in a capillary. These layers make up the **respiratory membrane**. It is here where blood and alveolar air exchange gases.

Air exchanges across the respiratory membrane occur by the diffusion process. Diffusion occurs from regions of higher pressure toward regions of lower pressure. The pressure of a gas determines how it diffuses from one region to another. Ordinary air consists of 78% nitrogen, 21% oxygen, 0.04% carbon dioxide, and traces of other gases. The amount of pressure each gas contributes is called the **partial pressure** of that gas. Because air is 21% oxygen, oxygen accounts for 21% of the atmospheric pressure, equivalent to 160 mm Hg of the atmospheric pressure of 760 mm Hg.

The resulting concentration of each gas is proportional to its partial pressure. Each gas diffuses between areas of higher partial pressure and areas of lower partial pressure, until the two areas reach equilibrium. Carbon dioxide diffuses from blood, because of higher partial pressure, across the respiratory membrane and into alveolar air. Oxygen diffuses from alveolar air into blood. Because of the large volume of air always present in the lungs, as long as breathing continues, alveolar partial oxygen pressure stays relatively constant, at 104 mm Hg. The partial pressure of oxygen is symbolized as P_{O_2}, and the partial pressure of carbon dioxide is symbolized as P_{CO_2}.

Dalton's law *of partial pressures* states that the total pressure from a mixture of gases is the sum of the pressure that each gas exerts independently. **Henry's law** states that when a gas contacts a liquid, it dissolves in the liquid in proportion to its partial pressure. During the gas phase, greater concentrations of a gas cause it to go into the solution in the liquid in higher quantities and at a faster rate.

The *solubility* of a gas in a liquid, along with the liquid's temperature, determines how much of the gas will dissolve in the liquid at a specific partial pressure. From the air, carbon dioxide and other gases have various solubilities in water or in blood plasma. Carbon dioxide has the highest solubility, with oxygen only 1/20th as soluble. Nitrogen is only half as soluble as this. Therefore, at a certain partial pressure, nearly no nitrogen will dissolve in water, but there is twice as much oxygen that will dissolve and 20 times more carbon dioxide than this amount.

Gas solubility decreases as the temperature of a liquid increases. For example, soda loses the carbon dioxide that it contains more rapidly at room temperature than it does in a refrigerator. Once all the carbon dioxide escapes from the solution, all that is left is flavored water, lacking any carbonation.

Alveolar Gas Movement

The mixture of gases in the atmosphere is very different from the mixture of gases in the alveoli of the lungs. **TABLE 19-4** compares these differences. The alveoli contain more carbon dioxide and water vapor and much less oxygen than the atmosphere, which also has abundant amounts of nitrogen.

Three primary factors influence the amounts of gases in the alveoli and atmosphere. In the lungs, gas exchanges include the diffusion of oxygen from the alveoli into the pulmonary blood and the diffusion of carbon dioxide in the opposite direction. The conducting passages humidify the air inside them. With each breath, alveolar gases mix. Only 500 mL of air enter with every tidal inspiration. Therefore, alveolar gas is really a mixture of new, inspired gases with those that remain in the respiratory passages between breaths. Increasing the depth and rate of breathing easily changes the alveolar partial pressures of oxygen and carbon dioxide. A high alveolar ventilation rate brings in more oxygen, and the alveolar partial pressure of oxygen therefore increases. Also, carbon dioxide is rapidly eliminated from the lungs.

External Respiration

External respiration is also referred to as *pulmonary gas exchange*. The blood in the pulmonary circuit is dark red in color. When it is returned to the heart and oxygenated for distribution to the body tissues, it becomes scarlet, which is much brighter red. This is because of the uptake of oxygen to hemoglobin in the red blood cells. The unloading or *exchange* of carbon dioxide also occurs at the same time, with the same speed. External respiration is influenced by three factors: the respiratory membrane's surface area and thickness, gas solubilities and partial pressure gradients, and the fact that alveolar ventilation is matched with pulmonary

TABLE 19-4				
Alveoli and Atmospheric Comparisons				
Component	Percentage in Alveoli	Partial Pressure in Alveoli	Percentage in Atmosphere (at sea level)	Partial Pressure in Atmosphere (at sea level)
Carbon dioxide	5.2%	40 mm Hg	0.04%	0.3 mm Hg
Water	6.2%	47 mm Hg	0.46%	3.7 mm Hg
Nitrogen	74.9%	569 mm Hg	78.6%	597 mm Hg
Oxygen	13.7%	104 mm Hg	20.9%	159 mm Hg

blood perfusion by ventilation-perfusion coupling. In a normal lung, gas exchange is extremely efficient, and the respiratory membrane is thin, only between 0.5 and 1 μm.

Internal Respiration

In *internal respiration*, gas is exchanged between the capillaries and body tissues. Diffusion gradients and partial pressure are reversed from those in external respiration and pulmonary gas exchange. The ways in which gas exchanges occur between the systemic capillaries and the body tissues are nearly the same, however, as those occurring in the lungs.

In the body tissue cells, carbon dioxide is produced while oxygen is continuously used for metabolic processes. The partial pressure of oxygen is always lower in the tissues, at 40 mm Hg, than in the systemic blood, in which it is 100 mm Hg. This means that oxygen quickly moves from the blood into the tissues, up to the point that equilibrium is reached. Simultaneously, carbon dioxide is quickly moved along its pressure gradient into the blood. Therefore, in the venous blood returning to the heart from the capillary beds, the partial pressure of oxygen is 40 mm Hg, whereas the partial pressure of carbon dioxide is 45 mm Hg. Gas exchanges occurring between the blood and alveoli and between the blood and body tissue cells occur via simple diffusion. This is influenced by the partial pressure gradients of oxygen and carbon dioxide on either side of the exchange membranes.

Oxygen Transport

As oxygen from the lungs and carbon dioxide from the cells enter the blood, they dissolve in the plasma or combine with blood components. About 98% of the oxygen transported by the blood binds the iron-containing protein **hemoglobin** in red blood cells. The remainder dissolves in the plasma. Because oxygen is poorly soluble in water, only approximately 1.5% of transported oxygen is carried in its dissolved form. This is why nearly all oxygen transported from the lungs to the body tissues occurs via its chemical combination with hemoglobin.

In the lungs, oxygen dissolves in blood and combines rapidly with the iron atoms of hemoglobin to form **oxyhemoglobin**, whose bonds are unstable. As PO_2 decreases, oxyhemoglobin molecules release oxygen, diffusing into nearby cells that have depleted their oxygen supplies in cellular respiration (**FIGURE 19-11**). Hemoglobin that has released oxygen is referred to as *reduced hemoglobin* or *deoxyhemoglobin*.

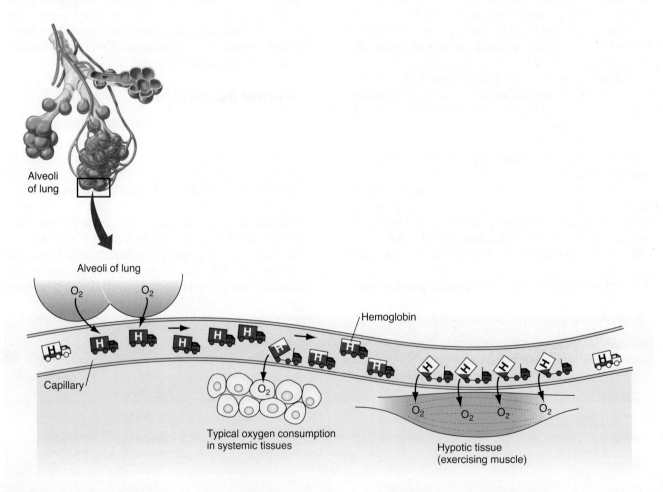

FIGURE 19-11 Cellular respiration.

The loading and unloading of oxygen is described in the following reversible equation:

$$HHb + O_2 \overset{\text{Lungs}}{\underset{\text{Tissues}}{\Leftrightarrow}} HbO_2 + H^+$$

where HHb is deoxyhemoglobin and HbO_2 is oxyhemoglobin. The hemoglobin molecule changes shape after the first oxygen molecule binds to iron. Then, it takes up two more oxygen molecules more easily, with uptake of the fourth molecule still easier. A hemoglobin molecule is *partially saturated* when one to three oxygen molecules are bound. It is *fully saturated* when all four of its heme groups are bound to oxygen. Unloading of a single oxygen molecule enhances unloading of the next molecule and then the next, meaning unloading and loading are functionally similar although opposite processes. The binding strength, or *affinity*, of hemoglobin for oxygen is altered based on how much oxygen saturation exists. Both loading and unloading processes are extremely efficient. The hemoglobin saturation and the partial pressure of oxygen saturation may be compared using a graph called an *oxygen-hemoglobin saturation curve*.

The partial pressure of oxygen, blood pH, temperature, the partial pressure of carbon dioxide, and blood concentrations of *2,3-bisphosphoglycerate* all regulate the rate of hemoglobin reversibly binding or releasing oxygen. These interacting determinants help deliver adequate amounts of oxygen to the body tissue cells.

As blood becomes more acidic or blood temperature rises, carbon dioxide increases in the blood, causing more release of oxygen. Therefore, during physical exercise, more oxygen is released to skeletal muscles. This increases carbon dioxide contraction, decreases pH, and raises temperature.

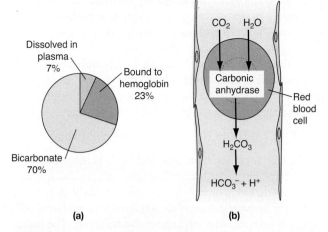

FIGURE 19-12 Carbon dioxide transport. (A) Most carbon dioxide transported in the blood travels as bicarbonate. (B) Bicarbonate is generated by carbonic anhydrase, which is present in red blood cells.

Carbon Dioxide Transport

Blood transports carbon dioxide to the lungs either as carbon dioxide dissolved in plasma, in quantities of 7% to 10%; as part of a compound formed by bonding to hemoglobin, which is slightly more than 20%; or as a bicarbonate ion, which is approximately 70%. **FIGURE 19-12** explains carbon dioxide transport. The amount of dissolved carbon dioxide in the plasma is determined by its partial pressure. The higher the partial pressure of carbon dioxide in the tissues, the more of it that will go into solution. Only about 7% of carbon dioxide transported by the blood is in this form. Approximately 200 mL of carbon dioxide are produced by active body cells every minute. This is exactly the same amount that is excreted by the lungs.

FOCUS ON PATHOLOGY

Hypoxia describes a deficiency of oxygen reaching the tissues, which may be due to decreased arterial oxygen partial pressure or *hypoxemia*, anemic hypoxia, inadequate blood flow, or cellular defects. Hypoxia is more easily seen in people with lighter skin, because the skin along with the mucosae become *cyanotic*, or bluish in color, when hemoglobin saturation is lower than 75%. Cyanosis is only visible in the mucosae and nail beds of people with darker skin. If hypoxia is complete and all oxygen is cut off, the condition is called *anoxia*.

Types of hypoxia include *anemic, ischemic* or *stagnant, histotoxic,* and *hypoxemic*. Anemic hypoxia results from insufficient amounts of red blood cells or those that lack hemoglobin or have abnormal hemoglobin. Ischemic hypoxia occurs from impaired or blocked blood circulation, such as in congestive heart failure. Histotoxic hypoxia is due to an inability of body cells to use oxygen, even though amounts are adequate; it is often caused by cyanide or other metabolic poisons. Hypoxemic hypoxia occurs from reduced arterial partial pressure of oxygen, which may be because of ineffective ventilation-perfusion coupling, air with too little oxygen, or impaired ventilation due to pulmonary diseases. A unique type of hypoxemic hypoxia is called *carbon monoxide poisoning*, which is often related to fires. Carbon monoxide has no odor or color and competes strongly against oxygen for heme binding sites. It can displace oxygen at very small partial pressures. Carbon monoxide poisoning causes confusion, severe headache, and sometimes a cherry red color of the skin. This condition is treated with 100% oxygen or hyperbaric therapy.

Carbon dioxide differs from oxygen in that it bonds with the amino groups of the "globin" or protein portion of these molecules. Oxygen and carbon dioxide do not compete for binding sites. Hemoglobin can transport both molecules at the same time. Carbon dioxide loosely bonds with hemoglobin to slowly form **carbaminohemoglobin**, which decomposes readily in regions of low carbon dioxide partial pressure. This can be better understood by the following equation:

$$CO_2 + Hb \Leftrightarrow HbCO_2 (carbaminohemoglobin)$$

where CO_2 is carbon monoxide and Hb is hemoglobin.

No catalyst is needed for this rapid reaction. Because carbon dioxide binds directly to the amino acids of globin and not to the heme, transport of carbon dioxide to red blood cells does not compete with oxyhemoglobin transport. The partial pressure of carbon dioxide and degree of hemoglobin oxygenation directly influence loading and unloading of carbon dioxide. It quickly dissociates from the hemoglobin in the lungs, where the partial pressure of carbon dioxide of air in the alveoli is lower than that in the blood. Deoxygenated hemoglobin can combine more quickly with carbon dioxide than oxygenated hemoglobin can combine with carbon dioxide.

The most important carbon dioxide transport mechanism forms **bicarbonate ions**. Carbon dioxide reacts with water to form carbonic acid. Most carbon dioxide molecules that enter the plasma quickly enter the red blood cells. It is unstable, dissociating into hydrogen and bicarbonate ions, as seen in this equation:

$$CO_2 + H_2O \Leftrightarrow H_2CO_3$$
$$\text{(carbon dioxide)} \quad \text{(water)} \quad \text{(carbonic acid)}$$
$$\Leftrightarrow H^+ + HCO_3^-$$
$$\text{(hydrogen ion)} \quad \text{(bicarbonate ion)}$$

In red blood cells, the enzyme **carbonic anhydrase** speeds the reaction of carbon dioxide and water, resulting in carbonic acid that releases hydrogen and bicarbonate ions. Nearly 70% of carbon dioxide transported by the blood is in this form. Because of carbonic anhydrase, the reaction shown in the equation above occurs thousands of times faster in red blood cells than it does in the plasma. The released hydrogen ions and the released carbon dioxide bind to hemoglobin and trigger the *Bohr effect*. Therefore, carbon dioxide loading enhances oxygen release.

Because hemoglobin acts as a buffer, freed hydrogen ions do not cause a significant change in pH under resting conditions. Therefore, blood only becomes slightly more acidic as it passes through tissues. Its pH declines only from 7.4 to 7.34 in this process.

Generated bicarbonate ions move fast, from red blood cells to the plasma, to be carried to the lungs. To balance this, chloride ions move from the plasma into red blood cells. This process of ion exchange is known as the *chloride shift*. It occurs because of facilitated diffusion, through a red blood cell membrane protein.

This process is reversed in the lungs. Blood moving through the pulmonary capillaries experiences a decline in its partial pressure of carbon dioxide, from 45 to 40 mm Hg. Carbon dioxide is first released from bicarbonate housings for this to occur. Bicarbonate ions reenter the RBCs, with chloride ions moving into the plasma. The bicarbonate ions bind with hydrogen ions, forming carbonic acid, which is then split by carbonic anhydrase to release water and carbon dioxide. This carbon dioxide, as well as the remainder released from hemoglobin and solution in plasma, diffuses along its partial pressure gradient, from the blood into the alveoli.

Carbon dioxide diffuses into the alveoli in response to relatively low partial pressure of carbon dioxide in alveolar air. Hydrogen and bicarbonate ions in red blood cells simultaneously recombine to form carbonic acid, quickly yielding carbon dioxide and water. **TABLE 19-5** summarizes how blood gases are transported.

TEST YOUR UNDERSTANDING

1. Define and explain hyperventilation.
2. How is oxygen transported from the lungs to the body's cells?
3. List potential causes of hypoxia.
4. Describe the effect of carbon dioxide and hydrogen upon oxygen unloading, and name this effect.
5. Identify the three ways carbon dioxide is transported in the blood, and name the most important of these ways.
6. Explain the relationship between carbon dioxide and pH in the blood.

TABLE 19-5

Blood Gas Transport

Gas	Substance Transported	Reaction
Oxygen	Oxyhemoglobin	1–2% dissolves in plasma
		98–99% combines with iron atoms of hemoglobin molecules
Carbon dioxide	Carbon dioxide	Nearly 7% dissolves in plasma
	Carbaminohemoglobin	Nearly 23% combines with amino groups of hemoglobin molecules
	Bicarbonate ions	Nearly 70% reacts with water to form carbonic acid; the carbonic acid then dissociates to release hydrogen ions and bicarbonate ions

Control of Breathing

Respiratory control has both involuntary and voluntary components. The involuntary centers of the brain regulate the respiratory muscles. They control respiratory minute volume by adjusting the depth and frequency of pulmonary ventilation. This occurs in response to sensory information that arrives from the lungs, various portions of the respiratory tract, and a variety of other sites.

The **respiratory areas** of the brain control inspiration as well as exhalation. The voluntary control of respiration reflects activity in the cerebral cortex that affects either the output of the respiratory center in the medulla oblongata and pons or the output of motor neurons in the spinal cord that control respiratory muscles. The most important parts comprise the **medullary respiratory center**, which consists of the dorsal and ventral respiratory groups and the respiratory group of the pons (**FIGURE 19-13**).

The dorsal respiratory group is located near the root of cranial nerve IX. It is important in stimulating the muscles of inspiration but is still not fully understood. Increased impulses result in more forceful muscle contractions and deeper breathing. Decreased impulses result in passive expiration. It is known that the dorsal respiratory group integrates input from chemoreceptors and peripheral stretch receptors. It communicates this information to the ventral respiratory group.

The ventral respiratory group controls other respiratory muscles, mostly the intercostals and abdominals, to increase the force of expiration and sometimes to increase inspiratory efforts. It is believed to be a center of integration and generation of rhythm. It is a network of neurons extending from the spinal cord, through the ventral brain stem, to the pons–medulla junction. Some neurons fire during inspiration, whereas others fire during expiration. The inspiratory neurons send impulses along the *phrenic and intercostal nerves*, exciting the diaphragm and external intercostal muscles, respectively. Therefore, damage to the phrenic nerves can increase

respiratory rate. The expiratory neurons cause the output to stop and passive expiration to occur, as the inspiratory muscles relax and the lungs then recoil.

This inspiratory and expiratory cycling is continuous, producing the normal respiratory rate of 12 to 15 breaths per minute. Inspiratory phases last about 2 seconds, whereas expiratory phases last about 3 seconds. *Eupnea* is the term describing this normal respiratory rate and rhythm. In severe hypoxia, the ventral respiratory group causes the individual to gasp for air. This may be a final effort to restore oxygen to the brain. When certain clustered neurons are completely suppressed, respiration stops. Causes of this include overdoses of alcohol or drugs such as morphine.

The basic rhythm of breathing may also be controlled by the pontine respiratory group in the pons. This consists of several centers influencing and modifying medullary neuron activities. The pontine group is believed to make the transitions between inspiration and expiration and the reverse, smoother processes. Lesions to the superior region of the pontine respiratory group cause prolonged inspirations to occur, which is called *apneustic breathing*.

However, the rhythmic quality of breathing is not fully understood. The most accepted theory is that normal respiratory rhythm is based on reciprocal inhibition of interconnected networks of neurons in the medulla. Instead of one set of "pacemaker neurons," two sets of neurons inhibit each other. Their activity occurs in cycles, and this generates respiratory rhythm.

Factors of Respiratory Rate and Depth

The depth of inspiration during breathing is based on the level of activity of the respiratory center and its stimulation of motor neurons that serve the respiratory muscles. With more stimulation, increased numbers of motor units are excited. Therefore, respiratory muscles contract with greater force. Respiratory rate is established by the length of time the inspiratory center is active or how fast it is turned off. Deep breathing is referred to as diaphragmatic breathing, while shallow breathing is known as costal breathing.

Certain chemicals also affect respiratory rate and depth. Important substances include carbon dioxide, hydrogen, and oxygen ions in the arterial blood. Other factors include emotional states, lung stretching capability, and levels of physical activity. Chemosensitive areas known as *central chemoreceptors*, located in the medulla oblongata, sense carbon dioxide and hydrogen ion changes in the cerebrospinal fluid. When these levels change, respiratory rate and tidal volume are signaled to increase. More carbon dioxide is exhaled, and both blood and cerebrospinal fluid levels of these chemicals fall, decreasing breathing rate.

Carbon dioxide is the most important chemical regulator of respiration. Arterial partial pressure of carbon dioxide is usually 40 mm Hg, maintained within 3 mm Hg of this level, mostly by how rising carbon dioxide levels affect the central chemoreceptors. *Hypercapnia* is a condition in which carbon dioxide accumulates in the brain. The accumulating carbon dioxide is hydrated, and carbonic acid is formed.

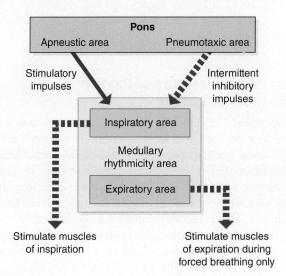

FIGURE 19-13 The medullary respiratory center.

When the acid is dissociated, hydrogen ions are freed and pH drops. This same thing happens when carbon dioxide enters red blood cells.

Increased hydrogen ions excite the central chemoreceptors, which extensively synapse with the respiratory regulatory centers. Breathing depth and rate therefore increase. Because alveolar ventilation is enhanced, carbon dioxide is quickly flushed out of the blood and pH rises. Alveolar ventilation is doubled with an elevation of only 5 mm Hg in arterial partial pressure of carbon dioxide. This is true even when there is no change in arterial oxygen levels or pH. The response to elevated partial pressure of carbon dioxide is even more extensive when partial pressure of oxygen and pH are lower than normal. Increased ventilation is usually self-limited. It stops when there is restoration of homeostatic blood partial pressure of carbon dioxide.

The rising levels of hydrogen ions within the brain increase the activity of the central chemoreceptors, even though rising blood carbon dioxide is the first stimulus. Although hydrogen does not easily diffuse across the blood–brain barrier, carbon dioxide accomplishes this with no problem. Therefore, control of breathing while resting mostly is based on regulation of hydrogen ion concentration in the brain.

However, *peripheral chemoreceptors* in the carotid bodies and aortic bodies also help and are able to sense changes in blood oxygen levels (**FIGURE 19-14**). They then increase the breathing rate, but this action requires extremely low levels of blood oxygen to occur.

The depth of breathing is regulated by the *inflation reflex*, which occurs when stretched lung tissues stimulate stretch receptors in the visceral pleura, bronchioles, and alveoli. The duration of inspiratory movements are shortened, preventing overinflation of the lungs during forceful breathing. Emotional upset, such as that caused by fear and pain, usually increase breathing rate. If breathing stops, even for a short time, blood levels of carbon dioxide and hydrogen ions rise and oxygen levels fall. Chemoreceptors are stimulated, and the urge to inhale increases, overcoming the lack of oxygen. The *deflation reflex* usually only functions during forced exhalation and inhibits the expiratory centers while stimulating the inspiratory centers when the lungs are deflating.

FOCUS ON PATHOLOGY

Hyperventilation consists of deep, rapid breathing that lowers blood carbon dioxide levels. After hyperventilation, it takes longer for carbon dioxide to rise back up to levels that produce the need to breathe in. Prolonged breath holding causes abnormally low blood oxygen levels. Hyperventilation should never be used to help hold the breath during swimming. It may cause loss of consciousness while under water.

Involuntary hyperventilation may be linked to an anxiety attack. Lowered carbon dioxide levels in the blood are referred to as *hypocapnia*. As blood vessels constrict, cerebral ischemia results in fainting or dizziness. Early symptoms of hyperventilation include tingling and tetany in the muscles of hands and face. Symptoms may be controlled by breathing into a paper bag, because air inspired from the bag is actually expired air and is rich in carbon dioxide. This causes carbon dioxide to be retained in the blood. Periods of *apnea*, which means "cessation of breathing" may occur when partial pressure of carbon dioxide is very low. Apnea usually lasts until this level rises enough to stimulate respiration.

How Partial Pressure of Oxygen Influences Breathing

The peripheral chemoreceptors contain cells that are sensitive to arterial levels of oxygen. These chemoreceptors lie in the *aortic bodies* of the aortic arch and the *carotid bodies* at the bifurcation of the common carotid arteries. Those in the carotid bodies are the main oxygen sensors. Normally, reducing partial pressure of oxygen only affects ventilation minimally. This primarily involves enhanced sensitivity of peripheral receptors to increased partial pressure of carbon dioxide. For oxygen levels to become a strong stimulus for increased ventilation, arterial partial pressure of oxygen must drop greatly, to at least 60 mm Hg.

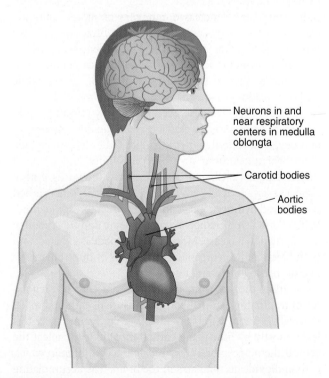

Neurons in and near respiratory centers in medulla oblongta

Carotid bodies

Aortic bodies

FIGURE 19-14 Stimulation of peripheral chemoreceptors.

How Arterial pH Influences Breathing

Even during normal levels of oxygen and carbon dioxide, changes to arterial pH can modify the rate and rhythm of breathing. Increased ventilation occurring because of reduced arterial pH is controlled via the peripheral chemoreceptors. This is in part because hydrogen ions do not cross the blood–brain barrier. Changes in partial pressure of carbon dioxide and hydrogen ion concentration are related yet different.

Reduced blood pH may be related to retention of carbon dioxide. However, it may also occur because of metabolic reasons. These include lactic acid accumulation because of exercise or fatty acid metabolite or *ketone body* accumulation because of uncontrolled diabetes mellitus. No matter what the reason, as arterial pH declines, the respiratory system will attempt to compensate and raise the pH. This occurs by the increase of respiratory rate and depth in an attempt to eliminate carbon dioxide and carbonic acid from the blood.

How Higher Brain Centers Influence Breathing

Respiratory rate and depth are modified when pain or strong emotions send signals to the respiratory centers. This occurs via the limbic system, including the hypothalamus. Changes in body temperature also affect respiration, with hotter temperatures increasing it and colder temperatures decreasing it.

Conscious control of breathing can also occur. The cerebral motor cortex sends impulses to the motor neurons, causing stimulation of respiratory muscles. This bypasses the medullary centers. Holding the breath is a limited function because the brain stem respiratory centers automatically reinitiate breathing once carbon dioxide levels in the blood become critical.

TEST YOUR UNDERSTANDING

1. Describe the medullary respiratory center.
2. Are peripheral chemoreceptors as sensitive to levels of carbon dioxide as they are to levels of oxygen?
3. Differentiate between the central and peripheral chemoreceptors and their actions.

Effects of Aging on the Respiratory System

Aging causes the lungs to lose elasticity, lowering their vital capacity. The ribs play a role in affecting breathing because they may become arthritic, and the costal cartilages may become less flexible. Respiratory volume is therefore impaired, resulting in the inability to exercise as long or as hard compared with earlier in life. Emphysema risk is much higher in smokers than in nonsmokers, but some evidence of the disease is present in most people over age 50

FOCUS ON PATHOLOGY

Chronic obstructive pulmonary disease, or *COPD*, has several components, which include *emphysema* and *chronic bronchitis*. Overall, most affected people are smokers, have *dyspnea*, coughing, frequent pulmonary infections, and then develop *hypoventilation, respiratory acidosis,* and *hypoxemia*. *Emphysema* results in the need for accessory muscles to be used to breathe, the development of a "barrel chest," and damage to the pulmonary capillaries. In *chronic bronchitis*, irritants that are inhaled cause chronic production of excessive mucus. Smoking and environmental pollution are major risk factors. Chronic bronchitis causes inflamed and fibrosed passageways, obstructed airways, frequent pulmonary infections, and moderate dyspnea. As a result of emphysema and chronic bronchitis, COPD patients often become either thin, with pink-tinged skin and excessive breathing, or bloated with cyanotic skin linked to pulmonary hypertension and right-sided heart failure. Treatment of COPD involves bronchodilators, inhaled corticosteroids, oxygen, and lung volume reduction surgery.

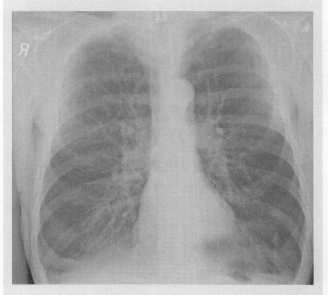

Chronic obstructive pulmonary disease. (Courtesy of Coastline Imaging.)

regardless of their history of smoking. Although aging affects the respiratory system of every adult, smokers experience greatly increased problems as aging continues.

FOCUS ON PATHOLOGY

FOCUS ON PATHOLOGY

Tuberculosis usually is transmitted by coughing and inhalation of infected air. The causative bacterium is *Mycobacterium tuberculosis*, which mostly affects the lungs but can also harm other body organs. Amazingly, nearly one-third of the world's population has the bacterium but does not develop the active form of the disease. Because the bacterium survives in lung nodules or *tubercles*, a weakened immune system may allow it to escape and cause the active disease. Symptoms of tuberculosis include fever, night sweats, severe coughing that often brings up blood, and weight loss. Although decreasing in incidence, deadly drug-resistant strains of tuberculosis have been discovered. Drug therapy usually requires a full year of antibiotics.

Lung cancer is the most common cause of death for men and women in the United States. Nearly all cases occur because of smoking, and, unfortunately, the disease is often not detected until highly advanced. Most patients die within 1 year of diagnosis. Other factors that cause lung cancer include exposure to air pollution or chemical substances and second-hand smoke. The three most common types are *adenocarcinoma, squamous cell carcinoma,* and *small cell carcinoma.* Without metastasis, total lung removal is preferred to prolong life and cure the patient. For diagnosis, chest x-ray and computed tomography are commonly performed. A malignant lung carcinoma forms a discrete nodule when viewed by these methods.

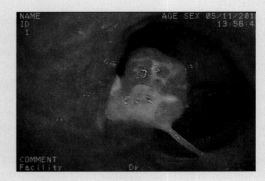

Carcinoma in the right upper lobe.

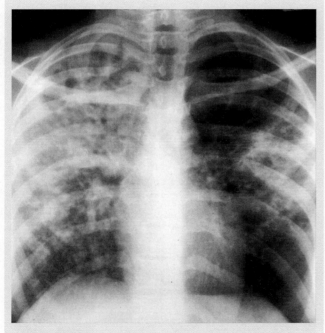

Tuberculosis. (Courtesy of Leonard V. Crowley, MD, Century College.)

SUMMARY

The respiratory system includes tubes that remove particles from incoming air. These tubes also transport air to and from the lungs and air sacs, where gas exchanges occur. Respiration is the entire process of gas exchange between body cells and the atmosphere. The organs of the respiratory system can be divided into the upper and lower respiratory tracts. The upper respiratory tract includes the nose, nasal cavity, paranasal sinuses, and pharynx. The lower respiratory tract includes the larynx, trachea, and lungs, which contain the bronchi, bronchioles, and alveoli. The pharynx connects the nasal cavity and mouth to the larynx superiorly and the esophagus inferiorly. The lungs are not symmetric, with the right lung having three lobes and the left lung having only two to accommodate the heart.

The four distinct respiratory volumes involved in respiration are tidal volume, inspiratory reserve volume, expiratory reserve volume, and residual volume. Also, four respiratory capacities are created by the combination of two or more of the respiratory volumes: total lung capacity, vital capacity, inspiratory capacity, and functional residual capacity. Pulmonary function was originally tested using a device called a spirometer, but today this has been replaced by an electronic measuring device into which the patient blows air.

The thoracic activity changes size of its capacity or volume as inspiration and expiration occur. Normal breathing is involuntary and rhythmic. Gas exchange between air and blood occurs in the alveoli. Blood transports gases between the lungs and body cells. Nearly all oxygen transported from the lungs to the body tissues occurs via its chemical combination with hemoglobin. Carbon dioxide bonds with the amino groups of the "globin" or protein portion of hemoglobin. The respiratory areas of the brain are the brain stem and portions of the medulla oblongata and pons. With aging, changes to the lungs, ribs, and costal cartilages combine to impair respiratory volume. Smoking is the most significant risk factor to respiratory impairment over our lifetimes.

KEY TERMS

Alveolar ducts
Alveolar sacs
Alveolar ventilation rate
Alveoli
Bicarbonate ions
Bronchial tree
Bronchioles
Carbaminohemoglobin
Carbonic anhydrase
Cricoid cartilage
Dalton's law
Diaphragm
Epiglottic cartilage
Epiglottis
Expiration
Expiratory reserve volume
Functional residual capacity
Glottis
Goblet cells
Hemoglobin
Henry's law

Hyperventilation
Hypoxia
Inspiration
Inspiratory capacity
Inspiratory reserve volume
Laryngopharynx
Larynx
Lingual tonsil
Lungs
Medullary respiratory center
Nasal cavity
Nasal conchae
Nasal septum
Nasopharynx
Oropharynx
Oxyhemoglobin
Palatine tonsils
Paranasal sinuses
Parietal pleura
Partial pressure
Pharyngeal tonsil

Pharynx
Pleural cavity
Primary bronchi
Residual volume
Respiration
Respiratory areas
Respiratory capacities
Respiratory membrane
Respiratory system
Respiratory volumes
Spirometer
Surface tension
Surfactant
Thyroid cartilage
Tidal volume
Total lung capacity
Trachea
Visceral pleura
Vital capacity

The following learning goals correspond to the objectives at the beginning of this chapter:

1. The primary functions of the respiratory system are the intake of oxygen and the removal of carbon dioxide.
2. The upper respiratory system consists of the
    A. *Nose:* allows air to enter and leave via the nostrils
    B. *Nasal cavity:* helps to warm and moisten air, using mucus to trap particles
    C. *Paranasal sinuses:* reduce the skull's weight and affect the quality of the voice
    D. *Pharynx:* carries food from the oral cavity to the esophagus and allows air to pass from the nasal cavity to the larynx; helps produce the sounds of speech
3. Outside of the lungs, the trachea or *windpipe* splits into the right and left bronchi. Branched airways leading from the trachea to the alveoli make up the bronchial tree. These branches begin with the right and left primary bronchi, with each dividing into a secondary bronchus, then into tertiary bronchi, and even finer tubes. Bronchioles are smaller tubes that continue to divide.
4. The alveoli are microscopic air sacs inside capillary networks of the lungs. They provide a large surface of epithelial cells that allow easy exchange of gases. Oxygen diffuses from the alveoli into the capillaries, and carbon dioxide diffuses from the blood into the alveoli.
5. External respiration is defined as gas exchange between air in the lungs and the blood. Internal respiration is defined as gas exchange between the blood and the cells.
6. External respiration consists of ventilation, which is the movement of air from outside of the body into and out of the bronchial tree and alveoli. During normal inspiration, when inside pressure decreases, atmospheric pressure pushes outside air into the airways. Phrenic nerve impulses stimulate the diaphragm to contract, moving downward. The thoracic cavity enlarges, internal pressure falls, and atmospheric pressure forces air into the airways. As the diaphragm contracts, the external intercostal muscles contract. The ribs raise and the sternum elevates. The lungs expand in response, and the thoracic wall moves upward and outward. There is an opposing effect in the alveoli.
7. The respiratory membrane is located in the alveoli. The inner lining is made up of simple squamous epithelium. Dense networks of capillaries are found nearby. At least two thicknesses of epithelial cells and a fused basement membrane layer separate the air in an alveolus from the blood in a capillary. These layers make up the respiratory membrane; it is here where blood and alveolar air exchange gases.
8. As oxygen from the lungs enters the blood, it dissolves in the plasma along with carbon dioxide from the cells or combines with blood components. About 98% of the oxygen transported by the blood binds the iron-containing protein hemoglobin in red blood cells. The remainder dissolves in the plasma. In the lungs, oxygen dissolves in blood and combines rapidly with the iron atoms of hemoglobin to form oxyhemoglobin. As the partial pressure of oxygen decreases, oxyhemoglobin molecules release oxygen, diffusing into nearby cells that have depleted their oxygen supplies in cellular respiration. When carbon dioxide increases in the blood, more oxygen is released.
9. Respiration rate is controlled by the respiratory areas of the brain, which include the brainstem, pons, and medulla oblongata. The medullar respiratory center consists of the dorsal and ventral respiratory groups and the respiratory group of the pons. The dorsal group is important in stimulating the muscles of inspiration. Increased impulses result in more forceful muscle contractions and deeper breathing. Decreased impulses result in passive expiration. The ventral group controls mostly the intercostal and abdominal muscles to increase the force of expiration and sometimes to increase inspiratory efforts. Certain chemicals also affect breathing rate and depth, as do emotional states, lung stretching capability, and physical activity.
10. The four distinct respiratory volumes are as follows:
    A. *Tidal volume:* approximately 500 mL; moved into or out of lungs during respiratory cycle
    B. *Inspiratory reserve volume:* approximately 3,000 mL; inhaled during forced breathing in addition to tidal volume
    C. *Expiratory reserve volume:* approximately 1,100 mL; exhaled during forced breathing in addition to tidal volume
    D. *Residual volume:* approximately 1,200 mL; remaining in lungs even after maximal expiration

CRITICAL THINKING QUESTIONS

A 52-year-old man with no history of smoking was diagnosed with primary lung cancer. He worked in the human resources section of his local health department. His sister died 7 years previously from breast cancer. The patient's wife had a history of smoking two packs of cigarettes a day for 20 years.

1. Explain the most common types of lung cancer.
2. How could this patient have contracted lung cancer without being a smoker?

REVIEW QUESTIONS

1. The openings of the nostrils are called the
   A. internal nares
   B. vestibules
   C. turbinates
   D. external nares

2. Which of the following cells secrete mucus in an airway?
   A. mast cells
   B. phagocytes
   C. goblet cells
   D. dust cells

3. Which of the following is the portion of the pharynx that receives both air and food?
   A. nasopharynx
   B. oropharynx
   C. laryngopharynx
   D. glottis

4. The vocal folds are located in the
   A. larynx
   B. trachea
   C. nasopharynx
   D. oropharynx

5. The trachea contains how many tracheal cartilages?
   A. 5
   B. 10
   C. 20
   D. 25

6. The airway between the larynx and the primary bronchi is the
   A. trachea
   B. pharynx
   C. bronchiole
   D. alveolar duct

7. The actual sites of gas exchange within the lungs are the
   A. bronchioles
   B. terminal sacs
   C. alveoli
   D. pleural spaces

8. Which of the following statements describes surfactant?
   A. It replaces mucus in the alveoli.
   B. It helps prevent the alveoli from collapsing.
   C. It protects the surface of the lungs.
   D. It replaces mucus in the alveoli.

9. When the external intercostal muscles and diaphragm contract,
   A. the volume of the lungs decreases
   B. the volume of the thorax increases
   C. the volume of the thorax decreases
   D. the lungs collapse

10. The residual volume of the lungs equals
    A. 500 mL
    B. 1,100 mL
    C. 1,200 mL
    D. 2,300 mL

11. The vital capacity plus the residual volume creates the
    A. total lung capacity
    B. functional residual capacity
    C. inspiratory capacity
    D. vital capacity

12. Ordinary air consists of mostly
    A. nitrogen
    B. hilum
    C. oxygen
    D. carbon dioxide

13. Most of the carbon dioxide in the blood is transported as
    A. carbonic acid
    B. carbaminohemoglobin
    C. solute dissolved in the plasma
    D. bicarbonate ions
14. The most important chemical regulator of respiration is
    A. the bicarbonate ion
    B. carbon dioxide
    C. oxygen
    D. the sodium ion

15. With aging,
    A. vital capacity increases
    B. the lungs become more elastic
    C. the lungs become more compliant
    D. pulmonary ventilation decreases

ESSAY QUESTIONS

1. Describe the route of air in the respiratory system.
2. List the laryngeal cartilages.
3. Describe the structures of the conducting and respiratory zones.
4. Describe the pleurae and their function.
5. Explain the inspiratory muscles and their actions.
6. Discuss how airway resistance, lung compliance, and alveolar surface tension affect pulmonary ventilation.
7. Explain Henry's law and Dalton's law.
8. Describe testing of pulmonary function.
9. Discuss how arterial pH influences breathing.
10. Describe age-related changes in respiratory function.

Urinary System

OBJECTIVES

After studying this chapter, the reader should be able to

1. Describe the location and structural features of the kidneys.
2. Describe the structure of the nephron.
3. Identify and describe the major factors responsible for the production of urine.
4. Describe how antidiuretic hormone and aldosterone influence the volume and concentration of urine.
5. List and describe the factors that influence filtration pressure.
6. Describe the structure and functions of the ureters, urinary bladder, and urethra.
7. Differentiate between the contents of different substances in the plasma and urine.
8. Describe the normal characteristics and composition of urine.
9. List the most important waste products that are excreted from the kidneys.
10. Describe the micturition reflex center.

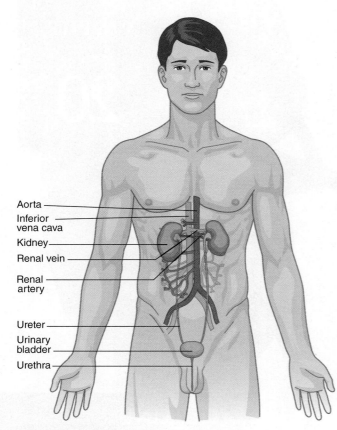

FIGURE 20-1 The urinary system.

Overview

The urinary system consists of two kidneys, two ureters, a **urinary bladder**, and a **urethra** (**FIGURE 20-1**). The urinary system has three major functions: (1) *excretion*, which is the removal of organic wastes from body fluids; (2) *elimination*, which is the discharge of these wastes into the environment; and (3) *homeostatic regulation* of the volume and solute concentration of blood plasma. The urinary system filters approximately 200 liters of fluid from the bloodstream every day.

The kidneys help to maintain homeostasis by regulating the composition, pH or *acid-base balance*, and volume of the extracellular fluid. This is accomplished by their removal of metabolic wastes and toxins from the blood and diluting them with water and electrolytes. This process forms urine, which the kidneys excrete. The other important functions of the kidneys are as follows:

- Secretion of the hormone erythropoietin, which helps to control red blood cell production
- Helping with the activation of vitamin D
- Helping to maintain blood volume and pressure via secretion of the enzyme renin
- Carrying out gluconeogenesis while fasting for long periods

Anatomy of the Kidneys

The **kidneys** are bean-shaped organs with a reddish-brown color. In adults, the kidneys are each enclosed in a tough,

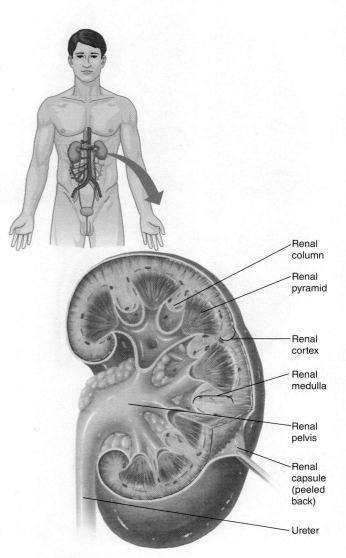

FIGURE 20-2 Gross anatomy of the kidney.

fibrous capsule (**FIGURE 20-2**). A thick layer of adipose tissue, known as the *perinephric fat capsule*, surrounds the fibrous capsule. The kidneys are about 11 cm long by 6 cm wide and 3 cm thick. The kidneys lie on either side of the vertebral column in depressions on the upper posterior wall of the abdominal cavity. Their upper border is near the 12th thoracic vertebra and their lower border near the 3rd lumbar vertebra; the left kidney is about 1.5 to 2 cm higher than the right one, because the right kidney is somewhat crowded downward by the liver. Each kidney weighs about 5.25 ounces or 150 grams.

The kidneys are positioned behind the parietal peritoneum, against the deep muscles of the back, which is described as **retroperitoneally**. They are surrounded and held in position by connective and adipose tissue. The *renal fascia* anchors the kidneys to surrounding structures and consists of a dense and fibrous outer tissue. Each kidney has a convex lateral surface and a concave medial side, resulting in a medial depression leading to a hollow **renal sinus**. This chamber's entrance is called the **hilum**, through which pass blood vessels, nerves, lymphatic vessels, and the *ureter*.

Internal Kidney Anatomy

The kidneys are organized into two major regions: an outer **renal cortex**, which is lighter in color, and an inner **renal medulla**, which is darker reddish-brown in color (Figure 20-2). Inside the renal sinus, the **renal pelvis**, a funnel-shaped sac, expands from the superior end of the ureter. It is subdivided into major calyces and minor calyces or *tubes*. Small elevations called *renal papillae* project into the renal sinus from the renal pelvis walls, and tiny openings leading into the minor calyces pierce each projection. Urine drains continuously from the papillae into the calyces, which empty it to the renal pelvis. It moves through the renal pelvis, into the ureter, and then to the bladder for storage. Urine is propelled by peristalsis via the walls of the calyces, pelvis, and uterine smooth muscles.

The renal medulla is made of conical tissue called *renal pyramids* and has striations. Each renal pyramid has a broad base that faces the cortex, whereas each apex or *papilla* faces internally. The renal cortex encloses the medulla, dipping into it between the renal pyramids to form *renal columns*. The cortex appears to have granules due to tiny tubules associated with the functional units of the kidneys, the **nephrons**. Each renal pyramid and the cortical tissue that surrounds it makes up a *lobe* of the kidney. Each kidney has approximately eight lobes.

Renal Blood Flow and Nerve Supply

The kidneys are continuously supplied with blood from the **renal arteries**, which arise from the abdominal aorta. These arteries transport large volumes of blood. While a person rests, the renal arteries carry between 15% and 30% of the total cardiac output, approximately 1,200 mL, into the kidneys every minute.

The renal arteries branch off at right angles inside the kidneys into *interlobar arteries*, *arcuate arteries*, and interlobular *cortical radiate* arteries (**FIGURE 20-3**). The final branches of the interlobular arteries lead to the nephrons and are called **afferent arterioles**. The microscopic blood vessels of the kidney are the main components of how it functions. The right renal artery is longest, because the aorta lies to the left side of the midline. Nearing a kidney, each renal artery is divided into five *segmental arteries*. Corresponding, in general, with the arterial pathways, the venous blood returns through a similar series of vessels. Nearly 90% of the blood that enters the kidney perfuses the renal cortex.

The **renal vein** then joins the inferior vena cava. Venous blood returns through a series of vessels that correspond generally to arterial pathways. Blood that leaves each kidney flows from the cortex through the cortical radiate vein, arcuate vein, interlobar vein, and, finally, the renal vein. Unlike renal arteries, there is no *segmental* component in the vein system. Exiting the kidney, the renal veins empty to the inferior vena cava. The *renal plexus* provides the kidney's nerve supply and also the nerve supply of the ureter. The renal plexus is a varied network of autonomic ganglia and nerve fibers that derives from the celiac plexus. It has many sympathetic fibers as its supply, from the inferior thoracic and

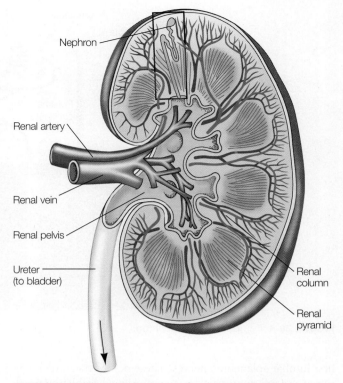

FIGURE 20-3 The main branches of a renal artery.

FOCUS ON PATHOLOGY

When the normal fatty casing of a kidney is reduced from starvation and rapid loss of weight, it may drop to a lower position. Known as *renal ptosis*, this can cause kinking of a ureter, resulting in restricting **urine**, increasing pressure on the renal tissues. Backup of urine is known as *hydronephrosis*, which can cause severe kidney damage, necrosis, and renal failure.

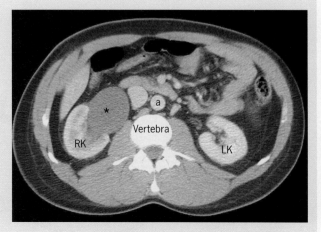

Hydronephrosis, computed tomography. (Courtesy of Dr. Myron Pozniak, Department of Radiology, University of Wisconsin School of Medicine and Public Health.)

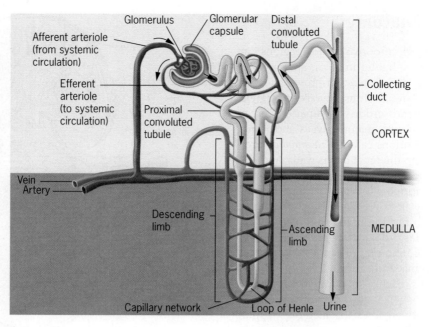

FIGURE 20-4 Components of a nephron.

first lumbar splanchnic nerves. These nerves trace the renal artery and are sympathetic vasomotor fibers regulating renal blood flow via adjustment of renal arteriole diameter. They also influence the nephrons' urine formation.

Structures of the Nephron

The functional units of the kidneys are the nephrons, in which 85% are *cortical nephrons*, located almost totally within the superficial cortex. There are about 1 million nephrons in a kidney, each consisting of a **renal corpuscle** and a **renal tubule** (**FIGURE 20-4**). The three major sections of each renal tubule are the **proximal convoluted tubule**, **nephron loop**, and **distal convoluted tubule**. The renal tubule leaves the **glomerular capsule** as the highly coiled proximal convoluted tubule (**FIGURE 20-5**). This makes a tight loop called the nephron loop. It then winds and twists some more to become the distal convoluted tubule, which empties into a collecting duct. The outer wall of the glomerular capsule is

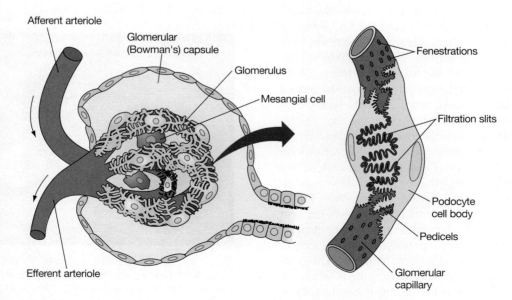

FIGURE 20-5 Structure of the renal corpuscle.

lined with a simple squamous *capsular epithelium* that is continuous with the *visceral epithelium* covering the glomerular capillaries. The capsular and visceral epithelia are separated by a *capsular space*.

The proximal convoluted tubule cells reabsorb water, ions, organic nutrients, and plasma proteins, when they are present, from the tubular fluid. They are released into the *peritubular* fluid, which is the fluid that surrounds the renal tubule. Filtrate moves from the renal corpuscle through the proximal convoluted tubule first, then the nephron loop, and finally the distal convoluted tubule. The many twists and turns of the renal tubules means they actually would be much longer if straightened out. These convolutions also increase their ability to process filtrate. Both the renal tubule and **collecting duct** are made up of just one layer of polar epithelial cells above a basement membrane, but they differ in their histology. The distal convoluted tubule passes between afferent and efferent arterioles and also comes into contact with them.

Parts of the Renal Tubule

The walls of the proximal convoluted tubule are made up of cuboidal epithelial cells that have large mitochondria. Dense microvilli are found on their luminal *apical* surfaces, forming a *brush border* that is similar to the one in the intestines. The brush border increases the surface area and reabsorption capabilities to a large degree. It easily reabsorbs water and solutes from the filtrate while secreting substances into it.

The proximal convoluted tubule dips toward the renal pelvis to form the descending limb of the U-shaped nephron loop, formerly called the *loop of Henle*. In this location, urine is concentrated. This structure is also described as having a "horseshoe shape." The proximal area of the descending limb is continuous with the proximal tubule and has similar types of cells. It then curves toward the renal corpuscle to form the ascending limb of the nephron loop. The ascending limb has a thick segment in most nephrons, but in others its thin segment extends around a bend to form the *ascending thin limb*. This returns to the renal corpuscle region, coiling tightly to become the distal convoluted tubule. This tubule's epithelial cells are similar to those of the proximal convoluted tubule in that they are cuboidal and only found in the cortex. However, they are thinner and have very few microvilli. These tubules, which receive filtrate from several nephrons, merge to form collecting ducts in the renal cortexes. They pass into the renal medulla, resulting in tubes that empty into the minor calyces through openings in the renal papillae. The exchanges between the ascending and descending limbs of the nephron loop are referred to as *countercurrent multiplication*, because the fluids are moving in opposite directions.

The collecting ducts are responsible for maintaining the water and sodium ion balance of the body. Their *type A* (principal cells) and *type B* (intercalated cells) play various roles in balancing acids and bases in the blood. Thousands of *collecting ducts* collect fluid, each one from many nephrons, and move it to the renal pelvis. The ducts run through medullary pyramids, causing them to appear striped. Nearing the renal pelvis, the collecting ducts become fused, delivering urine to the minor calyces through the papillae of the pyramids. Fusion of collecting ducts forms larger *papillary ducts*.

Capillary Beds of the Nephron

Each nephron's renal tubule is linked to a glomerulus and the peritubular capillaries. Also, juxtamedullary nephrons use the *vasa recta*, which are specialized capillaries. A **glomerulus** is a tangled cluster of parallel blood capillaries that comprises a *renal corpuscle*. All renal corpuscles are located in the renal cortex, but the renal tubules begin in the cortex and continue into the medulla, finally returning to the cortex. The glomerular capillaries are unique in that they are fed by an *afferent arteriole* and drained by an **efferent arteriole** (Figure 20-5). Blood, minus filtered fluids, is actually what drains out via the efferent arteriole. Having both types of arterioles keeps the pressure high in the glomerulus so filtration can be effective.

Efferent arterioles are smaller in diameter than afferent arterioles and resist blood flow slightly. They branch into complex, interconnected capillary networks, each called a **peritubular capillary**, which surrounds the renal tubule. The low-pressure blood inside eventually enters the venous system of the kidney. The *peritubular capillaries* are tightly located to renal tubules, emptying into local venules. Their pressure is low, because they arise from efferent arterioles, which have high resistance. The porous peritubular capillaries can therefore easily absorb water and solutes from renal tubule cells during their reclamation from the filtrate. Because the renal tubules are so closely aligned together, each nephron's peritubular capillaries absorb substances from several nearby nephrons.

A lot of fluid is produced by filtration. Approximately 99% of it is reabsorbed by renal tubule cells to be returned to the blood via the beds of the peritubular capillaries. The *cortical radiate arteries* running through the renal cortex give rise to the afferent arterioles. The peritubular capillaries or vasa recta are fed by various efferent arterioles.

The efferent arterioles that serve the juxtamedullary nephrons usually do not divide into peritubular capillaries but form bundles of long and straight *vasa recta*. The vasa recta are vessels extending deeply into the medulla, parallel to nephron loops, which are the longest found there. The vasa recta have very thin walls, helping to form concentrated urine.

Juxtaglomerular Complex

The **juxtaglomerular apparatus** or *complex* of each nephron is where the ascending limb of the nephron loop's most distal portion lies against an afferent arteriole supplying the glomerulus (**FIGURE 20-6A** and **B**). It may also lie against an efferent arteriole. Modifications of structure exist where the ascending limb and afferent arteriole meet. Each juxtaglomerular apparatus has three types of cells regulating filtrate formation rates and systemic blood pressure: the **macula densa**, **granular cells**, and *extraglomerular mesangial cells*.

The *macula densa* is a thickening in the wall of the distal tubule of the kidney nephron, at a point where it is in contact with the afferent glomerulus. The macula densa cells act as chemoreceptors. They monitor the filtrate's sodium chloride

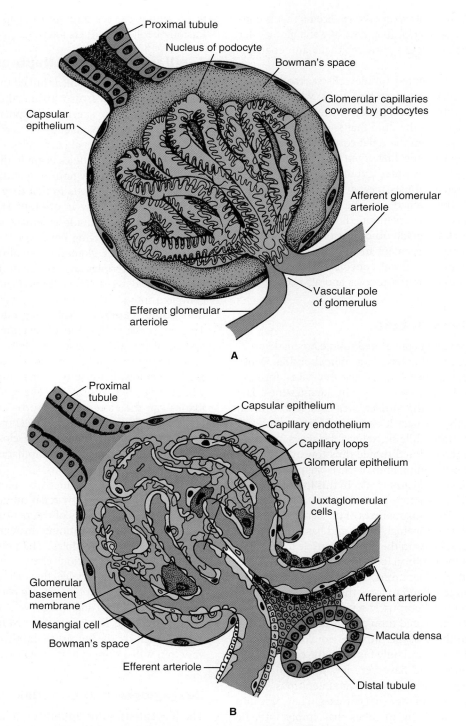

FIGURE 20-6 The structure of the glomerulus and Bowman's capsule. A. Anterior half of Bowman's capsule removed to reveal capillary tuft covered by podocytes (schematic). B. Cross section through glomerulus to reveal structure of glomerular filter and juxtaglomerular apparatus.

content as it enters the distal convoluted tubule. The *granular* or *juxtaglomerular cells* in the arteriolar walls are enlarged smooth muscle cells. They have large secretory granules containing *renin*, an enzyme. Granular cells act as mechanoreceptors. They monitor blood pressure of the afferent arteriole. *Extraglomerular mesangial cells* between the arteriole and tubule cells are interconnected via gap junctions. They are believed to pass signals that have regulatory functions between the macula densa and granular cells.

TABLE 20-1

Concentrations of Different Substances

Substance	Glomerular Filtrate	Plasma	Urine
Concentrations in mEq/L			
Sodium	142	142	128
Chloride	103	103	134
Bicarbonate	27	27	14
Potassium	5	5	60
Calcium	4	4	5
Magnesium	3	3	15
Phosphate	2	2	40
Sulfate	1	1	33
Concentrations in mg/100 mL			
Glucose	100	100	0
Urea	26	26	1,820
Uric acid	4	4	53

Formation of Urine

The purposes of urine formation are to cleanse the blood and balance the body's chemical substances. Three steps are involved in urine formation and the regulation of blood composition: glomerular filtration, tubular reabsorption, and tubular secretion.

Glomerular Filtration

Glomerular filtration is a passive process that initiates urine formation in the renal corpuscle. It uses hydrostatic pressure to force fluids and solutes through membranes. The plasma is filtered by the glomerular capillaries, producing *filtrate* that is free of cells and proteins. Most of this fluid is reabsorbed into the bloodstream via the colloid osmotic pressure of the plasma. Using two capillaries in series, the nephrons use glomerular filtration to help produce urine. The first capillary bed filters forming interstitial fluid but does not form it. The filtrate, which is derived from the plasma, moves into the renal tubule to form urine. Every 24 hours, glomerular filtration produces 180 liters or 47 gallons of fluid—this is more than four times the amount of total body water. Less than 1.5 liters, which is lower than 1% of the fluid, leaves the body as urine.

The filtration membrane is located between the interior glomerular capsule, also called **Bowman's capsule**, and the blood. It is a porous membrane, allowing water and solutes that are smaller than plasma proteins to freely pass through. Any macromolecules caught in the filtration membrane are engulfed by *glomerular mesangial cells*, which are specialized **pericytes**. Any molecules smaller than 3 nm in diameter can

pass through freely, from the blood into the capsule. These molecules include amino acids, glucose, nitrogenous wastes, and water. An example of a substance that is too large to pass through the filtration membrane is *albumin*.

Because of this, these substances are similar in concentration to blood and *glomerular filtrate*. Glomerular filtrate is mostly water with the same components as blood plasma, except for large protein molecules. **TABLE 20-1** compares concentrations of substances in glomerular filtrate, plasma, and urine. Molecules larger than 5 nm usually cannot enter the tubules, so plasma proteins remaining in the capillaries helps to regulate the oncotic or *colloid osmotic* pressure of glomerular blood. Therefore, all water cannot be lost to the capsular spaces. The filtration membrane is probably functioning abnormally when proteins or blood cells become present in the urine.

The outward pressure that affects filtration is the **hydrostatic pressure** in the glomerular capillaries. This is basically the same as glomerular blood pressure and the strongest force moving water and solutes from the blood across the filtration membrane. Here, the blood pressure is high in the glomerulus, at about 55 mm Hg. In other capillary beds, the pressure is only 26 mm Hg. The reason for the difference is that the glomerular capillaries drain via a high-resistance efferent arteriole with a smaller diameter than the afferent arteriole supplying them. Filtration then occurs along all the length of every glomerular capillary. Reabsorption does not occur as it does in other capillary beds. The *colloid osmotic pressure* in the glomerular capsular space is nearly zero, because practically no proteins enter the capsule.

The *osmolarity* of a solution is its osmotic concentration, or the total number of solute particles per liter. This is usually

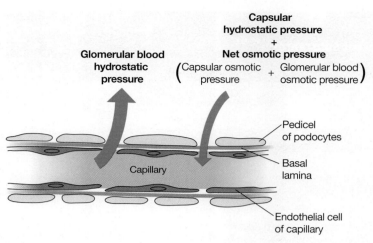

FIGURE 20-7 Net filtration pressure.

expressed in *osmoles per liter* (Osm/L) or *milliosmoles per liter* (mOsm/L). Body fluids have an osmolarity of approximately 300 mOsm/L, whereas fresh water is 5 mOsm/L and seawater 1,000 mOsm/L.

Glomerular Filtration Rate

The **glomerular filtration rate** (GFR) is defined as the volume of filtrate that forms every minute by the activities of the 2 million glomeruli in the kidneys. It is directly proportional to the **net filtration pressure**, the total surface area that is available for filtration, and the permeability of the filtration membrane (**FIGURE 20-7**). The net filtration pressure forces substances out of the glomerulus and is usually positive pressure. Tiny openings called *fenestrae* in glomerular capillary walls make them more permeable than the capillaries of other tissues. Cells called *podocytes* cover these capillaries, helping to make them impermeable to plasma proteins. The feet of the podocytes are called *pedicels*. Materials that pass from the blood, at the glomerulus, must be tiny enough to move through *filtration slits* between adjacent pedicels.

Net filtration pressure is directly proportional to the GFR. All factors related to GFR affect net filtration pressure. Any changes in afferent or efferent arteriole diameters alter the GFR. During filtration through capillary walls, proteins in the plasma raise colloid osmotic pressure with the glomerular capillaries. Anything that decreases plasma colloid osmotic pressure increases the filtration rate. The kidneys consume up to 25% of all oxygen the body uses while resting.

Regulation of Glomerular Filtration

The GFR is regulated by intrinsic controls, or *renal autoregulation*, and extrinsic controls via *the nervous and endocrine systems*. The intrinsic controls occur within the kidneys, whereas the extrinsic controls maintain blood pressure. The GFR must be relatively constant so the kidneys can manufacture filtrate and maintain extracellular homeostasis. The body's overall blood pressure must also be relatively constant. If nothing else changes, when the GFR increases, urine output also increases. This reduces blood volume and blood pressure. When the GFR decreases, the opposite occurs.

Extreme changes to mean arterial pressure, less than 80 mm Hg or higher than 180 mm Hg, causes the extrinsic controls to dominate to stop damage to the brain and other vital organs. Changing only the glomerular hydrostatic pressure can control the GFR. Therefore, the major mechanisms of pressure control focus on changing the glomerular hydrostatic pressure. When it rises, so do both the net filtration pressure and the GFR. The GFR will be reduced to zero if the glomerular hydrostatic pressure falls by 18% or greater, meaning it must be controlled precisely.

The GFR is kept relatively constant by autoregulatory mechanisms over the 80 to 180 mm Hg arterial pressure range. Normal daily changes in exercise activity, posture, or sleep do not result in significant changes in excretion of water and solutes. However, serious hemorrhage that causes extremely low systemic blood pressure will result in *hypovolemic shock*, which cannot be stopped by the intrinsic controls. Therefore, when mean arterial pressure is lower than 80 mm Hg, extrinsic controls take over and the autoregulatory mechanisms stop working.

The hormonal and neural mechanisms used in extrinsic controls include the *sympathetic nervous system* and the *renin-angiotensin-aldosterone mechanism*. Although the neural kidney controls help the whole body, the kidneys may suffer as a result. The kidney blood vessels are dilated, with their autoregulatory mechanisms dominating control when extracellular fluid volume is normal. At this time, the sympathetic nervous system is resting. Once the extracellular fluid volume becomes lower than 80 mm Hg, blood must be moved or *shunted* to vital organs. At that point, neural controls override autoregulatory mechanisms, which may reduce kidney blood flow enough to damage these organs.

Falling blood pressure causes the sympathetic nerve fibers to release norepinephrine and the adrenal medulla to release epinephrine. As a result, vascular smooth muscles constrict. This increases peripheral resistance, returning blood pressure to normal. This is the *baroreceptor reflex*. The GFR decreases from constriction of the afferent arterioles, assisting blood volume and pressure to return to normal. The *renin-angiotensin-aldosterone mechanism* is the primary control that increases blood pressure, yet it regulates GFR indirectly. Inadequate blood pressure means glomerular filtration cannot occur. It causes the granular cells in the juxtaglomerular complex to release renin. This occurs by either *direct stimulation of granular cells, stimulation of granular cells via input from activated cells of the macula densa,* or *reduced stretching of granular cells.*

Secretion of renin responds to three types of stimuli:

- When special afferent arteriole cells sense a drop in blood pressure
- In response to sympathetic stimulation
- When the macula densa senses decreased chloride, potassium, and sodium ions that reach the distal tubule

Renin in the bloodstream reacts with the plasma protein angiotensinogen, forming angiotensin I. In the lungs and blood plasma, angiotensin-converting enzyme converts angiotensin I to angiotensin II. Angiotensin II helps maintain sodium and water balance as well as blood pressure. It vasoconstricts the efferent arteriole, raising glomerular capillary hydrostatic pressure. This helps the decrease in GFR. Angiotensin II stimulates the kidneys to secrete aldosterone, encouraging *tubular reabsorption* of sodium.

FOCUS ON PATHOLOGY

Diabetic kidney disease causes chronic *glomerulonephritis*, in which there is reduction in the mass of nephrons and reduced GFR. When the GFR is decreased, there are increases in blood urea nitrogen and serum creatinine. Once the GFR is significantly decreased, outcomes include anemia, hypocalcemia, secondary hyperparathyroidism, hyperphosphatemia, acidosis, hyperkalemia, hypertension, edema, and increased chance of bleeding. Toxic wastes accumulate in most organ systems, resulting in uremia. The patient then requires dialysis of the kidneys or transplantation.

TEST YOUR UNDERSTANDING

1. Explain which types of molecule are trapped by the glomerular filtration membrane and which ones are not.
2. Contrast how glomerular filtration is regulated by intrinsic and extrinsic controls.
3. Describe the two types of extrinsic controls involved in glomerular filtration.

Tubular Reabsorption

Two other processes contribute to urine formation. **Tubular reabsorption** selectively moves substances from the tubular fluid into the blood, within the peritubular capillary (**FIGURE 20-8**). This occurs in the renal tubules and collecting ducts and is a transepithelial process. The kidney reclaims the correct amounts of water, electrolytes, and glucose as required by the body. All amino acids and glucose that were filtered are reabsorbed. Approximately 99% of water, sodium, and components are also reabsorbed. What is left over becomes urine.

Tubular reabsorption begins as soon as filtrate enters the proximal tubules. If not for tubular reabsorption, all the body's plasma would drain out as urine in under 30 minutes. In healthy adults, the total plasma volume filters into the renal tubules nearly every 22 minutes. Reabsorbed substances use either a paracellular or transcellular route to reach the blood. The paracellular route between the tubule cells is less extensive, because tight junctions connect these cells. These tight junctions are, however, not as tight in the proximal nephron and allow water and certain ions to pass through via the paracellular route. These ions include calcium, magnesium, potassium, and less amounts of sodium.

Nearly all organic nutrients such as glucose or amino acids are totally reabsorbed by healthy kidneys. This can maintain or restore normal plasma concentrations. However, water and specific ion reabsorption is regularly controlled as a result of signals from hormones. The reabsorption process is either *active* or *passive*, based on the actual substances transported. Adenosine triphosphate is required for **active tubular reabsorption**. This may be direct, as in primary active transport, or indirect, as in secondary active transport. The process of **passive tubular reabsorption** uses diffusion, facilitated diffusion, and osmosis. In these processes, substances move down their own electrochemical gradients.

Substances remaining in the renal tubule become more concentrated as water from the filtrate is reabsorbed by osmosis. Water reabsorption increases if sodium reabsorption increases, and vice versa. Active transport reabsorbs nearly 70% of sodium ions in the proximal renal tubule. Passive, negatively charged ions move along with the sodium ions. This is a form of passive transport because it does not require cellular energy expenditure. Movement of solutes and water into the peritubular capillary reduces fluid volume inside the renal tubule. Active transport reabsorbs sodium ions continually as tubular fluid moves through the nephron loop, distal convoluted tubule, and collecting duct. Nearly all sodium ions and water from the renal tubule via the glomerular filtrate are reabsorbed before urine excretion. Tubular reabsorption of sodium, nutrients, water, and ions is explained in **TABLE 20-2**.

All of the renal tubule is involved in reabsorption in varying degrees. However, the proximal convoluted tubule cells are the most active in this regard. These cells normally reabsorb all amino acids and glucose in the filtrate. They also normally absorb 65% of the water and sodium in the filtrate. By the time filtrate reaches the nephron loop, most electrolytes have been reabsorbed. In the proximal tubule, almost all *uric acid* and about 50% of *urea* are reabsorbed. However, both substances are eventually secreted back into the filtrate.

Once reaching the nephron loop, permeability of tubule epithelia changes greatly. At this point, water reabsorption is no longer related to solute reabsorption. Although water can leave the nephron loop's descending limb, it cannot leave the

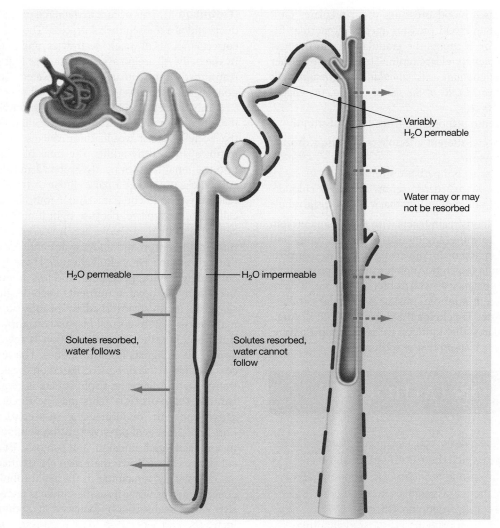

FIGURE 20-8 Tubular reabsorption of water.

TABLE 20-2	
Tubular Reabsorption of Various Substances	
Type of Tubular Reabsorption	**Mechanisms**
Sodium	**Primary Active Transport** Almost always uses active reabsorption, via the transcellular route. Sodium ions are the most abundant cations in the filtrate. Nearly 80% of energy used for active transport is involved in reabsorbing sodium ions. Sodium reabsorption by primary active transport releases energy and mechanisms for reabsorption of most other substances, including water.
Nutrients, water, and ions	**Secondary Active Transport** The gradient created by sodium and potassium ion pumping, at the basolateral membrane, causes secondary active transport to occur. Substances reabsorbed include amino acids, glucose, certain ions, and vitamins. **Passive Tubular Water Reabsorption** A strong osmotic gradient is established by movement of sodium ions and other solutes. Water moves via osmosis into peritubular capillaries. Aquaporins (transmembrane proteins) help by acting as water channels across cell membranes. **Passive Tubular Solute Reabsorption** When water leaves the tubules, solute concentrations in filtrate increase. If possible, they also follow their own concentration gradients into peritubular capillaries. This explains passive reabsorption of many solutes in the filtrate, including certain ions, lipid-soluble substances, and some urea.

TABLE 20-3

Hormones Affecting Filtrate in the Distal Convoluted Tubule and Collecting Duct

Hormone	Effects
Antidiuretic hormone (ADH)	Inhibits diuresis (urine output), causing the principal collecting duct cells to be more permeable to water, via aquaporin insertion into their apical membranes. Quantities of ADH determine numbers of aquaporins and amounts of water reabsorbed there. Overhydration causes osmolality of extracellular fluid to decrease. This decreases ADH secretion by the posterior pituitary, making the collecting ducts nearly impermeable to water. ADH also increases urea reabsorption by the collecting ducts.
Aldosterone	Controls reabsorption of remaining sodium ions. The adrenal cortex releases aldosterone to the blood because of decreased blood volume or pressure, or hyperkalemia. Decreased blood volume or pressure promotes the renin-angiotensin-aldosterone mechanism. Hyperkalemia directly stimulates the adrenal cortex to secrete aldosterone. Aldosterone enhances sodium reabsorption, helping to increase blood volume, and then blood pressure. When aquaporins are present, water usually follows sodium. Aldosterone also reduces blood potassium because its reabsorption of sodium is coupled with potassium secretion in the principal collecting duct cells. As sodium enters the cells, potassium moves into the lumen.
Atrial natriuretic peptide	Reduces blood sodium ions, to decrease blood volume and pressure. It is released by cardiac atrial cells when blood volume or pressure is elevated. It acts to lower blood sodium content, including direct inhibition of sodium reabsorption at the collecting ducts.
Parathyroid hormone	Increases the reabsorption of calcium ions. It acts mostly at the distal convoluted tubule.

ascending limb. This is where the aquaporins are at very low levels, or absent, in the tubule cell membranes. These differences in permeability are vitally important parts of how the kidneys form urine that is either concentrated or dilute. For solutes, a reverse situation compared with that of the water is true. They leave the ascending limb of the nephron loop but not the descending limb. Nearly no reabsorption of solutes occurs in the descending limb, yet they are both actively and passively reabsorbed in the ascending limb.

Reabsorption in the distal convoluted tubule and collecting duct is different. It is adjusted by hormones. Because most filtered water and solutes have already been reabsorbed, only a small part of the filtrate is affected. Approximately 10% of originally filtered sodium chloride and 25% of water experience hormonal adjustment. The hormones that are involved include *antidiuretic hormone, aldosterone, atrial natriuretic peptide,* and *parathyroid hormone.* These hormones are explained in greater detail in **TABLE 20-3**. **TABLE 20-4** summarizes how antidiuretic hormone helps regulate urine concentration and volume.

Tubular Secretion

Tubular secretion selectively moves substances from the blood in the peritubular capillary via the filtrate into the renal tubule. These substances include hydrogen, ammonia, and potassium ions, creatinine, and various organic acids and bases. Certain substances synthesized in the tubule cells, such as bicarbonate, are also secreted. Although essentially the opposite of tubular reabsorption, it also occurs along the length of the renal tubule and collecting duct. Some substances that the body must excrete, such as hydrogen ions and some toxins, are removed more quickly than through filtration. The proximal convoluted tubule is the main site of excretion, except for potassium. The cortical sections of the collecting ducts are also active in secretion.

Tubular secretion is important for four major processes: *disposing* of substances, *eliminating* undesirable substances, *removing* excessive potassium, and *controlling* blood pH. Tubular secretion disposes of certain drugs and metabolites

TABLE 20-4

Antidiuretic Hormone (ADH) and Urine

Component	Function
Plasma volume	Concentration of water decreases
Body fluids	Increase in osmotic pressure stimulates osmoreceptors in hypothalamus
Hypothalamus	Signals posterior pituitary to release ADH
Blood	Carries ADH to kidneys
ADH	Causes distal convoluted tubules and collecting ducts to increase water reabsorption by osmosis
Urine	Becomes concentrated, and urine volume decreases

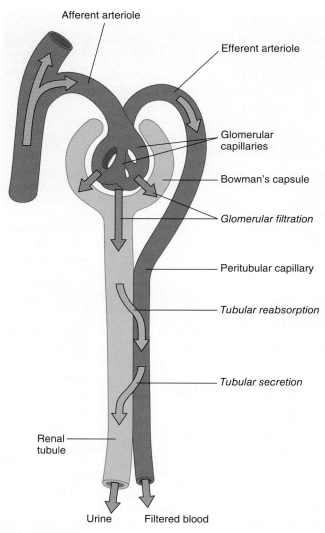

Afferent arteriole

Efferent arteriole

Glomerular capillaries

Bowman's capsule

Glomerular filtration

Peritubular capillary

Tubular reabsorption

Tubular secretion

Renal tubule

Urine   Filtered blood

FIGURE 20-9 Tubular secretion.

that may be tightly bound to plasma proteins. Because these proteins are usually not filtered, the bound substances are also not filtered and therefore must be secreted. Tubular secretion eliminates undesirable substances or end products that have been passively reabsorbed (**FIGURE 20-9**). Examples include the nitrogenous wastes, including urea and uric acid. Nephron processing of urea is complicated, but basically up to 50% of filtrate urea is excreted.

Tubular secretion also removes excessive potassium from the body. Nearly all potassium ions in the filtrate are reabsorbed in the proximal convoluted tubule and ascending nephron loop. Therefore, almost all potassium in the urine is derived from active tubular secretion into the last portions of the distal convoluted tubule and collecting ducts. This secretion is controlled by aldosterone. When blood pH drops toward being acidic, renal tubule cells actively secrete more hydrogen ions into the filtrate. They retain and generate more bicarbonate, which is a base. Therefore, blood pH rises, and the urine drains off any excess hydrogen. In the opposite situation, blood pH approaching alkalinity causes chloride ions to be reabsorbed instead of bicarbonate. The bicarbonate then leaves the body via the urine.

FOCUS ON PATHOLOGY

Polycystic kidney disease is a genetic disorder in which the renal tubules become "ballooned" outward. Multiple cysts develop on the renal cortex, and the kidney enlarges in size. Over time, the cysts replace the renal parenchyma, and renal failure results that requires dialysis. Polycystic kidney is associated with aneurysms of the aorta and brain, diverticula of the colon, and cysts of the pancreas, liver, and testes. This condition is diagnosed via abdominal computed tomography, magnetic resonance imaging, or ultrasound and by intravenous pyelogram.

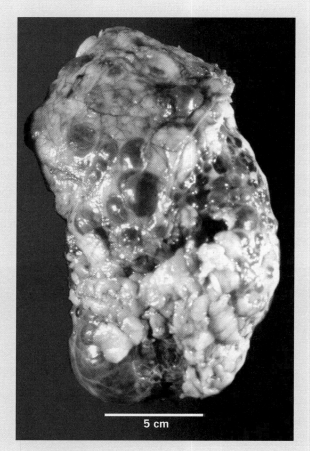

5 cm

Adult polycystic kidney.

At the distal convoluted tubule, potassium ions are removed from the peritubular fluid in exchange for sodium ions from the tubular fluid. The potassium ions then diffuse through potassium leak channels. Hydrogen ions generated by carbonic acid dissociation are secreted in exchange for sodium ions in the tubular fluid. This acidifies the tubular fluid while blood pH is elevated. Because production of lactic acid and ketone bodies during postabsorption can cause acidosis, both the proximal and distal convoluted tubules deaminate amino acids to strip off the amino groups. The reaction sequence binds hydrogen ions and yields ammonium and bicarbonate ions. The ammonium ions are pumped into the tubular fluid, whereas the bicarbonate ions enter the bloodstream via the peritubular fluid. Therefore, tubular deamination provides carbon chains for catabolism while generating bicarbonate ions to increase the plasma's buffering capacity.

Composition of Urine

Urine is the final product of glomerular filtration, tubular reabsorption, and tubular secretion and contains both filtered and secreted substances. Every minute, about 1,200 mL of blood pass through the glomeruli. Of this, 650 mL are plasma and approximately 125 mL are filtrate, forced into the glomerular capsules. At this rate, the entire plasma volume is filtered more than 60 times every day. **Urea** is a result of amino acid catabolism, and its plasma concentration reflects the amount of protein in the diet. Urea filters into the renal tubule, with about 80% reabsorbed, whereas the remainder is excreted in the urine. **Uric acid** is a result of metabolism of certain organic bases in nucleic acids. Active transport reabsorbs most of the uric acid present in the glomerular filtrate. **TABLE 20-5** summarizes some specific functions of the nephron segments and the collecting duct.

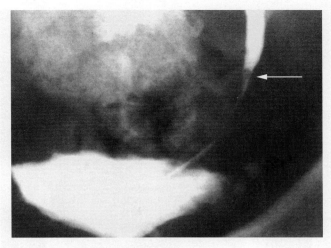

FIGURE 20-10 Intravenous pyelogram.

The chemical composition of urine is related to water volume and the amount of solutes the kidneys must eliminate or retain to maintain homeostasis. Urine is about 95% water and usually contains urea and uric acid. It may have traces of amino acids and electrolytes. Urine production varies between 0.6 and 2.5 liters per day. Urine production of 50 to 60 mL per hour is normal, with output of less than 30 mL per hour possibly indicating kidney failure. In decreasing concentrations, urine contains mostly urea, followed by sodium, potassium, phosphate, sulfate, creatinine, and uric acid. Tiny yet variable amounts of calcium, magnesium, and bicarbonate are also present. The analysis of urine samples is called *urinalysis*. An image of the urinary system, called an *intravenous pyelogram*, may be made via x-rays of the kidneys after administration of an intravenous radiopaque dye (**FIGURE 20-10**). A newer procedure called a *computed tomography urogram* is used more commonly today. It allows three-dimensional images to be reconstructed of portions of the urinary system (**FIGURE 20-11**).

TABLE 20-5

Functions of the Nephrons and Collecting Duct

Structure	Function
Renal corpuscle	
Glomerulus	Filters water and dissolved substances from plasma
Glomerular capsule	Receives glomerular filtrate
Renal tubule	
Proximal convoluted tubule	Reabsorbs glucose, amino acids, creatine, acids, and ions by active transport; reabsorbs water by osmosis; reabsorbs chloride and other negative ions by electrochemical attraction; actively secretes penicillin, histamine, creatinine, and hydrogen ions
Descending limb of nephron loop	Reabsorbs water by osmosis
Ascending limb of nephron loop	Reabsorbs sodium, potassium, and chloride ions by active transport
Distal convoluted tubule	Reabsorbs sodium ions by active transport, reabsorbs water by osmosis, and secretes hydrogen and potassium ions by electrochemical attraction
Collecting duct	Reabsorbs water by osmosis

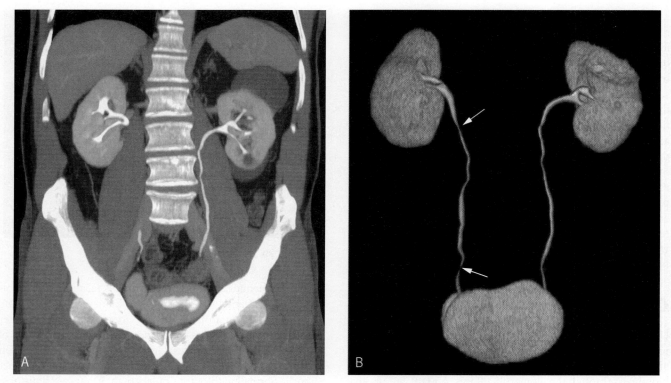

FIGURE 20-11 Computed tomography urogram. (A) In this coronal view, the left ureter can be followed from the kidney to the bladder. The central portion of the right ureter is not filled with contrast. (Courtesy of Dr. Myron Pozniak, Department of Radiology, University of Wisconsin School of Medicine and Public Health.) (B) The relationship of the kidneys, ureters, and bladder is rendered in three dimensions. Even small cysts can be seen on the surface of the kidney. Two strictures are present in the right ureter (arrows), and the segment of ureter above them is slightly dilated in comparison to the left ureter. (Courtesy of Dr. Myron Pozniak, Department of Radiology, University of Wisconsin School of Medicine and Public Health.)

The physical characteristics of urine include color, transparency, odor, pH, and specific gravity. When freshly voided, normal urine is clear, with a color between pale and deep yellow. The color is caused by the pigment **urochrome**, which results from the destruction of hemoglobin. Higher concentrations cause the urine to be deeper yellow. When fresh, urine is slightly aromatic, but after standing for a while, it develops an odor of ammonia. This is because of bacteria that metabolize the urea solutes. Normally, urine is slightly acidic, with a pH of 6. However, dietary or metabolic changes may cause its pH to change, ranging from 4.5 to 8. The *specific gravity* of urine is slightly higher than that of distilled water. This is because of the solutes it contains. Normal urine specific gravity is between 1.001 and 1.035, whereas distilled water's specific gravity is 1. Specific gravity is defined as the ratio of the mass of a substance to the mass of an equal volume of distilled water. Abnormal substances in the urine are explained in **TABLE 20-6**.

TABLE 20-6

Abnormal Substances in Urine

Abnormal Substance	Condition	Causes
Proteins	Proteinuria, albuminuria	Pathologic causes (over 150 mg/day) include heart failure, glomerulonephritis, and severe hypertension. These conditions are often a sign of asymptomatic renal disease. Nonpathologic causes include excessive physical exertion and pregnancy.
Ketone bodies	Ketonuria	Starvation or untreated diabetes mellitus causes excessive formation and accumulation of ketone bodies.
Bile pigments	Bilirubinuria	Obstruction of bile ducts from the liver or gallbladder or liver diseases such as cirrhosis or hepatitis.
Erythrocytes	Hematuria	Cancer, infection, kidney stones, or trauma that result in bleeding inside the urinary tract.
Glucose	Glycosuria	Diabetes mellitus.
Hemoglobin	Hemoglobinuria	Hemolytic anemia, severe burns, transfusion reaction, and a variety of other causes.
Leukocytes (pus)	Pyuria	Urinary tract infections.

TEST YOUR UNDERSTANDING

1. How is urine formed?
2. How are uric acid and urea excreted?
3. Explain why urine is yellow in color.

Renal Clearance

The volume of plasma from which the kidneys completely remove a particular substance over a specific time period, usually 1 minute, is known as **renal clearance**. Tests are performed to determine the GFR. This allows detection of glomerular damage and renal disease. For any substance the renal clearance rate, abbreviated "C," is calculated in milliliters per minute, using this equation:

$$C = UV / P$$

where U is the concentration of the substance in urine, calculated in milligrams per milliliter; V is the flow rate of urine formation, calculated in milliliters per minute; and P is the concentration of the substance in plasma, calculated in milligrams per milliliter.

To determine the GFR, the substance used is *inulin*. This is because inulin is filtered freely and the kidneys do not reabsorb or secrete it. Inulin is a plant polysaccharide with a renal clearance value that is equal to the GFR. When infused so the inulin plasma concentration is 1 mg/mL, this means its plasma concentration (P) is 1 mg/mL. Usually, its urine concentration (U) is 125 mg/mL and its flow rate (V) is 1 mL/min. Its renal clearance is calculated as follows:

$$C = (125 \times 1) / 1 = 125 \text{ mL/min}$$

This means that within 1 minute, the kidneys have cleared all the inulin that was present in 125 mL of plasma. We can then determine how the kidneys are handling the net amount of a certain substance.

There are three different outcomes to this determination:

1. If the substance has a clearance value that is less than the clearance value of inulin, the substance is reabsorbed.
2. If the renal clearance rate (C) is equal to that of inulin, there is no net reabsorption or secretion of the substance.
3. If C is greater than that of insulin, the substance is secreted by the tubule cells into the filtrate. This usually occurs with most drug metabolites.

It is essential to know a drug's renal clearance rate. If the rate is high, the drug dosage must also be high, and the drug must be administered frequently to maintain therapeutic levels.

Ureters

Once formed in the nephrons, urine passes from the collecting ducts to enter the calyces of the kidney and then through the renal pelvis and one of the ureters into the bladder. The urethra passes urine to outside of the body via the *ureteral openings*, which are slit-like in appearance. Each thin **ureter**

FOCUS ON PATHOLOGY

Chronic renal disease is defined as a GFR of less than 60 mL/min for at least 3 months. This disease often develops without symptoms over many years and is most often caused by diabetes mellitus. *Renal failure* is defined as a GFR of less than 15 mL/min. In renal failure, filtrate formation is decreased or totally stopped. It is associated with *uremia*, which means "urine in the blood," signified by anorexia, fatigue, mental changes, nausea, and muscle cramps. Uremia is now known to be caused by many factors, including imbalances of ions and hormones, metabolic abnormalities, and accumulation of toxins. Treatment options include hemodialysis or artificial blood filtering and kidney transplant.

is about 30 cm long, descending behind the parietal peritoneum to run parallel to the vertebral column. The ureters begin at the spinal L2 level, continuing from the renal pelvis. They descend behind the peritoneum and join the urinary bladder by running obliquely through its posterior wall, from underneath.

The wall of each ureter has three layers, the mucous coat (transitional epithelium), muscular coat, and fibrous coat. Urine is propelled by the muscular walls of the ureters. A flap-like fold of mucous membrane covers the opening through which urine flows from each ureter into the bladder. These folds keep urine from backing up and flowing back into ureters from the bladder. Backflow of urine is also stopped by any increase in bladder pressure, which compresses and closes the distal ureter ends.

The ureters are distended by incoming urine, which stimulates their musculari to contract. This propels the urine into the bladder, assisted by gravity. Peristaltic waves vary in strength and frequency according to the urine formation rate. Neural control of the peristaltic waves is believed to be insignificant in comparison with how the smooth muscles of the ureters stretch. Each ureter is innervated by both sympathetic and parasympathetic fibers.

Urinary Bladder

The *urinary bladder* is a hollow, muscular organ that stores urine and forces it into the urethra. It is found in the pelvic cavity behind the symphysis pubis, beneath the parietal peritoneum. In males, the prostate gland is inferior to the neck of the bladder, which empties into the urethra. In females, the bladder is anterior to the uterus and vagina. The wall of the bladder has many folds or *rugae* when it is empty, but these smooth out as it fills. The bladder is

Renal calculi, commonly called *kidney stones,* may be formed by calcium, magnesium, or uric acid salts in the urine that crystallize and collect in the renal pelvis. Although most are less than 5 mm in diameter and pass without any problems, larger stones can cause ureter obstruction and block urine flow. Extreme pain results, radiating from the flank to the anterior abdominal wall on the same side of the body. Kidney stones may be related to frequent bacterial urinary tract infections, retention of urine, high calcium levels in the blood, and urine that is usually alkaline. *Shock wave lithotripsy* is the standard treatment procedure, which uses ultrasonic shock waves to shatter the stones. Once shattered, they can easily pass through the urine. If a patient has a history of kidney stones, he or she should drink plenty of water each day to keep the urine diluted.

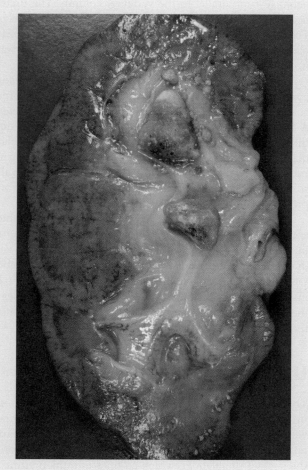

Kidney stones.

pear-shaped when full, rising superiorly in the abdominal cavity. The rugae disappear as the bladder walls become thinner due to stretching to contain urine. Because of the flexibility of its walls, there is no large rise in internal pressure as the bladder fills.

The bladder's internal floor has a triangular area or *trigone,* which has an opening at each of its three angles. **FIGURE 20-12** shows both the male and female urinary bladder and related structures. The urinary bladder wall has four layers, the mucous coat, submucous coat, muscular coat, and serous coat, and its cellular thickness changes based on how much urine it holds. The smooth muscle fibers of the muscular coat are interlaced, comprising the *detrusor muscle,* part of which surrounds the neck of the bladder to form the internal urethral sphincter. This muscle is innervated with parasympathetic nerve fibers that function in the micturition reflex. The mucous coat of the urinary bladder contains transitional epithelium. The urinary bladder is held in place by the *median and lateral umbilical ligaments.*

Micturition, also called urination or voiding, is the process of expelling urine from the urinary bladder. The detrusor muscle contracts along with the abdominal wall and pelvic floor muscles, and the external urethral sphincter relaxes. The micturition reflex center in the spinal cord sends parasympathetic motor impulses to the detrusor muscle, causing it to rhythmically contract. In infants and young children, micturition is reflexive. However, training to control micturition usually is successful between ages 2 and 3, because descending brain circuits have matured sufficiently to take control of micturition, replacing reflexive micturition. In older children and adults, the normal urge to urinate usually occurs before urine volume in the bladder exceeding 500 mL. After urination, there is usually only approximately 10 mL of urine left over.

The urinary bladder may hold up to nearly 1,000 mL or 2 pints of urine if necessary. However, the urge to urinate usually occurs once it contains around 200 mL. When approximately half full, the bladder is about 12 cm or 5 inches long, although it can greatly increase in size. The external urethral sphincter is under conscious control, allowing the micturition reflex to occur once the person decides to urinate. The detrusor muscle contracts and urine flows through the urethra.

Urethra

The urethra is a relatively thin-walled, muscular tube that conveys urine from the urinary bladder to outside of the body. It is lined with mucous membrane known as pseudostratified columnar epithelium and a thick layer of smooth muscle tissue. The portions of the urethra nearer the urinary bladder become transitional epithelium. The wall of the urethra has many mucous glands, also called *urethral glands,* which secrete mucus into the urethral canal. In females, the urethra is only about 3 to 4 cm or 1.5 inches long, opening via the *external urethral orifice* or urinary meatus.

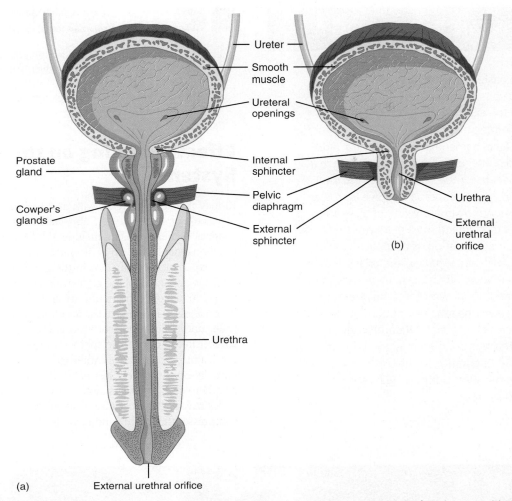

Prostate gland

Cowper's glands

Ureter

Smooth muscle

Ureteral openings

Internal sphincter

Pelvic diaphragm

External sphincter

Urethra

External urethral orifice

(a)

Urethra

External urethral orifice

(b)

FIGURE 20-12 Longitudinal sections of (A) the male urinary bladder and related structures and (B) the female urinary bladder and related structures.

FOCUS ON PATHOLOGY

When an individual is *incontinent* in adulthood, it is most commonly caused by weakening of the pelvic muscles due to childbirth or surgery, nervous system abnormalities, or the physical pressure of pregnancy. *Stress incontinence*, laughing or coughing, which causes a sudden increase in pressure throughout the abdomen, may force urine through the external sphincter. In *overflow incontinence*, urine drips from the urethra as soon as the bladder becomes overfull. *Urinary retention* is a condition in which the bladder cannot expel urine. It is often a result of general anesthesia or, in males, hypertrophy of the prostate. Chronic urinary retention problems may require insertion of a *catheter* or drainage tube through the urethra to drain the urine.

In males, the urethra is about 20 cm or 8 inches long. It functions as part of both the urinary and reproductive systems, extending from the bladder to the tip of the penis. In both males and females the portion of the urethra near the external opening becomes protective stratified squamous epithelium. There are three regions of the urethra in males: the *prostatic, membranous,* and *spongy* urethra. The **prostatic urethra** is inside the prostate gland and is about 2.5 cm or 1 inch in length. The **membranous urethra** is its intermediate portion, located inside the urogenital diaphragm. It extends from the prostate for about 2 cm to the beginning of the penis. The **spongy urethra** is about 15 cm in length, continuing throughout the penis up to its opening at the tip.

The **detrusor muscle** originating in the bladder becomes thicker, forming the *internal urethral sphincter* at the junction of the urethra and the bladder. This sphincter is involuntary and is controlled by the autonomic nervous system to prevent leaking of urine. As the urethra passes through the *urogenital diaphragm*, it is surrounded by the *external urethral sphincter*. This sphincter is voluntarily controlled. Another muscle, the *levator ani*, helps in voluntary constriction of the urethra.

FOCUS ON PATHOLOGY

It is much easier for females to contract urinary tract infections, because their urethras are very short and the external opening is near the anal opening. Wiping incorrectly, from back to front, can carry fecal bacteria into the urethra. Most urinary tract infections occur in sexually active women, because intercourse causes external genital and vaginal bacteria to move up toward the bladder. Approximately 40% of all women get urinary tract infections. Their symptoms include painful urination or *dysuria*, fever, urinary frequency and urgency, and changes in urine appearance. When the kidneys become involved, additional symptoms include backache and severe headache. Antibiotics are usually effective for treatment. Related conditions include *urethritis* or inflammation of the urethra, *cystitis* or inflammation of the bladder, and kidney inflammatory conditions such as *pyelonephritis* and *pyelitis*.

TEST YOUR UNDERSTANDING

1. Describe the structures needed for urination.
2. What is the amount of urine in the bladder that usually triggers the urge to urinate?
3. Contrast the female and male urethra.

Effects of Aging on the Urinary System

Kidney problems increase with age, including the formation of calculi or *kidney stones*, also called *nephrolithiasis*. Other changes because of aging include a decline in the number of functional nephrons, up to 40% in some individuals. Patients may experience a reduction in the glomeruli, damage to the filtration apparatus of the glomeruli that remain, and lessened renal blood flow. The nephrons and collecting system may become less responsive to the antidiuretic hormone, and both water and sodium reabsorption is lower. More sodium ions are lost in the urine. The sphincter muscles lose tone, which can lead to incontinence. Ability to control urination may be partially or completely lost after Alzheimer's disease, stroke, or other central nervous system events. Urinary retention in males may develop because of an enlarged prostate gland that compresses the urethra and restricts urine flow.

SUMMARY

The urinary system is made up of the kidneys, ureters, urinary bladder, and urethra. The kidneys maintain homeostasis by removing metabolic wastes from the blood and excreting them. They are made up of an outer cortex and an inner medulla. The nephron is the functional unit of the kidney. There are about 1 million nephrons in each kidney. Nephrons remove wastes from blood and regulate water and electrolyte concentrations, with urine as the end product.

Urine is about 95% water and also usually contains urea and uric acid. Glomerular filtration initiates urine formation in the renal corpuscle. The GFR is the volume of filtrate that forms every minute via the actions of the kidneys' glomeruli. Urine formation is also influenced by tubular reabsorption and tubular secretion. Tubular reabsorption selectively moves substances from the tubular fluid into the blood. Tubular secretion selectively moves substances from the blood in the peritubular capillary via the filtrate into the renal tubule.

The other primary structures of the urinary system include the ureters, urinary bladder, and urethra. The ureters connect each renal pelvis to the urinary bladder. The urinary bladder stores urine and forces it through the urethra during micturition, which is the act of expelling urine. The urethra conveys urine from the urinary bladder to outside of the body.

KEY TERMS

Active tubular reabsorption
Afferent arterioles
Bowman's capsule
Collecting duct
Detrusor muscle
Distal convoluted tubule
Efferent arteriole
Glomerular capsule
Glomerular filtration
Glomerular filtration rate
Glomerulus
Granular cells
Hilum
Hydrostatic pressure
Juxtaglomerular apparatus
Kidneys

Macula densa
Membranous urethra
Micturition
Nephron loop
Nephrons
Net filtration pressure
Passive tubular reabsorption
Pericytes
Peritubular capillary
Prostatic urethra
Proximal convoluted tubule
Renal arteries
Renal clearance
Renal corpuscle
Renal cortex
Renal medulla

Renal pelvis
Renal sinus
Renal tubule
Renal vein
Retroperitoneally
Spongy urethra
Tubular reabsorption
Tubular secretion
Urea
Ureter
Urethra
Uric acid
Urinary bladder
Urine
Urochrome

LEARNING GOALS

The following learning goals correspond to the objectives at the beginning of this chapter:

1. The kidneys are located on either side of the vertebral column in depressions on the upper posterior wall of the abdominal cavity. They are smooth, bean-shaped organs with a reddish-brown color. Adult kidneys are enclosed in tough, fibrous capsules. The kidneys are about 12 cm long by 6 cm wide and 3 cm thick. Each kidney has a convex lateral surface and a concave medial side resulting in a medial depression.

2. The nephron is the functional unit of the kidney. Each consists of a renal corpuscle and a renal tubule. Fluid moves through the renal tubules as it moves toward exiting the body. A glomerulus is a tangled cluster of blood capillaries that comprises a renal corpuscle, where fluid is filtered. The glomerulus is surrounded by a sac-like glomerular capsule at the proximal end of a renal tubule. The renal tubule leads away to coil into the proximal convoluted tubule. This structure dips toward the renal pelvis to form the descending limb or *loop of Henle* and then curves to form the ascending limb. It returns to the renal corpuscle region, coiling to become the distal convoluted tubule. The loop of Henle has a horseshoe shape. Tubules from several nephrons form collecting ducts, which pass into the renal medulla, and tubes that empty into the minor calyces.

3. Urine formation is initiated by glomerular filtration. The plasma is filtered by the glomerular capillaries, with most of this fluid reabsorbed into the bloodstream via the colloid osmotic pressure of the plasma. Using two capillaries in series, the nephrons help produce urine. The first capillary bed filters instead of forming interstitial fluid, with the filtrate moving into the renal tubule to form urine. Glomerular filtration produces 180 liters of fluid every 24 hours. Tubular reabsorption and tubular secretion also contribute to urine formation. Reabsorption moves substances from the tubular fluid into the blood, and secretion moves substances from the blood into the renal tubule.

4. Urine volume and concentration are affected by antidiuretic hormone and aldosterone hormone in differing ways. Antidiuretic hormone causes distal convoluted tubules and collecting ducts to increase water reabsorption by osmosis. This concentrates the urine, and volume decreases. Aldosterone may stimulate additional reabsorption of sodium and secretion of potassium from the distal convoluted tubule.

5. Net filtration pressure forces substances out of the glomerulus and is usually positive pressure. It is directly proportional to the GFR. Anything that decreases plasma colloid osmotic pressure increases the filtration rate. Blockages may significantly decrease filtration rate.

6.

A. *Ureters:* About 25 cm long each, they descend behind the partial peritoneum to run parallel to the vertebral column, joining the urinary bladder from underneath; each has three layers, propelling urine via their muscular walls. Flap-like membrane folds keep urine from backing up and flowing back into the ureters from the bladder.

B. *Urinary bladder:* A hollow, muscular organ that stores urine and forces it into the urethra; it lies in the pelvic cavity behind the symphysis pubis, with folded walls that smooth out as it fills. Its internal floor has a trigone with an opening at each of its three angles. The bladder wall has four layers, with a detrusor muscle surrounding the neck of the bladder to form the internal urethral sphincter.

C. *Urethra:* A tube that conveys urine to outside of the body; it is lined with mucous membrane and thick smooth muscle tissue. It has many urethral glands that secrete mucus into the urethral canal. The urethra of a male is much longer than that of a female; in males, it also functions as part of the reproductive system, conducting sperm as well as urine.

7.

A. The most important component of plasma is sodium. Its main substances include chloride, glucose, bicarbonate, and urea, with lesser amounts of potassium, calcium, uric acid, magnesium, phosphate, and sulfate.

B. The most important component of urine is urea. Its main substances include chloride, sodium, potassium, uric acid, phosphate, and sulfate, with lesser amounts of magnesium, bicarbonate, and calcium. When normal, the urine contains no glucose.

8. Normal urine is composed via glomerular filtration, tubular reabsorption, and tubular secretion. The amount of a given substance in urine is calculated as follows: amount filtered at the glomerulus – amount reabsorbed by the tubule + amount secreted by the tubule. Glomerular filtrate is received by the glomerular capsule, which is mostly water with the same components as blood plasma, except for large protein molecules.

9. The most important waste products excreted by the kidneys include urea, uric acid, and other nitrogenous wastes.

10. The micturition reflex center is in the spinal cord. Parasympathetic motor impulses are transmitted to the detrusor muscle, causing it to rhythmically contract.

CRITICAL THINKING QUESTIONS

A 35-year-old man who was born with one kidney was brought to the emergency department after a severe car accident. He was diagnosed with hypovolemic shock.

1. A person must have at least one functioning kidney to survive. Why do you believe a person cannot live without kidneys?

2. During hypovolemic shock, how does the body regulate blood pressure?

1. Which of the following is not a part of the urinary system?
   - A. kidney
   - B. gallbladder
   - C. ureter
   - D. urethra

2. Which of the following is the innermost layer of kidney tissue?
   - A. major calyx
   - B. renal pelvis
   - C. renal cortex
   - D. renal medulla

3. Bowman's capsule and the glomerulus make up the
   - A. renal corpuscle
   - B. renal papilla
   - C. renal pyramid
   - D. loop of Henle

4. The portion of the nephron nearest to the renal corpuscle is the
   - A. loop of Henle
   - B. collecting duct
   - C. distal convoluted tubule
   - D. proximal convoluted tubule

5. The process of filtration occurs at
   - A. the collecting duct
   - B. the loop of Henle
   - C. glomerulus
   - D. the proximal convoluted tubule

6. Which of the following portions of the nephron is able to concentrate urine?
   - A. collecting duct
   - B. loop of Henle
   - C. proximal convoluted tubule
   - D. urinary bladder

7. Which of the following types of epithelium lines the urinary bladder?
   - A. pseudostratified columnar
   - B. stratified squamous
   - C. simple cuboidal
   - D. transitional

8. When antidiuretic hormone level in the blood increases,
   - A. less urine is produced
   - B. more urine is produced
   - C. more salt is removed from the urine
   - D. less water is reabsorbed from the collecting duct

9. The glomerulus is located within the
   - A. renal capsule
   - B. renal pelvis
   - C. renal corpuscle
   - D. renal tubule

10. Which of the following substances is not normally allowed to pass through the filtration membrane?
    - A. amino acids
    - B. albumin
    - C. glucose
    - D. urea

11. Conical structures in the renal medulla are called
    - A. calyces
    - B. nephrons
    - C. renal pelvises
    - D. pyramids

12. Which of the following is not the normal function of the urinary system?
    - A. elimination of organic wastes
    - B. secretion of excess glucose molecules
    - C. regulation of blood volume
    - D. regulation of plasma concentrations of electrolytes

13. Which of the following segments of the nephron is horseshoe-shaped?
    - A. minor calyx
    - B. collecting duct
    - C. loop of Henle
    - D. proximal convoluted tubule

14. Which of the following hormones is secreted from the kidneys?
    - A. erythropoietin
    - B. aldosterone
    - C. thymosin
    - D. prolactin

15. The bladder's internal floor has a triangular area called the
    - A. mucous coat
    - B. detrusor muscle
    - C. urethral gland
    - D. trigone

ESSAY QUESTIONS

1. Describe the structures of the nephron.
2. Explain the important differences between blood plasma and glomerular filtrate.
3. Explain how the peritubular capillaries reabsorb substances.
4. Describe tubular secretion.
5. Describe the effects of antidiuretic hormone, aldosterone, and atrial natriuretic peptide in the kidneys.
6. Explain the processes of urine formation.
7. Describe renal clearance.
8. Explain how the urinary bladder anatomy supports its storage functions.
9. Define micturition, and describe the micturition reflex.
10. Describe the effects of aging that occur in the kidneys and urinary bladder.

Fluid, Electrolyte, and Acid-Base Balance

OBJECTIVES

After studying this chapter, the reader should be able to

1. Explain what is meant by the terms *fluid balance* and *electrolyte balance*.
2. Compare the composition of intracellular and extracellular fluids.
3. Identify the hormones that play important roles in regulating fluid balance and electrolyte balance.
4. Describe the movement of fluid within the extracellular and intracellular fluids.
5. Discuss the mechanisms by which sodium and potassium ion concentrations are regulated to maintain electrolyte balance.
6. Explain the buffering systems that balance the pH of the intracellular and extracellular fluids.
7. Identify the most frequent threats to acid-base balance.
8. Explain how the body responds when the pH of body fluids varies outside normal limits.
9. Describe metabolic alkalosis.
10. Compare respiratory acidosis with metabolic acidosis.

Overview

The maintenance of fluid, electrolyte, and acid-base balance is crucial for life. Our cells require physical and chemical homeostasis of surrounding tissues to function. **Electrolytes** are ions released through the dissociation of inorganic compounds able to conduct an electrical current in a solution. The amount of water and electrolytes gained from food and beverages, on a daily basis, is equal to the amount the body loses to the environment. The body replaces lost water and electrolytes and excretes any excess. Electrolytes are dissolved in the water of body fluids. When electrolyte concentrations are altered, water concentrations are also altered by adding or removing solutes. The reverse is also true, by either concentrating or diluting electrolyte concentrations. This chapter provides information about fluid composition and distribution in the internal environment and discusses the ways our organs function to balance fluids, electrolytes, acids, and bases.

Body Fluid Distribution

Total body water changes with age, body mass, and relative amount of body fat. It is also different between the sexes. Infants have approximately 73% of their bodies made up of water, in part because they have low body fat and low bone mass. Their skin is extremely soft because of this high water content. Once the infant grows into childhood, the decline in total body water has already begun. Healthy young boys have about 60% body water and girls about 50%. By the time an individual is elderly, only about 45% of the body mass consists of water. Gender differences in body water are related to the general fact that females have more body fat and less skeletal muscle than males. The least hydrated type of body tissue is adipose tissue, which contains no more than 20% water. All other types of tissue, including bone, have higher water contents. People with greater muscle mass have more body water because skeletal muscle is made up of about 75% water.

Fluid Compartments

Regions or *compartments* of the body contain different volumes of fluids, with varying compositions. Movement of water and electrolytes between compartments is regulated so they are stable. The two major compartments are an intracellular fluid compartment and an extracellular fluid compartment. The **intracellular fluid compartment** includes all water and electrolytes enclosed by cell membranes. In an adult, intracellular fluid represents about 63%, by volume, of total body water. Therefore, the intracellular fluid compartment in an adult man of approximately 150 pounds accounts for about 25 of 40 total liters of body water.

The **extracellular fluid compartment** includes all fluid outside of cells, making up about 37%, by volume, of total body water. This includes the plasma in the blood vessels, the lymph in the lymphatic vessels, and the interstitial fluid

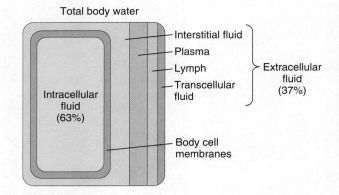

FIGURE 21-1 Cell membranes separate intracellular and extracellular fluids.

in the tissue spaces. This compartment is referred to as the body's *internal environment*. Some extracellular fluid is separated from other types of fluid and is known as **transcellular fluid** and includes

- *Aqueous and vitreous humors:* in the eyes
- *Cerebrospinal fluid:* in the central nervous system
- *Secretions:* from the exocrine glands
- *Serous fluid:* in body cavities
- *Synovial fluid:* in the joints

FIGURE 21-1 shows how cell membranes separate intracellular and extracellular fluids.

Fluid Composition

Many different types of solutes are dissolved in water, the *universal solvent*. Solutes are basically classified as *electrolytes* or *nonelectrolytes*. Electrolytes include inorganic salts, some proteins, acids, and bases. The acids and bases may be organic or inorganic. Nonelectrolytes have mostly covalent bonds, although other types of bonds exist, which means they cannot dissociate in a solution. No electrically charged particles are created when they dissolve in water. Most nonelectrolytes are organic molecules such as creatinine, glucose, lipids, and urea.

Electrolytes have much more osmotic power than nonelectrolytes, because their molecules dissociate into two or more ions. For example, although the nonelectrolyte *glucose* remains undissociated and contributes one solute particle, a sodium chloride ($NaCl$) molecule contributes two and a magnesium chloride ($MgCl_2$) contributes three. Both sodium chloride and magnesium chloride are examples of electrolytes. Sodium chloride dissociates into a sodium particle and a chloride particle. Magnesium chloride dissociates into a magnesium particle and two chloride particles.

Water always moves according to *osmotic gradients*, regardless of the type of solute particles contained, meaning water always moves from an area of lesser *osmolality* to an area of greater *osmolality*. As a result, electrolytes have more ability to cause fluid shifts than nonelectrolytes. In the body fluids, electrolyte concentrations are commonly expressed in *milliequivalents per liter (mEq/L)*. This measures the number of

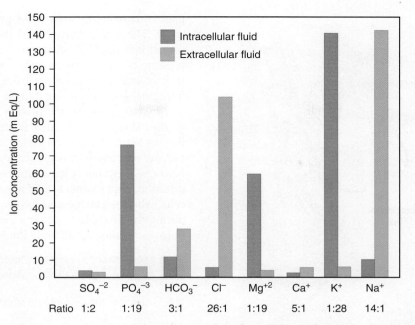

FIGURE 21-2 Concentration of various ions in extracellular and intracellular fluid. (Adapted from Shier, D. N., Butler, J. L., and Lewis, R. Hole's *Essentials of Human Anatomy & Physiology*, Tenth edition. McGraw-Hill Higher Education, 2009.)

electrical charges in 1 liter of solution. Any ion's concentration can be calculated in solution by using the following equation:

$$mEq/L = \frac{\text{Concentration of ions (mg/L)}}{\text{The ion's atomic weight (mg/mmol)}}$$
$$\times \text{Number of electrical charges on one ion}$$

Notice in the equation the concentration of ions is calculated in milligrams per liter. Also, the ion's atomic weight is calculated in milligrams per *millimole*. One millimole is one-thousandth of a mole. One mole is the base unit of amount of matter, which means a substance's amount that contains as many elementary entities as there are carbon atoms in 0.012 kg of carbon 12.

Therefore, to understand how this works, using sodium and calcium as examples, we need to calculate the mEq/L for each. We determine the normal concentrations of these ions in the plasma. Then we find their atomic weights by using the *periodic table*. By using the equation, we find the following for each:

$$\text{Sodium} = \frac{3,300 \text{ mg/L}}{23 \text{ mg/mmol}} \times 1 \text{ particle} = 143 \text{ mEq/L}$$

$$\text{Calcium} = \frac{100 \text{ mg/L}}{40 \text{ mg/mmol}} \times 2 \text{ particles} = 5 \text{ mEq/L}$$

Differences Between Extracellular and Intracellular Fluids

Most extracellular fluids contain high amounts of chloride, bicarbonate, and sodium ions. They have a greater concentration of calcium and less magnesium, phosphate, potassium, and sulfate ions than are found in intracellular fluid. Blood plasma has much higher levels of protein than interstitial

fluid or lymph (**FIGURE 21-2**). In extracellular fluids, the primary *cation* is sodium and the primary *anion* is chloride. Plasma contains fewer chloride ions than the interstitial fluid because plasma is electrically neutral, and nonpenetrating plasma proteins are usually anions.

Intracellular fluid differs in that it has high amounts of magnesium, phosphate, and potassium ions and low amounts of sodium and chloride; it is basically opposite in its ion content to extracellular fluid. In intracellular fluids, the primary cation is potassium and the primary anion is hydrogen phosphate. The cells additionally contain large quantities of soluble proteins, in amounts that are about triple to those found in plasma. The ion content of intracellular and extracellular fluid is based on activity of the cells' sodium-potassium pumps, which require adenosine triphosphate. These pumps maintain a balance in which intracellular sodium concentration is low and potassium concentration is high. The kidneys assist in this balance by secreting potassium into the filtrate, whereas sodium is reabsorbed from the filtrate.

Electrolytes are the most abundant solutes in the fluids of the body and control most chemical and physical reactions. However, they do not make up most dissolved solutes in the fluids. In the extracellular fluid, proteins and certain nonelectrolytes such as cholesterol, phospholipids, and triglycerides are large molecules that are present. In the plasma, these make up approximately 90% of the mass of dissolved solutes and 60% in the interstitial fluid. In the intracellular fluid, they make up 97%.

Fluid Movement Between Compartments

Hydrostatic pressure and osmotic pressure regulate the movement of water and electrolytes from one fluid compartment

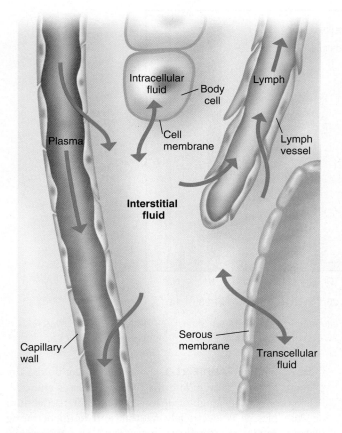

FIGURE 21-3 Blood plasma has much higher levels of protein than interstitial fluid or lymph. (Adapted from Shier, D. N., Butler, J. L., and Lewis, R. Hole's Essentials of Human Anatomy & Physiology, Tenth edition. McGraw-Hill Higher Education, 2009.)

to another (**FIGURE 21-3**). Hydrostatic pressure inside cells and surrounding interstitial fluid is normally equal and stable. Therefore, a change in osmotic pressure usually causes net fluid movement. The net inward force is known as *colloid osmotic pressure*. When the levels of sodium in the extracellular fluid decrease, this causes movement of water from the extracellular compartment into the intracellular compartment, via osmosis. Cells swell as a result. The opposite is true when sodium ion concentration in interstitial fluid increases, causing the cells to shrink.

Although water moves freely between the compartments, solutes are not equally distributed. This is due to their electrical charges, sizes, or need to use transport proteins. Basically, substances must pass through the plasma and interstitial fluid to reach the intracellular fluid. Exchanges between the plasma and "outside" environment are nearly continuous in the gastrointestinal tract, kidneys, and lungs. Plasma composition and volume are both altered. The plasma is the medium that allows substances to be delivered to all areas of the body. Balance is quickly restored by the body's adjustments between the plasma, extracellular fluid, and intracellular fluid.

There are two key points: Exchanges between plasma and interstitial fluid occur across capillary walls, and exchanges between the interstitial fluid and intracellular fluid occur across plasma membranes. For exchanges between plasma and interstitial fluid, the blood's hydrostatic pressure forces

plasma that almost totally lacks proteins into the interstitial space. The highly filtered fluid then is almost totally reabsorbed into the bloodstream because of the colloid osmotic pressure of the plasma proteins. Normally, lymphatic vessels pick up small amounts of net leakage remaining behind in the interstitial space, returning it to the blood.

Exchanges across the plasma membranes are based on permeability. Generally, there is substantial two-way osmotic flow of water. Restriction of ion changes is based on ions moving selectively through channels or by active transport. Nutrients, respiratory gases, and wastes usually move in one direction. An example is how metabolic wastes move out of cells, whereas glucose and oxygen move into them. Except during the first minutes after a change in one type of body fluid, osmolalities of all body fluids are equal.

Fluid Balance

Water is the primary fluid in the human body. When **water balance** exists, it means total water intake equals total water output, maintained by homeostatic mechanisms. Every individual differs in how much water they take in. In the United States, the average adult consumes about 2,500 mL of water per day, broken down as follows:

- *60% of intake:* water and beverages
- *30% of intake:* moist foods
- *10% of intake:* a byproduct of the oxidative metabolism of nutrients, also known as **water of metabolism**

Thirst is primarily responsible for the regulation of water intake. Intense thirst comes from osmotic pressure affecting extracellular fluids on the *thirst center* in the hypothalamus. Loss of body water increases osmotic pressure to stimulate osmoreceptors in the thirst center. Whenever total body water decreases by as small an amount as 1%, thirst is triggered. Drinking fluids triggers nerve impulses that inhibit the *thirst mechanism*, stopping drinking before the swallowed fluids are absorbed. This keeps a person from consuming too many liquids.

The body loses water in urine and feces; in sweat, as *sensible perspiration*; by evaporation from the skin, known as *insensible perspiration*; and from the lungs during breathing, known as **insensible water loss**. Water balance requires that 2,500 mL be eliminated each day, so water output is basically broken down as follows:

- *Lost in urine:* 60%
- *Lost by evaporation from skin and lungs:* 28%
- *Lost in feces:* 4%
- *Lost in sweat:* 8%

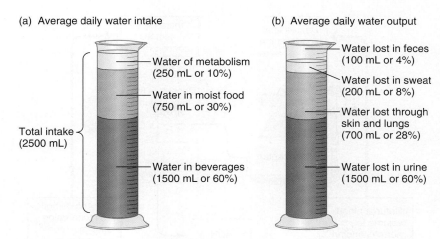

FIGURE 21-4 Water balance. (A) Major sources of body water and (B) routes by which the body loses water.

The above percentages may vary due to environmental temperature, relative humidity, and physical exercise. **FIGURE 21-4** depicts two components: major sources of body water and routes by which the body loses water.

The distal convoluted tubules of the nephrons and collecting ducts are most important in the regulation of water excreted in the urine. Their epithelial linings are mostly impermeable to water unless antidiuretic hormone (ADH) is present. When present, ADH increases water reabsorption to reduce urine production.

In a healthy individual, the osmolality of the body fluids is maintained strictly between 280 and 300 mOsm. Increased plasma osmolality triggers thirst and causes the release of ADH. The kidneys conserve water, excreting concentrated urine. Oppositely, a decrease in osmolality inhibits thirst and the release of ADH. The kidneys excrete large amounts of dilute urine. Sodium attracts water, yet the ADH and thirst mechanisms that control osmolality regulate water independently of sodium's effects.

Fluid Losses and Gains

The human body loses about 2,500 mL of water every day through urine, feces, and insensible perspiration, which involves gradual movement across the epithelia of the skin and respiratory tract. Other losses occur via sensible respiration, which is secretion through the sweat glands. Maximum perspiration rates can reach 4 liters per hour in extreme circumstances. Fever can also increase water loss, so a patient with fever should drink plenty of fluids to offset this condition.

The human body gains about 2,500 mL of water every day. Via liquids, 1,500 mL are lost; via foods, 750 mL are lost; and via metabolic generation, 250 mL are lost. Metabolic generation of water is defined as the production of water within cells. For example, when 1 g of a lipid is broken down, 1.7 mL of water are generated. This is higher than the amount generated by the breakdown of proteins or carbohydrates. **TABLE 21-1** lists sources of water input and methods of water output.

Water Intake Regulation

Water intake is regulated by several major types of stimuli: the effects of *osmoreceptors*, dryness of the mouth, and a decrease in blood volume or blood pressure. In the hypothalamus, the osmoreceptors monitor osmolality of the extracellular fluid by identifying changes in the stretching of plasma membranes, which are caused by the gain or loss of water. Only a 1% to 2% change will activate them. Dry mouth develops when the osmotic pressure of the blood increases, causing the salivary glands to produce less saliva. They do this because the osmotic gradient that pulls water from the blood into the salivary glands is reduced. A large decrease in blood volume or blood pressure, of between 5% and 10%, also triggers thirst. Changes are based on signaling from baroreceptors, directly activating the thirst center, and from the effects of angiotensin II. Altogether, thirst increases because of these events. Thirst is influenced by

TABLE 21-1	
Water Input and Output	
Source of Water Input	**Daily Amount**
Water from liquids	1,500 mL
Water from foods	750 mL
Water from metabolic generation	250 mL
Total water input	2,500 mL
Method of Water Output	**Daily Amount**
Via urination	1,500 mL
Via skin and lungs	700 mL
Via sweat	200 mL
Via defecation	100 mL
Total water output	2,500 mL

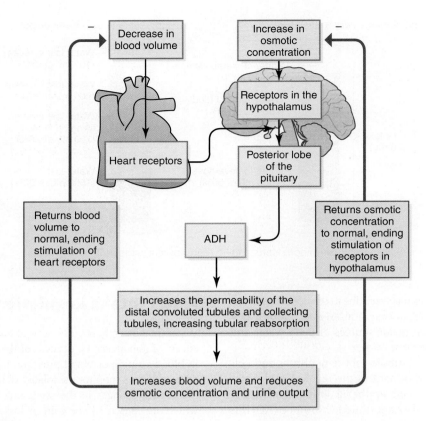

FIGURE 21-5 ADH secretion.

consuming sodium, such as in a snack food, because sodium influences the events.

Water Output Regulation

Water output occurs on a regular basis, and we cannot survive for long without consuming water. The kidneys are powerful but cannot compensate for a lack of water intake. Obligatory water loss includes insensible water loss, water in undigested food residue in the feces, and the minimum daily **sensible water loss**. The kidneys must flush 600 mmol of urine solutes, which are the end products of metabolism and other activities, out of the body via the urine every day. Because the maximum concentration of urine is approximately 1,200 mOsm, at least 500 mL of water need to be excreted.

In addition to obligatory loss of water, urine volume and solute concentration are based on intake of fluids, the diet, and other forms of water loss. Excessive sweating causes the kidneys to excrete much lower quantities of urine to maintain water balance. In normal individuals, the kidneys start to eliminate excess water about 30 minutes after drinking. This is the amount of time required to inhibit the release of ADH. About 1 hour after drinking water, diuresis has reached its peak. This declines to the lowest level after about 3 hours.

Role of ADH

The release of ADH is proportional to the amount of water reabsorbed in the collecting ducts of the kidneys. Low ADH levels mean that most water that reaches the collecting ducts

will not be reabsorbed. This is because a lack of aquaporins in principal cells' apical membranes prevents water movement. The water flows by without being reabsorbed. The urine is dilute, and there is reduced body fluid volume. High ADH levels cause aquaporins to be inserted in principal cell apical membranes. Almost all water that is filtered is reabsorbed. Only a small volume of urine, highly concentrated, is excreted. ADH secretion is regulated by two receptors, one in the brain and one in the heart (**FIGURE 21-5**).

In the hypothalamus, osmoreceptors sense the solute concentration of the extracellular fluid, triggering or inhibiting release of ADH from the posterior pituitary. Increased osmolality of the extracellular fluid causes the hypothalamic osmoreceptors to be stimulated, and ADH is released. Oppositely, decreased extracellular fluid osmolality slows ADH release. More water is excreted in the urine, and the blood osmolality is restored to normal. Significant blood volume or blood pressure changes also affect ADH secretion. If blood pressure is decreased, ADH release increases. This may be direct, because of baroreceptors in the atria and certain blood vessels, or indirect, because of the renin-angiotensin-aldosterone mechanism.

The changes that cause this must be significant because extracellular fluid osmolality changes are greatly important as daily stimulatory or inhibitory factors. Release of ADH may occur because of excessive sweating, diarrhea, or vomiting as well as hemorrhaging, severe burns, or a prolonged fever. When any of these occur, high ADH levels cause arteriole constriction, which directly increases blood pressure. This is where the alternate name for ADH, *vasopressin*, is derived.

1. What is the effect of ADH when you drink water?
2. What is water of metabolism?
3. Differentiate between sensible and insensible perspiration.
4. List the primary factors that regulate water intake and output.

Role of Aldosterone

Aldosterone helps in the regulation of water balance. Produced by the adrenal glands, aldosterone is a steroid hormone. Its levels in the blood are controlled by blood pressure and by the volume of the fluid in the nephrons of the kidneys. **FIGURE 21-6** illustrates the mechanisms involved in aldosterone secretion. Specific cells in the kidneys produce the enzyme known as **renin** when they are stimulated by a decline in blood pressure and in the volume of nephron filtrate.

When renin contacts the large plasma protein known as *angiotensinogen* in the bloodstream, it removes a segment of this protein. This process produces *angiotensin I*, a small peptide molecule. Because angiotensin I is inactive, it must be converted into its active form, *angiotensin II*. This requires enzymes found in the blood inside the lungs. Angiotensinogen is produced in the liver.

The secretion of aldosterone from the adrenal glands is stimulated by angiotensin II. When aldosterone moves through the blood to reach the kidneys, it stimulates nephron cells to increase how much sodium they reabsorb, increasing the tubular reabsorption of sodium. Water then follows the sodium ions, moving out of the nephron into the peritubular capillaries, increasing blood volume and blood pressure. These processes then shut the feedback loop off. Water balance is additionally affected by chemicals found in the diet, of which the most influential are caffeine and alcohol.

The Role of Atrial Natriuretic Peptide

Atrial natriuretic peptide (ANP) is a hormone produced by specialized myocardial cells. ANP is secreted by neurons originating in the hypothalamus. It acts as both hormone and neurotransmitter. Atrial natriuretic peptide increases the glomerular filtration rate and inhibits the release of renin. This hormone also reduces thirst, blocks the release of ADH and inhibits the release of aldosterone, resulting in decreased blood pressure.

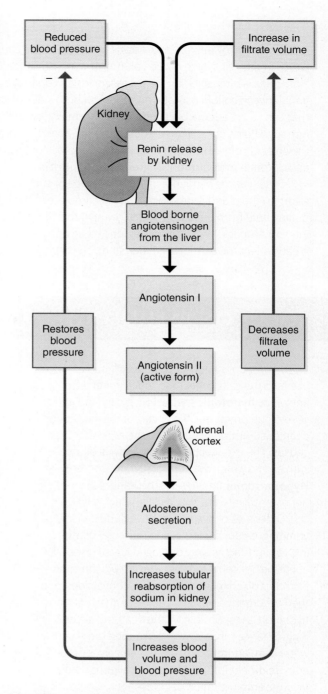

FIGURE 21-6 Aldosterone secretion.

Edema is defined as an abnormal accumulation of fluid in the interstitial spaces. The tissues swell, whereas the cells do not, and edema is actually an increase in volume only of the interstitial fluid. When fluid flows out of the blood in higher than normal amounts or cannot sufficiently return to the blood, edema occurs. These conditions may be caused by increased capillary permeability and hydrostatic pressure. Increased permeability is usually caused by ongoing inflammatory response conditions. Large amounts of exudate form because the capillaries become too porous from the effects of inflammatory chemicals. The exudate contains clotting proteins, other plasma proteins, immune elements, and nutrients.

Increases in capillary hydrostatic pressure can be caused by localized blockage of blood vessels, incompetent valves in the veins, high blood volume, or congestive heart failure. No matter what the cause, filtration at the capillary beds is intensified by the excessively high capillary hydrostatic pressure. Sometimes, edema is caused by an imbalance in colloid osmotic pressures on both sides of capillary membranes. **Hypoproteinemia** is a condition that can cause edema because of an abnormally low colloid osmotic pressure in plasma that is deficient in protein. Although fluids are still forced out of capillary beds at ends of arteries, they may not be able to return to the blood at the ends of veins. The interstitial spaces become congested with fluid. Causes of hypoproteinemia include liver disease, protein malnutrition, or **glomerulonephritis**.

Other causes of edema include blockage or surgical removal of lymphatic vessels. Plasma proteins cannot return to the blood normally. As they accumulate in the interstitial fluid, colloid osmotic pressure continually builds, pulling fluid from the blood and allowing it to collect. Tissue function can be impaired because excess fluid in the interstitial spaces makes it harder for oxygen and nutrients to diffuse between cells and the blood. Edema can greatly affect the cardiovascular system, causing blood pressure and volume to decline and impairing circulation.

FOCUS ON PATHOLOGY

Overhydration is another problem of fluid balance, in which the cells collect too much water. Also known as **hypotonic hydration**, it can lead to severe outcomes. Insufficiencies of the kidneys or overconsumption of water are the most common causes. The extracellular fluid becomes diluted, with excess water but normal sodium content. **Hyponatremia** signifies overhydration, promoting net osmosis into the tissue cells, which swell.

Outcomes of overhydration include nausea, vomiting, cerebral edema, and muscular cramping. Neurons are greatly damaged, and if cerebral edema is not corrected, the affected person soon becomes disoriented, experiences convulsions, and then becomes comatose, leading to death. Overhydration is responsible for the deaths of several long-distance runners, who consumed too much water in an attempt to hydrate themselves properly. Treatment for sudden, severe hyponatremia involves administration of intravenous hypertonic saline solution. This reverses the osmotic gradient, moving water out of the swollen cells.

Electrolyte Balance

When the quantities of electrolytes the body gains equal those it loses, **electrolyte balance** exists. This is also maintained by homeostasis. The most important electrolytes needed for cellular functions are sodium, potassium, calcium, magnesium, chloride, sulfate, phosphate, bicarbonate, and hydrogen ions. These are mostly provided in food but also are present in water and other beverages and as byproducts of metabolic reactions. Of all the electrolytes, sodium imbalance is most significant.

A severe deficiency of electrolytes may produce a desire to eat salty foods known as a *salt craving*. Salts help to control fluid movement in the body and provide needed minerals for excitability, membrane permeability, and secretory activities. Potassium and calcium are also among the most important electrolytes.

More electrolytes are lost by sweating on warm days and during strenuous exercise. Additional amounts are lost in the feces, but the greatest electrolyte output occurs because of kidney function and urine production. The kidneys control electrolyte output to maintain balance. Positive ions such as calcium, potassium, and sodium are essential for maintenance of cell membrane potential, muscle fiber contraction, and nerve impulse conduction. Nearly 90% of positively charged ions in the extracellular fluids are sodium ions, which are regulated by the kidneys and the hormone aldosterone. Electrolyte imbalances are summarized in **TABLE 21-2**.

Sodium Balance

Salts primarily enter the body in foods and fluids, but lesser amounts are due to metabolic activity. During catabolism of bone matrix and nucleic acids, phosphates are liberated. It is not difficult for us to obtain the amounts of electrolytes we need, however. Most Americans eat much more sodium than they actually need. Natural foods contain plenty of sodium, whereas processed foods contain too much sodium. Table salt or *sodium chloride* is used to excess.

Salts are mostly lost from the body via sweating, vomiting, and in the urine and feces. Sweat is usually hypotonic, but large amounts of salt can be lost when sweating becomes profuse. Large losses of salt in vomit or feces may be linked to disorders of the gastrointestinal tract. To balance salts in the body, the kidneys must be healthy.

Potassium Balance

The intracellular fluid contains nearly 98% of the body's potassium. This electrolyte diffuses out of the cellular cytoplasm into the extracellular fluid and therefore requires the cells to expend energy to recover its ions. The potassium ion

TABLE 21-2

Electrolyte Imbalances

Electrolyte	Condition	Causes and Outcomes
Sodium	Hypernatremia (>145 mEq/L)	**Dehydration**, excessive intravenous administration of sodium. Although uncommon in healthy people, it may occur in infants or elderly individuals who cannot indicate thirst because of confusion. It results in thirst, central nervous system dehydration (leading to confusion, lethargy, coma), and increased neuromuscular irritability (twitching and convulsions).
	Hyponatremia (<135 mEq/L)	Loss of solutes and/or retention of water, aldosterone deficiency, kidney disease, excess release of ADH, excess ingestion of water. There may be excessive sodium loss because of diarrhea, vomiting, burns, tubal drainage of the stomach, or excessive diuretic use. Aldosterone deficiency may be linked to Addison's disease.
Potassium	Hyperkalemia (>5.5 mEq/L)	Kidney failure, aldosterone deficiency, rapid intravenous infusion of potassium chloride, burns, or severe injuries to tissues, causing potassium to leave the cells. Outcomes include nausea, vomiting, diarrhea, bradycardia, cardiac arrhythmias, cardiac depression, and cardiac arrest. May also cause skeletal muscle weakness and flaccid paralysis.
	Hypokalemia (<3.5 mEq/L)	Vomiting, diarrhea or other gastrointestinal tract disturbances, Cushing's syndrome, gastrointestinal suctioning, starvation or inadequate dietary intake, hyperaldosteronism, and diuretic therapy. Outcomes include cardiac arrhythmias, flattened T wave, metabolic alkalosis, muscular weakness, mental confusion, nausea, vomiting.
Calcium	Hypercalcemia (>5.2 mEq/L or 10.5 mg/100 mL)	Hyperparathyroidism, excessive vitamin D, prolonged immobilization, malignancies, or renal disease (decreased excretion).
	Hypocalcemia (<4.5 mEq/L or 9 mg/100 mL)	Burns (causing calcium to be trapped in the damaged tissues), hypoparathyroidism, renal tubular disease, vitamin D deficiency, hyperphosphatemia, kidney failure, alkalosis, or diarrhea. Outcomes include increased neuromuscular excitability (tingling fingers, skeletal muscle cramps, tremors, convulsions, tetany, depressed excitability of the heart, fractures, or osteomalacia).
Phosphate	Hyperphosphatemia (>2.9 mEq/L)	Decreased urinary loss because of kidney failure, hypoparathyroidism, increased intestinal absorption, or major tissue trauma. Outcomes (for both hyperphosphatemia and hypophosphatemia) arise because of reciprocal changes in calcium levels rather than directly from changes in plasma phosphate concentrations.
	Hypophosphatemia (<1.6 mEq/L)	Decreased intestinal absorption, hyperparathyroidism, or increased urinary output.
Chloride	Hyperchloremia (>105 mEq/L)	Dehydration, increased retention or intake, hyperparathyroidism, or metabolic acidosis. Outcomes (for both hyperchloremia and hypochloremia) have no direct clinical symptoms because they are usually associated with the underlying cause, which is often related to abnormalities in the pH.
	Hypochloremia (<95 mEq/L)	Metabolic alkalosis, such as caused by vomiting or excessive ingestion of alkaline substances, and aldosterone deficiency.
Magnesium	Hypermagnesemia (>2.2 mEq/L)	Although rare, it occurs in kidney failure when magnesium is not excreted normally. May also be caused by excessive ingestion of antacids that contain magnesium. Outcomes include lethargy, impaired central nervous system functioning, respiratory depression, coma, and cardiac arrest.
	Hypomagnesemia (<1.4 mEq/L)	Alcoholism, chronic diarrhea, diuretic therapy, or severe malnutrition. Outcomes include tremors, increased neuromuscular excitability, convulsions, and tetany.

concentration in the extracellular fluid is based on a balance between the rate at which the ions are gained across the digestive epithelium and the rate at which they are lost into the urine. The actions of the ion pumps in the distal parts of nephrons and the collection system regulate potassium loss in the urine. When a sodium ion is reabsorbed from the tubular fluid, there is usually an exchange between it and a cation, most commonly potassium, from the peritubular fluid.

Normally, between 50 and 150 mEq of urinary potassium ions are lost, whereas the same amount is absorbed across the digestive epithelium. There is only a small amount of potassium lost in the perspiration and feces. In the extracellular fluid, potassium ion concentration is controlled by regulating active secretion rates along the distal convoluted tubule and nephron collecting system.

Three factors relate to how the rate of tubular secretion of potassium ions varies: changes in the potassium ion concentration of the extracellular fluid, changes in pH, and aldosterone levels. Basically, the higher the concentration of potassium in the extracellular fluid, the higher the rate of secretion. When pH falls in the extracellular fluid, the pH of the peritubular fluid also falls. There is then a decline in the rate of potassium secretion. This is because hydrogen ions, not potassium ions, are secreted as part of an exchange with sodium ions in the tubular fluid.

Aldosterone greatly affects the rate at which potassium ions are lost in the urine. This results from the ion pumps being sensitive to aldosterone and therefore reabsorbing sodium ions from the filtrate, exchanged for potassium ions from the peritubular fluid. Angiotensin II stimulates aldosterone secretion as part of blood volume regulation. Aldosterone secretion is also directly stimulated by high plasma potassium ion concentrations. The ways aldosterone influences the amounts of conserved sodium and the amounts of potassium excreted via the urine are closely related. Once plasma concentrations of potassium fall below 3.5 mEq/L *hypokalemia* develops, with extensive muscular weakness being followed by paralysis. Hypokalemia may cause death by affecting normal cardiac function.

Calcium Balance

There is more calcium in the body than any other mineral, and 99% of body calcium is deposited in the skeleton. This makes up 1 to 2 kg, or 2.2 to 4.4 pounds, of body calcium. Calcium is vital for controlling muscular and neural activities, for blood clotting, for forming the crystalline components of bones, as a cofactor for enzymatic reactions, and because of its *second messenger* functions. Calcium homeostasis is maintained in the extracellular fluid by parathyroid hormone and calcitriol but also by calcitonin to a smaller degree. Calcium ion concentrations are raised by parathyroid hormone and calcitriol, whereas calcitonin opposes their actions. Calcitriol is produced by the kidneys.

Although a small amount of calcium is lost every day in the bile, only tiny amounts are lost via the urine or feces. Therefore, an adult must absorb only 0.8 to 1.2 g/day of calcium, which is only approximately 0.03% of the amount of calcium stored in the skeleton. Calcium absorption is stimulated by parathyroid hormone and calcitriol. It is absorbed in the digestive tract and reabsorbed in the distal convoluted tubule.

Hypercalcemia is present when the extracellular fluid calcium ion concentration is higher than 5.3 mEq/L. In adults, it is usually caused by *hyperparathyroidism*, which is over-secretion of parathyroid hormone. Additional causes include malignant cancers of the breast, kidneys, bone marrow, or lungs. Excessive use of supplements containing calcium or vitamin D may also cause hypercalcemia. Hypercalcemia is considered severe when calcium ion concentration exceeds 12 to 13 mEq/L in the extracellular fluid. Signs and symptoms include confusion, fatigue, calcification of soft tissues such as the kidneys, and cardiac arrhythmias.

The opposite condition is *hypocalcemia*, in which there is a calcium ion concentration under 4.3 mEq/L. Much less common than hypercalcemia, this is usually caused by *hypoparathyroidism*, which is under-secretion of parathyroid hormone, chronic renal failure, or vitamin D deficiency. Signs and symptoms include osteoporosis, weak heartbeat, muscle spasms that may be accompanied by generalized convulsions, and cardiac arrhythmias.

Phosphate Balance

Phosphate ions are essential for the mineralization of bones. The mineral salts of the skeleton store approximately 740 g of phosphate ions. Phosphate most significantly affects the intracellular fluid, where it helps to activate enzymes, form high-energy compounds, and synthesize nucleic acids. In the plasma the normal concentration of phosphate ions is 1.8 to 3.0 mEq/L. It is reabsorbed from the tubular fluid in the proximal convoluted tubule. This reabsorption is stimulated by calcitriol. Via the urine and feces, approximately 30 to 45 mEq, or 0.8 to 1.2 g of phosphate, is lost every day.

Chloride Balance

Chloride ions are the most common ions found in the extracellular fluid, with normal plasma concentrations between 100 and 108 mEq/L. Chloride is usually very low in the intracellular fluid, approximately 3 mEq/L. Chloride is absorbed across

FOCUS ON PATHOLOGY

A salt or "sour" craving may develop because of a severe electrolyte deficiency. *Addison's disease* is a disorder involving the adrenal cortex not producing enough mineralocorticoid hormone and is commonly related to these cravings. Mineral deficiencies may also produce some rather bizarre cravings. If a person lacks sufficient iron, he or she may "crave" chalk, clay, or starch—a condition known as *pica*.

the digestive tract along with sodium. In the renal tubules, chloride and sodium ions are absorbed by several carrier proteins. Very little loss of chloride ions occurs via the urine and perspiration. Therefore, only 48 to 146 mEq, or 1.7 to 5.1 g/day, are required to maintain a chloride ion balance.

TEST YOUR UNDERSTANDING

1. Define the terms *electrolytes*, *water balance*, and *electrolyte balance*.
2. List the causes and symptoms of dehydration.
3. Describe how salts are lost and gained by the body.

Acid-Base Balance

Electrolytes that dissociate in water to release hydrogen ions are called **acids**. Electrolytes that release ions that combine with hydrogen ions are called **bases**. Homeostasis requires control of acid and base concentrations in body fluids. Most hydrogen ions in body fluids begin as byproducts of metabolic processes. The major sources of hydrogen ions are as follows:

- *Aerobic respiration of glucose:* produces carbon dioxide and water, forms carbonic acid, and releases hydrogen and bicarbonate ions
- *Anaerobic respiration of glucose:* produces lactic acid, adding hydrogen ions to body fluids
- *Incomplete oxidation of fatty acids:* produces acidic ketone bodies to increase hydrogen ion concentration
- *Oxidation of sulfur-containing amino acids:* yields sulfuric acid, releasing hydrogen ions
- *Hydrolysis of phosphoproteins and nucleic acids:* produces phosphoric acid, releasing hydrogen ions

Strong acids dissociate to release hydrogen ions more completely, whereas *weak acids* release them less completely. An example of a strong acid is hydrochloric acid and of a weak acid is carbonic acid. Bases release ions, such as hydroxide ions, that combine with hydrogen ions, lowering their own concentration. Examples of bases include sodium hydroxide and sodium bicarbonate. Strong bases dissociate to release more hydroxide ions than weak bases. Negative ions are often referred to as bases. They may combine with strong acids; for example, bicarbonate ions may combine with hydrogen ions from hydrochloric acid to form carbonic acid.

All functioning proteins, including enzymes, cytochromes, and hemoglobin, are influenced by hydrogen concentrations. This is true because of their abundant hydrogen bonds. Therefore, nearly all biochemical reactions are influenced by fluid environment pH, and there is close regulation of acid-base balance. Variations in optimal pH are not excessive. Although the normal pH of intracellular fluid is on average 7.0, in the arterial blood it is 7.4 and in the venous blood and interstitial fluid, 7.35. The lower pH in venous blood and the cells is because of their larger amounts of carbon dioxide and acidic metabolites. Carbon dioxide combines with water to form carbonic acid.

FOCUS ON PATHOLOGY

Alkalosis is signified by arterial blood pH above 7.45 and is also known as *alkalemia*. **Acidosis**, also called *acidemia*, is signified by arterial blood pH below 7.35. Although a pH of 7.0 is neutral, in terms of chemicals, a number such as 7.35 is not really a sign of an acidic state. However, because it is higher than the optimal hydrogen concentration for most cells, a pH between 7.0 and 7.35 is called *physiologic* acidosis.

The three sequential regulators of hydrogen ion concentration in the blood are chemical buffers, brain stem respiratory centers, and renal mechanisms. The first line of defense consists of chemical buffers, which act in less than a second to resist changes in pH. In 1 to 3 minutes, respiration changes in rate and depth, compensating for acidosis or alkalosis. The kidneys are the slowest to act, requiring several hours to days to alter the blood pH, but are the strongest regulators of acid-base balance.

Acid-base buffer systems consist of chemicals that combine with excess acids or bases. Buffer system chemicals can combine with strong acids, which release more hydrogen ions, to convert them into weak acids, which release fewer hydrogen ions. The three most important acid-base buffer systems in the body's fluids are as follows:

- *Bicarbonate buffer system:* This system is present in both intracellular and extracellular fluids, using the bicarbonate ion as a weak base and carbonic acid as a weak acid. It is sometimes called the *carbonic acid–bicarbonate buffer system*. Carbonic acid is formed when hydrogen ions are excessive and dissociates when conditions are basic or alkaline. The body maintains a readily available *bicarbonate reserve*.
- *Phosphate buffer system:* This system also operates in both intracellular and extracellular fluids and is very important in controlling hydrogen ion concentrations in the fluid of the nephrons and in urine. It consists of monohydrogen phosphate and dihydrogen phosphate.
- *Protein buffer system:* Consists of plasma proteins and certain cell proteins. When the solution pH falls, amino groups accept hydrogen ions; when it rises, carboxyl groups release hydrogen ions. For red blood cells, which are densely packed with hemoglobin molecules that buffer hydrogen ions, a *chloride shift* occurs. This involves dissociation of carbonic acid and bicarbonate ions diffusing into the plasma in exchange for chloride ions. In the lungs this occurs in reverse and is known as the *hemoglobin buffer system*.

TABLE 21-3

Three Major Acid-Base Buffer Systems

System	Components	Functions
Bicarbonate buffer system	Bicarbonate ion (HCO_3^-)	Under acidic conditions, it combines with a hydrogen ion.
	Carbonic acid (H_2CO_3)	Under alkaline conditions, it releases a hydrogen ion.
Phosphate buffer system	Monohydrogen phosphate (HPO_4^{-2})	Under acidic conditions, it combines with a hydrogen ion.
	Dihydrogen phosphate ($H_2PO_4^-$)	Under alkaline conditions, it releases a hydrogen ion.
Protein buffer system with amino acids	NH_2 group of an amino acid or protein	In the presence of excess acid, it combines with a hydrogen ion.
	COOH group of an amino acid or protein	In the presence of excess base, it releases a hydrogen ion.

TABLE 21-3 summarizes the three major buffer systems. Carbonic acid production increases when cells increase carbon dioxide production. As carbonic acid dissociates, hydrogen ions increase and the internal environment pH drops. These actions stimulate chemoreceptors in the medulla oblongata, increasing breathing so the lungs can excrete more carbon dioxide. If cells are less active, production of these components is low and breathing may be closer to resting levels. Nephrons excrete hydrogen ions in urine to help regulate hydrogen ion concentration. Epithelial cells in the renal tubules secrete hydrogen ions into the tubular fluid.

TEST YOUR UNDERSTANDING

1. Explain the difference between an acid and a base.
2. List the body's major chemical buffer systems.
3. Describe two additional ways the body balances acids and bases.

Acid-Base Imbalances

The pH of arterial blood is usually between 7.35 and 7.45. Abnormal values below 7.35 produce *acidosis*, whereas values above 7.45 produce *alkalosis*. Shifts in pH can be life threatening. Survival may be impossible if blood pH is below 6.8 or above 8.0 for more than a few hours (**FIGURE 21-7**). The partial pressure of carbon dioxide (P_{CO_2}) is the most important indicator of normal respiratory function. Normal levels are between 35 and 45 mm Hg. Dangerous acidosis and alkalosis conditions may be linked to cardiovascular, respiratory, urinary, digestive, or nervous system abnormalities. To correctly diagnose these conditions, most blood tests include screenings of pH and buffer system function. Blood pH, P_{CO_2}, and bicarbonate ion levels are measured. Additional tests include measuring the *anion gap* and using *nomograms* or *diagnostic charts* to plot test results. These steps help to correctly identify the condition, its severity, its causes, and whether it is compensated or uncompensated.

FOCUS ON PATHOLOGY

For life to continue, the blood pH cannot be lower than 6.8 or higher than 7.8. Below pH 6.8, central nervous system depression is severe, resulting in coma and a quick death. Above pH 7.8, over-excitation of the nervous system leads to extreme nervousness, muscle tetany, and convulsions, followed by death often because of respiratory arrest.

Respiratory Acidosis

The two major types of acidosis are *respiratory acidosis* and *metabolic acidosis*. Respiratory acidosis may be caused by increased carbon dioxide concentration as well as carbonic acid or *respiratory acid* and may result in the following conditions:

- Injury to the brain stem's respiratory center, decreasing breathing
- Obstruction of air passages and interference with air movement into alveoli
- Diseases decreasing gas exchange, such as pneumonia, or reducing respiratory membrane surface area, such as emphysema; also linked to cystic fibrosis

Respiratory acidosis is generally indicated by a P_{CO_2} that is above 45 mm Hg, known as *hypercapnia*, and lowered blood pH. It is usually caused by *hypoventilation*, which is an abnormally low respiratory rate. When the P_{CO_2} rises in the extracellular fluid compartment, hydrogen and bicarbonate ion concentrations also rise. This occurs as carbonic acid forms and dissociates. When buffer systems cannot keep up, the pH falls rapidly. Just a few minutes of hypoventilation may result in acidosis. The pH of the extracellular fluid may reduce to as low as 7.0.

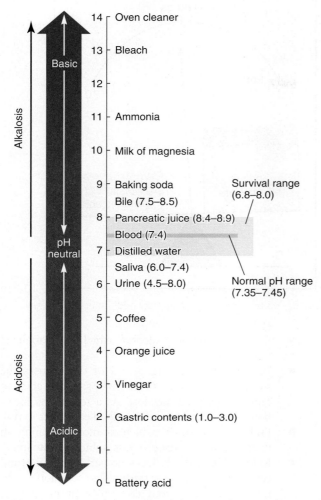

Typical pHs of common substances

14	Oven cleaner
13	Bleach
12	
11	Ammonia
10	Milk of magnesia
9	Baking soda / Bile (7.5–8.5)
8	Pancreatic juice (8.4–8.9)
	Blood (7.4)
7	Distilled water
	Saliva (6.0–7.4)
6	Urine (4.5–8.0)
5	Coffee
4	Orange juice
3	Vinegar
2	Gastric contents (1.0–3.0)
1	
0	Battery acid

Survival range (6.8–8.0)

Normal pH range (7.35–7.45)

FIGURE 21-7 Normal pH range and the survival range

When the body's chemical and physiological buffers return pH to normal, the acidosis is *compensated*. This is normally accomplished by chemoreceptors that stimulate an increase in breathing rate. In *uncompensated acidosis*, the pH continues to drop, and the patient can become comatose and eventually die. *Acute respiratory acidosis* develops when the decline in pH is severe. It is an especially dangerous condition when the patient's tissues generate large amounts of carbon dioxide or when normal respiratory activity is not possible. Therefore, for victims of cardiac arrest or drowning, reversing acute respiratory acidosis is the major goal. As a result, cardiopulmonary resuscitation, first aid, and life-saving courses teach *Airway, Breathing, and Circulation* as the "ABCs" of emergency care.

Chronic respiratory acidosis occurs because normal respiratory function is compromised but compensatory mechanisms have not completely failed. In a patient with central nervous system damage, normal respiratory compensation may not occur even when stimulated by chemoreceptors. People whose respiratory centers are desensitized by barbiturates or alcohol may also be unable to achieve normal respiratory compensation. These individuals often develop

acidosis because of chronic hypoventilation. Other factors, such as congestive heart failure, emphysema, pneumonia, pneumothorax, and respiratory muscle paralysis, can influence the development of chronic respiratory acidosis.

When normal pulmonary responses are disabled, the kidneys increase hydrogen ion secretion into the tubular fluid, slowing the rate of pH change. Unfortunately, the kidneys are not able to return pH to normal levels on their own. The underlying circulatory or respiratory problems must be corrected. Breathing efficiency may be temporarily improved with bronchodilators or mechanical devices providing air that is under positive pressure. Artificial respiration or mechanical ventilation are required once breathing has ceased. If the respiratory acidosis was not severe or prolonged, normal pH can still be restored. Respiratory acidosis treatment is made more difficult because the condition also causes *metabolic acidosis* as lactic acid is generated in tissues that do not have sufficient oxygen. The effects of respiratory acidosis and the compensation for the condition are shown in **FIGURE 21-8**.

Respiratory Alkalosis

Respiratory alkalosis is a less common condition that results from excessive carbon dioxide and carbonic acid loss. Called **hypocapnia**, this condition is signified by a $P_{CO_2} <$ 35 mm Hg, with raised blood pH. A temporary hypocapnia can be produced by *hyperventilation*, often in response to anxiety, pain, fever, or poisoning due to salicylates. Hyperventilation depletes carbon dioxide and increases body fluid pH to as high as 8.0. Fortunately, respiratory alkalosis is usually self-corrected, because chemoreceptor stimulation stops and the urge to breathe reduces. Carbon dioxide levels then return to normal.

Hyperventilation often results from pain or other physical stressors and extreme anxiety or other psychological stressors. It gradually elevates the pH of the cerebrospinal fluid, affecting central nervous system function. There are initial tingling sensations in the lips, hands, and feet. The individual may be light-headed and lose consciousness if the condition continues. Because unconsciousness stops perception of causative psychological stimuli, breathing rate declines and the condition is self-corrected. The effects of respiratory alkalosis and compensation for the condition are shown in **FIGURE 21-9**.

Hyperventilation is easily treated by having the patient rebreathe air that has been exhaled into a small paper bag. Rising P_{CO_2} in the bag results in similar rises in the arterial and alveolar carbon dioxide concentrations. The pH is then restored to normal levels. Rare situations that may involve respiratory alkalosis include high altitudes that cause hyperventilation, use of mechanical respirators, and those with brain stem injuries that cause them to be unable to respond to changes in plasma carbon dioxide concentrations.

Metabolic Acidosis

Metabolic acidosis is the second most common type of acid-base imbalance. Metabolic imbalances such as this are indicated by bicarbonate levels below or above the normal

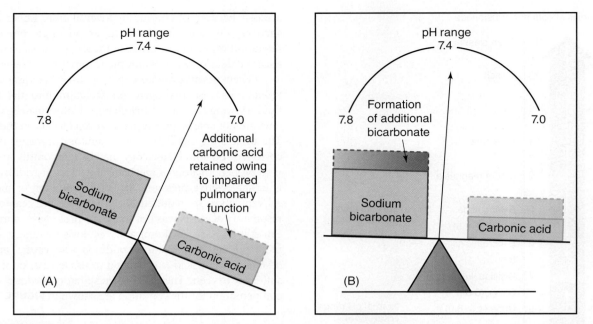

FIGURE 21-8 (A) Derangement of acid-base balance in respiratory acidosis. (B) Compensation by formation of additional bicarbonate.

range, which is 22 to 26 mEq/L. Metabolic acidosis may be caused by accumulation of nonrespiratory acids or loss of bases, such as in the following conditions:

- **Lactic acidosis**, which can develop after strenuous exercise or prolonged tissue hypoxia, known as oxygen starvation, as active cells rely on anaerobic respiration.
- Diabetes mellitus, which converts some fatty acids into ketone bodies such as acetoacetic acid, beta-hydroxybutyric acid, and acetone, causing ketonuria or **ketoacidosis**. This conversion of some fatty acids into ketone bodies also occurs during starvation.

- Overconsumption of alcohol, which is metabolized to acetic acid.
- Vomiting over a long period of time causes the stomach to continue to generate stomach acids to replace those that are lost. As a result, the bicarbonate concentration of the blood continues to rise.
- Prolonged diarrhea, which is more common in infants, causing excessive loss of bicarbonate ions.
- Kidney disease that reduces glomerular filtration and causes uremic acidosis; this is a less common condition. It may occur from glomerulonephritis and use of diuretics. When the reabsorption of sodium ions stops, secretion of hydrogen ions also stops.

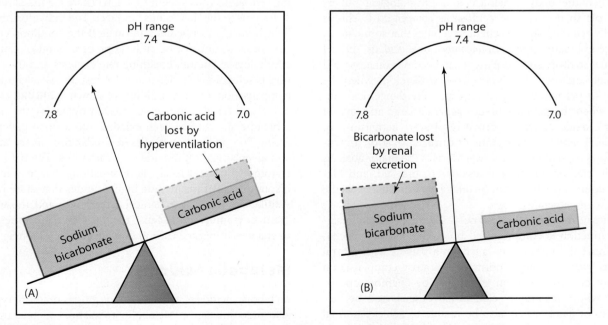

FIGURE 21-9 (A) Derangement of acid-base balance in respiratory alkalosis. (B) Compensation by excretion of bicarbonate.

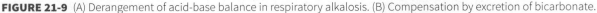

Diagnosis and treatment of metabolic acidosis is based on the cause. Although it can be easily linked to lactic acidosis after extreme physical activity, there may be many more complicated causative factors. The body generally compensates for metabolic acidosis via the lungs and kidneys. The lungs eliminate carbon dioxide molecules formed by the interaction of hydrogen ions with bicarbonate ions. The kidneys excrete additional hydrogen ions into the urine while generating bicarbonate ions, which are released into the extracellular fluid.

Metabolic and respiratory acidosis are often linked because oxygen-starved tissues generate lactic acid in massive amounts and because sustained hypoventilation results in decreased arterial partial pressure of oxygen. Examples include near-drownings, in which there is high P_{CO_2} and low partial pressure of oxygen in the body fluids. Lactic acid dominates the muscles because of the attempts of the drowning person to stay above water. Dissociation of lactic acids releases lactate and hydrogen ions. Emergency treatment is vital, including artificial or mechanical respiratory assistance and intravenous administration of an isotonic solution. This solution contains sodium bicarbonate, sodium gluconate, or sodium lactate.

Metabolic Alkalosis

Metabolic alkalosis results from excessive loss of hydrogen ions or gain of bases or *bicarbonate ions*. It is much less common than metabolic acidosis. In metabolic alkalosis, there is in an increase in blood pH, called alkalemia, after gastric drainage or *lavage*, use of certain diuretics, overuse of antacids, or prolonged vomiting. Loss of acidic gastric juice leaves body fluids more basic. A condition called *alkaline tide* may occur, caused by many bicarbonate ions moving into the extracellular fluid. This movement is related to secretion of hydrochloric acid from the gastric mucosa. Temporary elevation of bicarbonate ions in the extracellular fluid occurs during eating, but serious metabolic alkalosis may occur because of repeated vomiting as the stomach generates more stomach acids to replace those regurgitated. This means bicarbonate ion concentrations in the extracellular fluid rise continually. Metabolic alkalosis may also develop from taking excessive quantities of antacids.

Symptoms include decreased breathing rate and depth and increased blood carbon dioxide. The compensatory factors for metabolic alkalosis include reduced breathing rate, with a loss of bicarbonate ions in the urine. For mild cases, treatment usually is focused on controlling vomiting or treating other causative factors. Solutions that may be administered include sodium chloride or potassium chloride. Acute metabolic alkalosis is treated with ammonium chloride. As the ammonium ions are metabolized in the liver, hydrogen ions are liberated, which basically means hydrochloric acid is generated in greater quantities. As it diffuses into the bloodstream, the pH falls to normal levels. The effects of respiratory and metabolic acidosis and alkalosis are described in **TABLE 21-4**.

Compensations for Imbalances

If the lung or kidney buffer systems become insufficient, the acid-base balance is disrupted. As a result, the undisturbed system tries to compensate. The respiratory system is responsible for compensation of metabolic acid-base imbalances and works relatively quickly. The urinary system, although slower, is responsible for compensation of respiratory-related acid-base imbalances. The ways these systems compensate are reflected in changes in the P_{CO_2} and

TABLE 21-4

Effects of Respiratory and Metabolic Acidosis and Alkalosis

Respiratory Acidosis	Metabolic Acidosis	Respiratory Alkalosis	Metabolic Alkalosis
Respiratory congestion, slow and shallow respirations	Diabetic ketoacidosis, diarrhea, renal failure	Hyperventilation	Excessive antacid use, vomiting
P_{CO_2} is increased	Decreased bicarbonate, rapid and deep respirations, tissue hypoxia	Decreased levels of P_{CO_2}	Increased bicarbonate, slow and shallow respirations
More hydrogen excreted by kidneys and more bicarbonate reabsorbed	More hydrogen excreted by the kidneys; if the kidneys are not involved, there is increased bicarbonate absorption	Less hydrogen excreted by the kidneys and less bicarbonate reabsorbed	Less hydrogen excreted by the kidneys; if the kidneys are not involved, there is decreased bicarbonate absorption
High P_{CO_2} and bicarbonate levels	Low P_{CO_2} and bicarbonate levels	Partial pressure of oxygen low; bicarbonate levels low	High P_{CO_2} and bicarbonate levels
Compensated pH 7.35–7.4; decompensated pH < 7.33	Compensated pH 7.35–7.4; decompensated pH < 7.33	Compensated pH 7.4–7.45; decompensated pH > 7.47	Compensated pH 7.4–7.45; decompensated pH > 7.47

concentrations of bicarbonate ions. A patient can have a serious medical condition and still show a normal pH because of how these systems compensate.

Respiratory Compensation

When the respiratory system compensates for a metabolic acid-base imbalance, respiratory rate and depth change. They are usually elevated in metabolic acidosis. This is because high hydrogen ion levels stimulate the respiratory centers. Blood pH is below 7.35, and bicarbonate ion levels are below 22 mEq/L. The P_{CO_2} falls below 35 mm Hg as carbon dioxide is removed and excess acid leaves the blood. In respiratory acidosis, respiratory rate is often depressed, which is the immediate cause of the acidosis. This is not true for conditions of gas exchange impairment, such as pneumonia or emphysema.

For metabolic alkalosis, respiratory compensation involves slow and shallow breathing. This allows carbon dioxide to accumulate in the blood. Evidence of this compensation includes a pH above 7.45 at first, and sometimes longer; bicarbonate levels over 26 mEq/L; and a P_{CO_2} above 45 mm Hg.

Urinary Compensation

The kidneys speed up compensatory actions when an acid-base imbalance is of respiratory cause. Acidosis is shown when a person is hyperventilating. Although the kidneys are compensating, the levels of the P_{CO_2}, as well as bicarbonate ions, are high. The raised P_{CO_2} causes the acidosis. The increasing bicarbonate ion level shows the kidneys are retaining bicarbonate to compensate for the acidosis.

Oppositely, an individual who has respiratory alkalosis compensated for by the kidneys has a high blood pH and a low P_{CO_2}. As the kidneys eliminate more bicarbonate by not reclaiming it or by secreting it, its levels begin to fall. However, the kidneys cannot compensate for either alkalosis or acidosis if the condition is linked to a renal problem.

Effects of Aging on Water, Electrolyte, and Acid-Base Balance

Total body water decreases gradually as we age, predominantly from the intracellular compartment. These decreases reduce the dilution of waste products, toxins, and administered medications. The glomerular filtration rate declines, and the body cannot regulate pH via the urinary system as efficiently. More water begins to be lost because of an increased inability to concentrate the urine. As the skin becomes thinner, the rate of insensible perspiration increases. Older adults should increase their daily water intake to combat this condition. They are less able to conserve body water than younger people and are also less responsive to thirst cues. When homeostasis is interrupted, the body takes longer to return to normal.

Body mineral content is lower as muscles and bones decrease in mass. Body fat increases, however. Exercise and increased ingestion of dietary minerals can help in this regard. Because respiratory compensation decreases with age, the risk of respiratory acidosis increases, compounded by arthritic conditions and other conditions such as emphysema. As the other systems in the body decline in function, they affect fluid, electrolyte, and acid-base balances as well. Conditions that make the elderly more prone to acid-base imbalances include congestive heart failure with edema and diabetes mellitus. Nearly all disorders of the body systems, with increased aging, partially affect the balances of fluids, electrolytes, acids, and bases.

SUMMARY

The maintenance of fluid, primarily water, and electrolyte balance requires equal quantities of these substances to enter and leave the body. When water balance is altered, the electrolyte balance is affected. The intracellular fluid compartment includes the fluids and electrolytes enclosed by cell membranes. The extracellular fluid compartment includes all the fluids and electrolytes outside the cell membranes. Many different types of solutes are dissolved in water, which is the universal solvent. Most extracellular fluids contain high amounts of chloride, bicarbonate, and sodium ions. Most intracellular fluids contain high amounts of magnesium, phosphate, and potassium ions. Hydrostatic and osmotic pressure regulate fluid movements. Exchanges between plasma and interstitial fluid occur across capillary walls, whereas exchanges between interstitial and intracellular fluids occur across plasma membranes. Water balance requires equal intake and output. Water intake is mostly regulated by thirst. The distal convoluted tubules of the nephrons and collecting ducts regulate water output.

The release of ADH is proportional to the amount of water reabsorbed in the collecting ducts of the kidneys.

In the hypothalamus, osmoreceptors sense the solute concentration of the extracellular fluid, triggering or inhibiting release of ADH from the posterior pituitary. The hormone aldosterone stimulates water reabsorption in the kidneys. Dehydration is the loss of water or solutes, occurring when water output exceeds water intake over time. The most important electrolytes for cellular functions dissociate in body fluids to release ions of sodium, potassium, calcium, magnesium, chloride, sulfate, phosphate, bicarbonate, and hydrogen. Most electrolytes are lost through the kidneys. Concentrations of sodium, potassium, and calcium ions are the most important of all.

Acids are electrolytes that dissociate to release hydrogen ions. Bases release ions that combine with hydrogen ions. Body fluid pH must remain within a certain range. Acids and bases may be strong or weak. Buffer systems convert strong acids into weaker acids or strong bases into weaker bases. Respiratory or metabolic acidosis results from increases in concentrations of acids or loss of certain bases. Respiratory or metabolic alkalosis results from decreases in concentrations of certain acids, loss of hydrogen ions, or gain of bases.

KEY TERMS

Acid-base buffer systems
Acidosis
Acids
Aldosterone
Alkalosis
Bases
Dehydration
Edema
Electrolyte balance

Electrolytes
Extracellular fluid compartment
Glomerulonephritis
Hypocapnia
Hyponatremia
Hypoproteinemia
Hypotonic hydration
Insensible water loss
Intracellular fluid compartment

Ketoacidosis
Lactic acidosis
Renin
Sensible water loss
Transcellular fluid
Water balance
Water of metabolism

LEARNING GOALS

The following learning goals correspond to the objectives at the beginning of this chapter:

1.
   A. *Fluid balance:* Referring mainly to water balance, it means that total water intake equals total water output, maintained by homeostatic mechanisms.
   B. *Electrolyte balance:* When the quantities of electrolytes that the body gains equal those that it loses; also maintained by homeostasis.

2. Intracellular fluid is made up of water and electrolytes enclosed by cell membranes and contains more magnesium, phosphate, potassium, and sulfate ions than extracellular fluid. Extracellular fluid is made up of all fluid outside of cells, which includes the plasma, lymph, interstitial fluid, and transcellular fluid. It contains high amounts of chloride, bicarbonate, and sodium ions, as well as more calcium than is found in intracellular fluid.

3. The hormones important for regulating fluid and electrolyte balance include ADH and aldosterone.

4. Hydrostatic pressure and osmotic pressure regulate the movement of water and electrolytes from one fluid compartment to another. A change in osmotic pressure usually causes net fluid movement. When sodium ions decrease in the extracellular fluid, water moves from the extracellular compartment into the intracellular compartment via osmosis. The opposite is true when sodium ion concentration in interstitial fluid increases.

5. Many electrolytes are lost by sweating on warm days and during strenuous exercise. The greatest electrolyte output occurs because of kidney function and urine production. Nearly 90% of the positively charged ions in the extracellular fluids are sodium ions, regulated by the kidneys and aldosterone. Potassium ions are also regulated by aldosterone. Rising concentrations stimulate aldosterone secretion from the adrenal cortex. This enhances sodium ion tubular reabsorption and causes potassium ion tubular secretion.

6.
   A. *Bicarbonate buffer system:* Uses the bicarbonate ion as a weak base and carbonic acid as a weak acid.
   B. *Phosphate buffer system:* Very important in controlling hydrogen ion concentrations in the fluid of the nephrons and in urine.
   C. *Protein buffer system:* Consists of plasma proteins and certain cell proteins. When the solution pH falls, amino groups accept hydrogen ions; when it rises, carboxyl groups release hydrogen ions.

7. The most common threats to acid-base balance include acidosis, when the pH of arterial blood is below 7.35, and alkalosis, when pH is above 7.45. The two major types of acidosis are respiratory acidosis and metabolic acidosis. Likewise, the two major types of alkalosis are respiratory alkalosis and metabolic alkalosis.

8. When normal pH levels of arterial blood are not maintained, the body responds by producing acidosis or alkalosis. Survival may be impossible if pH is below 6.8 or above 8.0 for more than a few hours.

9. Metabolic alkalosis results from excessive loss of hydrogen ions or gain of bases or bicarbonate ions. This results in an increase in blood pH or alkalemia. It may follow gastric drainage or lavage, use of certain diuretics, or prolonged vomiting. It also may develop from taking too many antacids.

10. The differences between respiratory and metabolic acidosis are as follows:
   A. *Respiratory acidosis:* May be caused by increased carbon dioxide concentration as well as carbonic acid; may result in injury to the brain stem's respiratory center, obstruction of air passages, pneumonia, emphysema, or other respiratory conditions
   B. *Metabolic acidosis:* May be caused by accumulation of nonrespiratory acids or loss of bases; may result in kidney diseases, diabetes mellitus, long-term vomiting, prolonged diarrhea, or lactic acidosis

CRITICAL THINKING QUESTIONS

A 40-year-old firefighter was brought to the emergency department after being overcome by the intense heat of a large apartment fire. He was seriously dehydrated and had experienced some second-degree burns while saving an elderly resident of the building.

1. Why does prolonged sweating increase plasma sodium ion levels?
2. Why do burn patients consistently show elevated levels of potassium in their urine?

REVIEW QUESTIONS

1. Antidiuretic hormone
   A. stimulates water conservation by the kidneys
   B. stimulates the kidneys to retain sodium ions
   C. results in the loss of more sodium ions
   D. is secreted by the anterior pituitary gland
2. The primary regulator of water intake is
   A. pH of urine
   B. acidity of stomach
   C. thirst
   D. thalamus
3. Aldosterone
   A. regulates the blood pH
   B. increases the concentration of potassium in urine
   C. decreases blood volume
   D. promotes sodium retention in the kidneys
4. Which of the following is not a cause of acidosis?
   A. peripheral vasoconstriction
   B. prolonged vomiting
   C. diabetes mellitus
   D. kidney failure
5. The amount of potassium secreted by the kidneys is regulated by
   A. cortisol
   B. aldosterone
   C. progesterone
   D. antidiuretic hormone
6. Prolonged vomiting can result in
   A. metabolic alkalosis
   B. respiratory alkalosis
   C. respiratory acidosis
   D. metabolic acidosis
7. Renal failure can result in
   A. hypokalemia
   B. hyponatremia
   C. hyperkalemia
   D. decreased urea

8. Intracellular fluid has high concentrations of
   A. sodium
   B. potassium
   C. bicarbonate ions
   D. chloride
9. Nearly 90% of positively charged ions in extracellular fluids are
   A. potassium ions
   B. calcium ions
   C. sodium ions
   D. all of the above
10. When the amount of sodium ions in the extracellular fluid increases,
    A. thirst decreases
    B. osmoreceptors are stimulated
    C. aldosterone secretion increases
    D. the volume of urine produced increases
11. Intracellular fluid is found in
    A. the interstitial spaces
    B. lymph
    C. blood
    D. the cells of the body
12. Changes in the pH of body fluids are compensated for by all the following, *except*
    A. the phosphate buffer system
    B. an increase in urine output
    C. the carbonic acid–bicarbonate buffer system
    D. protein buffer
13. The primary components of extracellular fluid are
    A. interstitial fluid and plasma
    B. lymph and cerebrospinal fluid
    C. plasma and serous fluids
    D. all of the above

14. The most important factor affecting the pH of body tissues is the concentration of
    A. lactic acid
    B. hydrochloric acid
    C. ketone bodies
    D. carbon dioxide

15. Consuming a meal high in salt will
    A. cause hypotension
    B. decrease thirst
    C. result in a temporary increase in blood volume
    D. increase the release of renin

ESSAY QUESTIONS

1. Describe the body fluid compartments and the approximate fluid volume in each.
2. Define the terms electrolytes, solutes, and solvent.
3. Describe the thirst mechanism.
4. Explain hydrostatic and osmotic pressures.
5. Describe the percentages of average daily adult consumption of water.
6. Explain water intake and output regulation.
7. Describe the role of the respiratory system in controlling acid-base balance.
8. Explain the role of antidiuretic hormone and aldosterone in controlling body fluid balance.
9. Define the terms alkalosis, acidosis, and acid-buffer system.
10. Compare respiratory compensation with urinary compensation.

CHAPTER 22

Digestive System

OBJECTIVES

After studying this chapter, the reader should be able to

1. Identify the organs of the digestive system.
2. Explain the processes by which materials move through the digestive tract.
3. Describe the anatomy of the stomach and its roles in digestion and absorption.
4. Describe the anatomic characteristics of the small intestine.
5. Explain three hormones secreted from the digestive system to regulate digestion.
6. Describe the structure of the pancreas and secretory activities for digestion.
7. Describe the major functions of the liver.
8. Describe the regions of the large intestine.
9. Explain the significance of the large intestine in the absorption of nutrients.
10. Specify the nutrients required by the body.

Overview

Life is sustained by obtaining nutrients from the environment. Nutrients are the raw materials needed to synthesize essential compounds in the body. They may also be decomposed to provide energy required by the cells to continue functioning. The mechanical and chemical breakdown of foods and the *absorption* of resulting nutrients by the body's cells are known as **digestion**. The organs of the *digestive system* carry out the processes of mechanical digestion and chemical digestion. Mechanical digestion is the process of breaking large pieces of food into smaller ones without altering their chemical makeup. Chemical digestion uses chemicals to break food into simpler chemicals. The two major divisions of the digestive system are the **alimentary canal** and the *accessory digestive organs*.

The digestive system extends from the mouth to the anus and includes the mouth, pharynx, esophagus, stomach, small intestine, large intestine, rectum, and anus (**FIGURE 22-1**). Its associated **accessory organs** include the salivary glands, liver, gallbladder, and pancreas. The secretions from these accessory organs empty via ducts into the digestive tract. Glandular organ secretions are made up of water, enzymes, buffers, and other components. These secretions assist in preparing organic and inorganic nutrients for absorption across the epithelium of the digestive tract. The digestive system is basically a tube open at both ends that supplies nutrients for body cells. Its surface area in an adult is 186 square meters.

Alimentary Canal

The alimentary canal is an 8-meter-long continuous muscular tube passing through the thoracic and abdominopelvic cavities (**FIGURE 22-2**). This canal is also known as the *gastrointestinal tract* or *gut*. In a dead body the alimentary canal is longer, totaling 9 m in total, because it has lost its muscle tone. The digestive tube consists of four major layers, present from the esophagus to the anus (**FIGURE 22-3**): an internal mucosa and an external serosa, with a submucosa and a muscularis in between:

- The **mucosa (mucous membrane)**, *consisting of three layers:* (1) the inner mucous epithelium, which is made up of moist stratified squamous epithelium in the mouth, oropharynx, esophagus, and anal canal; (2) a loose connective tissue called the **lamina propria**; and (3) a thin outer layer of smooth muscle. It has projections extending into the **lumen** that increase its absorptive surface. The mucosa carries out secretion and absorption.
- *Submucosa:* Loose connective tissue with glands, blood vessels, lymphatic vessels, and nerves; it nourishes surrounding tissues and carries away absorbed materials.
- *Muscular layer:* Produces movements of the tube and is made of two smooth muscle tissue coats: circular fibers of the inner coat encircle the tube, causing contraction, and longitudinal fibers run lengthwise, causing shortening of the tube.

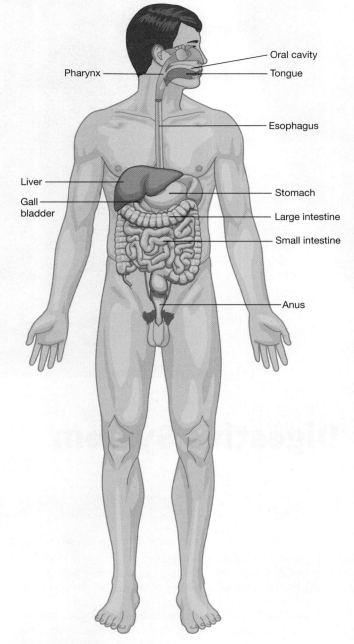

FIGURE 22-1 The digestive system.

- *Serosa:* Composed of a visceral peritoneum on the outside and connective tissue beneath; it protects underlying tissues and secretes serous fluid so abdominal organs slide freely against each other. The serosa is also called the *adventitia*.

Functions of the Digestive System

The functions of the digestive system consist of a series of seven essential steps:

1. *Ingestion:* Materials enter the digestive tract via the mouth.
2. *Propulsion:* The movement of food, which includes voluntary *swallowing* and involuntary *peristalsis*, which is

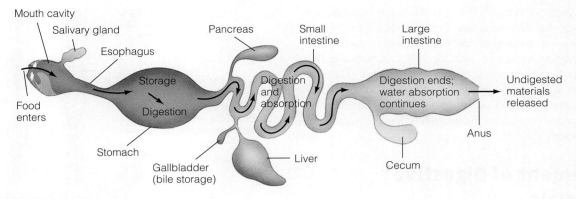

FIGURE 22-2 The alimentary canal.

the primary means of propulsion. Peristalsis involves alternating waves of muscular contraction and relaxation in the walls of the alimentary canal.

3. *Mechanical processing (breakdown):* Materials are crushed and broken into smaller fragments, making them easier to move through the digestive tract. Enzymes begin to attack the particles during chewing, as the teeth and tongue are used to tear and mash food. Additional mechanical processing is provided by the mixing motions of the stomach and intestines. Mechanical processing increases ingested foods' surface areas. *Segmentation* mixes foods with digestive juices, improving their absorption by moving various parts of the food mass over the intestinal wall repeatedly.

4. *Digestion:* The chemical breakdown of food into particles that are small enough to be absorbed by the digestive epithelium from the *lumen* or cavity of the canal;

simple molecules such as glucose are absorbed intact, whereas polysaccharides, proteins, and triglycerides must first be broken down before they can be absorbed. This is a catabolic process.

5. *Secretion:* Release of water, acids, buffers, enzymes and salts by the epithelium and glandular organs of the digestive tract.

6. *Absorption:* The movement of organic substrates, electrolytes, vitamins, and water across the epithelium of the digestive tract into the interstitial fluid. Organic substrates are molecules acted on by enzymes. Absorption occurs via active or passive transport into blood or lymph.

7. *Excretion:* The removal of waste products from body fluids via secretions from the digestive tract and glandular organs; after mixing with residue that cannot be digested, these waste products become *feces*, which are eliminated during the process of *defecation*.

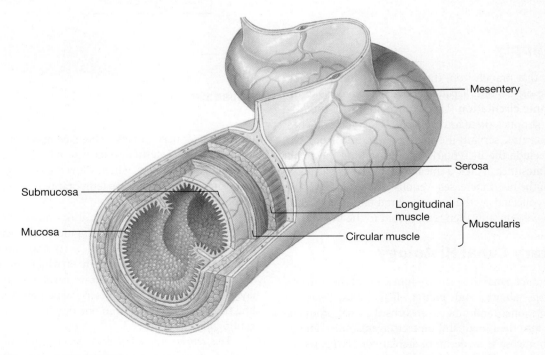

FIGURE 22-3 The layers of the alimentary canal.

The digestive system's lining protects surrounding tissues against digestive acids and enzymes that may corrode them, abrasion and other mechanical stress, and bacteria that may be consumed with food or that normally live inside the digestive tract. If bacteria reach areas of areolar tissue such as the *lamina propria*, immune cells such as macrophages attack them. The lamina propria lies beneath the epithelium and constitutes the mucosa or *mucous membranes* of the digestive tract.

Movement of Digestive Materials

There are two basic types of motor functions in the alimentary canal: mixing movements and propelling movements. When smooth muscles contract rhythmically, mixing occurs. Waves of contractions mix food with digestive juices. In the small intestine, mixing movements are aided by **segmentation**, involving alternating contraction and relaxation of smooth muscle in nonadjacent segments. Materials are not propelled along the tract in one direction because segmentation follows no set pattern. **Peristalsis** consists of the propelling, wave-like movements of the tube (**FIGURE 22-4**). Contraction appears in the wall of the tube in a "ring," whereas the muscular wall immediately ahead of the ring relaxes. The peristaltic wave moves along, pushing contents of the tube toward the anus.

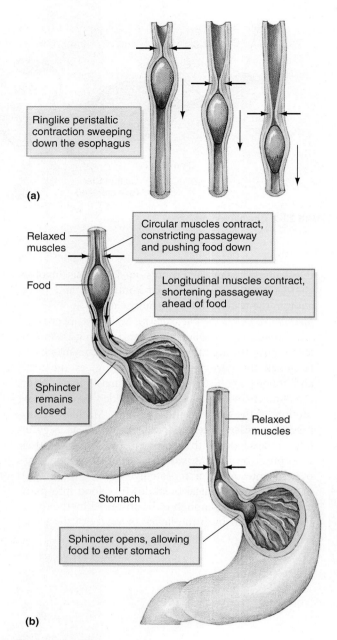

(a)

Ringlike peristaltic contraction sweeping down the esophagus

Relaxed muscles

Circular muscles contract, constricting passageway and pushing food down

Food

Longitudinal muscles contract, shortening passageway ahead of food

Sphincter remains closed

Relaxed muscles

Stomach

Sphincter opens, allowing food to enter stomach

(b)

FIGURE 22-4 Peristalsis.

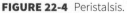

TEST YOUR UNDERSTANDING

1. Describe the organs of the alimentary canal, from beginning to end.
2. Describe the wall of the alimentary canal.
3. Define *peristalsis*.

Blood Supply

The arteries that branch from the abdominal aorta, serving the digestive organs and *hepatic portal circulation*, make up the **splanchnic circulation**. Usually, one-fourth of the cardiac output supplies these arteries, which include branches of the celiac trunk serving the liver, spleen, and stomach. They also include the mesenteric arteries serving the small and large intestines. After a meal the amount of blood needed from the heart increases. Venous blood that is rich in nutrients is collected by the hepatic portal circulation from the digestive viscera. It is then transported to the liver.

Alimentary Canal Histology

In the alimentary canal the primary functions of the mucosa are to *secrete, absorb,* and *protect*. It secretes digestive enzymes, hormones, and mucus; absorbs the final products of digestion into the blood; and protects against infections.

The submucosa is made up of areolar connective tissue that is rich in blood vessels, lymphatic vessels, lymphoid follicles, and nerve fibers. These components supply surrounding gastrointestinal tract wall tissues. The submucosa has many elastic fibers, which allow the stomach to return to its normal shape after it has temporarily held a large amount of food.

The muscularis externa, also known simply as the *muscularis*, functions in segmentation and peristalsis. The muscularis externa usually has a circular inner layer and a longitudinal outer layer, both of which are made up of smooth muscle cells. However, in certain areas the circular layer thickens to form *sphincters*, which are valves controlling the passage of food from one organ to the next and preventing backflow of food.

The *serosa* or *visceral peritoneum*, throughout most alimentary canal organs, is made up of areolar connective tissue, with a single layer of squamous epithelial cells that form the *mesothelium* covering it. However, the serosa is replaced by an *adventitia* in the portion of the canal known as the *esophagus*. The adventitia is ordinary fibrous connective tissue. It connects the esophagus to its surrounding structures. The retroperitoneal organs actually have both: an adventitia and a serosa. Here, the adventitia is located on the side that touches the dorsal wall of the body and the serosa is on the side that faces the peritoneal cavity.

Mouth

Digestion begins in the *mouth*, which is also known as the *oral cavity* or *buccal cavity*. It is encompassed superiorly by the palate, anteriorly by the lips, laterally by the cheeks, and inferiorly by the tongue. The *oral orifice* consists of the mouth's anterior opening. The mouth is continuous posteriorly with the *oropharynx*. Solid particles of food are reduced mechanically and mixed with saliva. The *vestibule* is the portion that lies between the teeth, cheeks, and lips.

Tongue

The **tongue** is covered by a mucous membrane and is connected to the floor of the mouth by a membranous fold called the **lingual frenulum**. The body of the tongue is made up of primarily interlaced, bundled skeletal muscle. It mixes food particles with saliva during chewing, moving food, in the form of a mass called a *bolus*, toward the pharynx during swallowing. The tongue also moves food underneath the teeth for chewing and helps to form consonant sounds when speaking.

The tongue contains intrinsic and extrinsic skeletal muscle fibers. Its *intrinsic muscles* are within the tongue itself and not attached to any bones. However, its *extrinsic muscles* originate on either the skull bones or soft palate, extending to the tongue. They change the tongue's position and are able to move it left and right and cause it to protrude or retract. There is a median septum of connective tissues, with each half containing identical muscle groups.

The tongue has rough **papillae** that project from its surface to provide friction (**FIGURE 22-5**). These peg-like projections emerge from the mucosa. The *filiform papillae* are cone-shaped and make the tongue's surface rougher. They aid in eating semisolid foods, providing friction so these foods can be manipulated. They are found in parallel rows on the dorsum of the tongue and are the smallest, most numerous type of papillae. Keratin is contained within the filiform papillae, causing the tongue to have a somewhat white appearance.

The keratin makes the filiform papillae stiff in comparison with other papillae.

Over much of the tongue's surface are scattered *fungiform papillae*, which are mushroom-shaped. They have a red appearance because of their vascular cores. In a V-shaped row on the posterior tongue are 10 to 12 *vallate papillae*. These papillae are very large, appear similar to the fungiform papillae, and have a furrow that surrounds them. On the lateral aspects of the posterior tongue are found *foliate papillae*, which appear as if they are folded into "pleats." The fungiform, vallate, and foliate papillae also contain the taste buds. In infancy and early childhood, the taste buds of the foliate papillae are most functional, with reduced function later in life. There are no papillae on the mucosa that covers the root of the tongue.

Tonsils and Palate

The root of the tongue is connected to the hyoid bone and covered with rounded lymphatic tissue masses called **lingual tonsils**, giving it a bumpy texture. The lingual tonsils lie just deep to the mucosa. The roof of the oral cavity is formed by the **palate**, which consists of a bony, anterior hard palate and a muscular, posterior soft palate. The soft palate arches posteriorly and downward into a cone-shaped projection called the **uvula**. In the back of the mouth, on either side of the tongue and near the palate, are masses of lymphatic tissue called the *palatine tonsils*. They lie beneath the epithelial lining of the mouth and help to protect against infection.

The *pharyngeal arches* lie on either side of the uvula, and the more anterior *palatoglossal arch* is located between the soft palate and the base of the tongue. The *fauces* is the arched opening between the soft palate and base of the tongue and is formed by a curved line connecting the palatoglossal arches and uvula. The fauces create the passage between the oral cavity and oropharynx. Extending from the soft palate to the pharyngeal wall is the more posterior *palatopharyngeal arch*. One palatine tonsil lies between the palatoglossal and palatopharyngeal arches on either side.

The *pharyngeal tonsils* are also known as the *adenoids*. They lie on the posterior pharynx, above the border of the soft palate. When the adenoids enlarge to block the passage between the nasal cavity and pharynx, they may be surgically removed, similar to the palatine tonsils.

Salivary Glands

Saliva is secreted by the **salivary glands**. It moistens food and begins the chemical digestion of carbohydrates. Saliva is also a solvent that dissolves foods so they can be tasted and helps to cleanse the mouth and teeth. Major salivary glands

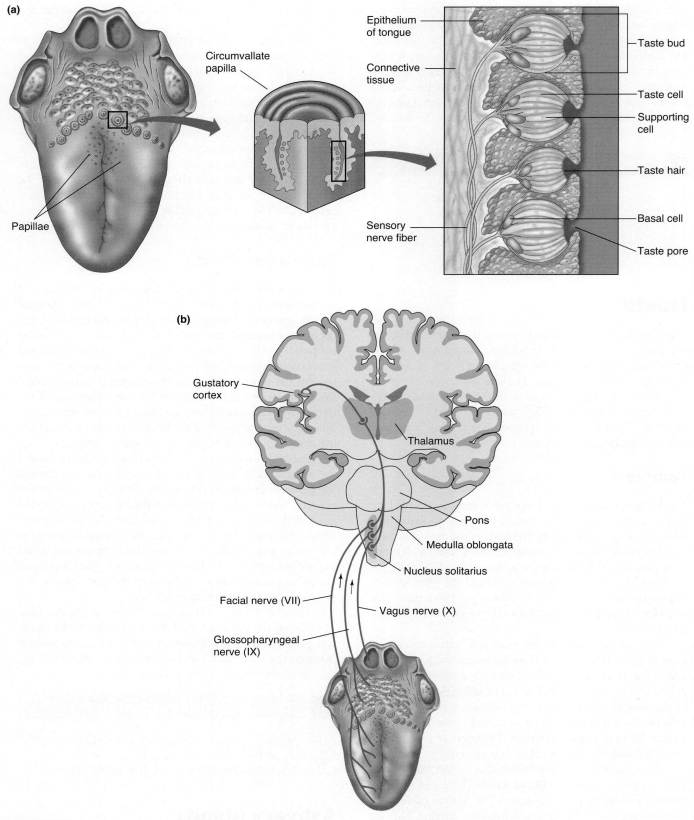

(a)

Circumvallate
papilla

Papillae

Epithelium
of tongue

Connective
tissue

Taste bud

Taste cell

Supporting
cell

Taste hair

Sensory
nerve fiber

Basal cell

Taste pore

(b)

Gustatory
cortex

Thalamus

Pons

Medulla oblongata

Nucleus solitarius

Facial nerve (VII)

Vagus nerve (X)

Glossopharyngeal
nerve (IX)

FIGURE 22-5 Surface of the tongue.

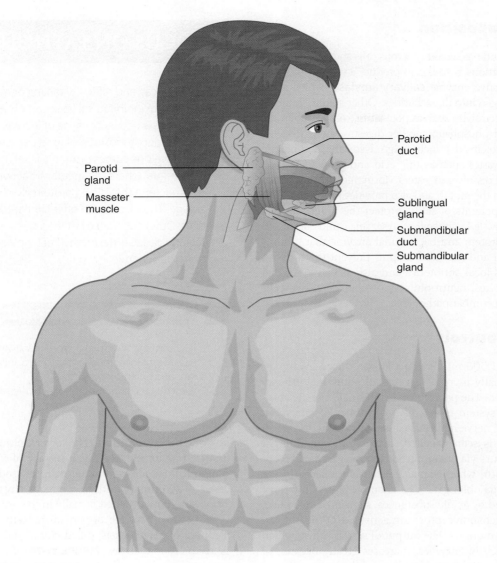

FIGURE 22-6 The major salivary glands.

are actually paired compound tubuloalveolar glands emerging from the oral mucosa and connecting to it via ducts. There are three pairs of major salivary glands:

- **Parotid glands**: The largest; they lie anterior and slightly inferior to each ear, between the cheek and masseter muscle, producing a clear and watery fluid rich in amylase (**FIGURE 22-6**). They are basically triangular in shape and have primary ducts parallel to the zygomatic arch. These ducts pierce the buccinator muscles, opening into the vestibule close to the second upper molar. Facial nerve branches pierce the parotid glands to connect to the muscles of facial expression. Facial paralysis can occur if surgery is performed on these glands. The parotid gland secretions are drained by a *parotid duct*, emptying into the vestibule near the second upper molar.
- *Submandibular glands*: Located in the floor of the mouth on the inside lower jaw surface; they secrete

a more viscous fluid than the parotid glands. The *submandibular ducts* open into the mouth, on both sides of the lingual frenulum, just posterior to the teeth.
- *Sublingual glands*: The smallest; they lie on the floor of the mouth inferior to the tongue and produce thick and stringy secretions. There are many *sublingual ducts*, opening along both sides of the lingual frenulum.

The submandibular and sublingual salivary glands are made up of serous and mucous secretory cells. *Serous cells* produce a watery secretion made up of ions, enzymes, and a small amount of mucin. Primarily, the submandibular and parotid glands contain serous cells. Mucous cells secrete **mucus**, a thick liquid that binds food particles and lubricates them during swallowing. Mucus is stringy and viscous in composition. Primarily, the sublingual glands contain mucous cells.

Saliva Composition

Each salivary gland has secretory serous cells and mucous cells, in varying proportions. Serous cells produce a watery fluid containing the digestive enzyme **salivary amylase**, which splits starch and glycogen into disaccharides. Other solutes found in saliva include electrolytes such as potassium, sodium, chloride, bicarbonate, and phosphate; another digestive enzyme called lingual lipase; proteins that include IgA, lysozyme, and mucin; and metabolic wastes such as uric acid and urea. *Mucin* is a glycoprotein that dissolves in water to form thick mucus, which hydrates foods in the mouth and also provides lubrication.

Three components of saliva protect the mouth against microorganisms: *IgA antibodies, lysozyme,* and *defensins.* Lysozyme is a protein and bactericidal enzyme that inhibits bacterial growth and may also help to prevent tooth decay. Defensins act as local antibiotics and also as cytokines that attract lymphocytes, neutrophils, and other defensive cells when needed to combat pathogens.

Salivary Controls

Approximately 1,500 mL of saliva are produced every day, but this can greatly increase because of additional salivary gland stimulation. The parasympathetic division of the autonomic nervous system is the main controller of salivation. Parasympathetic nerve impulses cause saliva secretion when appealing food is seen, smelled, tasted, or even thought about. This occurs via chemoreceptors and mechanoreceptors in the mouth, which signal the *salivatory nuclei* in the pons and medulla oblongata. The chemoreceptors are most strongly activated by acidic substances, such as orange juice, whereas the mechanoreceptors are activated by nearly any type of chewing motions. The output of serous saliva, which is watery and rich in enzymes, increases greatly because of impulses sent through the motor fibers of the *facial (VII)* and *glossopharyngeal (IX)* cranial nerves.

Unappealing food actually inhibits parasympathetic activity, producing less saliva and making swallowing difficult. The sympathetic division of the autonomic nervous system causes thick saliva that is rich in mucin to be released. Mostly, sympathetic fibers in the T1 to T3 regions are involved. When strongly activated, the sympathetic division inhibits saliva release by constricting blood vessels of the salivary glands. The mouth then becomes dry, which is called **xerostomia**. Salivation is also inhibited by dehydration, because filtration pressure at the capillary beds is reduced by lowered blood volume.

Teeth

Humans have two sets of **teeth** that form during their lifetimes. The *primary teeth,* also called *deciduous teeth*, erupt through the gums between the ages of 6 months and 4 years. These are also known as the *baby teeth* or *milk teeth*. There are a total of 20 deciduous teeth, 10 in each jaw, which is made up by the mandible and maxilla. Each tooth is clinically

TEST YOUR UNDERSTANDING

1. Contrast the three major types of salivary glands.
2. List the major components of saliva, including its antimicrobial components.
3. Describe the primary controller of the salivary gland functions.

described as a **dentition**. The lower central incisors are the first teeth to appear, usually at the age of 6 months. In 1- to 2-month intervals, additional pairs of teeth erupt. In most cases, all 20 primary teeth have emerged by the age of 2 years. They are eventually shed, usually in the order they appeared.

The *secondary teeth,* or permanent teeth, push the primary teeth out of their sockets, called *alveoli*, and usually consist of 32 teeth (16 in each jaw; **FIGURE 22-7A**). They lie more deeply than the primary teeth and absorb the roots of the primary teeth from below. The secondary teeth usually begin to appear at 6 years of age, but the final teeth, the third molars, may not appear until between ages 17 and 25. The third molars are commonly referred to as *wisdom teeth*. However, in some individuals wisdom teeth either never emerge or are totally absent. The primary and deciduous teeth are summarized in **TABLE 22-1**.

Teeth are classified by their shapes and functions and include incisors, canines, premolars, and molars. **Incisors** are shaped like chisels and are ideal for cutting food or for slicing off pieces of food. The **canines**, also known as the *cuspids* or *eyeteeth*, are cone-shaped and resemble fangs. The teeth best used for crushing or grinding are the **premolars**, or *bicuspids,* and **molars**. Both have broad crowns and rounded tips called *cusps*. Extra grinding ability is found with the molars because they have four to five cusps. Great crushing forces are developed as the upper and lower molars lock together during chewing.

Tooth Structure

Each tooth consists of a **crown** that projects beyond the **gum**, which is also called the *gingiva*, and a *root* that is anchored to

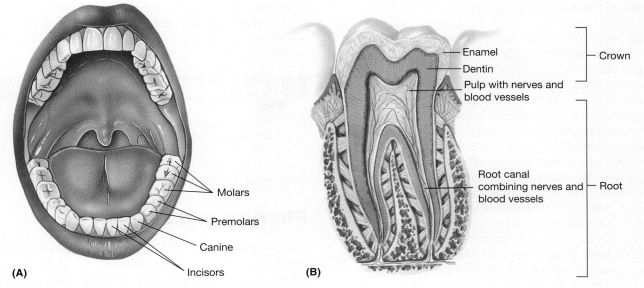

FIGURE 22-7 The teeth. (A) the oral cavity; (B) tooth structure.

the jaw's alveolar process. The crown of each tooth surrounds it tightly, like a collar. A *gingival sulcus*, which is a shallow groove, surrounds the neck of each tooth. Its mucosa is thin and not tightly connected to the periosteum. The epithelium is attached to the tooth at the base of the sulcus, preventing bacterial access to the lamina propria of the gingiva and to the cementum of the root, which is relatively soft. These attachments are strengthened and the epithelial cells stimulated when you brush and massage your gums.

The crown of each tooth is covered in glossy, white *enamel* that mainly consists of calcium salts. The enamel is the hardest substance in the body (**FIGURE 22-7B**), even harder than bone. However, it is brittle and similar to the substance called *ceramic*. It is only about as thick as a dime and bears the force of chewing directly on it. Enamel contains force-resisting columns of dense hydroxyapatite crystals, which are minerals aligned perpendicular to the surface of each tooth. When a tooth erupts, the cells producing the enamel degenerate. Therefore, when damaged by abrasion or injury, enamel is not replaced, and it

wears away with age. This requires artificial fillings to replace the lost areas of enamel.

The *neck* of the tooth is constricted, connecting the crown and the root. The *root* is enclosed in thin, bone-like *cementum* surrounded by a periodontal ligament, meaning the root is actually embedded in the jawbone. The cementum is a calcified connective tissue. The periodontal ligament contains blood vessels and nerves, along with thick collagenous fibers passing between the cementum and bone of the alveolar processes. The periodontal ligament anchors the tooth in its *alveolus*, and a fibrous joint or *gomphosis* is formed. One root is found in each of the canines, incisors, and premolars. However, the first upper premolars usually have two roots. There are three roots to the first two upper molars, but the corresponding lower molars only have two. Although the roots of the third molars vary, a fused single root is most commonly seen.

The bulk of a tooth below the enamel is the **dentin**, which is harder than bone but similar in structure. It surrounds the

TABLE 22-1

Primary and Secondary Teeth

Primary (Deciduous)	Secondary (Permanent)	Function
Central incisor: 4 Lateral incisor: 4	Central incisor: 4 Lateral incisor: 4	To bite off pieces of food
Canine (cuspid): 4	Canine (cuspid): 4	To grasp and tear food
First premolar (bicuspid): 0 Second premolar (bicuspid): 0	First premolar (bicuspid): 4 Second premolar (bicuspid): 4	To grind food particles
First molar: 4 Second molar: 4 Third molar: 0	First molar: 4 Second molar: 4 Third molar: 4	To grind food particles
Total: 20	Total: 32	

tooth's central **pulp cavity** that contains blood vessels, connective tissue, and nerves. Collectively, these components are called *pulp*. Blood vessels and nerves reach the pulp cavity through root canals extending into the root. The dentin is rich in proteins, acting as a shock absorber when chewing and biting. It contains unique radial striations known as *dentinal tubules*. Dentin, cementum, and enamel are calcified. They differ from bone in that they are avascular. Also, dentin and cementum contain collagen, whereas enamel does not and is almost all mineral in content. The pulp supplies nutrients to the tissues of the tooth and provides sensation. At the point where the pulp cavity extends into the tooth root, it becomes the *root canal*. The proximal end of each root canal has an *apical foramen*, which allows blood vessels, nerves, and other structures to enter into the pulp cavity. The superior and inferior alveolar nerves, which are branches of the trigeminal nerve, serve the teeth. Blood is supplied by branches of the maxillary artery called the superior and inferior alveolar arteries.

Tooth Disease

When bacteria eventually demineralize enamel and dentin, *cavities* or *dental caries* result. The decay starts when a film of bacteria, sugar, and various debris adheres to the teeth. This is known as *dental plaque*. Acids are produced, which dissolve the calcium salts in the teeth. Bacterial enzymes can then easily digest the rest of the organic teeth matrices. Plaque can be removed by frequent brushing and daily flossing.

Gum Disease

When plaque is not removed from the gums, it calcifies, forming a *calculus*, which is also known as *tartar*. This condition is more serious than tooth decay. The extremely hard calculi disrupt the seals between the gums and teeth. The sulci are deepened, and the gums may become infected by pathogenic anaerobic bacteria, a condition called *gingivitis*. The gums become red, swollen, sore, and often bleed. If the calculi are removed, gingivitis is reversible. If not, inflamed pockets of infected tissue develop. Immune system cells and neutrophils then attack the pathogens as well as the gum tissues. Deep pockets develop around the teeth, the periodontal ligament is destroyed, and bone is dissolved by activated osteoclasts. This condition, known as *periodontitis (periodontal disease)*, affects nearly 95% of people over the age of 35. In adults, periodontal disease causes between 80% and 90% of tooth loss.

However, intervention is still possible. The teeth are scraped, the infected pockets cleaned, and the gums are cut to shrink the size of the pockets. Anti-inflammatory and antibiotic therapies are initiated. The surrounding tissues can then reattach to the teeth and bone. Home regimens follow, including consistent brushing, flossing, and rinsing with hydrogen peroxide mixtures. It is also believed that untreated periodontal disease may be linked to heart disease and stroke. This is because the existing, chronic inflammation promotes atherosclerotic plaques, and bacteria that enter the blood from the infected gums result in clots to form, clogging cerebral and coronary arteries. Periodontal disease is commonly linked to diabetes mellitus, smoking, and piercings of the tongue or lips.

Pharynx and Esophagus

The **pharynx** allows food, liquids, and air to pass through its cavity, which lies posterior to the mouth. From the pharynx, the tubular esophagus leads to the stomach. These structures do not digest food but are important in that their muscular walls aid in swallowing. The nasal and oral cavities are connected to the larynx and esophagus by the pharynx, which consists of the following structures:

- *Nasopharynx:* Communicates with the nasal cavity to provide a passageway for air during breathing.
- *Oropharynx:* Lies posterior to the soft palate and inferior to the nasopharynx; it is a passageway for food from the mouth and for air from the nasal cavity. Food passes posteriorly into the oropharynx, followed by the laryngopharynx.
- *Laryngopharynx:* Lies inferior to the oropharynx; it is a passageway to the esophagus. Like the oropharynx, it also allows the passage of fluids and air.

The pharynx is similar in its histology to the oral cavity. Its mucosa contains a stratified squamous epithelium that resists friction and has many mucous-producing glands.

The **esophagus** is a hollow muscular tube, about 25 cm or 10 inches in length, with a diameter of about 2 cm. Basically a straight but collapsible tube, the main function of the esophagus is to pass solid food and liquids to the stomach. Food passes through the esophagus from the laryngopharynx to the stomach, descending posteriorly to the trachea. The esophagus passes through the mediastinum, penetrating the diaphragm through the **esophageal hiatus**, and is continuous with the stomach on the abdominal side of the diaphragm. It actually joins the stomach at the *cardial orifice*, which is surrounded by the *gastroesophageal* or *cardiac sphincter*. This sphincter is known by a third name, the **lower esophageal sphincter**. It is formed by a thickening of circular smooth muscle fibers.

This sphincter prevents stomach contents from regurgitating into the esophagus but temporarily relaxes to allow food to enter the stomach from the esophagus. The esophagus is different from the mouth and pharynx in that its wall has the same four basic layers as the rest of the alimentary canal: a mucosa, submucosa, muscularis externa, and a *fibrous adventitia* instead of a serosa. Throughout the submucosa of the esophagus there are many mucous glands that moisten and lubricate the inner lining of the tube.

Heartburn is a burning substernal pain that radiates. It is the first symptom of *gastroesophageal reflux disease*, commonly known as *GERD*. Heartburn occurs when stomach acid is regurgitated up into the esophagus. Symptoms are similar to those of a myocardial infarction or *heart attack*. It is usually linked to excessive eating or drinking, extreme obesity, pregnancy, and running. GERD may result in *Barrett's esophagus,* in which the tissue that lines the esophagus becomes replaced with tissue that is similar to the lining of the intestines. **Hiatal hernia** is also linked, which is a structural abnormality of the gastroesophageal sphincter. In hiatal hernia, the superior stomach protrudes just above the diaphragm so the diaphragm cannot reinforce the sphincter.

TEST YOUR UNDERSTANDING

1. What occurs when the soft palate and larynx elevate and the glottis closes?
2. What is a bolus?
3. Describe the layers of the esophagus.

Processes of Digestion

Most processes of digestion involve the mouth and its accessory digestive organs. In the mouth, food is ingested, chewing begins the mechanical breakdown of the food, swallowing initiates propulsion of food, and polysaccharides begin to be digested. Nearly no absorption occurs in the mouth, except for drugs such as nitroglycerine, which are absorbed through the oral mucosa. The pharynx and esophagus only function as conduits of food passage, from the mouth to the stomach.

The process of chewing or **mastication** involves opening and closing the jaws and moving them from side to side. The tongue moves food between the teeth, which grind and tear the food. This process breaks food down into smaller fragments so it can be more easily swallowed. The food is moved back and forth over the biting or *occlusal* surfaces. Mastication is a voluntary and a reflexive process.

Swallowing or **deglutition** occurs in three stages: chewing, physical swallowing, and peristalsis in the esophagus to the stomach. In the *voluntary stage*, the food is chewed and mixed with saliva, rolled into a mass or **bolus** by the tongue, and forced into the pharynx. The tip of the tongue is placed against the hard palate, and tongue contraction is the movement that actually forces the bolus into the oropharynx. This phase is also known as the *buccal phase*. Over 22 separate muscle groups are used in swallowing.

The second stage of swallowing begins as food stimulates sensory receptors, which trigger the swallowing reflex, momentarily inhibiting breathing. It is involuntary and known as the *pharyngeal–esophageal phase*. This phase is controlled by the swallowing center of the medulla oblongata and lower pons.

The third stage of swallowing is peristalsis, as the food is transported in the esophagus to the stomach. It only takes about 8 seconds for solid foods to pass from the oropharynx to the stomach. Because fluids are assisted by gravity, they are passed within 1 to 2 seconds. Before the wave of peristalsis reaches the end of the esophagus, the gastroesophageal sphincter relaxes reflexively. This allows food to enter the stomach. The sphincter closes after the food enters, which prevents regurgitation back into the esophagus.

Stomach

The **stomach** is a pouch-like organ shaped like the letter "J." It hangs inferior to the diaphragm, in the upper left abdominal cavity, and is partially obscured by the liver and diaphragm. The stomach is approximately 15 to 25 cm or 6 to 10 inches in length, although its volume and diameter change based on how much food is contained. When empty, its volume is about 50 mL, and it has a cross-sectional diameter just a little larger than the large intestine. The organ collapses inward when empty. Its capacity is approximately 4 liters or 1 gallon, and its inner lining consists of thick folds of mucosal and submucosal layers, called **rugae**. When the stomach is distended these folds disappear, and it can extend downward almost to the pelvis. The stomach is very movable in its middle regions but fixed at either end. The stomach mixes food from the esophagus with gastric juice, begins protein digestion and limited absorption, and moves food into the small intestine (**FIGURE 22-8**). It is divided into the cardiac, fundic, body, and pyloric regions:

- *Cardiac region:* A small area near the esophageal opening. This portion of the stomach that attaches to the esophagus is called the *cardia* or *cardial part*. It surrounds the cardial orifice, which is where food enters from the esophagus.
- *Fundic region:* Balloons superior to the cardiac portion and acts as a temporary storage area. It is also called the *fundus* and is dome-shaped. The fundus is located beneath the diaphragm. It bulges superolaterally to the cardia.
- *Body region:* The dilated, main portion of the stomach. It is the middle portion, commonly called the *body*, and is continuous inferiorly with the next portion.
- *Pyloric region:* Narrower than the rest of the stomach, this funnel-shaped region begins with a wider and superior *pyloric antrum*, becoming the *pyloric canal* as it nears the small intestine. This terminates at the *pylorus*. At its end the muscular wall thickens to form a powerful, circular **pyloric sphincter**, which acts as a valve controlling gastric emptying. The pylorus is actually continuous with the duodenum.

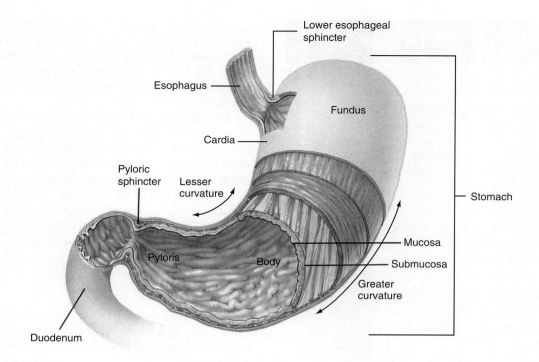

Lower esophageal sphincter

Esophagus

Fundus

Cardia

Pyloric sphincter

Lesser curvature

Stomach

Pyloris

Body

Mucosa

Submucosa

Greater curvature

Duodenum

FIGURE 22-8 The stomach.

The *greater curvature* of the stomach is its convex lateral surface. The stomach's *lesser curvature* is its concave medial surface. Two mesenteries extend from these curvatures. Known as *omenta*, they help tie the stomach to the body wall and other digestive organs. The two omenta are individually named the *lesser omentum* and the *greater omentum*.

The lesser omentum links the lesser curvature of the stomach to the liver. It is continuous with the visceral peritoneum that covers the stomach. The greater omentum is draped inferiorly from the greater curvature, covering the small intestine's coiled structure. It continues dorsally and superiorly to wrap the spleen and transverse large intestine. It then blends with the *mesocolon*, which is a dorsal mesentery securing the large intestine to the parietal peritoneum of the posterior abdominal wall. The *mesentery proper* is a thick sheet that suspends all of the small intestine except for the first 25 cm or 10 inches. It allows movement yet provides stability.

The autonomic nervous system serves the stomach. Thoracic splanchnic nerves relay sympathetic fibers through the celiac plexus. The vagus nerve supplies parasympathetic fibers. The gastric and splenic branches of the splenic trunk provide the stomach's arterial supply. Its corresponding veins are part of the hepatic portal system. They eventually drain into the hepatic portal vein.

Microscopic Anatomy of the Stomach

Like most of the alimentary canal, the wall of the stomach contains four tunics. However, its muscularis and mucosa have specialized functions. The muscularis externa has an incomplete, innermost, smooth muscle fibril layer, which runs obliquely. This is in addition to the usual longitudinal and circular layers of smooth muscle of the rest of the alimentary canal.

The stomach mucosa has a simple columnar epithelium made up only of mucous cells. A two-layer coat of cloudy alkaline mucus protects the stomach. The top layer of mucus is viscous and insoluble. It keeps the second layer trapped beneath it, which consists of rich amounts of bicarbonate. The stomach's inner lining of mucous membranes is thick, with many small *gastric pits* at the ends of tubular **gastric glands**. These glands have three main types of secretory cells, mucous, chief, and parietal cells. Mucous cells lie in the necks of the glands near the gastric pit openings; chief and parietal cells are in the deeper areas. The gastric pits have walls that are mostly formed by mucous cells. Together, the three types of secretory cells produce **gastric juice**. Mucus is secreted primarily from the cells in the glands of the cardia and pylorus. In the pyloric antrum, the cells produce mucus as well as several hormones, which include most of the **gastrin**, a stimulatory hormone. Gastric juice denatures proteins and inactivates most enzymes found in food. Gastric juice components are summarized in **TABLE 22-2**.

The glands of the fundus and body are much larger than in other areas and produce most of the secretions from the stomach. Most digestion occurs in these areas. The glands here contain many different secretory cells, which include mucous neck, parietal, chief, and enteroendocrine cells. The *mucous neck cells* are located in the neck and more basal regions of the stomach glands. They produce a thinner, more soluble mucus than the mucous cells of the surface epithelium. This acidic mucus is not fully understood in its function but helps to prevent the stomach from digesting itself.

The *parietal cells* are found mostly in the more apical region of stomach glands and are scattered among the

TABLE 22-2

Major Components of Gastric Juice

Component	Function	Source
Hydrochloric acid	Provides acid environment needed to convert pepsinogen into pepsin and for the action of pepsin	Parietal cells of gastric glands
Intrinsic factor	Aids in absorption of vitamin B_{12}	Parietal cells of gastric glands
Mucus	Provides an alkaline, viscous protective layer on inside stomach walls	Mucous cells
Pepsin	A protein-splitting enzyme that digests almost all types of dietary protein	Formed from pepsinogen in presence of hydrochloric acid
Pepsinogen	The inactive form of pepsin	Chief cells of gastric glands

chief cells. The parietal cells secrete both *hydrochloric acid* (*HCl*) and the glycoprotein known as **intrinsic factor**. HCl causes the contents of the stomach to be very acidic, with a pH between 1.5 and 3.5, a condition needed so *pepsin* can be activated effectively. HCl, and the environment it creates, is able to denature proteins, break down plant food cell walls, break down connective tissues from meats, and kill most bacteria ingested with foods and is of significant importance for digestion. For vitamin B_{12} to be absorbed in the small intestine, intrinsic factor is required. Negative feedback is used to regulate the concentration of HCl in the stomach (**FIGURE 22-9**).

Chief cells are most abundant near the base of a gastric gland. Cuboidal chief cells secrete **pepsinogen**, an inactive proenzyme that is converted by the acid in the gastric lumen to **pepsin**, an active *proteolytic* or *protein-digesting* enzyme. Stimulation of these cells results in the first-released pepsinogen molecules to be activated by HCl in the apical region of the gland. When pepsin becomes present, it additionally catalyzes pepsinogen conversion into more pepsin. This activation requires a small fragment of peptide from pepsinogen. When the fragment is removed, the pepsinogen changes shape, and its active site is exposed. This is a positive feedback process that is unlimited, except for the amount of available pepsinogen. The chief cells also secrete fat-digesting enzymes known as lipases, which are believed to handle nearly 15% of all lipolysis in the gastrointestinal tract.

Usually found deep inside gastric glands, *enteroendocrine cells* release many chemical messengers into the interstitial fluid of the lamina propria. Some act locally as paracrines, such as *serotonin* and *histamine*. *Somatostatin* and other messengers act locally as paracrines and also as hormones, which diffuse into blood capillaries, influencing several digestive system target organs. *Gastrin* is one of the hormones vital for regulating stomach secretion and motility. **TABLE 22-3** explains the hormones and paracrines involved in digestion.

Pepsin is most able to function in strongly acidic conditions, which are indicated by a pH of 1.5 to 2.0. In newborn infants but not in adults, the stomach also produces **renin** or *chymosin* and gastric lipase. These enzymes are important for the digestion of milk. Renin coagulates milk proteins and gastric lipase initiates the digestion of milk fats.

Acid triggers sympathetic nerve impulses to inhibit gastric juice secretion as food enters the small intestine. The peptide hormone **cholecystokinin** is released by proteins

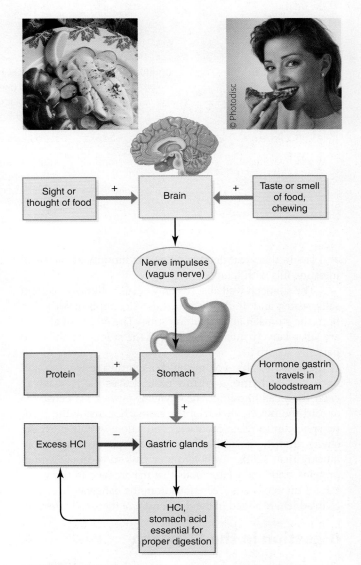

FIGURE 22-9 Pathway leading to the release of the HCl by the stomach. (Left photo: Courtesy of Len Rizzi/National Cancer Institute.)

TABLE 22-3

Hormones and Paracrines Involved in Digestion

Hormone or Paracrine	Production Site	Actions
Gastrin	G cells of the stomach mucosa	Increases HCl secretion from the parietal cells of the stomach, has a minor effect of stimulating gastric emptying, stimulates contraction of small intestine muscles, relaxes the ileocecal valve, stimulates mass movements in the large intestine
Gastric inhibitory peptide (or glucose-dependent insulinotropic peptide)	Duodenal mucosa	Inhibits HCl production in the stomach (a minor effect) and stimulates insulin release from the beta cells of the pancreas
Histamine	Stomach mucosa	Activates parietal cells of the stomach to release HCl
Serotonin	Stomach mucosa	Causes stomach muscle constriction
Somatostatin	Stomach and duodenal mucosa	Inhibits gastric secretion in the stomach of all products, inhibits pancreatic secretions, inhibits gastrointestinal blood flow and small intestine absorption, inhibits gallbladder and liver contraction and bile release
Motilin	Duodenal mucosa	Stimulates migrating motor complex of the proximal duodenum
Secretin	Duodenal mucosa	Inhibits gastric gland secretion in the stomach and gastric motility during the gastric phase of secretion, increases the pancreas' output of pancreatic juice rich in bicarbonate ions while potentiating action of cholecystokinin, increase the liver's bile output
Cholecystokinin	Duodenal mucosa	Inhibits secretory activity of the stomach, potentiates actions of secretin on the liver and pancreas, increases output of enzyme-rich pancreatic juice, stimulates the gallbladder to contract and expel stored bile, and relaxes the hepatopancreatic sphincter to allow bile and pancreatic juice to enter the duodenum
Intestinal gastrin	Duodenal mucosa	Stimulates the gastric glands of the stomach and motility
Vasoactive intestinal peptide	Enteric neurons	In the small intestine, it stimulates buffer secretion, dilates capillaries, and relaxes smooth muscle; in the pancreas, it increases secretion; in the stomach, it inhibits acid secretion

and fats in this area, decreasing gastric motility as the small intestine fills with food.

The stomach wall absorbs only small volumes of certain salts, water, and lipid-soluble drugs. Alcohol is absorbed in both the stomach and small intestine. The effects of alcohol are felt relatively quickly because of the stomach's ability to partially absorb it.

The stomach's volume increases during eating and decreases as **chyme**, a creamy paste, leaves the stomach to enter the small intestine. The chyme is pushed via peristalsis toward the pyloric region of the stomach, causing the pyloric sphincter to relax. Stomach contractions slowly push the chyme into the small intestine. Liquids pass through more quickly than solids. Carbohydrates pass most quickly, then proteins, and finally fatty foods that may remain in the stomach for up to 6 hours. Secretions from the pancreas, liver, and gallbladder are added in the duodenum of the small intestine.

Digestion in the Stomach

The stomach not only holds ingested foods but physically and chemically degrades them. Chyme is then moved from the stomach to the small intestine. The primary type of enzymatic breakdown in the stomach is protein digestion. HCl denatures dietary proteins so enzymes can digest them. The amino acid chains in dietary proteins are unfolded so digestive enzymes become more effective.

Pepsin is the most important protein-digesting enzyme produced by the gastric mucosa, but in infants *rennin* is another stomach enzyme that is needed. Rennin converts milk protein or *casein* into a curd-like substance. Lingual lipase from salivary glands also helps to digest certain triglycerides in the stomach, until the lipase also becomes digested. Lipid-soluble substances, such as aspirin or alcohol, easily pass through the mucosa of the stomach into the blood. Both of these substances are prone to causing gastric bleeding and should not be used if a gastric ulcer is present.

However, the secretion of intrinsic factor is actually the only stomach function that is *essential* for life. Intrinsic factor is vital for the intestines to absorb vitamin B_{12}, which is required for production of mature erythrocytes. Without this, *pernicious anemia* develops. Even after a complete surgical removal of the stomach, known as a *total gastrectomy*, injected vitamin B_{12} minimizes digestive problems.

Gastritis is acute or chronic inflammation of the stomach. It may be caused by nonsteroidal anti-inflammatory medications, alcohol, *Helicobacter pylori* infection, and smoking. Chronic gastritis when mainly caused by *H. pylori* can cause gastric ulcers, which are erosions of stomach tissue. Untreated chronic ulcers may be linked to stomach cancer. Although this type of cancer is not common in the United States, it is most common in Korea, Mongolia, Japan, Guatemala, and China.

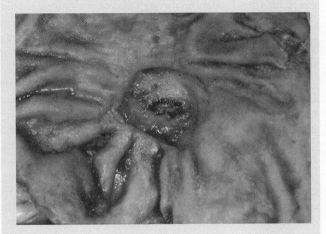

Gastric ulcer.

TEST YOUR UNDERSTANDING

1. List and name the various portions of the stomach.
2. What are pepsin and pepsinogen and the substances needed for their production?
3. Which types of stomach epithelial cells secrete pepsin and pepsinogen?
4. Explain how the mucosal barrier of the stomach is created.

Gastric Secretion

Gastric secretion is controlled by neural and hormonal mechanisms. Normally, about 3 liters of gastric juice are released by the gastric mucosa every day. This acidic mixture is so strong it can dissolve metal objects. Nervous control of gastric secretion is provided by long and short nerve reflexes. Long reflexes are mediated by the vagus nerve, and short reflexes are local, enteric reflexes. Nearly all stomach glands experience increased secretory action when the stomach is stimulated by the vagus nerve. Secretory activity is reduced by activation of the sympathetic nerves.

Gastrin is the primary hormonal controller of gastric secretion. It stimulates secretion of both HCl and enzymes. Small intestine hormones also help to control gastric secretion

and are primarily gastrin antagonists. The three phases of gastric secretion are the *cephalic, gastric,* and *intestinal phases.* For all of these, the stomach acts as the effector site. Once begun, one or all phases may occur simultaneously.

Cephalic (Reflex) Phase

The cephalic (reflex) phase is the first to occur, happening before food enters the stomach. It lasts for a few minutes and is triggered by the smell, sight, taste, or even thought of food. This phase prepares the stomach for digestion.

Gastric Phase

When food enters the stomach, the gastric phase is started by local neural and hormonal processes. The gastric phase lasts for 3 to 4 hours. About two-thirds of the gastric juice that is released is provided by this phase. Protein-rich foods in the stomach cause the pH to usually rise, because proteins buffer hydrogen ions. The higher pH stimulates gastrin secretion, then the release of HCl. This provides the required amount of acid needed to digest the proteins. Higher amounts of proteins in food cause more gastric juice and HCl to be released. During digestion, the gastric contents eventually become more acidic. This inhibits the gastrin-secreting cells once again, a negative feedback mechanism that maintains desired pH needed for gastric enzymes to work. Besides gastrin, acetylcholine and histamine also stimulate this phase. When just one of these three chemicals binds to parietal cells, secretion of HCl is minimal. When all three of them bind, however, HCl secretion is extensive. Histamine is most critical in this regard, and therefore antihistamines such as cimetidine are used to treat gastric ulcers caused by hyperacidity. This is because they bind to and block the histamine receptors of the parietal cells.

Intestinal Phase

There are both stimulatory and inhibitory components of the intestinal phase. As partly digested foods fill the duodenum of the small intestine, the excitatory or *stimulatory* actions begin. The intestinal mucosal cells are stimulated to release *intestinal* or *enteric gastrin.* This hormone keeps the gastric glands continually secreting. However, the effect is short as the intestine is distended with chyme that has many fats, hydrogen ions, partially digested proteins, and various irritants. The *enterogastric reflex* then triggers the inhibitory actions.

The enterogastric reflex is made up of three actions: inhibition of the vagal nuclei in the medulla oblongata, inhibition of local reflexes, and activation of sympathetic fibers, causing tightening of the pyloric sphincter. This tightening prevents additional entry of food into the small intestine. Several intestinal hormones called *enterogastrones* are then

TEST YOUR UNDERSTANDING

1. Explain the most important substances required for normal digestion.
2. What are the three phases of gastric secretion?
3. Describe how eating a large meal, in comparison with a smaller one, affects stomach emptying.

released, which include *secretin, cholecystokinin,* and *vasoactive intestinal peptide*. They inhibit gastric secretion while the stomach is highly active and play various other roles.

Small Intestine

Extending from the pyloric sphincter to the large intestine, the *small intestine* is a tubular organ with many loops and coils filling much of the abdominal cavity. It receives secretions from the liver and pancreas, completing digestion of the nutrients in chyme. It also absorbs the products of digestion and transports the remaining residues to the large intestine. The small intestine is the longest portion of the alimentary canal, yet its diameter is only about half that of the large intestine. It is approximately 6 to 7 m or about 20 feet in length but only about 2.5 to 4 cm or 1 to 1.6 inches in diameter. Because of loss of muscle tone, the small intestine is smaller in a cadaver, only 2 to 4 m or 7 to 13 feet.

The small intestine plays *the major role* in the digestion and absorption of nutrients, with 90% of nutrient absorption occurring there. Most of the remaining absorption of nutrients occurs in the large intestine. The small intestine consists of three portions: duodenum, jejunum, and ileum (**FIGURE 22-10**). The duodenum is mostly retroperitoneal, whereas the other portions are intraperitoneal. The lining of the small intestine has approximately 800 transverse folds known as *plicae circulares*. They do not disappear when the small intestine is filled, unlike the rugae of the stomach.

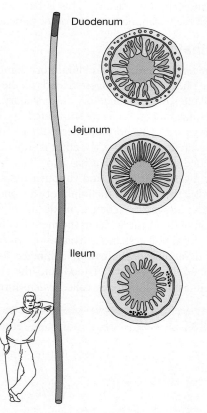

FIGURE 22-10 The three portions of the small intestine.

The plicae circulares increase the absorptive surface area of the small intestine.

The **duodenum** is about 25 cm or 10 inches long and 5 cm or 2 inches in diameter and relatively immovable. It is located posterior to the parietal peritoneum, following a C-shaped path by passing anterior to the right kidney and upper three lumbar vertebrae. The duodenum is curved around the head of the pancreas. It functions as a mixing area, receiving chyme from the stomach and digestive secretions from the pancreas and liver. The duodenum is the shortest portion of the small intestine yet has the most interesting functions. The bile duct delivers bile from the liver. The main pancreatic duct brings pancreatic juice from the pancreas. These ducts unite in the duodenal wall at the **hepatopancreatic ampulla**, which resembles a bulb and opens into the duodenum through the *major duodenal papilla*. The *hepatopancreatic sphincter* is a smooth muscle valve that controls entry of the substances from the liver and pancreas. The remainder of the small intestine is more mobile, lying free inside the peritoneal cavity.

Specialized *duodenal glands* secrete mucus. They are found in the submucosa of the duodenum and produce alkaline mucus that helps to neutralize the chyme, which is acidic, moving inward from the stomach. If inadequate, this mucous barrier is unable to protect the intestinal wall from erosion, resulting in *duodenal ulcers*. The submucosa is made up of typical areolar connective tissue. Also, the muscularis is typical and has two layers. Most of the duodenum is retroperitoneal, with an adventitia. This differs from the external intestinal surface of the other portions of the small intestine, which are covered with a visceral peritoneum or serosa.

The submucosa has an outer network of intrinsic nerve fibers and neurons known as the *submucosal plexus*, or *plexus of Meissner*. Digestive tract movements are primarily controlled by sensory neurons, interneurons, and the motor neurons of the *enteric nervous system*. This system is mostly innervated by the parasympathetic nervous system, although sympathetic postganglionic fibers also synapse within it. Many enteric fibers innervate the mucosa and *myenteric plexus*, also known as the *plexus of Auerbach*. This plexus lies between the circular and longitudinal layers of muscle.

The **jejunum** is the proximal two-fifths of the small intestine and is about 2.5 m or 8 feet in length and about 4 cm or about 1.5 inches in diameter. It links the duodenum with the ileum. Most chemical digestion and nutrient absorption occurs in the jejunum. The jejunum, along with the next segment, appears like coiled sausage in the central, lower abdominal cavity.

The final segment of the small intestine is called the called the **ileum**, which is not distinctly separate from the jejunum but has a smaller diameter, with a thinner, less vascular, and less active wall. It is the longest portion of the small intestine, totaling about 3.6 m or 12 feet in length. Also differentiating the ileum from the jejunum are Peyer's patches, which are defined as *organized lymphoid tissue* that are similar in appearance to lymph nodes. They function to protect the ileum from invasive, pathogenic microorganisms. Peyer's patches

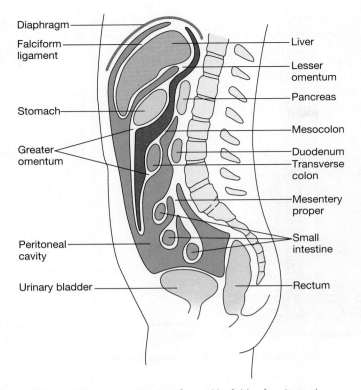

Diaphragm

Falciform
ligament

Stomach

Greater
omentum

Peritoneal
cavity

Urinary bladder

Liver

Lesser
omentum

Pancreas

Mesocolon

Duodenum

Transverse
colon

Mesentery
proper

Small
intestine

Rectum

FIGURE 22-11 The mesentery, formed by folds of peritoneal membrane, suspends portions of the small intestines from the posterior abdominal wall.

are also called *aggregated lymphoid nodules*. They are mostly located in the lamina propria but sometimes protrude into the submucosa. They increase in number toward the distal small intestine, meaning this area has higher amounts of bacteria that must be kept out of the bloodstream. The mucosa contains lymphoid tissue with proliferating B-lymphocytes. These cells move from the intestine to the blood and then target the intestinal lamina propria. Here they release IgA to help fight intestinal pathogens.

The **mesentery** is a double-layered fold of peritoneal membrane that suspends the jejunum and ileum from the posterior abdominal wall (**FIGURE 22-11**). The mesentery supports the blood vessels, lymphatic vessels, and nerves that supply the intestinal wall. A double fold of peritoneal membrane called the *greater omentum* drapes from the stomach over the transverse colon and folds of the small intestine. If the alimentary canal walls become infected, the greater omentum's cells may adhere to the inflamed area, helping to prevent the infection from spreading to the peritoneal cavity.

The small intestine is served by parasympathetic nerve fibers from the vagus nerve and sympathetic nerve fibers from the thoracic splanchnic nerves. Both types are relayed via the superior mesenteric and celiac plexuses. Arterial blood is supplied mostly from the superior mesenteric artery. The similarly routed veins mostly drain into the superior mesenteric vein. Nutrient-rich blood from the small intestine drains through these veins to the hepatic portal vein and is then carried to the liver.

The length of the small intestine provides a large surface area for absorbing nutrients. This is increased by more than 600 times by the presence of its circular folds, villi, and microvilli. These specialized structures are more numerous near the distal small intestine, so it is here where most absorption occurs. The total intestinal surface area of the small intestine is approximately 200 square meters.

The small intestine's *circular folds* of the mucosa and submucosa are deep and do not change. Each fold is about 1 cm or about 4/10 inch in height and functions to force chyme into a spiraling movement through the lumen of the small intestine. This slows down its movement so full nutrient absorption has time to occur.

The inner wall of the small intestine has many tiny finger-like projections of the mucous membrane called **intestinal villi** (**FIGURE 22-12**). The villi are slightly more than 1 mm or about 4/100 inch in length and give the inner wall a soft texture similar to velvet fabric. They are most numerous in the duodenum and proximal jejunum, decreasing in size along the way from the duodenum to the ileum. The villi help to contract the intestinal contents and increase the surface area of the intestinal lining to aid in absorption of digestive products. In the duodenum, the villi appear like leaves.

Each villus has a layer of absorptive, simple columnar epithelium consisting of *enterocytes*, a core of connective tissue with capillaries, a lymphatic capillary called a *lacteal*, and nerve fibers. The cores have dense capillary beds. The lacteals are actually wide lymphatic capillaries. Nutrients are carried away by blood capillaries and lacteals. Extremely long and densely packed *microvilli* are found in the absorptive mucosal cells. Therefore, the mucosal surface appears "fuzzy" and is referred to as the *brush border*.

Intestinal glands are located between the bases of adjacent villi and extend downward into the mucous membrane. Goblet cells, which secrete mucus, exist throughout the mucosa of the small intestine. Specialized mucous-secreting glands in the proximal duodenum secrete thick, alkaline mucus when specifically stimulated to do so. At the bases of the villi, intestinal glands secrete high volumes of a watery fluid with a nearly neutral pH. This fluid lacks digestive enzymes. The enzymes in the luminal surfaces of the intestinal mucosa break down food just before absorption. These enzymes include peptidases, sucrose, maltase, lactase, and intestinal lipase. **TABLE 22-4** summarizes these enzymes, their sources, and their actions. When stimulated by chyme, goblet cells and intestinal glands secrete their products. As the intestinal wall distends, it activates nerve plexuses, stimulating parasympathetic reflexes that trigger release of small intestine secretions.

Remember the small intestine is the most important absorbing organ of the alimentary canal. Very little absorbable material reaches its distal end. The digestion of carbohydrates begins in the mouth and is completed by enzymes from the intestinal mucosa and pancreas. Monosaccharides that result from this process are absorbed by the villi, and simple sugars are absorbed by active transport or facilitated diffusion. For carbohydrate metabolism, glucose is broken down to *pyruvic acid* or *pyruvate* via the process

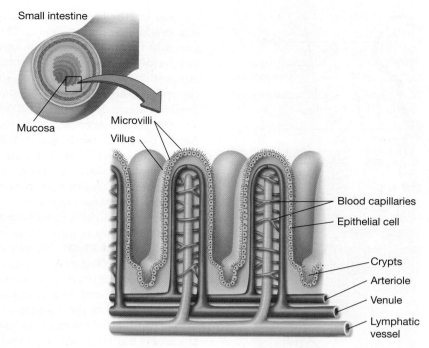

FIGURE 22-12 The small intestine mucosa is folded into villi and crypts. The epithelium covers the lamina propria, connective tissue containing abundant blood vessels and lymphatic vessels.

TABLE 22-4	
Major Digestive Enzymes	
Enzyme and Source	**Action**
Gastric enzyme (from chief cells)	
Pepsin	Begins protein digestion
Intestinal enzymes (from mucosal cells)	
Enterokinase	Converts trypsinogen into trypsin
Intestinal lipase	Breaks down fats into fatty acids and glycerol
Peptidase (primarily *dipeptidases*)	Breaks down (catabolizes) peptides into amino acids
Sucrase, maltase, lactase	Breaks down disaccharides into monosaccharides
Pancreatic enzymes (from pancreas)	
Nucleases	Break down nucleic acids into nucleotides
Pancreatic amylase	Breaks down starch and glycogen into disaccharides
Pancreatic lipase	Breaks down fats into fatty acids and glycerol
Proteolytic enzymes Trypsin Chymotrypsin Carboxypeptidase	Each of these enzymes breaks down proteins or partially digested proteins into peptides.
Salivary enzyme (from salivary glands)	
Salivary amylase	Begins carbohydrate digestion by breaking down starch and glycogen into disaccharides

of *glycolysis*. Glycolysis requires glucose molecules, cytoplasmic enzymes, *adenosine triphosphate*, *adenosine diphosphate*, inorganic phosphates, and *nicotinamide adenine dinucleotide*, which is a coenzyme.

Protein digestion via pepsin activity begins in the stomach and is completed via intestinal mucosa and pancreatic enzymes in the small intestine. Large protein molecules break down into amino acids and are actively transported into the villi to be carried away by the blood. Fat molecules are nearly entirely digested by intestinal mucosa and pancreatic enzymes. The fatty acids and molecules of glycerol that result diffuse into the epithelial cells of the villi.

Fatty acids are resynthesized into fats encased in proteins to form chylomicrons, which move to the bloodstream. Some fatty acids are absorbed directly into the capillaries of the villi without being resynthesized to fat. Chylomicrons transport dietary fats to muscle and adipose cells. Very-low-density lipoprotein (VLDL) molecules, formed in the liver, transport triglycerides from excess dietary carbohydrates. When VLDL molecules reach adipose cells, the enzyme lipoprotein lipase helps to convert VLDL to low-density lipoprotein (LDL). Because most triglycerides have been removed, LDL molecules have higher cholesterol than VLDL. Cholesterol is obtained for the body's needs by peripheral tissue cells, which use endocytosis to remove LDL from the plasma. **FIGURE 22-13** shows digestion, absorption, and transportation of lipids.

High-density lipoprotein (HDL) has high levels of protein and low levels of lipids. It removes cholesterol from tissues and sends it to the liver. HDL molecules containing cholesterol enter liver cells via receptor-mediated endocytosis. The liver excretes the cholesterol into the bile or uses it to create bile salts. The intestine reabsorbs much of the cholesterol and bile salts and repeats the cycle. Each time, some cholesterol and bile salts reach the large intestine and are excreted in the feces. The intestinal villi also absorb electrolytes via active transport and water via osmosis. **TABLE 22-5** summarizes the absorption of nutrients.

In the small intestine, the major mixing movement is segmentation, meaning small, ring-like contractions occur periodically to cut the chyme into segments and move it back and forth. This slows its movement through the small intestine. These weak peristaltic waves result in chyme taking between 3 and 10 hours to move through the small intestine.

Over-distention or irritation of the small intestine results in a peristaltic rush, which moves the small intestine's contents into the large intestine quickly. Normal absorption of nutrients, water, and electrolytes therefore does not occur in this situation. Peristaltic rush results in diarrhea, and prolonged diarrhea results in water and electrolyte imbalances.

The small intestine connects to the large intestine via a valve called the **ileocecal sphincter**. This sphincter is usually constricted to keep the contents of each intestine separate. After eating, peristalsis in the ileum relaxes the sphincter to force some small intestine contents into the **cecum** of the large intestine.

Intestinal Juice

Nearly 1 to 2 liters, or about 1 to 2 quarts, of intestinal juice are secreted by the intestinal glands every day. Hypertonic or acidic chyme is the major causative factor for this secretion, because it causes the intestinal mucosa to be distended or irritated. In normal conditions the intestinal juice is isotonic with the blood plasma and slightly alkaline, between 7.4 and 7.8 pH. Although mostly made of water, it also contains mucus secreted by the duodenal glands and mucosal goblet cells. Intestinal juice does not have high enzyme content because intestinal enzymes are mostly found at the brush border.

The brush border enzymes function in the breakdown of disaccharides and trisaccharides into simple sugars known as *monosaccharides* before absorption. *Maltase* is the enzyme that splits the bonds between the two glucose molecules of the disaccharide called *maltose*. The enzyme *sucrose* breaks down the disaccharide *sucrose* into both glucose and fructose, which is another sugar containing six carbons. The enzyme *lactase* hydrolyzes the disaccharide called *lactose* into one molecule of glucose and one molecule of *galactose*. Lactose is the primary carbohydrate found in milk, so lactase is very important in early life for its breakdown. When the intestinal mucosa stop its production, the individual becomes *lactose intolerant*. This leads to many unpleasant digestive symptoms.

TEST YOUR UNDERSTANDING

1. Explain the actions of the circular folds, villi, microvilli, and brush border.
2. What is the importance of the mesenteries?
3. Describe the three portions of the small intestine.
4. Differentiate between VLDL, LDL, and HDL.

Liver

The upper right quadrant of the abdominal cavity, inferior to the diaphragm, contains the **liver**, which is the largest gland in the body. It is reddish-brown, well supplied with blood vessels, and extends from the level of the fifth intercostal space to the lower margin of the ribs. The liver is enclosed in a fibrous capsule and divided into lobes by connective tissue. The liver weighs about 1.4 kg or 3 pounds in an average adult. This wedge-shaped organ occupies most of the right hypochondriac and epigastric abdominal regions. It is well protected by the ribs, which nearly completely encase it.

The right lobe of the liver is larger than its left lobe (**FIGURE 22-14**). A deep fissure separates the right and left lobes. There are also two other lobes known as the *caudate* and *quadrate* lobes that are only visible when the liver is viewed inferiorly. The **falciform ligament** is a mesentery separating the right and left lobes anteriorly. It suspends the liver from the anterior abdominal wall and diaphragm.

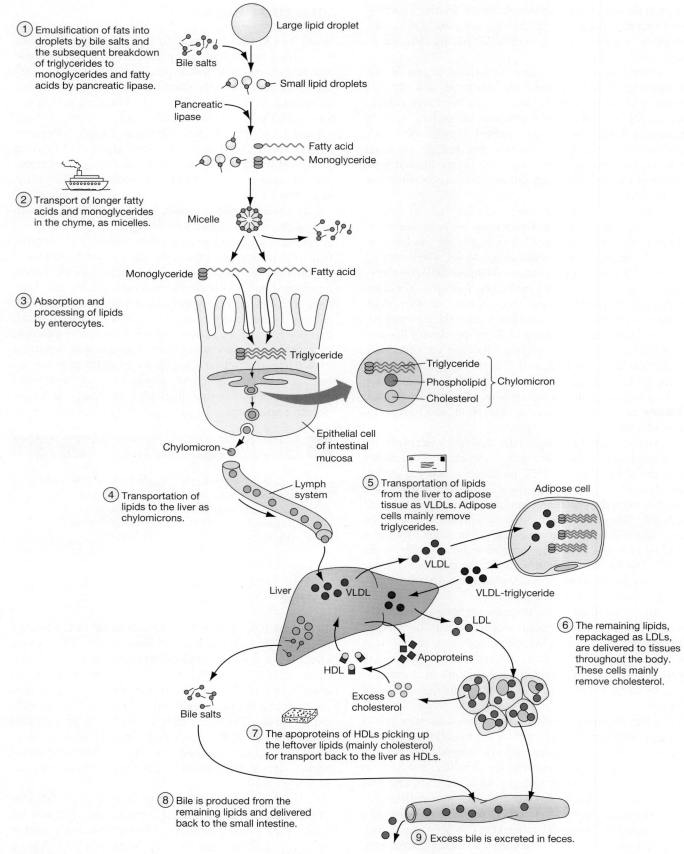

① Emulsification of fats into droplets by bile salts and the subsequent breakdown of triglycerides to monoglycerides and fatty acids by pancreatic lipase.

Large lipid droplet

Bile salts

Small lipid droplets

Pancreatic lipase

Fatty acid
Monoglyceride

② Transport of longer fatty acids and monoglycerides in the chyme, as micelles.

Micelle

Monoglyceride   Fatty acid

③ Absorption and processing of lipids by enterocytes.

Triglyceride

Triglyceride
Phospholipid ⎫ Chylomicron
Cholesterol ⎭

Epithelial cell of intestinal mucosa

Chylomicron

④ Transportation of lipids to the liver as chylomicrons.

Lymph system

⑤ Transportation of lipids from the liver to adipose tissue as VLDLs. Adipose cells mainly remove triglycerides.

Adipose cell

VLDL

Liver   VLDL   VLDL-triglyceride

LDL

⑥ The remaining lipids, repackaged as LDLs, are delivered to tissues throughout the body. These cells mainly remove cholesterol.

Apoproteins

HDL

Bile salts

Excess cholesterol

⑦ The apoproteins of HDLs picking up the leftover lipids (mainly cholesterol) for transport back to the liver as HDLs.

⑧ Bile is produced from the remaining lipids and delivered back to the small intestine.

⑨ Excess bile is excreted in feces.

FIGURE 22-13 Digestion, absorption, and transportation of lipids.

TABLE 22-5

Nutrient Absorption in the Intestines

Nutrient	Mechanism of Absorption	Mechanism of Transport
Amino acids	Active transport	Capillary blood
Electrolytes	Active transport and diffusion	Capillary blood
Fatty acids and glycerol	Facilitated diffusion of fatty acids into cells; facilitated diffusion of glycerol	
	1. Most fatty acids are resynthesized into fats and incorporated into chylomicrons for transport.	1. Lymph in lacteals
	2. Some fatty acids with relatively short carbon chains are transported without being changed back into fats.	2. Capillary blood
Monosaccharides	Active transport and facilitated diffusion	Capillary blood
Water	Osmosis	Capillary blood

Around the inferior edge of the falciform ligament is the **round ligament** or *ligamentum teres*, which is a fibrous remnant formed from the fetal umbilical vein. The entire liver is enclosed by the visceral peritoneum, except for its bare, most superior area, which touches the diaphragm. At a point called the **porta hepatis**, the *hepatic artery* and *hepatic portal vein* enter the liver. The common hepatic duct also enters here and runs inferiorly from the liver. All these vessels travel through the lesser omentum.

Liver cells or *hepatocytes* adjust circulating levels of nutrients through selective absorption and secretion. Blood from the liver returns to the systemic circuit through the hepatic veins, which open into the inferior vena cava. Many tiny **hepatic lobules** make up each lobe, and these lobules

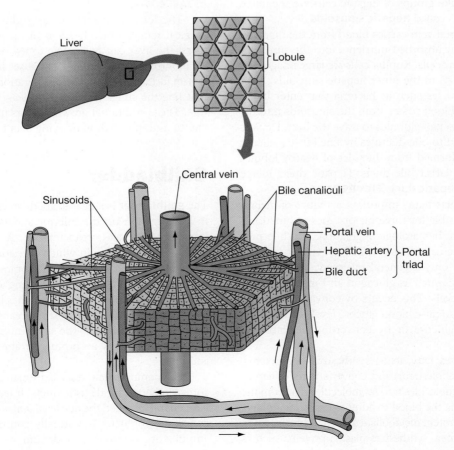

FIGURE 22-14 The liver.

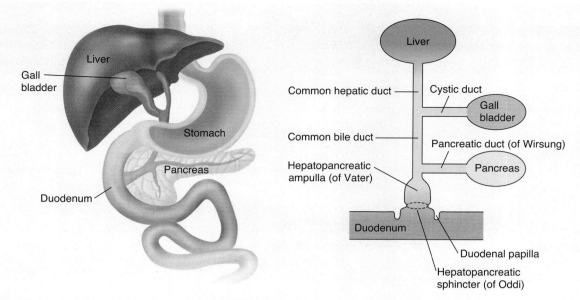

FIGURE 22-15 Gross anatomy of the human liver and gallbladder.

are the functional cells of the liver. These lobules are about the size of sesame seeds, with six sides. At each of the six corners, there is a *portal triad* or *portal tract region* that contains three primary structures: a bile duct, a branch of the hepatic artery, and a branch of the hepatic portal vein. Each lobule consists of many hepatic cells that radiate out from a central vein. Plate-like groups of hepatic cells are separated by vascular channels called **hepatic sinusoids**.

The hepatic portal vein carries blood from the digestive tract, bringing newly absorbed nutrients into the sinusoids to nourish the hepatic cells. Kupffer cells are large phagocytic macrophages attached to the inner hepatic sinusoids. They remove foreign particles such as bacteria that enter blood via the portal vein. Blood passes from the sinusoids into the central veins of the hepatic lobules to leave the liver. Hepatic secretions are carried to bile ductules by fine bile canaliculi. **Hepatic ducts** are formed from ductules of nearby lobules that unite to create larger bile ducts. Hepatic ducts merge into the **common hepatic duct** (**FIGURE 22-15**).

The liver conducts many important activities of metabolism and is responsible for three major types of functions: metabolic regulation, hematologic regulation, and bile production. The liver actually has over 200 functions, but this discussion provides only a general overview. Hepatic cells respond to hormones such as glucagon and insulin, lowering blood glucose levels. This occurs by converting glucose to glycogen. They also raise blood glucose levels by breaking down glycogen to glucose or by converting noncarbohydrates into glucose.

The liver oxidizes fatty acids; synthesizes lipoproteins, phospholipids, and cholesterol; and converts parts of carbohydrate and protein molecules into fat molecules. Fat from the liver is transported via the blood to adipose tissue for storage. The liver is vital for protein metabolism as well. It breaks down amino acids, forms urea, synthesizes plasma proteins such as albumin, and converts some amino acids into others.

The liver stores glycogen, iron, and various vitamins, including B_{12}, A, and D. Liver macrophages or *stellate macrophages* destroy damaged erythrocytes and engulf foreign antigens. Toxic substances are removed from the blood during *detoxification*, and bile is secreted, which is important to digestion. The major functions of the liver are summarized in **TABLE 22-6**.

The liver is amazing in its ability to regenerate. After surgical removal or other loss of up to 80% of its original mass, the liver can regenerate to its former size within 6 to 12 months. Injury to the liver causes hepatocytes to secrete *growth factors*. These cause proliferations of endothelial cells that line the sinusoids and the release of other growth factors. These additional growth factors influence the hepatocytes to multiply so dead or dying liver tissue can be replaced.

Gallbladder

The **gallbladder** is a pear-shaped, green-colored sac located in a depression on the inferior surface of the liver, which is mainly a storage organ for bile. A rounded *fundus* protrudes from the fossa in which it resides. It is connected to the **cystic duct**, which joins the common hepatic duct. The gallbladder has a thin epithelial lining and strong muscles in its wall and is about 10 cm or 4 inches long. It stores bile not immediately needed for digestion, reabsorbs water, and contracts to release bile into the small intestine. The gallbladder concentrates bile by absorbing certain amounts of its water and ions.

The common bile duct is formed by the joining of the common hepatic and cystic ducts. It leads to the duodenum via a chamber called the *duodenal ampulla*, where the hepatopancreatic sphincter is normally contracted. The duodenal ampulla opens into the duodenum at a small mound called the *duodenal papilla*. As bile collects in the common bile

TABLE 22-6

Principal Liver Functions

General	Specific
Blood filtering	Uses phagocytosis to remove damaged red blood cells and foreign substances
Carbohydrate metabolism	Changes glucose to glycogen and back again, as needed; changes noncarbohydrates to glucose
Detoxification	Removes blood toxins and wastes
Lipid metabolism	Converts portions of carbohydrates and proteins into fats, oxidizes fatty acids; synthesizes cholesterol, lipoproteins, and phospholipids
Protein metabolism	Removes amine groups from amino acid molecules; forms urea; forms plasma proteins; changes some amino acids to others
Secretion	Generates bile
Storage	Stores iron; vitamins A, D, and B_{12}; and glycogen

duct, it backs up into the cystic duct and flows into the gallbladder for storage. This occurs because of contraction of the gallbladder's muscular walls.

Bile usually enters the duodenum once cholecystokinin stimulates gallbladder contraction. The hepatopancreatic sphincter is contracted until a peristaltic wave in the duodenal wall influences its relaxation, passing bile into the small intestine. The hormones that help control digestion are listed in **TABLE 22-7**.

Bile

Bile is a fat emulsifier that is continuously secreted from hepatic cells. This yellow-green liquid contains water, bile salts, the bile pigments *bilirubin* and *biliverdin*, cholesterol, and electrolytes. It is alkaline in its pH. Bile salts make up most of these elements and have a unique digestive function. Bile pigments develop from the breakdown of hemoglobin in red blood cells and are normally excreted in the bile. Up to 900 mL of bile can be secreted or generated by the hepatocytes every day.

Only the bile salts and phospholipids play any role in the digestive process. *Bile salts* are derivatives of cholesterol that physically separate large fat globules that enter the small intestine into millions of smaller fatty droplets in a process known as **emulsification**. These more accessible droplets create large surface areas for fat-digesting enzymes to work with. The tiny fat droplets then mix with water, and lipases digest them more effectively as a result. Bile salts enhance absorption of cholesterol, fatty acids, and fat-soluble vitamins A, D, E, and K. They also help to solubilize cholesterol. When there is a lack of bile salts, lipids are poorly absorbed and vitamin deficiencies occur. The mixture of fatty acids and monoglycerides formed when pancreatic lipase breaks down triglycerides interacts with bile salts from the chime. This forms small lipid-bile salt complexes called *micelles* that allow absorption to occur and synthesis or *anabolism* of new triglycerides. These triglycerides combine with phospholipids, absorbed steroids, and fat-soluble vitamins. They are then coated with protein to become *chylomicrons*.

Bilirubin

Bilirubin is a waste product of the heme of hemoglobin formed during breakdown of erythrocytes that have become older and worn out. It is the primary bile pigment. Although bilirubin is absorbed from the blood by hepatocytes, excreted into the bile, and metabolized by resident

TABLE 22-7

Digestive Tract Hormones

Hormone	Function	Source
Gastrin	Causes gastric glands to increase secretions	Gastric cells, in response to food
Secretin	Stimulates pancreas to secrete fluid with high bicarbonate ion concentration	Cells in duodenal wall, in response to acidic chyme entering the small intestine
Cholecystokinin	Causes gastric glands to decrease secretions and inhibits gastric motility; stimulates pancreas to secrete fluid with high digestive enzyme concentration; stimulates gallbladder contraction to release bile	Cells of the intestinal wall, in response to proteins and fats in the small intestine

Cirrhosis of the liver is an irreversible, chronic disease in which normal hepatocytes are replaced with fibrous scar tissue. The appearance of the liver becomes nodular, and the blood circulation in the liver becomes abnormal. Cirrhosis is caused by consumption of alcohol, various types of viral hepatitis, and congestive heart failure. Most patients with cirrhosis suffer from splenomegaly, **ascites**, jaundice, hemorrhage, edema, varicosities, and hepatic encephalopathy. When the portal system backs up with blood, the pressure in the portal vein increases. This is known as **portal hypertension**.

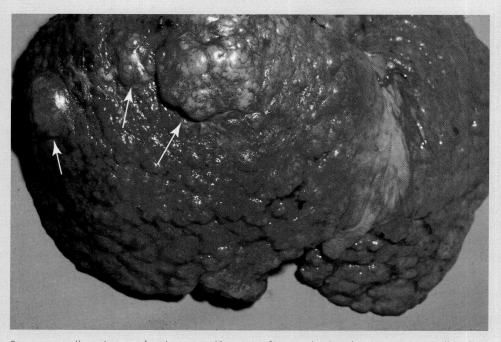

Squamous cell carcinoma of oral mucosa. (Courtesy of Leonard V. Crowley, MD, Century College.)

bacteria in the small intestine, the iron and globin from hemoglobin are saved and reused. In the large intestine, bilirubin is converted by bacteria to *urobilinogens* and *stercobilinogens*. Some urobilinogens are absorbed into the bloodstream for excretion via the urine. The remaining urobilinogens in the colon are converted to *urobilins*, and the remaining stercobilinogens are converted to *stercobilins*. Both of these conversions occur from exposure to oxygen. In varying proportions, these pigments give the feces its yellowish-brown or brown color. The metabolic activities of bacteria in the colon create small amounts of intestinal gas, which is known as *flatus*.

TEST YOUR UNDERSTANDING

1. Describe the function of the hormone secretin.
2. What are Kupffer cells?
3. List and name the functions of the liver.
4. Describe the importance of the enterohepatic circulation.

Pancreas

The **pancreas** lies posterior to the stomach, extending laterally from the duodenum toward the spleen. It is an elongated, tadpole-shaped organ, about 15 cm in length and weighing about 80 g or 3 ounces. The broad *head* of the pancreas lies within the loop that is formed by the duodenum of the intestine. The thinner *body* of the pancreas extends toward the spleen, whereas the *tail* appears short and bluntly rounded and abuts the spleen (**FIGURE 22-16**).

The pancreas is *retroperitoneal*, firmly bound to the posterior abdominal cavity wall. It acts as an endocrine gland but also has an exocrine function—it secretes the digestive juice known as **pancreatic juice**. Pancreatic acinar cells produce pancreatic juice and make up most of the pancreas. Smaller pancreatic tubes form larger ones, and eventually the *main pancreatic duct,* connected with the duodenum at the same place where the bile duct, from the liver and gallbladder, joins the duodenum (Figure 22-15). A smaller *accessory pancreatic duct* empties into the duodenum, proximal to the main pancreatic duct. The movement of pancreatic juices is controlled by a hepatopancreatic sphincter.

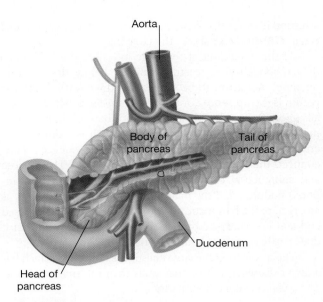

Aorta

Body of
pancreas

Tail of
pancreas

Duodenum

Head of
pancreas

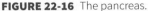

FIGURE 22-16 The pancreas.

The secretions of the pancreas are regulated mostly by hormones from the duodenum. When chyme arrives in the duodenum, the hormone *secretin* is released, triggering pancreatic secretion of a watery buffer solution with a pH between 7.5 and 8.8. This secretion contains bicarbonate and phosphate buffers that help to raise the pH of the chyme. Another duodenal hormone, cholecystokinin, stimulates production and secretion of pancreatic enzymes. These enzymes are able to digest carbohydrates, fats, nucleic acids, and proteins. **Pancreatic amylase** digests carbohydrates, splitting starch or glycogen molecules into disaccharides or *double sugars*. **Pancreatic lipase** digests fat, breaking triglycerides into fatty acids and glycerol. Two **nucleases** are also contained in pancreatic juice. These enzymes break down nucleic acids into nucleotides.

Proteolytic or *protein-splitting* enzymes such as trypsin, chymotrypsin, and carboxypeptidase split bonds between certain combinations of amino acids in proteins. Complete digestion of proteins requires different enzymes because no single enzyme can split all possible combinations of amino acids. The clusters of secretory acinar cells surrounding ducts in the pancreas are known as *acini*. They are filled with rough endoplasmic reticulum and have deeply staining *zymogen granules,* which are tiny structures that store proteolytic enzymes in cells. These enzymes are inactive until activated by other enzymes in the small intestine. For example, inactive trypsinogen is activated into trypsin when it contacts the enzyme called *enterokinase*.

Lightly staining *pancreatic islets* are scattered among the acini. They are actually mini-endocrine glands that release glucagon and insulin. Both of these hormones are important in the metabolism of carbohydrates.

Pancreatic Juice

Pancreatic juice is released by nervous and endocrine system regulation. It is clear in appearance and contains mostly water as well as enzymes, bicarbonate ions, and lesser amounts of other electrolytes. Between 1,200 and 1,500 mL of pancreatic juice is produced every day. The component of pancreatic juice that is rich in enzymes is produced by the acinar cells. In the smallest pancreatic ducts, the epithelial cells lining them release bicarbonate ions, making pancreatic juice alkaline, with a pH near 8.

When gastric juice secretion is stimulated, the pancreas is stimulated to release digestive enzymes. There is a nearly exact balance between HCl production in the stomach and bicarbonate ions production in the pancreas. As bicarbonate is secreted into the pancreatic juice, hydrogen ions enter the blood. The pH of venous blood flowing to the heart is basically unchanged, because acidic blood from the pancreas neutralizes the alkaline blood draining from the stomach.

As acidic chyme enters the duodenum, the peptide hormone **secretin** is released from the duodenal mucous membrane into the bloodstream. Secretin stimulates pancreatic juice with high concentrations of bicarbonate ions to be released, neutralizing acidic chyme. Proteins and fats in chyme stimulate cholecystokinin release from the intestinal wall, which travels through the bloodstream to the pancreas. Pancreatic juice then secreted has a high concentration of digestive enzymes.

In the duodenum, *enteropeptidase* activates *trypsinogen* to become *trypsin*. Enteropeptidase is an intestinal brush border protease. Once trypsin is activated, it then activates more trypsinogen as well as the pancreatic proteases known as *procarboxypeptidase* and *chymotrypsinogen*. Once active, they are respectively known as *carbodypeptidase* and *chymotrypsin*. Pancreatic enzymes that are secreted in active form include *amylase, lipases,* and *nucleases*. However, these require ions or bile to be present in the intestinal lumen to work effectively. *Proelastase* is an inert precursor protein of *elastase*, which is the enzyme that catalyzes the hydrolysis of elastin.

Pancreatic alpha-amylase is a *carbohydrase*, which is a type of enzyme that breaks down certain types of starches and is nearly identical to salivary amylase. *Pancreatic lipase* breaks down specific complex lipids. It releases fatty acids and other products that are easily absorbed. *Nucleases* break down DNA and RNA. *Proteolytic enzymes* break down certain proteins. These enzymes include *proteases* and *peptidases*. Proteases break down large protein complexes. Peptidases break down small peptide chains into individual amino acids.

FOCUS ON PATHOLOGY

Pancreatic cancer is the fourth leading cause of cancer-related death in the United States. The risk factors are family history, smoking, increased age, and diabetes mellitus. Symptoms are often vague, resembling other conditions, and may include pain, jaundice, weight loss, nausea, loss of appetite, and changes in bowel habits. No methods are available to detect pancreatic cancer in its early stages. Once diagnosed, it is usually too late to surgically remove the tumor.

Digestion in the Small Intestine

Fat digestion has only just started by the time food reaches the small intestine, even though proteins and carbohydrates have been already greatly degraded. It takes chyme between 3 and 6 hours to move through the small intestine, and the digestive process accelerates during this time. Nearly all nutrients and most of the water are absorbed here. The small intestine has no part in ingestion or defecation, similar to the stomach.

Intestinal juice does not provide much of what is needed to perform the breakdown of chyme. Bile, digestive enzymes, and bicarbonate ions are mostly imported from the liver and pancreas. The *brush border enzymes* are not involved here. We are unable to normally digest food and absorb nutrients when anything impairs the function of the liver or pancreas or their juices being delivered to the small intestine. Absorption in the small intestine is accomplished by its absorptive cells, using their large amounts of apical microvilli. Chyme entering the small intestine is usually hypertonic. Therefore, if large amounts were brought into the small intestine, there would be dangerously low blood volume because of osmotic water loss from the blood into the intestinal lumen.

Chyme is thoroughly mixed with bile, pancreatic juices, and intestinal juices by the intestinal smooth muscle. It moves food residues through the ileocecal valve into the large intestine. Therefore, *segmentation* is the most common motion of the small intestine and not peristalsis. Intrinsic pacemaker cells located in the circular smooth muscle layer influence the segmenting movements. Unlike the peristalsis of the stomach, these duodenal pacemakers depolarize more often than those in the ileum. In this way, intestinal contents are moved slowly, but steadily, toward the ileocecal valve. They have plenty of time to be digested and absorbed.

TEST YOUR UNDERSTANDING

1. Describe the exocrine functions of the pancreas.
2. Explain the actions of pancreatic amylase and pancreatic lipase.
3. Identify the types of fluids found in the pancreatic, cystic, and bile ducts.

Large Intestine

The diameter of the **large intestine** is much greater than that of the small intestine, although its length is only about 1.5 m. It begins in the lower right side of the abdominal cavity at the point where the ileum joins the cecum. It then ascends on the right side, crosses to the left, and descends into the pelvis. Its distal end opens to the outside of the body as the anus. The large intestine lies inferior to the stomach and liver and almost completely *frames* the small intestine. The large intestine's function is to absorb water and electrolytes from chyme and also to form and store feces. It also absorbs vitamins that are freed by bacterial action. The large

intestine is made up of the cecum, colon, rectum, and anal canal. **FIGURE 22-17** shows the large intestine.

At the beginning of the large intestine, the *cecum* is a dilated, pouch-like structure hanging below the ileocecal opening. A narrow tube projecting downward from the cecum is the **appendix** or *vermiform appendix*, which is usually about 9 cm in length. The size and shape of the appendix may vary greatly. A small *mesentery,* which is a double-layered suspending peritoneal tissue called the *mesoappendix,* connects the appendix to the ileum and cecum. The mucosa and submucosal of the appendix are dominated by lymphoid nodules, and the main function of the appendix is as an organ of the lymphatic system. This structure has a closed end and no established function related to digestion, but it does partly consist of lymphatic tissue.

The next part of the large intestine is the **colon**, which has a larger diameter and thinner walls than the small intestine. The colon consists of four parts:

- *Ascending colon:* Begins at the cecum, continues upward against the posterior abdominal wall, inferior to the liver, and then turns to the left sharply, at the *right colic flexure* or *hepatic flexure.*
- *Transverse colon:* The longest, most movable part, it is suspended by a fold of peritoneum and sags in the middle, below the stomach; near the spleen, it turns abruptly downward at the *left colic flexure* or *splenic flexure.*
- *Descending colon:* A mostly vertical section that makes an *S*-shaped curve near its lowest portion, at the *sigmoid flexure.*
- *Sigmoid colon:* The final portion, which is only 15 cm or 6 inches long, which becomes the rectum. The sigmoid colon lies posterior to the urinary bladder.

The *rectum* is next to the sacrum and resembles its curvature. It is attached to the sacrum by peritoneum. The rectum ends about 5 cm below the tip of the coccyx, becoming the **anal canal**, which consists of the last 2.5 to 4 cm of the large intestine. *Colorectal cancers* are the third most common cause of cancer-related death in men and women older than age 60. After age 50 a *colonoscopy* is recommended every 10 years. Early diagnosis of colorectal cancer may be made by *endoscopy*, specialized computed tomography *colonography*, and *barium enema* (**FIGURE 22-18**).

In the anal canal, the mucous membrane is folded into between six and eight longitudinal anal columns. The distal end of the canal opens to the outside as the **anus**, controlled by two sphincter muscles. The internal anal sphincter muscle is composed of smooth muscle and is under involuntary control. The external anal sphincter muscle is composed of skeletal muscle and is under voluntary control.

The large intestine does not have the villi found in the small intestine. Also, its longitudinal muscle fibers are not uniformly distributed throughout. The large intestine's muscle fibers form three distinct bands called *teniae coli* that extend the entire length of the colon and exert tension, creating a series of pouches called *haustra*, which cut into the intestinal lumen. Creases between the haustra affect the

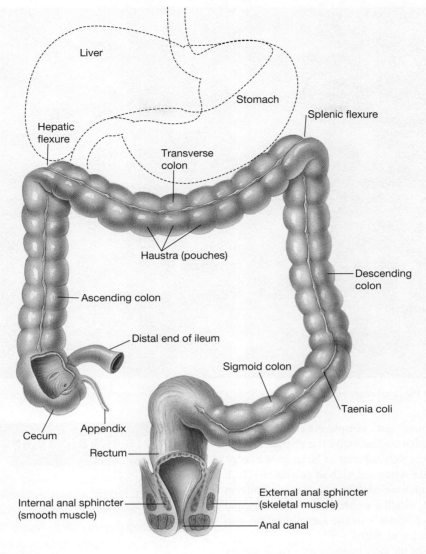

FIGURE 22-17 The large intestine.

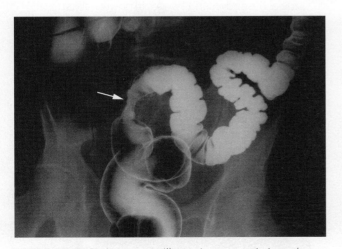

FIGURE 22-18 Barium enema illustrating a constricting colon cancer (arrow) with proximal dilation of the colon resulting from obstruction of the lumen by the cancer.

mucosal lining and produce a series of internal folds. The haustra permit the expansion and elongation of the colon. *Epiploic appendages* are small fat-filled pouches of the visceral peritoneum hanging from the surface of the large intestine. They are of unknown function.

The large intestine has little or no digestive function. It contains many tubular glands composed almost entirely of goblet cells (**FIGURE 22-19**). Mucus is the only important secretion of the large intestine and protects the intestinal wall against abrasion and binds particles of fecal matter. The mucus is alkaline, helping to control pH of the large intestine.

Chyme in the large intestine contains undigested or unabsorbed materials as well as electrolytes, mucus, bacteria, and water. In the proximal half of the large intestine, water and electrolytes normally are absorbed. Substances that remain form feces, which is stored in the distal portion of the large intestine. Intestinal flora, which are normal bacteria, break down some of the molecules that have not

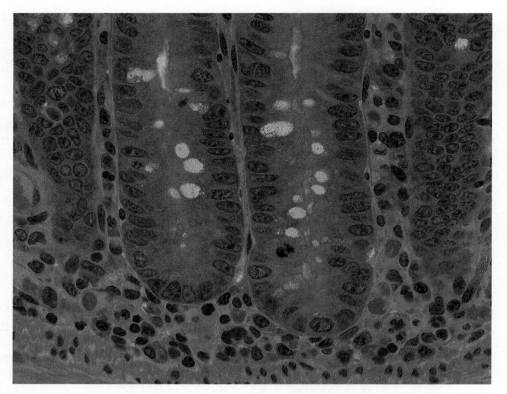

FIGURE 22-19 Crypts in the large intestine. (© Donna Beer Stolz, PhD, Center for Biologic Imaging, University of Pittsburgh Medical School.)

been digested by enzymes. An example is cellulose, which moves through the small intestine with little change but can be broken down by the colon bacteria to be used as energy. These bacteria synthesize vitamins such as cobalamin (B_{12}), the K vitamins *phylloquinone* and *menaquinone*, riboflavin (B_2), and thiamine (B_1), which are absorbed by the intestinal mucosa. The actions of bacteria in the large intestine also may produce intestinal gas or flatus.

The mixing actions of the large intestine are usually slower than those of the small intestine. The peristaltic waves of the large intestine happen only between two and three times per day. The intestinal walls constrict vigorously in *mass movements* to force contents toward the rectum. These movements usually follow a meal but may also be caused by irritations of the intestinal mucosa. Conditions such as colitis or *inflamed colon* may also cause frequent mass movements.

A defecation reflex can usually be voluntarily initiated by holding a deep breath and contracting the abdominal wall muscles. As the rectum fills, its wall distends, triggering the defecation reflex. The internal anal sphincter relaxes, diaphragm lowers, glottis closes, and abdominal wall muscles contract. Abdominal pressure increases, and the rectum is squeezed. The external anal sphincter relaxes, and the feces are forced to the outside. Defecation may be inhibited by voluntarily contracting the external anal sphincter.

Undigested materials, unabsorbed materials, water, electrolytes, mucus, discarded intestinal cells, and bacteria comprise **feces**. Water makes up about 75% of fecal matter; its color is derived from bile pigments that have been affected by bacterial action. The pungent odor of feces results from compounds produced by bacteria.

FOCUS ON PATHOLOGY

In about half of all people older than 60 years of age, multiple outpouchings of the colon develop, which is called *diverticulosis*. Usually, the outpouchings occur in the sigmoid colon. This condition is rarely symptomatic. However, when a diverticulum becomes inflamed, the condition is called *diverticulitis*. There is pain that is usually localized to the left side of the abdomen, changes in bowel habits, fever, and nausea. If the inflamed diverticulum ruptures, peritonitis may develop, requiring emergency surgery and intensive use of antibiotics.

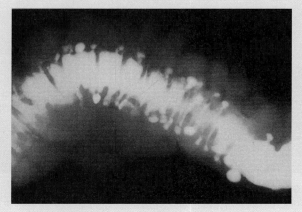

Diverticulosis.

1. Describe the four portions of the large intestine.
2. Which vitamin or vitamins do the normal bacteria in the large intestine synthesize?
3. Describe the components in feces.

Digestion and Absorption of Nutrients

Typical meals contain carbohydrates, lipids, proteins, water, electrolytes, and vitamins. The digestive system handles each of these components differently. Digestion involves breaking down large organic molecules before absorption can occur. Water, electrolytes, and vitamins can be absorbed without preliminary breakdown but may require special transport mechanisms. Discussion of the various types of nutrients is essential in understanding their actions within the digestive system.

The study of nutrients and how the body uses them is known as *nutrition*. **Nutrients** include carbohydrates, lipids, proteins, vitamins, minerals, and water. They are grouped as follows:

- *Macronutrients*: Those required in large amounts, which include carbohydrates, lipids, and proteins; they provide energy and have other specific functions. Potential energy is expressed in calories, which are units of heat.
- *Micronutrients*: Those required in much smaller amounts, such as vitamins and minerals; they do not directly provide energy but allow biochemical reactions that extract energy from macronutrients.

A **calorie** is the amount of heat needed to raise the temperature of a gram of water by 1°C. The calorie used to measure food energy is greater, by 1,000 times. Although referred to commonly as a *calorie*, it is technically referred to as a *kilocalorie*. Cellular oxidation causes the following calorie releases:

- One gram of carbohydrate yields about 4 calories.
- One gram of protein yields about 4 calories.
- One gram of fat yields about 9 calories.

Digestion breaks down nutrients so they can be absorbed and transported via the bloodstream. *Essential nutrients* are those that human cells cannot synthesize, such as certain amino acids.

Carbohydrates include sugars and starches and are organic compounds. Energy from carbohydrates mostly is used to power cellular processes. They are ingested in forms that include grains; vegetables; glycogen from meats; disaccharides from cane sugar, beet sugar, and molasses; and monosaccharides from fruits and honey. Digestion breaks carbohydrates down into monosaccharides, which include fructose, galactose, and glucose, for easy absorption. Liver enzymes convert fructose and galactose into glucose, which is the form of carbohydrate most commonly oxidized for use as cellular fuel.

Cellulose is a complex carbohydrate not digestible by humans. It provides bulk, also known as fiber or roughage, which helps the muscular digestive system walls to push food through its tubes. Many cells get their energy by oxidizing fatty acids, although neurons require continuous glucose to survive. The nervous system can be seriously impaired by lack of glucose. When carbohydrates are not consumed sufficiently, the liver may convert amino acids, from proteins, into glucose.

Some excess glucose is changed to glycogen, which is stored in the liver and muscles. Glucose can be rapidly mobilized from glycogen, but only a certain amount of glycogen can be stored. Excess glucose is usually converted into fat and stored in adipose tissue. For energy, the body first metabolizes glucose, then glycogen into glucose, and finally fats and proteins.

Carbohydrates are used by cells to synthesize vital biochemicals such as ribose and deoxyribose, which are needed to produce the nucleic acids RNA and DNA. They are also needed to synthesize the disaccharide lactose or *milk sugar* during breast milk secretion. Physically active people need more fuel than others, but eating excess carbohydrates may cause obesity and increased cardiovascular disease risks. Carbohydrate intake differs for each person, but current estimates state that between 125 and 175 g of carbohydrates should be consumed daily to avoid protein breakdown as well as metabolic disorders that result from the utilization of excess fat.

Lipids include fats, fat-like substances, and oils; cholesterol; and phospholipids. They supply energy for body processes and building of certain structures. The most common lipids found in the diet are fats known as *triglycerides*, found in both plant and animal-based foods. Saturated fats are found mostly in meats, eggs, milk, animal fat or *lard*, palm oil, and coconut oil. These fats, when consumed excessively, are a risk factor for cardiovascular disease. Unsaturated fats exist in nuts, seeds, and plant oils. Monounsaturated fats are found in olive, peanut, and canola oils and are the healthiest type of fats. Cholesterol is found in animal products, including liver, egg yolk, whole milk, butter, cheese, and meats. It is not present in foods of plant origin.

Lipids have many functions, but mostly they supply energy. Triglyceride molecules must first undergo hydrolysis, which is breakdown in the presence of water, before they can release energy. When this occurs, fatty acids and glycerol are released, absorbed, and transported in lymph and blood to the tissues. Some fatty acid portions react to form molecules of acetyl coenzyme A via reactions known as **beta-oxidation**. Excess amounts of this coenzyme convert into ketone bodies such as acetone, acetoacetate, or beta-hydroxybutyrate and can be reconverted in reverse. The presence of ketone bodies in the urine is known as *ketonuria*.

Certain fatty acids, known as *essential fatty acids*, cannot be synthesized by the liver. For example, linoleic acid, which is needed for phospholipid synthesis, cell membrane formation, and transport of lipids, is an essential fatty acid found in corn, cottonseed, and soy oils. Another essential fatty acid is linolenic acid.

Free fatty acids are used by the liver to synthesize triglycerides, phospholipids, and lipoproteins. Lipids are less dense than proteins; therefore, the proportion of lipids in a lipoprotein increases as the density of the particle decreases. The reverse is also true. VLDLs have a relatively high concentration of triglycerides. LDLs have a relatively high concentration of cholesterol. HDLs have a relatively high concentration of proteins.

The liver controls cholesterol in the body. It synthesizes cholesterol and releases it into the bloodstream or removes it from the bloodstream to be excreted via bile or to produce bile salts. Cholesterol does not create energy but provides structural materials for cell membranes and helps to synthesize certain sex hormones and adrenal hormones. Triglycerides are stored in adipose tissue and may be hydrolyzed into free fatty acids and glycerol when blood lipid concentration drops, such as during fasting.

Lipids vary in how they may be required for health. Fat intake must be enough to carry the fat-soluble vitamins. Lipids also make foods taste more appetizing. It is recommended that lipid intake not exceed 30% of daily calories.

Proteins are created from amino acids and include enzymes, plasma proteins, the muscle components *actin* and *myosin*, hormones, and antibodies. After digestion breaks proteins down into amino acids, they may also supply energy. They are transported to the liver, where deamination occurs, which is the loss of their nitrogen-containing portions. They react to form the waste urea, excreted in urine.

Foods rich in protein include meats, fish, poultry, cheese, nuts, milk, eggs, cereals, and, in lesser amounts, legumes, which include beans and peas. All except nine of the required amino acids can be synthesized by an adult's body. *Essential amino acids* are those that the body is unable to synthesize. **TABLE 22-8** lists the amino acids in foods, indicating the essential and nonessential amino acids. The body requires all these amino acids for proper growth and tissue repair.

The three classes of proteins are complete, incomplete, and partially complete proteins. **Complete proteins,** found in milk, meats, and eggs, have adequate amounts of the essential amino acids. **Incomplete proteins**, such as those found in corn, have too little tryptophan and lysine to maintain human tissues or support growth and development. A **partially complete protein**, such as gliadin, found in wheat, does not have enough lysine to promote growth but does have enough to maintain life.

Proteins supply the essential amino acids and provide nitrogen and other elements. Protein requirements differ based on body size, metabolism, activity levels, and other factors. Nutritionists recommend a daily protein intake of 0.8 g/kg of body weight; therefore, most average adults should consume 60 to 150 g of protein per day.

Vitamins are other organic compounds required for normal metabolism. Body cells cannot synthesize adequate amounts of vitamins, so they must come from foods. Vitamins are classified by their solubility. Fat-soluble vitamins include A, D, E, and K, and water-soluble vitamins include the B vitamin group and vitamin C.

TABLE 22-8
Amino Acids Found in Foods

Amino Acid	Most Common Source
Essential amino acids	
Histidine	Dairy products
Isoleucine	Nuts
Leucine	Beans
Lysine	Cheese
Methionine	Meats
Phenylalanine	Bananas
Threonine	Cottage cheese
Tryptophan	Meats
Valine	Peanuts
Nonessential amino acids	
Alanine	Meats
Arginine	Dairy products
Asparagine	Dairy products
Aspartic acid	Meats
Cysteine	High-protein foods
Cystine	High-protein foods
Glutamic acid	Meats
Glutamine	Meats
Glycine	Sweeteners
Hydroxyproline	Beans and vegetables
Proline	Meats
Serine	Soybeans
Tyrosine	Meats

Bile salts in the small intestine promote absorption of fat-soluble vitamins. They accumulate in various tissues and intake must be controlled. For example, when too much vitamin A is consumed, the body receives too much beta-carotene, and the skin may appear orange in color. **TABLE 22-9** explains the fat-soluble vitamins, including their adult recommended daily allowance (RDA).

The water-soluble vitamins include the B vitamins and vitamin C. The *B vitamins* consist of compounds essential for normal metabolism and help to oxidize carbohydrates, lipids, and proteins. They are often present together in foods; hence, they are referred to as the *vitamin B complex*. Cooking and food processing destroy some of these vitamins. *Vitamin C* (ascorbic acid) is one of the least stable vitamins. Found in

TABLE 22-9

Fat-Soluble Vitamins

Vitamin	Source	Adult RDA	Characteristics	Functions
A	Liver, fish, whole milk, butter, eggs, leafy green vegetables, yellow and orange vegetables, and fruits	4,000–5,000 international units (IU)	Several forms; synthesized from carotenes; stored in liver; stable in heat, acids, and bases; unstable in light	Necessary for synthesis of visual pigments, mucoproteins, and mucopolysaccharides; for normal development of bones and teeth; and for maintenance of epithelial cells
D	Produced when skin is exposed to ultraviolet light; also exists in milk, egg yolk, fish liver oils, and fortified foods	400 IU	A group of steroids; resistant to heat, oxidation, acids, and bases; stored in liver, skin, brain, spleen, and bones	Promotes absorption of calcium and phosphorus and the development of teeth and bones
E	Oils from cereal seeds, salad oils, margarine, shortenings, fruits, nuts, and vegetables	30 IU	A group of compounds; resistant to heat and visible light; unstable in presence of oxygen and ultraviolet light; stored in muscles and adipose tissues	An antioxidant; prevents oxidation of vitamin A and polyunsaturated fatty acids; may help maintain stability of cell membranes
K	Leafy green vegetables, egg yolk, pork liver, soy oil, tomatoes, cauliflower	55–70 µg	Occurs in several forms; resistant to heat but destroyed by acids, bases, and light; stored in the liver	Required for synthesis of prothrombin, which functions in blood clotting

many plant foods, it is necessary for the body to produce collagen, convert folacin to folinic acid, and metabolize certain amino acids. Vitamin C also promotes synthesis of hormones from cholesterol and is vital for iron absorption. **TABLE 22-10** explains the water-soluble vitamins, including their RDA.

Minerals are inorganic elements essential for human metabolism. Humans obtain minerals from plant foods or from animals that have eaten plants. Minerals are most concentrated in the bones and teeth and make up about 4% of body weight. Certain minerals are often incorporated into organic molecules, such as phosphorus from phospholipids, iron from hemoglobin, and iodine from thyroxine. Others are part of inorganic compounds, such as calcium phosphate in bone. Still others are free ions, including sodium, chloride, and calcium, in the blood.

Minerals make up part of every cell's structure and are present in enzymes, affect osmotic pressure, and are required for nerve impulse conduction. Other functions that rely on minerals include blood coagulation, muscle fiber contraction, and pH of body fluids. The minerals calcium and phosphorus make up almost 75%, by weight, of the body's mineral elements. These are called **major minerals**. **TABLE 22-11** lists and describes the major minerals and their RDAs.

Trace elements are essential minerals found in very small amounts. Each makes up less than 0.005% of adult body weight. **TABLE 22-12** explains the trace elements and their RDAs.

When a person's diet lacks essential nutrients, malnutrition results. This may be due to either under-nutrition or over-nutrition. Causes can include lack of food, poor-quality food, overeating, or taking too many vitamin supplements. Overeating, as well as insufficient exercise, results in the body becoming *overweight* and potentially *obese*. Obesity is defined as having a body mass index of 30 or more. A person's body mass index is used to determine adequate weight, overweight, or obesity. Body mass index is calculated by dividing a person's weight in kilograms (1 kg = 2.2 pounds) by height in meters squared (1 foot = 0.3 m). For example, a person who is 5 feet 6 inches tall is equivalent to 1.65 m tall. If this person weighs 180 pounds, that is equivalent to 82 kg. By dividing 82 kg by 1.65 m², a body mass index of 29 is found, which is considered overweight but not obese.

Effects of Aging on the Digestive System

Although the digestive system remains almost completely functional throughout life, a few age-related changes are connected to the effects of aging on other body systems. The digestive epithelium becomes more susceptible to damage, with the likelihood of peptic ulcers increasing. Tissue repair is less efficient, and the stratified epithelium of the mouth, esophagus, and anus becomes more fragile. Peristaltic contractions become weaker and general motility decreases. Fecal movement slows as a result, so constipation becomes more common. Straining to eliminate compacted feces can

TABLE 22-10

Water-Soluble Vitamins

Vitamin	Source	Adult RDA	Characteristics	Functions
B_1 (thiamine)	Lean meats, liver, eggs, whole-grain cereals, leafy green vegetables, legumes	1.5 mg	Destroyed by heat and oxygen, especially in alkaline environment	Required to oxidize carbohydrates; required for ribose synthesis
B_2 (riboflavin)	Meats, dairy products, leafy green vegetables, whole-grain cereals	1.7 mg	Stable to heat, acids, and oxidation; destroyed by bases and ultraviolet light	Required to oxidize glucose and fatty acids, and for cellular growth
B_3 (niacin; nicotinic acid)	Liver, lean meats, peanuts, legumes	20 mg	Stable to heat, acids, and bases; converted to niacinamide by cells; synthesized from tryptophan	Required to oxidize glucose and to synthesize proteins, fats, and nucleic acids
B_5 (pantothenic acid)	Meats, whole-grain cereals, legumes, milk, fruits, vegetables	10 mg	Destroyed by heat, acids, and bases	Required to oxidize carbohydrates and fats
B_6 (pyridoxine)	Liver, meats, bananas, avocados, beans, peanuts, whole-grain cereals, egg yolk	2 mg	A group of three compounds; stable to heat and acids; destroyed by oxidation, bases, and ultraviolet light	Required to synthesize proteins and some amino acids, to convert tryptophan to niacin, to produce antibodies, and to synthesize nucleic acids
B_7 (biotin)	Liver, egg yolk, nuts, legumes, mushrooms	0.3 mg	Stable to heat, acids, and light; destroyed by oxidation and bases	Required to metabolize amino acids and fatty acids, and to synthesize nucleic acids
B_9 (folic acid; folacin)	Liver, leafy green vegetables, whole-grain cereals, legumes	0.4 mg	Occurs in several forms; destroyed by oxidation in acid environment or by heat in alkaline environment; stored in liver, where it is converted into folinic acid	Required for metabolism of certain amino acids and for DNA synthesis; promotes red blood cell production
B_{12} (cyanocobalamin)	Liver, meats, milk, cheese, eggs	3–6 μg	Complex, cobalt-containing compound; stable to heat; inactivated by light, strong acids, and strong bases; absorption regulated by intrinsic factor from gastric glands; stored in liver	Required to synthesize nucleic acids and to metabolize carbohydrates; plays role in myelin synthesis; needed for normal red blood cell production
C (ascorbic acid)	Citrus fruits, tomatoes, potatoes, leafy green vegetables	60 mg	Chemically similar to monosaccharides; stable in acids but destroyed by oxidation, heat, light, and bases	Required to produce collagen, to convert folacin to folinic acid, and to metabolize certain amino acids; promotes absorption of iron and synthesis of hormones from cholesterol

TABLE 22-11

Major Minerals

Mineral	Source	Adult RDA	Locations	Functions
Calcium (Ca)	Milk, milk products, leafy green vegetables	800 mg	Mostly in inorganic salts of bones and teeth	Structure of bones and teeth; essential for nerve impulse conduction, muscle fiber contraction, and blood coagulation; increases permeability of cell membranes; activates certain enzymes
Chlorine (Cl)	Same as for sodium	No RDA established	Closely associated with sodium (as chloride); most highly concentrated in cerebrospinal fluid and gastric juice	Helps maintain osmotic pressure of extracellular fluids, regulate pH, and maintain electrolyte balance; essential in formation of HCl; aids transport of carbon dioxide by red blood cells
Magnesium (Mg)	Milk, dairy products, legumes, nuts, leafy green vegetables	300–350 mg	Abundant in bones	Required in metabolic reactions that occur in mitochondria and are associated with adenosine triphosphate (ATP) production via aerobic metabolism or cellular respiration; plays role in the breakdown of ATP to adenosine diphosphate
Phosphorus (P)	Meats, cheese, nuts, whole-grain cereals, milk, legumes	800 mg	Mostly in the inorganic salts of bones and teeth	Structure of bones and teeth; component in nearly all metabolic reactions; constituent of nucleic acid, many proteins, some enzymes, and some vitamins; occurs in cell membrane, ATP, and phosphates of body fluids
Potassium (K)	Avocados, dried apricots, meats, nuts, potatoes, bananas	2,500 mg	Widely distributed; tends to be concentrated inside cells	Helps maintain intracellular osmotic pressure and regulate pH; promotes metabolism; required for nerve impulse conduction and muscle fiber contraction
Sodium (Na)	Table salt, cured ham, sauerkraut, cheese, graham crackers	2,500 mg	Widely distributed; mostly in extracellular fluids and bound to inorganic salts of bone	Helps maintain osmotic pressure of extracellular fluids and regulate water movement; needed for conduction of nerve impulses and contraction of muscle fibers; aids in regulation of pH and in transport of substances across cell membranes
Sulfur (S)	Meats, milk, eggs, legumes	No RDA established	Widely distributed; abundant in skin, hair, and nails	Essential part of various amino acids, thiamine, insulin, biotin, and mucopolysaccharides

produce hemorrhoids. The haustra of the colon can sag and become inflamed. Muscular sphincters can weaken, leading to esophageal reflux and increased occurrence of heartburn.

The teeth can be gradually lost due to cavities or gingivitis. Erosion of tooth sockets because of a reduced calcium content in bones can also lead to tooth loss. Alcohol use can damage the digestive tract and liver, potentially leading to liver diseases such as cirrhosis. Rates of colon cancer and stomach cancer rise with age. Elderly smokers are more prone to oral and pharyngeal cancers. Olfactory and gustatory sensitivities decline, leading to dietary changes that can affect the whole body.

TABLE 22-12
Trace Elements

Trace Element	Source	Adult RDA	Locations	Functions
Chromium (Cr)	Liver, lean meats, wine	0.05–2 mg	Widely distributed	Essential for use of carbohydrates
Cobalt (Co)	Liver, lean meats, milk	No RDA established	Widely distributed	Component of cyanocobalamin; needed for synthesis of several enzymes
Copper (Cu)	Liver, oysters, crabmeat, nuts, whole-grain cereals, legumes	2–3 mg	Most highly concentrated in liver, heart, and brain	Essential for hemoglobin synthesis, bone development, melanin production, and myelin formation
Fluorine (F)	Fluoridated water	1.5–4 mg	Primarily in bones and teeth	Component of tooth structure (enamel)
Iodine (I)	Food content varies with soil content in different geographic regions; present in iodized table salt	0.15 mg	Concentrated in thyroid gland	Essential component for synthesis of thyroid hormones
Iron (Fe)	Liver, lean meats, dried apricots, raisins, enriched whole-grain cereals, legumes, molasses	10–18 mg	Primarily in blood; stored in liver, spleen, and bone marrow	Part of hemoglobin molecule; catalyzes vitamin A formation; incorporated into many enzymes
Manganese (Mn)	Nuts, legumes, whole-grain cereals, leafy green vegetables, fruits	2.5–5 mg	Most concentrated in liver, kidneys, and pancreas	Activates enzymes required for fatty acid and cholesterol synthesis, urea formation, and normal nervous system functioning
Selenium (Se)	Lean meats, fish, cereals	0.05–2 mg	Concentrated in liver and kidneys	Component of certain enzymes
Zinc (Zn)	Meats, cereals, legumes, nuts, vegetables	15 mg	Most concentrated in liver, kidneys, and brain	Component of enzymes involved in digestion, respiration, bone metabolism, liver metabolism; necessary for normal wound healing and maintaining skin integrity

SUMMARY

Digestion mechanically and chemically breaks down foods and absorbs them. The digestive system consists of an alimentary canal and several accessory organs. Regions of the alimentary canal perform specific functions. It consists of four major layers: mucosa, submucosa, muscular layer, and serosa. Seven essential steps make up the functions of the digestive system: ingestion, propulsion, mechanical processing, digestion, secretion, absorption, and excretion. The two basic types of motor functions in the alimentary canal are mixing and propelling movements.

The mouth receives food and begins digestion. The tongue mixes food particles with saliva during chewing. Salivary glands secrete saliva, which moistens food, helps bind food particles, begins chemical digestion of carbohydrates, makes taste possible, and helps clean the mouth. Humans have a primary and a secondary set of teeth that form during their lifetimes. The dentin that makes up a tooth is harder than bone. The pharynx and esophagus are important passageways, allowing food, liquids, and air to pass.

The stomach receives food, mixes it with gastric juice, carries on a limited amount of absorption, and moves food into the small intestine. Pepsin is the most important protein-digesting enzyme produced by the gastric mucosa. The small intestine extends from the pyloric sphincter to the large intestine and is the longest portion of the alimentary canal. It plays the major role in the digestion and absorption of nutrients. The pancreas produces pancreatic juice with enzymes that can split carbohydrates, fats, nucleic acids, and proteins. The liver metabolizes these substances, storing some of them, filters the blood, destroys toxins, and secretes bile. The small intestine receives secretions from the pancreas and liver, completes nutrient digestion, absorbs the products of digestion, and transports the residues to the large intestine. The gallbladder is mainly a storage organ for bile, which is a fat emulsifier. Bilirubin is a waste product of the heme of hemoglobin. The large intestine reabsorbs water and electrolytes and forms and stores feces.

Nutrition is the study of nutrients and how the body uses them. The macronutrients, which include carbohydrates, lipids, and proteins, are required in large amounts. Carbohydrates are organic compounds and include sugars and starches. Lipids include fats, fat-like substances, and oils. Proteins are created from amino acids and include enzymes, plasma proteins, muscle components, hormones, and antibodies. The micronutrients, including vitamins and minerals, are not required in large amounts. Vitamins are organic compounds required for normal metabolism. Minerals are inorganic elements also required for metabolism. Calories measure potential energy in foods.

KEY TERMS

Accessory organs
Alimentary canal
Anal canal
Anus
Appendix
Ascending colon
Ascites
Beta-oxidation
Bile
Bilirubin
Bolus
Calorie
Canines
Carbohydrates
Cecum
Cholecystokinin
Chyme
Cirrhosis

Colon
Common hepatic duct
Complete proteins
Crown
Cystic duct
Deglutition
Dentin
Dentition
Digestion
Duodenum
Emulsification
Esophageal hiatus
Esophagus
Falciform ligament
Feces
Gallbladder
Gastric glands
Gastric juice

Gastrin
Gum
Halitosis
Hepatic ducts
Hepatic lobules
Hepatic sinusoids
Hepatopancreatic ampulla
Hiatal hernia
Ileocecal sphincter
Ileum
Incisors
Incomplete proteins
Intestinal glands
Intestinal villi
Intrinsic factor
Jejunum
Lamina propria
Large intestine

Lingual frenulum
Lingual tonsils
Lipids
Liver
Lower esophageal sphincter
Lumen
Macronutrients
Major minerals
Mastication
Mesentery
Micronutrients
Minerals
Molars
Mucosa (mucous membrane)
Mucus
Nucleases
Nutrients
Palate

Pancreas
Pancreatic amylase
Pancreatic juice
Pancreatic lipase
Papillae
Parotid glands
Partially complete protein
Pepsin
Pepsinogen
Peristalsis
Pharynx
Porta hepatis
Portal hypertension
Premolars
Pulp cavity
Pyloric sphincter
Renin
Round ligament

Rugae
Salivary amylase
Salivary glands
Secretin
Segmentation
Serosa (serous layer)
Sigmoid colon
Splanchnic circulation
Stomach
Submucosa
Teeth
Tongue
Trace elements
Uvula
Vitamins
Xerostomia

LEARNING GOALS

The following learning goals correspond to the objectives at the beginning of this chapter:

1. The digestive system consists of the mouth, pharynx, esophagus, stomach, small intestine, large intestine, rectum, and anus. The accessory organs include the salivary glands, liver, gallbladder, and pancreas.

2. In the small intestine, peristalsis consists of the propelling, wave-like movements of the tube. Contraction appears in the wall of the tube in a "ring," whereas the muscular wall immediately ahead of the ring relaxes. The peristaltic wave moves along, pushing the contents of the tube toward the anus.

3. The stomach is a pouch-like organ shaped like a *J*. It hangs inferior to the diaphragm, in the upper left abdominal cavity. Its capacity is approximately 4 liters, and its inner lining consists of thick folds or *rugae* of mucosal and submucosal layers that disappear when the stomach is distended. The stomach mixes food from the esophagus with gastric juice, begins protein digestion and limited absorption, and moves food into the small intestine.

4. The small intestine extends from the pyloric sphincter to the large intestine. It is a tubular organ with many loops and coils filling much of the abdominal cavity. It consists of three portions: the duodenum, jejunum, and ileum. The duodenum is 25 cm long and *C*-shaped. The jejunum is the proximal two-fifths of the small intestine. The ileum is thinner and leads to the large intestine.

5. Gastrin is a peptide hormone released by certain stomach cells. It increases gastric gland secretory activity. Secretin is a peptide hormone released from the duodenal mucous membrane into the bloodstream when acidic chyme enters the duodenum. It stimulates pancreatic juice with high concentrations of bicarbonate ions to be released, neutralizing acidic chyme. Cholecystokinin is a peptide hormone released by proteins and fats in the small intestine. It decreases gastric motility as the small intestine fills with food.

6. The pancreas acts as both an endocrine and exocrine gland. For exocrine function, it secretes pancreatic juice. It is closely associated with the small intestine, extending horizontally across the posterior abdominal wall in the duodenum's *C*-shaped curve. Pancreatic acinar cells produce pancreatic juice and make up most of the pancreas. The pancreatic duct usually connects with the duodenum at the same place where the bile duct joins. Pancreatic juice has enzymes such as pancreatic amylase, pancreatic lipase, and two nucleases, able to digest carbohydrates, fats, nucleic acid, and proteins.

7. The liver functions to remove foreign particles such as bacteria that enter blood via the portal vein. It also conducts many important activities of metabolism. Hepatic cells respond to hormones such as glucagon and insulin, lowering blood glucose levels by converting glucose to glycogen. They also raise blood glucose levels by breaking down glycogen to glucose or by converting noncarbohydrates into glucose. The liver oxidizes fatty acids, synthesizes lipoproteins as well as phospholipids and cholesterol, and converts parts of carbohydrate and protein molecules into fat molecules. It breaks down amino acids, forms urea, synthesizes plasma proteins such as albumin, and converts some amino acids into others. The liver stores glycogen, iron, and various vitamins. It also secretes bile.

8.
   A. *Ascending colon:* Begins at the cecum, continues upward against the posterior abdominal wall, inferior to the liver, and then turns to the left.
   B. *Transverse colon:* The longest, most movable part, it is suspended by a fold of peritoneum and sags in the middle, below the stomach; near the spleen, it turns abruptly downward.
   C. *Descending colon:* A mostly vertical section that makes an *S*-shaped curve near its lowest portion.
   D. *Sigmoid colon:* The final portion, it become the rectum.

9. The large intestine has little or no digestive function. It contains many tubular glands composed almost entirely of goblet cells. In the proximal half of the large intestine, water and electrolytes are normally absorbed. Bacteria synthesize vitamins such as cobalamin, the K vitamins, riboflavin, and thiamine, which are absorbed by the intestinal mucosa.

10. The body requires macronutrients, which are those needed in large amounts, which include carbohydrates, lipids, and proteins. It also requires micronutrients in smaller amounts), which include vitamins and minerals.

CRITICAL THINKING QUESTIONS

A 56-year-old man who has had nausea, vomiting, and vague pain in his abdomen develops severe jaundice. He has smoked two packs of cigarettes per day for the past 20 years. His father had diabetes mellitus.

1. According to this scenario, which organ would be most likely linked to these symptoms?
2. If this patient was diagnosed with cancer, what would be the prognosis?

REVIEW QUESTIONS

1. Which of the following is not a function of the oral cavity?
   A. lubrication
   B. digestion of cholesterol fats
   C. digestion of carbohydrates
   D. mechanical processing of food

2. Blood vessels and lymphocytes are found in which of the following layers of the digestive system?
   A. mucosa
   B. submucosa
   C. muscularis
   D. serosa

3. Which of the following organs is not a component of the digestive system?
   A. colon
   B. stomach
   C. spleen
   D. pharynx

4. The crown of a tooth is covered by
   A. enamel
   B. pulp
   C. dentin
   D. cementum

5. The connection of the anterior portion of the tongue to the underlying epithelium is the
   A. glossal connection
   B. labial frenulum
   C. uvula
   D. lingual frenulum

6. Parietal cells secrete
   A. secretin
   B. hydrochloric acid
   C. gastrin
   D. pepsinogen

7. Which of the following is the portion of the stomach that connects to the esophagus?
   A. fundus
   B. antrum
   C. pylorus
   D. cardia

8. Peyer's patches are characteristic of the
   A. colon
   B. ileum
   C. duodenum
   D. jejunum

9. The middle portion of the small intestine is the
   A. cecum
   B. duodenum

C. ileum
D. jejunum

10. Which of the following intestinal hormones stimulates the pancreas?
    A. cholecystokinin
    B. gastrin
    C. secretin
    D. gastric inhibitory peptide

11. The Kupffer cells of the liver
    A. are phagocytic
    B. produce bile
    C. form urea
    D. store cholesterol

12. Which of the following is not a function of the liver?
    A. formation of plasma proteins
    B. formation of bile
    C. production of antibodies
    D. detoxification

13. A *haustra* is
    A. a gland in the large intestine that secretes enzymes
    B. an external pouch of the colon
    C. a ridge in the mucosa of the large intestine
    D. a hormone of the colon

14. Digestion of carbohydrates begins in the
    A. mouth
    B. stomach
    C. duodenum
    D. jejunum

15. The teniae coli are
    A. three longitudinal bands of muscle located beneath the serosa of the colon
    B. ridges in the mucosa of the colon
    C. external pouches of the large intestine
    D. the sigmoid colon and rectum

ESSAY QUESTIONS

1. Describe the major functions of the digestive system.
2. Describe the structure of a tooth.
3. List the layers of the alimentary canal *wall*.
4. Describe the mesocolon and greater omentum.
5. Describe parietal, chief, and mucous neck cells.
6. Name the three hormones produced by the digestive system and describe the function of each one.
7. Describe the main functions of the liver.
8. Describe the anatomy of the small intestine and list its main functions.
9. Explain the five sections of the colon and the function of the large intestine.
10. Describe the role of the pancreas in completion of digestion.

UNIT

VI

CONTINUITY OF LIFE

Reproductive System

OBJECTIVES

After studying this chapter, the reader should be able to

1. Describe the components of the male reproductive system.
2. Specify the normal composition of semen.
3. Explain the hormonal mechanisms that regulate male reproductive functions.
4. Outline the process of spermatogenesis.
5. Describe the structure of the penis.
6. Describe the components of the female reproductive system.
7. Identify the phases and events of the female reproductive cycle.
8. Identify and describe the ligaments that support the uterus and hold it in place.
9. Describe the structure of a mammary gland.
10. List the general symptoms of sexually transmitted infections.

Overview

The reproductive system is the only body system that is not essential to the survival of an individual but is needed to ensure the continued existence of the human species. The reproductive systems of both males and females contain organs and glands that create sex cells and transport them to areas where fertilization can occur. The male and female reproductive systems are functionally very different, but the primary sex organs of both are called **gonads**. The gonads of the male are the testes and of the female, the ovaries. The reproductive systems of both genders become functionally active at puberty.

Sex cells, regardless of gender, are called **gametes**. Male sex cells are called **sperm**, and female sex cells are called **oocytes** or eggs. Sex cells carry genetic instructions via 23 chromosomes. Other types of cells in the body carry 46 chromosomes. When sex cells from a male and female unite during fertilization, the 23 chromosomes from each partner unite to form 46 chromosomes. Certain reproductive organs secrete **sex hormones**, which are actually steroid hormones needed for development and maintenance of secondary sex characteristics and for reproduction. In males, sex hormones are called *androgens*. In females, they are *estrogens* and *progesterone*.

The *accessory reproductive organs* include various ducts, glands, and the external genitalia. When sexual intercourse results in fertilization, a sperm and an egg unite to form a fertilized egg, which is called a *zygote*. This is the original cell of a new human being, and all other cells form from it. After fertilization, the female uterus protects the embryo as it develops.

Anatomy of the Male Reproductive System

The structures of the male reproductive system include two epididymides, two ductus deferentia, two ejaculatory ducts, the urethra, two seminal vesicles, the prostate gland, and two bulbourethral glands. Sperm cells are produced and maintained by the male reproductive organs, which also transport these cells outside of the body and secrete male sex hormones. The primary sex organs or *gonads* of the male consist of the two testes, in which sperm cells and male sex hormones are formed. The accessory sex organs are the internal and external reproductive organs (**FIGURE 23-1**).

Scrotum

The male external reproductive organs consist of the **scrotum**, which encloses the testes, and the penis. The scrotum consists of a fleshy pouch of skin and subcutaneous tissue suspended below the perineum and anterior to the anus. Sparse hairs cover it externally. Internally, the medial septum or *raphe* subdivides it into two chambers, each enclosing a testis. The scrotum protects and controls the temperature of the testes, which is important for sex cell production.

When environmental temperatures are cold, the scrotum contracts and wrinkles, moving the testes closer to the pelvic cavity to absorb heat. When it is warmer outside, the scrotum relaxes and hangs loosely to ensure the testes are about 3°C lower than body temperature. This is better for the sperm cells to be produced and to survive. Viable sperm

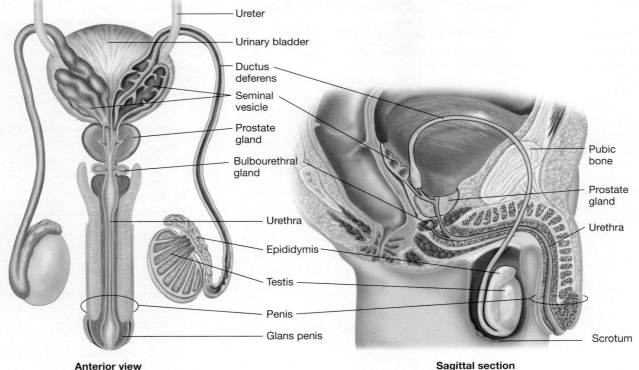

Anterior view

Ureter
Urinary bladder
Ductus deferens
Seminal vesicle
Prostate gland
Bulbourethral gland
Urethra
Epididymis
Testis
Penis
Glans penis

Sagittal section

Pubic bone
Prostate gland
Urethra
Scrotum

FIGURE 23-1 The male organs of reproduction.

cannot be produced at normal core body temperature, which is 98.6°F (37°C).

The scrotum contains two sets of muscles that respond to temperature changes. Each **dartos muscle** is a smooth muscle layer in the superficial fascia that acts to wrinkle the scrotal skin. Bands of skeletal muscle arising from the internal oblique muscles of the body's trunk are known as the **cremaster muscles**, which act to elevate the testes.

Testes

The **testes** are oval-shaped structures about 4 cm (1.5 inches) long and 2.5 cm (1 inch) wide located within the cavity of the scrotum. Each testis is also enclosed in two tunics. The outer is the **tunica vaginalis**, which has two serous layers and is formed from a peritoneal outpocket. The inner tunic is the **tunica albuginea** and is a fibrous capsule. Thin septa extend inward from the tunica albuginea and divide the testis into approximately 250 lobules. Each wedge-shaped lobule contains one to four highly coiled **seminiferous tubules** that, when uncoiled, may reach 80 cm in length. It is here where sperm are actually formed. The seminiferous tubules are made up of a thickened stratified epithelium that surrounds a central lumen filled with fluid. *Spermatogenic cells* are found in larger columnar cells known as *sustenocytes*. These cells play a variety of roles in sperm formation. Sperm are generated continuously.

A normal testis contains nearly one-half of a mile of seminiferous tubules. Each of these tubules forms a loop connected to a network of passageways known as the **rete testis**. Fifteen to 20 large *efferent ductules* connect the rete testis to the *epididymis*. This tube coils on the outer surface of the testis and becomes the ductus deferens (**FIGURE 23-2**). Three to five layers of **myoid cells**, which resemble smooth muscle cells, surround each seminiferous tubule. Rhythmic contractions of the myoid cells aid in squeezing sperm and testicular fluids through the seminiferous tubules and out of the testes. The rete testis receives sperm through a **straight tubule** formed by the seminiferous tubules of each lobule. The epididymis wraps around the posterior external surface of each testis. Immature sperm pass through the head and body of the epididymis to be stored in its "tail" portion until ejaculation.

Interstitial endocrine cells, also known as *Leydig cells*, lie inside the soft connective tissue that surrounds the seminiferous tubules. They produce testosterone and less important types of androgens. These substances are secreted into the surrounding interstitial fluid. The testes are supplied by long

FOCUS ON PATHOLOGY

Testicular cancer affects 1 in every 50,000 males. However, it is the most common cancer in men between the ages of 15 and 35. The most significant risk factor for testicular cancer is *cryptorchidism*, in which a testis does not fully descend into the scrotum. Risks for testicular cancer are also increased by history of orchitis or mumps as well as significant maternal exposure to environmental toxins. The testes should be self-examined on a regular basis. Testicular cancer is signified by a solid yet painless mass. Early detection is related to a very good prognosis. If there is no metastasis, more than 90% of testicular cancers are cured by *orchiectomy*, which is surgical removal of a cancerous testis. This procedure may be performed alone or along with radiation therapy or chemotherapy.

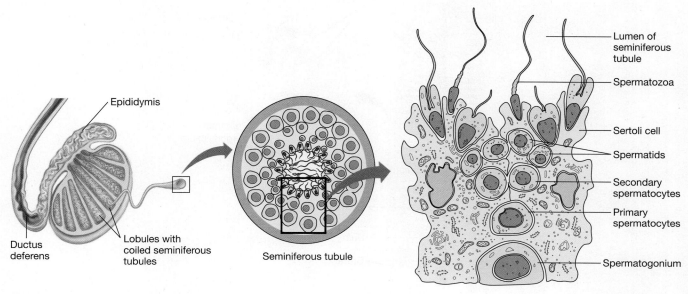

FIGURE 23-2 Internal structure of the testes.

testicular arteries that branch from the abdominal aorta, superior to the pelvis. The testes are drained by the *testicular veins*, which arise from a network known as the *pampiniform venous plexus*. This network surrounds each testicular artery inside the scrotum, winding around it. In each pampiniform plexus, cooler venous blood absorbs heat from arterial blood. Therefore, this blood becomes cooler before entering the testes, which helps to keep the testes at their normal, cool homeostatic temperature.

The testes are served by the sympathetic and parasympathetic divisions of the autonomic nervous system. Forceful trauma to the testes transmits impulses, causing intense pain and nausea. In the testes, blood vessels, nerve fibers, and lymphatics are enclosed by a connective tissue sheath. Together, these structures comprise the **spermatic cord**, passing through the inguinal canal.

TEST YOUR UNDERSTANDING

1. Explain the role of the scrotum in protection of the testes.
2. Describe the two major functions of the testes.
3. Identify the structures in which sperm are actually formed.

Penis

The **penis** is cylindrical in shape and conveys urine and semen through the urethra. When erect, it stiffens and enlarges, enabling insertion into the vagina during sexual intercourse. The penis is divided into three regions: the root, body, and *glans* or **glans penis**. The root of the penis is the fixed portion that attaches the penis to the body wall. At birth, skin that covers the penis is loose. It slides distally

over the head, forming the *foreskin* or **prepuce** around the glans. The prepuce is often removed surgically soon after birth in a procedure called a *circumcision*. This practice is more common in the United States, where at least 65% of males are circumcised. In the rest of the world, about 30% of males experience this procedure. Many cultures are not familiar with circumcision, including some Hispanic cultures and many European and Asian cultures. Most males from Muslim and Jewish cultures are circumcised. It is widely believed that circumcision reduces risk of acquiring HIV or other reproductive system infections.

The dorsal and ventral surfaces of the penis are actually named in relation to the penis being erect, not flaccid. The shaft or *body* of the penis is the tubular, movable portion of the organ. It contains three columns of erectile tissue. It has two dorsal **corpora cavernosa** and one ventral **corpus spongiosum** (**FIGURE 23-3**). The urethra is surrounded by the corpus spongiosum. Dense connective tissue surrounds each column in a capsule. The penis is enclosed by a layer of connective tissue, a thin layer of subcutaneous tissue, and skin. The erectile tissue of the penis contains many vascular spaces. These spaces fill with blood during sexual stimulation.

Male Duct System

When sperm are produced by the testes, they move out of the body via a system of ducts. These ducts are the epididymis, ductus deferens, ejaculatory duct, and urethra.

Epididymis

The cup-shaped **epididymis** can be felt through the skin of the scrotum. It is coiled and twisted to take up only a small amount of space, about 3.8 cm (1.5 inches). The head of the epididymis contains efferent ductules and lies above the

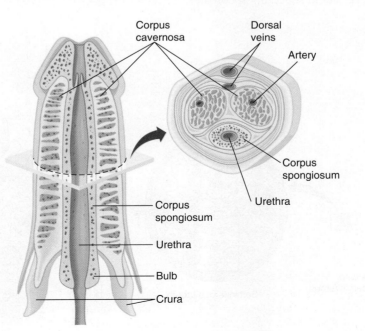

FIGURE 23-3 The penis.

superior aspect of each testis. The body and tail of the epididymis are found on the posterolateral area of each testis.

The epididymis controls the composition of the fluid produced by the seminiferous tubules. It also absorbs and recycles damaged spermatozoa and absorbs cellular debris. The products of the breakdown of enzymes are released into the surrounding interstitial fluids for pickup by the epididymal blood vessels. The epididymis also stores and protects spermatozoa and facilitates their functional maturation.

Most epididymides are tightly coiled tubes about 6 m (20 feet) in length, connected to the posterior border of the tests. These tubes are also described as the *ducts of the epididymides*. They course upward to become the ductus deferens. In the duct mucosa, certain pseudostratified epithelial cells have *stereocilia*, which are long, nonmoving microvilli. Having a large surface area, the stereocilia can absorb extra testicular fluid and pass nutrients to the millions of sperm cells temporarily stored in the lumen.

Immature sperm cells are nonmotile when they reach the epididymis; therefore, rhythmic peristaltic contractions move them through the duct as they mature. The surrounding fluid contains antimicrobial proteins such as defensins. The transfer of sperm from the testes and through the epididymides takes approximately 20 days. Once mature, sperm cells can move independently to fertilize egg cells but usually do not actually "swim" until after ejaculation. This occurs from the epididymides and not the testes. The secretions of the seminal vesicles are discharged into the ejaculatory duct at *emission*. This is when peristaltic contractions are occurring in the ductus deferens, seminal vesicles, and prostate gland. These contractions are controlled by the sympathetic nervous system. Although sperm are normally stored in the epididymides for several months, longer storage results in them being phagocytized by the epithelial cells there.

Ductus Deferens and Ejaculatory Duct

The **ductus deferentia**, also called the *vasa deferentia*, are muscular tubes approximately 45 cm (18 inches) in length. Singularly, each ductus deferens is called a *vas deferens*. They each pass upward, as part of the spermatic cord, along the medial side of a testis, through the inguinal canal in the lower abdominal wall to enter the pelvic cavity. They end behind the urinary bladder, uniting just outside the prostate gland with the duct of a seminal vesicle. This forms an **ejaculatory duct**, which is a short structure passing through the prostate gland to empty into the urethra. The vas deferens is the duct that is altered when a male undergoes a *vasectomy*.

Each ductus deferens can easily be felt as it passes anterior to the pubic bone, looping medially over the ureter and descending along the posterior wall of the bladder. The terminus portion expands to form an **ampulla**, joining the duct of a seminal vesicle. The mucosa of the ductus deferens is, like the epididymis, pseudostratified epithelium. It differs in that its muscular layer is very thick. During ejaculation, the smooth muscle of its walls creates peristaltic waves, quickly squeezing sperm forward, into the urethra.

Male Accessory Glands

The male accessory glands consist of a pair of seminal glands and bulbourethral glands, plus a single prostate gland.

Seminal Glands

The seminal glands are also called **seminal vesicles** and are sac-like structures lying on the posterior bladder surface. They are approximately 5 cm long, attached to the ductus deferens near the base of the bladder. Each seminal vesicle is a tubular gland having a total uncoiled length of about 15 cm. However, these glands are normally coiled back on themselves, making their coiled size only 5 to 7 cm. During ejaculation, they are emptied by a thick layer of smooth muscle that contracts inside their fibrous capsules. They have glandular tissue linings that contribute nearly 60% of semen volume.

The seminal vesicles secrete a slightly alkaline fluid that is yellowish in color and viscous. This fluid helps to regulate the pH of the tubular contents as sperm cells travel to outside the body. The yellow color of seminal fluid comes from a pigment that becomes fluorescent under ultraviolet light, a fact that is used for the investigation of certain crimes. Seminal fluid contains fructose, a monosaccharide that provides energy for sperm cells, as well as prostaglandins that stimulate muscular contractions within the female reproductive organs. These contractions aid the movement of sperm cells toward the egg cell. The fluid from the seminal glands also contains citric acid and a coagulating enzyme known as *vesiculase*.

Remember that the duct of each seminal gland joins the duct of the ductus deferens on the same side, forming the ejaculatory duct. Here, seminal fluid mixes with sperm, entering the prostatic urethra simultaneously during ejaculation. *Semen*, therefore, is 70% made up by seminal gland secretions.

Prostate

The **prostate gland** surrounds the proximal portion of the urethra, slightly inferior to the urinary bladder. It is a chestnut- or doughnut-shaped, muscular structure that is approximately 4 cm wide and 3 cm thick. It is surrounded by a thick connective tissue capsule and made up of 20 to 30 branched tubular glands with ducts that open into the urethra. These glands are embedded in a stroma, which is a mass of dense connective tissue and smooth muscle.

The prostatic smooth muscle contracts during ejaculation. Prostatic secretions are squeezed into the prostatic urethra through several ducts. The secretions consist of a milky fluid that is slightly acidic. Prostatic fluid enhances the motility of the sperm cells and helps neutralize the vagina's highly acidic secretions. It makes up to one-third of the volume of the semen. Prostatic fluid contains citrate, which provides nutrients, prostate-specific antigen, and enzymes such as fibrinolysin, acid phosphatase, and hyaluronidase.

A variety of conditions can affect the prostate on a fairly common basis. *Prostatitis* is inflammation that may be acute, chronic, or coupled with pelvic pain syndrome. Acute bacterial prostatitis is usually related to a bacterial infection, most commonly with *Escherichia coli*. Chronic bacterial prostatitis is usually from the same cause but recurs as prostate bacteria reinvade the bladder. It may be coupled with pelvic pain syndrome, and together these conditions are the most common form of prostatitis, being either inflammatory or noninflammatory. *Benign prostatic hyperplasia* is seen in nearly every elderly man. It causes distortion of the urethra and problems in urination. It is treated by surgery, microwave treatments, drugs that shrink the prostate, insertion of a small balloon to compress prostate tissue, or inserting a catheter to instill radiofrequency radiation. *Prostate cancer* is the second most common cause of cancer death in males, after lung cancer. Because of this fact, screening must be performed regularly, generally starting at age 45 if the patient has a history of the disease or by age 50 if there is no history. Screening involves digital examination, serum prostate-specific antigen level testing, and transrectal ultrasound imaging. There is a new blood test that has been shown to have more diagnostic accuracy than the commonly used *prostate specific antigen test*. The new test may reduce unnecessary biopsies and false positive results. It is known as the *Prostate Health Index (PHI) test*, and utilizes three prostate-specific markers. After diagnosis, treatments include surgery with or without radiotherapy.

Bulbourethral Glands

The **bulbourethral glands**, also known as Cowper's glands, are about 1 cm in diameter and lie inferior to the prostate gland surrounded by the external urethral sphincter muscle's fibers. These glands have tubes with epithelial linings secreting a thick, clear mucous-like fluid as a response to sexual stimulation. The fluid lubricates the end of the penis to prepare for sexual intercourse, even though females secrete most of the lubricating fluid needed for sexual intercourse. The fluid from the bulbourethral glands also neutralizes any urine, which is acidic.

Semen

The milky white, slightly sticky fluid the male urethra conveys to outside of the body during ejaculation is known as **semen**. It is made up of sperm cells from the testes and secretions of the seminal vesicles, prostate gland, and bulbourethral glands. Semen has an alkaline pH of between 7.2 and 8.0 and includes prostaglandins and nutrients. It helps to neutralize the acidic environment of the male urethra and the female vagina. Under acidic conditions, the sperm "swim" more slowly than normal.

Between 2 and 5 mL of semen are released at one time, with between 20 and 150 million sperm/mL. However, sperm only make up about 10% of the semen. Sperm cells begin to swim as they mix with accessory gland secretions. They acquire the ability to fertilize a female egg cell once they are inside the female reproductive tract in a process called capacitation, which is due to the weakening of the sperm cells' acrosomal membranes.

Mature sperm do not contain significant amounts of stored nutrients or cytoplasm. Nearly all energy needed for sperm adenosine triphosphate synthesis is provided by catabolism of the fructose in seminal gland secretions. The prostaglandins in semen decrease cervical viscosity in the female uterus, stimulating *reverse peristalsis*. This speeds up the movement of sperm through the female reproductive tract. Semen also contains the hormone *relaxin*, various enzymes, ingredients that suppress the immune response in the female reproductive tract, antibiotics that destroy certain bacteria, and clotting factors. Just after ejaculation, the clotting factors coagulate the semen, which causes the sperm to stick to the vaginal walls of the female so they do not drain out of the vagina. Fibrinolysin then liquefies the sticky mass, allowing the sperm to swim along their journey to the ovum.

Physiology of the Male Reproductive System

The physiology of the male reproductive system involves primary phases of sexual response. These include erection of the penis for penetration of the female vagina and ejaculation, which allows semen and the sperm it contains to be propelled into the vagina.

Male Sexual Response

When sexual stimulation occurs, parasympathetic nerve impulses from the sacral area of the spinal cord release nitric oxide, which dilates the arteries leading into the penis. Arterial pressure in the erectile tissue compresses the veins to reduce blood flow away from the penis.

Erection

The erectile tissues expand with blood and the penis swells and elongates to produce an **erection**. Before sexual arousal, arterioles that supply the erectile tissue are constricted and the penis is flaccid. Sexual arousal triggers the *parasympathetic reflex* that causes nitric oxide to be released locally, relaxing the smooth muscle in the walls of the penile blood vessels. The arterioles dilate, and the erectile bodies become filled with blood. As the corpora cavernosa expand, their drainage veins become compressed. The engorgement of the penis is maintained because outward blood flow cannot occur. The corpus spongiosum only slightly expands in comparison and functions to keep the urethra open when ejaculation occurs. When erect, the penis should not bend excessively. This is prevented by the way the collagen fibers surrounding the penis are arranged in longitudinal and circular fashion.

Ejaculation

Male orgasm is accompanied by emission and ejaculation, which is the propulsion of semen from the duct system. The movement of sperm cells from the testes and secretions of the prostate gland and seminal vesicles into the urethra is known as **emission**. In the urethra, all these components mix to form semen. Emission occurs as a result of spinal *sympathetic nerve impulses* that stimulate peristaltic contractions in the testicular ducts, epididymides, ductus deferentia, and ejaculatory ducts. The sympathetic nerves involved are mostly at the level of L1 and L2. Other sympathetic impulses simultaneously cause rhythmic contractions of the seminal vesicles and prostate gland.

The urethra fills with semen as sensory impulses pass into the sacral portion of the spinal cord. The bladder sphincter muscle constricts to prevent urine expulsion or semen reflux into the bladder. Contraction of the reproductive ducts and accessory glands helps to fill the urethra with semen. Somatic motor impulses are then transmitted to certain skeletal muscles, causing a reflex in which the penile erectile columns contract rhythmically because of the actions of the bulbospongiosus muscles. This increases pressure inside the erectile tissues, helping to force semen through the urethra to outside of the body, which is the process of **ejaculation**. Semen is propelled at a speed of nearly 11 miles per hour! Physiological and psychological release, known as an **orgasm**, is the culmination of sexual stimulation. Intense pleasure is experienced, and systemic changes include elevated blood pressure, rapid heartbeat, and generalized muscle contraction.

Fluid from the bulbourethral glands is expelled first during emission and ejaculation, followed by fluid from the prostate gland, passage of sperm cells, and, finally, fluid from the seminal vesicles. After ejaculation, the arteries of the erectile tissue immediately constrict. Smooth muscles in the vascular spaces contract partially, and veins of the penis carry away excess blood, gradually returning the penis to its flaccid state. **TABLE 23-1** summarizes the functions of the male reproductive organs.

After orgasm, a period of **resolution** quickly occurs, in which muscles relax. The internal pudendal arteries and penile arterioles are constricted by activity of the sympathetic nerve fibers. Blood flow is reduced into the penis. Small muscles are activated, squeezing the cavernous bodies to force blood from the penis into the general circulation. The penis eventually becomes flaccid again. There is a

TABLE 23-1

Male Reproductive Organs

Organ	Function
Testis (testes)	
Interstitial cells	Produce and secrete sex hormones
Seminiferous tubules	Produce sperm cells
Epididymis	A coiled duct that connects the rete testis to the ductus deferens; it is the site of functional maturation of spermatozoa
Ductus deferens	Transfers sperm cells to the ejaculatory duct
Seminal vesicle	Generates an alkaline fluid that contains prostaglandins and nutrients; this fluid helps to neutralize the acidic components of the semen
Prostate gland	The alkaline fluid secreted helps to neutralize the acidity of the semen to enhance motility of sperm cells
Bulbourethral gland	Located at the base of the penis, it secretes fluids into the penile urethra
Scrotum	Regulates the temperature of the testes by enclosing and protecting them
Penis	The copulatory organ that surrounds the urethra and serves to introduce semen into the female vagina

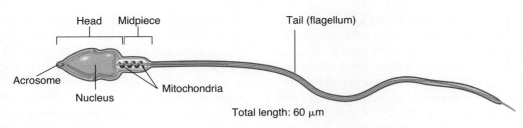

FIGURE 23-4 A mature sperm cell.

latent, refractory period after ejaculation in which the male is unable to achieve another orgasm. This period lengthens because of aging.

FOCUS ON PATHOLOGY

The inability to attain an erection when desired is known as *erectile dysfunction (ED)*. It commonly occurs because of a lack of adequate nitric oxide release from the penile parasympathetic nerves. About half of the men in the United States over age 40 have various degrees of ED. The condition may also be linked to alcohol use, psychological factors, or the use of drugs such as antidepressants and antihypertensives. Chronic ED is often related to abnormalities of blood vessels, hormones, or the nervous system. Varicose veins may also be implicated. Newer treatments for ED include drugs such as Viagra, Cialis, and Levitra, which potentiate the effect of the existing levels of nitric oxide. They must be used carefully in men with diabetes mellitus or preexisting heart disease.

TEST YOUR UNDERSTANDING

1. Explain the structures of the male reproductive duct system.
2. Describe the functions of the prostate gland.
3. Explain the processes involved in erection and ejaculation.

Spermatogenesis

Spermatogenesis is the process by which sperm cells or *spermatozoa* are formed. **Spermatogenic cells** form sperm cells and line the seminiferous tubules. **Interstitial cells**, also known as the *Leydig cells*, lie in spaces between the seminiferous tubules. Male sex hormones are produced and secreted by these interstitial cells.

The epithelium that makes up the seminiferous tubules contains supporting sustentacular or *Sertoli* cells and spermatogenic cells. These cells provide a framework that nourishes and regulates sperm cells, which are continually produced beginning at puberty, usually around age 14. Sperm cells collect in the lumen of each tubule, pass to the epididymis, and then mature. Each mature sperm cell is about 0.06 mm (60 μm) in length and appears like a tiny tadpole. It has a flattened "head," a cylinder-shaped "body," and a long "tail" (**FIGURE 23-4**). Approximately 400 million sperm are produced daily by a healthy male.

The head of a sperm cell has a nucleus and compacted chromatin containing its 23 chromosomes. The acrosome is a small protrusion that contains enzymes needed to help it to penetrate an egg cell during fertilization. The midpiece, or body of the sperm cell, has a filamentous core and spiraled mitochondria. The tail, or flagellum, consists of microtubules in an extension of the cell membrane. The tail moves via adenosine triphosphate from the mitochondria, propelling the sperm cell through its containing fluid. Normal development of spermatozoa in the testes requires temperatures that are about 1.1°C or 2°F lower than temperatures found elsewhere in the body.

A mature spermatozoan lacks an endoplasmic reticulum, a Golgi apparatus, lysosomes, peroxisomes, and many other intracellular structures. The loss of these organelles reduces the cell's size and mass. Spermatozoa are basically mobile carriers for the enclosed chromosomes and can be slowed down by an extra weight. Because the sperm cell lacks glycogen and other energy reserves, it must absorb fructose and other nutrients from the surrounding fluid.

In a male embryo, spermatogenic cells are undifferentiated. Also called **spermatogonia**, they contain 46 chromosomes. During embryonic development, spermatogonia undergo mitosis, creating two daughter cells. One of these is a new "type A" spermatogonium that maintains supplies of undifferentiated cells, whereas the other is a "type B" spermatogonium that enlarges to become a primary spermatocyte.

During puberty, primary spermatocytes reproduce via **meiosis**, a type of cell division that includes first and second meiotic divisions (**FIGURE 23-5**). It is different from *mitosis*, which is the process by which most body cells divide. Meiosis I is the first division, which separates chromosome pairs that are *homologous*, meaning "gene for gene." This does not mean they are identical, because genes may vary because of hereditary factors. Meiosis is also called *reductional division* because 46 chromosomes are reduced to 23. Each homologous chromosome is replicated before meiosis I occurs, so it consists of two complete DNA strands called *chromatids*.

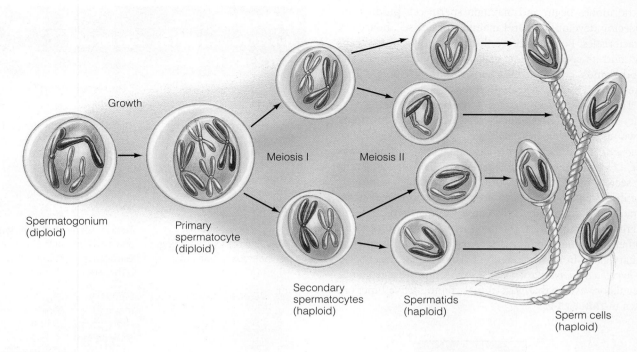

Growth

Spermatogonium
(diploid)

Meiosis I

Primary
spermatocyte
(diploid)

Meiosis II

Secondary
spermatocytes
(haploid)

Spermatids
(haploid)

Sperm cells
(haploid)

FIGURE 23-5 Meiosis.

These attach at areas called centromeres and carry all the genetic information associated with that specific chromosome. Each of the four daughter cells produced have half as many chromosomes as a typical *diploid* body cell. In meiosis, corresponding maternal and paternal chromosomes unite during *synapsis*.

Meiosis II causes one member of each homologous pair, via a condition called **haploid**, to separate its chromatids. This produces other haploid cells, with one set of chromosomes, but with the chromosomes no longer in the replicated form. Meiosis II causes each of the chromatids to become an independent chromosome. Each primary spermatocyte divides into two secondary spermatocytes; these divide again to form two spermatids, which mature. For each primary spermatocyte that undergoes meiosis, four sperm cells, with 23 chromosomes in each of their nuclei, are formed. A matched set of four chromatids is known as a *tetrad*. Meiosis II is also known as *equational division* because the number of chromosomes is not changed.

The final part of spermatogenesis is called *spermiogenesis*, in which each spermatid matures into a single sperm or *spermatozoon*. The Sertoli cells are also called *nurse cells* because they assist in the steps of spermatogenesis. A summary of these steps is as follows: (1) maintenance of the blood–testis barrier, (2) support of mitosis and meiosis, (3) support of spermiogenesis, (4) secretion of inhibin, (5) secretion of androgen-binding protein, and (6) secretion of müllerian-inhibiting factor. *Müllerian-inhibiting factor* is a hormone that causes regression of the *paramesonephric ducts* in the fetus, which eventually form the uterine tubes and uterus in females. When there is not enough of this hormone, the testes fail to descend into the scrotum.

FOCUS ON PATHOLOGY

Mostly because of sperm quantity or quality, about one in seven couples in the United States seek treatment for infertility. Factors widely believed to contribute to male infertility include xenobiotics from environmental toxins, solvents, polyvinyl chlorides, herbicides, pesticides, and compounds that act like estrogens, blocking actions of male sex hormones. Other factors may include tetracycline and other antibiotics, lead, radiation, selenium deficiencies, marijuana, and excessive alcohol use. Additional causes of male infertility may include calcium channel abnormalities, anatomic obstructions, oxidative stress, hormonal imbalances, overuse of hot tubs, and fever.

TEST YOUR UNDERSTANDING

1. Summarize the events of spermatogenesis.
2. List the major structural and functional regions of sperm.
3. Define the term *meiosis* and contrast it with mitosis.

Hormonal Regulation

Male reproductive functions are controlled by hormones from the hypothalamus, anterior pituitary gland, and testes.

The hormones begin and maintain sperm cell production, overseeing development and maintenance of secondary sex characteristics. Before puberty, the male body cannot reproduce, and its spermatogenic cells are undifferentiated. The hypothalamus controls the changes during puberty that make a male's body able to reproduce.

The hypothalamus secretes gonadotropin-releasing hormone, and the anterior pituitary secretes the **gonadotropins** known as *luteinizing hormone (LH)* and *follicle-stimulating hormone (FSH)*. Also known as *interstitial cell stimulating hormone*, LH promotes development of testicular interstitial cells that secrete male sex hormones. FSH stimulates seminiferous tubule cells to respond to the male sex hormone testosterone. These supporting cells cause spermatogenic cells to undergo spermatogenesis, creating sperm cells (**FIGURE 23-6**). Another hormone, inhibin, is secreted, keeping the anterior pituitary gland from oversecreting FSH via negative feedback. The *hypothalamic-pituitary-gonadal axis* comprises a sequence of regulatory events that govern male reproductive function, shown in **TABLE 23-2**.

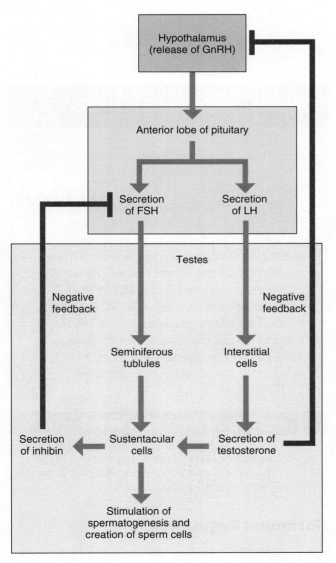

FIGURE 23-6 The hypothalamic-pituitary-gonadal axis.

TABLE 23-2

Hypothalamic-Pituitary-Gonadal Axis

Event	Result
Hypothalamus releases GnRH	Controls release of FSH and LH
GnRH binds to pituitary gonadotropic cells	These cells secrete FSH and LH into the blood
FSH stimulates spermatogenesis by stimulating release of androgen-binding protein	Keeps testosterone concentration near spermatogenic cells high, stimulating spermatogenesis
LH binds to interstitial endocrine cells surrounding seminiferous tubules	Tubules secrete testosterone and small amounts of estrogen; spermatogenesis is triggered
Testosterone enters the bloodstream	Stimulates sex organ maturation, secondary sex characteristics, and sex drive (libido)
Testosterone feeds back to inhibit hypothalamic release of GnRH	Acts directly on the anterior pituitary to inhibit gonadotropin release
High sperm count causes more inhibin to be released	Inhibits anterior pituitary release of FSH and hypothalamic release of GnRH

Androgens are the male sex hormones. They are mostly produced by the testicular interstitial cells, although the adrenal cortex synthesizes small amounts of them. **Testosterone** is the most important androgen, loosely attaching to plasma proteins for secretion and transport via the blood. Secretion begins during fetal development, continues for several weeks after birth, and almost stops completely during childhood. Between ages 13 and 15 it restarts, producing testosterone at a rapid rate and making the body reproductively functional. This period is known as **puberty**. Secretion continues after puberty throughout the life of males.

Testosterone enlarges the testes and accessory reproductive organs and develops the male secondary sex characteristics, as follows:

- Increased body hair on the face, chest, armpits, and pubic region
- Sometimes, decreased hair growth on the scalp
- Enlargement of the larynx and thickening of vocal folds, which lower the pitch of the voice
- Thickening of the skin
- Increased muscular growth, broadening of shoulders, and narrowing of waist
- Thickening and strengthening of the bones

Testosterone also increases cellular metabolism and red blood cell production. Males usually have more red blood cells in a microliter of blood than females do because of the actions of testosterone. It also affects the brain, stimulating sexual activity.

The more testosterone received by the interstitial cells, the greater the speed at which the male secondary sex characteristics develop. Testosterone output is regulated by a negative feedback system in the hypothalamus. More testosterone in the blood inhibits the hypothalamus, decreasing gonadotropin-releasing hormone (GnRH) secretion from the anterior pituitary. As LH secretion also falls, testosterone release from the interstitial cells decreases. Decreasing blood testosterone causes the hypothalamus to stimulate the anterior pituitary to release LH. Then the interstitial cells release more testosterone, and the blood testosterone levels increase again. A period in a man's life known as the *male climacteric* marks a decrease in testosterone level and a decline in sexual function.

The amount of testosterone and sperm produced reflects a balance among GnRH, FSH, and LH. GnRH indirectly stimulates the testes through its effect on FSH and LH release. Both FSH and LH directly stimulate the testes. Testosterone and inhibin exert negative feedback controls on the hypothalamus and anterior pituitary.

In puberty, this balance is achieved over about 3 years. Then, produced testosterone and sperm remain in basically constant amounts throughout life. When GnRH and gonadotropins are absent, the testes atrophy. Sperm and testosterone production then stops. Near puberty, higher levels of testosterone are needed to suppress GnRH release from the hypothalamus. More GnRH release causes more testosterone to be secreted by the testes. However, the hypothalamic inhibition threshold continually rises until the adult levels of hormone interaction are developed.

Testosterone, like all other steroid hormones, is synthesized from cholesterol. It works by activating certain genes, resulting in increased protein synthesis in target cells. This may require testosterone to be transformed into other steroid hormones in some target cells. In the prostate, it is converted to *dihydrotestosterone* and in certain brain neurons to *estradiol*. Throughout puberty, testosterone also has a variety of anabolic effects in the body. It causes accessory reproductive organs to mature. Without it, all accessory organs atrophy, erection and ejaculation are impaired, and semen volume decreases greatly. The results are impotence and sterility. However, testosterone replacement therapy is very successful.

The *male secondary sex characteristics* occur in the nonreproductive organs because of the effects of testosterone and other androgens. These are development of hair in the facial, axillary, and pubic regions; increased hair growth elsewhere on the body; a deepening of the voice due to larynx enlargement; skin thickening; increased oil production that may result in *acne*; increased bone density and size; and increased skeletal muscle mass. In males, testosterone increases the basal metabolic rate and changes behavior. Male libido is based on the effects of testosterone.

Anatomy of the Female Reproductive System

The anatomy of the female reproductive system is highly complex in comparison with that of the male, and the female reproductive and urinary tracts are totally separated. The female reproductive organs produce and maintain the egg cells or *oocytes*, which are the female sex cells. The organs also transport them to the site of fertilization, provide a strong environment for the developing fetus, give birth to a fetus, and produce female sex hormones. The principal organs of the female reproductive system, besides the ovaries, are the uterine tubes, uterus, vagina, and the components of the *external genitalia*. The primary sex organs or *gonads* are the two ovaries, which reproduce female sex cells and sex hormones. The accessory sex organs are the internal and external reproductive organs (**FIGURE 23-7**). As in males, a variety of accessory glands releases secretions into the female reproductive tract. The female internal genitalia are primarily located in the pelvic cavity and include the ovaries and duct system. The accessory ducts include the uterine tubes, uterus, and vagina.

Ovaries

The female gonads or **ovaries** are oval-shaped, solid structures about 3.5 cm long, 2 cm wide, and 1 cm thick. They lie in shallow depressions in the lateral pelvic cavity wall, on either side of the uterus. The ovaries are suspended by several ligaments in the peritoneal cavity, where the iliac blood vessels split into a "fork." Each ovary is anchored medially to the uterus by an **ovarian ligament** and laterally to the pelvic wall by the **suspensory ligament**. Also, a **mesovarium** suspends each ovary in between these points. The mesovarium and suspensory ligament are part of a **broad ligament**, which folds over the uterus to support the uterus, uterine tubes, and vagina. The ovarian ligaments are enclosed by the broad ligament.

The *ovarian arteries* serve the ovaries and are branches of the abdominal aorta. The ovaries are also served by the ovarian branch of the uterine arteries. To reach the ovaries, the ovarian blood vessels must travel through the mesovaria and suspensory ligaments.

Each ovary is externally surrounded by a fibrous *tunica albuginea*. This structure is then covered by a cuboidal epithelial cell layer that is known as the *germinal epithelium*. This epithelium is a continuation of the peritoneum. Each ovary additionally has an outer cortex enclosing the developing gametes. An inner medulla contains the primary blood vessels and nerves. However, the relative area of each region is not well defined.

Many small structures called **ovarian follicles** resemble sacs and are embedded in the cortex of each ovary, which is highly vascular and made of connective tissue. One oocyte is found in each follicle, incased in a variety of cells. If only

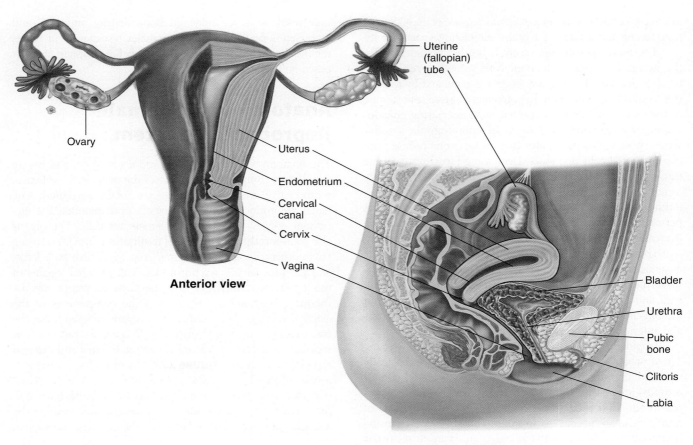

FIGURE 23-7 The female reproductive organs.

a single layer is present, these are called **follicle cells**, but if more than one layer is present, they are called **granulosa cells** (**FIGURE 23-8**).

In women of childbearing age, one ripening follicle ejects its oocyte from an ovary every month in a process called *ovulation*. The ruptured follicle then changes its appearance, becoming a glandular structure, the *corpus luteum*. This structure soon degenerates. The surfaces of the ovaries show pits and scars in older women because they have released many oocytes over a lifetime.

Ovarian tissues consist of an inner medulla and an outer cortex. The medulla is made up of loose connective tissue

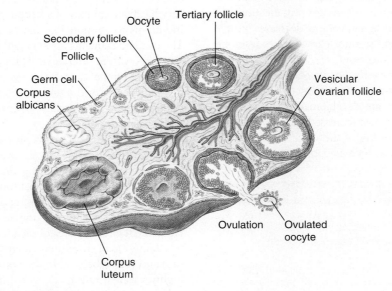

FIGURE 23-8 Ovarian follicle development.

with many blood and lymphatic vessels as well as nerve fibers. The cortex has more compact tissue with a granular appearance because of masses of ovarian follicles. The ovary's free surface is covered with cuboidal epithelium above a layer of dense connective tissue. The almond-shaped ovaries perform three main functions: production of immature female gametes called *oocytes*; secretion of female sex hormones, including estrogens and progestins; and secretion of inhibin, which is involved in the feedback control of pituitary FSH production. The most common form of estrogen is *estradiol*, followed by *estrone* and *estriol*.

Before birth, a female fetus develops small cell groups in the outer ovarian cortex that form several million **primordial follicles**. Each follicle consists of a primary oocyte surrounded by follicular cells. The primary oocytes begin to undergo meiosis early in development, but then the process stops and does not restart until puberty. No new primordial follicles form after the initial ones form, and oocytes degenerate. Although several million oocytes form in the female embryo, only about 1 million remain at birth, with only 400,000 left at puberty. The ovary releases less than 400 to 500 oocytes during a female's reproductive life.

Female Duct System

The female duct system has no or very little contact with the ovaries. The female reproductive system includes accessory structures, including two uterine tubes, a uterus, and a vagina.

Uterine Tubes

The **uterine tubes**, also called the *fallopian tubes* or *oviducts*, receive the ovulated oocytes from the ovaries and are each about 10 cm (4 inches) long. The uterine tubes are the sites where fertilization usually occurs. Each uterine tube empties into the superolateral area of the uterus via a constricted **isthmus**. As it curves around the ovary, each uterine tube's distal end expands to form an *ampulla*. Near the ovaries, each tube expands into a funnel-shaped **infundibulum** that partially encircles the ovary. Finger-like fimbriae surround its margin with one of the larger extensions connecting with the ovary.

The epithelium lining the uterine tube is composed of ciliated columnar epithelial cells, with scattered mucin-secreting cells. The mucosa is surrounded by concentric smooth muscle layers. The transport of oocytes involves a combination of ciliary movement and peristaltic contractions in the uterine tube walls. Nonciliated mucosal cells have dense microvilli and produce secretions that keep oocytes as well as any present sperm nourished and moist. The uterine tubes are externally covered by peritoneum, supported by a short mesentery called the **mesosalpinx**. This structure is actually part of the broad ligament.

Uterus

If the secondary oocyte is fertilized to become a zygote, the **uterus** receives the developing embryo, sustaining

FOCUS ON PATHOLOGY

Ectopic pregnancies may occur because the uterine tubes are not continuous with the ovaries. If an oocyte is fertilized elsewhere instead of the uterine tubes, such as the peritoneal cavity or distal part of the uterine tubes, it starts to develop there. Without enough mass and blood supply to support a full-term pregnancy, ectopic pregnancies often result in natural spontaneous abortion, causing hemorrhaging.

Infections can also spread from other reproductive tract areas into the peritoneal cavity. A condition known as *pelvic inflammatory disease* may develop if sexually transmitted microorganisms cause infection here. Broad-spectrum antibiotics are required immediately because pelvic inflammatory disease can scar the uterine tubes and ovaries, leading to sterility. Female infertility is often linked to scarring and closure of the uterine tubes.

its development. The uterus is hollow and muscular, shaped slightly like an inverted pear. Its size changes during pregnancy, from about 7.5 cm by 5 cm by 2.5 cm to much larger, able to hold the developing baby up until birth. At this point, it weighs 30 to 40 g. The uterus is located in the anterior pelvic cavity, superior to the vagina, usually bending over the urinary bladder. The uterine body is also called the *corpus*, the largest portion of the uterus. The **fundus** is the rounded portion of the corpus and is superior to the attachment of the uterine tubes. It ends at the constriction known as the *isthmus*. The **cervix** is the inferior portion of the uterus, extending from the isthmus to the vagina. The cervix surrounds the cervical orifice, where the uterus opens to the vagina. The uterine wall is thick, with three layers. The **endometrium** is the inner mucosal layer, covered with columnar epithelium and many tubular glands. It is made up of a *functional zone*, which is the layer nearest to the uterine cavity, and a *basilar zone*, which is near the myometrium.

Normally, the uterus is *anteverted*, which means *inclined forward*. In older women, it is often *retroverted*, which means *inclined backward*. The **cervical canal** communicates with the vagina through the *external os* and also with the uterine body cavity through the *internal os*. Cervical glands exist in the mucosa of the cervical canal and secrete mucus that fills the cervical canal and also covers the external os. This is believed to block bacteria from spreading into the uterus from the vagina. In most times during the uterine cycle, this cervical mucus blocks sperm entry. However, it allows sperm to pass through at the midpoint of the cycle, which is when it becomes less viscous.

Uterine Supporting Structures

Additional supports of the uterus include the *mesometrium*, laterally, and other ligaments. The **cardinal ligaments**, also called *lateral cervical ligaments*, extend from the cervix and superior vagina to the lateral pelvic walls more inferiorly than the mesometrium. Two **uterosacral ligaments** secure the uterus to the sacrum, posteriorly. Fibrous **round ligaments** bind the uterus to the anterior body wall. They pass through the inguinal canals, anchoring in the labia majora's subcutaneous tissue. Collectively, these ligaments allow the uterus to be quite movable, accommodating filling and emptying of the bladder and rectum.

Layers of the Uterine Wall

The three layers of the wall of the uterus are the **perimetrium**, **myometrium**, and endometrium. The perimetrium is the outer, incomplete, serous layer. The myometrium is the thick middle layer. It is made of interlaced smooth muscle bundles, and contracts rhythmically during childbirth, expelling the baby from the uterus.

The endometrium is the mucosal lining, made of simple columnar epithelium above an underlying, thick lamina propria. Fertilization causes the embryo to implant into the endometrium for the entire pregnancy. There are two chief layers or *strata* in the endometrium. The functional layer is the *stratum functionalis*, which changes based on ovarian hormone levels in the blood. This layer is shed during menstruation, about every 28 days. The basal layer is the *stratum basalis*, which is thinner. It forms a new stratum functionalis after menstruation. This layer does not respond to ovarian hormones. Many uterine glands in the endometrium change, lengthwise, along with the endometrial thickness changes that occur.

The cyclic changes of the uterine endometrium is linked to its vascular supply. From the internal iliacs of the pelvis arise the *uterine arteries*. They ascend along the sides of the uterus, branching into the uterine wall. The branches split into several *arcuate arteries* inside the myometrium. These arteries continue as *radial arteries* into the endometrium. Here, *straight arteries* supply the stratum basalis, whereas *spiral, coiled arteries* supply the stratum functionalis. The spiral arteries degenerate and regenerate continuously. When they spasm, these actions cause the functionalis layer to be shed during the menstrual cycle. In the endometrium, the veins have thin walls. They form an extensive network with small amounts of sinusoidal enlargements.

Painful menstruation is known as *dysmenorrhea*. It may be caused by inflammation of the uterus, myometrial contractions commonly known as *cramps*, or conditions that involve nearby pelvic structures.

Vagina

The **vagina** is a thin-walled fibromuscular tube, about 8 to 10 cm (3 to 4 inches) in length, extending from the cervix to the outside of the body. It conveys uterine secretions, receives the erect penis during intercourse, and provides the

open channel for offspring. The vagina extends up and back into the pelvic cavity and lies posterior to the urinary bladder and urethra but anterior to the rectum. The urethra is parallel to the course of the vagina anteriorly. The vagina is attached to these other structures by connective tissues.

The **hymen** is a thin membrane of connective tissue and epithelium that partially covers the vaginal orifice in females who have not had sexual intercourse. It has a central opening that allows uterine and vaginal secretions to pass to the outside of the body. The hymen is extremely vascular and may bleed when it stretches or ruptures during initial sexual intercourse. It can also be ruptured by insertion of tampons, sports activities, or pelvic examinations. In rare cases, it is tougher than normal and requires a surgical procedure for normal intercourse to occur.

The three major functions of the vagina are to serve as a passageway for the elimination of menstrual fluids, to receive the penis during sexual intercourse, and to hold the spermatozoa before their passage into the uterus. The vagina forms the interior portion of the *birth canal*, through which the fetus passes during delivery.

The vaginal wall has three layers:

- *Inner mucosal layer (mucosa):* Stratified squamous epithelium with no mucous glands. Dendritic cells act as antigen-presenting cells. They may be the route of HIV transmission from an infected male. This layer has no glands but is lubricated by the cervical mucous glands. It also has a mucosal transudate that leaks from the vaginal walls. Large amounts of glycogen are released by its epithelia, which are metabolized anaerobically by bacteria to form lactic acid. Therefore, the pH is very acidic, which helps to fight infections but is harmful to sperm. Because this fluid is alkaline instead of acidic in adolescent girls, they are predisposed to STIs if they are sexually active.
- *Middle muscular layer (muscularis):* Mostly smooth muscle fibers; helps to close the vaginal opening.
- *Outer fibrous layer (adventitia):* Dense connective tissue and elastic fibers.

The **vaginal fornix** is a recess produced at the upper end of the vaginal canal, which loosely surrounds the cervix. The *posterior fornix* is much deeper than the *lateral and anterior fornices*. The lumen of the vagina is basically small, and its posterior and anterior walls touch each other, except where the cervix keeps it open. During sexual intercourse and childbirth, the vagina can stretch considerably. However, ischial spines and the sacrospinous ligaments limit its lateral distention. When various microorganisms cause inflammation and infection of the vagina, it is known as *vaginitis*.

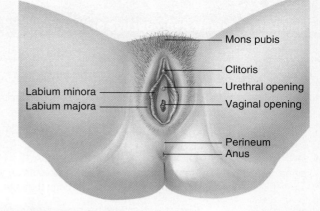

FIGURE 23-9 Female external genitalia.

The **labia minora** are flattened, hairless longitudinal folds composed of connective tissue. They contain the external openings of the urethra and vagina. They have a rich blood supply and therefore a pinkish appearance. They merge posteriorly with the labia majora to form a ridge called the **fourchette**. Anteriorly, they converge to form the hood-like covering of the clitoris.

The **clitoris** projects from the anterior end of the vulva between the labia minora. It is usually about 2 cm in length and 0.5 cm in diameter. It corresponds to the penis in males, with a similar structure. It is made up of two columns of erectile tissue called the *corpora cavernosa* and forms a glans at its anterior end that has many sensory nerve fibers. The exposed portion is called the *glans of the clitoris*, and the hooded fold is called the *prepuce of the clitoris*. The clitoris has a rich innervation of sensory nerve endings and swells with blood, becoming erect during tactile stimulation and sexual arousal.

The labia minora encloses the **vestibule**, into which the vagina opens posteriorly. The urethra opens into the vestibule in the midline, about 2.5 cm posterior to the glans of the clitoris. One pea-sized **vestibular gland** lies on each side of the vaginal opening, which is similar to the bulbourethral glands of males. They release mucus into the vestibule, moistening and lubricating it for intercourse. Under the vestibule's mucosa, on either side, is a mass of vascular erectile tissue called the **vestibular bulb**. These bulbs are similar to the single penile bulb and corpus spongiosum in males. They engorge with blood during sexual stimulation, helping the vagina to grip the penis and causing the urethral orifice to shut. This prevents semen and bacteria from moving superiorly into the bladder as intercourse occurs. **TABLE 23-3** summarizes the functions of the female reproductive organs.

External Genitalia

The external accessory organs of the female reproductive system include the **mons pubis**, labia majora, labia minora, clitoris, and vestibular glands (**FIGURE 23-9**). They surround the openings of the urethra and vagina, composing the **vulva** or *pudendum*. The *mons pubis* is a rounded area made of fatty tissue that overlies the pubic symphysis. This area becomes covered with pubic hair after puberty.

The **labia majora** enclose and protect the other external reproductive organs. They are made up of rounded folds of adipose tissue and thin smooth muscle covered by skin and hair. They lie close together, with a cleft that includes the urethral and vaginal openings separating the labia longitudinally. The labia majora are analogous to the male scrotum and enclose the labia minora.

Mammary Glands

The **mammary glands** are specialized to secrete milk after pregnancy. They are located in the subcutaneous tissue of the anterior thorax, within the breasts. The breasts are above the pectoralis major muscles, extending from the second to the sixth ribs, from the sternum to the axillae. They lie within the superficial fascia, also known as the *hypodermis*.

TABLE 23-3

Functions of Female Reproductive Organs

Organ	Function
Ovaries	Female reproductive organs that produce oocytes and sex hormones
Uterine tubes	Transport secondary oocytes in the direction of the uterus; fertilization occurs here, with the developing embryo conveyed to the uterus
Uterus	Muscular organ of the female reproductive tract, in which implantation, placenta formation, and fetal development occur
Vagina	Transports uterine secretions to outside of the body, receives the erect penis during intercourse; the fully developed fetus passes through the vagina during normal delivery
Labia majora	Protect and enclose the external reproductive organs
Labia minora	Protect the openings of the vagina and urethra
Clitoris	Gives pleasurable sensations during sexual stimulation
Vestibule	Contains the vaginal and urethral openings
Vestibular glands	Moisten and lubricate the vestibule with a secretion

The subcutaneous tissue of a *pectoral fat pad*, which is deep to the skin of the chest, contains each mammary gland.

Just below the center of each breast is an **areola**, which is a ring of pigmented skin. The areola is slightly bumpy because of large sebaceous glands and produces sebum to reduce cracking and chapping of the **nipple**, which is located near the tip of each breast, within the areola surrounding it (**FIGURE 23-10**). Smooth muscle fibers in the areola and nipple are controlled by the autonomic nervous system. This can cause the nipple to become erect when it is stimulated by touch or cold temperatures. Although present in males, the mammary glands have no function.

Each mammary gland is a modified sweat gland, made up of 15 to 25 lobes that contain alveolar glands and an alveolar duct, which leads to a lactiferous duct. This leads to the nipple. The lobes are separated by dense adipose and connective tissues. Dense suspensory ligaments extend inward to help support the weight of the breast. *Lobules* are smaller units inside the lobes. They contain glandular *alveoli*, which produce milk during lactation. Milk is passed from these compound alveolar glands into **lactiferous ducts**, which open to the outside of the nipple. Each duct, just below the areola, has a dilated *lactiferous sinus*, where milk accumulates during nursing. As female children reach puberty, their mammary glands develop because of ovarian hormones. The alveolar glands and ducts enlarge. Fatty tissue deposits around and within the breasts.

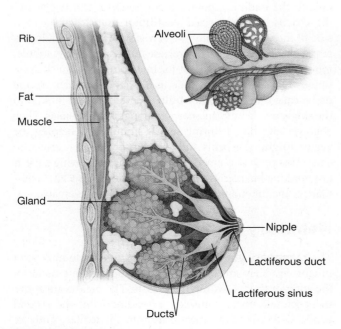

FIGURE 23-10 The mammary gland.

FOCUS ON PATHOLOGY

Invasive breast cancer is the second most common malignancy and also the second most common cause of cancer death in American women. It affects about 13% of the female population, arising from the epithelial cells of the smallest breast ducts. Cancer cells form a lump, and cells metastasize from this. Risk factors include family history, early onset menstruation, late menopause, no pregnancies, first pregnancy later in life, and no periods or only short periods of breast-feeding.

Unfortunately, more than 70% of women who develop breast cancer have no known risk factors. It is diagnosed by skin texture changes, puckering of the skin, and nipple leakage. Simple, regular breast self-examinations can find abnormalities before they have progressed significantly.

Mammography, the x-ray examination that detects very small breast cancers, should be performed in women over 40 years of age every year. When diagnosed, breast cancer is treated with radiation therapy, chemotherapy, and/or surgery. Drug therapies are used for estrogen-responsive breast cancers. Surgically, most physicians now recommend *lumpectomy*, which removes just the cancerous lump, or *simple mastectomy*, which removes only breast tissue and, sometimes, a portion of the axillary lymph nodes.

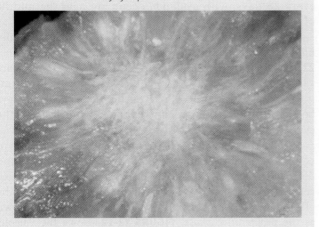

Breast biopsy. (Courtesy of Leonard V. Crowley, MD, Century College.)

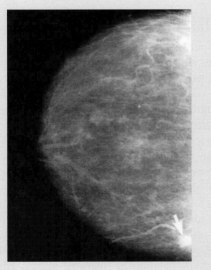

Mammogram. (Courtesy of Dr. Dwight Kaufman, National Cancer Institute.)

TEST YOUR UNDERSTANDING

1. Describe the structures of the external genitalia.
2. Explain the components of the mammary glands.
3. Identify risk factors for breast cancer.

Physiology of the Female Reproductive System

Females release egg cells only from puberty to menopause, which occurs, on average, at around age 51. Although today we know that egg stem cells continue to survive throughout life, it has not yet been proven that the cells are viable for reproduction. Physiology of the female reproductive system includes the processes of oogenesis, the ovarian cycle, hormonal regulation, the uterine or *menstrual* cycle, and the female sexual response.

Oogenesis

Oogenesis is the process of egg cell formation, producing female sex cells. During the fetal period, the diploid stem cells of the ovaries or *oogonia* multiply quickly, via mitosis. Eventually, *primordial follicles* appear, whereas the oogonia change into *primary oocytes*. They are surrounded by one layer of flattened *follicle cells*. The first meiotic division is begun by the primary oocytes. However, they stall in the late part of *prophase I* and do not complete their division.

At birth, a female infant is believed to have a certain finite amount of primary oocytes. Although there were 7 million oocytes originally, at birth about 1 million have survived programmed death. They are located in the cortical region of each immature ovary. By puberty, approximately 300,000 oocytes remain. Primordial follicles change into an enlarging collection of primary follicles over time. This process starts during the fetal period and continues until there are no more primordial follicles. At this time, *menopause* begins. In rare conditions, menopause occurs before age 40 and is known as *premature menopause*.

Oogenesis in the ovaries at puberty takes years for completion. During this time, some primary oocytes continue meiosis, with 23 chromosomes in their nuclei like their parent cells. When they divide, the distribution of the oocyte cytoplasm is unequal. The cells that result are different in size. FSH protects small numbers of growing follicles from programmed cell death every month. In every cycle, one of these follicles becomes the *dominant follicle* and continues meiosis I. This eventually produces two haploid cells, each of which have 23 replicated chromosomes, which are very different in size.

The secondary oocyte is large, whereas the *first polar body* is small (**FIGURE 23-11**). The large *secondary oocyte* can be fertilized by a sperm cell. Maturing follicles that were not selected undergo atresia. These events mean that the polar body receives nearly no cytoplasm or organelles. A spindle forms at the edge of the oocyte, and a small nipple-like structure also appears. The chromosomes from the polar body move into it.

The first polar body may continually develop and undergo meiosis II, with two smaller polar bodies being produced. The secondary oocyte stops functioning in metaphase II, and this is the cell that is ovulated. When no sperm

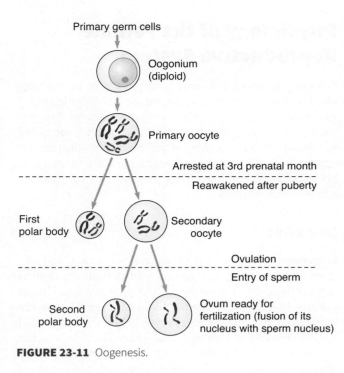

Primary germ cells

Oogonium
(diploid)

Primary oocyte

Arrested at 3rd prenatal month

Reawakened after puberty

First
polar body

Secondary
oocyte

Ovulation

Entry of sperm

Second
polar body

Ovum ready for
fertilization (fusion of its
nucleus with sperm nucleus)

FIGURE 23-11 Oogenesis.

penetrates an ovulated secondary oocyte, it deteriorates. However, if penetration by a sperm occurs, the oocyte completes meiosis II quickly. This produces a tiny *second polar body* and a large fertilized egg cell called a **zygote**. The joining of the egg and sperm nuclei constitutes *fertilization*.

The polar bodies soon degenerate. They allow for production of egg cells with massive amounts of cytoplasm and abundant organelles that carry the zygote through its first cell divisions, still with the right number of chromosomes.

During puberty, the anterior pituitary gland secretes higher amounts of FSH, enlarging the ovaries. The primordial follicles mature into **primary follicles**. During maturation, a primary oocyte enlarges and the surrounding follicular cells proliferate via mitosis. They organize into layers, with a cavity called the *antrum* appearing in the cellular mass. Clear follicular fluid fills the cavity to bathe the primary oocyte. The cavity moves the primary oocyte to one side.

Eventually, the mature follicle becomes 10 mm or greater in diameter, bulging outward on the ovary surface. The secondary oocyte is large and round, surrounded by a glycoprotein called the *zona pellucida*. The secondary oocyte is attached to follicular cells called the corona radiata. The follicular cells have processes extending through the zona pellucida that supply the secondary oocyte with nutrients. Up to 20 primary follicles mature at once, but 1 follicle usually grows larger than the others. Usually just the dominant follicle develops fully, whereas the others degenerate. Enlargement and multiplication of the granulosa cells cause adjacent cells in the ovarian stroma to form a *thecal cell layer* around the follicle. These cells, along with granulosa cells, produce estrogens.

Ovarian Cycle

The female reproductive cycle involves regular, recurring changes in the uterine lining and menstrual bleeding or *menses*. This monthly cycle usually begins around 13 years of age, continues into middle age, and then ceases during *menopause*. A female's first reproductive cycle is called **menarche**. It occurs once the ovaries and other reproductive organs have matured and started responding to specific hormones. Secretion of GnRH stimulates threshold levels of FSH and LH to be released. FSH stimulates maturation of ovarian follicles. Follicular cells produce increased estrogens and some progesterone. LH stimulates some ovarian cells to secrete precursors, such as testosterone, which are used to produce estrogens. This *ovarian cycle* occurs every 28 days, with *ovulation* occurring near the middle of the cycle.

Interestingly, only 10% to 15% of women actually have 28-day cycles. The ovarian cycle may range between 21 and 40 days in actuality. When this is the case, there are variations in the length of the follicular phase and the timing of actual ovulation. However, the luteal phase always begins on the 14th day after ovulation and lasts to the cycle's end.

In younger females, estrogens stimulate development of the secondary sex characteristics. They maintain and develop these characteristics as time passes. Increased estrogens during the first week of a reproductive cycle thicken the glandular endometrium of the uterine lining. This is known as the *proliferative phase*. **FIGURE 23-12** shows the various phases of the female reproductive cycle.

Follicular Phase

The first part of the *follicular phase* is known as the *preantral phase*, which is not dependent on gonadotropin. This is when cytokines, growth factors, and other intrafollicular paracrines control development of oocytes and follicles. The second *antral phase* is controlled by FSH and LH. Activated follicles grow greatly, and the primary oocyte in the dominant follicle restarts meiosis I.

In the *follicular phase* the developing follicle matures, and by approximately day 14 of the cycle it appears on the surface of the ovary as a blister-like bulge. Follicular cells inside the follicle loosen and follicular fluid accumulates. The maturing follicle secretes estrogens that inhibit the anterior pituitary from releasing LH but allow it to be stored. Anterior pituitary cells become more sensitive to GnRH secreted from the hypothalamus in rhythmic pulses. The stored LH is released, weakening and rupturing the bulging follicular wall. This sends the secondary oocyte and fluid from the ovary, in the process of *ovulation*. The space containing the follicular fluid fills with blood, which clots.

Near the end of follicle maturation, the primary oocyte finishes meiosis I. A secondary oocyte and first polar body are formed, readying the cycle for ovulation. The granulosa cells signal the oocyte to stop the completion of meiosis. Follicle growth from the primordial stage to this point is believed to

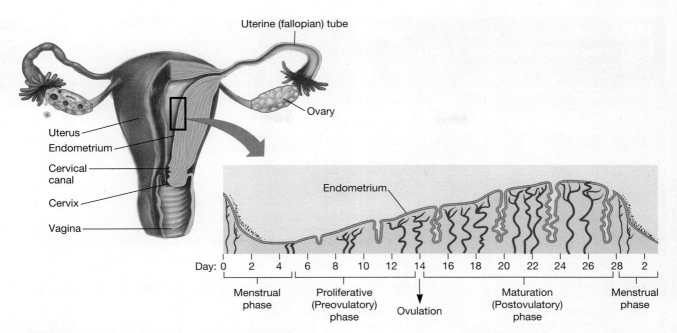

FIGURE 23-12 Endometrial changes during the female reproductive cycle.

take about 1 year. Therefore, each follicle that ovulates was actually beginning to grow between 10 and 12 ovarian cycles previously.

Ovulation

The primary oocyte undergoes oogenesis, developing a secondary oocyte and first polar body. This is known as **ovulation**. This process releases these developed structures along with one or two layers of follicular cells from the mature follicle. Anterior pituitary gland hormones trigger ovulation, swelling the mature follicle while weakening its wall. The wall ruptures, allowing the fluid and secondary oocyte to be expelled into the peritoneal cavity while still surrounded by the corona radiata. There may be a slight pain in the lower abdomen at the moment this occurs. Although the cause is actually unknown, it may be due to extreme stretching of the ovarian wall and irritation of the peritoneum by blood or fluid from the ruptured follicle.

Every adult women has several follicles that are continually at different stages of maturation. Because of this, one follicle is at the perfect stage of maturation when LH stimulates ovulation. Antral follicles survive because of FSH, which helps to select the dominant follicle, although this actual process is not fully understood. It is believed to add the largest amount of gonadotropin receptors, attaining the most FSH sensitivity at the fastest rate. Other follicles undergo apoptosis and are reabsorbed by the body.

Luteal Phase

The follicular cells enlarge to form a temporary **corpus luteum** after the ruptured follicle or *corpus hemorrhagicum* is absorbed. This *luteal phase* is when the corpus luteum

is active. Corpus luteum cells secrete large amounts of progesterone and estrogens during the last half of the cycle, and blood progesterone concentration increases sharply. Progesterone causes the endometrium to become more vascular and glandular while stimulating uterine gland secretion of more lipids and glycogen. This is known as the *secretory phase*. Endometrial tissues fill with fluids that are made up of nutrients and electrolytes, which support embryo development.

LH and FSH release is then inhibited, and no other follicles develop when the corpus luteum is active. If no egg cell is fertilized, on the 24th day of the cycle the corpus luteum begins to degenerate, to be replaced by connective tissue. The leftover remnant is called a *corpus albicans*. Then, estrogens and progesterone decline in level, and the endometrium constricts its blood vessels. The uterine lining starts to disintegrate and slough off. Damaged capillaries create a flow of blood and cellular debris, which passes through the vagina. This is called the *menstrual flow*. It usually begins approximately on the 28th day of the cycle, continuing for 3 to 5 days while estrogen concentrations are low. **TABLE 23-4** summarizes the female reproductive cycle. However, if the oocyte is fertilized, resulting in pregnancy, the corpus luteum continues to develop until the placenta assumes its hormone production duties. This occurs in approximately 3 months.

TEST YOUR UNDERSTANDING

1. Distinguish the function of estrogens and progesterone in the female reproductive system.
2. What is menarche?
3. What is a corpus luteum?

TABLE 23-4

Steps of the Female Reproductive Cycle

Structure	Function
Anterior pituitary gland	Secretes FSH and LH
Follicle	Maturation is stimulated by FSH
Follicular cells	Produces and secretes estrogens
	Estrogens maintain secondary sex characteristics.
Endometrium	Estrogens cause it to thicken.
Anterior pituitary gland	Releases a surge of LH, stimulating ovulation
Follicular cells	Become corpus luteum cells, secreting estrogens and progesterone
Uterine wall	Estrogens continue to stimulate its development.
Endometrium	Progesterone stimulates it to become more glandular and vascular.
Anterior pituitary gland	Estrogens and progesterone inhibit it from secreting LH and FSH.
Corpus luteum	If the egg cell is not fertilized, the corpus luteum degenerates and no longer secretes estrogens and progesterone.
Blood vessels in the endometrium	As concentrations of estrogens and progesterone decline, these vessels constrict.
Uterine lining	Disintegrates and sloughs off, producing menstrual flow
Anterior pituitary gland	No longer inhibited, it again secretes FSH and LH—and the reproductive cycle repeats.

Hormonal Regulation of the Ovarian Cycle

The female reproductive system is controlled by hormones, involving an interplay between pituitary gland and gonadal secretions. Female hormonal regulation is much more complicated than male hormonal regulation because it coordinates both the ovarian and uterine cycles.

The maturation of female sex cells, development and maintenance of secondary sex characteristics, and changes during the monthly reproductive cycle are controlled by the hypothalamus, anterior pituitary gland, and ovaries. Until about age 10, the female body is reproductively immature. When the hypothalamus begins to secrete more GnRH, the anterior pituitary releases FSH and LH, controlling female sex cell maturation and producing female sex hormones. The ovaries, adrenal cortices, and placenta secrete sex hormones during pregnancy that include **estrogens** and **progesterone**. The most abundant of the estrogens is *estradiol*, followed by *estrone* and *estriol*. Also, onset of puberty is linked to amounts of adipose tissue. *Leptin* is the hormone that informs the hypothalamus about these amounts. Puberty is delayed if blood levels of lipids and leptin are low.

In childhood, the ovaries are growing, with continuous secretion of only a small amount of estrogens. These keep the hypothalamus from releasing GnRH. With normal leptin levels, the hypothalamus becomes less sensitive to estrogen as puberty approaches. It starts to release GnRH rhythmically, with this hormone stimulating the anterior pituitary to release FSH and LH. As a result, the ovaries begin to secrete estrogens and other hormones in higher quantities. Gonadotropin levels increase continuously for approximately 4 years. Females at this stage are still not ovulating and pregnancy is not possible. In nonpregnant females, the ovaries are the main source of estrogens. Hormonal interactions stabilize eventually, and the adult ovarian cycle begins.

Estrogens and related hormones stimulate enlargement of accessory sex organs and develop and maintain the female secondary sex characteristics:

- Development of breasts and the mammary gland ductile systems
- Increasing adipose tissue deposition in the subcutaneous layer, breasts, thighs, and buttocks
- Increasing skin vascularization

The ovaries are also the main source of progesterone in nonpregnant females. Progesterone promotes uterine changes during the monthly cycle, affects the mammary glands, and helps regulate gonadotropin secretion. Concentrations of androgen in females at puberty produce different changes, including increased hair growth in the pubic region and armpits. The female skeleton responds to low androgen concentration by narrowing the shoulders and widening the hips.

Uterine Cycle

Controlled by estrogen, the uterine glands, blood vessels, and epithelium change with the phases of the **menstrual cycle**,

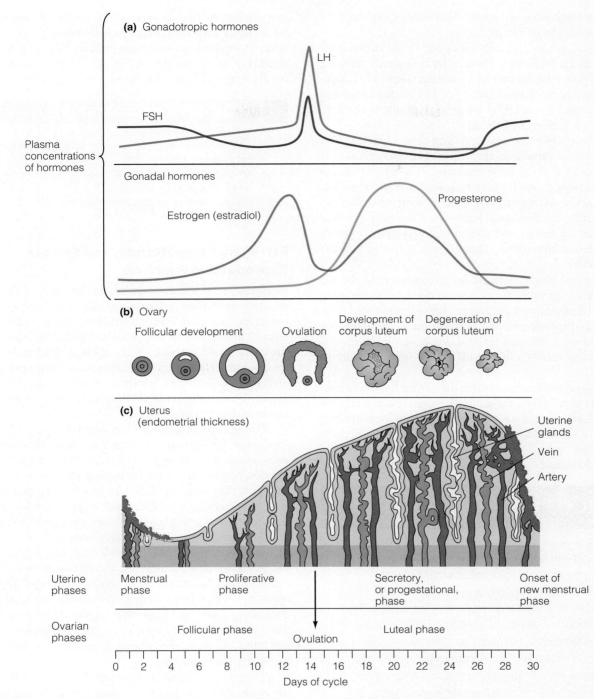

FIGURE 23-13 The menstrual cycle. (A) Hormonal cycles. (B) The ovarian cycle. (C) The uterine cycle.

which is also called the *uterine cycle*. It is coordinated with the ovarian cycle. The changes in this cycle can be divided up into a menstrual phase, proliferative or preovulatory phase, and a secretory, postovulatory phase (**FIGURE 23-13**).

The *menstrual phase* occurs during days 1 to 5. The uterus sheds all except the deepest part of its endometrium. Ovarian hormones are at their lowest normal levels, but gonadotropins are increasing. The functional layer of the endometrium is thick and depends on hormones. It detaches from the uterine wall, resulting in bleeding for 3 to 5 days.

Blood and detached tissue flow out through the vagina. By day 5, more estrogen is being produced by the ovarian follicles as they grow.

The *proliferative phase* occurs during days 6 to 14. The endometrium is rebuilt, influenced by the rise of estrogens in the blood. Its basal layer generates a new functional layer, which thickens. Its glands increase in size and the spiral arteries become more numerous. As a result, the endometrium returns to its earlier state: It is soft, smooth, thick, and well supplied with blood vessels. Estrogens cause the endometrial cells to synthesize progesterone receptors. This makes them ready for interaction with progesterone.

Cervical mucus is usually sticky and thick. However, as estrogen levels increase, it thins to form channels allowing sperm to pass into the uterus. Ovulation takes only 5 minutes, occurring on or about day 14 in the ovary as a response to a sudden release of LH by the anterior pituitary. The ruptured follicle is converted by LH to a corpus luteum.

The *secretory phase* occurs during days 15 to 28. This phase is not as variable as the others. The endometrium is readied for an embryo to be implanted. The corpus luteum increases progesterone levels, which affect the endometrium by causing the spiral arteries to become more extensive and by converting the functional layer into a secretory mucosa. In an effort to sustain an embryo, the endometrial glands become larger and coiled. They secrete nutrients into the uterine cavity.

A *cervical plug* is formed as progesterone levels rise and make the cervical mucus viscous once more. The plug helps to block entry of pathogens, other foreign materials, and sperm. Progesterone also helps to ready the uterus for the task of supporting an embryo. Increasing levels of progesterone and estrogen inhibit LH release from the anterior pituitary.

When no fertilization occurs, the corpus luteum degenerates, LH blood levels are reduced, progesterone levels are decreased, and the endometrium no longer has the hormones it needs to support a pregnancy. Its spiral arteries become kinked and spasm. The ischemic endometrial cells die because of a lack of oxygen and nutrients. The glands regress,

FOCUS ON PATHOLOGY

Menarche in girls can be delayed by highly strenuous physical activity. In adult women, such activity can disrupt normal menstruation and even result in *amenorrhea*, which is cessation of menstruation. Adipose cells help to convert adrenal androgens to estrogens and are the source of leptin, which is critical in the onset of puberty. However, female athletes have lower amounts of adipose tissue because they are leaner than less active females. The hypothalamus is signaled by leptin about stores of energy in the body. If there is not sufficient energy to support reproduction, the reproductive cycles slow or stop altogether.

However, when discontinuing regular strenuous physical activity, amenorrhea is usually reversed. Unfortunately, there is a negative outcome as well. In young, healthy female adults, there will be dramatic losses in bone mass. This is usually only seen in old age. Once the estrogen levels drop and the menstrual cycle stops, the loss of bone starts.

preparing menstruation to begin on day 28. The spiral arteries constrict for a final time, suddenly relaxing and opening wide. Blood flows into the weak capillary beds and they fragment. The functional layer is then sloughed off, and the uterine cycle begins again with this new menstrual flow.

TEST YOUR UNDERSTANDING

1. List the hormones most important for the regulation of the ovarian cycle.
2. Which hormone, if lower than normal, will delay the onset of puberty?
3. Explain the three phases of the uterine cycle.

Estrogen, Progesterone, and Female Reproductive Function

Estrogens are to females what testosterone is to males. Both of these hormones generate reproductive function. Two things happen when estrogen levels rise during puberty in a female's body: Oogenesis is promoted with follicle growth in the ovaries, and anabolic effects occur in the female reproductive tract. The tract is readied for supporting a pregnancy, with enhanced motility occurring in the uterine tubes and uterus. There is thickening of the vaginal mucosa and maturation of the external genitalia.

Because of estrogens, girls between the ages of 11 and 12 experience "growth spurts," which are more dramatic than those seen in boys. However, this is a shorter-term process for females, because increasing estrogen levels also cause a faster closure of the epiphyses of the long bones. Girls usually reach their full height between the ages of 13 and 15, whereas boys usually reach their full height between the ages of 15 and 19.

Secondary sex characteristics included by estrogen include breast development; widening and lightening of the pelvis, for future childbirth; and increased deposition of subcutaneous fat, mostly in the breasts and hips. The various types of estrogen also help to maintain low total blood cholesterol levels and high high-density-lipoprotein levels. They facilitate calcium uptake, keeping the skeleton's density intact. All these effects begin in puberty yet are not true secondary sex characteristics.

Progesterone helps to establish and regulate the uterine cycle. It causes changes to occur in the cervical mucus. Mostly in pregnancy, but in other times as well, progesterone inhibits uterine motility and assists estrogen in preparing the breasts for lactation. The term *progesterone* actually means "for gestation." In the majority of a pregnancy it is the placenta, and not the ovaries, that supplies most progesterone.

Female Sexual Response

The erectile tissues of the clitoris and vaginal entrance respond to sexual stimulation. Parasympathetic nerve impulses release nitric oxide to dilate the erectile tissues, increase blood inflow, and swell the tissues. The nipples become erect, and the vagina expands and elongates. If sexual stimulation is sufficiently intense, parasympathetic impulses cause the vestibular glands to secrete mucus into the vestibule, moistening and lubricating the surrounding tissues and lower vagina. This facilitates insertion of the penis.

Just as in males, touch and psychological stimulation increase sexual excitement along autonomic nerve pathways. The clitoris responds to local stimulation, culminating in an orgasm if stimulation is sufficient. Females do not ejaculate but do experience increased muscle tension, raised blood pressure and pulse rate, and uterine contractions. Just before orgasm, the outer one-third of the vagina is engorged with blood. This increases friction on the penis, with orgasm initiating reflexes directed by the sacral and lumbar spinal cord. The muscles of the perineum and walls of both the uterus and uterine tubes contract rhythmically. This helps transport sperm through the female reproductive tract toward the upper uterine tubes.

Females experience intense pleasure that is followed by relaxation, which is the same for males, but do not have a refractory period after orgasm. Therefore, females can experience multiple orgasms during one sexual experience.

TEST YOUR UNDERSTANDING

1. Which hormones generate reproductive function in females?
2. Explain why girls experience growth spurts that are more dramatic but shorter in overall duration than boys.
3. Describe the female sexual response, and identify differences between it and the male sexual response.

However, orgasm is not required for conception. It is now understood that female libido is not primarily influenced by the male sex hormone testosterone. It is instead influenced by dehydroepiandrosterone, which is an androgen produced by the adrenal cortex.

Birth Control

Birth control requires a method of **contraception**. It regulates whether an offspring is produced as a result of sexual intercourse, called *coitus*, and regulates the time at which it is conceived. Contraception stops fertilization of an egg cell or prevents the development of a ball of cells known as a *blastocyst* into an embryo. There are several quite different methods of contraception:

- *Coitus interruptus:* The withdrawal of the penis from the vagina before ejaculation; not the most reliable method because the male may not be able to withdraw just before ejaculation, and sperm cells in the semen may leave the penis before ejaculation occurs.
- *Rhythm method:* Also known as timed coitus, or natural family planning; abstaining from sexual intercourse 2 days before and 1 day after ovulation; however, it is not reliable because accurately identifying periods when the female is infertile is difficult.
- *Mechanical barriers:* Contraceptives that prevent sperm cells from entering the female reproductive tract (**FIGURE 23-14**):
  - *Male condom:* A thin latex or natural substance sheath placed over the erect penis

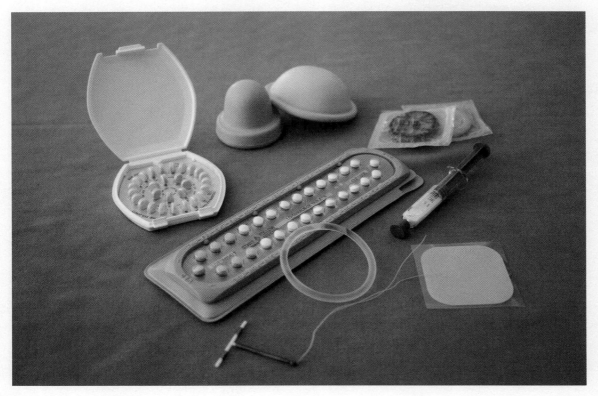

FIGURE 23-14 Various types of birth control.

before intercourse; male condoms are generally inexpensive.

- *Female condom:* A bag-like device inserted into the vagina before intercourse; both forms of condoms may decrease sensations but can prevent STIs.
- *Diaphragm:* A cup-shaped device with a flexible ring that forms a rim; it is inserted into the vagina to cover the cervix and prevent sperm cells from entering the uterus. It must be fitted by a physician and used with a spermicide that kills sperm cells. Diaphragms are inserted up to 6 hours before intercourse and must be left in place several hours afterward.
- *Cervical cap:* Similar to a diaphragm, it adheres to the cervix via suction and is inserted by the female before intercourse. Similar devices have been used for centuries throughout the world.

■ *Chemical barriers:* Creams, foams, and jellies with spermicidal properties; most effective when used along with a condom or diaphragm.

■ *Combined hormone contraceptives:* Estrogen and progestin administered in a variety of ways; these include a monthly insertion into the vagina such as ethinyl estradiol/etonogestrel (NuvaRing), a plastic skin patch such as ethinyl estradiol/norelgestromin (Ortho Evra), and various oral contraceptives in pill forms. These contain synthetic estrogen-like and progesterone-like chemicals that disrupt FSH and LH secretion to interfere with normal ovulation. They are nearly always effective, but have a variety of potentially serious adverse effects.

■ *Injectable contraception:* Medroxyprogesterone acetate (Depo-Provera) injected intramuscularly protects against pregnancy for 3 months by stopping maturation and release of a secondary oocyte. It has potential side effects for women with certain medical conditions.

■ *Hormonal implant:* The insertion of matchstick-sized capsules that contain a potent form of progesterone (Norplant) under the skin of a woman's arm (**FIGURE 23-15**).

■ *Intrauterine device (IUD):* A small solid object placed into the uterine cavity by a physician that interferes with implantation of a blastocyst. IUDs may be spontaneously expelled or can cause pain and excessive bleeding, requiring regular monitoring by a physician.

■ *Surgical methods:* Used to sterilize either the male or female without changing hormonal concentrations or sex drives; they may be reversible via microsurgery.

- *In males:* A vasectomy is performed, removing a small part of each ductus

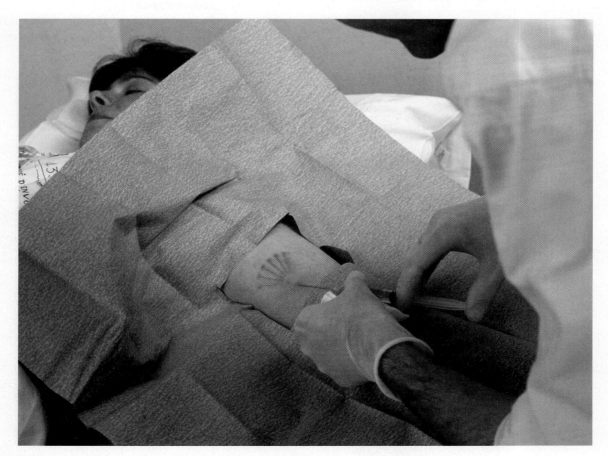

FIGURE 23-15 The site of a subcutaneous progesterone implant. (© Hattie Young/Science Source)

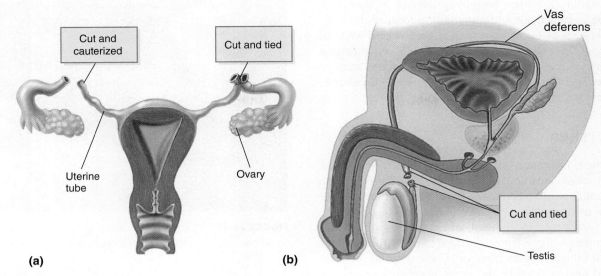

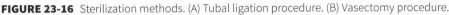

FIGURE 23-16 Sterilization methods. (A) Tubal ligation procedure. (B) Vasectomy procedure.

deferens or *vas deferens* and tying the cut ends of the ducts; this *ligating* of the ducts prevents sperm cells from leaving the epididymis, making the semen sperm-free. It may take several weeks after surgery for the sperm count in the semen to reach zero.

- *In females:* A tubal ligation is performed, cutting and ligating the uterine tubes so that sperm cells cannot reach an egg cell. **FIGURE 23-16** shows surgical methods of birth control in both sexes.

TEST YOUR UNDERSTANDING

1. How does an IUD prevent pregnancy?
2. What is the method that has the highest success rate in preventing pregnancy?
3. List three trade names of combined hormone contraceptives.

Sexually Transmitted Infections

Sexually transmitted infections (STIs), formerly known as *sexually transmitted diseases* and *venereal diseases*, are so named because they are spread by sexual contact. The highest rates of STIs, in developed countries, occur in the United States. Of the approximately 12 million Americans who get an STI, 3 million of these are adolescents. Latex condoms protect against STIs, and their use is encouraged widely.

Most reproductive disorders occur because of STIs. Viral diseases have now become the most common types of STIs; previously, bacterial diseases were most common. The most deadly STI is *AIDS*, which is caused by *HIV*. Many recognized

STIs are called "silent infections" because they may persist, in their early stages, without any symptoms. Often, once symptoms occur, it is too late to prevent complications or spread of the disease to sexual partners. Common symptoms are as follows:

- A burning sensation during urination
- Lower abdominal pain
- Fever
- Swollen neck glands
- Discharge from the vagina or penis
- Genital or anal pain, itching, or inflammation
- Pain during intercourse
- Oral or genital sores, blisters, bumps, or rash
- Itchy, runny eyes

Chlamydia

Chlamydia is the most common *bacterial* STI in the United States, infecting between 4 and 5 million Americans every year and increasing in prevalence in people of college age. Between 25% and 50% of diagnosed cases of pelvic inflammatory disease are caused by chlamydia. More than 150,000 infants are born to women with chlamydia every year. The causative agent, *Chlamydia trachomatis*, is present in 20% of men and 30% of women who also have gonorrhea. *Chlamydia trachomatis* has a dependence on host cells that is similar to a virus. It incubates within body cells in about 7 days. In 2010, there was a record high amount of reported cases of chlamydia: 1.2 million people.

Symptoms of chlamydia include urethritis, vaginal discharge, painful intercourse, irregular menses, and pain in the abdomen, rectum, or testicles. Urethritis is signified by painful, frequent urination and, in males, a thick penile discharge. Males may also experience a widespread urogenital tract infection as well as arthritis. Although 80% of infected women have no symptoms, it is a primary cause of female sterility. An infant born to an infected mother often develops conjunctivitis and, especially, a form of this condition known as *trachoma*, which is painful and leads to scarring of the cornea if not treated. Other complications in infants include respiratory tract inflammations such as pneumonia. Diagnosis of chlamydia requires cell cultures. Treatment with tetracycline is simple and effective.

Gonorrhea

Gonorrhea, commonly known as "the clap," occurs most often in adolescents and young adults. It is caused by the bacterium *Neisseria gonorrhoeae*. This bacterium invades the mucosae of the reproductive and urinary tracts. It is spread by contact with genital, pharyngeal, and anal mucosal surfaces.

Symptoms of gonorrhea in men are usually those of urethritis. If untreated, gonorrhea can cause urethral constriction and inflammation of the entire male duct system. In females, gonorrhea causes symptoms in 80% of cases, which include abdominal discomfort, abnormal uterine bleeding, vaginal discharge, and occasional urethral abnormalities similar to those that affect males. Gonorrhea in females leads to pelvic inflammatory disease and sterility. This disease has dropped to its lowest levels ever recorded in the United States, primarily because of antibiotic use. Ceftriaxone is the most commonly used antibiotic for gonorrhea. Unfortunately, antibiotic-resistant strains of gonorrhea are becoming more prevalent.

FOCUS ON PATHOLOGY

Pelvic inflammatory disease may be a complication of gonorrhea or chlamydia. In this disease, bacteria enter the vagina, spreading throughout the reproductive organs. Symptoms begin as intermittent cramps, then sudden fever, chills, weakness, and severe cramps. The infection can be stopped but requires hospitalization and intravenous antibiotics. It often scars the uterus and uterine tubes, resulting in infertility or increased risk of ectopic pregnancy, wherein an embryo develops inside a uterine tube instead of the uterus. Ectopic pregnancies occur one in four times in a female with pelvic inflammatory disease.

Syphilis

Syphilis is less common than chlamydia or gonorrhea in the United States but is increasing in prevalence. It is caused by a corkscrew-shaped bacterium called *Treponema pallidum*. Syphilis is usually transmitted by sexual contact but may also be transmitted by an infected mother to her fetus. When this

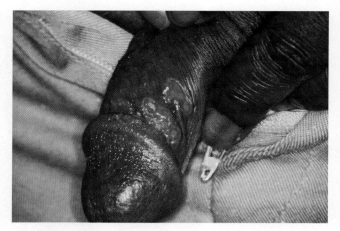

FIGURE 23-17 The chancre of primary syphilis as it occurs on the penis. The chancre has raised margins and is usually painless. (Courtesy of M. Rein, VD/CDC.)

occurs, the fetus is usually stillborn or dies soon after birth. The bacterium can easily penetrate abraded skin as well as intact mucosae. Just a few hours after exposure a systemic infection develops, but without any initial symptoms.

Within 2 to 3 weeks, a *chancre* appears at the site where the bacterium invaded the body. A chancre is a red, painless primary region (**FIGURE 23-17**). It usually appears on the penis in males, but in females it may be inside the vagina or on the cervix, making it nearly undetectable. The chancre ulcerates and crusts. Within a few weeks, it heals spontaneously and disappears.

Without treatment, secondary signs of syphilis appear in several more weeks. One of the initial symptoms of this phase is a pink skin rash over most of the body. Fever and joint pain commonly follow. All these signs and symptoms disappear on their own within 3 to 12 weeks. The disease then enters a *latent period*. The only way to detect it at this time is via a blood test. This stage may be killed by the immune system or may last for the rest of the person's life. It also may be followed by *tertiary syphilis*. This phase is characterized by destructive lesions known as *gummas*, which appear on the skin, blood vessels, bones, and structures of the central nervous system. For all stages of syphilis, penicillin is the treatment of choice.

Genital Herpes

Genital herpes is caused by the *herpes simplex virus 2*. The herpes simplex viruses are extremely difficult to control, remaining silent for weeks, months, or years and then flaring up suddenly. When they appear, there is a quick development of blister-like lesions. Herpes simplex is transmitted by direct skin-to-skin contact, when the virus is shedding, or via infectious secretions. The lesions appearing on the genitals are painful. If the condition is congenital, it can cause severe fetal malformations.

Most Americans with genital herpes are unaware they are infected. As many as 25% to 50% of all adults in the United States have the herpes simplex virus 2. Only 15% of these people have actual signs of the infection. Once infected, genital herpes remain forever in a person's body. The treatment of choice is the antiviral drug *acyclovir*. This medication heals lesions more quickly and reduces frequency of flare-ups.

Genital Warts

Genital warts are the second most common STI in the United States. They are caused by *HPV*, which is actually a group of more than 60 different viruses. Every year, about 6.2 million new cases of genital warts occur in America. It is believed that HPV infection increases cancer risks in areas of the body affected. The HPV virus is linked to 80% of all cases of invasive cervical cancer. However, most viral strains causing genital warts do not cause cervical cancer.

Genital warts usually recur, and treatment is difficult and under heavy debate. Unless widespread, many health professionals prefer not to treat genital warts. Others use laser therapy or cryosurgery to remove them. Another treatment involves the use of alpha-interferon.

Trichomoniasis

In sexually active young females in the United States, **trichomoniasis** is the most common curable STI. It is a parasitic infection that accounts for approximately 7.4 million new cases every year (**FIGURE 23-18**). Signs and symptoms

include a yellow-green vaginal discharge with a strong odor, although many infected women have no symptoms. It is easily and inexpensively treated with either metronidazole or tinidazole.

TEST YOUR UNDERSTANDING

1. Describe the most commonly seen *bacterial* STI in the United States.
2. Which STIs are listed as potentially resulting in sterility?
3. Which pathogen is commonly linked with cervical cancer?

Effects of Aging on the Reproductive System

In women, **menopause** signifies the end of reproductive life. Menopause usually occurs between ages 45 and 55, with menstrual cycles becoming irregular in the years before it occurs. Called *perimenopause*, this period is signified by the number of primordial follicles dropping every month, causing estrogen levels to decline and ovulation to eventually cease.

Progesterone levels also decline, and GnRH, FSH, and LH levels rise sharply. The uterus and breasts decrease in size, and the epithelia of the urethra and vagina thin. Reduced estrogen is linked to osteoporosis. Neural effects of menopause include "hot flashes," anxiety, and depression. Risks of atherosclerosis and other cardiovascular diseases also increase. Hormone replacement therapy may be required for women with severe menopausal symptoms. Menopause results in atrophy of the breasts, drying of the vagina, and an increase in vaginal infections. The menopausal woman may become irritable and have extremely dilated blood vessels in her skin, thinning of the skin, and loss of bone mass.

In recent years hormone replacement therapy has been linked to significant increases in heart disease, invasive breast cancer, stroke, and dementia. However, new data show that the smallest possible dose of hormone replacement therapy, for the shortest possible time, does reduce menopausal symptoms in women without existing breast cancer or the mutated *BRCA* gene or genes linked to the disease.

In men, changes due to aging occur more gradually than in women. Declining reproductive function is referred to as *andropause* or the *male climacteric*. Testosterone levels decline between ages 50 and 60, whereas FSH and LH levels increase. Although sperm production may continue past age 80, sexual activity gradually decreases. Sperm motility decreases with aging, slowing their movement greatly. Although a younger man's sperm move through the uterine tube in 20 to 50 minutes, the sperm of a 75-year-old man require 2 to 3 days for this. Although testosterone replacement therapy can be used to enhance sexual drive, it may increase the risk of prostate disease.

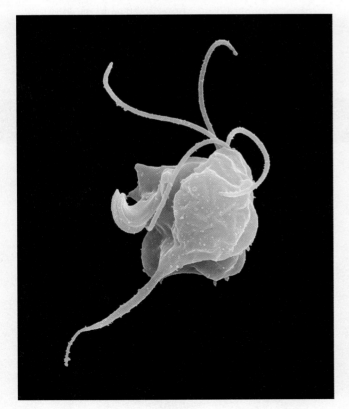

FIGURE 23-18 *Trichomonas vaginalis*. False-color scanning electron micrograph of a *T. vaginalis* trophozoite. (Bar = 5 μm.) (© Dr. Dennis Kunkel/Visuals Unlimited)

The reproductive organs produce sex cells and hormones, sustain them, or transport them. The primary male sex organs are the testes, which produce sperm cells and male sex hormones. A sperm cell consists of a head, midpiece, and tail. The male internal accessory organs include the epididymides, ductus deferentia, seminal vesicles, prostate gland, and bulbourethral glands. The male external reproductive organs include the scrotum, testes, and penis. Orgasm is the culmination of sexual stimulation. Emission and ejaculation accompany male orgasm. Male reproductive functions are controlled by hypothalamic and pituitary hormones, FSH, and LH. Male sex hormones are called androgens, with testosterone the most important.

The primary female sex organs are the ovaries, which produce female sex cells and sex hormones. Ovulation is the release of a secondary oocyte from an ovary. The release of an oocyte involves structures, including the primordial follicles, and the processes of oogenesis and follicle maturation. The female internal accessory organs include the uterine tubes, uterus, and vagina. The female external reproductive organs include the labia majora, labia minora, clitoris, and vestibule. The hypothalamus, anterior pituitary gland, and ovaries secrete hormones that control sex cell maturation. They also control development and maintenance of female secondary sex characteristic and changes that occur during the monthly reproductive cycle. The most important female sex hormones are estrogens and progesterone. The female reproductive cycle is approximately 28 days in length. A female's reproductive life is shorter than that of a male, beginning with menarche during puberty and ending with menopause.

Birth control is voluntary regulation of the production of offspring and when they are conceived. It usually involves some method of contraception. Popular methods include coitus interruptus, the rhythm method, condoms, diaphragms, cervical caps, chemical barriers, combined hormone contraceptives, injectable contraception, IUDs, and surgery. Some forms of contraception also protect against STIs. STIs often do not show symptoms until they have become very serious. Most reproductive diseases are caused by STIs. Chlamydia, trichomoniasis, HIV, gonorrhea, and syphilis are examples of diseases that may be transmitted sexually. Pelvic inflammatory disease may be a complication of gonorrhea or chlamydia and can lead to female sterility or ectopic pregnancy. Genital herpes is a common STI that may be present in 25% to 50% of all American adults. Genital warts are caused by HPV, which is linked to the development of cervical cancer. The end of reproductive life in women is signaled by menopause, but in men this does not occur as significantly, with some men able to father children into their later years.

KEY TERMS

Ampulla
Androgens
Areola
Broad ligament
Bulbourethral glands
Cardinal ligaments
Cervical canal
Cervix
Chlamydia
Clitoris
Contraception
Corpora cavernosa
Corpus luteum
Corpus spongiosum
Cremaster muscles
Dartos muscles
Ductus deferentia

Ejaculation
Ejaculatory duct
Emission
Endometrium
Epididymis
Erection
Estrogens
Follicle cells
Fourchette
Fundus
Gametes
Genital herpes
Genital warts
Glans penis
Gonadotropins
Gonads
Gonorrhea

Granulosa cells
Haploid
Hymen
Infundibulum
Interstitial cells
Isthmus
Labia majora
Labia minora
Lactiferous ducts
Mammary glands
Meiosis
Menarche
Menopause
Menstrual cycle
Mesosalpinx
Mesovarium
Mons pubis

Myoid cells
Myometrium
Nipple
Oocytes
Oogenesis
Orgasm
Ovarian follicles
Ovarian ligament
Ovaries
Ovulation
Pelvic inflammatory disease
Penis
Perimetrium
Prepuce
Primary follicles
Primordial follicles
Progesterone
Prostate gland

Puberty
Resolution
Rete testis
Round ligaments
Scrotum
Semen
Seminal vesicles
Seminiferous tubules
Sex hormones
Sexually transmitted infections
  (STIs)
Sperm
Spermatic cord
Spermatogenesis
Spermatogenic cells
Spermatogonia
Straight tubule
Suspensory ligament

Syphilis
Testes
Testosterone
Trichomoniasis
Tunica albuginea
Tunica vaginalis
Uterine tubes
Uterosacral ligaments
Uterus
Vagina
Vaginal fornix
Vestibular bulb
Vestibular gland
Vestibule
Vulva
Zygote

LEARNING GOALS

The following learning goals correspond to the objectives at the beginning of this chapter:

1. The components of the male reproductive system include sperm cells, male sex hormones, testes, seminiferous tubules, epididymides, ductus deferentia, spermatogenic cells, interstitial cells, ejaculatory duct, seminal vesicles, prostate gland, bulbourethral glands, semen, scrotum, and penis.

2. Semen is the fluid the male urethra conveys to outside of the body during ejaculation. It is made up of sperm cells from the testes as well as secretions of the seminal vesicles, prostate gland, and bulbourethral glands. It has an alkaline pH of 7.5 and includes prostaglandins and nutrients.

3. Male reproductive functions are regulated by the hormones from the hypothalamus, anterior pituitary gland, and testes. They begin and maintain sperm cell production, overseeing development and maintenance of secondary sex characteristics. The hypothalamus controls the changes during puberty that make a male's body able to reproduce. It secretes GnRH. The anterior pituitary secretes the gonadotropins known as LH and FSH. LH promotes development of testicular interstitial cells, and FSH stimulates seminiferous tubule cells to respond to testosterone, which is the most important androgen, or male sex hormone.

4. Spermatogenesis is the process by which sperm cells are formed. During embryonic development, undifferentiated spermatogenic cells called *spermatogonia* undergo mitosis, creating two daughter cells, a "type A" and a "type B" cell. The type A cell maintains supplies of undifferentiated cells, whereas the type B cell enlarges to become a primary spermatocyte. This cell reproduces via meiosis I, which separates chromosome pairs, and meiosis II, which causes one member of each pair to separate its chromatids to become independent chromosomes. Each primary spermatocyte divides into two secondary spermatocytes and then again into spermatids, which mature. For each primary spermatocyte that undergoes meiosis, four sperm cells with 23 chromosomes each are formed.

5. The penis is cylindrical in shape. When erect, it stiffens and enlarges, enabling insertion into the vagina during sexual intercourse. The shaft or body of the penis contains three columns of erectile tissue. It has two dorsal corpora cavernosa and one ventral corpus spongiosum. Dense connective tissue surrounds each column in a capsule. The penis is enclosed by a layer of connective tissue, a thin layer of subcutaneous tissue, and skin. The urethra extends through the corpus spongiosum, a structure that, at its distal end, forms the cone-shaped glans penis. This structure covers the ends of the corpora cavernosa and opens as the external urethral orifice. Males are born with a loose fold of skin called the foreskin or prepuce, which extends to cover the glans as a sheath.

6. The female reproductive system consists of the egg cells or *oocytes*, ovaries, primordial follicles, primary follicles, uterine tubes, uterus, cervix, vagina, hymen, labia majora and minora, clitoris, vestibule, and vestibular glands.

7. In the female reproductive cycle, the following steps occur:
   A. The anterior pituitary gland secretes FSH and LH.
   B. Maturation of the follicle is stimulated by FSH.
   C. The follicular cells maintain the secondary sex characteristics and cause the endometrium to thicken.
   D. The anterior pituitary gland releases a surge of LH, stimulating ovulation.
   E. The follicular cells become corpus luteum cells, releasing estrogens and progesterone.
   F. The uterine wall develops.
   G. Progesterone causes the endometrium to become more glandular and vascular.
   H. The anterior pituitary ceases secreting LH and FSH.
   I. If the egg cell is not fertilized, the corpus luteum degenerates and secretions stop.

A. Blood vessels in the endometrium constrict.
B. The uterine lining disintegrates and sloughs off, producing menstrual flow.
C. The anterior pituitary restarts the process by beginning to secrete LH and FSH again.

8. The uterus is supported and held in place by suspensory ligaments that include
   - The broad ligaments connected laterally to the entire body of the uterus, attaching to the walls of the pelvis and superiorly to the walls of the fallopian tubes
   - The uterosacral ligaments, extending from the lateral surfaces of the uterus to the anterior face of the sacrum
   - The round ligaments, which arise on the lateral margins of the uterus, posterior and inferior to the attachments of the uterine tubes
   - The lateral ligaments, extending from the base of the uterus and vagina to the lateral walls of the pelvis

9. The mammary glands, located inside the breasts, are specialized to secrete milk after pregnancy. Each mammary gland is made up of 15 to 20 lobes that contain alveolar glands and an alveolar duct that leads to a lactiferous duct. This leads to a nipple on the outside of the breast. The lobes are separated by dense connective and adipose tissues, which offer support and attach them to the fascia of the underlying pectoral muscles. Dense suspensory ligaments extend inward from the dermis of the breast to the fascia to help support its weight. In females, the mammary glands are stimulated by hormones to produce and secrete milk.

10. The general symptoms of STIs include a burning sensation during urination; lower abdominal pain; fever; swollen neck glands; discharge from the vagina or penis; genital or anal pain, itching, or inflammation; pain during intercourse; oral or genital sores, blisters, bumps, or rash; and itchy, runny eyes.

CRITICAL THINKING QUESTIONS

A 17-year-old boy felt a small nodule on the anterior part of his testes after showering. Because there was no pain, he ignored this nodule. Three years after, he experienced a severe heaviness in one side of his testes, especially when walking. His physician examined him, and after biopsy diagnosed him with testicular cancer.

1. Explain the structures of the testes and penis.
2. Describe the treatment of choice for testicular cancer without metastasis.

REVIEW QUESTIONS

1. A bundle of tissue that contains the ductus deferens, blood vessels, and nerves is called
   A. a straight tubule
   B. an efferent duct
   C. a spermatic cord
   D. an ejaculatory duct

2. Interstitial cells of the testis produce
   A. nutrients
   B. sperm
   C. androgens
   D. inhibin

3. Sperm production occurs in the
   A. epididymis
   B. rete testis
   C. ejaculatory ducts
   D. seminiferous tubules

4. Which of the following structures are located at the base of the penis, and produce a lubricating substance?
   A. bulbourethral glands
   B. preputial glands
   C. prostate glands
   D. seminal vesicles

5. The fold of skin that covers the tip of the penis is the
   A. corpus spongiosum
   B. corpus cavernosa
   C. prepuce
   D. penile urethra

6. The inferior portion of the uterus that projects into the vagina is the
   A. fornix
   B. cervix
   C. fundus
   D. isthmus

7. The structure that transports the ovum to the uterus is the
   A. infundibulum
   B. uterine tube
   C. endometrium
   D. fundus

8. During menses,
   A. the old functional layer of tissue is sloughed off
   B. the secretory glands and blood vessels develop in the endometrium
   C. a new uterine lining is formed
   D. the corpus luteum is formed

9. Which of the following is incorrect?
   A. The head of a human spermatozoa contains a nucleus.
   B. The tail of a human spermatozoa is called a flagellum.
   C. The middle piece of a human spermatozoa contains acrosome.
   D. The human spermatozoa contains many mitochondria.

10. Which of the following is incorrect?
   A. An ovary releases FSH.
   B. An ovary produces estrogen.
   C. An ovary produces progesterone.
   D. An ovary is located in the peritoneal cavity.

11. A membranous fold sometimes found at or near the vaginal canal opening is called the
   A. cul-de-sac
   B. fornice
   C. hymen
   D. ampulla

12. The erectile tissue located on the ventral surface of the penis is the
    A. prepuce
    B. corpora cavernosa
    C. membranous urethra
    D. corpus spongiosum

13. A typical ejaculation releases approximately _____ sperm.
    A. 200,000
    B. 800,000
    C. 100 million
    D. 250 million

14. Which portion of the uterine tube is closest to the ovary?
    A. infundibulum
    B. ampulla
    C. isthmus
    D. anterior segment

15. The principal hormone secreted by the corpus luteum is
    A. estrogen
    B. LH
    C. FSH
    D. progesterone

ESSAY QUESTIONS

1. Describe the male duct system.
2. Which hormones are released from the testes and ovaries? Describe their functions.
3. Describe spermatogenesis and oogenesis.
4. Explain the anatomy of the uterus and its function.
5. Describe the ovarian cycle and ovulation.
6. Describe the female sexual response.
7. Explain the most effective types of birth control.
8. Discuss the four stages of syphilis.
9. Describe the drug of choice for chlamydia, genital herpes, trichomoniasis, and syphilis.
10. Briefly describe the effects of aging on the male reproductive system.

Pregnancy and Development

OBJECTIVES

After studying this chapter, the reader should be able to

1. Describe the process of fertilization.
2. Describe the major events of cleavage.
3. Differentiate between an embryo and a fetus.
4. Describe the hormonal changes in the maternal body during pregnancy.
5. Describe the major events of the early periods of embryonic development.
6. Discuss the birth process and explain the role of hormones in this process.
7. List the three blood vessels in the umbilical cord and the basic umbilical cord functions.
8. Describe the length of the neonatal period.
9. Define the terms *chromosomes, genes, autosomes, alleles,* and *homozygous.*
10. Distinguish between dominant and recessive alleles.

Overview

A basic understanding of human development promotes understanding of anatomical structures. Additionally, human development and growth mechanisms are similar to the mechanisms used in the repair of injured tissues. When a sperm cell unites with a secondary oocyte, a **zygote** is formed. Normal pregnancy lasts for 38 weeks, with a human **embryo** developing and growing continually before birth. **Growth** means an increase in size and occurs as a result of increased numbers of cells and enlargement of newly formed cells. **Development** includes growth and is defined as the continuous process of an individual changing from one life phase to another. The period beginning with fertilization and ending at birth is known as the **prenatal period**. The period beginning at birth and ending at death is known as the **postnatal period**.

Fertilization

Fertilization is the union of a sperm cell with an egg cell. Also called *conception*, it usually occurs in a uterine tube. Once the developing offspring is implanted into the lining of the uterus, **pregnancy** begins. It consists of three trimesters, each about 3 months long.

Once ovulation occurs, the egg cell usually enters a uterine tube. During sexual intercourse the male deposits semen into the vagina, near the cervix. The sperm cells in the semen must "swim" upward through the uterus and uterine tube. The female reproductive tract secretes a thin fluid that promotes sperm transport and survival. This secretion increases the chance that sperm will reach an egg cell at the time when a woman is most fertile. Within 1 hour after intercourse, sperm cells reach the upper uterine tube, where the secondary oocyte is located. Only one sperm actually fertilizes this egg cell.

Fertilization actually occurs once a sperm cell binds with the zona pellucida surrounding the oocyte cell membrane. The sperm cell's acrosome releases enzymes such as *hyaluronidase* and *acrosin*, which aid penetration of the sperm head (**FIGURE 24-1**). At least several hundred sperm cells must be present to produce enough enzymes to allow one of them to penetrate. This is why men with very low sperm counts are termed *subfertile*.

When the head of a sperm enters the oocyte, the remainder stays outside, triggering vesicles beneath the oocyte membrane to strengthen the zona pellucida. This keeps additional sperm heads from entering. Entry of more than one would cause the zygote to be abnormal because of an overload of genetic material.

Once a sperm cell head enters the oocyte's cytoplasm and activates it, the sperm cell divides to form a large cell with a nucleus containing the female's genetic information (**FIGURE 24-2**). It also holds a tiny second polar body, which is expelled. Meiosis is now complete, and the approaching nuclei from the two sex cells are called *pronuclei*. They later meet and merge, with their nuclear membranes disintegrating and their chromosomes mingling. Fertilization is now complete. *Polyspermy*, or fertilization by more than one sperm, is prevented by a cortical reaction that releases enzymes that inactivate sperm receptors while hardening the zona pellucida.

The male and female each provide 23 chromosomes. A human body's somatic cells require 46 chromosomes—hence the contributed chromosomes from each partner combine. The cell this produces is called the *zygote*—the first cell of the future offspring. Once the oocyte has been activated and meiosis has finished, the nuclear material that is still inside the ovum reorganizes into the *female pronucleus*. Meanwhile, the nucleus of the spermatozoon swells to form the *male pronucleus*, as the remainder of the sperm cell breaks down. The two pronuclei join during *amphimixis* to form the zygote.

Prenatal Development

The time spent in prenatal development is called **gestation**. The *gestation period* occurs from the last menstrual period until birth, which takes approximately 280 days. A gestation time of less than 37 weeks is referred to as "premature." If gestation continues beyond 42 weeks, it is considered "postmature," regardless of the size of the **fetus** or other factors. A developing offspring is referred to as a variety of names based on the period of development. The fertilized egg is called a *conceptus* or, more commonly, a zygote. It undergoes mitosis about 30 hours after it has formed. The period from fertilization through the eighth week of gestation is known as the **embryonic period**, with the zygote now being called an *embryo*. The period from the ninth week of gestation through birth is known as the **fetal period**, with the embryo now being called a *fetus*. At birth, the fetus is then called an *infant*.

Cleavage and Blastocyst Formation

From the initial single fertilized egg cell, there is division into two **blastomeres** (**FIGURE 24-3**). These, in turn, mitotically divide into four cells, then eight, and so on. These divisions are rapid, yielding smaller cells because of lack of time for any cell growth. This phase of early cell division is called **cleavage**. During this period, the tiny cell mass moves through the uterine tube to the uterine cavity. This takes about 3 days, with the structure consisting of a solid "ball" of 16 or more cells that is called a **morula**. The tiny dividing cells have a high surface-to-volume ratio, allowing

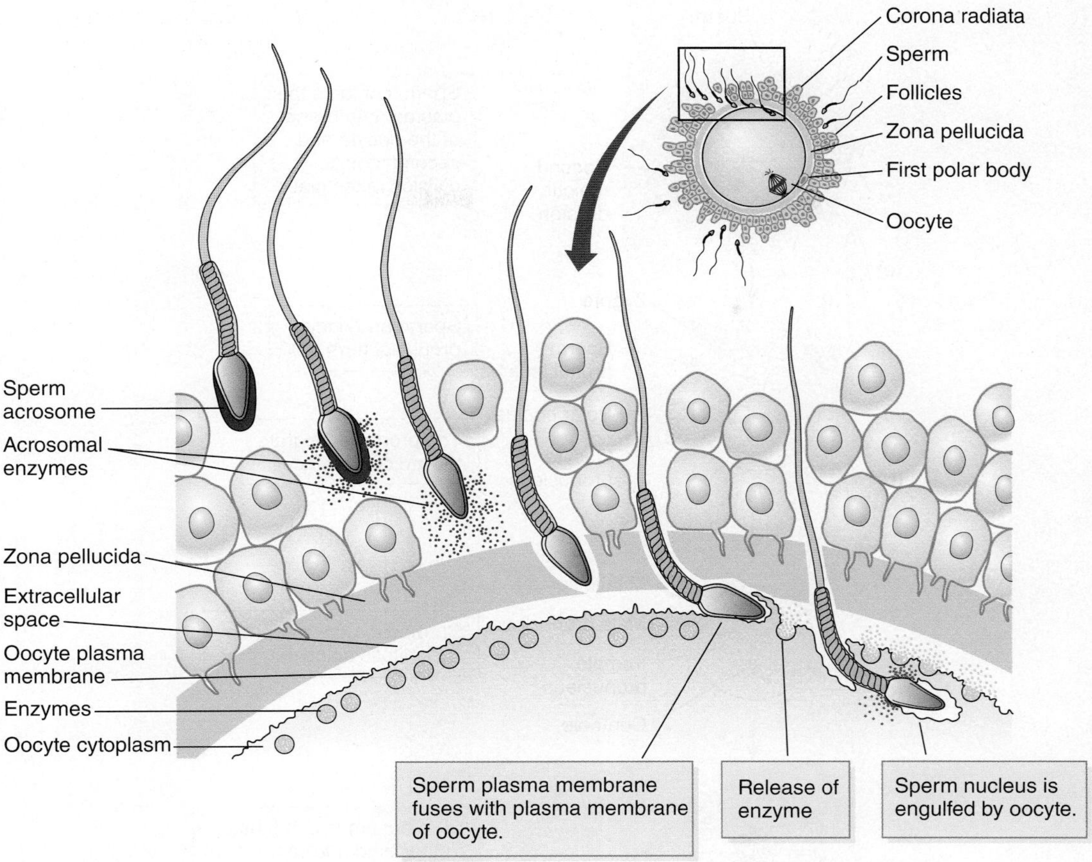
Corona radiata
Sperm
Follicles
Zona pellucida
First polar body
Oocyte
Sperm acrosome
Acrosomal enzymes
Zona pellucida
Extracellular space
Oocyte plasma membrane
Enzymes
Oocyte cytoplasm
Sperm plasma membrane fuses with plasma membrane of oocyte.
Release of enzyme
Sperm nucleus is engulfed by oocyte.

FIGURE 24-1 The steps of fertilization.

them to uptake oxygen and nutrients while disposing of wastes. The quickly dividing cells begin to build embryonic structures.

By the fifth day after fertilization, the embryo is made up of approximately 100 cells. It has begun accumulating fluid within an internal cavity and floats freely inside the uterus. During this time, the zona pellucida degenerates. The morula becomes a hollow **blastocyst**, which is basically a ball of cells that attaches to the endometrium. The blastocyst is filled with fluid and made up of one layer of large flat **trophoblast cells** as well as an inner cell mass of 20 to 30 rounded, clustered cells.

Soon, the trophoblast cells develop L-selectin adhesion surface molecules. They aid in the formation of the placenta and secrete several immunosuppressive factors, which protect the trophoblast and embryo from being attacked by the mother's cells. The embryo forms from the inner cell mass after it forms the **embryonic disc**. Three extraembryonic membranes also form from the embryonic disc. The fourth membrane, called the **chorion**, is formed from the trophoblast.

Implantation

After about 1 week, the developing offspring has become superficially implanted in the endometrium (**FIGURE 24-4**). Until this point, the cells that will form the developing offspring, known as pluripotent stem cells, can give rise to specialized cells, including additional stem cells. Uterine secretions, rich in glycoproteins, steroids, vitamins, and other nutrients, nourish the blastocyst. The *window of implantation* describes how receptive the endometrium is to implantation. This occurs because of surging ovarian hormone levels, estrogens and progesterone, in the blood.

When the endometrium is receptive, integrin and selectin proteins located on the trophoblast cells bind to respectively extracellular matrix components and selectin-binding carbohydrates located on the inner uterine wall. The extracellular matrix components are collagen, fibronectin, laminin, and other components. The blastocyst is implanted in the upper area of the uterus. In cases wherein the endometrium is not matured sufficiently, the blastocyst will detach, floating to a lower level of the uterus and implanting when it locates a site that has sufficient receptors and chemical signals. When the blastocyst is implanted in an area other than the uterus, the condition is called an *ectopic pregnancy*.

Successful implantation occurs in approximately 5 days. It is usually finished by the 12th day after ovulation, which is when the endometrium normally begins its sloughing-off process. Obviously, menstruation must be prevented to continue the pregnancy, because it would cause the embryo to be lost along with the endometrium. This is known as *spontaneous abortion*.

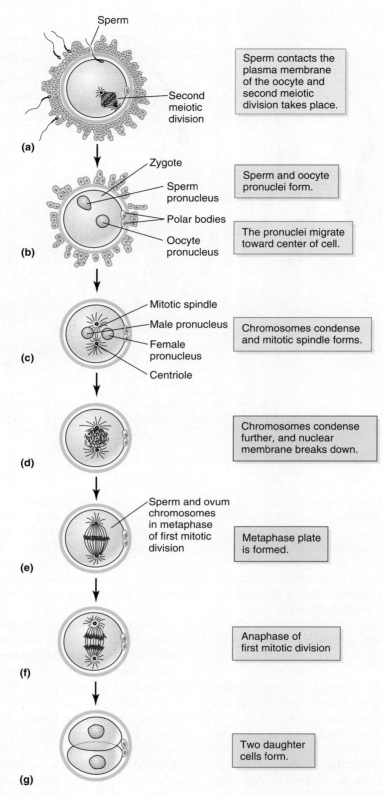

FIGURE 24-2 Fertilization and the first mitotic division.

The placenta produces several hormones during pregnancy. **Human chorionic gonadotropin (hCG)**, estrogen, and progesterone are the main hormones. hCG is secreted by trophoblast cells and maintains viability of the corpus luteum. It bypasses the effects of the hypothalamus, pituitary, and ovaries, prompting the corpus luteum to continually secrete progesterone and estrogen. This is controlled by the *chorion*. Therefore, the developing offspring assumes hormonal control of the uterus in this period. hCG is similar to *luteinizing hormone* in its effects but also has protease activity,

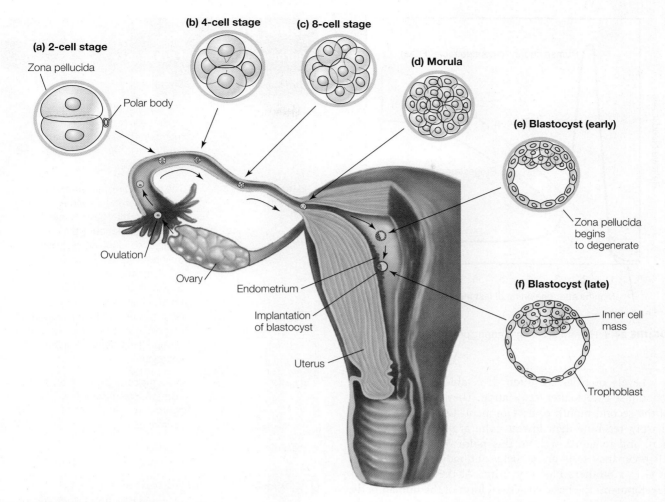

FIGURE 24-3 Cleavage. From zygote to blastocyst.

promoting development of the placenta by acting as an autocrine growth factor. In areas where the trophoblast "faces" the endometrium, hCG levels are higher. The placenta also releases *human placental lactogen*, which is also called *human chorionic somatomammotropin*. This polypeptide hormone functions similarly to growth hormone. It modifies the mother's metabolism to facilitate the energy supply of the fetus, and also has anti-insulin properties.

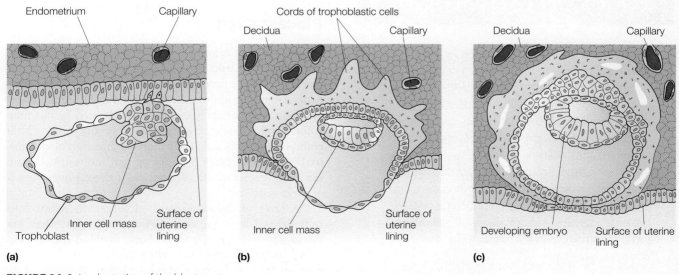

FIGURE 24-4 Implantation of the blastocyst.

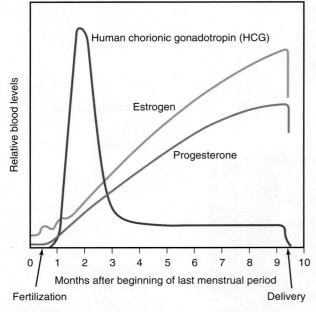

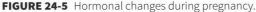

FIGURE 24-5 Hormonal changes during pregnancy.

Levels of hCG are often detectable in the mother's blood just 1 week after fertilization. They rise until the end of the second month of development. Levels then decline sharply, reaching their lowest point at 4 months of gestation, and remain low from this point on (**FIGURE 24-5**). All pregnancy tests are actually antibody tests, detecting hCG in a mother's blood or urine. At the eighth week of development, the basic structural form of the human body is recognizable, and the embryo is renamed a fetus. Simple versions of all organs are present. These organs and other structures enlarge and become specialized as the fetus develops. The hormonal changes of pregnancy are summarized in **TABLE 24-1**.

FOCUS ON PATHOLOGY

Ectopic pregnancy occurs when the fertilized egg transplants in a location other than in the uterus. In most cases, the egg implants inside one of the fallopian tubes. This may be life threatening to the mother. Ectopic pregnancy may be caused by history of the condition, defective formation of the fallopian tubes, scarring after a ruptured appendix, endometriosis, or scarring from past infections or surgery of the female organs. Common signs and symptoms of ectopic pregnancy include nausea, breast tenderness, abnormal vaginal bleeding, lower back pain, mild pelvic cramping, and abdominopelvic pain.

TABLE 24-1

Hormonal Changes of Pregnancy

Hormone	Changes
hCG	After implantation, hCG is secreted by the cells of the embryo; it maintains the corpus luteum, which continues to secrete estrogens and progesterone.
Estrogens and progesterone	The developing placenta secretes abundant amounts of these hormones; they have many effects: stimulation of the uterine lining to continue development, maintenance of the uterine lining, inhibiting the anterior pituitary's secretion of FSH and LH, stimulating mammary gland development, inhibiting uterine contractions (progesterone), and enlarging reproductive organs (estrogens).
Relaxin	From the corpus luteum, this hormone inhibits uterine contractions and relaxes the pelvic ligaments.
Placental lactogen	Secreted from the placenta to stimulate breast development.
Aldosterone	Secreted from the adrenal cortex to promote renal reabsorption of sodium.
Parathyroid hormone	Secreted from the parathyroid glands to help maintain high concentrations of maternal blood calcium.

FSH, follicle-stimulating hormone; LH, luteinizing hormone.

Placentation

Placentation is the formation of the **placenta** (**FIGURE 24-6**). This temporary structure takes over production of progesterone and estrogen production for the remainder of the pregnancy, beginning in between the second and third months of gestation. The corpus luteum has degenerated by this time, and the ovaries are inactive until birth occurs. Although the embryo begins obtaining nutrition via digestion of endometrial cells, the placenta provides oxygen and nutrition starting in the second month of gestation. It also assumes the role of waste removal.

A layer of extraembryonic mesoderm develops from cells derived from the original inner cell mass. They line the inner surface of the trophoblast, forming the chorion, which develops **chorionic villi**. These finger-like structures are more elaborate in structure where they contact the

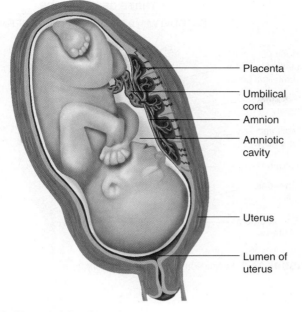

FIGURE 24-6 The placenta.

maternal blood. Blood vessels form in their cores, extending to the embryo to form the umbilical arteries and vein. Blood-filled **lacunae** are formed in the stratum functionalis of the endometrium. The villi are continually nourished by extravascularized maternal blood. During placentation, the distal parts of the allantois and blood vessels carrying blood in and out of the placenta are contained in the *body stalk*, which connects the embryo and chorion. The *yolk stalk* connects the endoderm of the embryo with the yolk sac.

Beneath the embryo, the present endometrium becomes the **decidua basalis**, whereas the endometrium surrounding the uterine cavity in the area of implantation becomes the **decidua capsularis**. The placenta is actually formed by the combination of the decidua basalis and the chorionic villi. The decidua capsularis expands to accommodate the fetus, filling and stretching the uterine cavity over time. The villi in the decidua capsularis become compressed and degenerate. The villi in the decidua basalis proliferate and become more branched.

By the third month of gestation, the placenta is usually fully functional. It supplies nutrition, oxygen, hormones, and also removes wastes. Barriers exist that prevent free passage of substances between the two blood supplies: the chorionic villi membranes and the embryonic capillaries of the endothelium. Normally, the maternal and embryonic blood supplies do not mix.

Blood levels of estrogens and progesterone continually increase throughout pregnancy. The uterine wall is maintained during the second and third trimesters by placental estrogens and placental progesterone. The placenta also secretes the hormone known as **placental lactogen**, which helps to stimulate breast development and prepares the mammary glands for milk secretion. The **relaxin** hormone is also produced by the placenta. After birth, the placenta detaches and sloughs off.

FOCUS ON PATHOLOGY

A *hydatidiform mole* is an abnormal growth of placental tissue with malignant characteristics. It may be diagnosed after a miscarriage or termination of pregnancy. Also referred to as a *molar pregnancy*, it may be caused by a genetic abnormality during fertilization. Usually, no fetus is present, and the placenta develops as a mass of clear vesicles with a grape-like structure. The mother experiences symptoms similar to a normal pregnancy, but there may be increased nausea and vomiting and vaginal bleeding. A blood test for hCG is highly elevated compared with what it should be for a normal pregnancy.

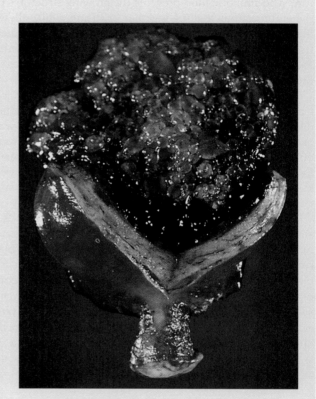

Hydatidiform mole.

TEST YOUR UNDERSTANDING

1. What is cleavage?
2. Differentiate an embryo from a fetus.
3. What is a morula?
4. Which hormone suppresses uterine contractions until the birth process begins?
5. What are lacunae?

Embryonic Development

The process of embryonic development, during and after implantation, involves many significant steps. The blastocyst is converted to a **gastrula**, and the three **primary germ layers** form. The **extraembryonic membranes** develop. Before developing three layers, the inner cell mass divides into two layers known as the upper *epiblast* and the lower *hypoblast*. The inner cell mass is then called the *embryonic disc*. The extraembryonic membranes form during weeks 2 and 3 of development and are the **amnion**, **yolk sac**, **allantois**, and chorion.

The amnion is a transparent, membranous sac that develops from cells of the epiblast and fills with **amniotic fluid**. As the embryonic disc eventually curves and forms the tubular body, the amnion also curves. The sac eventually extends entirely around the embryo, with its only break being the **umbilical cord**. The amnion protects the embryo against trauma and maintains a constant temperature. The amniotic fluid prevents the growing structures of the embryo from sticking together or fusing, while allowing freedom of movement. Amniotic fluid is first formed from maternal blood, but the growing functionality of the embryo's kidneys means that fetal urine later contributes to the amniotic fluid.

From cells of the primitive gut, the yolk sac forms, which hangs from the embryo's ventral surface. With the embryonic disc being the point of contact, the amnion and yolk sac appear like two balloons that touch each other. Human eggs contain only small amounts of yolk, with nutritive functions being assumed by the placenta. The yolk sac is important for two main reasons: It forms part of the embryo's digestive tube, and it is the source of the first blood cells and vessels that form.

The allantois forms at the caudal end of the yolk sac as a small formation of embryonic tissue. It is the structural basis for the umbilical cord, which links the embryo to the placenta. The allantois eventually becomes part of the urinary bladder. When fully formed, the umbilical cord has a core of embryonic connective tissue that is also called *Wharton's jelly*. The core also contains the umbilical arteries and vein and is covered by amniotic membrane externally. As previously described, the chorion helps to form the placenta. It is the outermost membrane, enclosing the embryonic body and each of the other membranes.

Gastrulation

The processes of **gastrulation** begin with a **primitive streak** appearing on the embryonic disc's dorsal surface. This groove with raised edges creates the longitudinal axis of the embryo. Epiblast cells on the surface of the embryonic disc move medially over other cells to enter the primitive streak. The first cells entering the groove displace the yolk sac's hypoblast cells to form the inferior germ layer, known as the **endoderm** (**FIGURE 24-7**). The cells that follow move laterally between the cells at the upper and lower surfaces to form the **mesoderm**. Mesodermal cells just beneath aggregate to form a rod of cells known as the *notochord*. This is the

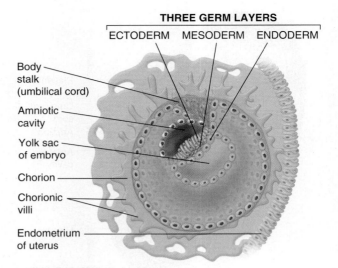

FIGURE 24-7 Formation of the three primary germ layers.

first axial support of the embryo. Cells that remain on the dorsal surface of the embryo make up the **ectoderm**. The embryo is now about 2 mm long.

In **organogenesis**, the primary germ layers of the embryo begin to develop the organs. Organogenesis is the primary event of embryonic development (**TABLE 24-2**). The formation of the spinal cord and brain are among the first events of organogenesis. These structures arise from the ectoderm of the inner cell mass. **FIGURE 24-8** shows how the spinal cord forms during this period. The ectoderm folds inward, creating the *neural groove* along the

TABLE 24-2		
Early Periods Of Embryonic Development		
Period	Occurrence	Events
Zygote	12–24 hours after ovulation	Fertilization of secondary oocyte occurs; completion of meiosis; zygote becomes genetically distinct, with 46 chromosomes.
Cleavage	30 hours to third day	Mitosis increases the number of cells.
Morula	Third to fourth day	Solid, ball-like mass of cells has developed.
Blastocyst	Fifth day through second week	A trophoblast is formed outside a hollowed cavity and an inner cell mass develops; it is implanted and flattened to form the embryonic disc.
Gastrula	End of second week	Formation of primary germ layers.

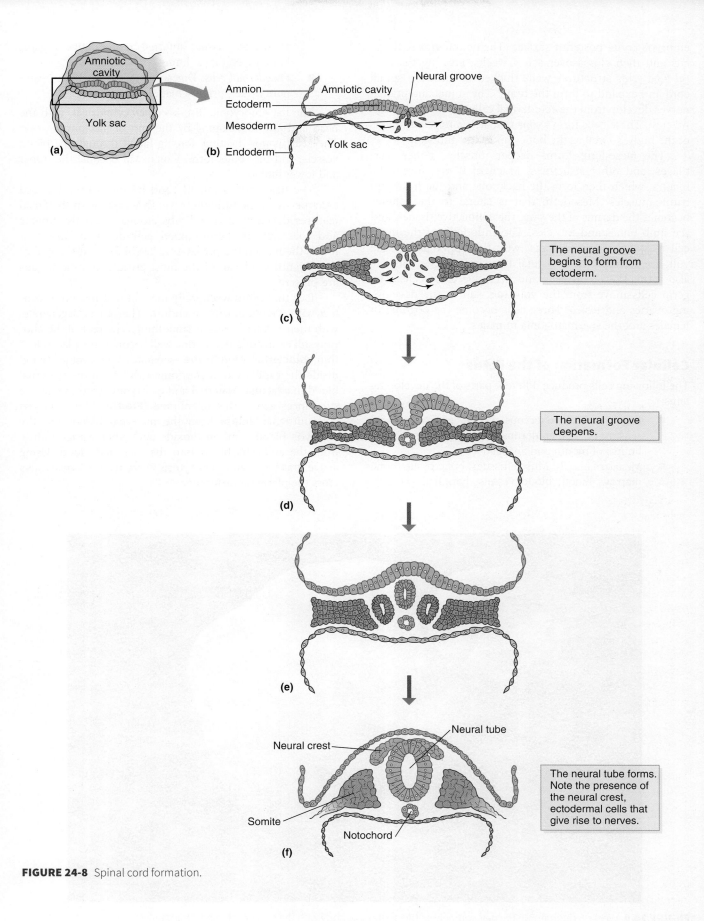

Labels in figure:

(a) Amniotic cavity, Yolk sac

(b) Amnion — Amniotic cavity — Neural groove
Ectoderm
Mesoderm
Endoderm — Yolk sac

(c) The neural groove begins to form from ectoderm.

(d) The neural groove deepens.

(e)

(f) Neural crest — Neural tube
Somite
Notochord — The neural tube forms. Note the presence of the neural crest, ectodermal cells that give rise to nerves.

FIGURE 24-8 Spinal cord formation.

embryo's entire posterior surface. The neural groove deepens and then closes over a few weeks, creating the *neural tube*. This structure's walls thicken to form the spinal cord and expand to form the brain. The spinal and cranial nerves develop from the ectodermal cells that form the *neural crest*. These cells form axons that attach to other organs of the body, as well as the bones, muscles, and skin.

The mesoderm forms deeper muscles, bones, cartilages, and other structures. Much of it first forms the *somites*, which then form the backbone and the head and trunk muscles. Mesoderm that is lateral to the somites becomes the dermis of the skin, the connective tissues, and the limb bones and muscles. The endoderm of the inner cell mass forms the yolk sac, with the upper part of the yolk sac forming the intestinal tract lining. The yolk sac also forms the blood cells and primitive germ cells. The germ cells move from the yolk sac wall to the developing ovaries and testes. These cells become the oogonia in females and the spermatogonia in males.

Cellular Formation of the Fetus

The following cells produce different parts of the developing fetus:

■ *Ectodermal cells:* Nervous system, parts of special sensory organs, epidermis, hair, nails, skin glands, linings of mouth and anal canal
■ *Mesodermal cells:* Muscle tissues, bone tissue, bone marrow, blood, blood vessels, lymphatic vessels, connective tissue, internal reproductive organs, kidneys, epithelial linings of body cavities
■ *Endodermal cells:* Digestive tract epithelium, respiratory tract, urinary bladder, urethra.

The flat embryonic disc becomes cylindrical, with the head and jaws developing by the end of the fourth week. The heart is now beating, forcing blood through the blood vessels, and tiny buds form, which will become the upper and lower limbs.

The head grows quickly and becomes rounded and erect between the fifth and seventh weeks, with the facial features developing. The limbs elongate and the fingers and toes appear. Programmed cell death or *apoptosis* forms them from the preexisting "webbing." At the end of the seventh week, all of the most critical internal organs are present.

Past the eighth week, only the villi that remain in contact with the endometrium endure. The others degenerate, with their former locations smoothing. The part of the chorion still contacting the uterine wall becomes the placenta. A thin **placental membrane** separates embryonic blood inside the capillary of a chorionic villus from the maternal blood in a lacuna. Maternal and embryonic blood exchange substances across this membrane (**FIGURE 24-9**). Oxygen and nutrients diffuse from the maternal blood into the embryo's blood. Carbon dioxide and other wastes diffuse from the embryo's blood into the maternal blood. Using active transport and pinocytosis, various substances also cross the placental membrane.

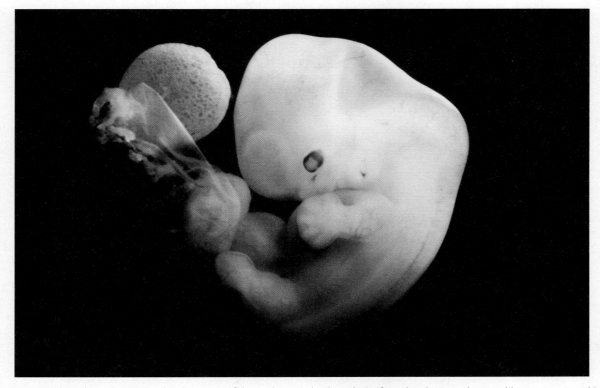

FIGURE 24-9 Weeks 5 through 7 in the development of the embryonic body with the face developing a human-like appearance. (© Ralph Hutchings/Visuals Unlimited)

Growth During the Fetal Period

Teratogens are environmental factors that cause congenital malformations by interfering with prenatal growth or development. The *fetal period* begins at the end of the eighth week and lasts until birth. Growth occurs rapidly during this period, with body proportions beginning to appear more like those of a normal infant. Growth of the head begins to slow as growth of the body increases. By the 12th week, the external reproductive organs may be distinguished as either male or female. **FIGURE 24-10** shows fetal development at 5 to 6 weeks, 4 months, and 5 months.

The fetus grows rapidly during the fourth month, reaching up to 20 cm in length as the limbs lengthen and the skeleton continues to ossify. Ultrasound may be used to assess a fetus in utero during pregnancy (**FIGURE 24-11**). Tests show that 4-month-old fetuses turn away from bright lights if flashed on the mother's belly and show reactions to loud noises. Growth slows during the fifth month, and the lower limbs have reached their final relative proportions. The mother may feel movement beginning around this time. The fetus begins to grow hair on its head, and the skin of the body is covered in fine hair and a mixture of dead epidermal cells and sebum from the sebaceous glands.

During the sixth month, the fetus gains substantial weight, and the eyebrows and eyelashes grow. The skin is wrinkled, translucent, and reddish in appearance because of many blood vessels. In the seventh month, fat is deposited in subcutaneous tissues, smoothing the skin. The eyelids, which were fused during the third month, reopen. By the end of the seventh month, the fetus is about 40 cm long.

During the final trimester, brain cells form networks, organs specialize and grow, and fat continues to develop beneath the skin. The testes of the male fetus descend into the scrotum. The final systems to mature are the digestive and respiratory systems; hence, many babies have difficulty breathing and digesting milk from the mother. At the end of the ninth month or, more accurately, after 266 days, the fetus is considered full term. By now it is nearly 50 cm long and weighs between 2.7 and 3.6 kg. The skin has lost its fine hair but is still coated with sebum and dead epidermal cells. The scalp is usually covered with hair. Nails have developed on the fingers and toes, and the skull bones are largely ossified. The fetus is normally positioned upside down with the head toward the mother's cervix (**FIGURE 24-12**).

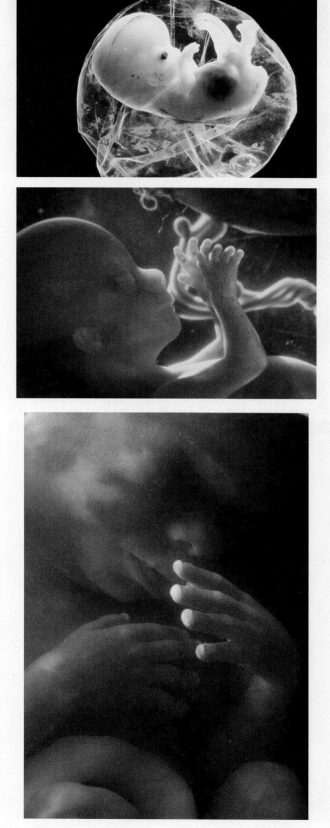

FIGURE 24-10 Fetal development. (A) Fetus at 5 to 6 weeks, (© Biophoto Associates/Science Source) (B) fetus at 4 months, (© Nestle/Petit Format/Science Source) and (c) fetus at 5 months. (© Neil Bromhall/Science Source)

FOCUS ON PATHOLOGY

Preeclampsia, also called *toxemia*, is a serious disease during pregnancy signified by hypertension and proteinuria. It usually occurs during the third trimester but may occur anytime after 20 weeks of gestation. Preeclampsia occurs in 7% of pregnancies in the United States, with unknown causes. It is most common in younger women during their first pregnancies. Risk factors include women with multiple fetuses, age over 35, and history of hypertension or vascular diseases, diabetes, or lupus. Signs and symptoms of preeclampsia include excessive weight gain that is often noticed as edema or peripheral swelling. However, edema does not always manifest. Another significant sign is elevation of blood pressure to more than 140/90. *Eclampsia* is a seizure condition that may develop as a result of preeclampsia.

FOCUS ON PATHOLOGY

Abruptio placentae is premature detachment of a normally positioned placenta from the uterine wall. It is a medical emergency for both the mother and the fetus. The detachment may be partial or complete. It may be linked to hypertension, preeclampsia, trauma, the use of cocaine, infection, and multiple fetuses. This condition causes hemorrhage, abdominal pain, and fetal distress or death.

Placenta previa is a condition of pregnancy in which the placenta is implanted abnormally in the uterus and covers the uterine cervix. It is the most common cause of painless bleeding in the third trimester of pregnancy. Its cause is unknown. Before hemorrhage, placenta previa may be diagnosed by ultrasonography and treated with complete bed rest under close observation.

Fetal Circulation

Maternal blood supplies oxygen and nutrients while carrying away wastes, diffusing these substances through the placental membrane. The first blood cells develop in the yolk sac. Before week 3, spaces appear in the splanchnic mesoderm that are soon lined by endothelial cells and covered with mesenchyme. They are linked together with quickly growing

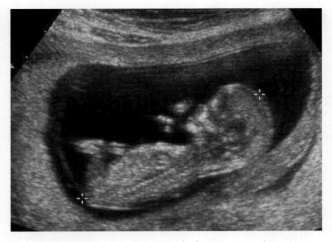

FIGURE 24-11 Ultrasound image of a fetus in utero. (Courtesy of Dr. Myron Pozniak, Department of Radiology, University of Wisconsin School of Medicine and Public Health.)

vascular networks that will form the heart, blood vessels, and lymphatics.

By the end of the third week, the embryo has a paired blood vessel system. The two vessels that form the heart have fused and are not bent to form an "S" shape. Just 3 to 4 days later the heart is already pumping blood, although the embryo is less than one-fourth inch in length. The umbilical arteries and vein as well as three vascular shunts form. They are all occluded when birth eventually occurs. The umbilical vein carries freshly oxygenated blood from the placenta into the embryo's body, bringing it to the developing liver.

Fetal blood contains about 50% more oxygen-carrying hemoglobin than maternal blood. Fetal hemoglobin can carry up to 30% more oxygen than adult hemoglobin. The path of blood in the fetal cardiovascular system is shown in **FIGURE 24-13**.

Nearly half the blood carried to the fetus via the umbilical vein passes into the liver, with the rest entering the **ductus venosus**, which bypasses the liver. This vessel extends to join the inferior vena cava, where oxygenated blood from the placenta mixes with deoxygenated blood from the lower areas of the fetal body. This blood then continues on to the right atrium. Because fetal lungs are nonfunctional, blood largely bypasses them. Much of the blood entering the fetal right atrium is moved directly into the left atrium through an opening in the atrial septum called the **foramen ovale**. Blood pressure is slightly greater in the right atrium than the left atrium. A small valve helps prevent blood flow from reversing. In the liver, blood flow is important to ensure the health of the liver cells. After birth, the infant's liver assumes the functions of nutrient processing that are handled by the mother's liver during gestation.

The rest of the right atrium blood passes into the right ventricle and out through the pulmonary trunk. The pulmonary blood vessels have a high resistance to blood flow during this period of development, but enough blood reaches them to sustain them. Most of the pulmonary trunk blood enters a fetal vessel called the **ductus arteriosus**, connecting to the descending portion of the aortic arch. Blood low in

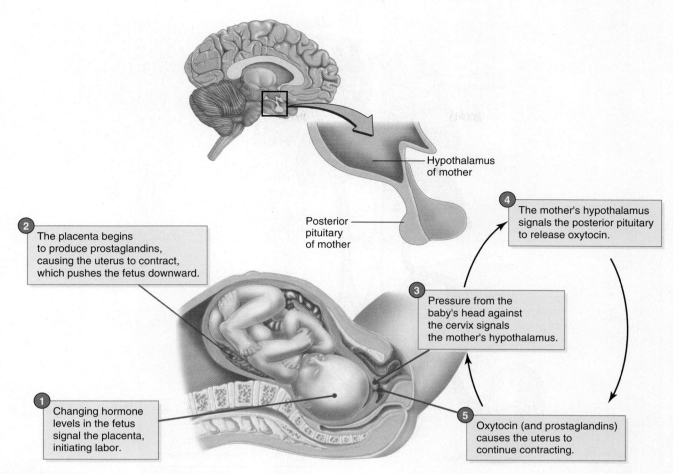

Hypothalamus
of mother

Posterior
pituitary
of mother

4 The mother's hypothalamus signals the posterior pituitary to release oxytocin.

2 The placenta begins to produce prostaglandins, causing the uterus to contract, which pushes the fetus downward.

3 Pressure from the baby's head against the cervix signals the mother's hypothalamus.

1 Changing hormone levels in the fetus signal the placenta, initiating labor.

5 Oxytocin (and prostaglandins) causes the uterus to continue contracting.

FIGURE 24-12 Full-term fetus positioned upside down with head near cervix.

oxygen is prevented from entering the portion of the aorta branching to the heart and brain.

A mixture of highly oxygenated blood entering the left atrium and a small amount of deoxygenated blood from the pulmonary veins moves into the left ventricle and is pumped into the aorta. Some reaches the myocardium and some reaches the brain. Blood from the descending aorta moves to the lower regions of the body, with the rest passing into the umbilical arteries, leading to the placenta. There, it is reoxygenated. **TABLE 24-3** summarizes fetal circulation. At birth, the fetal cardiovascular system must adjust when the placenta stops functioning and the newborn begins to breathe.

Parturition (Birth)

Pregnancy ends with the birth process, which begin hours or days before birth. The act of giving birth is called *labor*. Progesterone declines, and contractions are no longer suppressed. A prostaglandin is synthesized that promotes these contractions as the cervix thins and opens. Late in pregnancy, the uterine and vaginal tissues stretch. Nerve impulses are initiated to the hypothalamus, signaling **oxytocin** to be released from the posterior pituitary gland. This hormone stimulates powerful uterine contractions, aiding in the later

stages of labor. A *false labor* occurs when irregular spasms occur in the uterine musculature.

Stages of Labor

Rhythmic muscular contractions begin moving from the top to the bottom of the uterus, which is the beginning of *true labor*. In normal position, the fetus' head is forced against the cervix (**FIGURE 24-14**). This stimulates even stronger labor contractions. A positive feedback system is used to increase uterine contraction strength. The cervix continues to dilate, and more oxytocin is released. Abdominal wall muscles contract, helping to force the fetus through the cervix and vagina. **FIGURE 24-15** illustrates the three stages of childbirth: dilation of the cervix, expulsion of the fetus, and placental birth.

The first stage of labor is the dilation of the cervix. The second stage, called the expulsion stage, is when the fetus emerges from the vagina. The final or placental birth stage is when the placenta is expelled from the uterus.

If the fetus cannot pass through the vaginal canal because it is too narrow, an *episiotomy* may be performed, which temporarily enlarges the passageway by cutting through the perineal musculature. The episiotomy prevents the mother from experiencing jagged perineal tearing and

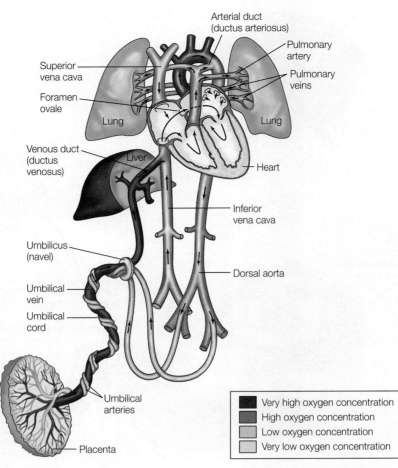

Labels on figure:
- Arterial duct (ductus arteriosus)
- Superior vena cava
- Pulmonary artery
- Pulmonary veins
- Foramen ovale
- Lung
- Lung
- Venous duct (ductus venosus)
- Liver
- Heart
- Inferior vena cava
- Umbilicus (navel)
- Dorsal aorta
- Umbilical vein
- Umbilical cord
- Umbilical arteries
- Placenta

Legend:
- Very high oxygen concentration
- High oxygen concentration
- Low oxygen concentration
- Very low oxygen concentration

FIGURE 24-13 General pattern of fetal circulation.

TABLE 24-3

Fetal Circulation

Structure	Function
Fetal blood	Hemoglobin has more oxygen-carrying capacity than adult hemoglobin.
Umbilical vein	Carries oxygen-rich blood from the placenta to the fetus.
Ductus venosus	Bypasses the liver to conduct nearly half of the umbilical vein blood directly to the inferior vena cava.
Foramen ovale	Bypasses the lungs to conduct much of the blood that enters the right atrium (from the inferior vena cava) through the atrial septum and into the left atrium.
Ductus arteriosus	During intrauterine life, it bypasses the lungs to conduct some pulmonary trunk blood to the aorta; this structure usually closes after birth.
Umbilical arteries	Carry blood from the mother to the placenta.

can be sutured back together easily after the birthing process is complete. When complications occur during dilation or expulsion, the infant can be delivered by *cesarean section (C section)*. An incision is made through the wall of the abdomen, and the uterus is opened wide enough to allow the infant's head to pass. Cesarean sections today represent nearly one-third of all live births.

Once the fetus has been born, the placenta separates from the uterine wall and is expelled through the birth canal. This expulsion is known as *afterbirth* and is accompanied by bleeding because of the separation from the uterine wall, which damages vascular tissues. Oxytocin compresses the bleeding vessels and minimizes blood loss. Later, breast-feeding also contributes to returning the uterus to its original size, via stimulation of oxytocin release from the posterior pituitary.

After the birth of a newborn, health is assessed in five ways: breathing, heart rate, skin color, muscle tone, and reflex response. These are assessed in an *Apgar score*, with each component given a score of between 0 and 2. A total score of 8 to 10 indicates the baby is healthy. In only 3% to 4% of deliveries, a *breech birth* occurs, in which the infant's legs or buttocks enter the vaginal canal before the head. Breech births have higher risks of harm to the infant. This is primarily because the umbilical cord can become constricted and cut off placental blood flow.

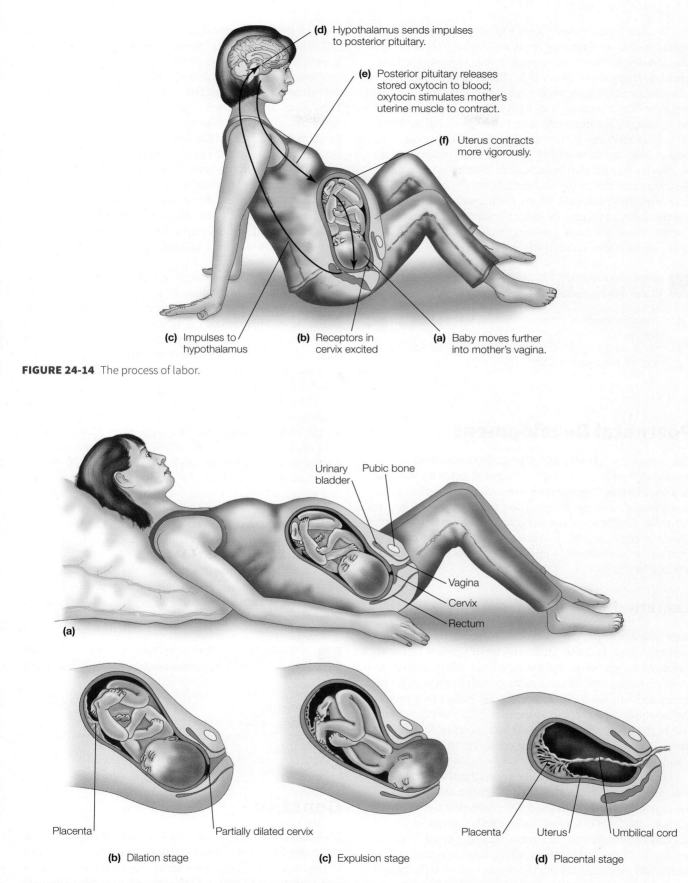

(d) Hypothalamus sends impulses to posterior pituitary.

(e) Posterior pituitary releases stored oxytocin to blood; oxytocin stimulates mother's uterine muscle to contract.

(f) Uterus contracts more vigorously.

(c) Impulses to hypothalamus

(b) Receptors in cervix excited

(a) Baby moves further into mother's vagina.

FIGURE 24-14 The process of labor.

Urinary bladder   Pubic bone

Vagina

Cervix

Rectum

(a)

Placenta   Partially dilated cervix

Placenta   Uterus   Umbilical cord

(b) Dilation stage

(c) Expulsion stage

(d) Placental stage

FIGURE 24-15 Stages of labor. (A) Fetal position before labor, (B) dilation of cervix, (c) expulsion stage, and (d) placental stage.

Multiple births include twins, triplets, quadruplets, quintuplets, and more. Fraternal twins are clinically termed *dizygotic* and develop when two separate oocytes are ovulated and fertilized. Dizygotic twins occur in 70% of twin births. Identical twins are clinically termed *monozygotic* and develop when either the blastomeres separate early in cleavage or because of the splitting of the inner cell mass before gastrulation. These twins have identical genetic makeups because they are both formed from the same pair of gametes. Less commonly, *conjoined twins* may develop because of an incomplete splitting of blastomeres or the embryonic disc. Formerly known as *Siamese twins*, the conjoined infants often share certain organs, and the ability of them to be surgically separated is uncertain. Overall, twins are more common than triplets, which are more common than quadruplets, and so on.

TEST YOUR UNDERSTANDING

1. Describe the developmental milestones of the fetal period.
2. What are the significant components of fetal blood?
3. Explain the stages of labor.

Postnatal Development

The mammary glands are continually stimulated during pregnancy. Estrogens extend the ductile systems and deposit fat around them. Progesterone stimulates the alveolar gland development, assisted by placental lactogen. Breast size is normally doubled during pregnancy, and the mammary glands become capable of secreting milk. However, milk production is temporarily inhibited by placental progesterone and lactogen.

Lactation

After childbirth, placental hormones decline rapidly in the mother's blood. Prolactin stimulates the mammary glands to secrete milk, but before this a watery fluid called *colostrum* is secreted. Colostrum contains more protein but less carbohydrates and fat than milk. It contains antibodies that protect the newborn from various infections. Milk becomes available to the infant through the *milk letdown reflex*, which continues to function until the infant is *weaned*, usually between 1 and 2 years after birth.

The ejection of milk requires specialized myoepithelial cells around the alveolar glands to contract. Stimulation of the nipple or areola elicits the reflex action that controls milk ejection. Oxytocin is released and the cells contract within 30 seconds of stimulation. As long as milk is ejected from the breasts, prolactin and oxytocin release continues and milk is continually produced. If milk is not removed from the breasts regularly, the mammary glands are signaled to stop producing milk. Human milk is the best possible food for human babies, containing exactly the right balance of required nutrients.

The **neonatal period** begins at birth, extending to the end of the first 4 weeks. Newborns must quickly adapt to respiration, digestion, excretion, and regulation of body temperature. The first breath of a newborn must be forceful enough to begin to expand the lungs, which eases breathing. Their lungs are collapsed initially, and the tiny airways are very resistant to air movement. Surface tension tends to hold the moist membranes of the lungs together. Secretion of surfactant occurs, reducing surface tension.

A newborn's liver is unable to supply enough initial glucose to support metabolism, so stored fat is used for energy. Their kidneys excrete a dilute fluid because they cannot yet process concentrated urine. Newborns often become dehydrated as a result and develop a water and electrolyte imbalance. Their temperature-regulating system may also not be normally functional.

After birth, the umbilical vessels constrict, with the umbilical arteries closing first. If not clamped or severed for a minute or more, blood continues to flow from the placenta to the newborn through the umbilical vein. The foramen ovale closes due to blood pressure changes as fetal vessels constrict. Blood pressure in the right atrium falls. Resistance to blood flow through the pulmonary circuit decreases, and blood pressure in the left atrium increases.

The valve on the left side of the atrial septum closes the foramen ovale. It gradually fuses with the tissues along the margin of the foramen. Adults have a depression called the *fossa ovalis* marking the site of the previous opening. The ductus arteriosus also constricts after birth, and blood can no longer bypass the lungs by moving from the pulmonary trunk into the aorta. Constriction of the ductus arteriosus may be complete within 15 minutes, but permanent closure of the foramen ovale may take up to 1 year. Within 4 months after birth, most of the circulating hemoglobin has become of the adult type (**FIGURE 24-16**).

TABLE 24-4 summarizes major events during the neonatal period and later life, **TABLE 24-5** explains changes related to aging, and **TABLE 24-6** lists normal physical growth for females and males during childhood.

TEST YOUR UNDERSTANDING

1. Explain the hormones involved in milk production and secretion.
2. How long does the neonatal period last?
3. Describe the major events that occur in the neonatal period.

Genetics

Children inherit traits from their parents and relatives as determined by DNA. When a gene's DNA sequence changes or *mutates*, an illness may result. *Spontaneous mutations* occur because of random DNA replication errors. The field of **genetics** investigates how genes confer certain characteristics affecting health or contributing to natural variation.

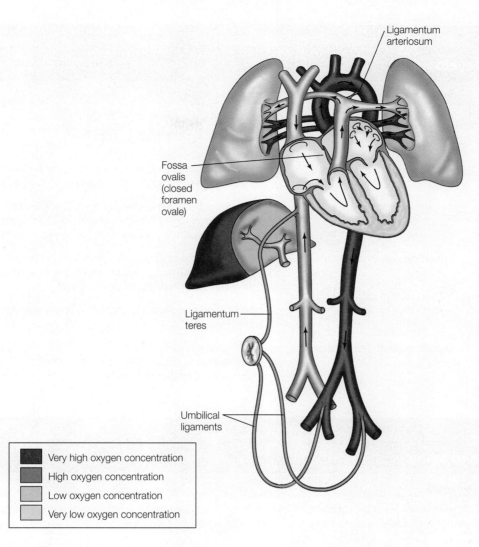

Ligamentum
arteriosum

Fossa
ovalis
(closed
foramen
ovale)

Ligamentum
teres

Umbilical
ligaments

Very high oxygen concentration

High oxygen concentration

Low oxygen concentration

Very low oxygen concentration

FIGURE 24-16 Major changes in the newborn's cardiovascular system.

It also focuses on how genes are passed from generation to generation. Fetal chromosome checks provide clues to a child's future health. A gene's position on a chromosome is called a *locus*. The *Human Genome Project* was created to develop a written copy of the entire human *genome*—the entire set of genetic material or DNA within human chromosomes.

Karyotypes are charts that display the 23 chromosome pairs of human somatic cells (**FIGURE 24-17**). **Autosomes** are pairs 1 through 22 and do not carry genes that determine sex. Only pair 23, the X and Y chromosomes, are **sex chromosomes**. Females have two X chromosomes, and males have one X and one Y chromosome.

Somatic cells have two copies of each autosome and therefore two copies of each gene. Gene copies can be identical or slightly different in a DNA sequence. Such varying forms of a gene are called **alleles**. An individual with two identical alleles of a gene is **homozygous** for that gene. A person with two different alleles is **heterozygous** for that gene. A heterozygote is also called a *carrier*.

The combination of alleles constitutes a person's **genotype**. *Penetrance* is the percentage of people with a certain genotype

that show the *expected* phenotype. Associated with a particular genotype, the appearance, health condition, or other characteristics make up the **phenotype**. A certain inherited trait may be anticipated to occur in the offspring of two individuals when their genes and chromosomes are considered.

Patterns of inheritance through families are known as *modes of inheritance*. A **dominant** allele masks expression of a **recessive** allele. Capital letters are used to designate dominant alleles. The extent to which a certain allele is expressed when it is present is called its *expressivity*. The following generalizations describe modes of inheritance:

- *Autosomal conditions that affect both sexes:* X-linked characteristics affect males much more often than females. Y-linked characteristics are only passed from father to son.
- *Autosomal recessive conditions from two healthy carrier parents:* Recessive conditions can "skip" generations.
- *Dominant condition with at least one affected parent:* Generations are not skipped in these cases.

Three major modes of inheritance are autosomal recessive, autosomal dominant, and X-linked recessive. In autosomal

TABLE 24-4

Periods of Development

Period	Duration	Events
Neonatal period	Birth to end of week 4	Newborn begins respiration, eating, digestion, excretion of wastes, regulation of body temperature, and adjustments to cardiovascular system.
Infancy	End of week 4 to 1 year	High growth rate; teeth start to erupt; muscular and nervous systems mature, allowing coordinated activities; communication begins.
Childhood	1 year to puberty	High growth rate; deciduous teeth erupt and are replaced by permanent teeth; high degree of achieved muscular control; bladder and bowel controls are established; maturation of intellectual abilities.
Adolescence	Puberty to adulthood	Reproductively functional; emotionally more mature; growth spurts occur in skeletal and muscular systems; high levels of motor skills developed; intellectual abilities increase.
Adulthood	Adolescence to old age	Anatomical and physiological states change very little; degenerative changes begin.
Senescence	Old age to death (geriatric period)	Degenerative changes continue; body becomes less able to cope with demands; death often results from mechanical disturbances to cardiovascular system or free disease processes affecting vital organs.

TABLE 24-5

Changes Due to Aging

Body System	Changes
Integumentary	Degenerative loss of collagenous and elastic dermis fibers; decreased production of hair pigment; reduced activity of sweat and sebaceous glands; skin thins, wrinkles, and dries out; hair turns gray, then white
Skeletal	Degenerative loss of bone matrix; bones thin, become less dense, are more likely to fracture; intervertebral disc and vertebrae compression may shorten stature
Muscular	Skeletal muscle fiber loss; degenerative changes in neuromuscular junctions; loss of muscular strength
Nervous	Degenerative changes occur in the neurons, dendrites and synaptic connections are lost, lipofuscin accumulates in the neurons, sensations decrease, mental faculties decrease, communication ability decreases, smell and taste sensations diminish, close vision is lost due to less eye elasticity of the lenses
Endocrine	Reduced hormonal secretions; decreased metabolic rate; reduced stress-coping ability; reduced ability to maintain homeostasis
Cardiovascular	Degenerative cardiac muscle changes; decrease in artery lumen diameters; decreased cardiac output; increased blood flow resistance; increased blood pressure
Lymphatic	Decrease in immune system efficiency; increased infections and neoplastic diseases; increased autoimmune diseases
Digestive	Decreased gastrointestinal tract motility; reduced digestive juice secretion; reduced digestion efficiency
Respiratory	The lungs experience a degenerative loss of elastic fibers, the number of alveoli decreases, vital capacity is reduced, dead air space increases, the ability to cough productively decreased
Urinary	Kidneys degenerate, with fewer functional nephrons—there are 35% fewer functional nephrons by age 70; filtration rate reduced; tubular secretion and reabsorption reduced
Reproductive	
Male	Sex hormone secretion is reduced; prostate gland enlarges; sexual energy decreases
Female	Ovaries degenerate; sex hormone secretion is reduced; menopause occurs; secondary sex characteristics reduce

TABLE 24-6		
Normal Physical Growth (Height and Weight)		
Age (yr)	Average Height (inches)	Average Weight (pounds)
2	33½ (girls) to 34 (boys)	26½ (girls) to 27 (boys)
3	37 (girls) to 37½ (boys)	31 (girls) to 32 (boys)
4	39½ (girls) to 40 (boys)	35 (girls) to 36 (boys)
5	42½ (girls) to 43 (boys)	39 (girls) to 40 (boys)
6	45 (girls) to 45½ (boys)	44 (girls) to 45 (boys)
7	47 (girls) to 47½ (boys)	49½ (girls) to 50 (boys)
8	49½ (girls) to 50 (boys)	55 (both sexes)
9	52 (girls) to 52½ (boys)	62½ (both sexes)
10	54 (both sexes)	70 (both sexes)

recessive inheritance, two recessive alleles, one from each parent, transmit a trait. For example, with cystic fibrosis, if half of a heterozygous male's sperm have the trait causing this disease and half of the female's secondary oocytes also have the trait, the random combination of sperm and oocytes can cause the following:

- A 25% chance of each offspring inheriting two "wild-type" alleles, which are those that are not mutations but normal alleles with observable characteristics different from the standard form.
- A 50% chance of inheriting a disease-causing allele from either parent and therefore being a *carrier*.
- A 25% chance of inheriting a disease-causing allele from each parent.

An autosomal dominant condition requires only one disease-causing allele for inheritance. An example is Huntington's disease, wherein an affected person has an affected parent. X-linked recessive inheritance differs in how it affects females and males. For a female, it is similar to autosomal recessive inheritance because she has two X chromosomes—she can be a heterozygote or a homozygote. Males, with only one X chromosome, express recessive alleles on that chromosome, inheriting an X-linked recessive condition from a mother who is a carrier or is affected. Examples are colorblindness and hemophilia. Patterns of inheritance are predicted by using a *Punnett square*, which is a simple diagram that shows various combinations of parental alleles the offspring may inherit. Gene interactions may determine certain phenotypic traits in interactions described as *polygenic inheritance*.

Sometimes, meiotic changes occur in the structure of chromosomes, with the gametes having different chromosomes

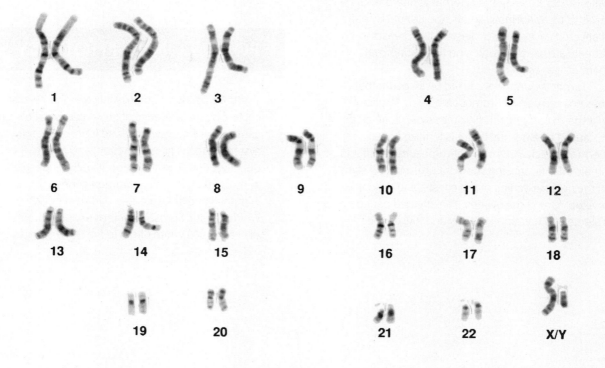

Normal Karyotype

FIGURE 24-17 The 23 pairs of the human karyotype. (Courtesy of National Cancer Institute.)

from those of either parent. This *genetic recombination* increases the range of possible variations among the gametes and later generations, because the genotypes are formed by combinations of gametes during fertilization. In one type of recombination, parts of chromosomes become rearranged. When tetrads form and adjacent chromatids overlap, the process is called *crossing over*. The chromatids can break, with overlapping segments trading places. Usually, genetic exchange between homologous chromosomes is called crossing over, whereas genetic exchange between nonhomologous chromosomes is called *translocation*.

Genomic imprinting is very important during early embryonic development. It usually causes specific but reversible chemical DNA and protein modifications, which control whether the gene is expressed or silenced. *Imprinting patterns* are developed, which can determine if derived genes are transcribed during embryo development. Genomic imprinting is most often implicated in *Angelman syndrome*, a hyperactivity-retardation-seizure disorder, and *Prader-Willi syndrome*, which causes short stature, reduced skin pigmentation and muscle tone, degrees of mental retardation, and underdeveloped gonads. **TABLE 24-7** lists a number of human traits and diseases related to chromosomes.

Environmental factors may affect inherited traits and conditions. These factors include nutrition, exposure to toxins or pathogens, and physical activity. Environmental factors hold great importance for polygenic traits, which are those determined by more than one gene, such as height, skin color, and intelligence.

FOCUS ON PATHOLOGY

The most common conditions related to chromosomal abnormalities include Down syndrome, Klinefelter syndrome, and Turner syndrome. *Down syndrome*, also called *trisomy 21*, affects approximately 1 of every 700 infants in the United States. They usually are short in stature with rounded faces, a protruding tongue, slanted eyes, and mental retardation. Life span may be shorter than normal, and many Down syndrome babies die in infancy from heart abnormalities or respiratory infections. Incidence increases dramatically with a maternal age over 35 years.

Klinefelter syndrome is caused by an ovum containing an extra X chromosome that is fertilized by a sperm carrying a Y chromosome. It affects male infants, causing the external genitalia and testes to be abnormally small. Approximately half of affected cases develop female-like breasts. Patients are usually sterile and have abnormal spermatogenesis.

Turner syndrome is caused by an ovum that does not carry an X chromosome being fertilized by a sperm carrying this chromosome. It can also be caused by a normal ovum is fertilized by a sperm that lacks an X or a Y chromosome. It affects female infants, causing short stature, a fold of skin on the neck, widening of the chests, and lack of development of the ovaries. The affected patient is sterile and has small breasts and low estrogen levels.

FOCUS ON PATHOLOGY

Cystic fibrosis is an autosomal recessive disease caused by the presence of two recessive alleles. It causes abnormal sweat gland function, respiratory system mucous gland function, and pancreatic duct function. The condition usually leads to an early death. It is a very common genetic disease, with the gene being carried by 1 of every 22 Whites. Cystic fibrosis develops in approximately 1 of every 2,000 White births in the United States.

TABLE 24-7

Human Traits and Diseases Related to Chromosomes

Disorders	Descriptions
Autosomal dominant	
Achondroplasia	Dwarfism caused by a defect in the epiphyseal plates of long bones as they form
Brachydactyly	Shortened fingers and disfiguration of the hands
Freckles	Permanent melanin aggregations in the skin
Huntington's disease	Progressive nervous system deterioration that begins in the late twenties or early thirties; results in mental deterioration and early death
Marfan's syndrome	Connective tissue defect that causes excessive growth and aortic rupture
Widow's peak	Hairline that comes to a point on the forehead.
Autosomal recessive	
Albinism	Lack of pigment in the eyes, hair, and skin
Attached earlobe	Earlobes remain attached to the skin of the neck instead of separated from it
Cystic fibrosis	Buildup of mucus in the lungs and pancreatic failure
Hyperextendable thumb	Able to bend thumb past a 45-degree angle
Phenylketonuria	Phenylalanine accumulates in the blood, resulting in mental retardation
Sickle-cell anemia	Abnormal hemoglobin causes sickle-shaped red blood cells, which obstruct vital capillaries
Tay-Sachs disease	Improper metabolism of chemicals known as gangliosides in the nerve cells, causing early death

SUMMARY

Pregnancy is the presence of a developing offspring in the uterus. The production of fertilization is a zygote with 46 chromosomes. The developing offspring moves down the uterine tube to the uterus, where it implants in the endometrium. The most important hormones involved in pregnancy include hCG, estrogens, progesterone, and relaxin. The embryonic period extends from the beginning of the second week through the eighth week of development. The embryo is encircled almost entirely by the amniotic sac, except for a break that allows passage of the umbilical cord. Embryonic development proceeds from gastrulation, in which the first structures form, through organogenesis, when the organs develop. By the beginning of the eighth week, the embryo is recognizable as human.

The fetal period extends from the end of the eighth week until birth. Placentation is the formation of the placenta, a temporary structure that controls production of progesterone and estrogen, beginning between the second and third months of gestation. The fetus is full term at the end of 38 weeks. Birth is also known as parturition and involves three stages of labor: dilation of the cervix, expulsion of the fetus, and placental birth.

During postnatal development, the mammary glands of the mother begin to secrete milk. The neonatal period extends from birth to the end of the fourth week. The newborn's respiratory and digestive systems are the least well developed of all body systems. In regards to human development, growth is defined as an increase in size. Development is the process of changing from one life phase to another. The five stages of postnatal development are the neonatal period, infancy, childhood, adolescence, and maturity. The periods from infancy to adolescence fall under the medical specialty known as *pediatrics*.

The field of genetics studies how children inherit traits from their parents and relatives, as determined by DNA. The combination of varying forms of genes, called alleles, make up a person's genotype. Patterns of inheritance through families are called modes of inheritance, which include autosomal recessive, autosomal dominant, and X-linked recessive.

KEY TERMS

Allantois	Endoderm	Organogenesis
Alleles	Extraembryonic membranes	Oxytocin
Amnion	Fertilization	Phenotype
Amniotic fluid	Fetal period	Placenta
Autosomes	Fetus	Placental lactogen
Blastocyst	Foramen ovale	Placental membrane
Blastomeres	Gastrula	Placentation
Chorion	Gastrulation	Postnatal period
Chorionic villi	Genetics	Pregnancy
Cleavage	Genotype	Prenatal period
Decidua basalis	Gestation	Primary germ layers
Decidua capsularis	Growth	Primitive streak
Development	Heterozygous	Recessive
Dominant	Homozygous	Relaxin
Ductus arteriosus	Human chorionic gonadotropin	Sex chromosomes
Ductus venosus	(hCG)	Teratogens
Ectoderm	Lacunae	Trophoblast cells
Embryo	Mesoderm	Umbilical cord
Embryonic disc	Morula	Yolk sac
Embryonic period	Neonatal period	Zygote

LEARNING GOALS

The following learning goals correspond to the objectives at the beginning of this chapter:

1. Fertilization is the union of a sperm cell with an egg cell. Also called conception, it usually occurs in a uterine tube. During sexual intercourse, the male deposits semen into the vagina, near the cervix. The sperm must reach the uterine tube, where the secondary oocyte is located. Only one sperm actually fertilizes this egg cell. Fertilization occurs once a sperm cell binds with the zona pellucida surrounding the oocyte cell membrane. Enzymes aid the sperm head's penetration; several hundred sperm cells must be present to produce enough needed enzymes. The head of a sperm enters the oocyte, but the remainder stays outside. The oocyte membrane strengthens to keep additional sperm heads from entering. Inside the oocyte's cytoplasm, the sperm head causes the oocyte to divide to form a large nucleated cell and a tiny second polar body. The sperm provides 23 chromosomes and the oocyte provides the same amount.

2. The zygote undergoes mitosis about 30 hours after it has formed. This gives rise to two blastomeres that in turn divide into four cells, then eight, and so on. These divisions are rapid, yielding smaller cells because of

lack of time for any cell growth. This phase of early cell division is called cleavage. During this period, the tiny cell mass moves through the uterine tube to the uterine cavity. This takes about 3 days, with the structure consisting of a solid ball of nearly 16 cells, called a morula.

3. Until the end of the eighth week of development, the offspring is called an embryo. At this point, the basic structural form of the human body is recognizable. Starting with the eighth week and lasting until birth, the offspring is called a fetus, with simple versions of all organs present. These organs and other structures enlarge and become specialized as the fetus develops.

4. After implantation, hCG is secreted by the cells of the embryo. It maintains the corpus luteum, which continues to secrete estrogens and progesterone. The developing placenta secretes estrogens and progesterone, which have many effects on the uterine lining, other hormones' secretion, mammary gland development, control of contractions, and also enlarge reproductive organs. From the corpus luteum, relaxin inhibits uterine contractions and relaxes the pelvic ligaments. Placental lactogen is secreted from the

placenta to stimulate breast development. Aldosterone is secreted from the adrenal cortex to promote renal absorption of sodium. Parathyroid hormone is secreted from the parathyroid glands to help maintain high concentrations of maternal blood calcium.

5. Twelve to 24 hours after ovulation, a secondary oocyte may be fertilized. Meiosis is completed, with the zygote having 46 chromosomes and being genetically distinct. Cleavage occurs from 30 hours after fertilization up to 3 days, with cell number increasing by mitosis. Between the third and fourth day, a solid morula has developed. Between the fifth day and second week, a hollowed ball called a blastocyst has formed an outer trophoblast and inner cell mass; this implants and flattens to form an embryonic disc. By the end of the second week, primary germ layers form a gastrula.

6. The birth process begins hours or days before birth, and the act of giving birth is called labor. Progesterone declines, and contractions are no longer suppressed. A prostaglandin is synthesized that promotes these contractions as the cervix thins and opens. Late in pregnancy, the uterine and vaginal tissues stretch. Nerve impulses are initiated to the hypothalamus, signaling oxytocin to be released from the posterior pituitary gland, stimulating powerful uterine contractions. Rhythmic muscular contractions begin moving from the top to the bottom of the uterus. In normal position, the fetus' head is forced against the cervix, stimulating even stronger labor contractions. The cervix continues to dilate, and more oxytocin is released. Abdominal wall muscles contract, helping to force the fetus through the cervix and vagina.

7. The umbilical cord contains two arteries and one vein. The cord transports blood between the embryo and placenta and suspends the embryo in the amniotic cavity.

8. The neonatal period begins abruptly at birth and extends to the end of the first 4 weeks.

9.
    A. *Chromosomes:* Thread-like structures in cell nuclei that contain protein and genes that control DNA functions.
    B. *Genes:* The basic units of heredity in living organisms.
    C. *Autosomes:* Chromosomes that do not carry genes that determine sex.
    D. *Alleles:* Variant forms of a gene, which can be identical or slightly different in DNA sequence.
    E. *Homozygous:* A condition related to genes wherein there are two identical alleles.

10. Dominant alleles mask expression of recessive alleles. Gene copies can be identical or slightly different in a DNA sequence. Such varying forms of a gene are called alleles.

CRITICAL THINKING QUESTIONS

A couple that has been trying to have a baby for 3 years goes to see a fertility specialist. After testing, the woman tests normal, but the man is shown to be "subfertile." He has a very low sperm count.

1. How can this affect the couple's chances of having a baby?
2. What can the physician suggest to this couple that may help the woman become pregnant?

REVIEW QUESTIONS

1. The union of a sperm cell and an egg cell is called
    A. cleavage
    B. implantation
    C. plantation
    D. fertilization

2. The process of cell division that occurs after fertilization is called
    A. blastulation
    B. cleavage
    C. embryogenesis
    D. implantation

3. The inner cell mass of the blastocyst will form
    A. the embryo
    B. the placenta
    C. the morula
    D. blood vessels of the placenta

4. The solid ball of cells after several rounds of cell division is called a
   A. blastocyst
   B. morula
   C. blastula
   D. chorion
5. A blastocyst is a
   A. solid ball of cells
   B. hollow ball of cells
   C. portion of the ovary
   D. part of the penis
6. Most of the blood in the pulmonary trunk bypasses the lungs by entering a fetal vessel called the
   A. foramen ovale
   B. ductus venosus
   C. ductus arteriosus
   D. umbilical vein
7. What substance fills the space between the amnion and embryonic disc?
   A. amniotic fluid
   B. aqueous fluid
   C. allantois
   D. colostrum
8. The hormone that increases the flexibility of the symphysis pubis and causes dilation of the cervix during pregnancy is
   A. estrogen
   B. luteinizing hormone
   C. human placental lactogen
   D. relaxin
9. The first stage of labor is the
   A. dilation stage
   B. expulsion stage
   C. decidual stage
   D. neonate stage
10. The time spent in prenatal development is referred to as
   A. implantation
   B. embryogenesis
   C. plantation
   D. gestation
11. An individual who has two identical alleles of a gene is referred to as
   A. homozygous
   B. homologous
   C. heterozygous
   D. autosome
12. Chromosomes that are not sex chromosomes are referred to as
   A. heterozygous
   B. homozygous
   C. homologous
   D. autosomes
13. An implantation occurring somewhere other than in the uterus is called
   A. placenta previa
   B. an ectopic pregnancy
   C. an abortion
   D. hydramnios
14. A developing fetus may be distinguished as either male or female at
   A. 8 weeks of development
   B. 12 weeks of development
   C. 4 months of development
   D. 6 months of development
15. Which of the following hormones is involved in milk production?
   A. estrogen
   B. progesterone
   C. relaxin
   D. prolactin

ESSAY QUESTIONS

1. Describe the process of fertilization.
2. Describe cleavage and blastocyst formation.
3. What is the function of gastrulation?
4. Describe the major functions of the placenta.
5. Explain which body system and other parts of the body develop from ectodermal cells.
6. Describe fetal circulation.
7. Explain the stages of labor.
8. Define the terms karyotypes, autosomes, and heterozygous.
9. Describe the three major modes of inheritance.
10. Explain environmental factors that may affect inherited traits and conditions.

Glossary

A bands: The areas between I bands of a sarcomere; they are marked by partial overlapping of actin and myosin filaments and appear dark.

A-V bundle: The bundle of His; a large structure that receives the cardiac impulse from the distal atrioventricular node; it enters the upper part of the interventricular septum.

Abduction: Moving a part away from the midline (longitudinal axis), or median plane, of the body.

Absolute refractory period: The period from the opening of sodium channels until they begin to reset to their original resting state.

Accessory organs: In the digestive system, these include the salivary glands, liver, gallbladder, and pancreas.

Accommodation: Adjustment of the lens of the eye for close or distant vision.

Acetabular labrum: A circular rim of fibrocartilage of the hip joint that increases the depth of the acetabulum.

Acetylcholine: The neurotransmitter that stimulates skeletal muscle to contract.

Acetylcholinesterase: The enzyme that causes muscle relaxation by the decomposition of acetylcholine.

Acid-base buffer systems: Chemicals that combine with excess acids or bases.

Acid mantle: A slightly acidic film on the skin surface that acts as a barrier to bacteria, viruses, and other potential contaminants that could penetrate the skin.

Acidosis: Also known as acidemia; the accumulation of acid and hydrogen ions or depletion of the bicarbonate content in the blood and body tissues, decreasing the pH.

Acids: Electrolytes that dissociate in water to release hydrogen ions.

Acromegaly: A disorder marked by progressive enlargement of the head, face, hands, and feet because of excessive secretion of growth hormone from the anterior lobe of the pituitary gland, occurring after puberty.

Actin: The component that makes up most of the thin protein filaments of the myofibrils.

Action potential: The basis for a nerve impulse, based on the cell membrane reaching its threshold potential; it is a brief reversal of membrane potential with a change in voltage of approximately 100 millivolts.

Activation energy: The amount of energy required to start a reaction.

Active site: The part of an enzyme molecule that binds a substrate.

Active transport: The movement of particles through membranes from regions of lower concentration to regions of higher concentration.

Active tubular reabsorption: A selective process that reclaims materials from the tubular fluid and returns them to the bloodstream; it can move a solute against an electrochemical gradient and requires energy derived from metabolism.

Adaptive (specific) defense: Immunity; it targets specific pathogens and acts more slowly than innate defenses.

Addison's disease: A disorder caused by lower than normal amounts of adrenal gland hormones being produced; these hormones include the glucocorticoids, mineralocorticoids, and sex hormones.

Adduction: Moving a part toward the midline of the body.

Adenosine triphosphate: An adenine-containing RNA nucleotide to which two additional phosphate groups have been added; also known as ATP, it is the primary energy-transferring molecule in body cells, providing a form of energy that can be immediately used by them.

Adiponectin: A hormone produced exclusively in adipose tissue that is involved in many metabolic processes, including glucose regulation and the metabolism of fat for energy production.

Adipose tissue: Fat tissue that lies beneath the skin, between muscles, around the kidneys, behind the eyes, in certain abdominal membranes, on the heart's surface, and around certain joints.

Adrenal androgens: Sex hormones from the adrenal cortex; may be converted to estrogens, progesterone, or testosterone.

Adrenergic fibers: Sympathetic postganglionic neurons that secrete norepinephrine (noradrenalin).

Adrenocorticotropic hormone (ACTH): Also known as corticotropin, it controls hormone secretion from the adrenal cortex; it may also be secreted in larger quantities due to stress.

Aerobic respiration: The release of energy from glucose or another organic substrate in the presence of oxygen.

Afferent arterioles: The final branches of the interlobular arteries of the kidneys; they lead to the nephrons.

Afferent (sensory) division: The part of the peripheral nervous system that carries impulses to the central nervous system from the body's sensory receptors.

Agglutination: The clumping of red blood cells after a transfusion reaction.

Agonist: A prime mover; a muscle that contracts to provide most of a desired movement.

Agranulocytes: Leukocytes without granular cytoplasm.

Albumins: The smallest of plasma proteins; they make up around 60% of these proteins by weight.

Aldosterone: A mineralocorticoid produced by the adrenal cortex that helps the kidneys to balance sodium and potassium as well as stimulating water retention via osmosis.

Alimentary canal: The mouth, pharynx, esophagus, stomach, small intestine, large intestine, rectum, and anus.

Alkalosis: Also known as alkalemia; the accumulation of bases, or loss of acids from the blood and body tissues, increasing the pH.

All-or-none phenomenon: The description of how an action potential occurs, which is either completely or not at all; the action potential is generated and propagated once it reaches threshold whether or not the stimulus continues, and it cannot occur if threshold is never reached, even only by a slight amount.

Allantois: A structure that forms during the third week of development as a tube extending from the early yolk sac into the connecting stalk of the embryo.

Alleles: Variant forms of a gene, which can be identical or slightly different in DNA sequence.

Allergens: Antigens; chemicals that stimulate B cells to produce antibodies or allergies.

Alveolar ducts: Thin ducts leading to the alveolar sacs.

Alveolar sacs: Outpouchings that lead to the alveoli.

Alveolar ventilation rate: A measurement of the flow of gases in and out of the alveoli during a certain time interval; it includes the air in the dead space and is based on millimeters of air per minute.

Alveoli: Microscopic air sacs inside capillary networks of the lungs; they are composed mainly of simple squamous epithelial cells called pneumocytes.

Ammonia: A compound of nitrogen and hydrogen that is secreted by the kidneys to neutralize excess acid; however, in sufficient quantities, it is toxic to body cells.

Amnion: A membrane that develops, during the embryonic period, around the embryo; it appears during the second week.

Amniotic fluid: A liquid that fills the space between the amnion and embryonic disc.

Amphiarthrotic: A joint that is slightly movable; mostly found in the axial skeleton, along with synarthrotic joints.

Ampulla: An expansion at the end of each semicircular canal containing a crista ampullaris.

Amygdaloid body: An almond-shaped nucleus on the tail of the caudate nucleus and is part of the limbic system.

Anabolism: The synthesis of larger molecules from smaller ones.

Anaerobic: Able to function without oxygen.

Anal canal: The last 2.5 to 4 cm of the large intestine, located at the lower portion of the rectum.

Anastomoses: Communications between vessels via collateral channels.

Anatomists: Experts or students in the study of anatomy.

Anatomy: The study of body parts, forms, and structures.

Androgens: Male sex hormones mostly produced by the testicular interstitial cells.

Angiotensin II: The most potent known vascular constricting agent; it also causes the release of aldosterone, another agent that increases blood pressure.

Angiotensinogen: A serum globulin formed by the liver that is cleaved by renin to form angiotensin I.

Anions: Ions with a negative charge.

Annular ligament: The ligament that surrounds the heat of the radius and is part of the elbow joint.

Antagonists: Muscles that cause movement in the opposite direction of prime movers.

Anterior cruciate ligament: The ligament attached to the tibia's anterior intercondylar area that passes upward, laterally, and posteriorly to attach to the femur; it attaches to the medial side of the femur's lateral condyle and prevents the tibia from sliding forward on the femur to control hyperextension of the knee.

Antibodies: Immunoglobulins or aggluitinins; they are gamma globulin proteians that react to destroy antigens or antigen-containing particles and are produced from B cells.

Antibody monomer: A molecule formed by each antibody's four looped polypeptide chains and connected by sulfur-to-sulfur (disulfide) bonds.

Antidiuretic hormone: Abbreviated as ADH, it regulates the water concentration of body fluids by reducing water excretion by the kidneys.

Antigen-binding site: An area made up by the V regions of heavy and light chains of an antibody; it has a shape fitting a certain antigenic determinant or epitope. In each monomer arm, each antibody monomer has two antigen-binding sites or regions.

Antigen-presenting cell: An accessory cell, which may be a macrophage, B cell, or other type of cell that has processed antigen fragments on its surface.

Antigens: Also called agglutinogens, they are proteins, polysaccharides, glycoproteins, or glycolipids commonly found on red blood cell surfaces; cells learn to recognize antigens as either "self" or "nonself" (foreign).

Anus: The opening of the distal end of the anal canal; feces pass out of the anus to outside of the body.

Aorta: The largest artery in the body, it originates from the left ventricle of the heart and extends down to the abdomen, where it branches off and sends oxygenated blood to all body tissues.

Aortic arch: The second section of the aorta; it branches into the brachiocephalic trunk, left common carotid artery, and left subclavian artery.

Aortic valve: Located at the base of the aorta, it has three cusps and opens to allow blood to leave the left ventricle during contraction.

Apex: The lowest superficial part of the heart, formed by the inferolateral part of the left ventricle.

Apocrine glands: Exocrine glands that lose parts of their cell bodies during secretion.

Aponeuroses: Broad sheets of fibers that may attach to bones or to the coverings of other muscles.

Appendicular skeleton: The pectoral girdle, upper limbs, pelvic girdle, and lower limbs.

Appendix: A tube-like structure emerging from the first part of the large intestine that contains many lymphoid follicles; its actions are not fully understood.

Aqueous humor: Watery fluid filling the anterior eye cavity.

Arachidonic acid: A 20-carbon fatty acid in all cell membranes from which eicosanoids are derived; it is abundant in the brain, muscles, and liver.

Arachnoid mater: The thin, web-like middle layer of the meninges.

Arcuate popliteal ligament: The ligament that reinforces the joint capsule posteriorly; it has a superior arc from the head of the fibula over the popliteus muscle.

Areola: The colored ring of tissue around the nipple.

Areolar tissue: The type of tissue that binds skin to underlying organs and fills in spaces between muscles.

Arrhythmias: Irregularities in the force or rhythm of the heartbeat.

Arteries: Elastic vessels able to carry blood away from the heart under high pressure.

Arterioles: Subdivisions of arteries; they are thinner and have muscles that are innervated by the sympathetic nervous system.

Arthritis: Inflammation in a joint.

Arthroscopic surgery: A type of surgery used to remove damaged cartilage from joints; an arthroscope is used, which is very small and contains a lens and fiberoptic light source.

Ascending colon: Begins at the cecum and continues upward and left.

Ascites: An abnormal intraperitoneal accumulation of a fluid containing large amounts of protein and electrolytes.

Astrocytes: Neuroglia of the central nervous system, usually found between neurons and blood vessels.

Atlas: The first cervical vertebra, supporting the head.

Atomic number: A whole number representing the number of positively charged protons in the nucleus of an atom.

Atomic weight: The total number of protons and neutrons in the nucleus of an atom.

Atoms: The smallest complete units of an element that have the element's properties, varying in size, weight, and interaction with other atoms.

ATPase: An enzyme that catalyzes the breakdown of adenosine triphosphate to both adenosine diphosphate and phosphate, releasing energy.

Atria: The upper chambers of the heart; they receive blood returning to the heart.

Atrioventricular node (A-V node): A specialized mass of cardiac muscle fibers in the interatrial septum of the heart; it transmits cardiac impulses from the sinoatrial node to the A-V bundle.

Auditory ossicles: The bones of the middle ear.

Auditory tube: Eustachian tube; it connects the middle ear cavity to the pharynx.

Auricle: The funnel-shaped structure of the outer ear.

Autoantibodies: Those produced by the body in reaction to any of its own cells or cell products.

Autocrine: Denoting self-stimulation through cellular production of a factor and a specific receptor for it.

Autoimmunity: An abnormal immune response in which the body attacks its own tissues.

Automaticity: The capacity of a cell to initiate an impulse without an external stimulus such as neural or hormonal regulation; also known as autorhythmicity.

Autonomic nervous system: The part of the nervous system that handles involuntary effectors such as the heart, certain glands, and smooth muscle in blood vessels.

Autonomic reflex: A reflex that activates visceral effectors such as smooth or cardiac muscle or glands; it is also known as a visceral reflex.

Autosomes: The chromosomes that do not carry genes that determine sex.

Avascular: Lacking blood vessels.

Axial skeleton: The skull, hyoid bone, vertebral column, and thoracic cage.

Axis: The second vertebra.

Axon collaterals: Structures of axons that project back toward the cell to which the axon is attached; they easily form synapses with the cell itself, or other nearby cells, and serve as regulation systems.

Axon terminals: Also called terminal boutons; they are enlarged endings of axons that make synaptic contacts with other nerve cells or with effector cells.

Axons: Extensions from neurons that send out electro-chemical messages.

B cells: Lymphocytes that produce and secrete antibodies that bind and destroy foreign antigens.

Baroreceptors: Nerve endings that are stimulated by pressure changes, including increased arterial blood pressure; they are located in the aortic arch and carotid sinuses.

Basal lamina: A thin, noncellular layer of ground substance lying under epithelial surfaces that separates the epidermis from the areolar tissue of the adjacent dermis.

Basal nuclei: Help to control skeletal muscle activity; they filter out inappropriate responses and are involved in cognition and emotion.

Base: The portion of the heart opposite the apex; it is superior and medially located and forms the upper border of the heart. The base mostly involves the atria and proximal portions of the great vessels.

Basement membrane: Anchors epithelial tissue to connective tissue.

Bases: Electrolytes that release ions that bond with hydrogen ions.

Basophils: Leukocytes that have fewer granules than eosinophils; they become deep blue in basic stain.

Beta-oxidation: When fatty acids are broken down in the mitochondria or peroxisomes.

Bicarbonate ions: Those related to carbonic acid; they are formed from carbon dioxide transport mechanisms.

Bile: A yellow-green fluid secreted from hepatic cells that contains water, bile salts, bile pigments (bilirubin and biliverdin), cholesterol, and electrolytes.

Bilirubin: An orange pigment formed from biliverdin that has potent antioxidant activity; a waste product of the heme of hemoglobin that is formed during breakdown of worn-out erythrocytes, it is excreted along with biliverdin in the bile.

Biliverdin: A green pigment created from decomposing heme, which is converted into bilirubin.

Blastocyst: The embryonic form that follows the morula in human development.

Blastomeres: Cells resulting from the cleavage of a fertilized ovum during early embryonic development.

Blood: The liquid pumped by the heart through all arteries, veins, and capillaries.

Blood flow: The amount (volume) of blood that flows through blood vessels, organs, or the systemic circulation, in milliliters per minute (mL/min).

Blood pressure: The force that blood exerts against the inner walls of blood vessels. It most commonly refers to pressure in arteries supplied by the aortic branches, even though it actually occurs throughout the vascular system.

Blood volume: The sum of formed elements and plasma volumes in the vascular system; most adults have about 5 liters of blood.

Blood–brain barrier: The structure created by the endothelial cells that line the central nervous system capillaries, which controls exchange between the blood and interstitial fluid.

Bolus: A mass; for example, food is chewed, mixed with saliva, and rolled into a bolus by the tongue.

Bone lining cells: Flat cells on bone surfaces where bone remodeling does not occur; they are believed to also help maintain the bone matrix.

Bone: The most rigid type of connective tissue, with a high mineral content that makes it harder than other types.

Bony labyrinth: The rigid outer wall of the inner ear; it consists of the vestibule, semicircular canals, and cochlea.

Bowman's capsule: A thin, membranous double-walled capsule surrounding the glomerulus.

Brachial plexuses: Found in the shoulders between the neck and armpits, they supply the skin and muscles of the arms and hands, most importantly including the musculocutaneous, median, radial, ulnar, and axillary nerves.

Brachiocephalic trunk: One of the three arteries branching from the arch of the aorta, running about 5 cm and dividing into the right common carotid and right subclavian arteries.

Brachiocephalic vein: The vein feeding the superior vena cava, collecting blood from the subclavian and jugular veins.

Bradycardia: Slowness of the heartbeat, usually under 60 beats per minute in adults.

Brain stem: The section of the brain that contains the midbrain, pons, and medulla oblongata; its structure is similar to that of the spinal cord, and it produces controlled and automatic behaviors required for survival.

Brain waves: The patterns of neuronal electrical activity recorded on an electroencephalogram.

Broad ligament: The ligament that folds over the uterus to support the uterus, uterine tubes, and vagina. It encloses the ovarian ligaments.

Broca's area: A small posterior part of the inferior frontal gyrus of the left cerebral hemisphere that is an essential component of motor mechanisms needed for speech.

Bronchial tree: Consists of branched airways leading from the trachea to the alveoli.

Bronchioles: Small tubes that continue to divide, including terminal bronchioles, respiratory bronchioles, and alveolar ducts.

Bulbourethral glands: Cowper's glands; they lie inferior to the prostate gland and secrete a lubricating fluid that prepares the penis for sexual intercourse.

Burn: Tissue damage caused by intense heat, chemicals, electricity, or radiation that kills cells and denatures cell proteins.

Bursae: Closed sacs lined with a synovial membrane.

Bursitis: An inflammation of one or more bursae; it most often occurs in the shoulders, hips, or knees.

Calcaneus: The heel bone.

Calcarine sulcus: A groove of the medial surface of the occipital lobe that separates the wedge-shaped cuneus of the cerebrum from the lingual gyrus.

Calcitonin: A thyroid hormone that regulates the concentrations of blood calcium and phosphate ions.

Calmodulin: A calcium-binding messenger protein in eukaryotic cells that transduces calcium signals by binding calcium ions and then modifying interactions with target proteins.

Calorie: The amount of heat needed to raise the temperature of a gram of water by one degree.

Canines: The four teeth, one on each side of the upper and lower jaws, situated between the lateral incisors and first premolars.

Capillaries: The smallest diameter blood vessels, which connect the smallest arterioles to the smallest venules.

Carbaminohemoglobin: The bonding of carbon dioxide with hemoglobin.

Carbohydrates: Substances (including sugars) that provide much of the energy required by the body's cells and that help to build cell structures.

Carbonic anhydrase: An enzyme in red blood cells that speeds reaction of carbon dioxide and water, resulting in carbonic acid.

Cardiac conduction system: The initiation and distribution of impulses through the myocardium that coordinates the cardiac cycle.

Cardiac cycle: A heartbeat; it consists of a complete series of systolic and diastolic events.

Cardiac muscle: The muscle found only in the heart, comprising most of the heart walls; it is striated but not voluntary and contracts without nervous system stimulation.

Cardiac muscle tissue: A special striated muscle of the myocardium, containing dark intercalated discs at the junctions of abutting fibers.

Cardiac output: The volume discharged from the ventricle per minute, calculated by multiplying stroke volume by heart rate, in beats per minute.

Cardiac plexuses: The plexuses around the base of the heart, mostly in the epicardium; they are formed by cardiac branches from the vagus nerves and the sympathetic trunks and ganglia.

Cardinal ligaments: Parts of the thickenings of the visceral pelvic fascia beside the cervix and vagina; they pass laterally to merge with the upper fascia of the pelvic diaphragm.

Carotid bodies: Small structures in the carotid arteries that contain chemoreceptors that are involved in the control of respiration.

Carotid sinuses: Dilations of the arterial walls at the bifurcations of the common carotid arteries. They contain sensory nerves that respond to changes in blood pressure.

Carpals: The bones of the wrist; they include the scaphoid, lunate, triquetrum, pisiform, trapezium, trapezoid, capitate, and hamate bones.

Cartilage: A rigid connective tissue that supports, frames, and attaches to many underlying tissues and bones.

Cartilaginous joints: Those connected by hyaline cartilage, or fibrocartilage, such as the joints that separate the vertebrae.

Catabolism: The breakdown of larger molecules into smaller ones.

Catalysts: Atoms or molecules that can change the rate of a reaction without being consumed during the process.

Cations: Ions with a positive charge.

Cauda equina: The "horse's tail"; the collection of nerves at the end of the spinal cord. The spinal cord ends in the lumbar area and continues through the vertebral canal as this structure.

Caudate nucleus: An elongated, curved mass of gray matter lateral to the thalamus in the floor of the anterior horn and body of the lateral ventricle.

Cecum: A pouch-like structure at the beginning of the large intestine that receives waste material from the small intestine.

Cell: The functional and structural unit of life.

Cell membrane: The plasma membrane; it controls movement of substances into and out of the cell.

Cellular immune response: Cell-mediated immunity; it occurs when T cells attach to foreign, antigen-bearing cells such as bacterial cells, and interact with direct cell-to-cell contact.

Central nervous system (CNS): The brain and spinal cord.

Centrioles: Barrel-shaped, hollow organelles inside a centrosome.

Centrosome: A nonmembranous organelle consisting of two hollow centrioles.

Cerebellum: Processes inputs from the cerebral motor cortex, brain stem, and sensory receptors and then regulates skeletal muscle movements for many different activities, such as driving a car, playing a musical instrument, or using a computer. All cerebellar activity is subconscious.

Cerebral aqueduct: A narrow channel in the midbrain connecting the third and fourth ventricles.

Cerebral arterial circle: A vascular network at the base of the brain formed by the interconnection of the middle cerebral, anterior cerebral, posterior cerebral, basilar anterior communicating, and posterior communicating arteries.

Cerebral cortex: A thin layer of gray matter comprising the outer portion of the cerebrum that is nearly completely covered by an extensive layer of neural cortex.

Cerebral edema: Swelling of the brain, which may be caused by a traumatic head injury.

Cerebral hemispheres: The left and right divisions of the cerebrum.

Cerebral peduncles: The anterior halves of the midbrain, which are divided into the crus cerebri anteriorly and the tegmentum posteriorly.

Cerebrospinal fluid (CSF): A clear, watery liquid found in the subarachnoid space and other areas vital for central nervous system function.

Cerebrovascular accident: The most common nervous disorder, also called a stroke or a brain attack, occurs when the brain's blood circulation is blocked, causing the death of brain tissue.

Cerebrum: The largest part of the brain, responsible for many nervous system functions.

Cerumen: The yellow-brown waxy substance secreted in the ear canal that assists in cleaning and lubrication; it is commonly known as earwax.

Ceruminous glands: Specialized sudoriferous glands (sweat glands) located subcutaneously in the external auditory canal that produce cerumen by mixing their secretion with sebum and dead epidermal cells.

Cervical canal: The spindle-shaped canal extending from the isthmus of the uterus to the opening of the uterus into the vagina.

Cervical plexuses: Found deep in the neck, they are formed from branches of the first four cervical nerves.

Cervical vertebrae: The seven smallest vertebrae, found in the neck.

Cervix: The lower one-third of the uterus; it surrounds the cervical orifice, where the uterus opens to the vagina.

Chemical barriers: Innate defenses that include enzymes, other chemical substances, pepsin, hydrochloric acid, tears, lysozyme, salt from perspiration, interferons, or a complement.

Chemical reaction: A process in which molecules are formed, changed, or broken down.

Chemistry: The study of the composition of matter and changes in its composition.

Chemoreceptors: Located in the aortic arch and large neck arteries, they are stimulated by the binding of certain chemicals to send impulses to the cardioacceleratory center, increasing cardiac output.

Chemotaxis: A reaction to antigen–antibody coupling in which macrophages and neutrophils are attracted.

Chlamydia: Any of several common, often asymptomatic, sexually transmitted infections caused by the microorganism Chlamydia trachomatis.

Cholecystokinin: A peptide hormone released by proteins and fats in the small intestine that stimulates contraction of the gallbladder, increasing secretion of pancreatic juice and decreasing gastric motility.

Cholinergic fibers: Sympathetic and parasympathetic preganglionic fibers, secreting acetylcholine.

Chondrocytes: Cartilage cells; they lie totally inside the extracellular matrix.

Chordae tendineae: Strong fibers originating from the papillary muscles that attach to the cusps of the tricuspid valve.

Chorion: A structure formed from two layers of cells that line a trophoblast.

Chorionic villi: Highly branched structures that grow out from a trophoblast.

Choroid coat: The vascular layer that separates the fibrous and inner layers of the eye; it is covered by the sclera and attached to the outer layer of the retina.

Chromatin: Loosely coiled DNA and protein fibers that condense to form chromosomes.

Chromatophilic substance: Sac-like Nissl bodies throughout the cytoplasm of neurons.

Chromosomes: Structures formed from condensed DNA fibers and protein; they are thread-like and are contained within the nucleus of the cells.

Chyle: A milky fluid consisting of lymph and emulsified fat extracted from chyme by the lacteals during digestion and passed to the bloodstream through the thoracic duct.

Chyme: A semifluid paste made of food particles and gastric juice.

Cilia: Structures that extend from the surfaces of epithelial (lining) cells that move in a coordinated manner to move fluids over the cell surfaces.

Ciliary body: The structure associated with the vascular layer of the eye that secretes aqueous humor and contains the ciliary muscle.

Ciliary ganglia: The parasympathetic ganglia in the posterior parts of the eye orbits.

Ciliary zonule: A ring of fibrous strands connecting the ciliary body with the crystalline lens of the eye; it is also known as the zonule of Zinn or Zinn's membrane.

Circadian rhythms: Associated with environmental day and night cycles, these rhythms help the body to distinguish day from night.

Circulatory shock: Also known simply as "shock," it is a life-threatening condition in which blood does not circulate normally, and the organs and tissues do not receive enough blood.

Circumduction: Moving a part so its end follows a circular path, as if describing a cone in space. The distal end of a circumducting limb moves in a circle, whereas the "point" of the cone (the hip or shoulder joint) remains nearly stationary. Circumduction actually consists of the movements of flexion, then abduction, then extension, then adduction.

Circumferential lamellae: The layers of bone that underlie the periosteum and endosteum.

Circumvallate papillae: The large, round structures that have taste buds and lie near the back of the palatine section of the tongue, and are arranged in a V-shaped formation directed toward the throat.

Cirrhosis: A collective term for diseases that cause slowly progressive deterioration of liver function; it is characterized by damage to the functional cells of the liver and by scarring.

Cisterna chyli: An enlarged sac, where the thoracic duct arises anteriorly to the first two lumbar vertebrae; it collects lymph from the lumbar trunks and intestinal trunk.

Cisterns: Cavities filled with fluid inside the endoplasmic reticulum, where sugar groups are attached to proteins; different cisterns also exist in the Golgi apparatus.

Clathrin: A protein that plays a major role in the formation of coated vesicles.

Clavicle: The collarbone.

Cleavage: A phase of early rapid cell division, as the zygote undergoes mitosis.

Cleavage lines: Also known as tension lines or Langer's lines, these are lines in the skin with less flexibility than other areas; they correspond to alignment of collagen fibers in the dermis.

Clitoris: The structure that projects from the anterior vulva between the labia minora; it contains erectile tissue with many sensory nerve fibers.

Clone: A cell that is identical to the original cell from which it formed.

Coagulation: The formation of a blood clot.

Coccyx: The tailbone.

Cochlea: The portion of the inner ear that has hearing receptors.

Coenzymes: Organic cofactors derived from B vitamins or other vitamins; enzyme cofactors may be either a metal element ion, such as iron or copper, or an organic molecule that assists the reaction.

Cofactor: A part of an enzyme that assists with enzymatic reactions in a specific way; cofactors may be metal element ions such as iron or copper or organic molecules derived from B vitamins or other vitamins.

Collagen: The most abundant protein in the body; it is a type of fibrous protein with supporting functions.

Collateral ligament: One of the two strong capsular ligaments in the elbow joint that restrict horizontal movements; it is located medially.

Collecting duct: One of many small tubes inside the kidneys that funnel urine into the renal pelvis for drainage into the ureter. Also, the thoracic duct and right lymphatic duct.

Colloids: A type of mixture also known as emulsions; they are heterogeneous, meaning their composition is dissimilar in different areas, often appearing translucent or milky. Colloids consist of two separate phases: a dispersed (internal) phase and a continuous phase, which is also known as a dispersion medium, in which the colloid is dispersed. A colloidal system may be a solid, liquid, or gas.

Colon: The second part of the large intestine, consisting of four parts.

Colony-stimulating factors (CSFs): Glycoproteins that can cause the proliferation and differentiation of leukocytes.

Common hepatic duct: The large duct formed by the merging of the hepatic ducts.

Compact bone: Bone cells called osteocytes occupy small chambers (lacunae) that create concentric circles around central canals in bones.

Complement: A group of proteins in plasma and other body fluids that interact to cause inflammation and phagocytic activities.

Complete proteins: Those that have adequate amounts of essential amino acids.

Compounds: Molecules made up of different bonded atoms.

Concussion: An injury to the brain produced by violent trauma, followed by temporary or prolonged loss of function.

Conjunctiva: The membranous covering on the anterior surface of the eye that also lines the eyelids.

Connective tissues: Tissues that bind, support, protect, frame, and fill body structures; they also store fat, produce blood cells, repair tissues, and protect against infection.

Constant (C) region: A region at one end of an antibody's polypeptide chains that are nearly the same, or identical, in all antibodies of the same class.

Contraception: A method of birth control that stops fertilization of an egg cell after sexual intercourse or prevents a blastocyst from developing into an embryo.

Contractility: The ability to forcibly shorten when sufficiently stimulated; this ability makes muscle tissue different from all other tissue types.

Contusion: Also called cerebral contusion; a form of traumatic brain injury in which the brain tissue becomes bruised.

Conus medullaris: The terminal end of the spinal cord.

Coracohumeral ligament: The superior ligament that is the thickest area of the shoulder joint's capsule. It helps to support the weight of the arm.

Cornea: The transparent anterior portion of the outer layer of the eye wall.

Corona radiata: The radiating crown of projection fibers passing from the internal capsule to all parts of the cerebral cortex.

Coronary arteries: The first two aortic branches, which supply blood to the heart tissues.

Coronary sinus: The wide venous channel, about 2.25 cm long, which empties into the right atrium.

Coronary veins: Those that branch out and drain blood from the myocardial capillaries to join the coronary sinus.

Corpora cavernosa: The two dorsal columns of erectile tissue in the shaft of the penis.

Corpora quadrigemina: The largest nuclei of the midbrain; they create four round protrusions on its dorsal surface.

Corpus callosum: A deep bridge of nerve fibers connecting the brain hemispheres.

Corpus luteum: Yellow body; a temporary glandular structure created from enlarged follicular cells because of the release of luteinizing hormone.

Corpus spongiosum: The single ventral column of erectile tissue in the shaft of the penis.

Cortex: The outer surface layer of an organ.

Corticosteroids: A group of natural and synthetic analogues of hormones secreted by the pituitary gland; they include the glucocorticoids, mineralocorticoids, and corticotropins.

Cortisol: A glucocorticoid of the middle adrenal cortex that influences protein and fat metabolism and stimulates glucose to be synthesized from noncarbohydrates.

Covalent bond: A bond in which electrons are shared between atoms to produce molecules in which the shared electrons occupy a single orbital that is common to both atoms.

Cranium: The brain case; the part of the skull that holds the brain.

Creatine phosphate: Phosphocreatine; an organic compound in muscle tissue that can store and provide energy for muscle contraction.

Cremaster muscles: Two muscles, each of which has its origin from the internal oblique and inguinal ligament, enveloping the spermatic cord and testis; they act to raise the testicles.

Cricoid cartilage: A ring-like cartilage that forms the lower and rear parts of the larynx.

Crista ampullaris: The sensory organ in a semicircular canal that aids with dynamic equilibrium.

Crista galli: A thick, triangular process projecting superiorly from the cribriform plate of the ethmoid bone.

Crown: The upper portion of a human tooth; it is covered by enamel.

Crystals: Large collections of cations and anions held together by ionic bonds; they are commonly seen in salts, which are ionic compounds.

Cushing's syndrome: A relatively rare endocrine disorder resulting from excessive exposure to the hormone cortisol; it is usually caused by overuse of medications containing cortisol, but also may be caused by the body overproducing this hormone.

Cutaneous membrane: The skin; it covers the entire surface of the body.

Cuticle: Also known as the eponychium, it is the strip of hardened skin at the base and sides of a nail.

Cyclic adenosine monophosphate (cAMP): It is the second messenger associated with one group of hormones and causes changes in response to a first messenger hormone's binding.

Cystic duct: A channel connected to the gallbladder that joins the common hepatic duct.

Cytology: The study of cellular structure and function.

Cytoplasm: The gel-like material that fills out a cell; it makes up most of the cell's volume and suspends the cell's organelles.

Cytoskeleton: The cell skeleton; cellular scaffolding contained in the cytoplasm.

Cytosol: The semifluid material in living cells; it is part of the cytoplasm, surrounding organelles and other insoluble cytoplasmic structures. Many chemical reactions occur in the cytosol.

Dalton's law: The pressure exerted by a mixture of non-reacting gases, which is equal to the sum of partial pressures of the separate components, but only at very low pressures.

Dartos muscles: Two muscles, within the wall of the scrotum, that regulate the temperature of the testes by contracting to wrinkle the scrotal skin.

Decidua basalis: A structure formed from the part of the endometrium that lies beneath the embryo; along with the chorionic villi, this structure forms the placenta.

Decidua capsularis: A structure formed from the part of the endometrium surrounding the uterine cavity face of an implanted embryo; during development, this structure expands to accommodate the fetus.

Decomposition: A reaction that occurs when bonds with a reactant molecule break, forming simpler atoms, molecules, or ions.

Defensins: Natural substances secreted by skin cells that create holes in bacteria, helping to kill them.

Deglutition: Swallowing.

Dehydration: The loss of water and/or solutes; it occurs when water output exceeds water intake over time and is signified by thirst, decreased urine output, dryness or stickiness in the mouth, and dry flushing of the skin.

Dehydration synthesis: An anabolic process that joins small molecules by releasing the equivalent of a water molecule.

Dehydrogenases: Enzymes that catalyze redox reactions in which hydrogen atoms are removed.

Dendrites: Extensions from neurons that receive electro-chemical messages.

Dendritic cells: Also known as Langerhans cells, they are star-shaped protective cells that move from the bone marrow to the epidermis, phagocytizing antigens, migrating to lymph nodes, and presenting the antigen to T cells; they function to consume foreign substances and play a key role in activating the immune system.

Dense connective tissue: White fibrous tissue that makes up tendons and ligaments and exists in the eyeballs and deep skin layers.

Dentate nuclei: Large laminar nuclei of gray matter in the white matter of the cerebral hemispheres.

Denticulate ligaments: Saw-toothed shelves of pia mater in the spinal cord.

Dentin: The chief material of teeth; it surrounds the pulp and is situated inside the enamel and cementum. Harder and denser than bone, it consists of a solid organic substratum infiltrated with lime salts.

Dentition: The clinical description of a tooth; it also refers to the development and eruption of the teeth.

Deoxyribonucleic acid (DNA): One of the two classes of nucleic acids, DNA determines inherited characteristics such as hair color, eye color, and blood type; it affects all aspects of body structure and function, encodes information for protein building, and controls body shape and characteristics.

Depolarization: A decrease in membrane potential, in which the inside of the membrane becomes less negative (moves closer to zero) than the resting potential.

Depression: Lowering a part (moving it inferiorly); when you chew, your mandible is elevated and depressed repeatedly.

Dermcidin: A peptide that kills microbes.

Dermis: The inner layer of the skin, consisting of papillary and reticular regions.

Desmosomes: Cell structures specialized for cell-to-cell adhesion.

Detrusor muscle: Surrounding the neck of the bladder to form the internal urethral sphincter, this muscle functions in the micturition reflex.

Development: The continuous process by which an individual changes from one phase of life to another (including the prenatal and postnatal periods).

Developmental anatomy: The study of structural body changes occurring throughout the life span.

Diaphragm: Also known as the thoracic diaphragm, it is a sheet of internal muscle that extends across the bottom of the rib cage; the diaphragm expands and contracts to aid in breathing.

Diaphysis: The shaft of the long bones; it is a tubular structure forming the long bone axis, made of a thick collar of compact bone surrounding a central medullary cavity.

Diarthrotic: A joint that is freely movable; these joints are found in large numbers in the limbs.

Diastole: The relaxation of a heart structure.

Diastolic pressure: The minimum pressure that remains in the arteries before the next ventricular contraction.

Diencephalon: The core of the forebrain, surrounded by the cerebral hemispheres, and consisting of the thalamus, hypothalamus, and epithalamus.

Digestion: The mechanical and chemical breakdown of foods and the absorption of resulting nutrients by the body's cells.

Diploe: The spongy bone in flat bones

Dipole: A polar molecule having two electrical charges or magnetic poles.

Disaccharides: Double sugars formed when two mono-saccharides are joined by dehydration synthesis and a water molecule is lost; examples include sucrose (table sugar) and lactose (milk sugar).

Dislocation: Also known as a luxation, it occurs when bones are forced out of alignment, as commonly caused by falls or sports activities.

Distal convoluted tubule: The convoluted portion of the nephron that lies between the nephron loop and the non-secretory part of the nephron; it plays an important part in urine concentration.

Dominant hemisphere: The side of the cerebrum controlling the use and understanding of language.

Dominant: More influential than "recessive"; for example, a dominant allele masks expression of a recessive allele.

Dorsal root: Also called the posterior or sensory root; it is identified by an enlarged structure known as the dorsal root ganglion.

Dorsal root ganglion: Also called the spinal ganglion; it is a nodule on a dorsal root of the spine that contains cell bodies of neurons in afferent spinal nerves.

Dorsiflexion: Moving the ankle so the top of the foot comes closer to the shin or moving the wrist so the back of the hand comes closer to the arm (wrist extension).

Double helix: A spiral staircase-like structure that makes up a DNA molecule.

Ductus arteriosus: A fetal vessel through which most of the blood in the pulmonary trunk bypasses the lungs; it connects the pulmonary trunk to the descending portion of the aortic arch.

Ductus deferentia: The vasa deferentia; muscular tubes that pass upward, eventually entering the pelvic cavity of males.

Ductus venosus: A vessel that bypasses the liver and receives about half of the blood carried by the umbilical vein.

Duodenum: The first section of the small intestine, located posterior to the parietal peritoneum.

Dura mater: The outermost layer of the meninges.

Dynamic equilibrium: Maintenance of balance when the head and body are suddenly moved or rotated.

Dystrophin: An important structural protein that links thin filaments to proteins in the sarcolemma; these sarcolemma proteins are anchored to the extracellular matrix.

Eardrum: The tympanic membrane; it covers the auditory canal and separates the external ear from the middle ear.

Ectoderm: The outer primary germ layer that develops during gastrulation.

Edema: An abnormal accumulation of fluid in the interstitial spaces; it occurs when fluid flows out of the blood in higher than normal amounts or cannot sufficiently return to the blood.

Effectors: Response structures located outside the nervous system; they include muscles and glands.

Efferent arteriole: Receives blood that has had fluids filtered from it via the glomerular capillaries, which arise from the afferent arterioles.

Efferent (motor) division: The part of the peripheral nervous system that transmits impulses from the central nervous system to the muscles and glands (also known as the effector organs).

Eicosanoids: Lipids mostly derived from arachidonic acid that are important for blood clotting, inflammation, labor contractions, regulation of blood pressure, and many other body processes; they are considered "local hormones," with specific effects on target cells close to their site of formation.

Ejaculation: The forcing of semen through the urethra to outside of the body.

Ejaculatory duct: A structure formed by the ductus deferentia uniting with the duct of a seminal vesicle; this type of duct passes through the prostate gland to empty into the urethra.

Elastic arteries: Also known as conducting arteries; they are the arteries of largest diameter, and are also the most elastic, with large lumens. Their lumens offer low resistance as blood moves from the heart to the medium-sized arteries.

Elastic cartilage: A flexible type of cartilage that provides framework for the ears and larynx.

Elasticity: The ability of a muscle cell to recoil, resuming its resting length after stretching.

Electrocardiogram (ECG): The recording of electrical changes in the myocardium during the cardiac cycle; the ECG machine works by placing nodes on the skin that connect via wires and respond to weak electrical changes of the heart.

Electroencephalogram: A piece of electrical equipment used to record electrical activity in the brain by measuring voltage differences among various cortical areas.

Electrolyte balance: When the quantities of electrolytes that the body gains equal those that it loses.

Electrolytes: Molecules that release ions in water.

Electronegativity: The capability of an atom to attract electrons very strongly; examples of atoms with this ability include oxygen, nitrogen, and chlorine.

Electrons: Single, negatively charged particles that revolve around the nucleus of an atom.

Electropositive: The state of an atom in which there is only a low ability to attract electrons, causing the atom to often lose its valence shell electrons to other atoms; examples of electropositive atoms include potassium and sodium.

Elements: Fundamental substances that compose matter, such as carbon, hydrogen, and oxygen.

Elevation: Raising a part (lifting it superiorly).

Embolus: A clot that dislodges or fragments to be carried away in the blood flow.

Embryo: An offspring between the time of implantation until the end of the eighth week, when the basic form of the human body is recognizable.

Embryology: The study of developmental changes occurring before birth.

Embryonic disc: A flattened cell mass developed during the early embryonic period; it has an outer ectoderm and an inner endoderm.

Embryonic period: The period around the time of implantation, when certain cells on the inner face of a blastocyst organize to create an inner cell mass that will form the body of the developing offspring.

Emission: The movement of sperm cells from the testes and secretions of the prostate gland and seminal vesicles into the urethra.

Emulsification: The process of breaking fat globules into smaller droplets.

Endocardium: The inner layer of the heart wall.

Endocrine glands: Glands that secrete into tissue fluid or blood.

Endocytosis: The process of movement, via a cell membrane secretion, of particles too large to enter a cell by other processes within a cell vesicle.

Endoderm: The inner primary germ layer, formed during gastrulation from the first cells entering the groove that displace the hypoblast cells of the yolk sac.

Endolymph: The watery fluid in the membranous labyrinth of the ear.

Endometrium: The inner mucosal layer of the uterine wall.

Endomysium: A thin sheath of connective tissue that surrounds individual muscle fibers.

Endoplasmic reticulum (ER): An organelle composed of flat sacs, long canals, and fluid-filled vesicles; the ER transports molecules between cell parts.

Endorphins: Natural pain relievers produced by the hypothalamus and pituitary gland.

Endosteum: A fibrovascular membrane that lines the medullary cavity of a long bone.

Endothelium: The layer of epithelial cells that lines the cavities of the heart and blood vessels; it helps prevent blood clotting and may also help in regulating blood flow.

Energy: The capacity to do work, or to put matter into motion.

Enkephalins: Substances involved in pain reception.

Enzymes: Proteins that catalyze biochemical reactions; in the body, enzymes assist in digestion, protein formation, and drug metabolism. Absence of a single enzyme can lead to a serious deficiency disease.

Eosinophils: Leukocytes with coarse, same-sized granules that appear dark red in acid stain.

Ependymal cells: Neuroglia of the central nervous system that cover specialized brain parts and form inner linings enclosing spaces inside the brain and spinal cord.

Epicardium: The outer layer of the heart wall.

Epidermis: The outer layer of the skin, made up of stratified squamous epithelium.

Epididymis: A cup-shaped structure in the scrotum that is coiled and twisted; it controls the composition of the fluid that is produced by the seminiferous tubules, absorbs and recycles damaged spermatozoa, and absorbs cellular debris. It also stores and protects spermatozoa and facilitates their functional maturation.

Epidural space: The outermost part of the spinal canal, which lies outside the dura mater.

Epiglottic cartilage: The basic structural component of the epiglottis; it is attached to the thyroid cartilage of the larynx by the thyroepiglottic ligament.

Epiglottis: A flap-like structure that allows air to enter the larynx; during swallowing, it partially covers the larynx to prevent food and liquids from entering air passages.

Epimysium: A sheath of dense irregular connective tissue surrounding an entire muscle.

Epinephrine: Adrenaline; a hormone and neurotransmitter important for the body's fight-or-flight response.

Epiphyseal plate: Where the diaphyses meet the epiphyses; it is made of four cartilage layers: reserve cartilage, proliferating (hyperplastic) cartilage, hypertrophic cartilage, and the calcified matrix.

Epiphyses: The bone ends.

Epithalamus: The most dorsal portion of the diencephalon, it joins the pineal gland, which is important for sleep, wakefulness, and antioxidant release.

Epithelial membranes: Membranes that cover body surfaces and line body cavities.

Epithelial tissues: Body tissues that cover organs, form the inner lining of cavities, and line hollow organs.

Epithelium: An avascular layer of cells that forms a barrier providing protection and regulating permeability; glands are secretory structures derived from epithelia.

Equilibrium: Uniform distribution of molecules.

Erection: The swelling and elongation of the penis in preparation for sexual intercourse.

Erythropoietin: A glycoprotein hormone produced mainly by the kidneys that stimulates the production of red blood cells by stem cells in the bone marrow.

Esophageal hiatus: The opening in the mediastinum through which the esophagus passes, penetrating the diaphragm.

Esophageal plexuses: The plexuses surrounding the esophagus, formed by branches of the left and right vagi and the sympathetic trunks. They also contain visceral afferent fibers from the esophagus.

Esophagus: A straight, collapsible tube through which food passes from the pharynx to the stomach.

Estrogens: Female hormones that have many functions, including the enlargement of the vagina, uterus, uterine tubes, ovaries, and external reproductive structures.

Ethmoid bone: The main supporting structure of the nasal cavities; it also forms part of the eye orbits.

Eversion: Turning the foot so the plantar surface (sole) faces laterally.

Excitability: Responsiveness; the ability to receive and respond to a stimulus, which includes any changes inside or outside the body. For muscles, the stimulus is usually a chemical (such as a neurotransmitter or a local pH change).

Exocrine glands: Glands that open onto body surfaces or into the digestive tract.

Exocytosis: The opposite of endocytosis, wherein a substance stored in a cell vesicle is secreted from the cell.

Expiration: Exhalation.

Expiratory reserve volume: Supplemental air; additional air that is expelled from the lungs due to forced exhalation.

Extensibility: The ability to stretch or extend; muscle cells can stretch beyond their resting length when they are relaxed.

Extension: Straightening parts at a joint so that they move farther apart.

External acoustic meatus: The external ear canal, which extends from the auricle to the tympanic membrane.

External jugular veins: The more superficial and lateral of the large vessels of the neck that receive most of the blood from the exterior of the cranium and the deep tissues of the face.

Extracellular fluid compartment: All fluid outside of cells in the body.

Extraembryonic membranes: The amnion, yolk sac, allantois, and chorion; these membranes form during the first 2 to 3 weeks of development.

Extrinsic muscles: Those that do not originate in the body part to which they insert.

Eyelid: The thin fold of skin covering and protecting the eye.

Facial skeleton: The maxillae, zygomatic bones, nasal bones, vomer, inferior nasal conchae, lacrimal bones, palatine bones, and mandible.

Facilitated diffusion: The spontaneous transport of molecules or ions across a membrane via certain transport proteins.

Falciform ligament: A triangular body ligament, such as the broad ligament of the liver.

Fascia: Tissue that surrounds every muscle that may form cord-like tendons beyond each muscle's end.

Fascicles: Groups of muscle fibers within each skeletal muscles; they resembles bundles of sticks.

Feces: A mixture of undigested materials, unabsorbed materials, water, electrolytes, mucus, discarded intestinal cells, and bacteria.

Femur: The thighbone.

Fertilization: The union of an egg cell and a sperm cell.

Fetal period: The period that begins at the end of the eighth week of development and lasts until birth.

Fetus: An offspring after the eighth week of development up until birth.

Fibrillation: Arrhythmia marked by rapid, random contractions of various areas of cardiac tissue.

Fibrin: Insoluble threads of protein made from the plasma protein fibrinogen.

Fibrinogen: A plasma protein that is important for blood coagulation.

Fibroblast: A star-shaped fixed cell that produces fibers via protein secretion into the extracellular matrix.

Fibrocartilage: A tough type of cartilage that absorbs shock in the spinal column, knees, and pelvic girdle.

Fibronectin: A high-molecular-weight glycoprotein of the extracellular matrix that binds to receptor proteins called integrins; it binds collagen, fibrin, and other components.

Fibrosis: Formation of excessive fibrous bands of scar tissue between muscle fibers, commonly due to aging.

Fibrous joints: Those that lie between bones that closely contact each other, joined by thin, dense connective tissue.

Fibrous proteins: Strand-like, highly stable proteins that provide mechanical support and tensile strength for body tissues; they are insoluble in water.

Fibula: The lateral calf bone.

Filum terminale: A thread-like structure that extends from the lower end of the spinal cord.

Fissure: A deep groove in the cerebrum's surface.

Flaccid paralysis: An abnormal condition characterized by the weakening of muscles or loss of muscle tone.

Flagella: Singular form, flagellum; structures that extend from sperm cells that undulate, enabling the cells to "swim."

Flat bones: Those that resemble plates, with broad surfaces.

Flexion: Bending parts at a joint so they come closer together.

Flexure lines: Skin markings that occur close to joints, where the dermis is more tightly secured to deeper structures; they include the creases on the palms of the hands.

Folia: Fine gyri on the surface of the cerebellum that have a folded appearance and are transversely oriented.

Foliate papillae: The tongue structures that have taste buds embedded in their surfaces; these papillae are clustered into two groups positioned on each side of the tongue, just in front of the "V" of the circumvallate papillae.

Follicle cells: The term used to describe a single layer of cells that encase the oocyte in each follicle; if there is more than a single layer, these cells are called granulosa cells.

Follicle-stimulating hormone (FSH): A gonadotropin affecting the testes and ovaries; it stimulates the maturation of sex cells.

Fontanels: Also fontanelles; the soft spots on a baby's skull.

Foramen ovale: An opening in the atrial septum through which blood flows from the fetal right atrium into the left atrium.

Fornix: Fiber tracts that link regions of the brain.

Fourchette: The frenulum of the pudendal labia, which is the posterior union of the labia minora, anterior to the posterior commissure.

Fovea centralis: The region of the retina of the eye that has densely packed cones and provides the greatest visual activity.

Frontal bone: The bone that forms the forehead and part of the roof of the nasal cavity.

Functional residual capacity: Expiratory reserve volume plus residual volume.

Functional syncytium: A mass of merging cells that function as a unit.

Fundus: The rounded portion of the corpus (uterine body); it is superior to the attachment of the uterine tubes.

Fungiform papillae: The mushroom-shaped tongue structures that contain the taste buds that respond to both sweet and sour tastes.

Funiculi: Long, rope-like structures within the spinal cord.

Galactosemia: A rare genetic metabolic disorder that affects the ability to properly metabolize the sugar galactose; affected infants develop poor feeding, lethargy, jaundice, liver damage, and bleeding. This may lead to sepsis, shock, cataracts, and intellectual disability.

Gallbladder: A pear-shaped sac located in a depression on the inferior surface of the liver that stores bile, reabsorbs water, and contracts to release bile into the small intestine.

Gametes: The mature male germ cells (spermatozoa) or mature male female cells (ova) that unite during the process of fertilization.

Gamma globulin: The portion of blood proteins made up by antibodies (immunoglobulins).

Ganglia: Clusters of neuron cell bodies in the peripheral nervous system, which lie along the peripheral nerves.

Gastric glands: Those inside the stomach's inner lining that may have mucous, chief, or parietal cells with differing secretions (known as gastric juice).

Gastric juice: A substance produced by a combination of secretions from the mucous, chief, and parietal cells of the gastric glands.

Gastrin: A hormone secreted by the stomach that stimulates the production of gastric juice.

Gastrula: A term used to describe the blastocyst after the three primary germ layers form.

Gastrulation: Cellular rearrangements and migrations in which the three primary germ layers are developed, during week 3 of gestation.

Genetics: The field that investigates how genes confer specific characteristics that affect health or contribute to natural variation and how genes are passed from generation to generation.

Genital herpes: A sexually transmitted infection caused by a herpes virus that is characterized by the formation of fluid-filled, painful blisters in the genital area.

Genital warts: Condylomata acuminata or venereal warts; they are growths in the genital area caused by a sexually transmitted papillomavirus.

Genotype: A status of an individual that is based on the combination of alleles, for one gene or many.

Gestation: The period from the fertilization of the ovum until birth.

Ghrelin: A hormone secreted by the stomach that stimulates appetite, feeding, and growth hormone secretion from the anterior pituitary.

Gigantism: Excessive growth of the body or any of its parts, especially as a result of oversecretion of growth hormone from the pituitary gland prior to puberty.

Glandular epithelium: Specialized tissue that produces and secretes substances into ducts or body fluids.

Glans penis: The cone-shaped end of the penis that covers the ends of the corpora cavernosa and opens as the external urethral orifice.

Glenohumeral ligaments: The ligaments that slightly strengthen the front of the shoulder joint capsule. They are absent in some individuals.

Globular proteins: Spherical proteins that are chemically active, water soluble, and important in almost all biologic processes; they are also referred to as functional proteins.

Globulins: Antibodies made by the liver or lymphatic tissues that make up around 36% of the plasma proteins.

Globus pallidus: The smaller, more medial part of the lentiform nucleus.

Glomerular capsule: A sac-like structure that surrounds the glomerulus, from which it receives filtered fluid.

Glomerular filtration: The process that initiates urine formation.

Glomerular filtration rate: The volume at which blood passes through the glomeruli of the kidneys.

Glomerulonephritis: An inflammatory disease of both kidneys mostly affecting children between ages 2 and 12; it is inflammation of the glomeruli resulting in inefficient processing of waste products and filtering of water from the bloodstream.

Glomerulus: A tangled cluster of blood capillaries that comprises a renal corpuscle.

Glottis: A structure between the vocal cords that changes shape; when swallowing occurs, it closes to prevent food or liquid from entering the trachea.

Glucagon: Stimulates the liver to break down glycogen and convert certain noncarbohydrates into glucose.

Gluconeogenesis: A process in which new glucose is formed from noncarbohydrate molecules in the liver; it occurs when too little glucose is available for metabolic needs and glycerol and amino acids are converted to glucose.

Glycogenesis: A process in which glucose molecules are combined in long chains to form glycogen; it occurs when high levels of adenosine triphosphate begin to stop the process of glycolysis.

Glycogenolysis: A process in which lysis of glycogen occurs when blood glucose levels drop.

Glycolipids: Lipids that have sugar groups attached and are found only in the outer plasma membrane surface.

Glycolysis: A process that involves a series of enzymatically catalyzed reactions in which glucose is broken down to yield lactic acid or pyruvic acid.

Glycosomes: Granules of stored glycogen the provide glucose during muscle cell activity.

Goblet cells: Cells found throughout pseudostratified columnar epithelium; involved in secretion of mucus.

Golgi apparatus: An organelle that consists of approximately six flattened sacs dealing mostly with proteins synthesized on ribosomes.

Gomphoses: Fibrous joints with a peg-in-socket structure; the only example of these is the articulation of the teeth in their alveolar sockets.

Gonadocorticoids: Also called adrenal sex hormones, they may supplement sex hormones from the gonads and stimulate early reproductive organ development.

Gonadotropins: Hormones secreted by the anterior pituitary gland, which include luteinizing hormone and follicle-stimulating hormone.

Gonads: The sex organs, which produce sperm (testes) or eggs (ovaries).

Gonorrhea: A highly contagious sexually transmitted infection caused by the bacterium Neisseria gonorrhoeae; it is commonly referred to as "the clap."

Gouty arthritis: Also known as gout; it is a condition based on excessive, abnormal levels of uric acid deposited as needle-like urate crystals in soft tissues of joints, most commonly the great toe.

Granular cells: Also known as the juxtaglomerular cells of the kidney; they synthesize, store, and secrete the enzyme known as renin.

Granulocytes: Leukocytes with granular cytoplasm.

Granulosa cells: The term used to describe more than one single layer of cells that encase the oocyte in each follicle; if there is only a single layer of cells, these cells are called follicle cells.

Gray commissure: A horizontal bar of gray matter in the very middle of the spinal cord surrounds its central canal and contains cerebrospinal fluid; it has dorsal and ventral horns.

Gross (macroscopic) anatomy: The study of large body structures that can be seen without a microscope. Subdivisions include regional, systemic, and surface anatomy.

Ground substance: The noncellular components of the extracellular matrix, containing the fibers.

Growth hormone (GH): Stimulates cells to grow and divide more frequently and enhances the movement of amino acids to stimulate growth.

Growth: An increase in size.

Gum: A firm layer of flesh covering the alveolar processes of the jaws and the bases of the teeth.

Gyri: Ridges or convolutions in the cerebrum separated by grooves.

H zone: A narrow, less-dense zone of myosin filaments bisecting an A band in striated muscle.

Hair bulb: The lower expanded extremity of a hair that fits over the hair papilla at the bottom of the hair follicle.

Hair follicles: Tube-like structures in which hairs develop; they extend from the skin surface into the dermis.

Hair matrix: The actively dividing part of the hair bulb that produces the hair; it originates in the hair bulge, just slightly above the hair bulb.

Halitosis: Offensive breath resulting from poor oral hygiene.

Haploid: A condition involved in the second phase of meiosis wherein one member of each homologous pair separates its chromatids.

Hapten: A small molecule that cannot stimulate an immune response by itself; found in certain drugs, dust particles, animal dander, and various chemicals.

Haversian systems: Haversian canals and their concentrically arranged lamellae; these constitute the basic units of structure in compact bones.

Heart block: A delay in the normal flow of electrical impulses that cause the heart to beat.

Helicotrema: The cochlear apex; it is an opening that connects the vestibular canal and scala tympani.

Helix: The prominent rim of auricular portion of the external ear; the auricula is the rounded visible edge.

Hematocrit: The percentage of blood volume made up by red blood cells.

Hemoglobin: The iron-containing protein in red blood cells. It helps red blood cells to carry oxygen.

Hemopoiesis: The process of blood cell production.

Hemostasis: The stoppage of bleeding.

Henry's law: The solution of a gas in a liquid solution at a constant temperature is proportional to the partial pressure of the gas above the solution.

Hepatic ducts: Channels formed from lobules that create large bile ducts; they merge into the common hepatic duct.

Hepatic lobules: The functional cells of the liver.

Hepatic portal system: A series of vessels and two distinct capillary beds, lying between the arterial supply and the final venous drainage. Its initial capillary beds are found in the stomach and intestines, draining into vessels of the hepatic portal vein, and then to a second capillary bed inside the liver.

Hepatic sinusoids: Vascular channels that separate plate-like groups of hepatic cells.

Hepatopancreatic ampulla: The dilation formed by the junction of the pancreatic and bile ducts at their opening into the lumen of the duodenum.

Heterozygous: A condition related to genes wherein there are two different alleles.

Hiatal hernia: A protrusion of a portion of the stomach upward through the diaphragm.

Hilum: An indented region of a lymph node where blood vessels and nerves are attached. Also, the indented part of a kidney, where renal vessels, nerves, and the ureter pass.

Hip joints: Also known as the coxal joints; they are ball-and-socket joints with movements limited by the deep hip sockets as well as strong ligaments. Each hip joint is formed by the articulation of the femur's spherical head with the hip bone's acetabulum.

Histology: The study of body tissues.

Holocrine glands: Exocrine glands that release entire cells, which disintegrate to release secretions.

Holoenzyme: The name for the collective parts of an enzyme; this includes a protein portion (apoenzyme) and a cofactor.

Homeostasis: The maintenance of a relatively constant internal environment in the body.

Homeostatic mechanisms: Effectors, receptors, and the body's set point, which act together to maintain homeostasis.

Homocystinuria: An inherited disorder that affects metabolism of the amino acid methionine; symptoms include failure to thrive, visual problems, chest deformities, intellectual disability, and lengthening of the limbs, fingers, and overall body shape.

Homozygous: A condition related to genes wherein there are two identical alleles.

Hormones: Secretions from endocrine glands that enter the lymphatic fluid or blood, travel to specific target organs, and prompt them to act in a certain way.

Human chorionic gonadotropin (hCG): A hormone that normally prevents spontaneous abortion.

Humerus: The largest, longest bone of the upper arm.

Humoral immune response: When antibodies react to destroy antigens or antigen-containing particles.

Hyaline cartilage: The type of cartilage on the ends of bones in many joints, the soft portion of the nose, and in the respiratory passages' supporting rings; it is the most common type of cartilage.

Hydrogen bond: The attraction of the positive hydrogen end of a polar molecule to the negative nitrogen or oxygen end of another polar molecule.

Hydrolysis: Enzymatically adding a water molecule to split a molecule into smaller portions.

Hydrostatic pressure: The backpressure exerted by water against a cell membrane. Also, the outward pressure that affects filtration in the glomerular capillaries.

Hymen: A thin membrane of connective tissue and epithelium that partially covers the vaginal orifice.

Hyoid bone: The bone that supports the tongue.

Hyperextension: Extending the parts at a joint beyond the normal range of motion, often resulting in injury, because the anatomic position is exceeded.

Hyperpolarization: An increase in membrane potential, in which the inside of the membrane becomes more negative (moves further from zero) than the resting potential.

Hypertension: Chronically elevated blood pressure, in which the systolic pressure is usually above 140 mm Hg, and the diastolic pressure is usually above 90 mm Hg.

Hyperventilation: Deep, rapid breathing; it lowers blood carbon dioxide levels.

Hypocapnia: A state of reduced carbon dioxide in the blood, usually because of hyperventilation.

Hyponatremia: Lower than normal concentrations of sodium in the blood plasma; if excessively low, it can result in seizures and coma.

Hyponychium: Also known as the "quick" of a nail, it is the thickened epidermis beneath a nail's free distal end, especially its posterior part, in the region of the lunula.

Hypophyseal portal veins: Those that pass along the pituitary stalk to the anterior pituitary's capillary network.

Hypoproteinemia: Abnormally low levels of total protein in the blood; commonly linked to inadequate dietary supply of protein, dilation of lymphatic vessels in the intestines, renal failure, or as a result of burns.

Hypotension: Blood pressure below 90/60 mm Hg.

Hypothalamus: Located below the thalamus, this structure is the primary visceral control center of the body and vital for homeostasis.

Hypotonic hydration: Overhydration; the collection of excessive water by body cells.

Hypoxia: Low oxygen concentrations in the blood, often related to disease, high altitudes, or anemia.

I bands: Isotropic bands within striated muscle fibers; they appear dark in polarized light but light when stained.

Ileocecal sphincter: The muscle connecting the small intestine to the large intestine.

Ileum: The third part of the small intestine; it is thinner than the jejunum.

Iliofemoral ligament: One of the ligaments that reinforces the hip joint capsule; it lies anteriorly, is very strong, and has a V-shape.

Ilium: The uppermost, largest portion of the hipbone.

Immunity: Adaptive (specific) defense; it targets specific pathogens via specialized lymphocytes that recognize foreign particles.

Immunocompetent: Ability of the immune system to mobilize and deploy its antibodies because of stimulation by antigens.

Immunogenicity: The ability to stimulate certain lymphocytes to multiply.

Immunologic surveillance: The immune system's potential ability to recognize and remove malignant cells throughout a person's lifetime.

Incisors: One of the four anterior teeth in each dental arch.

Incomplete proteins: Those that have too little tryptophan and lysine to maintain human tissues or support growth and development.

Incretins: A group of gastrointestinal hormones that cause an increase in the amount of insulin released from the beta cells of the islets of Langerhans of the pancreas after eating.

Inferior colliculi: Two small, rounded elevations on the dorsal midbrain below the two superior colliculi; they are relay centers for auditory fibers.

Inferior hypogastric (pelvic) plexus: One of the bilateral mixed autonomic plexuses in the pelvis distributed to the pelvic viscera; it receives the hypogastric nerves and the pelvic splanchnic nerves and conveys visceral afferent fibers.

Inferior nasal conchae: Scroll-shaped bones attached to the lateral nasal cavity walls that support the mucous membranes.

Inferior vena cava: Along with the superior vena cava, one of the two largest veins in the body; it returns deoxygenated blood from areas of the body that are inferior to the diaphragm.

Inflammation: A tissue response to injury or infection that may include redness, swelling, heat, and pain.

Infundibulum: The funnel-shaped structure formed by the expansion of each uterine tube; it partially encircles the ovary. Also, the funnel-shaped, unpaired stalk at the base of the hypothalamus behind the optic chiasm; it is continuous below with the stalk of the pituitary gland.

Inhibiting hormones: Hormones from a body structure that inhibit hormone release from other structures.

Innate (nonspecific) defense: One that protects the body from pathogens involving mechanical barriers, chemical barriers, natural killer cells, inflammation, phagocytosis, fever, or species resistance.

Inorganic: Not having both carbon and hydrogen atoms.

Inorganic components: Made up of hydroxyapatites or mineral salts; they provide strength while keeping bones from becoming brittle.

Insensible water loss: The amount of fluid lost on a daily basis from the lungs, skin, respiratory tract, and water excreted in the feces; it is between 40 and 600 mL in a normal adult.

Insertion: A movable part of the body to which a skeletal muscle is fastened at a movable joint; its action opposes that of an origin.

Inspiration: Inhalation.

Inspiratory capacity: Tidal volume plus inspiratory reserve volume.

Inspiratory reserve volume: Complemental air; additional air that enters the lungs because of forced inspiration.

Insula: A brain lobe that is buried deep within the lateral sulcus and forms part of the floor of the brain.

Insulin: Opposes glucagon by stimulating the liver to form glycogen from glucose and inhibiting the conversion of noncarbohydrates into glucose.

Integral proteins: Types of proteins inserted into the lipid bilayer, which are mainly transmembrane proteins that protrude on both sides, that can interact with the nonpolar lipid tails buried in the membrane as well as the water inside and outside of the cell.

Integration: The process by which the nervous system processes and interprets sensory input.

Integumentary system: The body system made up of the skin and its accessory structures (hair, nails, glands, etc.).

Intercostal nerves: Supply the intercostal muscles and upper abdominal wall muscles while receiving sensory impulses from the skin of the abdomen and thorax.

Interferons: Hormone-like peptides or cytokines that bind to uninfected cells and stimulate them to make protective antiviral proteins.

Interleukins: Hormones upon which many of the effects of leukocytes depend.

Internal capsule: A mass of white fibers separating the lentiform nucleus of a cerebral hemisphere from the caudate nucleus and dorsal thalamus.

Interstitial cells: The cells of Leydig; they lie in spaces between the seminiferous tubules, producing and secreting male sex hormones.

Intervertebral joints: Articulations found between superior and inferior articular processes of adjacent vertebrae in the spine.

Intestinal glands: Those located between the bases of adjacent intestinal villi, extending downward into the mucous membrane.

Intestinal villi: Tiny projections of the mucous membrane of the inner wall of the small intestine.

Intracellular fluid compartment: All water and electrolytes enclosed by cell membranes in the body.

Intraperitoneal: Inside the peritoneum.

Intrinsic factor: A substance secreted by the parietal cells that helps the small intestine to absorb vitamin B12.

Inversion: Turning the foot so the plantar surface faces medially.

Involuntary nervous system: The autonomic nervous system, which is generally not under conscious control.

Ions: Atoms that either gain or lose electrons.

Iris: The colored, muscular portion of the eye surrounding the pupil that regulates its size.

Irregular bones: Those that may be of various shapes and often are attached to other bones.

Ischemia: Deprivation of blood to a body tissue.

Ischiofemoral ligament: One of the ligaments that reinforces the hip joint capsule; it spirals posteriorly.

Ischium: The strongest portion of the hipbone.

Isotonic: Any solution that has the same osmotic pressure as body fluids.

Isotope: One of two (or more) forms of an element having the same number of protons and electrons but different numbers of neutrons; they may or may not be radioactive.

Isthmus: A constricted area through which each uterine tube empties into the superolateral area of the uterus.

Jejunum: The second part of the small intestine; it makes up the proximal two-fifths.

Joint capsule: The outer layer of ligaments in a synovial joint.

Joints: Articulations; they act as junctions between bones.

Juxtaglomerular apparatus: Also called a juxtaglomerular complex; it is made up of enlarged smooth muscle cells along with the macula densa.

Keratinocytes: Older skin cells that have hardened with age in a process known as keratinization.

Ketoacidosis: Dangerously high level of ketones due to the body burning fat for energy instead of glucose.

Ketogenesis: The process in which the liver converts acetyl coenzyme A molecules to ketones, which are also called ketone bodies.

Ketones: Ketone bodies, which are organic compounds containing a carbonyl group that has a carbon atom joined to two other carbon atoms; this means the carbonyl group occurs within the carbon chain. Examples of ketones include acetone, acetoacetic acid, and β-hydroxybutyric acid.

Kidneys: The organs that help to maintain homeostasis by regulating the composition, pH, and volume of the extracellular fluid.

Labia majora: The structures that enclose and protect the other external reproductive organs of the female.

Labia minora: The structures that lie between the labia majora; they are flattened, longitudinal folds composed of connective tissue.

Lacrimal bones: Those that make up part of the eye orbits and contain the tear sacs.

Lacrimal gland: A tear-secreting gland of the eye.

Lacteals: Special lymphatic capillaries of the small intestine that take up lipids.

Lactic acidosis: A condition that may develop after strenuous exercise or prolonged tissue hypoxia (oxygen starvation).

Lactiferous ducts: Ducts conveying the milk secreted by the mammary lobes to and through the nipples.

Lacunae: Irregular spaces that form around and between the villi. Also, small spaces, cavities, or depressions in bones or cartilages that are occupied by cells.

Lamella: A layer, such as of bone matrix, in an osteon of compact bone.

Lamellar bone: Another name for compact bone; it is derived the term lamella.

Lamina propria: The loose connective tissue layer of the mucosa (mucous membrane) of the digestive tube.

Laminin: A major protein in the basal lamina that influences cell differentiation, migration, adhesion, phenotype, and cell survival.

Large intestine: Having a much greater diameter than the small intestine, it begins in the lower right side of the abdominal cavity where the ileum joins the cecum, with its distal end opening to the outside of the body as the anus.

Laryngopharynx: The portion of the pharynx below the upper edge of the epiglottis, opening into the larynx and esophagus.

Larynx: Also known as the voice box; an enlargement above the trachea and below the pharynx that conducts air while preventing foreign objects from entering. It houses the vocal cords.

Lateral ventricles: Two curved openings deep within the cerebrum that provide a pathway for cerebrospinal fluid; these ventricles are the largest of all brain ventricles.

Lens: Transparent eye structure that helps to refract light so the retina can focus on it.

Leptin: A hormone that plays a key role in regulating energy intake and expenditure, including appetite and metabolism; it is derived from adipose tissue.

Leukocytes: White blood cells; they protect the body against disease and develop from hemocytoblasts in red bone marrow.

Leukocytosis: A condition of white blood cells exceeding 10,000 per cubic millimeter, indicating an acute infection.

Ligaments: Collagenous fibers that bind two or more bones to a joint.

Limbic system: A group of structures on the medial aspect of each cerebral hemisphere and diencephalon that function in emotional response and memory processing.

Lingual frenulum: The membranous fold that anchors the tongue to the floor of the mouth.

Lingual tonsils: Rounded lymphatic tissue masses that cover the root of the tongue.

Lipid rafts: Dynamic structures of saturated phospholipids packed tightly together believed to concentrate certain receptor molecules or protein molecules required for membrane invagination (infolding), cell signaling, or other activities.

Lipids: Fats, fat-like substances (cholesterol and phospholipids), and oils that do not dissolve in water and supply energy for body processes and building of certain structures.

Lipogenesis: Triglyceride synthesis; it occurs when cellular adenosine triphosphate and glucose levels are high.

Lipolysis: The breakdown of stored fats into fatty acids and glycerol, which are then released to the blood.

Liver: The organ that filters the blood, synthesizes proteins, and produces biochemicals required for digestion.

Long bones: Those with long bone shafts and expanded ends.

Longitudinal fissure: The largest, deepest groove between the medial surfaces of the cerebral hemispheres.

Loose connective tissue: Adipose, areolar, and reticular connective tissue.

Lower esophageal sphincter: Cardiac sphincter; located above the area where the esophagus joins the stomach; it is made up of circular smooth muscle fibers.

Lower limbs: The femurs, tibias, fibulas, patellae, tarsals, metatarsals, and phalanges.

Lumbar puncture: Also called a spinal tap, this is a procedure in which cerebrospinal fluid is removed for analysis via a needle inserted into the subarachnoid space inside the meningeal sac inferior to the lumbar region of the spine.

Lumbar vertebrae: The five vertebrae of the lower back.

Lumbosacral plexuses: Made up of the last thoracic nerve and the lumbar, sacral, and coccygeal nerves and extend into the pelvic cavity; they are associated with the skin and muscles of the lower abdominal wall, buttocks, external genitalia, thighs, legs, and feet.

Lumen: A blood-containing cavity or channel within a vessel or tubular organ.

Lungs: Soft, spongy, cone-shaped structures used in breathing.

Luteinizing hormone (LH): A gonadotropin affecting the testes and ovaries; it stimulates secretion of sex steroids.

Lyme disease: An infection caused by a spirochete transmitted by the bite of infected ticks; joint inflammation, pain, and arthritis develop in half of cases as long as 2 years after transmission.

Lymph nodes: Specialized, bean-shaped organs that act as filters or traps for foreign particles.

Lymph nodules: Follicles that are the functional units of lymph nodes.

Lymph sinuses: Spaces inside lymph nodes that comprise complex channels through which lymph moves.

Lymph: The fluid inside the lymphatic capillaries or vessels; interstitial fluid.

Lymphatic capillaries: Microscopic vessels extending into interstitial spaces in complex networks.

Lymphatic pathways: Tiny tubes formed from lymphatic capillaries that merge to form larger vessels.

Lymphatic trunks: Structures that drain lymph from lymphatic vessels and join either the thoracic duct or the right lymphatic duct.

Lymphatic vessels: Those that conduct lymph; they are similar to veins, but with thinner walls, and have valves to prevent backflow.

Lymphocytes: Leukocytes with large, round nuclei inside a thin cytoplasm rim.

Lymphoid tissue: The cells and organs that make up the lymphatic system, including the leukocytes, bone marrow, thymus, spleen, and lymph nodes.

Lysosomes: Tiny sac-like organelles that dispose of cell wastes and worn-out cell parts.

Lysozyme: A family of enzymes that damage bacterial cell walls; various types of lysozymes are found in various body secretions.

M line: A fine dark band in the center of the H zone in the myofibrils of striated muscle fibers.

Macronutrients: Those required in large amounts (carbohydrates, lipids, and proteins).

Macrophages: Large, actively phagocytic cells of various types; fixed macrophages or histiocytes are found in certain tissues and organs, such as the microglia of the nervous system and Kupffer cells of the liver sinusoids; free macrophages travel throughout the body, such as alveolar macrophages, which monitor exchange surfaces of the lungs.

Macula densa: A group of modified epithelial cells in the distal convoluted tubule that control renin release by relaying information about sodium concentration to the juxtaglomerular cells.

Macula lutea: A yellowish depression in the retina where acute vision arises.

Maculae: Equilibrium receptor regions of the saccule and utricle, which are the two membranous sacs suspended in the perilymph of the vestibule of the inner ear; the maculae respond to gravity and transmit impulses concerning changes in head position.

Major minerals: Calcium, chlorine, magnesium, phosphorus, potassium, sodium, and sulfur.

Mammary glands: Accessory organs specialized to secrete milk after pregnancy.

Mammillary bodies: Two paired, small round masses in the fossa of the midbrain, forming part of the hypothalamus.

Mandible: The only movable bone in the face; it forms the lower jaw.

Maple syrup urine disease: An inherited disorder in which the body is unable to process certain amino acids normally; it is characterized by sweet-smelling urine, poor feeding, vomiting, lethargy, and developmental delays. The condition can lead to seizures, coma, and death.

Marrow: Soft connective tissue that fills the inner cavities of many bones.

Mast cells: Cells to which antibodies, formed in response to allergens, attach, bursting the cells and releasing allergy mediators, which cause symptoms.

Mastication: Chewing, tearing, or grinding of food with the teeth while it becomes mixed with saliva.

Matrix: A combination of connective tissue, blood vessels, and minerals that compose bone.

Matter: Liquids, gases, and solids both inside and outside of the human body; it takes up space and has weight.

Maxillae: The bones that make up the upper jaw.

Mechanical barriers: Innate defenses that include the skin, mucous membranes, hair, sweat, and mucus.

Mechanoreceptors: Receptors that sense mechanical stimulation such as changes in pressure or tension.

Mediastinum: The medial cavity of the thorax, which contains the heart, its large vessels, the trachea, esophagus, thymus, lymph nodes, and other structures and tissues.

Medulla: The central portion of certain organs.

Medulla oblongata: The most inferior part of the brain stem; it blends into the spinal cord and contains the cardiovascular center, respiratory centers, and various other brain centers.

Medullary respiratory center: The dorsal and ventral respiratory groups as well as the respiratory group of the pons.

Megakaryocytes: Red bone marrow cells that fragment to produce platelets.

Meiosis: A type of cell division that includes first and second divisions.

Melanin: A dark pigment that provides the skin with color.

Melanocytes: Skin cells that produce melanin; they are found in the stratum germinativum layer of the epidermis, just above the dermis.

Melanosomes: Granules within melanocytes that contain tyrosinase and synthesize melanin; they are transferred from the melanocytes to keratinocytes.

Melatonin: A catecholamine hormone synthesized and released by the pineal gland; it is involved in regulation of sleep, mood, puberty, and ovarian cycles.

Membranous labyrinth: The labyrinth of the ear that is lodged within the bony labyrinth and has the same general form; it is much smaller, however, and separated from the bony walls by the fluid known as the perilymph.

Membranous urethra: The part of the male urethra situated between the layers of the urogenital diaphragm; it connects parts of the urethra passing through the prostate gland and penis.

Memory cells: Cells that develop from any clone cells that do not become plasma cells; if they encounter the same antigen later, they can cause an almost immediate humoral response.

Menarche: A female's first reproductive cycle.

Meninges: Layered membranes that protect the brain and spinal cord.

Menisci: Shock-absorbing fibrocartilage pads in certain synovial joints.

Menopause: The period when a female's reproductive cycle ceases; also called the female climacteric.

Menstrual cycle: Also called the uterine cycle, it is coordinated with the ovarian cycle, and includes a menstrual phase, proliferative or preovulatory phase, and a secretory, postovulatory phase.

Merocrine glands: Exocrine glands that release fluid by exocytosis.

Mesentery: A double-layered fold of peritoneal membrane that suspends the jejunum and ileum from the posterior abdominal wall.

Mesoderm: The middle primary germ layer that develops during gastrulation.

Mesosalpinx: A short mesentery that supports the peritoneum that externally covers the uterine tubes; it is part of the broad ligament.

Mesovarium: The fold of peritoneum that suspends each ovary in between the uterus and pelvic wall; it is part of the broad ligament.

Metabolism: The cellular chemical reactions that break down and build up substances inside living cells.

Metacarpals: The bones of the palms of the hands.

Metatarsals: The bones of the soles of the feet; they form the foot arches.

Microfilaments: The smallest of the cytoskeletal elements, they provide cell movement.

Microglial cells: Neuroglia found throughout the central nervous system that have phagocytic actions.

Micronutrients: Those required in small amounts (vitamins and minerals).

Microscopic anatomy: The study of small body structures, requiring the use of a microscope.

Micturition: Urination; the process of expelling urine from the urinary bladder.

Midbrain: A portion of the brain stem between the diencephalon and pons.

Mineralocorticoids: Adrenal corticosteroids that are active in the retention of salt and in the maintenance of life; examples include aldosterone and deoxycorticosterone.

Minerals: Inorganic elements essential for human metabolism.

Mitochondria: Elongated, fluid-filled sacs that can move through the cytoplasm; they are the major sites of chemical reactions in the cell.

Mitosis: The division of chromosomes in a cell nucleus.

Mitral valve: The bicuspid valve; it lies between the left atrium and left ventricle, preventing blood from flowing back into the left atrium from the left ventricle.

Mixed nerves: The most common types of peripheral nerves; they contain both sensory and motor fibers, transmitting impulses to and from the central nervous system.

Mixtures: Substances composed of two or more components that are physically intermixed.

Molarity: The number of moles of solute per liter of solution. It is indicated by the abbreviation "M" and expressed in moles per liter.

Molars: The 12 teeth, 6 in each dental arch, that are located posterior to the premolars.

Mole: The atomic weight or molecular weight of an element or compound, weighed out in grams.

Molecular weight: The sum of an element or compound's atomic weights. The amount of each atom of the element or compound is multiplied by its individual atomic weight to find a total atomic weight for that atom. Then, all total atomic weights of the atoms in the element or compound are added together.

Molecules: Particles made up of two or more joined atoms.

Monocytes: Leukocytes that are the largest type of blood cells, with varied nuclei.

Mononuclear phagocytic system: Phagocytic cells that remove foreign particles from the lymph and blood.

Monosaccharides: Simple sugars, which have 6 carbon atoms, 12 hydrogen atoms, and 6 oxygen atoms; examples include glucose, fructose, galactose, ribose, and deoxyribose.

Mons pubis: The rounded fleshy prominence over the symphysis pubis in the female.

Morula: A solid, spherical mass of cells resulting from the cleavage of the fertilized ovum in the early stages of embryonic development.

Motor areas: The parts of the cerebrum, mostly in the frontal lobes, that control skeletal muscle functions.

Motor (efferent) nerves: Peripheral nerves that carry impulses only away from the central nervous system; they are relatively rare in the human body.

Motor end plate: The flattened end of a motor neuron that transmits neural impulses to a muscle.

Motor endings: The elements of the peripheral nervous system that activate effectors by releasing neurotransmitters.

Motor neurons: Those that control effectors, including skeletal muscles.

Motor output: Responses by the nervous system that activate the effector organs (muscles and glands).

Motor unit: A motor neuron and the muscle fibers it controls.

Mucosa (mucous membrane): The surface epithelium, connective tissue, and smooth muscle of the alimentary canal.

Mucous membranes: Membranes that line cavities and tubes that open to the outside of the body.

Mucus: Related to digestion, it is a thick liquid that binds food particles and lubricates them during swallowing.

Multiunit smooth muscle: Found in the irises of the eyes and walls of blood vessels, it has separated muscle fibers and contracts only when stimulated by nerve impulses or certain hormones.

Muscarinic receptors: Receptors of the autonomic nervous system's target organs that bind acetylcholine; they are named for activation by a toxin (muscarine) that comes from mushrooms.

Muscle fatigue: A state of physiologic inability for a muscle to contract, even though it may still be receiving stimuli.

Muscle fibers: Elongated skeletal and smooth muscle cells; muscle fibers do not include cardiac muscle cells because they are not elongated.

Muscle impulse: One that passes in many directions over a muscle fiber membrane after stimulation by acetylcholine.

Muscle tissues: Contractile tissue consisting of filaments of actin and myosin, which slide past each other, shortening cells.

Muscle tone: The phenomenon in which relaxed muscles are nearly always slightly contracted; it is caused by spinal reflexes that activate a group of motor units, and then another, in response to activated stretch receptors in muscles.

Muscular arteries: Also known as distributing arteries, they deliver blood to body organs via a tunica media that is primarily composed of circularly arranged smooth muscle.

Myelin: An electrically insulating material that forms a sheath, usually only around the axon of a neuron.

Myelin sheaths: Cells wound tightly around axons; they originate from Schwann cells.

Myoblasts: Embryonic cells that become muscle cells or fibers; also known as sarcoblasts.

Myocardium: The thick middle layer of the heart wall that is made mostly of cardiac tissue.

Myofibrils: Thread-like fibers that make up the sarcoplasm.

Myoglobin: A pigment synthesized in the muscles to give skeletal muscles their reddish-brown color.

Myoid cells: Cells, in three to five layers, that surround each seminiferous tubules; their rhythmic contractions aid in squeezing sperm and testicular fluids through the seminiferous tubules and out of the testes.

Myometrium: The thick muscular middle layer of the uterine wall.

Myosin: The component that makes up most of the thick protein filaments of the myofibrils.

Nail folds: The folds of palmar skin around the bases and sides of nails.

Nasal bones: The thin, delicate bones that join to form the bridge of the nose.

Nasal cavity: A hollow space located behind the nose, divided into right and left portions.

Nasal conchae: The bones and bone processes of the nasal cavity that divide it into passages known as the superior, middle, and inferior meatuses.

Nasal septum: A structure made of bone and cartilage that divides the nasal cavity into right and left portions.

Nasopharynx: The section of the pharynx that is posterior to the nasal cavity, inferior to the sphenoid bone, and superior to the level of the soft palate. It is a passageway only for air.

Natural killer (NK) cells: Cells that patrol blood and lymph during immunologic surveillance; they are able to lyse and kill both cancer and viral cells by releasing cytotoxins.

Negative feedback: The mechanism that controls hormone secretion, triggered by an internal or external stimulus; as hormone levels rise, it inhibits the system and secretion decreases. As hormones decrease, the system starts up again.

Neonatal period: The period beginning abruptly at birth and extending to the end of the first 4 weeks.

Nephron loop: Formerly called the loop of Henle; the U-shaped part of the nephron that functions in water resorption and urine concentration.

Nephrons: The functional units of the kidneys.

Nerve fibers: Long axons in the body; examples include the axons of the motor neurons controlling the skeletal muscles of the great toe, which extend for up to 4 feet from the lumbar region of the spine.

Nerve impulses: Electrochemical changes transmitted by neurons to other neurons and to cells outside the nervous system.

Nerve pathways: Those that carry nerve impulses.

Nerve tracts: Major nerve pathways made up of long bundles of myelinated nerve fibers.

Nerves: Bundles of neuron processes in the peripheral nervous system.

Nervous tissues: Neurons and neuroglia.

Net filtration pressure: Usually a positive pressure, it forces substances out of the glomerulus.

Neuroendocrine organ: An organ that is controlled by both nervous and hormonal stimulation.

Neurofibrils: Fine, thread-like organelles that help to make up a cell body.

Neuroglial cells: The supporting tissue cells of the nervous system. They provide insulation, physical support, and nutrients to neurons.

Neurohypophysis: The posterior lobe of the pituitary gland, along with the infundibulum.

Neurolemma: The area of Schwann cells containing most of the cytoplasm and nuclei, outside the myelin sheath; also spelled neurilemma.

Neuromuscular junction (end plate): The connection between a motor neuron and a muscle fiber.

Neurons: The basic nerve cells of the nervous system, containing a nucleus within a cell body and extending one or more processes.

Neurotransmitters: Biochemicals that make synaptic transmission possible.

Neutrons: Uncharged or "neutral" particles in the nucleus of an atom.

Neutrophils: Leukocytes with small granules that appear light purple in neutral stain; older neutrophils are called segs and younger neutrophils are called bands.

Nicotinic receptors: Receptors of the autonomic nervous system's target organs that bind acetylcholine; they are named for activation by nicotine.

Nipple: Mammillary papilla; the pigmented projection on the anterior surface of the breast, surrounded by the areola. In females, it gives outlet to the lactiferous ducts.

Nodes of Ranvier: Narrow gaps between Schwann cells.

Nonprotein nitrogenous substances: Amino acids, urea, and uric acid in the plasma.

Norepinephrine: Noradrenalin or noradrenaline; it assists epinephrine in managing the fight-or-flight response and is synthesized from dopamine.

Nucleases: Enzymes in the pancreatic juice that break down nucleic acids into nucleotides.

Nuclei: Clusters of neuron cell bodies in the central nervous system.

Nucleic acids: Macromolecules that carry genetic information or form structures within cells; the two classes of these are DNA and RNA.

Nucleolus: A "mini-nucleus" where ribosomes are formed; made up mostly of RNA and protein.

Nucleus: The central portion of an atom that contains protons and neutrons. Also, the inner part of the cell that houses its genetic material and controls cellular activities.

Nucleus pulposus: The central part of each intervertebral disk, consisting of a pulpy elastic substance that loses some of its resiliency with age.

Nutrients: Carbohydrates, lipids, proteins, vitamins, minerals, and water.

Oblique popliteal ligament: The ligament that partially stabilizes the posterior aspect of the knee joint; it is part of the tendon of the semimembranosus muscle and fuses with the joint capsule.

Occipital bone: The bone that forms the back and base of the cranium.

Olfactory bulbs: Structures in the forebrain needed to perceive odors.

Olfactory organs: Masses of epithelium covering the upper part of the nasal cavity, the superior nasal conchae, and part of the nasal septum.

Olfactory stem cells: Short cells at the base of the olfactory epithelium involved in the sense of smell; even in adults, these cells have the same ability as embryonic stem cells to develop into many other types of cells.

Oligodendrocytes: Neuroglia of the central nervous system found aligned along nerve fibers.

Omega-3 fatty acids: Types of fatty acids from cold-water fish that are known to decrease the risk of heart disease and certain inflammatory diseases.

Oocytes: Eggs; female sex cells; they are formed in the ovaries.

Oogenesis: The process of egg cell formation, which begins at puberty.

Opposition: Involving the saddle joint between the trapezium and metacarpal I, the thumb performs opposition when you touch it to the tips of the other fingers on the same hand.

Opsonization: A reaction in which the antigen–antibody complexes become coated, marking them for ingestion and destruction by phagocytes.

Optic disc: Area of the retina where nerve fibers (axons) exit to become part of the optic nerve; also referred to as the blind spot.

Optic nerve: Cranial nerve II; it transmits visual information from the retina to the brain.

Organ systems: Groups of organs coordinated to carry out specialized functions.

Organelles: Structures within cells that have specialized functions.

Organic: Having both carbon and hydrogen atoms.

Organic components: The components of bones that include osteogenic cells, osteoblasts, bone lining cells, osteocytes, osteoclasts, and osteoid.

Organism: An individual living thing, such as a human being.

Organogenesis: The formation of organs in an embryo; the organs form from the primary germ layers.

Organs: Structures consisting of groups of tissues with specialized functions.

Orgasm: Physiologic and psychological release that is the culmination of sexual stimulation; accompanied in males by emission and ejaculation—in females there is a lesser expulsion of fluid.

Origin: A relatively immovable part of the body where a skeletal muscle is fastened at a movable joint; its action opposes that of an insertion.

Oropharynx: The section of the pharynx continuous with the oral cavity via the arched isthmus of the fauces; it lies posterior to the oral cavity, allowing both air and food to pass.

Osmolarity: The total concentration of all solute particles in a solution.

Osmotic pressure: The tendency of water to move into the cell by osmosis.

Ossification: The formation of bone by osteoblasts.

Osteoarthritis: A slowly developing condition characterized by deterioration of cartilage in joints and overgrowth of bone tissue.

Osteoblasts: Cells involved in the formation of bony tissue.

Osteocalcin: A protein found in the extracellular matrix of bone and dentin that causes pancreatic beta cells to divide, secreting more insulin; it also restricts fat storage and triggers the release of adiponectin. Osteocalcin is also involved in regulating mineralization in the bones and teeth.

Osteoclasts: Macrophages of the bone surface that dissolve the matrix and return minerals to the extracellular fluid.

Osteocytes: Mature bone cells; they maintain protein and mineral content of the surrounding bone matrix and participate in the repair of damaged bone.

Osteogenic cells: Also known as osteoprogenitor cells, these mitotically active stem cells are found in the periosteum and endosteum. They are squamous or flattened cells when bones are growing. Stimulation of these cells causes them to often differentiate into osteoblasts or bone lining cells. Others may remain osteogenic cells

Osteoid: The organic part of the bone matrix; it makes up nearly one-third of the matrix and is composed of ground substance and collagen fibers.

Osteons: The structural units of compact bone, also known as Haversian systems; they are elongated cylinders oriented parallel to the long axes of bones.

Osteoprogenitor cells: Same as osteogenic cells.

Otic ganglia: The parasympathetic ganglia immediately below the foramen ovale; their postganglionic fibers supply the parotid gland.

Otolith membrane: Also called the otolithic membrane; it is a gelatinous membrane in the vestibular apparatus of the inner ear that plays an important role in the sense of equilibrium.

Oval window: The opening between the stapes and inner ear.

Ovarian follicles: Many small structures embedded in the cortex of each ovary that resemble sacs, in which primary oocytes develop.

Ovarian ligament: A ligament that anchors each ovary medially to the uterus; it is itself anchored laterally to the pelvic wall by the suspensory ligament.

Ovaries: Oval-shaped structures in a female's pelvic cavity that develop the oocytes (egg cells).

Ovulation: The development of a secondary oocyte and first polar body via oogenesis of the primary oocyte.

Oxidases: Enzymes that catalyze the transfer of oxygen.

Oxidation: The process by which oxygen combines with another chemical, is involved in the removal of hydrogen, or loses electrons.

Oxygen debt: The amount of oxygen that liver cells need to convert lactic acid into glucose and muscle cells need to restore adenosine triphosphate and creatine phosphate levels.

Oxyhemoglobin: The combination of oxygen that dissolves in blood and the iron atoms of hemoglobin.

Oxytocin: A hormone released by the posterior pituitary gland that stimulates powerful uterine contractions, helping in the later stages of labor; also involved in the milk production process.

Pacemaker: The term used to refer to the sinoatrial node.

Pacesetter cells: Cells that generate slow wave potentials through digestive smooth muscle sheets over gap junctions.

Pain receptors: Sensory nerve endings associated with pain.

Palate: The roof of the oral cavity, consisting of hard and soft palates.

Palatine bones: Those that form the posterior roof of the mouth or part of the hard palate.

Palatine tonsils: Small masses of lymphoid tissue between the pillars of the fauces on both sides of the pharynx.

Palatine tonsils: The largest tonsils, found on either side of the posterior end of the oral cavity; they are the tonsils that most often become infected.

Pancreas: A gland with both endocrine and exocrine function; related to digestion, it secretes pancreatic juice.

Pancreatic amylase: An enzyme in pancreatic juice that digests carbohydrates.

Pancreatic juice: A digestive juice secreted by the pancreas.

Pancreatic lipase: An enzyme in pancreatic juice that digests fat.

Papillae: Rough projections of the tongue that provide friction and contain the taste buds.

Papillary layer: A component of the dermis that consists of areolar tissue and contains capillaries, lymphatics, and sensory neurons.

Papillary muscles: Those that contract as the heart's ventricles contract, pulling on the chordae tendinae to prevent the cusps from swinging back into the atrium.

Paracrine: Relating to a kind of hormone function in which the effects of the hormone are restricted to the local environment.

Paralysis: Loss of motor function due to spinal cord trauma.

Paranasal sinuses: Air-filled spaces inside the skull bones that open into the nasal cavity; they affect the quality of the voice.

Paraplegia: Paralysis of both lower limbs, due to transection of the spinal cord between the T1 and L1 levels.

Parasympathetic: The part of the nervous system that decreases heart and breathing rates and is part of the "rest-and-digest" response.

Parathyroid hormone (PTH): Increases blood calcium concentration and decreases blood phosphate ion concentration, affecting the bones, intestines, and kidneys.

Paresthesias: Abnormal sensations caused by spinal cord trauma.

Parietal: Relating to the wall of a cavity.

Parietal bones: Those that form the upper sides and roof of the cranium.

Parietal pleura: A folded back portion of the visceral pleura that forms part of the mediastinum and lines the inner thoracic cavity.

Parotid glands: The largest type of salivary gland, lying anterior and slightly inferior to each ear.

Partial pressure: The amount of pressure each gas contributes to diffusion.

Partially complete protein: One, such as gliadin, that does not have enough lysine to promote growth but does have enough to maintain life.

Passive tubular reabsorption: The type of tubular reabsorption that utilizes diffusion, facilitated diffusion, and osmosis.

Patella: The kneecap.

Pathogen: A disease-causing agent, which may be a virus, bacterium, fungus, or protozoan.

Pathophysiology: The study of changes associated with or resulting from disease or injury.

Pectoral girdle: The scapulae and clavicles.

Pelvic girdle: The hipbones.

Pelvic inflammatory disease: A possible complication of gonorrhea or chlamydia in which bacteria enter the vagina and spread throughout the reproductive organs.

Pelvic splanchnic nerves: Also called the nervi erigentes; they are visceral branches from the ventral primary rami of the second, third, and fourth sacral spinal nerves, which join the inferior hypogastric plexus to form the pelvic plexuses. They convey both presynaptic parasympathetic and sensory fibers.

Pelvis: The structure formed by the hipbones, sacrum, and coccyx.

Penis: The cylindrical male sex organ, it conveys urine and semen through the urethra.

Pepsin: The most important digestive enzyme in the gastric juice, formed when pepsinogen contacts hydrochloric acid.

Pepsinogen: The inactive enzyme precursor that forms pepsin.

Perception: The conscious interpretation of sensations (stimuli).

Pericardium: A membranous structure that encloses the heart and proximal ends of the large blood vessels and consists of several different layers.

Pericytes: Cells resembling smooth muscle cells that function to regulate renal medullary blood flow.

Perilymph: An extracellular fluid located within the cochlea of the inner ear, in the scala tympani and scala vestibuli; it is similar in composition to plasma and cerebrospinal fluid.

Perimetrium: The outer serosal layer of the uterine wall.

Perimysium: A layer of fibrous connective tissue that surrounds each fascicle in muscles.

Periosteum: The fibrovascular membrane covering a bone.

Peripheral nervous system (PNS): The peripheral nerves connecting the central nervous system to other parts of the body.

Peripheral proteins: Proteins that are not embedded in the lipid bilayer, which may be enzymes, motor proteins, or proteins with cell-linking functions. Motor proteins are involved in changing cell shape during muscle cell contraction and cell division.

Peripheral resistance: A force produced by friction between blood and blood vessel walls.

Peristalsis: The wave-like motion of many tubular organs caused by the rhythmicity of visceral smooth muscle.

Peritoneal membranes: Smooth, transparent membranes that line the abdominal cavity and contain the internal organs of the abdomen.

Peritonitis: Inflammation of the peritoneal membranes of the abdomen; this condition may occur spontaneously (primary peritonitis) or result as a secondary condition, usually because of a bacterial infection or a chemical irritant.

Peritubular capillary: One of many complex, interconnected capillary networks that branch off of efferent arterioles.

Peroxisomes: Sac-like organelles that have enzymes that speed up many biochemical reactions.

Perpendicular plate: Flat portion of a bone that lies within or closely approximates a vertical plane.

Peyer's patches: Aggregated lymphoid nodules in the walls of the distal small intestine that resemble the tonsils; they act to destroy bacteria and generate memory lymphocytes.

pH: A value by which hydrogen ion concentrations may be measured.

Phagocytosis: The engulfing and digesting of particles, cells, and molecules.

Phalanges: The bones of the fingers and toes

Pharyngeal tonsil: Also called the adenoids, it is located high on the posterior wall of the nasopharynx. It traps pathogens from the incoming air and destroys them.

Pharyngeal tonsil: The tonsil located in the posterior nasopharynx; when enlarged, it is referred to as the adenoids.

Pharynx: The cavity lying posterior to the mouth connecting to the esophagus; it has both oral and nasal usages.

Pharynx: Throat; allows the passage of food from the oral cavity to the esophagus and air from the nasal cavity into the larynx.

Phenotype: The appearance, health condition, or other characteristics associated with a particular genotype.

Phenylketonuria: A birth defect caused by a gene mutation, in which the enzyme needed to break down phenylalanine is unable to do so; this results in high levels of phenylalanine, which leads to mental retardation, seizures, slowed growth, and pale skin.

Phospholipid: A modified triglyceride consisting of a glycerol portion with fatty acid chains; phospholipids are important parts of cell structures.

Phospholipids: Lipids that have both charged and uncharged sections that encourage biologic membranes to form closed, mostly round structures that reseal when torn. Components of phospholipids include a head, tail, saturated fatty acids, and unsaturated fatty acids.

Phosphorylation: The metabolic process of introducing a phosphate group into an organic molecule through the action of a phosphorylase or kinase.

Photoreceptors: Sensory receptors sensitive to light energy, including the rods and cones of the eyes.

Phrenic nerve: The nerve that conducts motor impulses to the diaphragm.

Physiology: The study of body functions.

Pia mater: The innermost layer of the meninges.

Pineal gland: Also called the pineal body or epiphysis cerebri; a small, conical structure attached by a stalk to the posterior wall of the third brain ventricle, it secretes melatonin.

Pituitary dwarfism: Decreased bodily growth because of deficiency of growth hormone secreted from the pituitary gland.

Pituitary gland: Also called the hypophysis; an endocrine gland at the base of the brain in the sella turcica, attached by a stalk to the hypothalamus.

Placenta: A complex vascular structure that attaches the embryo to the uterine wall and exchanges nutrients, gases, and wastes between maternal blood and the embryo's blood; it also secretes hormones.

Placental lactogen: A hormone secreted from the placenta that helps to stimulate breast development and prepares the mammary glands for milk secretion.

Placental membrane: A thin structure that separates embryonic blood in a capillary of a chorionic villus from maternal blood in a lacuna.

Placentation: The formation of a placenta from the chorionic villi and decidua basalis; the placenta is disc-shaped when it forms.

Plantar flexion: Moving the ankle so the foot moves farther from the shin, pointing the toes. This corresponds to wrist flexion.

Plasma cells: Antibody-producing cells that form when activated B cells proliferate.

Plasma cells: Those that produce antibodies (immunoglobulins) to destroy antigens or antigen-containing particles; plasma cells are formed from divided and differentiated B cells.

Plasma proteins: The most abundant solutes (dissolved substances) in the plasma.

Plasma: The liquid portion of blood.

Platelets: Thrombocytes; platelets are incomplete cells important in blood clotting.

Pleural cavity: The potential space between the visceral and parietal pleurae.

Pleurisy: Inflammation of the pleura, which is the membrane surrounding and protecting the lungs; it occurs when an infection or harmful agent irritates the pleural surface, usually resulting in sharp chest pains.

Plexuses: The main portions of the spinal nerves combine (except in the thoracic region) to form complex networks.

Polar: A molecule that uses a covalent bond in which electrons are not shared equally; this results in a shape that has an uneven distribution of charges.

Polysaccharides: Complex carbohydrates that contain many simple joined sugar units, such as plant starch; they are polymers of simple sugars linked together via dehydration synthesis, functioning as storage products.

Pons: The bulging brain stem region between the midbrain and medulla oblongata; it is mostly composed of conduction tracts that relay information.

Porta hepatis: A fissure on the visceral surface of the liver, along which the portal vein, hepatic artery, and hepatic ducts pass.

Portal hypertension: An increased venous pressure in the portal circulation caused by compression or occlusion in the portal or hepatic vascular system.

Posterior cruciate ligament: A strong ligament of the knee, it is attached to the tibia's posterior intercondylar area; it passes superiorly, medially, and anteriorly and prevents forward sliding of the femur or backward displacement of the tibia.

Postganglionic fiber: An axon of the neurons that receive impulses from preganglionic fibers.

Postnatal period: The period beginning at birth and ending at death.

Preganglionic fiber: An axon that leaves the central nervous system to synapse with neurons that have cell bodies inside an autonomic ganglion.

Pregnancy: The condition that begins when the developing offspring implants into the uterine lining; it consists of three trimesters (each about 3 months in length).

Premolars: One of eight teeth, four in each dental arch, located lateral and posterior to the canine teeth, in front of the molars.

Prenatal period: The period beginning at fertilization and ending at birth.

Prepuce: The male foreskin; also, a similar fold of skin around the female clitoris.

Presbycusis: Hearing loss that commonly occurs with aging; it is usually linked to heredity, chronic exposure to loud noises, earwax blockage, inner ear damage, infections, and a ruptured tympanic membrane.

Primary bronchi: Branches of the bronchial tree that divide into secondary bronchi, tertiary bronchi, and finer tubes.

Primary follicles: Matured primordial follicles.

Primary germ layers: Three cell layers that arise in the embryonic period from which all organs of the body form.

Prime mover: An agonist; a muscle that contracts to provide most of a desired movement.

Primitive streak: During gastrulation, a groove with raised edges that appears on the dorsal surface of the embryonic disc.

Primordial follicles: Structures in developing female fetuses that contain a primary oocyte surrounded by follicular cells.

Processes: Arm-like structures that extend from the cell body of all neurons.

Progesterone: A female hormone that promotes changes in the uterus during the reproductive cycle, affects the mammary glands, and helps regulate gonadotropin secretion.

Prolactin (PRL): Controls milk production in females after they give birth and may help to maintain sperm production in males.

Pronation: Turning the hand so the palm is downward, facing posteriorly. The forearm is rotated medially, moving the distal end of the radius across the ulna, forming an X between the two bones. The forearm remains in this position when a person is standing but relaxed. Pronation is not as strong a movement as supination.

Prostaglandins: Lipids made from arachidonic acid that usually act more locally than hormones, are very potent, stimulate hormone secretions, and help to regulate blood pressure.

Prostate gland: A structure that surrounds the proximal urethra; it secretes a milky, alkaline fluid that neutralizes the acidic fluid containing sperm cells.

Prostatic urethra: The part of the male urethra from the base of the prostate gland to the point where the urethra emerges from the apex of the prostate gland.

Proteins: Substances made up of amino acids that are vital for many body functions, including structures and their functions, energy, and hormonal requirements.

Prothrombin: An alpha globulin made in the liver that is converted into thrombin.

Protons: Single, positively charged particles inside the nucleus of an atom.

Protraction: Moving a part forward, which is a nonangular anterior movement in the transverse plane. For example, the mandible is protracted when you stick your jaw out.

Proximal convoluted tubule: The convoluted portion of the nephron between the Bowman's capsule and loop of Henle; it functions in the resorption of sugar, sodium, and chloride ions, as well as in the resorption of water from the glomerular filtrate.

Pseudostratified columnar epithelium: Tissue that is layered in appearance and is involved in secretion; lines respiratory system passages.

Puberty: The time during development when the body becomes reproductively functional.

Pubis: The part of the hipbone that is superior and partly anterior to the ischium.

Pubofemoral ligament: One of the ligaments that reinforces the hip joint capsule; it is a triangular thickening of the inferior area of the capsule.

Pulmonary circuit: The blood flow and blood vessels within the lungs and between the lungs and the heart.

Pulmonary plexuses: The plexuses formed by several trunks of the vagus nerve, joined at the root of the lung by branches from the sympathetic trunk and cardiac plexuses. These plexuses are divided into anterior and posterior parts.

Pulmonary valve: Lying at the base of the pulmonary trunk, this valve has three cusps and allows blood to leave the right ventricle while preventing backflow into the ventricular chamber.

Pulmonary veins: Four veins, two on each side, that convey oxygenated blood from the lungs to the left atrium of the heart.

Pulp cavity: The space in a tooth bounded by dentin and containing the dental pulp; it is divided into the pulp chamber and pulp canal.

Pulse pressure: The difference between the systolic and diastolic pressures.

Pulvinar: The prominent medial part of the posterior end of the thalamus.

Pupil: The opening in the iris through which light enters the eye.

Purkinje cells: Large, densely branching neurons in the cerebellar cortex of the brain.

Purkinje fibers: Consisting of branches of the atrioventricular bundle that spread and enlarge, these fibers are located near the papillary muscles; they continue to the heart's apex and cause the ventricular walls to contract in a twisting motion.

Pus: A thick fluid formed from masses of leukocytes, bacterial cells, and damaged tissue.

Putamen: The larger, more lateral part of the lentiform nucleus.

Pyloric sphincter: A circular muscle acting as a valve to control gastric emptying.

Quadriplegia: Paralysis of all four limbs because of transection of the spinal cord in the cervical region.

Radial collateral ligament: One of the two strong capsular ligaments of the elbow joint that restrict horizontal movements; it is triangular and located on the lateral side.

Radioisotopes: Also known as radioactive isotopes or radionuclides, they are atoms with unstable nuclei.

Radius: The shorter, lateral bone of the forearm.

Reactivity: The ability to react with activated lymphocytes and antibodies that are released via immunogenic reactions.

Recessive: Less influential than "dominant"; for example, a recessive allele's expression is masked by a dominant allele.

Red blood cells (erythrocytes): Those that transport gases, including oxygen.

Red marrow: A connective tissue within bones where blood cells are produced.

Red nucleus: An oval nucleus located centrally in the upper portion of the reticular formation of the brain.

Referred pain: Pain that feels as if it is originating from a body part other than the site being stimulated.

Reflex arc: Sensory impulses from receptors can reach their effectors without being processed by the brain. The five basic components of the reflex arc are a receptor, a sensory neuron, an integration center, a motor neuron, and an effector.

Reflexes: Involuntary, nearly instantaneous movements in response to stimuli; an example is the automatic withdrawing of the hand from an extremely hot surface.

Refraction: Bending of light as it passes between media of different densities.

Regional anatomy: The study of all structures in a certain body region, which are examined at the same time.

Relative refractory period: A period that follows the absolute refractory period; in this period, most sodium channels have resumed the resting state, some potassium channels are open, and repolarization is occurring.

Relaxin: A female hormone secreted by the corpus luteum that helps soften the cervix and relax the pelvic ligaments in childbirth.

Releasing hormones: Those that control the anterior pituitary gland's secretion.

Renal arteries: The vessels that supply the kidneys with blood; they arise from the abdominal aorta.

Renal clearance: The volume of plasma from which the kidneys completely remove a particular substance over a specific time period (usually one minute).

Renal corpuscle: The initial blood-filtering component of the nephron.

Renal cortex: The outer portion of each kidney; it forms renal columns and has tiny tubules associated with the nephrons.

Renal medulla: The inner portion of each kidney; it is made of conical renal pyramids and has striations.

Renal pelvis: A funnel-shaped sac inside the renal sinus that is subdivided into major and minor calyces (tubes).

Renal sinus: A hollow medial depression of each kidney into which passes blood vessels, nerves, lymphatic vessels, and the ureter.

Renal tubule: The portion of the nephron containing the tubular fluid filtered through the glomerulus.

Renal vein: The vessel from the kidneys that joins the inferior vena cava.

Renin: A protein enzyme released by certain kidney cells when the body has decreased sodium levels or low blood volume. It increases the amount of angiotensinogen in the blood.

Renin: An enzyme produced by specific cells in the kidneys in response to a decline in blood pressure and in the volume of nephron filtrate.

Renin: Chymosin; an enzyme that mediates extracellular volume and the mean arterial blood pressure.

Repolarization: The restoration of the internal negativity of a resting neuron; during repolarization, sodium ion channels are inactivating as potassium ion channels open.

Residual volume: The air that remains in the lungs regardless of the level of expiration (about 1,200 mL).

Resistin: A protein secreted by immune and epithelial cells that is believed to be linked to obesity, insulin resistance, and diabetes; it antagonizes the effects of insulin and is also known as adipose tissue–specific secretory factor.

Resolution: A period after orgasm, in which muscles relax and blood flow is reduced; in males, during this period, the penis eventually becomes flaccid again.

Respiration: The process of gas exchange between the atmosphere and cells.

Respiratory areas: Parts of the brain that control inspiration and expiration.

Respiratory capacities: The four capacities created by the combination of two or more of the respiratory volumes.

Respiratory membrane: Layers of an alveolus that separate air from blood in a capillary; it is where blood and alveolar air exchange gases.

Respiratory system: Regulates breathing via oxygen intake and removal of carbon dioxide; it includes tubes that filter incoming air and microscopic air sacs where gases are exchanged.

Respiratory volumes: Four distinct volumes involved in respiration (tidal volume, inspiratory reserve volume, expiratory reserve volume, and residual volume).

Resting potential: The difference in electrical charges on the inside and outside of a resting cell due to the flow of sodium and potassium ions.

Rete testis: A network of passageways formed by the looped seminiferous tubules in a testis; it is connected via the efferent ductules to the epididymis.

Reticular cells: Cells forming the stroma of bone marrow and lymphatic tissues that have processes contacting those of similar cells, forming a network.

Reticular connective tissue: The type of tissue that helps to create a framework inside internal organs such as the spleen and liver.

Retina: The inner layer of the eye wall, including the visual receptors.

Retraction: Moving a part backward, which is a nonangular posterior movement in the transverse plane. For example, the mandible is retracted when you pull your jaw back after sticking it out.

Retroperitoneal: Behind (posterior to) the peritoneum.

Retroperitoneally: Positioned behind the parietal peritoneum against the deep muscles of the back; the kidneys are positioned in this manner.

Rheumatoid arthritis: A chronic, painful inflammation of the joints that usually affects the hands and feet but may involve multiple joints in the body.

Rhinencephalon: The olfactory region of the brain, located in the cerebrum.

Rhodopsin: Visual purple; the light-sensitive pigment in the rods of the retina.

Ribonucleic acid (RNA): One of the two classes of nucleic acids, RNA manufactures specific proteins by using the information provided by DNA; human cells have three types of RNA (messenger, transfer, and ribosomal).

Ribosomes: Organelles responsible for protein synthesis; they are attached to the endoplasmic reticulum.

Ribs: The 12 pairs of bones that primarily make up the thoracic cage, connecting posteriorly to the thoracic vertebrae.

Right lymphatic duct: The smaller of the two collecting ducts; it receives lymph from the right side of the head and neck, right upper limb, and right thorax.

Rotation: Moving a part around its axis, either directed toward the midline or away from it. It is common at the hip, shoulder, and first two cervical vertebrae.

Rotator cuff: A group of four tendons of the shoulder joint that encircle this joint; the rotator cuff blends with the articular capsule. If the arm is strongly circumducted, the rotator cuff can be stretched severely, a common athletic injury.

Round ligament: A fibrous cord extending from the umbilicus to the anterior part of the liver.

Round ligaments: Fibromuscular bands attached to the uterus near the uterine tubes, passing through the inguinal ring to the labia majora.

Round window: A membrane-covered opening between the inner ear and middle ear.

Rugae: Ridges or folds, such as those in the mucous membrane of the stomach; they also exist in the mucous membrane covering the anterior part of the hard palate.

Rule of nines: A standardized method used to quickly assess how much body surface area has been burned on a patient; it is applied only to second- and third-degree burns.

Saccule: An enlarged region of the membranous labyrinth of the inner ear.

Sacrum: The bottom bone of the vertebral column, attached to the coccyx and pelvis.

Salivary amylase: The digestive enzyme that splits starch and glycogen into disaccharides.

Salivary glands: Those that secrete saliva to moisten food and begin digestion.

Sarcolemma: The thin membrane covering a striated muscle fiber.

Sarcomeres: The repeating patterns of striation units that appear along each skeletal muscle fiber.

Sarcoplasm: The cytoplasm of a muscle cell, which contains large amounts of glycosomes as well as myoglobin.

Sarcoplasmic reticulum: Smooth endoplasmic reticulum in muscle fibers that stores and releases calcium ions.

Satellite cells: Neuroglial cells in the peripheral nervous system that surround neuron cell bodies, with similar functions to the astrocytes of the central nervous system.

Scapula: The shoulder blade.

Schwann cells: Neuroglial cells in the peripheral nervous system that form a myelin sheath around axons.

Sclera: The white, fibrous outer layer of the eyeball.

Scrotum: A pouch of skin and subcutaneous tissue hanging from the lower abdominal region, posterior to the penis.

Sebaceous follicles: Large sebaceous glands that discharge sebum directly onto the epidermis via their ducts.

Sebaceous glands: Holocrine glands made up of specialized epidermal cells; they are primarily located near hair follicles and secrete sebum.

Sebum: An oily mixture of fatty material and debris from cells secreted by holocrine glands (sebaceous glands) through hair follicle ducts.

Secretin: A hormone from the duodenum that controls secretions into the duodenum as well as water homeostasis throughout the body.

Secretin: A peptide hormone that stimulates pancreatic juice with high concentrations of bicarbonate ions to be released, neutralizing acidic chyme.

Segmentation: Alternating contraction and relaxation of smooth muscle in nonadjacent segments of the small intestine.

Semen: The fluid that the male urethra conveys to outside of the body during ejaculation; it contains sperm cells.

Semicircular canals: The tubular inner ear structures housing receptors that provide the sense of dynamic equilibrium.

Seminal vesicles: Sac-like structures that attach to the ductus deferens near the base of the urinary bladder; they secrete an alkaline fluid that regulates pH.

Seminiferous tubules: Highly coiled structures inside each lobule of a testis; they form a network of channels, then ducts, which join the epididymis.

Semipermeable: Pertaining to the property of a membrane that allows water or solvents to pass through freely but restricts or prevents passage of materials dissolved in the fluid.

Sensation: The awareness of changes in the external and internal environments.

Sensible water loss: A measurable amount of fluid lost on a daily basis via the urine.

Sensory adaptation: Sensory receptors becoming unresponsive or inhibition along the central nervous system pathways leading to the sensory regions of the cerebral cortex.

Sensory (afferent) nerves: Peripheral nerves that carry impulses only toward the central nervous system; they are relatively rare in the human body.

Sensory input: The information gathered by the nervous system through the sensory receptors.

Sensory receptors: Structures located in the dermis that initiate nerve impulses, which can reach our conscious awareness.

Sensory receptors: The receptors that are specialized to respond to environmental changes (stimuli).

Sensory receptors: Those located at the ends of peripheral neurons; they provide the nervous system's sensory functions.

Septum pellucidum: Also called the septum lucidum; it is a thin membrane of nervous tissue that forms the medial wall of the lateral ventricles in the brain.

Septum: A solid, wall-like structure that separates the left atrium and ventricle from the right atrium and ventricle.

Serosa: The fourth level of the alimentary canal, it is composed of a visceral peritoneum and connective tissue.

Serotonin: A vasoconstrictor released from blood platelets when blood vessels break, controlling bleeding; it is also a neurotransmitter.

Serous membrane: The type of membrane that lines each body cavity; it is composed of a parietal membrane adhering to the cavity wall and a visceral membrane adhering to organs.

Serum: The clear, yellowish liquid that remains after clot formation; serum is plasma minus its clotting factors.

Sesamoid bones: Those enclosed in a tendon as well as fascial tissue, located near joints (articulations).

Sex cells: Germ (reproductive) cells; in males they are known as sperm and in females as oocytes (eggs).

Sex chromosomes: The X and Y chromosomes, which determine sex.

Sex hormones: Steroid hormones such as estrogens or testosterone produced by the ovaries, testes, or adrenal cortex, affecting growth or function of reproductive organs or development of secondary sex characteristics.

Sexually transmitted infections (STIs): Those that are transferred from one partner to another during sexual intercourse.

Short bones: Small, often cube-shaped bones such as those of the wrist and ankle.

Sigmoid colon: The final portion of the colon that becomes the rectum.

Simple columnar epithelium: Single-layer tissue found in female reproductive tubes, the uterus, and most digestive tract organs; involved in secretion and absorption.

Simple cuboidal epithelium: Single-layer tissue covering the ovaries and lining kidney tubules and glandular ducts; involved in secretion and absorption.

Simple squamous epithelium: Single-layer tissue lining the alveoli, capillary walls, blood and lymph vessels, and body cavities.

Sinoatrial node (S-A node): A small mass of specialized tissue just beneath the epicardium in the right atrium that initiates impulses through the myocardium to stimulate contraction of cardiac muscle fibers.

Skeletal muscle tissue: Voluntary muscle tissue attached to bones and composed of long thread-like cells that have light and dark striations.

Skull: The cranium and facial bones.

Sliding filament model: A method of action of muscle contraction involving how sarcomeres shorten, with thick and thin filaments sliding past each other toward the center of the sarcomere from both ends.

Smooth muscle tissue: Unstriated, involuntary muscle tissue with a "spindle"-shaped appearance; it composes hollow internal organ walls.

Solutes: Substances present in smaller amounts in a mixture.

Solutions: Homogeneous mixtures of components, meaning the mixture has exactly the same composition throughout; solutions may be gases, liquids, or solids.

Solvent: The substance present in the greatest amount in a mixture, usually a liquid.

Soma: The cell body of the neuron, consisting of a spherical nucleus with a conspicuous nucleolus surrounded by cytoplasm.

Somatic cells: All other cells in the human body besides the sex cells.

Somatic nervous system: The division of the peripheral nervous system providing motor innervation of skeletal muscles; it is also called the voluntary nervous system.

Somatic nervous system: The part of the nervous system that handles consciously controlled motor functions, including skeletal muscle movements.

Somatic reflex: A reflex that activates skeletal muscle.

Somatosensory system: The area of the sensory system that serves the limbs and body wall; it receives inputs from exteroceptors, interoceptors, and proprioceptors.

Somatotopy: The mapping of structures of the central nervous system.

Special senses: The senses of hearing, vision, equilibrium, smell, and taste.

Species resistance: An innate (nonspecific) defense wherein one species is resistant to certain diseases that may affect other species.

Sperm: Male sex cells; they are formed in the testes.

Spermatic cord: A structure that passes through the inguinal canal; it is formed by the testicular blood vessels, nerve fibers, and lymphatics, which are enclosed by a connective tissue sheath.

Spermatogenesis: The process by which sperm cells are formed.

Spermatogenic cells: Those that form sperm cells and line the seminiferous tubules.

Spermatogonia: Undifferentiated spermatogenic cells in a male embryo.

Sphenoid bone: The anterior portion of the base of the cranium.

Spinal cord: A thin column of nerves leading from the brain to the vertebral canal.

Spinal reflexes: Somatic reflexes that are controlled by the spinal cord and often do not directly involve the higher brain centers.

Spirometer: An instrument for measuring the air taken into and exhaled by the lungs.

Splanchnic circulation: The arteries that branch from the abdominal aorta, serving the digestive organs and hepatic portal circulation.

Spleen: The largest lymphatic organ, it is filled with blood instead of lymph and filters the blood via the actions of lymphocytes and macrophages.

Splenic cords: Areas of reticular connective tissue in the red pulp of the spleen.

Splenic sinusoids: Blood-filled structures in the red pulp of the spleen that are also known as venous sinuses; they are separated by the splenic cords.

Spongy bone: Similarly composed to compact bone, but its cells do not aggregate around the central canals. The cells in spongy bone lie inside the trabeculae (supporting structures of dense tissue) and take their nutrients from diffused substances that enter the canaliculi.

Spongy urethra: The part of the male urethra that is surrounded by erectile tissue; also called the penile urethra.

Sprain: Stretching or tearing of the ligaments reinforcing a joint, most commonly occurring in the ankle, knee, and lumbar region of the spine.

Static equilibrium: The maintenance of balance when the head and body are motionless.

Stem cells: Cells that retain the ability to divide repeatedly without specializing and that allow for continual growth and renewal.

Sternum: The breastbone.

Steroid: Molecules with four connected rings of carbon atoms, including cholesterol, estrogen, progesterone, testosterone, cortisol, and estradiol.

Stimuli: Changes in the environment to which the body's receptors respond.

Stomach: A pouch-like organ that mixes food from the esophagus with gastric juice, begins protein digestion and limited absorption, and moves food into the small intestine.

Straight tubule: A tubule through with the rete testis receives sperm; it is formed by the seminiferous tubules of each lobule.

Stratified columnar epithelium: Thick tissue found in the male urethra, ductus deferens, and areas of the pharynx.

Stratified cuboidal epithelium: Thick tissue that lines the mammary gland ducts, sweat glands, salivary glands, pancreas, ovaries, and seminiferous tubules.

Stratified squamous epithelium: Thick tissue that forms the epidermis and lines the mouth, esophagus, vagina, and anus.

Stratum basale: The deepest layer of the epidermis, also known as the stratum germinativum.

Stratum corneum: The outermost layer of the epidermis, consisting of dead and desquamating cells.

Stratum germinativum: The deepest layer of the epidermis, also known as the stratum basale; in this layer, cell division occurs.

Stratum granulosum: The epidermal layer between the stratum lucidum and stratum spinosum, in which keratin is accumulated.

Stratum lucidum: The clear, translucent layer of the epidermis just below the stratum corneum.

Stratum spinosum: The epidermal layer between the stratum granulosum and stratum basale, characterized by the presence of prickle cells.

Striate: Striped, grooved, or ridged; such as the primary visual (striate) cortex.

Striations: Areas of alternating, colored bands of skeletal muscle fiber.

Striatum: Also called the corpus striatum; a collective term for the caudate nucleus, putamen, and globus pallidus.

Stroke volume: The volume of blood discharged from the ventricle with each contraction; in adults, it is usually about 70 mL.

Stroma: The basic internal structural framework of an organ.

Subarachnoid hemorrhage: Bleeding into the subarachnoid space, which is between the arachnoid membrane and the pia mater.

Subcutaneous layer: The hypodermis; it is a loose connective tissue below the dermis that binds the skin to the organs underneath. It is mostly made up of adipose (fatty) tissue.

Subdural hemorrhage: Also called subdural hematoma; a form of traumatic brain injury in which blood gathers in the outermost meningeal layer, between the dura mater and arachnoid mater.

Submucosa: The second level of the alimentary canal, made up of loose connective tissue, glands, blood vessels, lymphatic vessels, and nerves.

Substantia nigra: The layer of gray matter separating the covering (tegmentum) of the midbrain from the crus cerebri.

Substrates: Substances upon which enzymes act.

Sulcus: A shallow groove in the cerebrum's surface.

Superior vena cava: Along with the inferior vena cava, one of the two largest veins in the body; the superior vena cava is formed by the joining of the brachiocephalic veins.

Superior vena cava: The second largest vein of the body, returning deoxygenated blood from the upper half of the body to the right atrium.

Supination: Turning the hand so the palm is upward, facing anteriorly. The forearm is rotated laterally. In the anatomic position, the hand is supinated while the radius and ulnae are parallel.

Surface anatomy: The study of internal body structures related to overlying skin surfaces.

Surface tension: An effect that makes it difficult for the alveoli to inflate; it is caused by attraction of water molecules.

Surfactant: A mixture of lipids and proteins synthesized to reduce the tendency of alveolar collapse and to ease alveolar inflation.

Suspensions: A type of mixtures with large, often visible solutes that usually settle; they are heterogeneous mixtures, an example of which is blood.

Suspensory ligament: The ligament that anchors the ovarian ligament laterally to the pelvic wall.

Sutural bones: Also known as Wormian bones, these are the small, flat, and irregular bones between the flat bones of the skull. They range in size from as large as a quarter to as small as a grain of sand.

Sutures: Seams that occur only between the bones of the skull; they are a type of fibrous joints.

Sweat glands (sudoriferous glands): Those that originate in the deep dermis or superficial subcutaneous layers and secrete sweat out of the skin through the pores; they include merocrine (eccrine) and apocrine glands.

Sympathetic: The part of the nervous system that increases heart and breathing rates; part of the "fight-or-flight" response.

Symphyses: Cartilaginous joints where fibrocartilage unites bones.

Synapse: A junction between any two communicating neurons; a synapse is the site of intracellular communications between neurons.

Synaptic cleft: A fluid-filled space between presynaptic and postsynaptic membranes.

Synaptic vesicles: Tiny membrane-bounded sacs on axon terminals of presynaptic neurons; they each contain thousands of neurotransmitter molecules.

Synarthrotic: A joint that is immovable; mostly found in the axial skeleton, along with amphiarthrotic joints.

Synchondroses: Cartilaginous joints in which plates or bars of hyaline cartilage unite bones; nearly all of these are synarthrotic.

Syndesmoses: Fibrous joints in which ligaments connect their related bones, and the connecting fibers are longer than those found in sutures.

Synergists: Muscles that work with a prime mover to make its action more effective.

Synostoses: Unions between adjacent bones or parts of single bones formed by osseous material.

Synovial fluid: The fluid secreted by synovial membranes that lubricates synovial joints.

Synovial joints: Complex joints that allow free movement and are lubricated with synovial fluid.

Synovial membrane: The inner layer of a joint capsule; it is made up of loose connective tissue.

Synthesis: A reaction that occurs when two or more reactants (atoms) bond to form a more complex product or structure.

Syphilis: An infectious systemic disease that may be either congenital or acquired through sexual contact or contaminated needles; acquired syphilis has four stages and can be spread by sexual contact during the first three of these four stages.

Systemic anatomy: The study of body structure in a system-by-system progression.

Systemic circuit: The general blood circulation of the body, not including the lungs. It is also called the greater circulation.

Systole: The contraction of a heart structure.

Systolic pressure: The maximum pressure during ventricular contraction.

T cells: Lymphocytes that interact directly with antigens, producing the cellular immune response; they also stimulate the B lymphocytes to produce antibodies.

T-tubule: The tubule that passes transversely from the sarcolemma across a myofibril of striated muscle.

Tachycardia: A heart rate over 100 beats per minute; tachycardia may or may not be accompanied by irregular heart rhythms or other forms of heart disease, such as heart failure. Tachycardia also occurs naturally during vigorous exercise.

Tactile cells: Also known as Merkel cells, they are located at the epidermal–dermal junction and have spiked shapes; they combine with disc-like sensory nerve endings to form tactile (Merkel) discs, which are receptors for the sense of touch.

Talus: A bone that articulates with the calcaneus and navicular bones to form the lower part of the ankle joint.

Target cells: Cells needed for specific action that are acted upon by hormones; a hormone may bind target cells in three ways: with endocrine action, paracrine action, or autocrine action.

Tarsals: The bones of the ankles; they include the medial cuneiform, intermediate cuneiform, lateral cuneiform, navicular, cuboid, talus, and calcaneus.

Taste buds: Organs having receptors associated with the sense of taste.

Taste hairs: Hair-like projections of the gustatory cells of taste buds.

Teeth: The structures used for chewing inside the mouth; humans have two sets—primary (deciduous) and secondary (permanent) teeth.

Temporal bones: Those that form the lower sides and base of the cranium.

Tendons: Collagenous fibers that connect muscles to bones.

Teratogens: Environmental factors that cause congenital malformations by interfering with prenatal growth or development.

Terminal branches: Structures of axons that allow information from the neuron to travel to more than cell at a time.

Terminal ganglia: The primarily parasympathetic ganglia situated on or close to an innervated organ; they are the sites of where preganglionic nerve fibers terminate.

Testes: Oval-shaped structures in the scrotum where sperm are formed.

Testosterone: The most important male sex hormone (androgen).

Thalamus: The deep region that makes up most of the diencephalon; it relays information coming into the cerebral cortex and has right and left halves.

Thermoreceptors: Sensory receptors sensitive to temperature changes.

Thoracic cage: The ribs, thoracic vertebrae, and sternum.

Thoracic duct: The larger and longer of the two collecting ducts; it receives lymph from the lower limbs, abdominal regions, left upper limb, and left side of the head, neck, and thorax.

Thoracic vertebrae: The 12 vertebrae located in the center of the vertebral column that (mostly) connect with the ribs.

Threshold potential: The point at which a cell membrane potential has sufficiently depolarized neurons.

Thrombin: A substance that causes fibrinogen to be cut into sections of fibrin and then joined into long threads as part of the clotting process.

Thrombocytes: See platelets.

Thrombopoietin: A hormone that causes megakaryocytes to develop from hemocytoblasts, resulting in eventual platelet (thrombocyte) formation.

Thrombus: A clot that forms abnormally in a vessel.

Thymosins: Hormones that affect early production and differentiation of lymphocytes.

Thymus: A lymphatic organ located in the thorax that is important in early immunity; it shrinks with age and is eventually replaced by other types of tissue.

Thyroglobulin: A protein produced by the thyroid gland's follicular cells; it is used by the thyroid gland to produce thyroxine and triiodothyronine.

Thyroid cartilage: Commonly known as the Adam's apple, it is the shield-shaped cartilage of the larynx.

Thyroid-stimulating hormone (TSH): Also known as thyrotropin, it controls the thyroid gland and is regulated by the hypothalamus's thyroid-releasing hormone.

Thyroxine: The thyroid hormone also known as T4 or tetraiodothyronine; it is weaker than T3 but has the same actions.

Tibia: The larger of the two bones of the lower leg; the shinbone.

Tibial collateral ligament: A wide, flat ligament running from the femur's medial epicondyle to the tibial shaft's medial condyle; it is fused to the medial meniscus of the knee.

Tibiofemoral joints: The lateral and medial joints of the knee that lie between the femoral condyles (above) and the semilunar cartilages of the tibia (below).

Tidal volume: The volume of air that enters or leaves during a single respiratory cycle (one inspiration and one expiration); this is usually about 500 mL.

Tissues: Cells that are organized into groups and layers; each type of body tissue is specialized for particular functions.

Titins: Also known as connectins, they are giant proteins that function as molecular springs and are responsible for the passive elasticity of muscle.

Tongue: The structure connected to the floor of the mouth that is covered by mucous membrane; used to mix and move food particles.

Tonsillar crypts: Areas in the tonsils that collect bacteria and other particles; they are formed by the epithelium over the tonsils as it continues deeply inside them.

Tonsils: A ring of lymphoid tissue surrounding the entrance to the pharynx; they collect and remove a variety of pathogens that enter the pharynx, in inhaled air, or in food.

Total lung capacity: Vital capacity plus residual volume.

Trabeculae: Small, flat, or needle-like pieces of bone.

Trace elements: Essential minerals found in very small amounts; include chromium, cobalt, copper, fluorine, iodine, iron, manganese, selenium, and zinc.

Trachea: Also known as the windpipe; a cylindrical tube extending downward anterior to the esophagus into the thoracic cavity; it splits into the right and left bronchi.

Tracts: Bundles of neuron processes in the central nervous system.

Trans fats: Oils used in margarines and baked products that are solidified by adding hydrogen atoms at the sites of carbon double bonds; they are known to increase risks for heart disease more significantly than solid animal fats.

Transcellular fluid: Extracellular fluid that is separated from other fluids (including the aqueous and vitreous humors, cerebrospinal fluid, exocrine gland secretions, serous fluid, and synovial fluid).

Transient ischemic attacks: Also called mini-strokes; changes in blood supply to particular brain areas, resulting in brief neurologic dysfunction that persists for less than 24 hours. If dysfunction persists longer, it is categorized as a stroke.

Transitional epithelium: Tissue that changes in appearance due to tension; it lines the urinary bladder, ureters, and superior urethra.

Transverse tubules: Also known as T-tubules; membranous channels extending inward and passing through muscle fibers.

Trichomoniasis: An infection of the genital and urinary tract; it is the most common sexually transmitted disease in younger, sexually active females and is caused by a protozoan, Trichomonas vaginalis.

Tricuspid valve: Lying between the right atrium and ventricle, this valve allows blood to move from the right atrium into the right ventricle while preventing backflow.

Triiodothyronine: The thyroid hormone also known as T3; it increases energy release from carbohydrates, increases protein synthesis, accelerates growth, and stimulates nervous system activity.

Trochlea: A loop of fibrocartilage on the superolateral eyeball that has pulley-like functions; the tendon of the superior oblique muscle passes through it, and it is the only cartilage found in the orbit. The trochlea is situated on the superior nasal aspect of the frontal bone.

Trophoblast cells: The mesectodermal cells that cover the blastocyst.

Tropomyosin: An actin-binding protein that regulates muscle contraction and other actin-related mechanical functions of the body.

Troponin: A regulatory protein in the actin filaments of skeletal and cardiac muscle that attaches to tropomyosin.

Tubular reabsorption: The process that moves substances from the tubular fluid into the blood, within the peritubular capillary.

Tubular secretion: The process that moves substances from the blood in the peritubular capillary into the renal tubule.

Tunica albuginea: In males, the inner tunic that encloses a testis; it is a fibrous capsule. In females, it is the fibrous structure that externally surrounds each ovary.

Tunica externa: The outermost layer of the three distinct layers that make up an artery's wall.

Tunica intima: The innermost layer of the three distinct layers that make up an artery's wall.

Tunica media: The middle layer of the three distinct layers that make up an artery's wall.

Tunica vaginalis: The outer tunic that encloses a testis; it has two serous layers.

Twitches: Fine movements of a small area of muscle.

Tympanic cavity: The middle ear, located inside the temporal bone; it is filled with air and contains the auditory ossicles. On its lateral surface, it meets the external auditory meatus, from which it is separated by the tympanic membrane (eardrum).

Tyrosinase: A copper-containing enzyme in the body tissues that catalyzes the oxidation of tyrosine into melanin and other pigments.

Ulna: The longer, medial bone of the forearm.

Ulnar collateral ligament: Strong capsular ligaments that restrict horizontal movements.

Umbilical cord: A structure that suspends the embryo in the amniotic cavity; it conducts substances between the mother and embryo.

Upper limbs: The humerus bones, radius bones, ulna bones, carpals, metacarpals, and phalanges.

Urea: Also known as carbamide; an organic compound that helps to metabolize nitrogen-containing compounds. It is the primary nitrogen-containing substance in the urine.

Urea: The result of amino acid catabolism; it filters into the renal tubule, with most of it reabsorbed and the balance excreted in the urine.

Ureter: One of two tubes that descend behind the parietal peritoneum to join the urinary bladder from underneath.

Urethra: A tube that conveys urine from the urinary bladder to outside of the body.

Uric acid: The result of metabolism of certain organic bases in nucleic acids, mostly reabsorbed via active transport from the glomerular filtrate.

Urinary bladder: A hollow, muscular organ that stores urine and forces it into the urethra.

Urine: The final product of tubular reabsorption and secretion; it is a clear, yellow-colored fluid that carries wastes out of the body.

Urochrome: The end product of hemoglobin breakdown, found in the urine and responsible for its yellow color.

Uterine tubes: Fallopian tubes, or oviducts; they open near the ovaries, penetrate the uterus, and open into the uterine cavity.

Uterosacral ligaments: Parts of the thickenings of the visceral pelvic fascia beside the cervix and vagina; also called Petit's ligaments.

Uterus: The structure that sustains the development of an embryo.

Utricle: An enlarged portion of the labyrinth of the inner ear.

Uvula: A cone-shaped projection from the soft palate.

Vaccine: A substance that includes antigens that stimulate an immune response against a particular pathogen.

Vagina: The female sex organ that conveys uterine secretions, receives the penis during intercourse, and provides the open channel for offspring.

Vaginal fornix: A recess in the upper part of the vagina caused by the protrusion of the uterine cervix into the vagina.

Variable (V) region: An area on one end of each antibody's polypeptide chains; extremely different V regions exist in antibodies that respond to different regions.

Varicose veins: The bluish bulges that are formed when the valves of a vein become incompetent and leak.

Vasa vasorum: A system of many tiny blood vessels that nourish the outer tissues of blood vessel walls.

Vascular anastomoses: Interconnections between blood vessels by collateral channels.

Vasoconstriction: The contraction of blood vessels, which reduces their diameter.

Vasodilation: The relaxation of blood vessels, which increases their diameter.

Vasomotor center: The part of the medulla oblongata that controls blood vessel diameter and peripheral resistance.

Vasomotor fibers: Sympathetic efferents used to transmit highly steady impulses from the vasomotor center of the medulla oblongata.

Vasomotor tone: A constant level of nervous stimulation to the muscles in the blood vessel walls that gives the muscles a resting level of contraction.

Vasopressin: A hormone that decreases the production of urine and also causes contraction of smooth muscle of blood vessels. It is also called antidiuretic hormone.

Vasospasm: An action of muscle contraction in a small blood vessel that occurs after it is cut or broken; this action can completely close the ends of a severed vessel.

Veins: Blood vessels that carry blood back to the atria; they are less elastic than arteries.

Venous valves: The valves of veins that prevent blood from flowing backward.

Ventral roots: The anterior or motor roots; they are made up of axons from motor neurons with cell bodies inside the spinal cord's gray matter.

Ventricles: Hollow chambers in the brain that are continuous with one another as well as with the central canal of the spinal cord; they are filled with cerebrospinal fluid.

Ventricles: The lower chambers of the heart; they receive blood from the atria, which they pump out into the arteries.

Venules: Microscopic vessels that link capillaries to veins.

Vermis: A worm-like structure of the cerebellum that connects its two hemispheres.

Vertebrae: The bones of the vertebral column (backbone).

Vertebral column: The backbone; it consists of 26 vertebrae separated by cartilaginous intervertebral discs, the sacrum, and the coccyx.

Vesicles: Vacuoles; membranous sacs formed by part of a cell membrane folding inward and pinching off. They are tiny, bubble-like structures containing either liquid or solid material that was formerly outside the cell.

Vestibular bulb: One of two aggregations of erectile tissue that are internal parts of the clitoris and can also be found in the vestibule; also called clitoral bulb.

Vestibular gland: One of two glands that lie on each side of the vaginal opening; it secretes mucus into the vestibule to moisten and lubricate the vagina for insertion of the penis.

Vestibule: The central part of the labyrinth, behind the cochlea and in front of the semicircular canals.

Vestibule: The structure into which the vagina opens posteriorly and the female urethra opens midline.

Viscera: Organs in the body cavities, especially in the abdomen.

Visceral: Relating to the membranous covering of an organ.

Visceral pleura: A layer of serous membrane attached to each lung surface.

Visceral smooth muscle: Muscle made up of sheets of spindle-shaped cells; it is found in the walls of the intestines, stomach, urinary bladder, and uterus.

Viscosity: The ability or inability of a fluid solution to flow easily. A solution that has high viscosity is relatively thick and flows slowly because of the adhesive effect of adjacent molecules.

Vital capacity: Inspiratory reserve volume plus tidal volume plus expiratory reserve volume.

Vitamins: Organic compounds required for normal metabolism.

Vitreous humor: The fluid between the lens and retina of the eye.

Volkmann's canals: Perforating canals that lie at right angles to long axes of bones and connect blood and nerve supplies of each periosteum to those in the central canals and medullary cavity.

Voluntary muscle: Striated muscle that can be controlled voluntarily.

Voluntary nervous system: The somatic nervous system, which is under conscious control.

Vomer bone: The flat bone making up the lower posterior nasal septum.

Vulva: The external accessory female organs, including the labia majora, labia minora, clitoris, and vestibular glands; they surround the openings of the urethra and vagina.

Water balance: Total water intake equaling total water output.

Water of metabolism: A byproduct of the oxidate metabolism of nutrients; it makes up only 10% of daily water intake.

Wernicke's area: A portion in the posterior temporal lobe of the left brain hemisphere that is involved in the recognition of spoken words.

White blood cells: Also called leukocytes); those that protect the body against disease, particularly infectious disease.

Xerostomia: Dryness of the mouth, caused by cessation of normal salivary secretion.

Yellow marrow: A fatty tissue inside the shafts of long bones where lipids are stored for potential energy needs of the body.

Yolk sac: A structure that forms during the second week of development, attaching to the underside of the embryonic disc; it forms blood cells in the early periods of development and gives rise to cells that will become sex cells eventually.

Z discs: Also called Z lines or Z bands, they are dark, thin protein bands to which actin filaments are attached in striated fibers; they mark the boundaries between adjacent sarcomeres.

Zygomatic bones: Also known as the malar bones; they form the prominence of each cheek.

Zygote: A large fertilized egg cell produced after contacting a male sperm cell.

Zygote: The first cell of a future offspring; it contains 23 chromosomes from the father and 23 chromosomes from the mother.

Index

Note: Page numbers followed by *f*, or *t* indicate materials in figures, or tables respectively.

brain centers, influence breathing, 465
brain control inspiration, respiratory areas of, 463
brain stem, 252–253, 253f
    medulla oblongata, 400
brain waves, 254
break test, 198
breast biopsy, 569
breast-feeding, 598
breastbone, 153
breastfeeding process, 329
breathing, 164, 446
    control of, 463–465, 463f, 464f
    mechanics of, 453–457, 454f
    rhythm of, 463
    thoracic cavity pressure, 423
breech birth, 598
broad ligament, 563
broad-spectrum antibiotics, 565
Broca's area, 249, 256
broken hip, 143
bronchi, 449–450, 450f
bronchial arteries, 406, 452
bronchial tree, 449, 452t
bronchiectasis, 456
bronchioles, 450
bronchoconstriction, 452
bronchodilation, 452
bronchogram, 456
bronchopneumonia, 455
bronchus dexter, 450
brown adipose tissue, 94
brown fat, 94
brush border, 529
brush border enzymes function, 531, 538
buboes, 426
buccal cavity, 517
buccal phase, 523
buffers, 31
buffy coat, 357
bulbar conjunctiva, 306
bulbourethral glands, 558, 559
bundle of His, 381
burns
    first-degree, 122, 123f
    second-degree or partial-thickness, 122, 123f
    third-degree or full-thickness, 122–123, 123f
bursae, 172, 173
bursitis, 183

C

C cells, 334
C1 inactivator, 363
C proteins, 190
calcaneus (heel bone), 159–160
calcarine sulcus, 250
calcification front, 141
calcitonin, 141, 334, 335t
calcitriol, 137, 341
calcium (Ca), 6, 545t
    balance, 501t, 502
calcium ions, 361, 382
    levels of, 141
calcium phosphate, 133

calculus, 522
calmodulin, 215, 323
calorie, 541
calorigenic effect, 332
cAMP. See cyclic adenosine monophosphate
canal, 163t
canal of Schlemm, 309
cancer
    cell division and, 61–63, 62f
    skin, 121–122
cancer cells, 63
cancer therapy, 63
canines, 520
capacitance vessels, 394
capillaries, 88, 372, 392–394, 393f, 395t
    blood pressure, 393–394, 398
    definition of, 391, 392f
    glomerular, 475, 477
    lymphatic, 420, 421f
    of muscles, 393
capillary barrier, 258
capillary beds, 394
capillary blood pressure, 398
capillary plexuses, 394
capsular epithelium, 475
capsular ligaments, 173
capsular space, 475
capsules, 425
carbaminohemoglobin, 353, 462
carbodypeptidase, 537
carbohydrates, 6, 33, 34, 526, 541
    metabolism, 529
carbon dioxide, 351, 459, 459t
    definition of, 32
    transport of, 461–462, 461f, 462t
carbon monoxide poisoning, 461
carbonic acid, 504
    production of, 504
carbonic anhydrase, 462
carcinoma, 466
cardia part, 523
cardiac conduction system, 380
cardiac cycle, 379, 383, 397
cardiac muscle, 189, 211t, 216f, 217–218, 379
    characteristics of, 218
    depolarization and contraction of, 380
cardiac muscle cells, 379
    death of, 385
cardiac muscle fibers, 383
cardiac muscle tissue, 98
cardiac notch, 451
cardiac output, 383–384
cardiac pacemaker cells, 380
cardiac plexuses, 281
cardiac region, 523
cardiac reserve, 384
cardiac skeleton, 383
cardiac sphincter, 522
cardiac tamponade, 372
cardiac veins, 409
cardial orifice, 522
cardinal ligaments, 566
cardioaccceleratory center, 382

epithelium, 85, 86*t*
epitympanic recess, 299
EPSP. *See* excitatory postsynaptic potential
equational division, 561
equilibrium, 55
    sense of, 303–305
ER. *See* endoplasmic reticulum
erectile dysfunction (ED), 560
erection, 558–559
erythrocytes, 97, 484*t*
erythropoiesis, 352, 354–356, 354*f*, 355*f*
erythropoiesis-stimulating hormone, 356
erythropoietin, 341, 354, 356–357
eschar, 122
esophageal arteries, 406
esophageal hiatus, 522
esophageal plexuses, 281
esophagus, 281, 517, 522–523
essential amino acids, 35, 36*t*, 542
essential fatty acids, 541
essential hypertension, 400–401
essential nutrients, 541
essentials for life, 5–7
estradiol, 563, 565, 572
estriol, 565, 572
estrogens, 337, 340, 414, 554, 572–574, 590*t*, 600
    blood levels of, 591
    secretion of, 143
estrone, 565, 572
ethmoid bone, 147, 148*f*
ethmoidal air cells, 147
ethmoidal labyrinth, 147
eupnea, 463
Eustachian tube, 300
eversion, 179
excess postexercise oxygen consumption. *See* oxygen debt
excessive catabolism, 70
exchange reactions, 30
exchange vessels, 372
excitability, 5
    smooth muscle, 216
excitable membranes, 234
excitation-contraction coupling, 194
excitatory, 279
excitatory postsynaptic potential (EPSP), 240
excitotoxin, 263
excretion, 6, 515
    epithelia, 85
"exiting" control center, 7
exocrine gland secretions, 89, 321
    types of, 90, 90*t*
exocytosis process, 59, 60, 89
expiration, 446, 453, 454*f*
expiratory cycling, 463
expiratory reserve volume, 456, 457*t*
expressivity, 601
expulsion stage, 597
extensibility, 190
extension, 179, 198
extensive capillary beds, 173
extensive wound, 120
extensor digitorum, 199
external acoustic meatus, 144, 299

external auditory canal, 299
external callus, 140
external carotid arteries, 403
external ear, 298–299, 299*f*
external elastic membrane, 391
external genitalia, 287, 563, 567
external iliac arteries, 408
external iliac vein, 413
external jugular veins, 409
external occipital crest, 144
external occipital protuberance, 144
external reduction, 139
external respiration, 446, 459–460
external urethral sphincter, 487
exteroceptors, 119, 231
extracapsular ligaments, 173
extracellular fluid compartment, 494, 494*f*, 495*f*
extracellular fluids, 48
    vs. intracellular fluids, 495, 495*f*
extracellular matrix components, 587
extraembryonic membranes, 592
extraembryonic mesoderm, layer of, 590
extraglomerular mesangial cells, 475, 476*f*
extrapyramidal system, 261
extrinsic eye muscles, 307, 307*f*, 307*t*
extrinsic muscles, 517
extrinsic pathway, clotting system activation, 361
exudate, 430
eye, 308, 308*f*
eye movement, muscles for, 200*t*
eyeball, anatomy of, 307–308, 308*f*
    inner layer, 310–313
    middle layer, 309–310
    outer layer, 308–309
eyebrows, 306
eyelash follicles, 306
eyelashes, 306
eyelid, 306
eyelid muscle functions, 307*t*
eyeteeth, 520

F
F cells, 340
facet, 163*t*
facial artery, 403
facial burn, 123
facial fibers, 275*t*
facial muscles, 199*t*, 213*f*
facial nerves (VII), 281, 298
facial paralysis, 519
facial skeleton, 147–148
facilitated diffusion, 55–57, 58*f*
facilitated neurons, 239
facilitation, 239
falciform ligament, 531
fallopian tubes. *See* uterine tubes
false labor, 597
false ribs, 153
false vocal cords, 449
falx cerebelli, 257
falx cerebri, 257
farmer's lung, 437
fascia, 189, 191, 191*f*

immediate hypersensitivities, 437
immune-complex hypersensitivities, 437
immune interferon, 429
immune system cells, 522
immune system homeostasis, imbalance of, 436–437, 437t
immune system, parts of, 420
immunity, 429
   active humoral, 432, 433t
   age-related changes, 438
   antibody-mediated, 433
   artificially acquired active, 433t
   artificially acquired passive, 433t
   cell-mediated, 435–436, 436t
   naturally acquired active, 433t
   naturally acquired passive, 433t
   passive humoral, 433
immunity (specific) defenses, 431
immunocompetent cells, 426
immunodeficiency, 436
immunogenicity, 431
immunoglobulins/Igs, 433
   groups, 434, 435t
immunologic surveillance, 430
immunological escape, 430
immunological memory, 431–433, 433t
impaired function, 430
implantation, 587–590
imprinting patterns, 604
impulses, 260
   processing of, 239–240
inactivated, ion distribution, 234
inadequate ACh stimulation, 287
incisors, 520
incomplete antigens, 431
incomplete fracture, 139
incomplete proteins, 542
incomplete tetanus, 197
incretins, 340
indirect renal mechanism, 400
indolamines, 239
infancy, 602t
infant, 586
infectious granulomas, 431
infectious mononucleosis, 358
inferior cerebral veins, 409
inferior colliculi, 253
inferior gluteal arteries, 408
inferior hypogastric (pelvic) plexus, 284
inferior mesenteric artery, 402–403, 407
inferior mesenteric vein, 412
inferior nasal conchae, 148
inferior oblique muscle, 307, 307t
inferior orbital fissure, 148
inferior part of body, 17t
inferior phrenic arteries, 402, 406
inferior rectus muscle, 307t
inferior sagittal sinuses, 257, 409
inferior suprarenal branches, 407
inferior vena cava, 375–376, 409
inflamed colon, 540
inflammation process, 99, 420, 429, 430
   of pleurae, 453
inflammatory response, 430

inflation reflex, 464
infraorbital foramen, 147
infraspinous fossa, 155
infundibulum, 251, 325, 565
ingestion, 514
inguinal region, 19t
inhalation, 453
inherited connective tissue disorder, 97
inhibiting hormones, 324, 325
inhibitory neurotransmitters, 237
inhibitory postsynaptic potential, 240
injectable contraception, 576
innate (nonspecific) defenses, 420, 429–430
inner adrenal cortex, 337
inner layer of eyeball, 310–313
inner mucosal layer (mucosa), 567
innervation, 236
innominate artery, 402
inorganic chemicals, 32
inorganic components of bones, 135
inorganic substances, 32, 32t
inositol triphosphate, 324
insensible perspiration, 111, 119, 496
insensible water loss, 496
insertion, 198, 198f, 199t–211t
insomnia, 255
inspiration, 446, 453, 454f
   depth of, 463–465
inspiratory capacity, 456, 458t
inspiratory cycling, 463
inspiratory reserve volume, 456, 457t
insula, 248
insulin, 341
insulin-like growth factors (IGFs), 326
integral proteins, 48
integration, nervous system, 226
integument, 108
integumentary system, 11, 108
   accessory structures, 114–118
   age-related changes, 120–121
   burns, 122–123
   components, 108
   definition of, 108
   functions, 118–119
   response to injuries/wounds, 120
   skin, 108–114
   skin cancer, 121–122
interaction, patterns of, 261–262
intercalated discs, 98, 218, 379
intercostal nerves, 277, 463
interferon-α, 429
interferon-β, 429
interferon-γ, 429
interferons, 429
interleukin-1, 430, 435
interleukin-2, 435
interleukins, 357–358
intermediate fibers, 191
intermediate filaments, 53t, 54
internal acoustic meatus, 147
internal callus, 140
internal capsule, 250
internal carotid arteries, 403

Klinefelter syndrome, 604
knee-jerk reflex, 177
knee joints, 176–177
    anatomy of, 177f
kneecap (patella), 159
Krebs cycle, 71, 73–74
Kupffer cells, 534
kyphosis, 152, 164

L

L-selectin adhesion surface molecules, 587
labia majora, 567
labia minora, 567
labor, 597
    process of, 599f
    stages of, 597–600, 599f
lacrimal apparatus, 306–307
lacrimal bones, 148
lacrimal canaliculi, 306
lacrimal caruncle, 306
lacrimal fossa, 144
lacrimal gland, 306, 307f
lacrimal (tear) gland, 144
lacrimal puncta, 306
lacrimal sac, 147, 306
lacrimal secretion, 306
lacrimal sulcus, 148
lactase, 531
lactate ion, 195
lactation, 600
lacteals, 420, 529
lactic acid, 73, 195, 196
lactic acidosis, 506
lactiferous ducts, 568
lactiferous sinus, 568
lactose intolerant, 531
lacunae, 95, 133, 591
lamella, 133
lamellae, 96
lamellar bone, 133
lamina propria, 99, 514, 516
laminae, 149
laminin, 91
Langerhans cells, 109, 112
language functions, 256
large granular leukocytes, 430
large hemispheric infarct, 262f
large hypertensive hemorrhage, 263f
large intestine, 538–540
laryngopharynx, 448, 522
larynx (voice box), 448–449, 448f, 452t
latent period, 197, 197f
lateral cervical ligaments, 566
lateral circumflex femoral arteries, 408
lateral epicondyles, 156
lateral femoral condyle, 177
lateral fornices, 567
lateral greater trochanter, 159
lateral horns, 260, 281
lateral malleolus, 159
lateral masses, 147
lateral nail grooves, 114
lateral part of body, 17t

lateral plantar arteries, 408
lateral plantar veins, 413
lateral rectus muscle, 307t
lateral rotation, 178
lateral thoracic artery, 405
lateral ventricles, 247
lateral white column, 260
lateralization, 249
latex condoms, 577
LDLs. *See* low-density lipoproteins
leakage (nongated) channels, 56
    ion distribution of, 234
left anterior descending artery, 379
left ascending lumbar vein, 411
left atrioventricular (A-V) valve, 374, 377
left coronary artery, 379
left gastric artery, 407
left hypochondriac region, 18t
left iliac (inguinal) region, 19t
left lumbar region, 19t
left renal arteries, 407
left ventricle, 375, 376
leg movement, muscles for, 209t, 215f, 216f
leg muscles, 216f
lens, 309, 310f, 311f, 314f
lens fibers, 309
leptin, 142, 341, 572
lesser cornua, 149
lesser wings, 147
leukemia, 359
leukocytes (white blood cells), 357, 484t
leukocytosis, 366
leukopoiesis, 358
leukotrienes, 324
levator ani, 487
levator palpebrae superioris muscle, 307t
Leydig cells, 560
LH. *See* luteinizing hormone
life, essentials for, 5–7
life-threatening disorder, 288
ligaments, 92, 93, 181
ligamentum flavum, 180
ligamentum nuchae, 151, 180
ligamentum teres, 176, 533
ligand-gated channels, 278
ligase enzymes, 61
light-adapted state, 313
light bands (I bands), 189f, 190
light-sensitive proteins, 312
light waves, 311
limbic system, 252, 252f, 286
limbs
    lower, 159–160, 160f–162f, 162t, 163t
    upper, 155–157, 156f–158f
lingual artery, 403
lingual frenulum, 517
lingual lipase, 520
lingual tonsils, 428, 448, 517
lipases, 39, 525
lipid monolayers, 60
lipid rafts, 48
lipid-soluble substances, 55, 119, 526
lipidemia, 366

metabolic reactions, 68
  anabolism, 68–69
  catabolism, 70
  control of, 70
metabolism, 6, 68
    of lipids, 77–78
    of proteins, 79–80
metacarpal arteries, 405
metacarpals, 157
metaphase, 61
metaphyseal vessels, 132
metaphysis, 131
metarterioles, 394
metastasis, 62
metatarsals, 160
MHC. *See* major histocompatibility complex
micelles, 535
microcirculation, 394
microfilaments, 51, 53*t*, 54
microglial cells, 228
micronutrients, 541
microphages, 358
microscopic anatomy, 4
microscopic atoms, 5
microscopic structures, 5
microtubules, 53*t*
microvilli, 50
micturition, 486
middle cerebral arteries, 404
middle colic artery, 407
middle ear, 299–300
middle layer of eyeball, 309–310
middle meningeal artery, 403
middle muscular layer (muscularis), 567
middle nasal conchae, 147
middle suprarenal arteries, 407
milia, 120
milk, ejection of, 600
milk letdown reflex, 600
milk teeth, 520
mineral salts, 135
mineralocorticoids, 336–337
minerals, 541, 543
  storage of, 138
minute ventilation, 458
mitochondria, 52, 52*f*, 53*t*, 229, 236
mitochondrial disease, 69
mitochondrion, 52, 52*f*
mitosis, 60*f*, 61, 560
mitral valve, 374, 377, 377*t*, 383
mixing movements, 516
mixtures, 27
modes of inheritance, 601
modified sweat glands, 118
molar pregnancy, 591
molarity, 27
molars, 520
molecular anatomy, 4
molecular formulas, 30
molecular weight, 27
molecules, 5, 27–28
moles, 27
monocyte macrophage system, 430

monocytes, 355*f*, 359
mononuclear phagocytic system, 430
monosaccharides, 33, 33*f*, 68, 529, 531
monosynaptic reflex, 280
monozygotic, 600
mons pubis, 567
morbidly obese, 94
morula, 586, 592*t*
motilin, 526*t*
motor areas, 249
motor end plate, 191, 192*f*
motor endings, 278
motor neurons, 191, 231
motor nuclei, 253
motor output, 226
motor proteins, 111
motor roots, 260
motor units, in skeletal muscles, 191,
      193*f*
mouth, 517, 543
movements
    of body, 5
    of bones, 138, 138*f*
MRI. *See* magnetic resonance imaging
mRNA. *See* messenger ribonucleic acid
mucin, 90, 429, 520
mucosa (mucous membrane), 449, 514
mucosa-associated lymphoid tissue, 424
mucosae, 99
mucous glands, 486
mucous membranes, 99, 516
mucous neck cells, 524
mucus, 296, 516, 519, 525*t*, 539
Müllerian-inhibiting factor, 561
Multi-CSF, 358
multiaxial movement, 178
multicellular exocrine glands, 91
multineuron pathways, 261
multineuronal pathways, 261
multiple sclerosis, 233, 437*t*
multipolar neurons, 231
multipotent stem cells, 354
multiunit smooth muscle, 215
muscarine, 286
muscarinic ACh receptors, 287
muscarinic receptors, 286
muscle cells, 189*f*, 193
muscle contraction, 192–214, 194*f*, 195*t*
muscle fatigue, skeletal muscles, 196
muscle fibers, 97, 190
    structure of, 190, 190*f*
    types of, 190, 216*f*
muscle impulse, 194, 218
muscle tendons, 173, 181
muscle tissues, 85, 86*t*, 97–98
muscle tone, 189
muscles, pterygoid, 147
muscular arteries, 392
muscular atrophy, 212
muscular dystrophy, 213
muscular layer, of alimentary canal, 514
muscular pump, 398
muscular sphincters, 546

ophthalmic artery, 404
ophthalmic veins, 409
opioids, 239
opposition, 180
opsin, 312
opsonization, 434
optic canals, 147
optic disc, 310
optic nerves, 274t, 308
optic radiations, 313
ora serrata, 309
oral cavity, 452t, 517, 521f
oral mucosa, squamous cell carcinoma of, 536
oral orifice, 517
orbicularis muscle, 306
orbicularis oculi muscle, 199, 307t
orbicularis oris muscle, 199
orbital complexes, 147
orbital fat, 308
orbital process, 148
orbitofrontal cortex, 250
orchiectomy, 555
organ systems, 5, 11
    cardiovascular system, 12–13
    digestive system, 13
    endocrine system, 12
    integumentary system, 11
    lymphatic system, 13
    muscular system, 11
    nervous system, 11–12
    reproductive system, 13, 16
    respiratory system, 13
    skeletal system, 11
    urinary system, 13
organelles, 46, 229, 230
    definition of, 5
    structures and functions of, 53, 53t
organic chemicals, 32
organic components, of bones, 134
organic solvents, 119
organic substances, 32–37
organism, 5
    levels of, 6
organization levels of body, 5, 5f
organization of body, 8
    abdominal regions, 17, 17f
    anatomic planes, 16, 16f, 16t
    body cavities and membranes, 8–9
    body regions, 17, 19t–20t
    diagnostic imaging, 10–11
    directional terms, 16, 17t
    organ systems. See organ systems
organization phase, 99
organized lymphoid tissue, 528
organogenesis, 592
organs, 5
    adrenergic and cholinergic effects on, 286t
orgasm, 559
origin, 198, 198f, 199t–211t
oropharynx, 448, 517, 522
Ortho Evra, 576
orthostatic hypotension, 288, 401
osmolality, 494

osmolarity, 56, 477
osmoles per liter, 56
osmoreceptors, 497, 498
    sense of, 331
osmosis, 56
osmotic pressure, 56
osseous spiral lamina, 300
osseous tissue, 96
ossicles, 300
ossification, 135
    endochondral, 135
    intramembranous, 135, 135f
    secondary, 136
osteitis fibrosa cystica, 335
osteoarthritis, 181–183
osteoblasts, 92, 96, 132–133
osteocalcin, 341, 342
osteoclast-activating factor, 164
osteoclasts, 133, 133f, 136, 141
osteocytes, 96, 132, 133, 133f, 135
osteogenesis, defined as, 135
osteogenic cells, 132, 133f, 136
osteogenic layer, 132
osteoid, 132
osteoid seams, 140–141
osteolysis, 133
osteomalacia, 142
osteons, 96, 133
osteopenia, 161
osteophages, 133
osteoporosis, 100, 143, 143f, 164
osteoprogenitor cells, 132
otic ganglia, 281
otitis media, 300
otolith membrane, 304
otoliths, 304
otosclerosis, 303
outer adrenal cortex, 336
outer fibrous layer (adventitia), 567
outer layer of eyeball, 308–309
oval window, 299
ovarian arteries, 402, 407, 563
ovarian cycle, 570–571, 573f
    hormonal regulation of, 572
ovarian follicles, 563
    development, 564f
ovarian ligaments, 563
ovarian tissues, 564
ovaries, 563–565, 572
    definition of, 563
    ovulation and, 564, 570, 571, 574
overhydration, 500
ovulation, 564, 570, 571, 574
oxaloacetic acids, 73, 78
oxidases, 70
oxidation, 74
    of amino acids, 79
    of glycerol and fatty acids, 77
    of sulfur-containing amino acids, 503
oxidation process, 70
oxidation reactions, 70
oxidation-reduction reactions, 70
oxidative phosphorylation, 71, 75

rotator cuff, 176
rough endoplasmic reticulum (RER), 50, 50f, 53t, 230
round ligaments, 533, 566
round window, 299
rubospinal tracts, 261
rugae, 485, 486, 523
rule of nines, 122, 122t

S

S-shaped tube, 299
S-T segment, 381–382
S wave, 381
saccule, 300
sacral canal, 151
sacral hiatus, 151
sacral plexus, 277, 278t
sacrificial bonds, 134–135
sacrum, 149, 151, 151f
saddle joint, 175
sagittal plane, 16t
saliva composition, 520
salivary amylase, 520
salivary controls, 520
salivary glands, 517–520
salivatory nuclei, 520
salt craving, 500
saltatory propagation, 234
sarcolemma, 189–190, 190f–192f, 218
sarcomeres, 189–193, 217, 219
sarcoplasm, 189, 191, 215, 217–219
sarcoplasmic reticulum, 190, 191, 192f, 194
satellite cells, 217, 228
saturated fats, 34, 34f, 35f
scala media, 300
scala tympani, 300
scala vestibuli, 300
scalae, 300
scapula (shoulder blade), 153, 155f
scar tissue, 120
Schwann cells, 228, 230f
sciatic nerve, 277, 278
SCID. See severe combined immunodeficiency disease
sclera, 308
scleral venous sinus, 309
scoliosis, 152
scotomas, 311
scrotum, 554–555
sebaceous follicles, 117
sebaceous gland duct, 118
sebaceous (oil) glands, 117, 117f
seborrhea, 118
seborrheic dermatitis, 117
sebum, 117
second-degree burn, 122, 123, 123f
second-order neurons, 261
second polar body, 570
secondary active transport, 57, 58
secondary bronchi, 450
secondary curves, 152
secondary hypertension, 401
secondary immune response, 432, 432f
secondary lymphoid organs, 424
secondary oocyte, 569

secondary ossification centers, 136
secondary polycythemia, 357
secondary sex characteristics, 574
secondary teeth, 520, 521, 521t
secretin, 91, 340, 341, 526t, 535t, 537
secretion, 89, 90, 515
secretory phase, 571, 574
secretory unit, 91
secretory vesicles, 51, 60
segmental arteries, 473
segmental bronchi, 450
segmentation, 515, 516, 538
seizure, 255
selective permeability, 46
selectively permeable channels, 234
selenium (Se), 546t
sella turcica, 147
semen, 557–558
semicircular canals, 300
semicircular ducts, 300
semiconservative replication, 61
semilunar cartilages, 177
semilunar valves, 377, 382
seminal glands, 557
seminal vesicles, 557
seminiferous tubules, 555, 557
semipermeable, 46
semispinalis capitis, 201t, 203t
semitransparent membrane, 299
senescence, 602t
senile cataracts, 309
sensation, 272
    epithelia, 85
sense organs, 272
senses
    age-related changes, 314–315
    equilibrium, 303–305
    general, 295–296
    hearing. See hearing, sense of
    overview, 295
    sight. See sight, senses of
    smell, 296–297
    special, 296
    taste, 297–298
sensible perspiration, 111, 496
sensible water loss, 498
sensorineural deafness, 303
sensors, 7
sensory adaptation, 295
sensory areas of cerebrum, 250
sensory fibers, 259
sensory inputs, 260
    nervous system, 226
sensory nerves, 180
sensory neurons, 230, 272
sensory receptors, 11, 119, 227, 231, 271–272, 295
sensory roots, 260
sensory stimuli, 85
separations, 113
sepsis, 122
septum, 374
septum pellucidum, 247
sequential multiple analysis test (SMAC), 366

survival, 6–7
suspensions, 28
suspensory ligaments, 309, 563
sustenocytes, 555
sutural bones, 129
sutures, 143–144, 163t, 170–171
swallowing, 514, 523
sweat (sudoriferous) glands, 117–118
swelling, 430
symmetry, 261
sympathectomy, 288
sympathetic activation, 280
sympathetic chain, 281
sympathetic division, 226, 280–281
  of ANS, 282f
  and parasympathetic divisions, differences between, 284t
sympathetic fibers, 281
sympathetic ganglia, 281
sympathetic innervation, 382
sympathetic motor fibers, 452
sympathetic nerve impulses, 559
sympathetic nervous system, 478
sympathetic postganglionic fibers, 286
sympathetic preganglionic fibers, 286
sympathetic stimulation, 287, 384
sympathetic (vasomotor) tone, 287
sympathetic trunk, 281
sympathetic trunk ganglion, 281
sympathetic venoconstriction, 398
sympathomimetic drugs, 287
symphyses, 171
symphysis pubis, 158
symport system, 57
synapses, 191, 192f, 236–237
synaptic boutons, 230
synaptic cleft, 194, 236
synaptic delay, 237
synaptic fatigue, 237
synaptic knobs, 230, 237
synaptic terminals, 230, 236
synaptic transmission, 236–239
synaptic vesicles, 194, 236
synarthrotic, 170
synchondroses, 171
syndesmoses, 171
syneresis, 363
synergism, 324
synergists, 198
synostoses, 171
synovial cavities, 8
synovial fluid, 173
synovial joints, 172–177, 173f
  types of, 175f
synovial membrane, 99, 173
synovitis, 183
synthesis reactions, 30, 34
syphilis, 578
systemic anatomy, 4
systemic blood pressure, 397
  function, 336t
systemic blood vessels, 401
systemic circuit, 372, 373f, 398
  definition of, 391, 391f

systemic circulation, 401
systemic lupus erythematosus, 437t
systole, 379, 397
systolic pressure, 397

T
T-lymphocytes (T cells)
  activation, 432
  antibody production by, 436t
  vs. B-lymphocytes, 433t
  cytotoxic, 430
  definition of, 359
  differentiation of, 432
  maturation, 426
T-tubule (transverse tubules), 190–191, 190f, 217
tachycardia, 385
tactile cells, 113
tactile discs, 113, 119
tactile receptors, 271
tailbone, 151, 151f
talus, 159
target cells, 321
  activation, 324
tarsal glands, 306
tarsal plates, 306
tarsals, 159
tartar, 522
tastant, 298
taste buds, 297, 297f, 298
taste hairs, 297
taste pores, 297
taste, sense of, 297–298
tears, 306
tectorial membrane, 301
tectospinal tracts, 261
tectum, 253
teeth, 520–522, 521f, 546
tegmentum, 253
telodendria, 230
telophase, 61
temperature-regulating system, 600
temporal bones, 144, 147
temporal summation, 240
temporalis muscle, 201t
tendon sheaths, 173
tendonitis, 183
tendons, 92, 93, 192
teniae coli, 538
tension lines, 113
tensor tympani, 300
tentorium cerebelli, 257
teratogens, 595
terminal arteriole, 394
terminal boutons, 230
terminal branches, 230
terminal bronchioles, 450
terminal cisternae, 190
terminal cisterns, 190
terminal ganglia, 281
terminal hair, 116
tertiary syphilis, 578
testes, 555–556
  internal structure of, 555f